DATE DUE

AUG 18 1987		
JUN 10 1988		
FEB 28 1989		
NOV 25 1989		
NOV 24 1989		
10-20-90		
FEB 14 1993		
SEP 29 1996		

DEMCO 38-297

Ervin Epstein, M.D.

Emeritus Professor of Dermatology
University of California at San Francisco
Oakland, California

Ervin Epstein, Jr., M.D.

Associate Clinical Professor of Dermatology
University of California at San Francisco
Oakland, California

SKIN SURGERY

SIXTH EDITION

1987

W. B. SAUNDERS COMPANY

Philadelphia   Rio de Janeiro
London   Sydney
Toronto   Tokyo
Mexico City   Hong Kong

W. B. Saunders Company: West Washington Square
Philadelphia, PA   19105

Library of Congress Cataloging-in-Publication Data

Skin surgery.

Includes bibliographies and index.

1. Skin—Surgery.   I. Epstein, Ervin, 1909–   .
II. Epstein, Ervin, 1941–   [DNLM: 1. Skin—surgery.
WR 650 S628]

RD520.S56 19   617'.477   86–6543

ISBN 0–721–1809–X

Editor: Bill Lamsback
Designer: Terri Siegel
Production Manager: Carolyn Naylor
Manuscript Editor: David Prout
Illustration Coordinator: Lisa Lambert

Skin Surgery   ISBN   0–7216–1809–X

Last digit is the print number: 9   8   7   6   5   4   3   2   1

Dedication

Since the fifth edition of this book was published, two very important leaders of dermatology and plastic surgery have died. Each has contributed important chapters to previous editions of this publication. Marion Sulzberger was acclaimed "Mr. Dermatology" by the *Journal of the American Medical Association.* He was considered to be the dermatologist of the twentieth century by colleagues all over the world. Dr. John Marquis Converse was the long-time Lawrence D. Bell Professor and Chief of Plastic Surgery at the New York University Medical School. In addition, he was the author of a prestigious two-edition, seven-volume text that is recognized as a standard text in the field of plastic surgery. It is with great pride that this sixth edition of *Skin Surgery* is dedicated to the memory of these two giants who contributed so much to previous editions of this work and who attained such preeminence in the specialties that joined to make cutaneous surgery a viable therapeutic approach to the conditions discussed on the pages of this volume.

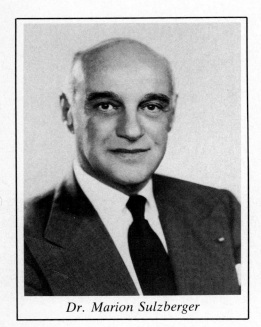

Dr. Marion Sulzberger

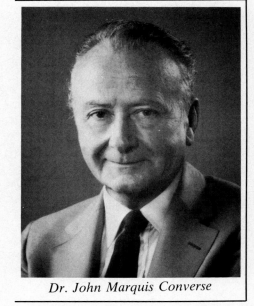

Dr. John Marquis Converse

Preface

This sixth edition of *Skin Surgery* attests to the ever increasing popularity of cutaneous surgery among dermatologists. When the first edition of this book was published in 1956, the *Journal of the American Medical Association* published a cartoon depicting a mousey-looking man sitting on a sofa holding a letter in his hands. He was reading it to his wife who was sitting nearby knitting. The caption read, "Somebody wants to buy the television rights to my book on skin surgery." To date, the letter making this offer has not arrived.

The fifth edition was a two-volume effort of approximately 1250 pages. It was decided that this was too long. In this sixth edition, the material has been streamlined, and every effort has been made to eliminate repetition. The latter is very difficult to accomplish when one is utilizing almost 60 contributors who do not see any part of the book other than their own until it is published.

In an attempt to update the material, 40% of the solo or senior authors have not been represented in this book previously. Most of the other chapters have undergone considerable rewriting. Therefore, while there are some features reminiscent of previous editions, this is a new book in many ways.

Some of the chapters are beyond the skills of dermatologists or even dermatologic surgeons. Chapters by McBride and Ketcham would fall into the latter category. They are included for educational purposes and to demonstrate what can be accomplished in serious, advanced cutaneous tumors by specialists more skilled in certain procedures than dermatologists. Many other chapters, such as those on blepharoplasty and advanced skin grafting, would certainly be beyond the ability of most skin specialists to perform. On the other hand, many dermatologic surgeons have proven their ability to utilize these modalities in their practice. Some might question the inclusion of liposuction, wondering what relevance it has to the diagnosis and treatment of skin diseases. Yet, it is a popular procedure being performed by a number of trained dermatologic surgeons.

This book must not be construed as a license for the reader to do more than he or she is qualified to do. The general practitioner should not perform neurosurgery; the dermatologist should not attempt major reconstructive procedures. Both specialties, dermatology and surgery, are blessed with advantages over the other. The surgeon has been trained in a technique that has been honed and sharpened to perfection by constant practice. He or she should be able to perform operations much more skillfully than the dermatologist. The dermatologist has been trained in the recognition and alleviation of cutaneous entities. This included instruction in not only recognizing the thousands of cutaneous entities, but knowledge of the prognosis of these conditions. As a rule, therefore, dermatologic surgery is more conservative than that practiced by the surgeon. Yet, it is as adequate. As a result, it produces less morbidity and often less cicatrization. Also, it is performed in the doctor's own office and therefore costs much less. This is an advantage for the patient as well as for the dermatologist who can operate on site and avoid the myriad of paperwork that accompanies hospital surgery.

In treating skin cancers, the dermatologist's conservatism offers many advantages to the patient including simplicity, lack of anxiety, speed, minimum scarring, and most important, cure rates that are just as high as those of the surgeon in uncomplicated cases. However, when we encounter complicated instances, then special procedures, including the enlistment of the manual skills and experience of the expert surgeon, should not be shunned . . . they should be sought.

It is with pride that this sixth edition is being published. When the first edition was produced in 1956, the senior editor did not dream that this publication would gain such success that it would lead to a fifth two-volume edition or to this sixth edition. We thank the publishers for their understanding and help, the contributors who have made all this possible by their unselfish cooperation, and most of all, we thank the readers who, after all, dictate the success of this treatise.

ERVIN EPSTEIN, M.D.
ERVIN EPSTEIN, JR., M.D.

Contributors

THOMAS H. ALT, M.D.

Assistant Clinical Professor, Department of Dermatology, School of Medicine, University of Minnesota; Courtesy Staff at Methodist Hospital, St. Louis Park, Minn., and at Unity Hospital, Fridley, Minn.

LOUIS C. ARGENTA, M.D., F.A.C.S.

Interim Section Head and Associate Professor, University of Michigan Hospitals; Staff Surgeon, Veterans Hospital; Ann Arbor, Mich.

SAMUEL AYRES, III, M.D.

Associate Clinical Professor of Dermatology, University of Southern California School of Medicine; Senior Attending Staff, Dermatology, Los Angeles County–University of Southern California Medical Center, Los Angeles, Calif.

THOMAS J. BAKER, M.D.

Assistant Clinical Professor Surgery (Plastic), University of Miami School of Medicine; Senior Attending, Mercy Hospital; Consultant at Cedars Medical Center; Courtesy Staff at Jackson Memorial Hospital; Miami, Fla.

ROBERT BARAN, M.D.

Head of the Dermatologic Division, General Hospital, Cannes, France.

KIRK A. BARBER, M.D., F.R.C.P.(C)

Clinical Lecturer, Department of Medicine (Dermatology), University of Calgary, Calgary, Alberta.

CROWELL BEARD, M.D.

Clinical Professor of Ophthalmology, Emeritus, University of California Medical School, San Francisco, Calif.

RICHARD G. BENNETT, M.D., F.A.C.C.

Adjutant Associate Professor, Division of Dermatology, University of California at Los Angeles; Consultant at Veterans Administration Wadsworth Medical Center, Veterans Administration, Sepulveda, and University of Southern California County Medical Center; Los Angeles, Calif.

ROGER I. CEILLEY, M.D.

Assistant Clinical Professor, Department of Dermatology, University of Iowa, College of Medicine; Chief, Dermatology Section, Iowa Methodist Medical Center; Senior Staff, Mercy Medical Center; Consultant at Des Moines Veterans Hospital and Broadlawns Polk County Hospital; Des Moines, Iowa.

MARVIN E. CHERNOSKY, M.D.

Clinical Professor, Department of Dermatology, University of Texas Medical School at Houston; Active Staff, Hermann Hospital; Staff Physician, Dermatology, Park Plaza Hospital; Consultant Staff, Shriners' Crippled Children Hospital; Consultant Staff, Memorial Hospital System; Houston, Texas.

REED O. DINGMAN, M.D., F.A.C.S.

Emeritus Professor, University of Michigan, Ann Arbor, Mich. (Dr. Dingman died in December 1985.)

JOHN H. DONOHUE, M.D.

Chief Surgical Resident, University of California, San Francisco, Calif.

DAVID J. DUGAN, M.D.

Associate Clinical Professor of Surgery, Stanford University School of Medicine, Palo Alto, Calif.

KENNETH EPSTEIN, Ph.D.

Cowell Student Health Center, University of California, Santa Cruz, Calif.

RIAD N. FARAH, M.D.

Vice Chairman, Department of Urology and Assistant Clinical Professor of Surgery (Urology), University of Michigan Medical School, Henry Ford Hospital, Detroit, Mich.

LAWRENCE M. FIELD, M.D., F.I.A.C.S.

Director, Advanced Cutaneous Surgery Clinic, Department of Dermatology, University of California, San Francisco, San Francisco, Calif.

ANDREW A. GAGE, M.D.

Professor of Surgery, State University of New York at Buffalo School of Medicine; Associate Institute Director for Clinical Affairs, Roswell Park Memorial Institute, Buffalo, N.Y.

LEON GOLDMAN, M.D.

Professor Emeritus Dermatology, College of Medicine, University of Cincinnati; Consultant in Dermatology, Children's Hospital of Cincinnati; Director, Laser Medicine and Surgery Treatment Center and Laser Laboratory, Jewish Hospital of Cincinnati; Director, Laser Treatment Center, University Hospital; Cincinnati, Ohio.

NORMAN GOLDSTEIN, M.D., F.A.C.P.

Associate Clinical Professor of Dermatology, John A. Burns School of Medicine, University of Hawaii–Manoa; Dermatology Consultant at Queens Medical Center (Oahu), St. Francis Hospital (Oahu), Kuakini Hospital (Oahu), Wilcox Memorial Hospital (Kauai), Maui Memorial Hospital (Maui), Tripler Army Medical Center; (Honolulu); Hawaii.

HOWARD L. GORDON, M.D.

Assistant Clinical Professor of Surgery (Plastic), University of Miami School of Medicine; Senior Attending, Mercy Hospital; Consultant, Cedars Medical Center; Courtesy Staff, Jackson Memorial Hospital; Miami, Fla.

DANIEL E. GORMLEY, M.D.

Assistant Clinical Professor, Division of Dermatology, UCLA Center for Health Sciences, Los Angeles, Calif.; Attending Dermatologist at Foothill Presbyterian Hospital, Glendora, Calif.; Glendora Community Hospital, Glendora, Calif.; Intercommunity Medical Center, Covina, Calif.; and San Dimas Community Hospital, San Dimas, Calif.

RONALD P. GRUBER, M.D.

Formerly Clinical Instructor, Division of Plastic Surgery, Stanford University Medical Center; Merritt Hospital; Providence Hospital; Oakland, Calif.

ECKART HANEKE, M.D.

Professor of Dermatology, University of Erlangen, Department of Dermatology; Head, Department of Dermatology, Ferdinand-Sauerbruch-Klinikum Elberfeld, Wuppertal; Federal Republic of Germany.

C. WILLIAM HANKE, M.D.

Associate Professor of Dermatology and Pathology, Indiana University School of Medicine; Active Medical Staff at Indiana University Hospital, Wishard Memorial Hospital, and Veterans Administration Hospital; Indianapolis, Ind.

HARRY J. HURLEY, M.D.

Clinical Professor of Dermatology, School of Medicine, University of Pennsylvania; Attending Physician at Hospital of the University of Pennsylvania and Mercy Catholic Medical Center; Philadelphia, Pa.

ROBERT JACKSON, M.D., F.R.C.P.(C)

Clinical Professor of Medicine (Dermatology), University of Ottawa; Consultant Dermatologist, Ottawa Civic Hospital; Ottawa, Ontario.

SHELDON S. KABAKER, M.D., F.A.C.S.

Associate Clinical Professor, University of California, San Francisco; Active Staff at Samuel Merritt Hospital, Providence Hospital, Peralta Hospital, San Francisco General Hospital and University of California Hospitals; San Francisco, Calif.

JEROLD Z. KAPLAN, M.D., F.A.C.S.

Assistant Clinical Professor of Surgery, University of California at Davis; Medical Director, Alta Bates Hospital Burn Center, Berkeley, Calif.

ALFRED S. KETCHAM, M.D., F.A.C.S.

Professor of Clinical Oncology, American Cancer Society; Professor of Surgery and Chief, Division of Oncology, Department of Surgery, University of Miami School of Medicine; Attending Surgeon at Jackson Memorial Hospital, Veterans Administration Hospital, and University of Miami Hospital and Clinic; Miami, Fla.

ROBERT W. KISTNER, M.D., F.A.C.S., F.A.C.O.G.

Associate Professor, Department of Obstetrics and Gynecology, Harvard Medical School; Senior Gynecologist, Brigham Women's Hospital, Boston, Mass.

DANIEL M. LASKIN, D.D.S., M.S.

Professor and Chairman, Department of Oral and Maxillofacial Surgery, School of Dentistry, and Professor of Surgery and Chairman, Division of Oral and Maxillofacial Surgery, School of Medicine, Medical College of Virginia; Attending Oral and Maxillofacial Surgeon at MCV Hospitals and Richmond Eye and Ear Hospital; Richmond, Va.

RONALD R. LUBRITZ, M.D., F.A.C.P.

Clinical Professor of Medicine (Dermatology), Tulane University School of Medicine; Visiting Staff, Charity Hospital of Louisiana at New Orleans; Active Staff at Forrest General Hospital and Methodist Hospital, Hattiesburg, Miss; Courtesy Staff at Anderson Hospital, Riley Hospital, and Rush Hospital, Meridian, Miss.

WILLIAM S. LYNCH, M.D.

Assistant Professor, Department of Dermatology, Case Western Reserve University School of Medicine; Assistant Dermatologist and Director, Mohs Micrographic Surgery, University Hospitals of Cleveland; Cleveland, Ohio.

CHARLES M. McBRIDE, M.D., C.M.

Surgeon, The University of Texas; Professor of Surgery, M. D. Anderson Hospital and Tumor Institute; Houston, Texas.

GEORGE R. MIKHAIL, M.D.

Associate Clinical Professor of Dermatology, University of Michigan Medical School, and Director, Mohs Chemosurgery Section, Henry Ford Hospital, Detroit, Mich.

FREDERICK L. MOFFATT, M.D., F.R.C.S.(C)

Instructor of Clinical Surgery and Fellow, Division of Oncology, Department of Surgery, University of Miami School of Medicine; Attending Surgeon and Fellow at Jackson Memorial Hospital and University of Miami Hospital and Clinic; Miami, Fla.

FREDERIC E. MOHS, M.D.

Emeritus Clinical Professor of Surgery, University of Wisconsin School of Medicine; Emeritus Director of Chemosurgery Clinic, University of Wisconsin Hospital and Clinics; Madison, Wis.

PATRICIA MYSKOWSKI, M.D.

Assistant Professor of Medicine, Cornell University Medical College; Assistant Attending Physician, Memorial Sloan-Kettering Cancer Center; Assistant Member, Memorial Hospital; New York, N.Y.

RHODA S. NARINS, M.D.

Formerly Assistant Professor of Dermatology and Chief of Dermatologic Surgery Department, Albert Einstein School of Medicine; Senior Attending, White Plains Hospital and Phelps Memorial Hospital, North Tarrytown, N.Y.

RICHARD B. ODOM, M.D.

Clinical Professor of Dermatology and Vice Chairman, University of California, San Francisco; San Francisco, Calif.

WILLIAM R. PANJE, M.D.

Professor and Chairman, Ear–Head and Neck Surgery, Pritzker School of Medicine, University of Chicago; Attending Physician at Mitchell Hospital, University of Chicago Medical Center, and Wyler's Childrens Hospital; Chicago, Ill.

LAWRENCE CHARLES PARISH, M.D.

Clinical Professor of Dermatology, Jefferson Medical College of Thomas Jefferson University; Visiting Professor of Dermatology, Yonsei University School of Medicine, Seoul, South Korea; Dermatologist, Thomas Jefferson University; Chief of Dermatology, Albert Einstein Medical Center—Mount Sinai Division; Attending Physician at Frankford Hospital of the City of Philadelphia and St. Agnes Medical Center; Philadelphia, Pa.

GEORGE L. POPKIN, M.D.

Professor of Clinical Dermatology, New York University School of Medicine; Attending Physician, New York University Hospital; New York, N.Y.

BIJAN SAFAI, M.D.

Assistant Professor of Biology, Sloan-Kettering Institute Division at Cornell University Graduate School of Medicine; Professor of Medicine, Cornell University Medical College; Chief, Dermatology Service and Attending Physician, Memorial Sloan-Kettering Cancer Center; Attending Physician, Division of Dermatology Department of Medicine, New York Hospital; Adjunct Member, Rockefeller University; New York, N.Y.

EUGENE P. SCHOCH, Jr., M.D.

Clinical Associate Professor, Southwestern Medical School, Dallas; Senior Staff, Brackenridge Hospital; Courtesy Staff at Seton Hospital, St. Davids Hospital, and Shoal Creek Hospital; Consultant at Austin State Hospital, Austin, Texas.

THEODORE R. SCHROCK, M.D.

Professor of Surgery, University of California, Medical School, San Francisco, Calif.

JAMES J. STAGNONE, M.D.

Clinical Professor, Dermatology Department, University of New Mexico School of Medicine; Attending Physician at UNM School of Medicine Hospital, Presbyterian Hospital, St. Joseph's Hospital, and University Heights Hospital; Albuquerque, N.M.

SAMUEL J. STEGMAN, M.D.

Associate Clinical Professor of Dermatology, University of California, San Francisco; San Francisco, Calif.

MARTIN G. UNGER, M.D., F.R.C.S.(C)

Lecturer, University of Toronto Medical School; Plastic Surgeon at One Medical Place Hospital, Orthopedic and Arthritic Hospital, and Wellesley Hospital; Toronto, Ontario.

WALTER P. UNGER, M.D., F.R.C.P.(C)

Assistant Professor of Dermatology. University of Toronto Medical School; Dermatologist, Wellesley Hospital; Toronto, Ontario.

CHARLES P. VALLIS, M.D., F.A.C.S.

Clinical Instructor in Plastic Surgery and Dermatology, Tufts Medical School; Clinical Instructor in Plastic Surgery, Harvard Medical School; Attending Surgeon, Atlanticare Medical Center, Lynn, Mass.

EUGENE J. VAN SCOTT, M.D.

Clinical Professor of Dermatology, Temple University Health Sciences Center, Philadelphia, Pa.

LARS M. VISTNES, M.D., F.R.C.S.(C), F.A.C.S.

Professor of Surgery, Stanford University School of Medicine; Head, Division of Plastic Surgery, Stanford University Medical Center; Stanford, Calif.

ERIC C. VONDERHEID, M.D.

Associate Professor of Dermatology, Temple University Health Sciences Center, Philadelphia, Pa.

RICHARD K. WINKELMANN, M.D., Ph.D.

Professor of Dermatology, Mayo Medical School; Consultant in Dermatology, Mayo Clinic; Rochester, Minn.

JOSEPH A. WITKOWSKI, M.D.

Clinical Professor of Dermatology, University of Pennsylvania School of Medicine; Professor of Medicine (Dermatology), Pennsylvania College of Podiatric Medicine; Senior Attending, Nazareth Hospital; Chief of Dermatology, Northeastern Hospital, Philadelphia, Pa.

J. NILAS YOUNG, M.D.

Associate Clinical Professor, University of California, Davis; Cardiothoracic Surgeon at Samuel Merritt Hospital and Children's Hospital, Oakland, Calif.

SETRAG A. ZACARIAN, M.D., F.A.C.P.

Clinical Professor of Dermatology, Tufts Medical School; Associate Clinical Professor of Dermatology, Yale Medical School; Chief of Dermatology Service, Baystate Medical Center, Springfield, Mass.

Contents

General Considerations

Psychology of Cosmetic Surgery

Cosmetic surgery is an ancient art; five thousand years ago, for example, rhinoplasties were performed by ceramic artists and tile makers in Egypt. Over the years procedures have gradually improved and become more precise, especially from the attempts to restore the appearance of people disfigured in wars. The range of application of these techniques has also expanded so that today's practitioner can alter the appearance of almost any part of the body.

The cost to the patient for cosmetic surgery can be considerable. Since third-party insurers usually do not cover these procedures, patients must often finance their own surgery and also undergo the pain, discomfort, and inconvenience associated with these techniques. Nevertheless, the demand for cosmetic surgery has increased dramatically during the last few decades. In the 1940s, approximately 15,000 of these procedures were performed annually. By the mid-1970s over one million plastic surgeries were performed each year—many of them for cosmetic purposes.[1] This sharp rise in popularity reflects a broadening of the patient population base. At one time the typical client was a celebrity or jet setter; today many people with moderate incomes and less glamorous lifestyles seek this medical service. Patients hope for, and frequently expect, miraculous transformations in their physical appearance that will significantly alter their social and psychological functioning.

In order to fully understand the increased popularity of cosmetic surgeries, one must be aware of the shifting patterns of our culture. Every age produces its own forms of personality and psychopathology. When Freud conducted his pioneering work, the typical psychiatric patient suffered from one of the classic neuroses. The presenting symptomatology often included compulsive hand-washing, phobias, a debilitating fixation, or a hysterical paralysis.

Although some patients still present with symptoms of classic neuroses, today's patients evidence more character disorders or borderline personalities. Instead of presenting with well-defined symptoms, patients in the last 50 years complain of more vague and pervasive feelings of loneliness, low self-esteem, narcissistic self-involvement, and unsatisfying interpersonal relationships. Lacking the necessary ego strengths to maintain an independent base of self-esteem, these patients depend on others for constant approval and admiration.

Psychohistory has demonstrated that psychopathology is influenced by a wide variety of social phenomena, e.g., political and economic movements or artistic and fashion styles.

It has been suggested that the narcissistic personality, so common at the present time, represents a reasonable way of coping with the conditions of modern life.[2] Howvever, as these people age they find it more difficult to command the external validation that sustained and supported them in their youth. The normal pleasures of old age, such as reflection upon past and present interpersonal relationships, pride over life-long accomplishments, expanding intellectual and artistic pursuits, or the growing awareness of spiritual issues, can do little for the narcissist. As Lasch has remarked, "In a society that dreads old age and death, aging holds a special terror for those whose self-esteem requires the admiration usually reserved for youth, beauty, celebrity, and charm."[3] For these people, cosmetic surgery can delay the devastating effects of aging.

PHYSICAL ATTRACTIVENESS

Just as the patterns of psychopathology tend to vary over time, so does the importance attached to physical appearance. Some societies routinely executed children who were deemed at birth to be physically deformed. Other societies ignored alterations in body configuration unless the defect interfered with the individual's capacity to function. Many societies have developed their own particular customs relating to physical appearance. For example, some Oriental cultures practiced painful techniques for reshaping feet while some South Pacific societies developed elaborate tatooing or scarring designs.

During the early period of American history, physical appearance did not play a paramount role in determining the value of a person in the eyes of another. The American frontier provided an opportunity for individuals of European descent to distinguish themselves through hard work, motivation, and the ability to survive in a new land. Those principles and values have been modified at an accelerating rate by contemporary realities. Information about what is desirable and appropriate in modern America is largely disseminated by the mass media. Conformity to these standards is elicited through the advertising genius of Madison Avenue. Even a casual perusal of advertisements reveals the overriding importance of physical attractiveness in selling products and people in our consumer-oriented society. Still, many of the earlier values continue to influence the way people sometimes think things "ought to be." Many well-known aphorisms express the minimal importance of physical appearance: "Don't judge a book by its cover," "Beauty is only skin deep," and "Beauty is in the eye of the beholder." Prevailing religious doctrines teach that the body is inferior to the mind and spirit and therefore stress the importance of moral conduct over physical appearance. Perhaps as a result, people are sometimes confused about the importance of physical attractiveness in our society and may feel guilty about their desire to have cosmetic surgery.

The systematic study of this subject has been widely neglected among social scientists until very recently. Aronson has suggested that the investigation of the role of physical attractiveness has been avoided out of fear of discovering that beautiful people, in fact, are better liked than homely people and that they possess a much greater chance of attaining success.[4] Recent research has demonstrated that these fears were well-justified.

Consistently large positive correlations have been found between physical attractiveness and popularity beginning in childhood and continuing through adulthood. In the nursery school unattractive children are perceived by their classmates and teachers as significantly less self-sufficient in behavior, less likely to possess socially desirable personality traits, and less likeable overall than their more physically appealing classmates.[5] Attractive children also receive preferential treatment; Clifford and Walster found that teachers are significantly more tolerant of disruptive behaviors in attractive children than in less attractive children.[6]

In adulthood physical attractiveness continues to be an important determiner of popularity. It is a potent factor in establishing dating preferences,[7] acceptance into college sororities and fraternities,[8] and marriage partners.[9] Many studies have shown that positive personality descriptions are assigned consistently to attractive individuals. Dion, Berscheid, and Walster, after a comprehensive review of the literature, reported that attractive adults are expected to be more kind, sensitive, modest, interesting, strong, poised, and socially adept, and to be more sexually warm and responsive than persons of lesser physical attractiveness. They are also assumed to have better personalities, to lead happier lives, and to gain greater social, economic, and professional success than less attractive people.[10] These studies clearly indicate that in contemporary America, most people do not believe that beauty is only skin deep and may regularly judge a book by its cover.

It is not surprising that there is a great demand for cosmetic surgery. People yearn for happiness and they believe that people who possess greater physical attractiveness are happier. So, they try to become more beautiful despite the financial sacrifice, pain, inconvenience, and physical trauma associated with cosmetic surgery.

PREOPERATIVE ASSESSMENT

Patients seek cosmetic surgery because they want to improve their appearance. They recognize that, if they are more attractive, other people will respond more favorably to them and that they will then have a better opportunity of getting more of what they want out of life. The research presented in the previous section indicates that these expectations are well-founded. Attractive individuals do receive preferential treatment in a wide variety of interpersonal situations. It is not surprising, therefore, that most people who undergo cosmetic surgery are pleased with the results. If patients are realistic about the potential and limitations of cosmetic surgery, and if they accurately assess the impact that these changes will have upon their psychosocial functioning, then the chances are good that they will be satisfied with the results of the operation. Indeed, only 2.7% of patients report dissatisfaction six months to four years after the operation.[11] One of the main purposes of the preoperative assessment is to estimate the likelihood that the presenting patient will be made happier by the contemplated surgery.

Young people are superior candidates for this type of surgery. The fact that they tend to heal better physically may contribute to their success. They also tend to be more flexible psychologically and may better integrate the social changes brought about by the change in appearance. Since physical appearance plays an important role in influencing interpersonal relationships, individuals who are less attractive may develop psychological difficulties secondary to the negative social feedback that they receive. It has been found, for example, that jailed convicts are less attractive physically than people with no criminal record.[12] Perhaps the effects of the negative interpersonal experiences have become less entrenched at an early age and therefore these people can benefit more from cosmetic surgery.

Other patients who respond well to cosmetic surgery include those who present with a substantial disfigurement that is correctable by surgery and that clearly inhibits them from fulfilling otherwise realistic social or vocational ambitions. Also, patients who are making other positive changes in their lives tend to make good candidates. These patients do not focus all their emotional problems on their physical appearance, but instead view surgery as an additional method of improving their lives, e.g., a reformed drug addict who wants the needle tracks eradicated from his skin as part of the total rehabilitation process. For this patient the removal of the identifying scars and the underlying thrombosed veins can help erase the memory as well as the social stigma of the patient's past. Similarly, patients who are involved in ongoing psychotherapy or vocational training may respond well to cosmetic surgery because they view the altered physical appearance as an adjunct to other positive changes.

Although most patients respond favorably to their cosmetic surgery, some pose a potential risk because of psychological factors. Emotional variables such as self-esteem, body image, and interpersonal style play an important role in the patient's decision to seek cosmetic surgery. These factors will also affect the patient's degree of satisfaction with the results. In order to maximize the possibility of the surgical intervention being successful from both the patient's and the doctor's point of view, the physician first needs to consider several psychological factors. Competent preoperative screening should allow the physician to detect most high-risk patients, and effective preoperative counseling will prevent much of their dissatisfaction.

In making the preoperative assessment the surgeon should listen carefully to the patient's account of his or her disfigurement, including the role that it has played in the person's life. The actual degree of deformity is not the only factor to be considered while performing this phase of the evaluation. The most important factor is the degree of realism possessed by the patient regarding the deformity. Although surgical procedures undertaken to correct gross deformities are more likely to effect strikingly beneficial results for both the patient and the surgeon, the correction of minor deformities can also produce postoperative satisfaction.[13]

If the patient's description of either the magnitude of the deformity or the effects of having the deformity seem exaggerated, then the surgical intervention may prove inadequate for the patient. Some patients overemphasize the importance of their disfigurement. Although in some cases this tendency may be the result of normal self-involvement and insecurity, in other cases the disfigurement may symbolize for the patient a more serious psychological conflict. Some people will use any external factor, even their own face, to account for their failures in life. In these circumstances, the surgery, no matter how successful from a technical or aesthetic point of view, will be unable to resolve adequately the patient's basic psychological issues. If the deformity is used as a crutch to relieve a sense of failure, then the sudden removal of that crutch may leave a patient undefended against his or her own inade-

quacy and may provoke psychological decompensation.[14] The greater the disparity between the physical conspicuousness of a disfigurement and the patient's subjective perception of it, the less likely cosmetic surgery will satisfy the patient.

The surgeon should assess how reasonably patients regard the changes that are likely to occur in their life as a result of the surgery. Although physical appearance is important, the surgeon needs to detect when patient's expectations for transformations in their lives are unrealistic. Cosmetic surgery is not a panacea for personal inadequacies. Patients who anticipate that surgical correction of an anatomic defect or the alteration of a socially unpopular look will lead to miraculous changes in their lifestyle will probably be dissappointed. They may attribute subsequent failures to inadequate or unsuccessful surgery, irrespective of an objective evaluation of the procedure. The best way to deal with this problem is to establish realistic expectations in the patient before surgery.

Interestingly, the presence of emotional disturbance, regardless of how severe it may be, does not necessarily contraindicate cosmetic surgery.[13] The incidence of emotional disturbance among people seeking cosmetic surgery is between 60% and 70%,[15] but most of these people benefit from their surgery. Working with a psychotic population, Clarksen and associates found that the best predictor of patient satisfaction among even these highly disturbed people "is the degree to which the patient's overall appreciation of the possibilities and limitations of the procedure are consonant with reality. . . ."[16]

Finally, the surgeon should assess the patient's awareness of the pain, swelling, discoloration, and scarring that may be experienced as a result of the surgery. The better prepared the patient is, the more likely that he or she will be tolerant of the recovery period.

If the patient's expectations seem unrealistic, the doctor should carefully explain what cosmetic surgery entails and what it can and cannot accomplish. If possible, the patient's spouse or another close relative or friend should be present for the discussion so the patient can be reminded of what the doctor said. The surgeon can show before and after pictures to illustrate what is likely to occur to the patient from the postoperative period to full recovery. After the surgeon presents an accurate and thorough description of the contemplated surgery, patients should be asked to put into their own words the salient points of the explanation in order to ensure that they have not distorted the information. After the doctor is satisfied that the patient possesses a realistic understanding of the anticipated surgery, patients should then be required to notify the doctor when they are ready for the operation. By leaving this step to the patient's initiative, his or her motivation for the surgery can again be assessed.

Only in the most unusual circumstances should a

patient's request for cosmetic surgery be refused. However, patients with potentially risky psychological factors require special screening and consideration. Patients' objective assessment of their physical defect as well as what the surgery can and cannot accomplish should be measured. Patients who do not possess realistic understanding should be educated by the physician, and then their ability to incorporate this new information should be evaluated.

PSYCHOLOGICAL CONSULTATION

Physicians who perform cosmetic surgery do not seek psychological consultations as a standard procedure. However, if the physician feels uncomfortable, for psychological reasons, about undertaking a cosmetic procedure, such a consultation may be useful. Davis[17] has specified six circumstances under which such a consultation would be advisable: (1) when a doctor feels uneasy about the patient's motivation; (2) when a doctor suspects that the patient's expectations are not reasonable; (3) when there is a history of previous psychiatric treatment; (4) when a doctor suspects paranoia, masochism, mania, or depression; (5) when the patient tries to flatter a doctor into doing a procedure that may not be strongly indicated or that has been refused by another surgeon; and (6) when the doctor suspects that the patient may be emotionally disturbed, although manageable by proper psychiatric assistance. Surgical procedures that are successful aesthetically or technically may not be considered successful by patients who fall into one or more of the above categories. In such instances the cooperation of a mental health professional with whom the patient already has a positive relationship can be useful in managing these high-risk patients. It is difficult for a therapist to establish such a relationship when a patient is referred after the operation has taken place. The patient may not be amenable to such a referral even before the operation. After all, many of these individuals have already decided to handle their dissatisfaction through nonpsychological techniques. Consequently, when the surgeon suspects that a therapist may be useful in managing a case, the referral is best made before the cosmetic procedure. Studies have shown that a patient's willingness to accept referral to a mental health professional is positively related to the patient's tendency to accept the surgical results. Patients who refuse consultation are likely to respond less favorably to the results of their cosmetic surgery.[18]

In making referrals the physician must be aware that not all mental health professionals are skilled in the issues relevant to cosmetic surgery. It may be useful to ask the consultant to answer the following questions:

1. Is the patient mentally ill? If so, should the surgery be done anyway? With what precautions?
2. Does the patient have hidden fantasies about the surgery so that it is unlikely he or she will be a satisfied patient? Is it impossible for the surgery to really accomplish the patient's objective?
3. Will the stress of surgery lead to decompensation (a breakdown of defenses with resulting psychological problems)? May surgery be done with special precautions?
4. Does the patient have tendencies to be litigious? Accusatory or angry at the surgeon and the hospital?
5. Will the patient change his mind and regret the surgery? Is his or her motivation too shaky or unrealistic?
6. Can the patient accept less than perfection? Will the patient be disappointed if the result is a little different from what he or she fancied?[19]

POSTOPERATIVE REACTIONS

Cosmetic surgery patients develop fewer emotional complications than other surgical cases.[20] This may be due to the fact that, since the procedures are not life-threatening, many of the patient's normal defenses against illness, helplessness, and trauma are not elicited. The majority of patients having cosmetic surgery adapt successfully and profit from the body changes. Most patients report satisfaction, improved self-esteem, relief from depressive symptoms, and improvement in interpersonal relationships following cosmetic surgery.[18] As a result the cosmetic operation has been called by some the "twenty-minute hour."

Nevertheless, psychological sequelae are the most common complications of cosmetic procedures. Reich[11] in a follow-up of 599 cosmetic surgery cases found that 31% of patients experienced a short-lived depression or reactive anxiety following surgery. The reasons for these postoperative reactions vary from patient to patient. In some individuals these reactions may represent a healthy response to a significant life change. Patients may mourn the loss of their old appearance or the lost opportunities, wasted times, and unnecessary struggles that patients may feel they have experienced as a result of their physical defect. The depression may be the result of the patient's inability to express or even to consciously acknowledge the anger of undergoing a costly and painful process in order to gain the acceptance of other people. The anxiety may represent a normal reaction to an uncertain future, which will hopefully be filled with new possibilities for securing more of what the patient desires.

For some, the postoperative period will involve more serious psychological complications. Many research studies have shown that any life change, even one which is considered advantageous, tends to be stressful for a person.[21] A variety of stressors can impinge upon the cosmetic surgery patient during the postoperative period.

Cosmetic surgery patients experience an alteration in their body image as a result of the surgery. This change can produce a major stress in some individuals. During the early stages of the postoperative period, while the discoloration, swelling, and pain persist, this factor can be of marked importance.

If an individual is in a strange environment, such as a hospital, many of the usual feedback cues that help a person maintain his or her identity and self-esteem may be absent. Patients may be unable to resume their occupation immediately or to maintain their regular social schedule. Any of these changes can be disorienting.

In addition, as a result of the surgery, patients may be unable to care for themselves adequately and may require the assistance of others. If other people are unavailable or if the patient has some conflicts about surrendering to these dependency needs, the situation may be unpleasant.

Also, to the degree that patients have harbored unrealistic expectations about the operation, they will have to face their unrealized expectations. When interpersonal relationships do not immediately improve, when new vocational opportunities do not suddenly emerge, or when they realize that their experiences have not changed in certain important ways despite an altered physical appearance, patients may react unfavorably.

If patients do not possess the psychological resources to cope successfully with the problems associated with cosmetic surgery, then they may decompensate. Although the characteristics of decompensation vary, the nature and severity of it can be predicted from a preoperative psychological assessment. More importantly, the presence of an ongoing psychotherapeutic relationship can help these patients to cope more successfully with the difficulties encountered during the postoperative period. For those patients who have grown up anticipating a certain kind of interpersonal feedback, psychological help may be useful in learning to adjust to new social realities of the successfully treated cosmetic surgery patient.

In working with individuals who may experience more stress during the postoperative period than they are normally able to tolerate, it is important to mobilize as many different support systems as possible to assist the person in getting through the recovery period and making an optimal adjustment. Psychologists, social workers, psychiatrists, and occupational therapists can provide assistance. If the patient is in a hospital, a warm attitude from as many staff members as possible will help alleviate patients' anxiety and make them feel more comfortable and trusting about the hospital personnel. Also, existing resources, including both the patient's own personality and his or her social support system, can be mobilized. In general, patients should receive as much external stimulation as possible to keep them oriented to their surroundings and to minimize the intrusion of internal fears and fantasies into their consciousness. Any pleasant form of sensory stimulation, such as television, radio, books, or magazines, can be useful in this regard. Visitors can help the person to cheer up and to provide emotional support. In some circumstances psychoactive medications may also be beneficial in the management of otherwise difficult patients.

It is common for patients to experience some dissatisfaction with their surgery in the absence of pronounced decompensation. At times, the patient's dissatisfaction is the result of physical complications that are a source of disappointment to the doctor as well. Although the patient may have been adequately informed prior to the surgery about possible complications, research has shown that cosmetic surgery patients deny their own vulnerability to untoward developments. Consequently, these unfortunate individuals may be not only disappointed but also highly emotional after an operation. In such instances the patient should be given the opportunity to express feelings of anger, sadness, of disappointment, regardless of how irrational these feelings may seem. It is an error for the physician to challenge the patient's view at this stage. Surgeons do not have to agree with the patient's reasoning, but they do need to convey the impression of being sympathetic and understanding of the patient's feelings. Usually, after expressing feelings in an accepting and supportive environment, the irrationality and emotionality is reduced. After these feelings have been adequately expressed, the patient and doctor can discuss what options are available. In some instances the possibility of another operation can be considered.

By dealing successfully with the patient's feelings, the possibility of maintaining a good rapport will be enhanced, and the patient will be more cooperative with the doctor. Also, the chances of avoiding litigation, regardless of the merits of the case, will increase. Research has shown that most malpractice cases are the result of patient grievances other than the specified complaints.[22] Two of the more common reasons for malpractice suits are that the patient is suit-conscious or trying to avoid paying the bill. It is probably true that in 90% of the cases where the patient sues there is no malpractice, and in 90% of the cases where malpractice does exist there is no suit. Most law suits originate out of personality conflicts or damaged feelings. The patient wants to feel that the physician understands and is interested in his or her complaints. Some patients may persist in their anger even after the doctor has adequately demonstrated understanding and concern. In these cases the patient's underlying motive may be to see if the doctor will set limits. In these instances the physician should adopt the role of a parent or relative and deal firmly with behaviors that even the patient probably knows are unacceptable. In extreme cases the doctor may offer to work with the patient only after all disruptive behaviors are discontinued. Doctors should not allow the patient to believe that they are afraid of litigation or feel guilty. This impression may serve to encourage the patient's tendency to sue.

CONCLUSION

The increased popularity of cosmetic surgery is one aspect of the personality pattern of our times. Alienated from the self, people look to others to supply the positive feedback that they are unable to generate for themselves. It is no wonder that people seek cosmetic surgery. The prevailing social and cultural emphasis upon appearance is widespread and apparent.

Almost all personality theories include the ability to fully experience pleasure through the body as a cornerstone of health. Although patients may be satisfied with their cosmetic surgery, they have not necessarily overcome their psychopathology.

Dissatisfaction with physical appearance, though fully understandable in the current social context, represents a symptom of the person's inability to maintain self-esteem. By improving one's appearance through cosmetic surgery, an individual's adjustment may be improved, but much remains unaltered.

REFERENCES

1. Chesnoff RZ: The kindest cuts. Geo, 2:98–110, 1980
2. Lasch C: The Culture of Narcissism. New York, W. W. Norton, 1979
3. Lasch, ibid., p 41
4. Aronson E: Some antecedents of interpersonal attraction. In Arnold WJ and Levine D (eds): Nebraska Symposium on Motivation. Lincoln, Neb.: University of Nebraska Press, 1969
5. Dion K, Berscheid E: Physical attractiveness and social perception of peers in preschool children. Mimeographed research report available for the authors, 1972
6. Clifford MM, Walster E: The effects of physical attractiveness on teacher expectations. Sociology of Education, 46(2):248–258, 1973
7. Cavior N, Dokecki PR: Physical attractiveness, perceived attitude similarity, and academic achievement as contributors to interpersonal attraction among adolescents. Developmental Psychology, 9:44–54, 1973
8. Roff M, Brody DS: Appearance and choice status during adolescence. Journal of Psychology, 36:347–356, 1953
9. Cavior N, Boblett PJ: Physical attractiveness of dating versus married couples. Proceedings of the 80th Annual Convention of the American Psychological Association, 1:175–176, (Summary), 1972
10. Dion K, Berscheid E, Walster E: What is beautiful is good. Journal of Personality and Social Psychology, 24(3):285–290, 1972
11. Reich J: The surgery of appearance: Psychological and related aspects. Medical Journal of Australia, 2:5, 1969
12. Masters FW, Greaves DC: The Quasimodo complex. British Journal of Plastic Surgery, 20:204–210, 1967
13. Hay E: Psychiatric Aspects of cosmetic nasal surgery. British Journal of Psychiatry, 116:85–97, 1970
14. Jacobsen WE, Meyer E, Edgerton MT, et al: Screening of rhinoplasty candidates from the psychological point of view. Plastic and Reconstructive Surgery, 13:279–281, 1960
15. Edgerton ME, Jacobsen WE, Meyer E: Surgical psychiatric study of patients seeking plastic (cosmetic) surgery: Ninety-eight consecutive patients with minimal deformity. British Journal of Plastic Surgery, 13:136–145, 1960
16. Clarksen P, Stafford-Clark D: Role of the plastic surgeon and psychiatrist in the surgery of appearance. British Medical Journal, 2:1768–1771, 1960
17. Davis DL: Psychiatric screening of patients for cosmetic surgery. Mimeographed research report, 1979.
18. Wright MR: Cosmetic procedures, the management of the dissatisfied patient. Mimeographed report available from the author.
19. Shulman BH: Psychiatric assessment of the candidate for cosmetic surgery. Presented at the meeting of the American Academy of Facial Plastic and Reconstructive Surgery, St. Louis April 1973
20. Gifford S: Cosmetic surgery and personality change: A review of some clinical observations. In Goldwyn RM (ed): The Unfavorable Result in Plastic Surgery: Avoidance and Treatment. Boston, Little, Brown & Co., 1972
21. Holmes TH, Rahe RH: The social readjustment rating scale. Journal of Psychosomatic Research, 11:213–218, 1967
22. Rosenthal GK: Preventing malpractice claims. Washington University Magazine, 47(4):7–13, 1977

2

MARVIN E. CHERNOSKY, M.D.

An Office Surgery

A well-equipped office allows one to perform dermatologic surgery without sacrificing quality. A patient may enter and leave the doctor's office more conveniently than the hospital. Records, already completed in the office, need not be duplicated. The minor nature of many procedures does not require a complete history, physical examination, and admission laboratory work as in a hospital. Because many surgeries are relatively brief, they can be performed when the patient comes for a routine office visit. Doing a procedure on the spur of the moment is desirable because it decreases preoperative apprehension and reduces the number of required visits. Surgery requiring greater amounts of time can be scheduled immediately for a special office period. Busy, office-oriented physicians do not have and should not take the time to go to hospitals to perform services that can be performed adequately in their own offices. Territorial familiarity with a single office means greater efficiency because it eliminates adapting to several hospitals, different types of operating rooms, instruments, and assisting personnel. The office dermatologic assistant is often more efficient and willing to be more helpful than the more broadly trained hospital assistant, who must also relate to other surgeons. Personally chosen instruments designed for dermatologic surgery and constant in design and size are also an asset.

Aside from the convenience to both patient and surgeon and the concomitant decrease in expense, medical advantages accrue when performing surgery in the office. The flora of microorganisms in most offices are usually different and less pathogenic than those found in hospitals. Ambulatory office patients return immediately to home environments where homeostasis with microorganisms has already been acquired.

THE SURGERY ROOM AND LARGE EQUIPMENT

The size of the operating room should be adequate for the people using it. Small or slim physicians and assistants require less floor space to deliver efficient service than do personnel with larger physiques. In certain types of surgery, blood and other debris may splatter nearby walls. They should be constructed of some smooth, easily washable material such as tile or plastic.

Adequate lighting is an important requirement. My two operating rooms have natural daylight from windows, as well as adjustable overhead lighting fixtures (Castle Ceiling Light) that provide concentrated, shadowless, white light throughout a field of adequate diameter. Spotlight fixtures should not be used because they produce excessive shadowing. Several types of lights are available and all of them have advantages and disadvantages.

An adjustable operating table is essential for proper positions during surgery, to adjust the height to accommodate the surgeon, and to use the Trendelenburg position at a moment's notice if syncope develops. The table should be equipped with an adjustable headrest, stirrups for the lithotomy position, and rail attachments for an arm rest. It should be covered with smooth, washable material. Side guardrails or restraining straps, or both, should be available. Some surgeons prefer a table with a very small headrest, which allows the operator to get closer to the patient. For some types of minor surgery and other treatments, a relatively inexpensive, small barber chair is convenient and can be purchased through barber supply houses. The shorter of two operators may be required to stand on a special metal platform with a nonskid surface.

An adequate tabletop cabinet (Fig. 2–1) is needed to hold sterile instrument pans, transfer forceps, and other supplies. A Mayo stand is used to present sterile instruments during the operation. Another stand or table, preferably with wheels for maneuverability, is needed for nonsterile instruments, such as the bipolar electrocoagulator used for hemostasis. Some surgeons prefer to sit on a stool mounted on casters during operations.

A call bell or interoffice communication system is needed at times to summon assistance to the operating room. In my operating and treatment rooms, I have an electrical system that, when activated by touching a button (with the elbow when wearing surgical gloves), activates a bell and lights outside the room door and is shown on numbered panels in the laboratory and front office. All rooms in my office are equipped with speakers with volume controls that provide suitable soothing background music.

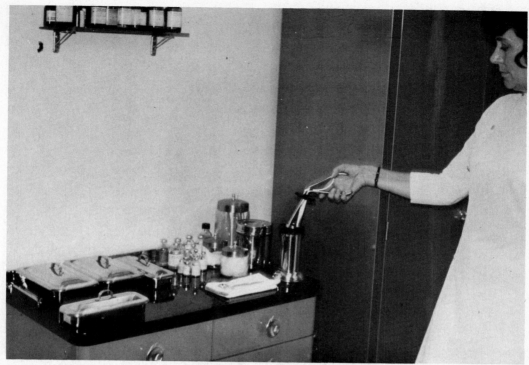

Figure 2—1. Tabletop cabinet for sterile instrument pans, transfer forceps, and other supplies. Note the wall shelf for medicines and chemical cauterants is placed out of reach of small children.

STERILIZATION EQUIPMENT AND DISPOSABLE MATERIALS

Equipment must be available to adequately clean, sterilize, store, and transfer surgical instruments and supplies. Instruments should be washed immediately after use with detergents and water. One timesaver is the ultrasonic instrument cleaner.

Bard-Parker transfer forceps are stored in Zephiran Chloride 1:1000 solution and are used only to handle sterilized materials. All instruments used in invasive skin procedures are sterilized by steam pressure or dry heat. A compact piece of equipment manufactured by Pelton and Crane provides both dry-heat and steam-pressure sterilization (Fig. 2–2).

Basic instrument packs used in closed surgery include drapes, eye sheets, towels, hemostats, and various forceps. All should be autoclaved and stored for instant use when needed. At the time of surgery, various sharp instruments are sterilized separately in stainless steel pans using dry heat and are added to this pack using transfer forceps. Dry-heat sterilization does not dull the edges of sharp instruments as does autoclaving. The lids of these pans are kept closed except when sterile instruments are removed. Office personnel should not breathe or cough into open pans. Instruments stored in this manner are used frequently and must be resterilized several times a week. Instruments used infrequently are wrapped individually (autoclave paper for steam or aluminum foil for dry heat sterilization). Time, temperature, and steam pressure requirements are available from sterilizer manufacturers. An appropriate autoclave sterilization indicator, such as Autoclave Tape (3-M Company), should be used to assure adequate sterilization.

Disposable materials include rubber gloves, needles, syringes, and paper eye sheets. For most cases, I still prefer cloth eye sheets because they conform better to the skin surface and do not tear or shed. Eye sheets should be made with tightly woven, 270-thread Pima cotton. Some operators prefer to use dental syringes (Cooke-Waite) with a disposable Carpule containing the anesthetic.

INSTRUMENTS AND EQUIPMENT FOR COLD STEEL SURGERY

In order to choose instruments best fitted for the individual physician's needs, I recommend actually using various instruments before any sizeable quantity is purchased. Such factors as the operator's skill, temperament, size and contour of the hands, and available assistance must be considered. The size and type of instruments should be standardized in order to avoid adaptations from operation to operation. High-quality stainless steel instruments should

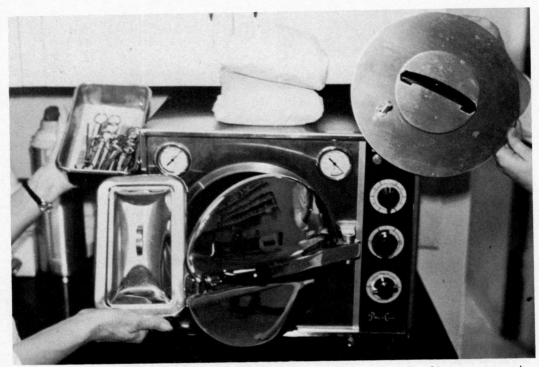

Figure 2–2. Combination dry-heat sterilizer and steam-pressure autoclave. Wrapped packs of instruments can be autoclaved. Instruments in stainless steel pans can be sterilized with dry heat when the unit is sealed with the door being held at right.

be selected. The following list of basic equipment and instruments should be of benefit to doctors who are planning or expanding their office.

1. Adjustable operating table (preferably electrically operated with stirrups, arm board, guardrails, and restraining straps)
2. Overhead adjustable lighting
3. Combination dry-heat sterilizer and steam pressure autoclave (Pelton and Crane)
4. Sponges, drapes, towels, towel clips, and suture materials
5. Transfer forceps
6. Razor
7. Bard-Parker handles, disposable blades (no. 10, 11, and 15)
8. Small, curved mosquito hemostats
9. Ochsner artery forceps
10. Sharp, single-prong skin hooks (double-prong hooks are occasionally used for large excisions)
11. Hudson (or Adson) forceps with and without teeth
12. Small mouse tooth forceps (iris forceps)
13. Curved, double-pointed, microscopic dissecting scissors (or the slightly smaller iris scissors)
14. Curved, blunt tenotomy scissors
15. Casteneri's rhytidectomy dissection scissors (6-inch)
16. Storz stitch scissors (ophthalmic)
17. Straight operating scissors, one end sharp, one end blunt
18. Bandage scissors
19. Bipolar electrocautery and electrosector with removable, sterilizable active electrodes
20. Monopolar electrodesiccator (such as the Hyphrecator by Birtcher)
21. Olser-Hegar needle holder and combined suture scissors with Ochsner diamond jaws.
22. Laschal Precision Suture Tome, Model 403, with a no. 15 slot
23. Littauer stitch scissors
24. Skin punches, sizes 1 to 8 mm
25. Dermal curettes, sizes 1, 2, and 3
26. Metal applicator sticks
27. Various sizes and types of comedo extractors
28. Microlance blood lances
29. Nail nippers (concave edge and double spring in handle)
30. Electric Moto-drill no. 1
31. Steel dental burrs (nos. 3 and 11)
32. Plastic face shield
33. Podiatric nail probe and packer
34. Freer elevator, blunt single-end
35. Jeweler's forceps (for delicate work or pinpoint coagulation).

Additional equipment and instruments that are nice to have for greater efficiency, for that "occasional" case, or for certain specialized procedures include:

1. Ultrasonic instrument cleaner
2. Electric hair shaver
3. Large self-retaining skin retractor
4. Small automatic skin retractor
5. Lucite lid plate (Jaeger, Storz)
6. Chalazion forceps (Lordan)
7. Nasal and ear specula with light source
8. Penberthy aspirator with straight and intraoral tips (or a more expensive electric-powered suction machine, such as Sorensen's)
9. Power-driven skin punches, sizes 1 to 8 mm
10. Dermoplaning machine with wire brushes and diamond fraises (such as the Kurtin dermoplaner or the Bell hand engine)
11. Heath curette, 1 mm size
12. Flexible lachrymal probes, double-end
13. Grafco-Standard ear piercer (Graham-Field Surgical Co.) utilizing stainless steel, temporary ear posts
14. Dermajet
15. Honing machine (Honing Machine Corp., Mishawaka, Indiana)
16. Auto Suture, Model SFM-2, with disposable loading units SM-25 and SM-25 W and staple remover or one of several brands of disposable staplers.
17. Microbipolar forceps (Birtcher Corp.).

Although some brand names are included above, this does not necessarily imply that similar instruments are unsatisfactory. The quantity of instruments purchased is related to the amount of dermatologic surgery to be performed.

Any details about the uses, advantages, or disadvantages of these listed items would not be feasible or appropriate in this chapter. Figure 2–3

illustrates a set of surgical instruments and drapes over an operative site prepared for excisional surgery and suture closure.

Nondisposable cutting instruments such as scissors, curettes, and skin punches must be kept sharp. An office assistant utilizing the Honing machine with various attachments can be very useful, but occasional professional sharpening and realignment are required. In an attempt to discourage pilferage and to monitor sharpening procedures, my instruments are marked with an electric vibrator tool showing the dates and my name. Scissors, after several sharpenings, are relegated to coarser work, such as trimming callouses.

Ochsner artery forceps are used only on tissue being excised. Only the nonmutilating skin hook is used on skin to be approximated. Hudson forceps with teeth are used on deep fascia and those without teeth to hold sutures or Steri-strips. The Storz stitch scissors, a very fine ophthalmologic instrument with small, double-pointed blades, are used when removing small suture material. I also use them to cut tissue when removing very small tumors on the eyelid margin or other delicate areas. The Olsen-Hegar needle holder and combination suture scissors with Ochsner diamond jaws are convenient to use when operating without an assistant. Before accepting this instrument from the supplier, each one should be tested for the holding power of the occluded, finely serrated jaws while stress is placed on 6-0 nylon suture, as when performing instrument ties.

Figure 2–4 shows a relatively new instrument, the Laschal Precision Suture Tome, Model 403, with a no. 15 slot. This instrument is used to safely cut sutures adjacent to the knots; its use is described in Chapter 10. The electric Moto-drill no. 1 or the

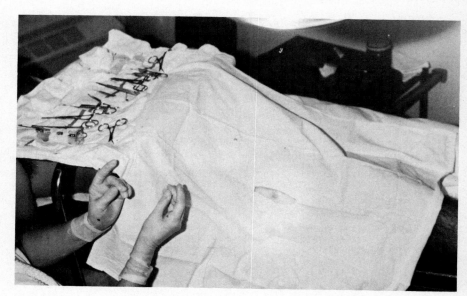

Figure 2–3. Instruments and drapes prepared for excisional surgery and wound closure by suturing.

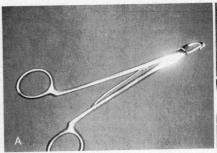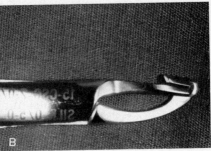

Figure 2—4. *A*, The Laschal Precision Suture Tome is used for cutting sutures adjacent to the knot in the depths of wounds. *B*, Detail of instrument tip.

dermoplaning machine is used as the power source for no. 3 and 11 steel dental burrs in drilling or removing diseased portions of nails.

Figure 2–5 displays three instruments used to immobilize skin and produce hemostasis when performing surgery on the eyelid, lip, or rim of naris. The Lucite lid plate is placed underneath the eyelid after appropriate topical conjunctival anesthesia and held in position by an assistant to provide a firm base upon which to operate. The chalazion forceps are useful when approaching a lesion percutaneously or by way of the palpebral conjunctiva.

The inexpensive Penberthy aspirator is useful with a straight or intraoral tip to suck saliva or blood out of a surgical field. The tip and tubing can be autoclaved.

Figure 2–6 shows the Auto-Suture, skin and fascia model, with disposable loading units and staple remover. Several other brands of disposable staplers are available.

Figure 2–7 shows the Birtcher microbipolar forceps, which I use to control hemostasis during closed surgical procedures. The instrument attaches to the bipolar terminals of the Hyphecator, and the surgeon controls coagulation of the grasped blood vessel with a foot pedal. More details concerning instruments used in cold steel surgery will be found in other chapters.

INSTRUMENTATION FOR ELECTROSURGERY

The basic instrument that should be in all treatment rooms for curettage and desiccation of tumors as well as other procedures is the monopolar electrodesiccator, such as the Birtcher Hyphrecator or the Bantam Bovie. Both can also provide bipolar coagulation. Some spark gap instruments as well as a vacuum tube apparatus can be used as a cold cautery scalpel for electrosection. Actual (hot) cautery is useful for preventing or treating surface hemorrhage and is found sometimes to be more controllable and less painful when removing a large number of small benign skin tumors (with or without the aid of a curette or scissors). Because its use causes no electric current to pass through the body, it is indicated for use on patients with cardiac pacemakers.

Epilation for superfluous hair is performed in my office by supervised technicians using an automatically timed, high-frequency electronic apparatus (Proteus Epilator, Model MWD-5B). Details of

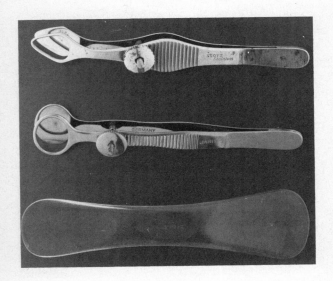

Figure 2–5. Lucite lid plate and chalazion forceps used to immobilize skin during surgery on the eyelid, lip, or rim of naris.

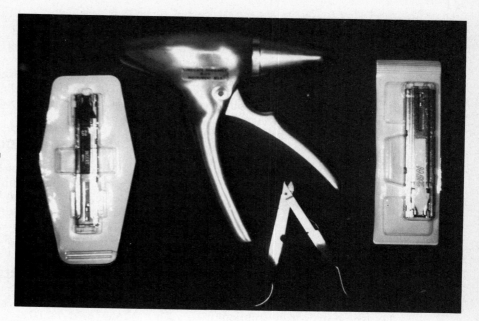

Figure 2–6. Auto-Suture with loading units and staple remover.

instrumentation, technique, and results have been previously described in an article.[1]

INSTRUMENTATION FOR CRYOSURGERY

Superficial cryotherapy or cryosurgery can be performed with dry ice: broken, sawed, or sculptured into appropriate shapes; dipped in acetone; and applied to the skin with varying pressures and lengths of time. The portable Kidde dry ice apparatus is easy to use on house or hospital calls, but the small quantity of ice produced limits its usefulness. Other freezing sources include sprays such as Fluoroethyl (75% dichlorotetra-fluoroethane and 25% ethyl chloride).

Liquid nitrogen used for superficial cryosurgery can be placed on the skin with various forms of cotton, copper, or polyurethane applicators. Thermos bottles or larger special containers can be used to store it.

Sophisticated equipment utilizing liquid nitrous oxide or liquid nitrogen have been developed for superficial and deep surgery. These instruments provide freezing by spraying the material on the skin or by using closed cryoprobe systems. I am currently using the Cryac (Owens Laboratories) liquid nitrogen spray. Details of cyrosurgery instrumentation are found in other chapters.

LASER AND LIPOSUCTION SURGERY INSTRUMENTATION

In recent years, a limited number of dermatologists have become proficient in laser or liposuction surgery or both. The specialized instrumentation required for these procedures is described in Chapters 25 and 27.

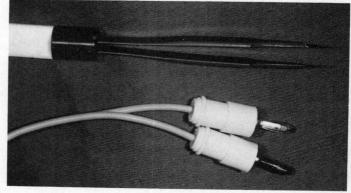

Figure 2–7. Birtcher microbipolar forceps for coagulation of blood vessels.

TOPICAL CHEMOTHERAPY AND CHEMOSURGERY SUPPLIES

Numerous types of chemicals are used in dermatologic chemosurgery. Because many of these are very caustic, proper precautions should be taken in the handling of them, both by the physician and office assistants. As illustrated in Figure 2–1, chemicals should be placed on high shelves, out of reach of small children. The choice of topical agents used is an individual matter. Materials in my rooms include the following:

1. Saturated solution phenol
2. 10% Silver nitrate
3. Betadine solution
4. Monsel's solution
5. 35% Aluminum chloride solution
6. Trichloroacetic acid (5%, 10%, 15%, 20%, 30%, and 50% saturated solutions)
7. Saturated solution of monochloroacetic acid
8. 1% Gentian violet solution
9. 10% Potassium hydroxide solution
10. Spirits of ammonia
11. Million reagent
12. 25% Podophyllin in compound tincture of benzoin
13. Zephiran Chloride 1:1000 solution
14. 4% Chlorhexidine skin cleanser (Hibiclens)
15. Tissue-marking dyes.

EMERGENCY EQUIPMENT AND DRUGS

This chapter cannot be concluded without stressing the fact that *all* physicians' offices should have emergency equipment and drugs, whether or not office surgery is performed. However, rather than summarize this vital subject here, the reader is referred to Chapters 8 and 9.

REFERENCE

1. Chernosky ME: Permanent removal of superfluous hair. Tex Med. 67:72–78, 1971

3

DANIEL E. GORMLEY, M.D.

Control of Surgical Infection

The physician who violates the cutaneous barrier must take appropriate steps to minimize the risk of infection. Although the skin is highly resistant to microorganisms, surgically related local or systemic sepsis is always possible. The high success rate of cutaneous surgery with its low frequency of complications should not engender a false sense of security. In the well-run surgical facility, commitment to infection control finds expression in adequately monitored standards and procedures that are designed to protect everyone connected with the operative process.

INFECTION

Patterns of Infection

Pathogens reaching the wound may originate from the surgical environment or may be native to the patient. Inflammation resulting from trauma and infection is the first change to occur after inoculation.[1] Abscess formation is a process of localization characterized by toxin-induced tissue liquefaction. A focus of purulent material is surrounded by a zone of inflammation and granulation tissue.[1] Extension to anatomic spaces or fistula formation may occur. Resolution occurs most rapidly with drainage of the abscess. Cellulitis, which is a more diffuse process of infection and inflammation, can involve subcutaneous tissue. It may spread rapidly and have poorly defined borders.[2] Lymphangitis, with its streaks of erythema and tenderness, is possible with either abscess formation or cellulitis.[2] Rarely occurring gangrenous processes, such as necrotizing fasciitis which can evolve from minor wounds, may be caused by obligate or facultative anaerobes.[3, 4] The synergistic action of more than one pathogen may be required. Streptococci are often present. Characterized by a rapidly advancing front of tissue necrosis, necrotizing fasciitis involves the subcutaneous fat and possibly the deep fascia. Skin at the edge of the involved area is erythematous. There is a central discoloration that may vary from gray to violet or black. Gangrene of the skin may occur. These infections, which may result from the synergistic interaction of multiple pathogens, resemble other entities such as anaerobic cellulitis and gas gangrene.[2]

Systemic sequelae of wound infections include bacteremia, metastatic spread of infection, and toxemia.[2] Bacterial, mycologic, or viral pathogens can spread over abraded surfaces.[5–7] Serious complications, while rare, can appear at any time to confront the unwary practitioner.

Bacteriology of Wound Infections

The skin is a selective environment that permits the growth of certain resident organisms. Although many of these bacteria are harmless if introduced into a wound, others can cause infection. There are some organisms that may be present only transiently or under certain circumstances. Humidity, hygiene, the presence of open lesions, antibiotic usage, and hospital confinement are among the factors that can affect the flora of the skin.[8, 9]

A list of some of the bacteria capable of causing wound infections must be headed by gram-positive cocci as the most common offenders. *Staphylococcus epidermidis,* a coagulase-negative microorganism, is a normal inhabitant of the skin that can cause abscesses, suture tract infections, bacteremia, and endocarditis.[10, 11] *Staphylococcus aureus*, often part of the flora of the skin, causes abscesses and cellulitis. These infections tend to be more aggressive than those of *S. epidermidis*. Bacteremia and metastatic spread are possible. Although they are irregular inhabitants of the skin,[12] beta-hemolytic streptococci are more prevalent when hygiene is poor and humidity is high.[2] Respiratory infections and carrier states that can occur in epidemics may be predisposing factors. The ability of these organisms to survive on the skin and to cause cellulitis, erysipelas, septicemia, and nephritis makes them important surgical pathogens. Enterococci, which can participate in synergistic infections,[4] have been isolated from the skin of the perineum[13] and from some chronic ulcers.[14]

Gram-negative wound infections are less prevalent in dermatologic surgical practice than they are in hospitals where operative procedures are done on the gastrointestinal and genitourinary systems. *Escherichia coli* does not survive for long on dry skin.[15] Most commonly found in the perineum and in intertriginous areas, *E. coli* colonizes moist ulcers.[16] It has been reported as a cause of cutaneous abscesses[17] and gangrenous septic processes.[2, 4] *Pseudomonas* cause wound infections, pyoderma, and septicemia. They are found in the toe webs, external auditory canal, chronic ulcers, and other moist surfaces.[15] *Enterobacter aerogenes,* which is a rare cause of skin wound infections (author's experience), has been isolated from the axillae.[15] *Proteus* sp. are found in the perineum and toe webs. Wound infections and endocarditis have been reported.[15] Gram-negative folliculitis caused by *Proteus* could conceivably set the stage for a surgical infection. *Mima* and *Herellea* spp. are regarded as normal skin flora with a predilection for toe webs and the axillary regions.[15] Cellulitis and wound infections among the debilitated have been reported.[18] Other gram-negative organisms capable of causing infections in other parts of the body only rarely cause cutaneous surgical wound infections. Agents such as *Haemophilus* sp. have been associated with cellulitis,[15] especially in children, and under the right circumstances might be dangerous in the skin surgery setting.

Anaerobic Organisms

Clostridial organisms can be found in the perineal area.[19] Spores found in soil will contaminate virtually any surface, including the skin. Clostridia are capable of replicating within apparently trivial wounds or injuries,[17, 20] especially in subcutaneous tissue,[2] as long as anaerobic conditions exist.[20] Conditions of diminished oxygen tension, which can evolve in some wounds, may conceivably favor anaerobic growth. Even if the local effects of an infection are inconsequential, the dissemination of exotoxins from organisms such as *Clostridium tetani* can have serious consequences. Other organisms are capable of replicating as facultative anaerobes and will sometimes cause synergistic infections as described above.

Aerobic Organisms

Mycobacteria, which are not normal skin inhabitants, are capable of infecting abrasions and wounds. Contaminated instruments have been implicated in epidemic infections.[19]

Viral Infections

Because herpes simplex is capable of spreading across an abraded surface, the presence of an active herpetic process in the skin is a contraindication for dermabrasion or chemical peeling.[5, 6]

Mycotic Infections

Cutaneous candidosis was reported in a group of dermabraded patients.[7]

Treatment

Treatment of infection should be based on appropriate antimicrobial therapy as determined by Gram staining, culture, and sensitivity studies. (Anaerobic organisms require special culturing techniques.) Until laboratory data are obtained, therapy must sometimes be initiated empirically. A knowledge of the pathogens prevalent in the community as well as their likely antibiotic susceptibilities can be obtained from a periodic review of office and hospital culture data. Incision and drainage of abscesses may be all that is necessary for resolution without antibiotic therapy.[17] Thorough débridement of necrotic, infected, and autolyzed tissue is essential.[2] Tetanus immunizations should be current.

SURGICAL ANTISEPSIS

Antisepsis is the process by which microorganisms are eliminated from a viable surface.[21, 22] There is, of course, no way to sterilize a living surface. Overzealous efforts to reduce the number of pathogens may compromise the ability of the skin to resist infection.[23] Since there is no such thing as a totally sterile procedure, some degree of wound contamination is inevitable. From a practical standpoint a surgical procedure is rendered reasonably safe as long as the magnitude of the bacterial inoculum is maintained at a sufficiently low level.[9] Relatively simple cleansing measures will ordinarily suffice to make this possible.

The process of antisepsis involves three steps: (1) the removal of as many microorganisms as possible from the surface of the skin, (2) the destruction of a maximum number of residual pathogens, and (3) the creation of a persistent bacteriostatic effect that retards the growth of organisms after the initial killing phase. The ideal antiseptic should accomplish all of this with a broad-spectrum killing power and without systemic or local toxicity. Rapid action, low cost, and aesthetic acceptability are also important.

As Table 3–1 shows, many antiseptics fall short of meeting all desired requirements. The following program appears to be adequate for a dermatologic surgical procedure.

Surgical preparation can begin several days in advance with daily washings of the operative area using an agent that leaves bacteriostatic residues on the skin. Before surgery the skin is scrubbed with a chlorhexidine gluconate or povidone-iodine scrubbing material with sufficient vigor and water to flush away soil, debris, and excess oil. Scrubbing should start in the center of an operative area and proceed to the peripheral areas (Fig. 3–1). It is sometimes easier to wash an entire area, such as the face, than to attempt to restrict the clean surface to a smaller subregion. If the center of the operative area is badly contaminated, the plan is revised so that the spread of bacteria into the area of the incision is avoided. After washing, the surface can be blotted

TABLE 3–1. Antiseptics and Disinfectants

1. **Antiseptics** (substances used to reduce the number of microorganisms on living surfaces).[21]
   a. *Soap and Water.* Little direct effect on bacteria in the absence of added bacteriostatic agents. The scrubbing and flushing effect mechanically removes bacteria as well as the dirt and oil that harbor them. This is particularly important with respect to spores and other forms that are resistant to chemical antisepsis.
   b. *Cationic Detergents.* Quaternary ammonium compounds (e.g., benzalkonium chloride, benzethonium chloride, and cetylpyridinium chloride are inoffensive and relatively nontoxic but not effective against spores, *Pseudomonas*, or tuberculosis. They are inactivated by soaps and organic material.
   c. *Organic Solvents.* Solvents such as isopropyl and ethyl alcohol are bacteriocidal and fungicidal but not sporicidal. Dilutions with water of 60 to 95% (70% concentration most popular) are more effective than pure alcohol. Solvents facilitate removal of bacteria-laden oil, but their overzealous use makes the skin more susceptible to infection.[23]
   d. *Phenol Derivatives.* Phenol derivatives such as hexachlorophene, dichlorophen, and chlorophenol must be used repeatedly for bacteriostasis. They leave residues on surfaces, including the skin, that are effective against staphylococci. They are not inactivated by soap or organic material and absorbed through intact skin. Evidence of neurotoxicity in infants and fear of teratogenesis has caused sharp reduction of their use in the United States.[44, 45]
   e. *Heavy Metal Compounds.* Such compounds as merbromin and thimerosal are inactivated by organic matter.
   f. *Iodine.* Tincture of iodine (2%) or Lugol's solution are rapidly bacteriocidal and sporicidal. They can irritate and discolor the skin and damage tissues in higher concentrations. (The concentration of tinctures may increase as a result of alcohol evaporation.) Reactivity of free iodine causes it to be inactivated by the presence of organic material. Nevertheless, tincture of iodine remains a valuable agent that can be applied to surfaces that may have been contaminated with spores or resistant forms.[25]
   g. *Iodophors.* Iodophors, such as polyvinylpyrrolidone, iodine, or povidone-iodine, are excellent agents for antiseptic preparation of the skin because of their broad spectrum of action.[25] This includes gram-negative organisms and comparatively sustained killing power (one hour) in the presence of organic material. It is not promptly sporicidal. As used in dermatologic surgery, toxicity is low. Aesthetically acceptable, it is available in a 10% solution that can be applied after scrubbing with a 2% cleansing scrubbing agent.
   h. *Chlorhexidine Gluconate.* Marketed for approximately 25 years in Europe, this compound has a broader spectrum of killing power than many agents. Poorly absorbed through the skin, it has a low level of toxicity. Deafness has occurred when it reached the middle ear through a perforated tympanic membrane.[24] Nonirritating and aesthetically pleasing, it provides a bacteriostatic effect on the skin in the presence of organic material.
   i. *Hydrogen Peroxide.* Little direct effect on bacteria, but its effervescent action provides a mechanical débriding effect. Good for cleansing blood from surfaces.
2. **Disinfectants** (used to eliminate pathogens from inanimate surfaces).[25]
   a. *Soap and Water.* (See above).
   b. *Sodium Hypochlorite.*[25] This material is too irritating for routine use on the skin but is an inexpensive and effective disinfectant for floors and work surfaces. It is bactericidal, sporicidal, and probably virucidal but corrodes metal and destroys cloth.

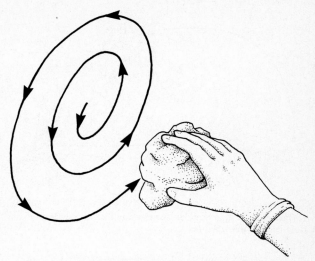

Figure 3–1. Scrubbing should start in the center of an operative area and proceed to the peripheral areas, as indicated by the arrows.

with a sterile towel or dried by evaporation. Scrubbing with Hibiclens will leave bacteriostatic residues on the skin. If povidone-iodine is used, the 2% scrub can be augmented by an application of the 10% solution with prepackaged swabs. If there is concern about unusual contamination with resistant organisms such as spores, treatment with 1% tincture of iodine[25] may be advisable after washing is completed. This can be followed after 15 minutes with the application of a more durable bacteriostatic agent.

Unless hair at the operative site is so thick as to interfere with the procedure, it should not be cut.[26] If hair must be removed, it should be clipped. Cellophane tape can be used to pick up pieces of hair before scrubbing. The area clipped should be kept as small as possible for both cosmetic and bacteriologic reasons. Shaving and close clipping are avoided because they produce infection-prone microscopic injuries.[9] Hair beyond the operative area can be parted away from the incision line and secured with sterilized barrettes or elastic bands.

After scrubbing, the area peripheral to the operative site is draped with sterile towels or disposable barriers over a wide enough area so that instruments, gloves, and sutures do not touch contaminated surfaces. Sterile drapes and barriers may either be of reusable cloth or disposable paper and plastic. Only sterile, waterproof, plastic-backed barriers should be used on the surgical tray in order to eliminate the risk of moisture-borne contamination. The operative field may be defined by the margins of three drapes placed in a triangular fashion (Fig. 3–2) or by an opening in the drape itself. Occlusive adhesive drapes may increase the incidence of wound infection.[9]

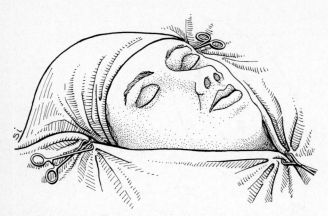

Figure 3–2. A triangular arrangement of three drapes that defines the operative field.

PROPHYLACTIC ANTIBIOTICS

The American Heart Association has recommended that prophylactic antibiotics be used in patients with valvular or other structural heart abnormalities (including prosthetic heart valves) whenever surgical manipulation of infected or contaminated tissue is undertaken (Table 3–2).* This reduces the risk of bacterial endocarditis, which may supervene if bacteremia occurs. Specific recommendations have been made for surgery in the mouth (Table 3–3). For surgery in other areas, the American Heart Association has three recommendations:

1. In susceptible patients, prophylaxis to prevent endocarditis is indicated for surgical procedures on any infected or contaminated tissues, including incision and drainage of abscesses. In these circumstances, regimens should be individualized but in most instances should include antibiotics effective against *Staphylococcus aureus*.

2. Antibiotic prophylaxis for the surgical and dental procedures indicated above should also be given to patients with documented previous episodes of bacterial endocarditis even in the absence of clinically detectable heart disease.

3. Patients with indwelling transvenous cardiac pacemakers appear to present a low risk of endocarditis; when such cases occur, they are predominantly due to staphylococci. However, physicians may choose to employ prophylactic antibiotics when surgical procedures are performed in these patients. The same recommendations apply to renal dialysis patients with arteriovenous shunt appliances. Endocarditis prophylaxis also deserves consideration in patients with ventriculoatrial shunts for hydrocephalus, because there are documented cases of bacterial endocarditis in these patients.[27]

A similar policy might be considered for patients who have implanted prostheses in other areas that

---

*It is recognized that it is not possible to make recommendations for all possible clinical situations. Practitioners must exercise their clinical judgment in determining the duration and choice of antibiotic when special circumstances apply.

TABLE 3–2. Recommendations of the American Heart Association for Antibiotic Prophylaxis in Patients Who Are at Risk for the Development of Bacterial Endocarditis[27]

Cardiac Conditions* for which Endocarditis Prophylaxis Is Indicated:
  Prosthetic cardiac valves (including biosynthetic valves)
  Most congenital cardiac malformations
  Surgically constructed systemic-pulmonary shunts
  Rheumatic and other acquired valvular dysfunction
  Idiopathic hypertrophic subaortic stenosis
  Previous history of bacterial endocarditis
  Mitral valve prolapse with insufficiency**
Endocarditis Prophylaxis Not Recommended:
  Isolated secundum atrial septal defect
  Secundum atrial septal defect repaired without a patch six or more months earlier
  Patent ductus arteriosus ligated and divided six or more months earlier
  Postoperative coronary artery bypass graft surgery

*This table lists common conditions but is not meant to be all-inclusive.
**Definitive data to provide guidance in management of patients with mitral valve prolapse are particularly limited. It is clear that, in general, such patients are at low risk of development of endocarditis, but the risk-benefit ratio of prophylaxis in mitral valve prolapse is uncertain.
(Modified from and reprinted with the permission of the American Heart Association.)

---

might serve as foci of infection in the event of bacteremia.[28, 29] Patients in these categories can be identified only if an adequate history is obtained. Consultation with the appropriate specialist is often helpful. Gram staining, culture, and sensitivity studies should be obtained as early as possible. Since blood-borne dissemination of pathogenic organisms may occur in spite of preventive efforts, adequate follow-up observation is mandatory. Patients should be advised to report signs and symptoms of infection immediately.

Immunoincompetence, advanced age, and poor circulation are among the factors used to justify preoperative antibiotics. Benefits must be weighed against the risk of adverse effects.[30]

SURGICAL TECHNIQUE AS IT RELATES TO INFECTION CONTROL

If infection is unavoidably present, it should not be invaded in order to produce local anesthesia.[31] Field or nerve block is preferable to local infiltration. If excision is undertaken, infected or inflamed areas are often best removed en bloc with margins and a minimum of manipulation. Incision should be made *from* clean areas *to* contaminated ones. Incision and drainage is accomplished with a minimum of manipulation. Careful surgical technique reduces the risk of sepsis by insuring that wounds are managed so that foreign material and necrotic tissue are kept to a minimum and that dead space, seromas,

TABLE 3–3. Recommendations of the American Heart Association Antibiotic Regimens for Oral and Respiratory Tract Procedures[27]

Standard Regimen	
For dental procedures that cause gingival bleeding, and oral or respiratory tract surgery	Penicillin V 2.0 gm orally one hour before, then 1.0 gm six hours later. For patients unable to take oral medications, 2 million units of aqueous penicillin G intravenously or intramuscularly 30 to 60 minutes before a procedure and 1 million units six hours later may be substituted
Special Regimens	
Parenteral regimen for use when maximal protection desired; e.g., for patients with prosthetic valves	Ampicillin 1.0 to 2.0 gm intramuscularly or intravenously *plus* gentamicin 1.5 mg/kg intramuscularly or intravenously 30 minutes before the procedure, followed by 1.0 gm oral penicillin V six hours later. Alternatively, the parenteral regimen may be repeated once eight hours later
Oral regimen for penicillin-allergic patients	Erythromycin 1.0 gm orally one hour before, then 500 mg six hours later
	For those who cannot tolerate either penicillin or erythromycin, an oral cephalosporin (1.0 gm one hour prior to the procedure plus 500 mg six hours after initial dose) may be useful, but data are lacking to allow specific recommendation of this regimen. Tetracyclines *cannot* be recommended for this purpose.
Parenteral regimen for penicillin-allergic patients	Vancomycin 1.0 gm intravenously, *slowly* over one hour, starting one hour before. No repeat dose is necessary*

*In unusual circumstances or in cases of delayed healing, it may be necessary to provide additional doses of antibiotics even though bacteremia rarely persists longer than 15 minutes after the procedure. Penicillin V is the preferred form of oral penicillin because it is relatively resistant to gastric acid. For those patients taking an oral penicillin for secondary prevention of rheumatic fever or for other purposes, viridans streptococci relatively resistant to penicillin may be present in the oral cavity. In such cases, the physician or dentist should select erythromycin or one of the parenteral regimens. Some patients with a prosthetic heart valve in whom a high level of oral health is being maintained may be offered oral antibiotic prophylaxis for routine dental procedures. Parenteral antibiotics are recommended, however, for patients with prosthetic valves who require extensive dental procedures, especially extractions, or oral or gingival surgical procedures.

Pediatric doses: Ampicillin 50 mg/kg per dose; erythromycin 20 mg/kg for first dose, then 10 mg/kg; gentamicin 2.0 mg/kg per dose; penicillin V full adult dose if greater than 60 lb (27 kg), one-half adult dose if less than 60 lb (27 kg); aqueous penicillin G 50,000 units/kg (25,000 units/kg for follow-up); vancomycin 20 mg/kg per dose. The intervals between doses are the same as for adults. Total doses should not exceed adult doses.

(Modified from and reprinted with the permission of the American Heart Association.)

and hematomas are avoided. If anaerobic conditions exist in any wound, tetanus immunization should be current. Studies indicate that general surgical procedures lasting more than an hour are more likely to be complicated by infection.[32] This is probably due to tissue and wound factors. Contamination of implements and sutures with time and handling may also play a role. Wounds, regardless of origin, are not ordinarily closed if they are heavily inoculated or infected or if they contain devitalized tissue.[33] Clean incisions are often protected best with a simple dry dressing. A mildly occlusive (nonsensitizing) ointment used judiciously may facilitate healing and prevent crust formation. Since moisture also promotes bacterial growth, wound dressings must be designed with regard to such variables as skin hydration, wound properties, and the degree of bacteriologic contamination.[34]

STERILIZATION

Sterilization is the process whereby a substance or surface is rendered totally free of *all* forms of microorganisms.[35] The concept is an absolute one that allows for no compromises. All instruments or supplies placed within the confines of the operative field should be sterile. Disposable items are purchased in a prepackaged sterile state. Reused equipment must be appropriately cleaned, sterilized, and stored between each use.

Cleaning must be done carefully to insure that blood and tissue fragments, which may be caked on the instruments, are removed. These residues are called soil and may protect organisms from the sterilization process. After a brush scrub, placing the instruments for five to seven minutes in an ultrasonic cleaner facilitates the process. Detergents of neutral pH have been recommended and must be completely rinsed from instruments before they are autoclaved. The grasping and friction surfaces of instruments are particularly likely to retain soil and require special care. Only gloved and experienced employees with the highest sense of responsibility should be allowed to clean instruments. After cleaning, instruments can be soaked in instrument milk before autoclaving.[35]

Autoclaving

Steam heat produced by an autoclave is the mainstay of office sterilization because it is dependable, simple, relatively fast, economical, space-efficient, and aesthetically acceptable. Other methods can and sometimes must be used, however, and are discussed later.

The autoclave is effective because of the penetrating power of wet heat. Steam under pressure will pass through resistant spore walls and destroy the chemical integrity of proteins and DNA. Sterilizing conditions are defined in terms of temperature, pressure, and time. Certain minimal conditions must be achieved at the *surface* of the instrument for sterilization to occur. These conditions are defined as a temperature of 121°C and an absolute pressure of 15 psi for 15 minutes. As Table 3–4 shows, the required time can be diminished at higher temperatures and pressures. If the instrument is wrapped in a surgical pack or if the autoclave is fully loaded, more time may be required. As previously noted, soil on the surface of an instrument may interfere with the sterilization process. The effects of altitude must also be appreciated. The pressure gauge on some autoclaves records the difference between the atmospheric and internal pressures. If so, an additional 0.5 psi should be added to the minimum 15 psi required for sterilization for every thousand feet of elevation above sea level. Practical considerations deriving from these basic principles are as follows:

1. Only a new or fully reconditioned autoclave should be purchased and then maintained in good condition. Defective gaskets and seals may result in insufficient pressure for sterilization. Gauges should be checked regularly to insure that they are working properly. The use of distilled water retards the buildup of salt deposits, but does not eliminate the need for cleaning or regular checkups by qualified service personnel. Most importantly, the performance of the autoclave should be monitored. Telltale tape strips that change color when a sterilizing cycle is complete can be placed on the surgical packs. A reliable but time-consuming monitor is commercially available in the form of spores, which if placed in the autoclave will later grow in culture if sterilizing conditions are not attained.

2. The autoclave should be used properly. The goal is to insure that every surface is reached by pressurized steam. Proper circulation of steam is less likely to occur in an overloaded autoclave. Concave surfaces (e.g., cups) should be pointed downward to prevent water pooling. Instrument packs should be dry when removed. Adequate drying time should be allowed in accordance with the manufacturer's instructions. The time of sterilization does not include the startup time (about 15 minutes). A cycle time of 35 to 45 minutes is usually required.

3. An autoclave of adequate size should be purchased. A small diameter (up to nine inches) may be adequate for many practices, but it may prove to be insufficient as the surgical part of a practice

grows. Under these circumstances a larger autoclave (9- to 12-inch diameter) is a prudent investment for reasons of safety and economy.

4. Metal, cloth, and heat-resistant plastic can be autoclaved. Heat-sensitive implements are best treated by gas sterilization.

Other Methods of Sterilization

Dry Heat. Implements can be sterilized by heat alone. The process is slower, generates heat, and shortens the life of some items, e.g., cloth. It offers no advantage over autoclaving for the office practitioner.

Gas Sterilization. Heat-sensitive implements can be sterilized with ethylene oxide. The process is slow and the required equipment is elaborate. Arrangements can often be made to sterilize heat-sensitive equipment at hospitals.

Chemiclave. The use of chemicals in the autoclave is becoming more popular and has made it possible to lower the humidity of the sterilization process. This lessens drying time and, purportedly, the potential for instrument corrosion. However, hepatitis eradication cannot be tested, and one must purchase, store, and properly use the chemicals.

Cold Sterilization. The concept of sterilizing instruments by immersing them in chemicals is not regarded as a safe method at this time.

Packaging and Storing of Instruments

Needs and methods vary greatly and only general comments can be made about the packaging and storing of instruments. After cleaning, instruments can be placed singly or in standardized groupings in labeled, dated packs. The wrapping used must be permeable to the sterilizing medium. Muslin, cotton, and paper are popular wrapping materials. Pieces of two-layered muslin can be used to form a double wrapping. It is cheap, is readily permeated by steam, and can be quickly formed into a neat surgical pack. With folding, many layers of material can be placed around the instruments. Crepe paper can be similarly used. Without a paper or polyethylene outer envelope, multiple (two or more) layers of muslin have a shelf life of approximately three weeks. With repeated washings (75 or more) muslin loses its effectiveness as a packing material.

Transparent paper, which is available in strips or preformed pouches, can also be used for instrument packs. Sealed with heat or tape, they form an elegant pack with a shelf life of approximately one year. Packs found to be wet are presumed to be contaminated and discarded.

Storing instruments in unsealed containers, which may or may not be filled with disinfectants, is

TABLE 3–4. Minimal Exposure Times for Steam Sterilization at the Surface Undergoing Sterilization

Temperature	Pressure	Time*
121°C	15.0 psi	15 minutes
126°C	20.0 psi	10 minutes
134°C	29.4 psi	3 minutes

*Additional time must be allowed for temperature and pressure buildup.[35]

becoming less popular because of the possibility of contamination and bacterial growth. This practice may also cause corrosion.

Power Instruments

The possibility of transmission of infection exists whenever nonsterilized surfaces, which are exposed to blood and tissue fragments, are brought into a contact pattern that reaches more than one patient. This hazard can be eliminated if portions of power instruments (including switches) that are brought into the operative field are sterilized in accordance with manufacturers' instructions. Switches external to the operative area can be foot-activated, controlled by an assistant, or protected by sterile adaptors. Instruments that are run by an external power source represent an interface between the general and operative environment. A demarcation point can be defined by a clip that secures the line at the edge of the operative field with sufficient slack distally for maneuvering. Sterilized portions of lines that enter the operative area should be allowed to contact only scrubbed skin or draped areas.

Electrosurgical implements are made in both disposable and reusable forms. The use of sterilized equipment has been advocated.[35] Presterilized packaged units are available for a nominal cost. Cutting and coagulating implements can be reused, provided they are cleaned and sterilized between uses. Gas sterilization probably prolongs the life of at least some of these units. Use of devices in which both handles and electrodes are sterilized eliminates the hazard of patient-to-patient contamination. A thin epilating needle can be sheathed with a sterile 20-gauge injection needle. Sterile implements such as clamps or clamp-held injection needles can be used as conductors for electrocoagulation if they are touched by an electrode which need not be sterile if it is not brought in contact with the wound. Such improvisations involving nonsterile components are best reserved for small procedures.

Gloves

Gloves are used for the mutual protection of the patient and operating personnel. A policy that requires only sterile gloves be used on hands that enter the wound is consistent with standards set for other surgical implements and supplies. Disposable, presterilized, packaged gloves of adequate quality and dexterity are available in different sizes for approximately $1.25 per pair. Although nonsterile examination gloves are more economical, quality and fit are variable and, if stored in open boxes, subject to contamination. The safety and better fit of individually packaged sterile gloves justify their cost. For very small procedures, especially those that do not require wound closure (i.e., incision and drainage), clean, nonsterile gloves can be used if glove-to-wound contact is avoided.

The following precautions should be observed: Sterile gloves are donned using the proper technique (Fig. 3–3) after the hands have been carefully dried. The glove envelope is peeled open and the inner sterile envelope is placed on a dry, clean surface before gloves are put on. Once gloved the hand touches only sterile surfaces or the surgically prepped skin of the patient. Starch is removed from the gloves with damp, sterile, saline-soaked gauze.

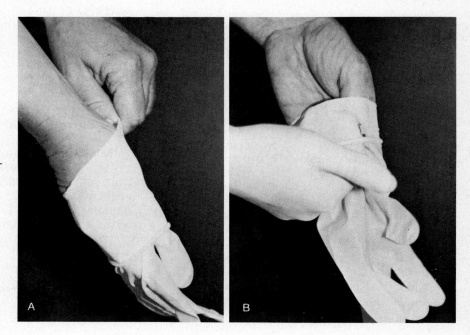

Figure 3–3. *A* and *B*, Proper technique for donning sterile gloves.

Punctured gloves are discarded immediately. These points, which are second nature to the physician, may be overlooked by less experienced assistants.

THE SURGICAL ENVIRONMENT

Operative Personnel

The risk of infection from operative personnel can be greatly reduced with precautions that need not be as elaborate as those in a hospital operating room. Evidence suggests that a brushless three-minute scrub with an agent that leaves bacteriostatic residues on the skin is adequate.[36] This can be done at the beginning of the operative day followed by shorter washings between procedures. Surgical masks and caps are inexpensive, are readily donned, and may reduce the theoretic risk of infection. Personnel with active skin infections are a recognized source of operative sepsis.[10]

The Surgical Facility

It is not possible, of course, to sterilize the operating room. Although a specialized, limited-access operatory with adequate space and ventilation is ideal, other areas can be used if the transition from general to surgical use is preceded by adequate housekeeping measures. Whether or not the operatory is a specialized unit, floors, walls, light fixtures, ceilings, and ventilators must be free of danders, dust, lint, and effects of deterioration. Surfaces likely to be contaminated by blood or tissue residues must be promptly and thoroughly disinfected with a solution of 0.5% sodium hypochlorite.

OCCUPATIONAL SAFETY

The number of infectious diseases transmitted from surgical patients to health care professionals is legion.

Hepatitis B

There is justifiable anxiety about the possibility of exposure to hepatitis B because of its prevalence and high degree of infectivity.[37] Active immunization against hepatitis B is available in a vaccine made from plasma that contains the hepatitis B surface antigen. Some health care institutions have recommended that personnel at risk for exposure to hepatitis B be vaccinated. The vaccine reportedly has a 95% protective efficacy but is derived from populations at increased risk to develop acquired immunodeficiency syndrome. The plasma is, how-

ever, subjected to extensive virucidal, denaturization, and separation procedures. So far, there is no evidence to suggest that recipients of hepatitis B vaccine are at risk for the development of AIDS, and there is reason to hope that a synthetic vaccine made from recombinant DNA techniques will be available in a few years.[38] Some authorities have recommended that the immune status of the professional be evaluated before the vaccine is administered, since some may already be protected by virtue of prior exposure.[37]

When exposure of personnel to blood or tissue fragments is likely, patients should be screened for hepatitis B carrier states. Elective procedures might best be deferred on those who do not meet the criteria for serving as safe blood donors. If during an operation the skin of an unvaccinated operator or assistant is broken and inoculated with potentially infectious material, the patient's status with respect to hepatitis B should be promptly evaluated. If there is evidence to suggest that exposure of an unimmunized worker* may have occurred, treatment with specific hepatitis B gamma globulin should be undertaken immediately. The same policy is also advisable for any injury from an uncleaned sharp implement removed from an individual patient's tray. Gloves should always be used. Face shields and full-length surgical gowns are desirable for procedures in which exposure to splashed blood and tissue fragments is difficult to avoid. Glasses and masks are also protective. Blood can become airborne in almost any procedure.

Non-A, Non-B Hepatitis

There is no laboratory test available for the screening of patients with non-A, non-B hepatitis.[37] Patients with a history of unexplained jaundice or liver disease should be approached with caution. Nonspecific pooled gamma globulin may be protective if exposure to non-A, non-B hepatitis is suspected.

Delta Agent Hepatitis

Delta agent hepatitis is a distinct, infectious process that occurs in association with hepatitis B.[39, 40] This entity is caused by an RNA virus and can be acquired at the same time or subsequent to inoculation with hepatitis B and can complicate the course of the illness. The possibility of exposure of surgical personnel to this virus while working cannot be

---

*Immunity can be evaluated by measuring levels of antibodies directed against the hepatitis B surface antigen, a measure that might be considered whether or not the individual has been vaccinated.

excluded. Methods used to prevent hepatitis B infection, if successful, are probably prophylactic.

Acquired Immunodeficiency Syndrome

There is little evidence to suggest that health care professionals are likely to contract AIDS as a result of occupational exposure.[41] Recently, however, there has been concern about a possible change in epidemiologic patterns of this disease.[42] Preventive measures are similar to those recommended for the avoidance of exposure to hepatitis.[43, 44]

Other Infections

If the history or findings suggests the existence of a particular infectious process, appropriate studies and treatment should be completed on the patient before any surgery is undertaken whenever possible. If the person is known or suspected of being infectious at the time of surgery, precautions such as gowns and double gloves should be used by operative and housekeeping personnel. When accidental inoculation occurs, prompt treatment of the exposed professional is indicated.

Instruments and Work Areas

Instruments should be cleaned by gloved personnel in regularly disinfected areas in which eating, drinking, smoking, and contact patterns with food and drink utensils are avoided. Spills on sinks and countertops must be rigorously cleaned and disinfected with 0.5% sodium hypochlorite.

Sharp disposable implements can be returned to the containers from which they came. They are then placed in receptacles for hazardous or infectious trash and later sealed in marked double-thickness bags for proper disposal. Hospital facilities for the disposal of hazardous or infectious materials can be used.

COST CONTROL

The surgical tray equipped with a combination of disposable and reusable items contributes to the cost of surgery. Since patients may sometimes be billed a reasonable tray charge, material and labor costs of assembly should be monitored. Standardization of packing, storing, and retrieval procedures help control costs. Economical bulk rates may sometimes be obtained by buying through a hospital or ambulatory surgical clinic.

CONCLUSION

Prevention of infection in the office requires a level of professionalism equal to that found in the hospital. This responsibility is readily accepted by staff members who with adequate training, equipment, and supervision derive no small measure of pride from their ability to meet and maintain high standards.

REFERENCES

1. Florey HW, Jennings MA: Chemotaxis, phagocytosis and the formation of abscesses: The reticulo-endothelial system. In Florey, HW (ed): General Pathology, 4 Ed. Philadelphia, W. B. Saunders, 1970, pp 151–152
2. Swartz MN, Weinberg AN: Infections due to gram positive bacteria. In Fitzpatrick TB, Eisen A, Wolf FK, et al: Dermatology in General Medicine, 2 Ed. New York, McGraw-Hill, 1979, p 17
3. Rea WJ, Wyrick WJ: Necrotizing Fasciitis, Ann Surg 172:957–964, 1970.
4. Giullano A, Lewis F, Hadley K, et al: Bacteriology of necrotizing fasciitis. Am J of Surg 134:52–57, 1972
5. Resnik SS, Lewis LA, Cohen BH: Trichloroacetic acid peeling. Cutis 17:127–129, 1976
6. Roenigk HH, Jr: Dermabrasion: State of the art. J Derm Surg and Oncol 11:306–311, 1985
7. Siegle RJ, Chiarmonte A, Knox DW, et al: Cutaneous candidosis as a complication of facial dermabrasion. J Derm Surg and Oncol 10:891–895, 1984
8. Noble WC, Somerville DA: Microbiology of Human Skin. Philadelphia, W. B. Saunders, 1974, pp 284–315
9. Cruse PJE, Foord R: Epidemiology of wound infections. Surgical Clinics of North America 60:27–39, 1980
10. Noble WC, Somerville DA: Microbiology of Human Skin. Philadelphia, W. B. Saunders, 1974, pp 144–159
11. Quinn EL, Cox F, Drake EH: Staphylococcic endocarditis. JAMA 196:815–818, 1966
12. Noble WC, Somerville DA: Microbiology of Human Skin. Philadelphia, W. B. Saunders, 1974, pp 160–171
13. Ibid., p 285
14. Ibid., p 261
15. Ibid., pp 172–184
16. Roenigk HH, Young JR: Leg ulcers. Medical and Surgical Management. Hagerstown, Md., Harper & Row, 1975, p 156
17. Meislin HW, Lerner SA, Graves ML, et al: Cutaneous abscesses. Ann Int Med 87:145–149, 1977
18. Reynolds RC, Cluff LE: Infection of man with Mimeae. Ann Int Med 58:759–767, 1963
19. Noble WC, Somerville DA: Microbiology of Human Skin. Philadelphia, W. B. Saunders, 1974, pp 185–205
20. Kerr JH: Tetanus. In Wyngaarden JB, Smith LH, Jr (eds): Cecil's Textbook of Medicine, 17 Ed. Philadelphia, W. B. Saunders, 1985, pp 1579–1582
21. Boyd RF, Hoerl BG: Basic Medical Microbiology. Boston, Little Brown & Co, 1977
22. Sebben JE: Surgical antisepsis. J Amer Acad Derm 9:759–765, 1983
23. Lacey RW: Antibacterial action of human skin. In vivo effect of acetone, alcohol and soap on behaviour of Staphylococcus aureus. Brit J Exp Path 49:209–215, 1968
24. Physicians' Desk Reference, 39 Ed. Oradell, NJ, Medical Economics Co, 1985, p 2037
25. Harvey SC: Antiseptics and disinfectants. In Gilman AG, Goodman LS, Gilman A (eds). The Pharmacologic Basis of

Therapeutics, 6 Ed. New York, MacMillan, 1980, pp 964–987

26. Simmons BP: Guidelines of Surgical Wound Infections. Guidelines for the Prevention and Control of Nosocomial Infections. Atlanta, Ga, U.S. Dept. of Health and Human Services, Public Health Service, Centers for Disease Control, Center for Infectious Diseases, 1982

27. Committee on Rheumatic Fever and Infective Endocarditis of the Council of Cardiovascular Disease in the Young of the American Heart Association: Prevention of bacterial endocarditis. Circulation 70:1123A–1127A, 1984

28. Hewitt WL: Diagnosis and management of deep hip sepsis. In The Hip: Proceedings of the 5th Open Scientific Meeting of the Hip Society. St. Louis, C. V. Mosby, 1977, pp 147–151

29. Lattimer G, Keblish P, Dickson T, et al: Hematogenous infection in total hip replacement: Recommendations for prophylactic antibiotics. JAMA 242:2213, 1979

30. Noud M: Antimicrobial prophylaxis in surgery. UCLA Medical Center Drug Information Bulletin, 1985

31. Moore D: Regional Block, 4 Ed. Springfield, Ill., Charles C Thomas, 1965, p 47

32. Ritter MA, Eitzen HE, French MLV, et al: The effect that time, touch and environment have on bacterial contamination of instruments during surgery. Ann Surg 184:642–644, 1976

33. Hill GJ: Outpatient Surgery. Philadelphia, W. B. Saunders, 1973, p 88

34. Bennett RG: The debatable benefit of occlusive dressings for wounds (editorial). J Derm Surg Oncol 8:166–167, 1982

35. Sebben JE: Sterilization and care of surgical instruments and supplies. J Amer Acad Derm 11:381–391, 1984

36. Galle PC, Homesley HD, Rhyne AL: Reassessment of the surgical scrub. Surg Gynec and Obstet 147:215–218, 1978

37. Smith JG, Jr, Chalker DK: Viral hepatitis: A hazard for dermatologists. Seminars in Dermatology 3:136–139, 1984

38. Sachs HS, Rose DN, Chalmers TC: Should the risk of acquired immunodeficiency syndrome deter hepatitis B vaccination? JAMA 252:3375–3377, 1984

39. Rizzetto M: The delta agent. Hepatology 5:729–737, 1983

40. Redeker AG: Delta agent and hepatitis B (editorial). Ann Int Med 98:542–543, 1983

41. Siegel L: Health care personnel and AIDS (letter). Arch Int Med 144:24–31, 1984

42. Needle Stick Transmission of HTLV-III from a patient infected in Africa (editorial). Lancet II, 1376–1377, 1984

43. Burrow GN: Caring for AIDS patients: The physician's risk and responsibility. Can Med Assoc Journ 129:1181, 1983

44. Acquired immune deficiency syndrome (AIDS): Precautions for clinical and laboratory staff. Morbid Mortal Weekly Rpt 31:577–579, 1982

45. Hexachlorophene and newborns. FDA Drug Bull, Dec 1971

46. Hexachlorophene: Interim caution regarding use in pregnancy. FDA Drug Bull, Aug–Sept 1978

Local Anesthetics

Pain and suffering have always accompanied human disease, and their relief has long been a goal of medical science. Although agents for general anesthesia were first employed in the nineteenth century, modern local anesthetics were developed only in the last 40 years.

Local anesthesia can be defined as the circumscribed loss of sensation achieved by the inhibition of impulse transmission in nerve endings, peripheral nerves, or spinal roots. Local anesthetics are pharmacologic agents that interrupt nerve conduction in a transient, predictable, and reversible manner without the loss of consciousness.

HISTORY

The beginnings of modern local anesthetic agents can be traced to the ancient Inca civilization of South America. The leaves of the indigenous coca plant (*Erythroxylon coca*) have long been known to produce circumoral numbness and a mood-elevating effect when chewed. In 1855, the active alkaloid, erythroxylin, was extracted from the leaves of this plant, and in 1860, cocaine was isolated from the erythroxylin extract by Albert Niemann.[1]

Cocaine acetate was first described as having important clinical potential in 1868 by a Peruvian army surgeon.[2] The actual clinical application of cocaine resulted from the work of two Viennese physicians, Carl Koller and Sigmund Freud.[3] The initial investigation began as an effort to aid a colleague who was addicted to morphine and resulted in the observation that 2% cocaine solution completely desensitized the cornea when applied topically. The use of cocaine solution as an effective ophthalmologic anesthetic quickly gained worldwide acceptance.[4] The versatility of cocaine was appreciated by William Halsted at Johns Hopkins University. He employed cocaine for more than 1000 cases of nerve conduction blockade and, ironically, became addicted to the drug himself.[5]

As clinical usage of cocaine became more widespread, an appreciation of its toxic properties also became apparent. This led to a search for less toxic compounds, and procaine, an ester of para-amino benzoic acid, was synthesized by Einhorn in 1905. Other ester derivatives, such as tetracaine and chloroprocaine, were subsequently developed.

Lidocaine, the prototype of the amino-amide group of local anesthetics, was discovered by Löfgren in 1948.[6] This category was found to possess potent anesthetic properties as well as high tissue penetrance and low toxicity. The past three decades have witnessed the refinement of this category of compounds with the development of prilocaine, etidocaine, mepivacaine, and bupivacaine. This family of local anesthetics has become the most commonly used in modern medical practice.

MECHANISM OF NERVE CONDUCTION

Anatomy

Nerve fibers convey impulses to various body areas via a complex electrochemical process that can be initiated by chemical, mechanical, or electrical stimuli. The impulses are conducted along nerve fibers or axons. The key structure for nerve impulse conduction is the cell membrane surrounding the axon, the axolemma. The physiochemical properties of this biologic membrane directly determine the diffusion characteristics of compounds in contact with it. The morphologic structure of this membrane is generally thought to consist of a lipoprotein matrix. A bimolecular phospholipid framework exists, with hydrophilic, polar ends facing outward and hydrophobic, nonpolar portions facing inward. This is surrounded by and perhaps intercalated with various protein complexes. Electron microscopy reveals the thickness of this membrane unit to be 70 to 80Å.

All nerve fibers have a surrounding nucleated cell, the Schwann cell (Fig. 4–1).[7] The functions of the Schwann cell include the synthesis of myelin, which forms a lamellated cylinder of fatty material that surrounds most larger nerve fibers. The Schwann cell is probably not directly involved with the physiochemical aspects of impulse conduction, but it may function in the synthesis of enzymes and other membrane components.

The myelin sheath provides insulation for the nerve fiber. It is interrupted at regular intervals by a gap known as the node of Ranvier. This interspace exposes the nerve membrane to the medium surrounding it and is actually the space between two adjacent Schwann cells and their myelin sheaths. As the diameter of the axon increases, the thickness of the myelin sheath increases. The relationship is a

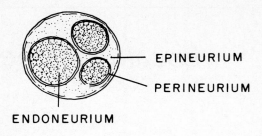

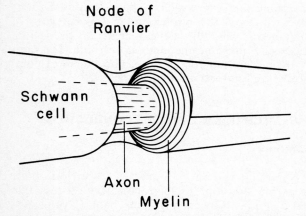

Figure 4–1. Cross section of peripheral nerve and a myelinated peripheral nerve depicting a Schwann cell, myelin sheath, and node of Ranvier.

constant one, with the myelin sheath accounting for approximately 40 percent of the diameter of the entire nerve fiber. The internodal distance is also proportional to the diameter of the axon by a factor of 100 to 1 (usually 0.2 mm to 3 mm). Therefore, the thicker the axon, the greater the distance between one node and the next. The insulating properties of myelin permit faster impulse conduction than in unmyelinated nerves of equal size.

Each individual axon is surrounded by a connective tissue membrane, the endoneurium. Groups of axons are encompassed by the perineurium, and a number of axonal groups are ensheathed in the epineurium (Fig. 4–1). Peripheral nerves contain a mixture of both sensory afferent and motor efferent fibers. The end result of impulse transmission is determined by both the pattern and proportion of different nerve fibers. A classification of the types and characteristics of nerve fibers is provided in Table 4–1.

Another critical anatomic structure of nerves is the transmembrane ion channel (Fig. 4–2).[8] Discrete ion channels are located along the membrane. In myelinated nerves, the channels are located at the nodes of Ranvier. The external opening of the sodium channel is guarded by a fixed aperture filter that selects cations according to size. At the axo-

plasmic mouth of the channel are the m-gates that control sodium activation. Further inward along the channel are the h-shutters that control sodium inactivation.

The potassium channel is also guarded by a selectivity filter, about 3Å in diameter, at the external surface. A single activation gate is situated along the internal surface. Measurements of transmembrane electrical activity have indicated that ionic fluxes of sodium and potassium are responsible for impulse transmission.

Impulse Transmission

Electric phenomena in nerve membranes depend on the concentrations of sodium and potassium in the axoplasm and in the extracellular fluid, and on the permeability of the nerve membrane to these ions. At rest, the intracellular concentration of potassium is 110 to 170 mEq/L and the extracellular concentration is 3 to 5 mEq/L. Conversely, the intracellular concentration of sodium is 5 to 10 mEq/L, and the extracellular concentration is 140 mEq/L. At rest, these gradients are maintained because of the selective permeability of the nerve membrane to potassium ions, with only slight permeability to sodium ions. Consequently, the resting membrane potential as measured by intracellular electrodes in nerve preparations is -60 to -90 mV. At rest, the nerve membrane functions essentially as a potassium electrode.

Stimulation of a nerve triggers permeability to sodium ions with an opening of sodium activation gates. This initiates depolarization from the resting level to the firing threshold of -50 to -60 mV. At this point, the sodium influx approximates the potassium efflux. At the firing threshold, there is an explosive increase in sodium permeability with maximum influx of sodium ions. Potassium begins to leave the cell, moving toward its outward concentration gradient. For practical purposes, the nerve has been transformed into a sodium electrode with a positive membrane potential of $+40$ mV. The net voltage change is termed the action potential[9] (see Fig. 4–2).

As the membrane potential rises, the sodium inactivation gates close and the permeability to sodium is diminished. High potassium permeability is restored, and potassium moves out of the cell. The membrane becomes repolarized with the aid of an energy-dependent sodium pump to restore electrochemical equilibrium. This is an active transport mechanism requiring energy from oxidative phosphorylation. Not only are sodium ions transported from inside to outside the nerve cell against a concentration gradient, but potassium ions move from outside to inside until the resting concentrations are restored. During this process of depolari-

TABLE 4–1. Nerve Fiber Classification

Class	Diameter (μm)	Myelination	Conduction Speed (msec)	Function
Aα	10–20	Heavy	70–120	Motor/proprioception
Aβ	5–12	Moderate	30–70	Pressure/touch
Aγ	4–8	Moderate	15–30	Proprioception
Aδ	1–4	Light	12–30	Pain/temperature
B	1–3	Light	3–15	Vasoconstriction (preganglionic autonomic)
C	0.5–1.0	None	0.5–2.5	Pain/temperature (postganglionic autonomic)

zation and repolarization, the membrane is refractory to activation by additional stimuli.

The generated impulse is then propagated along the nerve fiber. In myelinated nerves, the myelin sheath acts as an insulator. Conduction is enhanced by movement from one node of Ranvier to the next, which ensures a greater velocity of impulse transmission. This leapfrog transmission is known as saltatory conduction.[10]

LOCAL ANESTHETIC AGENTS

Classification

The ideal local anesthetic agent should possess a number of properties: (1) Its onset of action should be short, but the duration should be sufficiently long to complete any planned procedure. (2) It should be nonirritating and cause no irreversible damage to nerves. (3) The potential systemic toxicity of the agent should be low. The structure of most clinically effective local anesthetic agents has the general configuration:[11]

Aromatic portion--------------Intermediate chain------------
                               Amine portion
(Lipophilic)   (Hydrophilic)

Alteration of the aromatic or amine portion or the intermediate chain will influence the anesthetic properties of the compound. A change in the aromatic or amine portion of the agent will alter the lipid/water solubility coefficient and the protein-binding characteristics of the compound. Lipid solubility is the single most important determinant of intrinsic anesthetic potency.[12] The duration of effective anesthesia is determined by the extent of binding to proteins embedded in the nerve membrane. Also, increasing the size of the intermediate chain enhances anesthetic potency up to a critical point, above which a decrease in potency occurs.[13]

The two clinically useful classes of local anesthetics are the amino-esters (Fig. 4–3) and the amino-amides (Fig. 4–4).[14–16]

Cocaine is a benzoic acid ester and most of the other agents of the amino-ester category are derivatives of para-aminobenzoic acid. Benzocaine (ethyl 4-aminobenzoate) is a widely used topical agent,

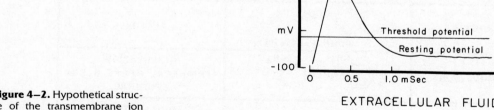

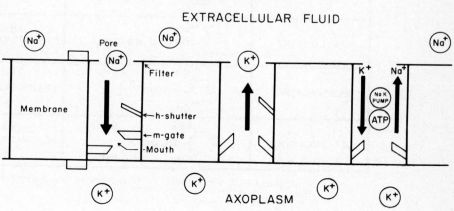

Figure 4–2. Hypothetical structure of the transmembrane ion channel in a myelinated peripheral nerve. The action potential and its relationship to sodium and potassium movement is also illustrated.

AGENT (PROPRIETARY NAME)	CHEMICAL STRUCTURE	PRINCIPAL USES
COCAINE	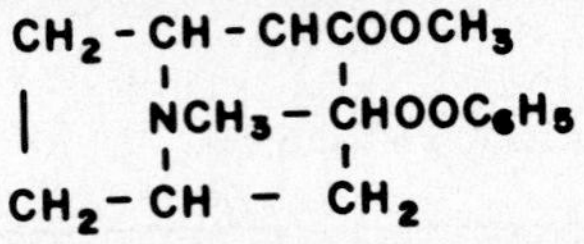 $CH_2-CH-CHCOOCH_3$ $\quad\quad NCH_3-CHOOC_6H_5$ $CH_2-CH-CH_2$	TOPICAL
BENZOCAINE	$H_2N\text{—}\bigcirc\text{—}\overset{O}{\overset{\|}{C}}-OC_2H_5$	TOPICAL
PROCAINE	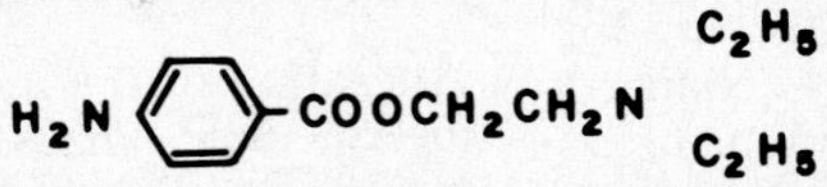 $H_2N\text{—}\bigcirc\text{—}COOCH_2CH_2N\overset{C_2H_5}{\underset{C_2H_5}{}}$	INFILTRATION SPINAL
TETRACAINE	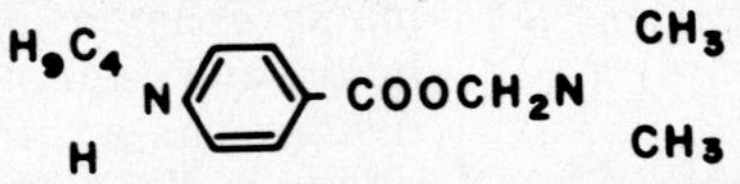 $\overset{H_9C_4}{\underset{H}{}}N\text{—}\bigcirc\text{—}COOCH_2N\overset{CH_3}{\underset{CH_3}{}}$	SPINAL TOPICAL
CHLOROPROCAINE	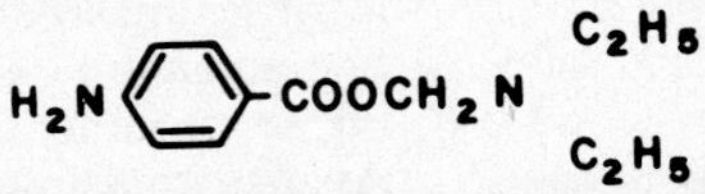 $H_2N\text{—}\bigcirc\text{—}COOCH_2N\overset{C_2H_5}{\underset{C_2H_5}{}}$	INFILTRATION PERIPHERAL NERVE BLOCK EPIDURAL

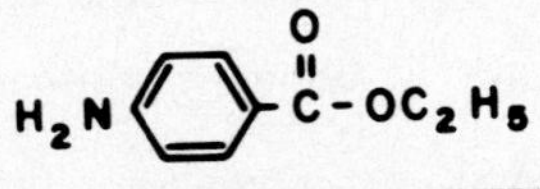

Figure 4–3. Clinically important amino-ester local anesthetic agents.

AGENT	CHEMICAL STRUCTURE	PRINCIPAL USES
LIDOCAINE	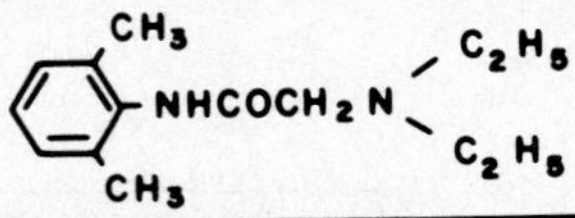 $\overset{CH_3}{\underset{CH_3}{}}\bigcirc\text{—}NHCOCH_2N\overset{C_2H_5}{\underset{C_2H_5}{}}$	INFILTRATION PERIPHERAL NERVE BLOCK SPINAL/EPIDURAL TOPICAL
DIBUCAINE	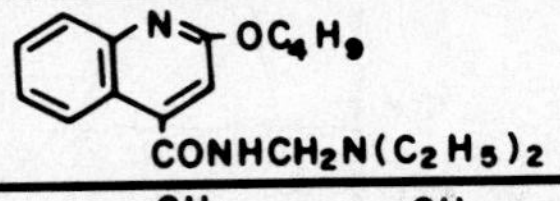 $\bigcirc\bigcirc\overset{N}{=}OC_4H_9$ $CONHCH_2N(C_2H_5)_2$	SPINAL
MEPIVACAINE	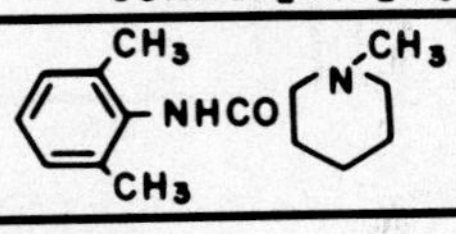 $\overset{CH_3}{\underset{CH_3}{}}\bigcirc\text{—}NHCO\overset{CH_3}{N}\bigcirc$	INFILTRATION PERIPHERAL NERVE BLOCK EPIDURAL
PRILOCAINE	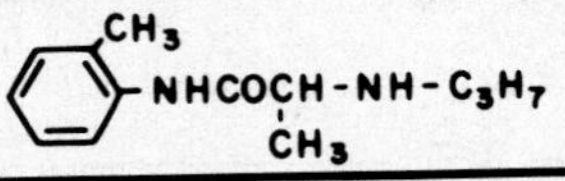 $\overset{CH_3}{}\bigcirc\text{—}NHCOCH-NH-C_3H_7$ $\quad\quad\quad CH_3$	INFILTRATION PERIPHERAL NERVE BLOCK EPIDURAL
BUPIVACAINE	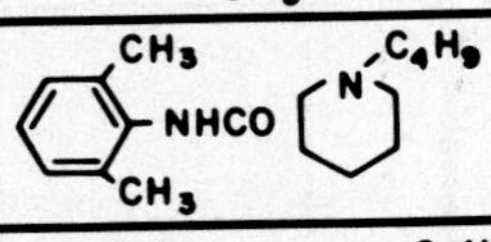 $\overset{CH_3}{\underset{CH_3}{}}\bigcirc\text{—}NHCO\overset{C_4H_9}{N}\bigcirc$	INFILTRATION PERIPHERAL NERVE BLOCK EPIDURAL
ETIDOCAINE	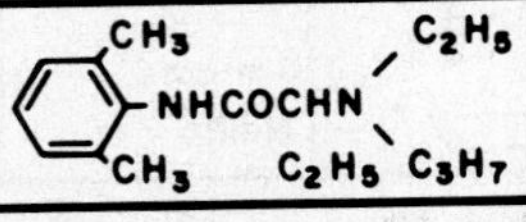 $\overset{CH_3}{\underset{CH_3}{}}\bigcirc\text{—}NHCOCHN\overset{C_2H_5}{\underset{C_2H_5\ C_3H_7}{}}$	INFILTRATION PERIPHERAL NERVE BLOCK EPIDURAL

Figure 4–4. Clinically important amino-amide local anesthetic agents.

particularly in nonprescription medications. Procaine (4-aminobenzoate acid 2-(diethylamine)ethyl ester) is principally used for infiltration procedures and has little topical anesthetic effect. Tetracaine (4-(butylamino)-benzoate acid 2-(dimethylamino)-ethyl ester) is a potent, injectable and topical agent commonly used as a spinal anesthetic. Tetracaine differs structurally from procaine by the addition of a butyl group to the aromatic portion of the procaine molecule. This results in a hundredfold increase in lipid solubility and a tenfold increase in protein binding. The resultant intrinsic anesthetic potency of tetracaine is 16 times greater than procaine, and its duration of action is four times longer. Finally, chloroprocaine (2-diethylaminoethyl 4-amino-2-chlorobenzoate) is an injectable agent with relatively little toxicity.

The prototype of amino-amide compounds is lidocaine (2-(diethylamino)-N-(2,6-dimethylphenyl)-acetamide), a xylidine derivative and a tertiary amine. It has replaced procaine as the most commonly used local anesthetic agent. Prilocaine (2-propylamino-2-propionotoluidide) is a toluidine derivative and a secondary amine with low systemic toxicity. Etidocaine (2-N-ethylpropylamino 2-6-butyroxylidide) is similar to xylocaine with the substitution of a propyl for an ethyl group on the amine position and the addition of an ethyl group at the alpha carbon in the intermediate chain. These changes double its duration of action and produce a 50-fold increase in lipid solubility and a fourfold increase in anesthetic potency.

Mepivacaine (1-methyl-2,6 hexahydropicolinlxylidide) is a clinically useful drug in the amino-amide series in which the amino chain is incorporated into a ring system by linking an amino-alkyl group with the intermediate acyl chain. The anesthetic properties of this compound resemble lidocaine, except that it is ineffective topically. Bupivacaine (1-butyl-2,6-hexahydropicolinlxylidide) is formed by the addition of a butyl group to the amine end of mepivacaine, resulting in a 35-fold increase in lipid solubility and a significant increase in protein binding. The new compound has a fourfold increase in anesthetic potency and a longer duration of action.

A third category of compounds, the guanidine-type structures, also possess potent local anesthetic properties. At present, these chemicals have not been sufficiently modified for safe clinical use. Tetrodotoxin, a compound derived from puffer fish, and saxitoxin, which is produced by certain marine dinoflagellates found in shellfish, are the most prominent members of this group.[17] They are potent biotoxins and are among the most potent inhibitors of nerve conduction known.

A fourth class of agents with local anesthetic properties is the tetraethylammonium (TEA) derivatives.[18, 19] In these compounds, an ethyl group is replaced by a C_6, C_8, C_{12}, C_{14} or C_{16} side chain.

These compounds have a hydrophilic amino group, a lipophilic carbon chain, but no aromatic group as in the amino-ester or amino-amide agents. Furthermore, the amino group is an ethylated quaternary amine, rather than a tertiary amine. Like conventional local anesthetics, potency and duration of action appear to increase with increasing compound length. Although these agents have been found to be potent local anesthetics, they are not yet clinically useful.

Mechanism of Action

Local anesthetic agents exert their primary effect on the cell membrane.[20] Theoretically, the drugs may have activity either at the external or internal (axoplasmic) surface of the nerve membrane. Except for benzocaine, most local anesthetics act predominantly in the ionized form on the axoplasmic surface of the nerve membrane. There is good evidence for a specific receptor theory to explain local anesthetic activity with the receptor being located at or near the internal opening of the sodium channel.[21–24] This receptor exhibits some degree of stereospecificity for the anesthetic agent, with a resultant effective blockade of the sodium channel. The normal electrophysiologic depolarization cascade cannot continue, and impulse transmission is halted. The sequence of events resulting in local anesthetic effect are outlined in Table 4–2.

The classic local anesthetic agents also block conduction of nerve transmission by membrane expansion.[25] This is a nonspecific action and may well be the principal mode of action for benzocaine. Apparently, the amino-ester and amino-amide agents

TABLE 4–2. Sequence of Local Anesthetic Action

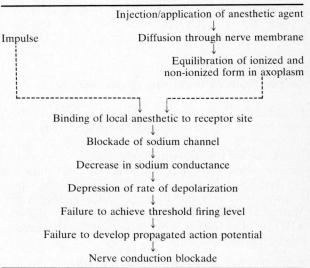

Injection/application of anesthetic agent
↓
Impulse   Diffusion through nerve membrane
↓
Equilibration of ionized and non-ionized form in axoplasm
↓
Binding of local anesthetic to receptor site
↓
Blockade of sodium channel
↓
Decrease in sodium conductance
↓
Depression of rate of depolarization
↓
Failure to achieve threshold firing level
↓
Failure to develop propagated action potential
↓
Nerve conduction blockade

increase the freedom of movement of the lipid molecules of the axonal membrane, causing an expansion of some portion of the membrane that is critical for impulse conduction. The most likely explanation is that there is an unfolding of membrane protein, together with some disordering of the lipid component of the cell membrane.[26] This conformational change in the membrane constricts the transmembrane ion channels, with resultant diminution of ionic flux and conduction blockade. Displacement of membrane-bound calcium ions may also be involved. Calcium is known to condense lipid layers and local anesthetics can displace it.

Two additional sites of action exist for the biotoxins and for TEA. The marine biotoxins, tetrodotoxin and saxitoxin, block the external pore of the sodium channel, inhibiting depolarization.[27] TEA and its derivatives appear to have two mechanisms of action. These compounds block a receptor site located at the internal opening of the potassium channel, thus inhibiting repolarization.[28, 29] They also appear to inhibit the sodium channel in a manner analogous to that described above for the clinically useful local anesthetic agents.

All types of nerve fibers are affected by the clinically useful local anesthetics (see Table 4–1). In general, the order of sensitivity to blockade appears to be: preganglionic, pain and temperature, touch, proprioception, and motor fibers (with preganglionic being the most sensitive and motor fibers the least sensitive). Specifically, it is known that myelinated preganglionic B-fibers are about three times more sensitive than nonmyelinated C-fibers. Large A-fibers are most resistant to local anesthetics. However, the smallest A-fibers (δ) are more sensitive than C-fibers, even though they conduct impulses more rapidly. Also, sensory A-fibers (α) are more sensitive than motor A-fibers (γ). Although the conduction velocity is the same, the sensory fibers conduct at a higher frequency. Finally, all local anesthetics block sensory fibers more rapidly than motor fibers. Each agent, however, will exhibit a relative selectivity for different types of fiber.[30]

Active Form of Local Anesthetic Agents

Most local anesthetic agents are weak bases with the free base being poorly soluble. The drugs, however, are administered clinically in the acidic form as HCl salts, which are highly ionized and water-soluble. These compounds exist in solution as an equilibrium mixture of the non-ionized, lipid-soluble base (B) and ionized, water-soluble conjugate acid (BH$^+$). The relationship between the base (B) and acid (BH$^+$) is expressed by the Henderson-Hasselbalch equation:

$$pH = pKa + \log (B/BH^+)$$

where pKa is the dissociation constant. Physiologic buffers increase the pH of the environment thereby increasing the amount of free base, with the lipid-soluble form diffusing through the nerve membrane. The free base then re-equilibrates with the acid form in the axoplasm, generating an abundant concentration of cation that becomes available as the active blocking component.[23]

Experimentally, the carbonated form of the local anesthetic appears to have an enhanced effect over the hydrochloride derivative.[31] The reasons for this include the fact that the pH is higher, therefore the concentration of available unchanged base is increased. Also, CO_2 is released and diffuses into the interior of the cell, lowering the pH and increasing the ionization of the agent at the site of action. Clinically, the superiority of carbonated derivatives varies with the particular agent and mode of administration. For example, carbonated lidocaine and prilocaine are superior to the hydrochloride form for epidural block.[16]

Anesthetic Profile of a Local Anesthetic

The anesthetic characteristics of a compound are dependent on (1) lipid solubility, (2) protein binding, (3) pKa, (4) non-nervous tissue diffusibility, and (5) intrinsic vasodilator activity. These characteristics are directly related to the structure-activity relationships of each compound.[22]

Lipid solubility is the primary determinant of intrinsic anesthetic potency. This is consistent with the composition of the nerve membrane, with approximately 90 percent of the axolemma composed of lipids. Therefore, agents with a high lipid solubility (partition coefficient) will penetrate easily and rapidly, which results in a potent blocking effect with a rapid onset of action.

The protein-binding characteristics of an anesthetic primarily influence its duration of action. Proteins account for approximately 10 percent of the nerve membrane. Agents that penetrate the axolemma and bind firmly to membrane protein will exhibit prolonged duration of action.

The dissociation constant (pKa) of an agent is the pH at which its ionized form (BH$^+$) is in complete equilibrium with its non-ionized form (B). The amount of a specific agent present in the base form when injected into tissue (pH 7.4) is inversely proportional to the pKa of that agent. The pKa values of the common local anesthetic agents are all greater than normal tissue pH; therefore, the drugs will exist predominantly in their ionized form. A high pKa yields less base at a given pH than other anesthetics having their pKa closer to the pH. Stated in different terms, the more alkaline the environment, the more non-ionized base is available for diffusion, thereby reducing the latent period of nerve blockade. Conversely, if the environment is more acidic (as in soft tissue infection) the ionized form will predominate, and the effectiveness of blockade will be diminished.

When a local anesthetic is injected into tissue, the agent must initially diffuse through connective tissue to reach the nerve. The non-nervous tissue diffusibility for each agent differs markedly. For example, lidocaine and prilocaine have the same pKa and onset of action in isolated nerve preparations in the laboratory, but in vivo lidocaine has a more rapid onset. The precise explanation for this is unknown.

Finally, it has become apparent that certain local anesthetic agents may possess intrinsic vasodilator activity.[13] In fact, all local anesthetics, with the exception of cocaine, have variable vasodilator effects. For example, the intrinsic anesthetic potency of lidocaine in vitro is greater than that of mepivacaine, although their durations of action are similar. In vivo, however, their anesthetic potency is equivalent, whereas mepivacaine has a longer duration of action. This is partly because of the greater vasodilator activity of lidocaine, resulting in greater vascular absorption and making less lidocaine available for nerve blockade.

Metabolism

The metabolism of local anesthetic agents varies according to their chemical structure.[17] The ester class of local anesthetics are hydrolyzed by the enzyme pseudocholinesterase. Cocaine is the only ester-type agent that is metabolized primarily in the liver. The rate of hydrolysis varies among the different agents in this class with chloroprocaine showing the most rapid rate of hydrolysis (4.7 μmol/ml/hr), compared to procaine (1.1 μmol/ml/hr) and tetracaine (0.3 μmol/ml/hr). The intensity of anesthesia and toxicity vary inversely with the rate of hydrolysis. The principal metabolite formed by the hydrolysis of procaine, chloroprocaine, and tetracaine is para-aminobenzoic acid (PABA). As will be seen, this may have sensitizing effects in some individuals.

The metabolism of the amino-amide compounds is more complex and occurs primarily in the liver. The rates of metabolism vary with prilocaine being the most rapid; lidocaine, mepivacaine, and etidocaine being intermediate; and bupivacaine the slowest.

Local anesthetic agents and their metabolites are excreted primarily via the kidney. Only small amounts of the ester-type compounds are excreted unchanged in the urine. For example, two percent of an administered dose of procaine appears unchanged in the urine, while its principal metabolite, PABA, is found in the urine. Likewise, the amino-amide agents undergo almost complete hepatic me-

tabolism prior to renal excretion, with less than five percent of unchanged drug present in the urine. More than 70 percent of administered lidocaine can be identified in the urine as the metabolite hydroxyxylidine.[17]

Vasoconstrictor Agents

Vasoconstrictor agents are frequently combined with local anesthetics to enhance their intensity and duration of action, to reduce peak plasma concentrations thereby diminishing potential systemic toxicity, and to minimize local bleeding.

Most vasoconstrictors used in local anesthetics are adrenergic or sympathomimetic amines. The most commonly used agents and their characteristics are listed in Table 4–3. Epinephrine, the most commonly used vasoconstrictor, is a potent stimulator of both alpha- and beta-receptors. In most soft tissues, vasoconstriction occurs.

The enhancement of local anesthesia by vasoconstrictors occurs partly because most local anesthetics have intrinsic vasodilator properties, which are negated by the vasoconstrictor agent. Systemic toxicity is decreased because systemic absorption is slowed and drug absorption can be balanced by drug metabolism.

Clinical Uses

Local or regional anesthesia can be classified as follows:
1. Topical anesthesia.
2. Infiltration anesthesia (extravascular or intravascular).
3. Peripheral nerve blockade (single or multiple nerve blockade).
4. Central neural blockade (epidural or subepidural blockade).

Dermatologic applications are usually limited to topical anesthesia, extravascular infiltration technique, and occasionally peripheral nerve blockade. Peripheral nerve blockade is reviewed in the next chapter, and central neural blockade is beyond the scope of this discussion.[34]

TABLE 4–3. Characteristics of Commonly Used Vasoconstrictor Agents

Vasoconstrictor	Concentration		Maximum Dose	
Epinephrine	1:50,000	(0.02 mg/ml)	0.20 mg	10 ml
	1:100,000	(0.01 mg/ml)	0.20 mg	20 ml
	1:200,000	(0.005 mg/ml)	0.20 mg	40 ml
Norepinephrine	1:30,000	(0.033 mg/ml)	0.33 mg	10 ml
Levonordefrin	1:20,000	(0.05 mg/ml)	1.0 mg	20 ml
Phenylephrine	1:2,500	(0.40 mg/ml)	4.0 mg	10 ml

TABLE 4–4. Topical Anesthetic Agents

Anesthetic	Concentration (%)	Form	Use	Onset (min)	Duration (min)
Benzocaine	1–5	Cream	Skin, mucous membranes	Slow	Prolonged
	20	Ointment	Skin, mucous membranes		
	20	Aerosol	Skin, mucous membranes		
Cocaine	4–10	Solution	Ear, nose, throat	2.5–10	10–30
Dibucaine	0.25–1.0	Cream, ointment, aerosol	Skin	2.5–5	30–60
	0.25	Solution	Ear		
	2.5	Suppositories	Rectum		
Lidocaine	2.0–4.0	Solution	Ear, nose, throat	5	15–30
	2	Viscous jelly	Oropharynx, GU		
	2.5–5.0	Ointment	Skin, mucous membranes, rectum		
	10	Suppositories, aerosol	Rectum, gingiva		
Tetracaine	0.5–1.0	Cream, ointment	Skin, mucous membranes, rectum	5–10	60
	0.25–1.0	Solution	Ear, eye, nose, throat		

Topical Anesthesia

Topical anesthesia can be provided by the ester and amide derivatives or by skin refrigerants. Intact skin usually impedes the absorption of most commercially available ester and amide anesthetics. They are more practical for mucous membranes, especially in surgical procedures around the eyes or nose. It should be noted that tetracaine and lidocaine can provide anesthesia by local injection or by topical application. Table 4–4 lists the agents that are commonly available and their characteristics.[35, 36] Skin refrigerants (Table 4–5) are used for many minor dermatologic procedures and for dermabrasion.[37, 38]

Extravascular Infiltration Anesthesia

There are three categories of local anesthetics based on anesthetic potency and duration of action.[39]

1. Low potency and duration of action—procaine and chloroprocaine.
2. Intermediate potency and duration of action—lidocaine, mepivacaine, and prilocaine.
3. High potency and duration of action—tetracaine, bupivacaine and etidocaine.[40]

The characteristics of the commonly used local anesthetic agents are listed in Table 4–6. The ideal local anesthetic has a rapid onset and a long duration of action. The newer amino-amide agents, bupivacaine and etidocaine, have exceedingly long durations of action, which is beneficial for lengthy or repetitive surgical procedures.[41-43] Mixtures of local anesthetics have been utilized in an attempt to maximize the desirable properties of each agent, but the ultimate result may depend on additional factors, such as the pH of the final solution.[44, 45]

Special consideration must be given to the administration of local anesthetics in certain diseases. The patient with scleroderma will generally have increased duration of action because of slow absorption from the tissue. If liver disease is present, the duration and potential toxicity of amide-type anesthetics will be increased so that it may be desirable to administer a lower dose of an amino-ester derivative. Likewise, if a patient has a pseudocholinesterase deficiency, ester-type local anesthetics will be hydrolyzed quite slowly, thereby markedly prolonging their anesthetic effects.

Injection of a local anesthetic into infected tissue may not produce as effective a blockade as desired. Infected tissue has an abundance of lactic acid and other acids producing an acidic pH. This enhances formation of the non-ionized base that is less diffusible, thereby delaying the onset of the action. Also, if epinephrine is employed as a vasoconstrictive agent, the solution is normally buffered to a lower pH with sodium pyrosulfite or sodium bisulfide to

TABLE 4–5. Skin Refrigerants

Agent	Chemical Components	Maximum Cooling Temperature (5 cm distance at 25 sec with a freestanding thermocouple) (°C)
Aerofreeze	Trichlorofluoromethane (Freon 11) Dichlorodifluoromethane (Freon 12)	−43.0 ± 0.5
Medi-Frig	Dichlorodifluoromethane (Freon 12)	−63.7 ± 0.9
Frigiderm	Dichlorotetrafluoroethane (Freon 114)	−40.5 ± 0.5
Fluro Ethyl	Dichlorotetrafluoroethane (Freon 114) Ethyl chloride (25%) (75%)	−41.9 ± 0.9

TABLE 4—6. Characteristics of Commonly Used Local Anesthetic Agents

Agent	Principal Uses and Concentration (%)	pKa	Lipid Solubility	Onset/Duration of Action	Maximum Single Dose	Primary Metabolic Site
Lidocaine	Infiltration 0.5–2%, peripheral nerve 1–2%, spinal 1–2%, topical 4%	7.9	Medium	Rapid onset, short to intermediate duration (60–120 min)	300 mg plain 500 mg with epinephrine	Liver
Mepivacaine	Infiltration 1–2%, peripheral nerve 1–2%, spinal 1.5–2%	7.6	Medium	Slow onset, intermediate to long duration (90–180 min)	300 mg plain 500 mg with epinephrine	Liver
Prilocaine	Infiltration 1%, peripheral nerve 1%, spinal 2–3%,	7.9	Medium	Slow onset, short to intermediate duration (60–120 min)	400 mg plain 600 mg with epinephrine	Liver
Bupivacaine	Infiltration 0.25–0.5%, peripheral nerve 0.25–0.5%, spinal 0.25–0.75%	8.1	High	Slow onset, long duration (4–8 hr)	175 mg plain 250 mg with epinephrine	Liver
Etidocaine	Infiltration 0.5–1%, peripheral nerve 0.5–1%, spinal 1.0–1.5%	7.7	High	Rapid onset, long duration (4–8 hr)	200 mg plain 300 mg with epinephrine	Liver
Cocaine	Topical 4–10%	–	Medium	Slow onset, medium duration (20–30 min)	150 mg	Liver
Benzocaine	Topical 0.4–5%	–	Medium	Rapid onset, short duration (10–20 min)	–	Plasma
Procaine	Infiltration 1–2%, spinal 2%	8.9	Low	Slow onset, short duration (30–45 min)	500 mg plain 600 mg with epinephrine	Plasma
Tetracaine	Topical 0.5–1%, infiltration 0.1–0.2%, spinal 0.25–1%	8.5	High	Slow onset, long duration (30–180 min)	100 mg	Plasma
Chloroprocaine	Infiltration 1–2%, peripheral nerve 1–2%, spinal 2%	8.7	Low	Rapid onset, medium duration (60–120 min)	600 mg plain 750 mg with epinephrine	Plasma

minimize oxidation of the epinephrine. This will further reduce anesthetic effectiveness.

Technique

Local infiltration can be effectively performed with Luer-Lok syringes and a 1 to 1½ inch (25- to 30-gauge) needle. The initial injection should be at the periphery of the planned surgical site, which will raise a small wheal. Before injection, the syringe should be aspirated to insure the extravascular placement of the needle. As the needle is advanced to spread the anesthetic field, it should be reintroduced through an area that was previously injected. This will minimize the pain and burning sensation produced by the infiltration. Also, there is a direct relationship between the speed of injection and pain, so that very slow injections are preferable. In general, it is best to infiltrate circumferentially around the site and to confirm the presence of anesthesia with pinprick tests prior to beginning the procedure.

Toxicity

In view of their enormous use, the local anesthetic agents have a remarkably good safety record.[46–49] Although the agents are injected locally, toxic levels of drug may occasionally be absorbed into the bloodstream. The response to this may be either systemic or local. As mentioned before, aspiration of the syringe should always be performed prior to injection to guard against inadvertent intravascular injection. A vasoconstrictive agent such as epinephrine (1:200,000) will slow the rate of absorption and reduce peak blood levels after absorption. Vasoconstrictive substances should be avoided in acral areas such as fingers, toes, and the penis as well as in patients with cardiac, thyroid, and ischemic arterial disease.

Allergic contact sensitivity is rare and usually related to the metabolic conversion of ester-type drugs into para-aminobenzoic acid or other derivatives. Contact sensitivity has been reported to procaine and tetracaine, and photocontact sensivitiy reactions have been reported to dibucaine and benzocaine.[50–53] It is felt that there is potential cross-reactivity between various ester compounds as well as a cross-reactivity with the sulfonamides.[54, 55]

Allergic contact reactions to amide type agents are extremely rare but may occur with lidocaine.[56] A unique type of toxic reaction is the development of methemoglobinemia following prilocaine anesthesia. The compound responsible for the reaction is o-toluidine, a metabolite of prilocaine.[21]

Anaphylactic reactions are rare but occur more commonly with the ester-type agents than with the amide-type, although deaths have been reported in association with both.[57] In the evaluation of an allergic reaction, the use of preservatives, usually methylparabens, in the solution must be considered. In a small percentage of patients, this agent can initiate allergic phenomena. If allergic reactions are well documented to both classes of local anesthetic agents, sufficient anesthesia for most minor surgical procedures can usually be achieved using normal saline or diphenhydramine.[58, 59]

Systemic toxicity to local anesthetics generally involves the cardiovascular and central nervous systems. At doses that produce nontoxic blood levels, either a slight increase or no change in blood pressure is noted. As blood levels approach toxic amounts, hypotension results from a direct relaxant effect on vascular smooth muscle. (Cocaine is the only local anesthetic agent that causes significant vasoconstriction). At massive doses, cardiovascular collapse may result from peripheral vascular vasodilatation, reduction in myocardial contractility, and decreased heart rate.

Toxic effects occur most frequently in the central nervous system. These include dizziness, tinnitus, light-headedness, circumoral numbness, and nystagmus. If the toxicity progresses, overt tonic-clonic convulsions develop that eventually terminate in shallow respiratory effort. Blood pressure falls dramatically, and a progressive bradycardia ensues, leading ultimately to cardiac arrest. It is imperative that this sequence of events be differentiated from a vasovagal reaction, a response to a vasoconstrictor, or from allergic sensitivity and that immediate appropriate therapy be initiated (Table 4–7).[60]

The use of vasoconstrictors may substantially reduce the likelihood of undesirable side effects of local anesthetics.[33] Epinephrine can significantly increase heart rate and norepinephrine can induce hypertension and reflex bradycardia when used in conjunction with local anesthetics, even in young and healthy people. In older individuals with cardiovascular disease, the effects may be more profound. Repeated injections with increased dosage magnify the potential toxicity.

Evidence is accumulating that significant drug interactions may occur with vasoconstrictor agents, particularly with phenothiazines, tricylic antidepressants, beta-blockers, adrenergic blocking agents, and thyroid hormones.[33]

Phenothiazines, especially chlorpromazine and thioridazine, can interact with vasoconstrictors. These drugs are alpha-receptor blockers, and the addition of epinephrine may compound orthostatic hypotension. The tricyclic antidepressants inhibit the uptake of natural adrenergic amines by the nerve terminal. The pressor effects of vasoconstrictor agents is therefore compounded. Likewise, vasoconstrictors, such as epinephrine, will have enhanced pressor effects if used in conjunction with beta-blocking agents (e.g. propranolol). Adrenergic blocking agents, such as guanethidine and reserpine, decrease the release of norepinephrine from adrenergic nerve terminals. These receptors thus become hypersensitive to sympathomimetics. Finally, thyroid hormone can induce a state of hypersensitivity of the cardiovascular system, so the effect of sympathomimetic agents may be exaggerated.

In conclusion, there are no absolute guidelines for selecting a local anesthetic agent. This must be individualized for the particular patient and circumstances. An understanding of the particular operative needs and of the pharmacologic principles involved will permit selection of the appropriate local anesthetic agent.

TABLE 4–7. Differentiation of Reactions During Local Anesthesia

Reaction	Clinical Features	Comments
1. Local anesthetic toxicity		
A. Intravascular injection	Immediate seizure	Have parenteral diazepam present
B. Overdose	CNS symptoms begin 5–15 min after injection	
2. Allergy		
A. Immediate	Anaphylaxis (hypotension, bronchospasm)	Usually secondary to ester-type agents
B. Delayed	Urticaria	
3. Reaction to vasoconstrictor	Apprehension, headache, tachycardia, palpitations	Have adrenoreceptors available (phentolamine and propranolol)
4. Vasovagal attack	Rapid onset, bradycardia, hypotension	May lose consciousness

REFERENCES

1. McAuley JE: The early development of local anesthesia. Br Dent J 121:139–142, 1966
2. Von Oettingen WF: The earliest suggestion of the use of cocaine for local anesthesia. Ann Med Hist (N.S.) 5:275–280, 1933
3. Liljestrand G: Carl Koller and the development of local anesthesia. Acta Physiol Scand (Suppl) 299:3–30, 1967
4. Pearman K: Cocaine: A review. J Laryngology otology 93:1191–1199, 1979
5. Olch PD: William S Halsted and local anesthesia: Contributions and complications. Anesthesiology 42:479–486, 1975
6. Löfgren N: Studies on Local Anesthetics. Xylocaine: A New Synthetic Drug. Stockholm: Haeggstroms, 1948
7. Bickers DR, Hazen PG, Lynch WS: Local anesthetic agents. In Clinical Pharmacology of Skin Disease. New York, Churchill Livingstone Inc, 1984, pp 252–269
8. Cousins MJ, Bridenbaugh PO (eds): Neural Blockade in Clinical Anesthesia and Pain Management. Philadelphia, J. B. Lippincott, 1980
9. Hodgkin AL, Huxley AF: A quantitative description of membrane current and its application to conductance and excitation in nerves. J Physiol (London) 117:500–544, 1952

10. Hodgkin AL: The Conduction of the Nervous Impulses. Liverpool: Liverpool University Press, 1965

11. Covino BG, Giddon DB: Pharmacology of local anesthetic agents. J Dent Res 60(8):1454–1459, 1981

12. Truant AP, Takman B: Differential physical-chemical and neuropharmacologic properties of local anesthetic agents. Anesth Anal 38:478–484, 1969

13. Covino BG, Vassallo HG: Local Anesthetics: Mechanisms of Action and Clinical Use. New York, Grune and Stratton, 1976

14. Ritchie JM, Greene NM: Local anesthetics. In Gilman AG, Goodman LS, Gilman A (eds): The Pharmacological Basis of Therapeutics. New York, MacMillan, 1980, pp 300–320

15. Cousins MJ, Mather LE: Clinical pharmacology of local anesthetics. Anaesth Intens Care 8:257–277, 1980

16. Reynolds FJM: The pharmacology of local anesthetic drugs. In Churchill Davidson HC (ed): A Practice of Anesthesia. Chicago, Yearbook Medical Publishers, 1984, pp 830–855

17. DeJong RH: Local Anesthetics. Springfield, Ill., Charles C Thomas, 1977

18. Scurlock JE, Curtis BM: Tetraethylammonium derivatives: Ultralong-acting local anesthetics. Anesthesiology 54:265–269, 1981

19. Curtis BM, Scurlock JE: The mechanism of action of local anesthesia by tetraethylammonium derivatives. Anesthesiology 54:270–277, 1981

20. Singer MA, Jain MK: Interaction of four local anesthetics with phospholipid bilayer membranes: Permeability effects and possible mechanisms. Can J Biochem 58:815–821, 1980

21. Mather LE, Cousins MJ: Local anesthetics and their current clinical use. Drugs 18:185–205, 1979

22. Strichartz GR: Molecular mechanisms of nerve block by local anesthetics. Anesthesiology 45:421–438, 1976

23. Covino BG: New developments in the field of local anesthetics and the scientific basis for their clinical use. Acta Anesth Scand 26:242–249, 1982

24. Courtney KR, et al: Frequency-dependent conduction block. Anesthesiology 48:111–117, 1978

25. Strichartz GR: Current concepts of the mechanism of action of local anesthetics. J Dent Res 60(8):1460–1467, 1981

26. Seeman P: Anesthetics and pressure reversal of anesthesia. Expansion and recompression of membrane proteins, lipids, and water. Anesthesiology 47:1–12, 1977

27. Adams HV, et al: The local anesthetic activity of tetrodotoxin alone and in combination with vasoconstrictors and local anesthetics. Anesth Analg (Cleve) 55:568–573, 1976

28. Armstrong CM, Hille B: The inner quaternary ammonium ion receptor in potassium channels of the node of Ranvier. J Gen Physiol 59:388–400, 1972

29. Hille B: The selective inhibition of delayed potassium currents in nerve by tetraethylammonium ion. J Gen Physiol 50:1287–1302, 1967

30. Gissen AJ, Covino BG, Gregus J: Differential sensitivities of mammalian nerve fibers to local anesthetic agents. Anesthesiology 53:467–474, 1980

31. Tucker GT, Mather LE: Pharmacokinetics of local anesthetic agents. Brit J Anesth 47:213–225, 1975

32. DiFazio CA: Local Anesthetics: action, metabolism and toxicity. Otolaryngologic Clin of N Amer 14:515–519, 1981

33. Jastak JT, Yagida JA: Vasoconstrictors and local anesthesia: A review and rationale for use. J Amer Dent Assoc 107:623–630, 1983

34. Moore DC: Regional Block, 4th Ed. Springfield, Ill., Charles C Thomas, 1971

35. Allen ED, Elkington AR: Local anesthesia and the eye. Br J Anaesth 52:689–694, 1980

36. Sabbahi MA, et al: Topical anesthesia: A possible treatment method for spasticity. Arch Phys Med Rehabil 62:310–314, 1981

37. Burks JW: Dermabrasion and Chemical Peeling. Springfield, Ill. Charles C Thomas, 1979

38. Hanke CW, O'Brian JJ, Solow EB: Laboratory evaluation of skin refrigerants used in dermatology. J Dermatol Surg Oncol 11:45–49, 1985

39. Gangarosa LP: Newer local anesthetics and techniques for administration. J Dent Res 60(8): 1471–1480, 1981

40. Hameroff SR, et al: Comparison of bupivacaine, etidocaine, and saline for trigger-point therapy. Anesth Analg 60:752–755, 1981

41. Lonick II, et al: Local anesthesia with bupivacaine and lidocaine. J Am Pod Assoc 67:9–93, 1977

42. Pederson H, et al: Pharmacokinetics of etidocaine in fetal and neonatal lambs and adult sheep. Anesth Analg 61:104–108, 1982

43. Jenson OT, et al: Advantages of long-acting local anesthesia using etidocaine hydrochloride. J Oral Surg 39:350–353, 1981

44. Galindo A, Witchen T: Mixtures of local anesthetics: Bupivacaine-chloroprocaine. Anesth Analg 59:683–685, 1980

45. DeJong RH, Bonin JD: Mixtures of local anesthetics are no more toxic than parent drugs. Anesthesiology 54:177–181, 1981

46. Moore DC: Local anesthetic drugs: Tissue and systemic toxicity. Acta Anaesthesiol Belg 32:283–300, 1981

47. DeJong RH: Toxic effects of local anesthetics. JAMA 239:1166–1168, 1978

48. DeJong RH, Bonin JD: Toxicity of local anesthetic mixtures. Toxic Appl Pharmacol 54:501–507, 1980.

49. Cloninger P: Reactions to local anesthetic agents. Western J Med 131:316–320, 1979

50. Prystowsky SD, et al: Allergic contact hypersensitivity to nickel, neomycin, ethylenediamine, and benzocaine. Arch Dermatol 115:959–962, 1979

51. Ryan ME et al: Contact urticaria and allergic contact dermatitis to benzocaine gel. J Am Acad Dermatol 2:221–223, 1980

52. Horio T: Photosensitivity reaction to dibucaine: Case report and experimental induction. Arch Dermatol 115:986–987, 1979

53. Kaidbey KH, Allen H: Photocontact allergy to benzocaine. Arch Dermatol 117:77–79, 1981

54. Fisher AA: Contact Dermatitis. Philadelphia, Lea & Febiger, 1973

55. Cronin E: Contact Dermatitis. New York, Churchill Livingstone, 1980

56. Fregert S, et al: Contact allergy to Lidocaine. Contact Dermatitis 5:185–188, 1979

57. Christie JL: Fatal consequences of local anesthesia: Report of five cases and a review of the literature. J Forensic Sci: 671–679, 1975

58. Wiener SG: Injectable sodium chloride as a local anesthetic for skin surgery. Cutis 23:342–343, 1979

59. Roberts EW, Loveless H: The utilization of diphenhydramine for production of local anesthesia: Report of a case. Texas Dental J 97:13–15, 1979

60. DeShazo RD, Nelson HS: An approach to the patient with a history of local anesthetic hypersensitivity: Experience with 90 patients. J Allergy Clin Immunol 63:387–394, 1979

5

WILLIAM R. PANJE, M.D.

Nerve Block Anesthesia of the Head and Neck

Regional anesthesia is a relatively safe and effective method to achieve a painless operative field for diagnostic or therapeutic purposes. Regional anesthesia, sometimes referred to as conduction anesthesia, is achieved by directly anesthetizing a single nerve, or several, that supplies an operative field. Local anesthesia differs from regional anesthesia in that in the former the anesthetic is injected along the line of incision and within the structures of the surgical wound. In this way, a large number of free nerve endings are anesthetized, sparing the specific sensory nerve trunk. Infiltrative local anesthesia is effective in achieving anesthesia to the specific injected area, but it often involves the infiltration of a large volume of an anesthetic solution that may distort tissue planes and cause unnecessary patient pain from tissue distention.

Regional anesthesia includes a number of methods for blocking nerve impulse conduction. The specific regional anesthetic methods dealt with in this chapter include nerve block, field block, and topical anesthesia.

To accomplish a specific nerve block, one must be familiar with the anatomic course of the nerve to be anesthetized. Concomitantly, familiarity with the various ostium and superficial bony landmarks is needed. The present chapter will try to outline the basic anatomy necessary to achieve regional anesthesia to the cutaneous structures of the head and neck. Knowledge of this basic neuroanatomy and a few simple techniques in the use of local anesthetics should permit the cutaneous surgeon to perform an almost unlimited number of painless operative procedures.

Premedication

Perception and reaction make up the two components of the pain stimulus. Pain perception is a noxious stimulus transmitted by the peripheral nervous system, i.e., free nerve endings. Pain perception is readily blocked by a number of infiltrative anesthetics. Pain reaction is the patient's response to remembrance of an unpleasant situation. This embraces complex neurophysiopsychological processes that involve the posterior thalamus and cerebral cortex. The patient's past experiences and learning influence the degree of pain reaction. The judicious use of various premedications that dull the patient's sensorium and past remembrances will, in most cases, offer a more pleasant and pain-free operative experience for the patient as well as the surgeon.

Diazepam (Valium), in combination with a narcotic, increases the pain threshold as well as providing amnesia in surgical patients. If the patient is of good health, the intravenous or intramuscular administration of 5–10 mg of diazepam 10 to 30 minutes prior to nerve block anesthesia will greatly reduce the patient's anxiety. The addition of a narcotic will increase the pain threshold. Nysentil, which is related to morphine, is a relatively fast-acting narcotic that lasts usually for 20 to 30 minutes. Repeated doses do not appear additive in side effects and can be easily reversed with a narcotic antagonist such as naloxone hydrochloride (Narcan).

Diazepam or a narcotic or both appear warranted in the highly emotional and anxious patient. Likewise, operative procedures lasting longer than 30 minutes would seem suitable for premedication.

NEUROANATOMY

The trigeminal nerve provides the principal sensory nerve supply to the face and scalp. The sensory fibers arise from the gasserian ganglion and supply the cutaneous areas anterior to a line drawn from the vertex of the skull to the upper part of the external ear, then caudally to the angle of the mandible and along its lower border to the meatus (Fig. 5–1). The three major nerves that supply the face include V_1 (ophthalmic nerve), V_2 (maxillary nerve), and V_3 (mandibular nerve). Knowledge of the courses of these nerves will allow one to selectively anesthetize areas of the face.

Ophthalmic Division

The ophthalmic division includes afferent fibers from the anterior scalp, forehead, upper eyelid, lateral angle to the eye, and the tip and alae of the

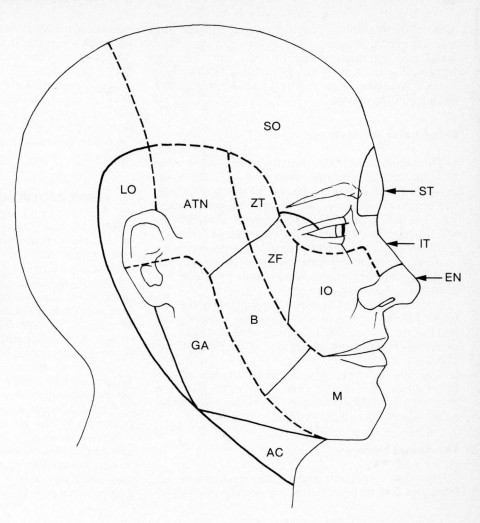

Figure 5–1. Zones of peripheral sensory innervation of the face (side view). V₁: SO is the supraorbital nerve; ST, the supratrochlear; IT, the infratrochlear; EN, the external nasal. V₂: ZT is the zygomatico-temporal; ZF, the zygomatico-facial; IO, the infraorbital. V₃: ATN is the auriculo-temporal; B, the buccal; M, the mental. Cervical nerves include LO, the lesser occipital; GA, the greater auricular; and AC, the anterior cervical. (Courtesy of *The Journal of Dermatologic Surgery and Oncology,* 5(4):311–315, April 1979. Copyright 1979, *The Journal of Dermatologic Surgery and Oncology,* Inc.)

nose. The ophthalmic nerve divides into three branches: the lacrimal, frontal, and nasociliary nerves, which exit the cranium through the superior orbital fissure. The lacrimal nerve supplies sensation to the lateral angle of the eye. The frontal nerve divides into the supratrochlear and supraorbital nerves. The supratrochlear passes anteriorly and medially toward the upper medial angle of the orbit to supply the skin of the upper eyelid and lower medial portion of the forehead. The supraorbital nerve passes lateral to the supratrochlear nerve in the supraorbital foramen. The supraorbital nerve passes cephalad approximately 2.5 cm from the midsagittal plane of the head. The supraorbital notch or foramen can usually be palpated at the middle part of the supraorbital rim. The supraorbital nerve provides cutaneous sensation to the upper eyelid, the forehead, and the anterior scalp region back to the vertex of the skull.

The nasociliary nerve is the third branch of the ophthalmic division. It divides into several branches, including the long root of the ciliary nerve, long ciliary nerve, posterior ethmoid nerve, and the anterior ethmoid nerve. These nerves are, in general, of little interest to the cutaneous surgeon except for the anterior ethmoid nerve. This nerve travels along the medial aspect of the orbit to enter the ethmoid labyrinth and cross the floor of the anterior cranial fossa to enter the nose at the crista galli. Two branches, the internal and external nasal branches, arise here. They both travel down and forward, with the latter exiting the internal nares through the junction of the upper lateral cartilage and the bony nasal dorsum to supply sensation to the tip and lateral ala of the nose.

Maxillary Division

The second division of the trigeminal nerve transmits sensory impulses from the skin over the anterior part of the temporal region, over the prominence of the zygomatic bone, the lower eyelid, the side of the nose, and the upper lip. The maxillary division passes through the foramen rotundum and divides into the principal afferents of the midfacial integument. The zygomatic nerve proceeds through the inferior orbital fissure to give rise to the zygomatic facial and zygomatic temporal branches. The infraorbital nerve travels along the bony orbital floor to exit onto the front of the maxilla through the infraorbital foramen.

Mandibular Division

The third division of the trigeminal nerve exits from the cranium at the foramen ovale. The principal mandibular nerve afferents to the face include the auriculo-temporal, buccal, and mental nerves. The auriculo-temporal nerve supplies sensation to the superior half of the pinna, tragus, and temporal scalp region. The auriculo-temporal nerve becomes somewhat superficial just anterior to the tragus coursing from behind the neck of the condyle of the temporomandibular joint.

The buccal nerve becomes superficial at the anterior border of the masseter muscle opposite the level of the second and third mandibular molars. Its principal integument sensation is to that of the cheek.

The mental nerve is a terminal branch of the inferior alveolar nerve that exits onto the face through the mental foramen. It provides sensation to the lower lip and chin region.

The Spinal Nerves

The sensory nerve supply of the neck is derived from the first three cervical nerves (Fig. 5–2). The superficial cervical branches of these nerves reach the neck's surface at the junction of the upper and middle third of the sternocleidomastoid muscle (Fig. 5–3). The ascending branches supply the occipito-mastoid region of the head and lower part of the auricle. The transverse branches are distributed to the anterior part of the neck between the lower border of the jaw and the sternum. The descending branches innervate the shoulder and upper pectoral region.

NERVE BLOCKING—GENERAL PRINCIPLES

Several basic fundamentals should be remembered and routinely practiced if one is to accomplish consistently successful nerve blocks.

A smaller syringe (3 to 5 cc) should be utilized for more optimum handling. This syringe may be disposable. The needle should be 2.5 to 3.75 cm long, depending upon the nerve to be blocked, and of a 25 to 27 gauge diameter.

A 1 to 2% solution of lidocaine (Xylocaine) is combined best with 1:100,000 epinephrine in order to achieve up to one hour of anesthesia per block. Lidocaine has a very low allergenicity and readily diffuses through tissues.

An intradermal wheal should be produced in the proximity of the nerve or nerves to be blocked in order to avoid pain on movement, reintroduction, and redirection of the needle.

The bevel side of the needle should be placed downward and steady traction applied to the skin. The traction will tighten the skin and allow for an

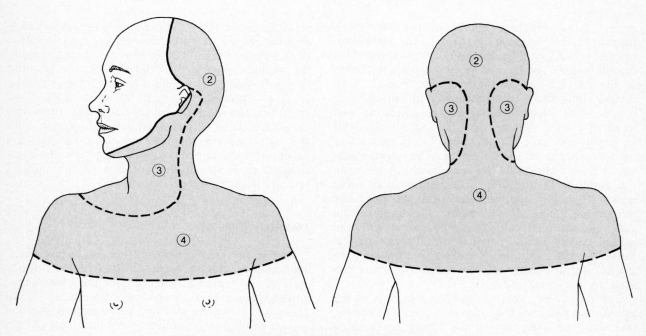

Figure 5–2. Sensory nerve supply of cervical nerves C_2, C_3, C_4.

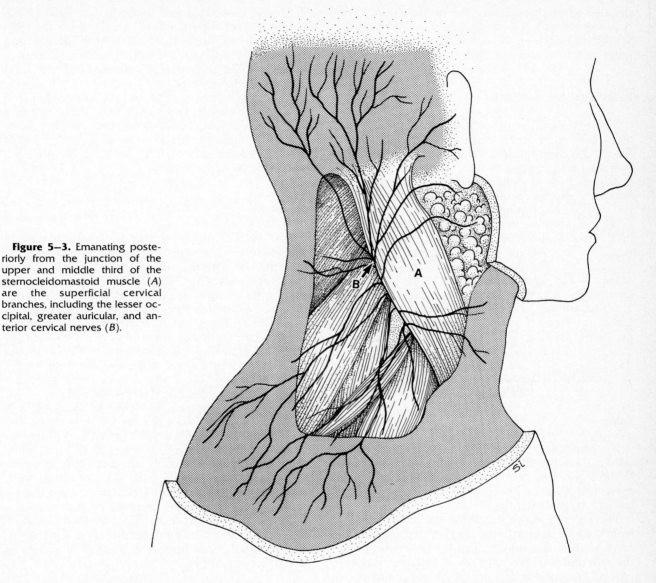

Figure 5–3. Emanating posteriorly from the junction of the upper and middle third of the sternocleidomastoid muscle (*A*) are the superficial cervical branches, including the lesser occipital, greater auricular, and anterior cervical nerves (*B*).

easier needle introduction. Likewise, the digital skin pressure will initiate sensory impulses that will partly mask the more painful impulses generated upon needle insertion.

A nerve block can be intraneural or extraneural. The former (i.e., depositing material within the nerve) should be avoided unless one is attempting a total nerve destruction, such as in an alcohol neurolysis. Direct intraneural injection, often followed by postoperative neuralgia, is usually quite painful. Extraneural blocks are not painful, and the degree of anesthesia reaches that of an intraneural block, provided the anesthetic material is placed in proximity to the nerve.

The nerve block has an added benefit over local infiltrative anesthesia in that the operative field is not distorted from the injection of an anesthetic solution. Conduction anesthesia can be repeated a

number of times successfully and, most importantly, can and should be used after loss of anesthesia in an operated area in which the tissues have been elevated. This is important because the elevated tissues are frequently bleeding and do not retain locally injected anesthetic solution long enough to achieve optimum anesthesia.

When establishing regional anesthesia, one should avoid striking the bone with the needle since the periosteum is quite sensitive. Too rapid instillation of an anesthetic solution should be avoided as well as injections into areas of skin tightly bound to underlying structures, i.e., the auricle and tip of the nose, because the pressure receptors are fairly insensitive to local anesthetics, especially at the immediate time of injection, and will elicit patient discomfort.

One should always inject on withdrawing the

needle rather than during the introduction. When depositing solution in a localized area, the operator should pull back on the syringe's plunger to test for possible intravascular needle position.

Individual Nerve Blocks

The peripheral sensory supply to the scalp, face, and neck have been outlined. Individual nerve blocks can anesthetize selected areas without distortion of the overlying tissues, and toxic anesthetic reactions from overdosage are reduced. Although adequate anesthesia can be achieved by injection of an anesthetic solution into the general area of the peripheral location of sensory nerves, the placement of the anesthetic more proximal to the nerve terminations will usually provide a more effective and reliable desensitization. The more frequently used nerve blocks in the head and neck include the infraorbital, mental, greater auricular, maxillary, and mandibular nerve blocks. Wide areas of anesthesia can be achieved with these blocks as well as providing for easier local infiltrative anesthesia.

CONDUCTION ANESTHESIA FOR SPECIFIC OPERATIVE SITES

Scalp

By employing the following specific techniques, one can achieve anesthesia to all or selected areas of the scalp. The cutaneous surgeon should consider using techniques when removing scalp lesions and for hair transplantation.

The sensory nerve supply to the scalp emanates from a number of different nerves that encircle the head along a line drawn through the eyebrows and that continues to the junction of the anterocephalic part of the auricle and temporal scalp and posteriorly to a point 2.5 cm below the occipital protuberance (Fig. 5–4). The forehead is supplied by the frontal nerve (supraorbital and supratrochlear) and the zygomatic temporal nerve (V_2), while the auriculo-temporal nerve (V_3) supplies the temporal region. The occipital and parietal regions are supplied by the greater and lesser occipital nerves (cervical).

To insensitize a selected area of the scalp, one would simply deposit an anesthetic solution along the line of origin of the sensory nerves to that area. For example, in performing hair transplantation, the injection of 1% lidocaine with 1:100,000 epinephrine along the line of origin of the lesser and greater occipital nerves will anesthetize the occipital donor area. Supplemental injection of the actual donor area primarily for hemostasis can then be done with minimal or no patient discomfort. The frontal scalp region is anesthetized by depositing an anesthetic along the eyebrows and glabella.

Muscle tissue is denser over certain areas of the cranium. This is particularly evident along the temporal region. One must inject both deeply and superficially in this area in order to achieve adequate anesthesia. Subperiosteal injections are not required and should be avoided.

The scalp is very vascular and therefore may bleed to a greater degree if only peripheral nerve blocking is performed. One should always inject the operative site with an anesthetic and a vasoconstrictor (at least 1:100,000 epinephrine) five minutes after injecting the principal nerve supply.

Nose

The external nose receives its innervation from the infratrochlear and external nasal nerves (V_1) and the infraorbital and anterior spinous nerves (V_2). As shown in Figure 5–5, one can secure anesthesia of the integument of the external nose by applying an anesthetic solution to the infraorbital foramen (1), the junction of the brow with the nasal root (2), the bridge of the nose at the bony cartilaginous junction (3), and at the base of the columella (4). The external nasal nerve can alternatively be blocked by applying a 4% cocaine solution to the anterior superior part of the internal nose.

When performing nerve blocks to the nose, it is more convenient and effective to field block the nasal pyramid. The needle is inserted at the location of the infraorbital foramen, and 0.5 cc of an anesthetic solution is injected. The needle is then advanced subcutaneously toward the root of the nose, returned to the infraorbital foramen, and then inserted inferiorly toward the base of the columella (anterior spinous process). The anesthetic solution is deposited upon return to the site of skin insertion. The external nasal branch is a separate block, as described previously.

Lips

The upper lip receives innervation from the infraorbital and anterior spinous nerves (V_2). The lower lip is innervated primarily via the mental nerve (V_3). Thus, by performing infraorbital nerve blocks, mental nerve blocks, and injection of the base of the columella (anterior spinous nerves), total perioral anesthesia can be achieved.

Eyelids

The eyelids receive cutaneous innervation from the supraorbital, supratrochlear, infratrochlear, and lacrimal nerves (V_1) and the infraorbital nerve (V_2). Primarily, these are terminal branches of the ophthalmic nerve, which more or less encircle the

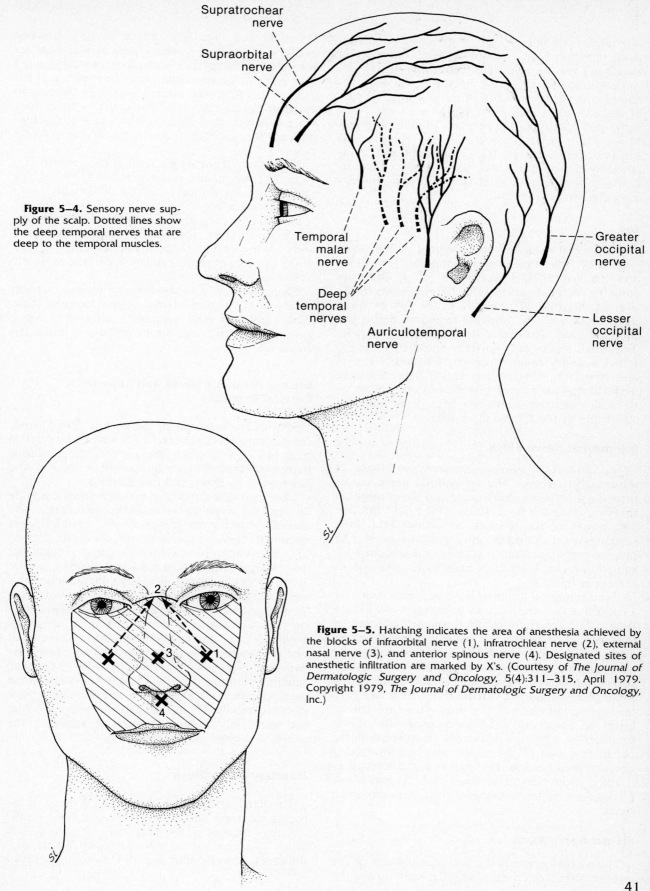

Supratrochear nerve

Supraorbital nerve

Figure 5–4. Sensory nerve supply of the scalp. Dotted lines show the deep temporal nerves that are deep to the temporal muscles.

Temporal malar nerve

Deep temporal nerves

Auriculotemporal nerve

Greater occipital nerve

Lesser occipital nerve

Figure 5–5. Hatching indicates the area of anesthesia achieved by the blocks of infraorbital nerve (1), infratrochlear nerve (2), external nasal nerve (3), and anterior spinous nerve (4). Designated sites of anesthetic infiltration are marked by X's. (Courtesy of *The Journal of Dermatologic Surgery and Oncology,* 5(4):311–315, April 1979. Copyright 1979, *The Journal of Dermatologic Surgery and Oncology,* Inc.)

orbit at its bony rim. Thus, by injecting an anesthetic along the outer bony limits of the orbit, outer eyelid anesthesia can be achieved. Tetracaine or 4% cocaine solution should be dropped into the conjunctiva to complete anesthesia of the conjunctival part of the lids. Individual nerve blocks are usually not warranted because of the necessity of multiple punctures. Deep orbital blocks are not required to achieve adequate periorbital anesthesia and, if incorrectly done, can cause undesirable complications—retroorbital hemorrhage, blindness, and extraocular muscle paresis.

Ear

The primary sensory nerve supply of the pinna originates from the auriculo-temporal nerve (V_1) and the greater auricular nerve (C_{2-4}). Branches from the occipital nerve supply the cutaneous region over the mastoid. Nerve block of the greater auricular nerve and the auriculo-temporal nerve will produce good anesthesia to the external auricle. These two blocks only partially anesthetize the external auditory canal, since the VII and X nerves also contribute sensory innervation here. Selective nerve blocks for auricular anesthesia are preferable to local infiltrative anesthesia because of the close adherence of the skin to the cartilage.

Infraorbital Nerve Block

The infraorbital nerve is the terminal branch of the maxillary nerve. The infraorbital nerve passes from the pterygomaxillary space into the infraorbital foramen along the floor of the orbit to exit into the soft tissues of the midface. It divides into three branches upon exiting the infraorbital foramen. The inferior palpebral branch supplies the conjunctiva, skin of the cheek, mucous membrane, and skin of the upper lip.

The infraorbital foramen is located approximately 1 cm below the inferior bony orbital rim and 2.5 cm from a line drawn vertically through the length of the nose. A depression is usually palpable in the infraorbital foramen area and is often noted by the patient to be more tender to digital pressure. The supraorbital notch, infraorbital foramen, and mental foramen all lie along a vertical line 2.5 cm lateral to the midsagittal plane of the head. It is sufficient to instill an anesthetic solution in proximity of the foramen to achieve satisfactory infraorbital nerve block. Insertion of the needle into the foramen is not indicated because subsequent paresthesias may develop if the nerve is injected directly, and it will provide no better anesthesia than a periforamen block.

Mental Nerve Block

The mental nerve is the terminal portion of the inferior alveolar nerve and supplies sensation to the lower lip and chin. The mental nerve is blocked easily at the mental foramen. The mental foramen is located at the anterior body of the mandible along a line drawn between the lower bicuspids perpendicular to the lower margin of the mandible. In children, the foramen is located closer to the inferior margin of the mandible. In the older edentulous patient, the foramen is located near the alveolar ridge.

The extraoral route of anesthesia is preferred. A 3 cm, 25 gauge needle is connected to a 3 ml syringe and introduced through the site of puncture until the bony mandible is contacted. The puncture site is located along a perpendicular line drawn through the infraorbital and supraorbital foramen that intersects a horizontal line located approximately a third of the distance from the caudal edge of the mandible to the lower lip.

Then, 2 to 3 cc of an anesthetic solution is injected slowly in the region of the mental foramen. One should inject at both mental foramen when doing lower lip and chin operations because of sensation crossover.

Greater Auricular Nerve and Superficial Cervical Branches

Sensory nerve supply of the neck is derived from the first four cervical nerves. The superficial cervical branches of C_{2-4} reach the neck at the posterior border of the sternocleidomastoid muscle at the junction of its upper and middle third.

The superficial cervical nerves are found easily by locating a few pertinent anatomic landmarks. The mastoid process and angle of the mandible are identified, then a line is drawn connecting them. This line is then bisected with a perpendicular line that extends inferiorly to cross the posterior border of the sternocleidomastoid muscle. Definition of this muscle can be increased by having patients turn their head away from the injection site while applying counterpressure to the chin. Using a 25 gauge needle, 3 cc of an anesthetic solution is injected at that point where the perpendicular line crosses the posterior border of the muscle (Fig. 5–6). The patient will notice a gradual loss of sensation to the lower auricle and neck skin. Supplemental anesthetic is usually needed around the operative site, but since only a small amount is required, the injection is more easily tolerated.

Maxillary Nerve Block

The maxillary nerve is the second division of the trigeminal nerve and leaves the cranial vault via the foramen rotundum to enter the sphenomaxillary fossa. The external cutaneous sensory supply is to the cheek, lower eyelid, side of the nose, and upper lip.

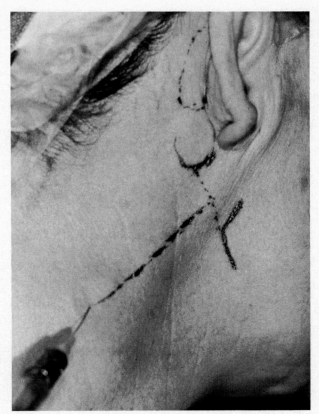

Figure 5—6. Needle points to the site of injection for blocking the greater auricular, lesser occipital, and anterior cervical nerves. (Courtesy of *The Journal of Dermatologic Surgery and Oncology,* 5(4):311—315, April 1979. Copyright 1979, *The Journal of Dermatologic Surgery and Oncology,* Inc.)

There are a number of different ways to approach the maxillary nerve at the foramen rotundum. The extraoral and greater palatine routes offer the easiest, most consistent, and relatively complication-free way of achieving anesthesia of the maxillary nerve.

The extraoral route is accomplished by first placing a wheal of anesthetic just inferior to the bisection of the zygomatic arch. An 8 cm, 22 gauge needle (spinal needle) that has been threaded with a rubber marker is introduced through the wheal. The needle is advanced at right angles to the zygomatic arch until striking bone, which is the lateral pterygoid plate. Bone is usually encountered at approximately 5 cm of needle depth. Upon striking bone, the rubber marker is set, 1 cm from the skin. The needle is then withdrawn until the tip reaches the subcutaneous tissues and then is redirected at approximately a 30 degree angle to the skin. The needle is inserted anteriorly to the marker; if no bone is encountered, the sphenomaxillary space has been entered. The syringe is aspirated and, if negative, 2 cc of an anesthetic solution is injected.

An alternative approach is to inject the spheno-maxillary space through the greater palatine foramen. The foramen is situated in the hard palate 1 cm medial to the last molar tooth. An initial injection of 0.5 cc of lidocaine solution is inserted into the region that will be probed for the greater palatine foramen. A 3.75 cm, 25 gauge needle is utilized for the block. The needle is bent to a 90 degree angle approximately 2.5 cm from the tip. The needle, which is attached to a 3 cc syringe with 1 cc of an anesthetic solution, is then gently inserted into the formen to a depth of 2.5 cm. It is important not to force the needle tip through the length of the foramen. The needle is aspirated and, if negative, 1 cc of solution is injected. If upon aspiration, air is encountered, the needle should be withdrawn and reinserted. Usually, the needle has been passed into the nasopharynx, and by bringing the needle a little forward, the foramen will be encountered.

The major complication with either of these routes for maxillary nerve block is that of blindness from injection of the ophthalmic nerve. This is avoidable by paying strict attention to limiting the depth of the injection to 5 cm for the extraoral route and a 2.5 cm for the intraoral route, always aspirating first, and never injecting more than 2 cc of anesthetic solution. Hemorrhage is usually not a problem with either of these two routes.

Mandibular Nerve Block

The mandibular nerve is the third division of the trigeminal nerve and leaves the cranial cavity through the foramen ovale, which lies posterior to the pterygomaxillary space. Sensory distribution is to the temporal region, the external auditory meatus and auricle, and the lower portion of the face, including the lower lip and chin.

The nerve is blocked best by an extraoral route, similar to the one described for the maxillary nerve. An 8 cm, 25 gauge needle with a rubber marker is used, which is inserted until the lateral pterygoid plate is encountered, as done for blocking of the maxillary nerve. The rubber marker is set 1 cm from the surface of the skin, and the needle is withdrawn into the subcutaneous tissue. The needle is then reintroduced approximately 1 cm posterior to where the needle struck the pterygoid plate. As mentioned before, the needle must not be inserted more than 5 cm, and one must always aspirate before injection and use no more than 1–2 cc of an anesthetic solution. Frequently, the maxillary and mandibular nerves will be blocked simultaneously.

REFERENCES

1. Covino BG, Vassallo HG: Local Anesthetics: Mechanisms of Action and Clinical Use. New York, Grune & Stratton, 1976
2. Adriani J: Labat's Regional Anesthesia: Techniques and Clinical Applications, 3rd Ed. Philadelphia, W B Saunders, 1967
3. Monheim LM: Local Anesthesia and Pain Control in Dental Practice. St. Louis, C V Mosby, 1969, pp 68–122
4. Panje WR: Local anesthesia of the face. J Dermatol Surg Oncol, 5(4): 311–315, 1979

6

Basic Principles of Cutaneous Surgery

TISSUE HANDLING

The sine qua non of successful cutaneous surgery is the utmost gentleness in handling all tissue. Damaged and injured tissue leads to necrosis, followed by fibrosis and scarring, the result of which may not be immediately evident but will manifest itself later. Dr. Sterling Bunnell, known to many as the father of modern hand surgery, remarked "One does not repair a watch with a sledgehammer" (Fig. 6–1).

In the handling of tissue, one must be aware of adjacent structures, lest they be damaged in enthusiastic attempts by the assistant to allow the surgeon to see what he is doing.

THE INSTRUMENTS

All surgical instruments have been designed for a particular use and are not necessarily interchangeable. Thus, surgical instruments suitable to the general surgeon, which must traverse the abdominal wall, are not necessarily suitable for use on the face. Figure 6–2 shows the relative sizes of typical instruments used in general surgery compared with those used in plastic surgery. It is primarily the smaller size that provides the delicacy in handling tissue that is mandatory for successful cutaneous surgery. It is not unlike the dissimilarity between the instruments an auto mechanic will use and those used by a jeweler. Both are essential to the size of the structure being worked upon.

Similarly, an instrument designed for one purpose should not be used for something else. Thus, a Kelly clamp is designed to grasp bleeding vessels, not the tips of cutaneous flaps. They are crushing instruments and achieve that purpose no matter where they are used. The tip of the flap illustrated in Figure 6–3 has been held by a Kelly clamp and is surely destined to necrose.

It is much simpler to manage skin edges by using a skin hook, such as the one in Figure 6–4. One might argue that such an instrument is not always available in the emergency room. However, it can easily be fashioned from a disposable no. 25 needle that is bent into an appropriately sized hook with a sterile cotton-tipped applicator jammed into the hub of the needle for a handle. Figure 6–5 shows the assembly of such a useful tool.

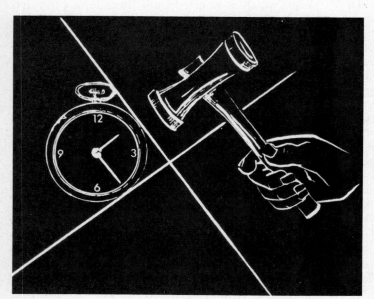

Figure 6–1. "One does not fix a watch with a sledgehammer."

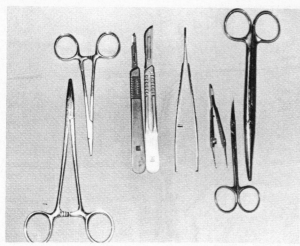

Figure 6–2. Typical sizes of instruments used ideally for plastic surgery, placed alongside identical instruments used for general surgery.

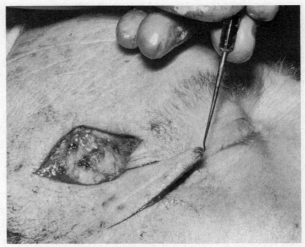

Figure 6–4. The tip of a flap handled with a skin hook.

DRAPING

All too often, particularly with surgery on the face, a small area of skin is prepared, and a drape with a small hole in it is placed over the rest of the face. As the patient becomes increasingly hot and claustrophobic, he or she will change position, the drapes will shift, the surgeon will move them back, and after this exercise has been repeated a few times, the entire field is contaminated (Fig. 6–6A). It is much more convenient and pleasant for the patient to have the entire face prepped and draped off using a head drape (Figs. 6–6B and C).

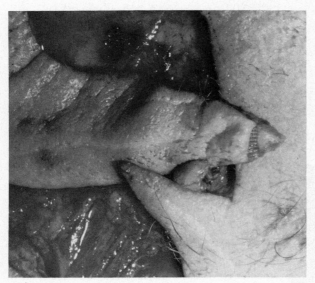

Figure 6–3. The tip of this flap has been grasped and held with a Kelly clamp. The marks from the clamp are visible and the tip of the flap is destined to necrose.

ANESTHESIA

Most cutaneous surgery can be performed with local infiltration anesthesia. A 0.5% or 1% solution of lidocaine (Xylocaine) with epinephrine (1:200,000 or 1:100,000) is slowly infiltrated in the area to be operated upon. A very small (27- or 30-gauge) hypodermic needle should be used whenever possible to minimize both the discomfort of the needle penetration and the rate of injection of the solution. It is the quick distension of tissue in a rapid infiltration that causes pain, not the solution itself or the needle penetration. It is best to use the smallest amount of anesthetic that can accomplish the purpose in order to avoid distortion of the tissues. The local anesthetic with epinephrine serves the dual purpose of providing excellent capillary hemostasis in addition to the anesthetic effect. For this reason, one should wait five to seven minutes to get the benefit of the epinephrine. A definite blanching of the skin is a clear indication of such effect. It should be noted that in individuals sensitive to epinephrine, a good hemostatic effect can be achieved with a solution as weak as 1:800,000.

In long procedures, reinjection of the anesthetic solution at the termination of the procedure will permit several hours of freedom from incisional discomfort. Longer-acting local anesthetics, such as bupivacaine hydrochloride (Marcaine), will achieve the same purpose.

THE INCISION

The incision and any plans for closure should be clearly marked on the skin before actually making the incision. Whether one uses the readily available prepackaged skin markers or the equally available (and usually cheaper) few drops of methylene blue

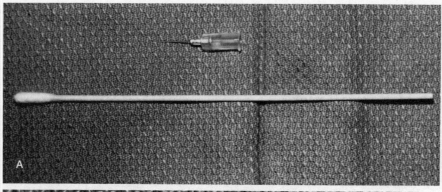

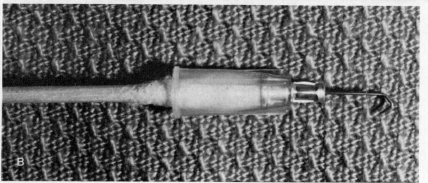

Figure 6–5. *A,* Commonly available items in any hospital setting: cotton-tipped applicator and disposable hypodermic needle. *B,* The end of a disposable 25-gauge needle can be bent into a small hook and made into a disposable skin hook by having the cotton-tipped applicator jammed into the hub of the needle.

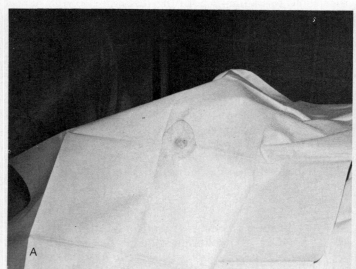

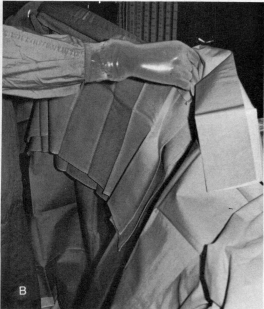

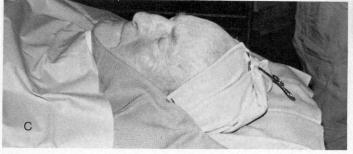

Figure 6–6. *A,* Draping the face and exposing the lesion through a small hole maximizes the patient's discomfort and may contaminate the operative field. *B,* Preparation of head drape with small half-sheet and two towels. *C,* Head drape in place with entire face prepped.

in a suture pack with a sharpened cotton-tipped applicator is immaterial. Proposed incisions should be marked and oriented so that the lines of incision and eventual lines of closure will lie in or be parallel to a crease of expression (Fig. 6–7). These lines are easy to see in older individuals (Fig. 6–8) but may be more obscure in younger people (Fig. 6–9A). Upon animation, however, the lines are readily seen (Fig. 6–9B) or can be produced by pinching the skin (Fig. 6–9C).

On occasion, a lesion is oriented in such a way that the ideal line of closure would produce a defect out of proportion to the size of the lesion (Fig. 6–10A). Excision of the lesion along its longitudinal axis would produce a suture line that is at right angles to the lines of expression (Fig. 6–10B). However, a suitable compromise is a sigma-shaped excision and resulting suture line that, as shown in Figure 6–10C, allows part of the incision to be parallel to the lines of expression and only a minor portion to cross them. The ideal proportion of length to width in the design of a lentiform excision is three to one or more. This distributes tension better along the entire wound, and there is less tendency for dog-earing at both ends. When the ratio is less than this, the tension is greater in the center of the wound, and there is a marked tendency to develop dog-ears (Fig. 6–11).

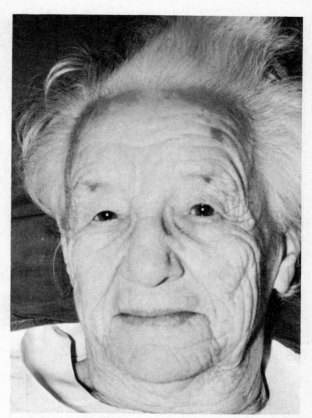

Figure 6–8. Creases of expression are readily visible in older people.

Now, and only now, is the incision ready to be made. Using a blade size designed for this purpose (e.g., a Bard-Parker no. 15), the incision is made at right angles to the skin using the bevel of the knife rather than the tip, which is neither designed nor ideally sharpened for cutting. All lesions sent to the pathology department must be clearly identified so that the margins of the specimen can be oriented to the margins of the incision. This is particularly important in malignant skin tumors. Marking at a given position (such as 12 o'clock or 3 o'clock, upper margin or medial margin) can be done by using a suture or by staining it with concentrated silver nitrate.

PREPARATIONS FOR CLOSURE

Undermining

In order to facilitate closure, to allow closure in layers, and to permit easy eversion of skin edges, a small to moderate amount of undermining of the skin edges must be performed. This can be achieved by using a scalpel in the subcutaneous layer while supporting the margin with a couple of skin hooks (Fig. 6–12) or by using small scissors.

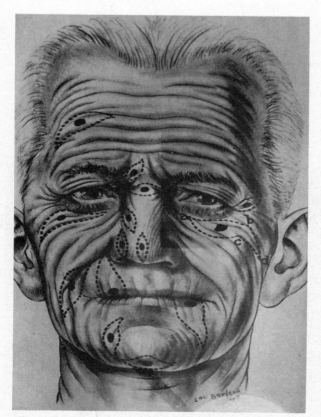

Figure 6–7. The long axis of any elliptical incision is arranged so that the resulting scar is in or parallel to creases of expression.

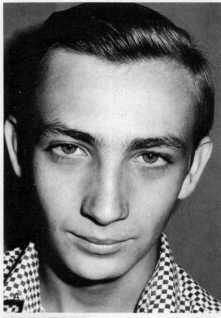

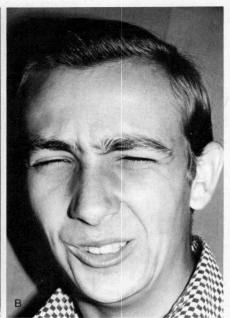

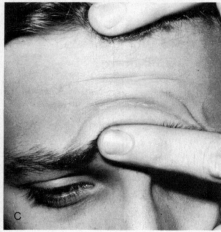

Figure 6–9. *A,* Creases of expression may be virtually absent in young individuals. *B,* Lines of expression can be demonstrated by having the patient animate the face. *C,* The same lines can also be reproduced by pressure on the skin.

Figure 6–10. A 3:1 length-to-width ratio excision of skin parallel to the lines of tension produces a longer eventual scar (*A*) than if the same lesion is created across the lines (*B*). A satisfactory compromise can often be reached by a sigma-shaped incision (*C*). (From Gorney M: Tissue Dynamics and Surgical Geometry, in Kernahan, DA, Vistnes LM: Biological Aspects of Reconstructive Surgery. Boston, Little, Brown & Co, 1977. Reproduced with permission.)

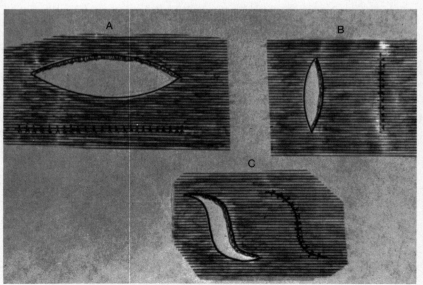

If proportion of wound is greater
than 3 x 1:

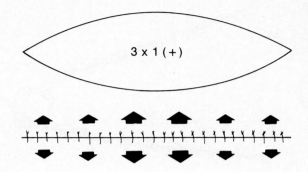

3 x 1 (+)

① tension better distributed
② dog ear less

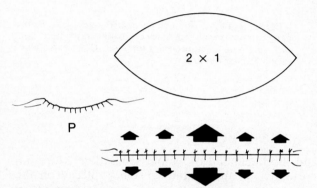

2 × 1

P

Figure 6–11. Ideal and less-than-ideal proportions of lenti-form skin excisions. (From Gorney M: Tissue Dynamics and Surgical Geometry, in Kernahan DA, Vistnes LM: Biological Aspects of Reconstructive Surgery. Boston, Little, Brown & Co, 1977. Reproduced with permission.)

Hemostasis

As Figure 6–13 indicates, lack of hemostasis in a wound often leads to hematoma, which in turn leads to dehiscence and frequently a wound infection.

As mentioned earlier, the use of a local anesthetic with epinephrine is effective for hemostasis. The use of a disposable battery-powered cautery will discourage minor bleeders, but more effective hemostasis is achieved with true electrocoagulation that uses either a monopolar or bipolar current. The latter destroys less of the surrounding tissue and produces more effective coagulation.

Exposure

In order to see what one is doing through all of these maneuvers, optimal exposure is mandatory. To quote Bunnell again, "It is difficult to repair a watch in an inkwell"; similarly, it is hard to perform delicate surgery in a pool of blood. In the emergency

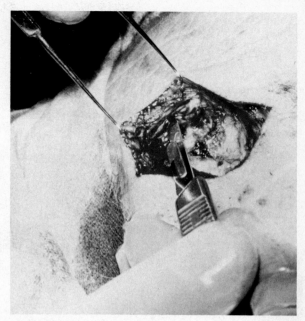

Figure 6–12. With skin edges supported by skin hooks, undermining of skin edges is performed with scalpel or scissors.

room or an office setting, a nurse or an assistant is not always available to provide exposure in the form of retraction. However, a sterile safety pin with the head removed and ends bent back provides an extremely useful self-retaining retractor (Fig. 6–14).

THE CLOSURE

Layer Closure Without Wound Tension

In a primary closure, a small amount of undermining will usually fulfill the dictum that wounds should be closed in layers without tension. If this is not possible, the wound should be closed without tension by the suitable rotation of local flaps or by the application of a split-thickness or full-thickness skin graft, depending on the area and location.

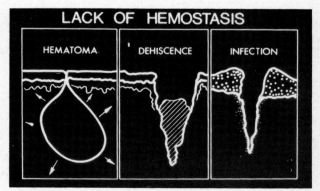

LACK OF HEMOSTASIS

| HEMATOMA | DEHISCENCE | INFECTION |

Figure 6–13. Schematic illustration showing the results from lack of hemostasis.

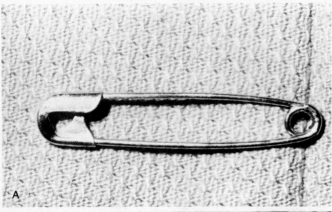

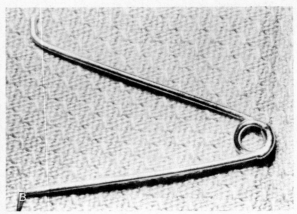

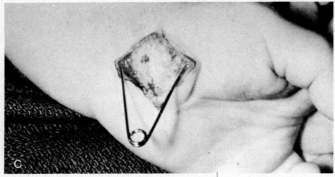

Figure 6–14. *A*, An ordinary sterile safety pin. *B*, The same safety pin with the head removed and the ends bent back to create a self-retaining retractor. *C*, An example of such a retractor in use.

Proper Selection of Suture Material

Just as instruments have been designed for specific uses, so have suture materials with swaged needles been similarly designed. As a general rule, the finer the suture material, the finer the needle. Just as small instruments are preferable for plastic surgery, so are fine suture materials with small needles. In addition to the surgical importance, this also has a financial implication, since a large needle on the end of a heavy suture grasped by a delicate instrument will ruin the instrument. Thus, the smooth-jawed Webster needle holder, which is so useful for instrument tying 6-0 suture material, is easily sprung when clamped down on a large needle at the end of a 3-0 suture. Virtually without exception, all suture materials used for cutaneous surgery should have cutting needles rather than tapered ones, which are more difficult to push through dense dermal tissue and fascia (Fig. 6–15).

Subcutaneous suture material should be selected for its desired purpose keeping in mind that catgut has an effective longevity of only four or more days, chromic catgut has an effective longevity of 14 or more days, and polyglycolic acid is somewhere in-between. Without the use of subcutaneous suture material in the closure of a wound, there is a tendency for inversion of the skin edge and the possibility of a hematoma in the so-called dead space, which increases scar deposition, infection,

and the likelihood of wound separation. More importantly, all the wound tension is placed on the skin suture, which must be left in place longer than desired and which often results in "railroad tracks" of scar tissue across the line of incision (Fig. 6–16). By using a subcutaneous suture, all these problems are avoided.

It should be noted that in areas of considerable natural tension (such as the forehead), in areas of thick skin (such as the back), or in areas where there is constant natural movement (such as the chest, abdomen, or extremities), delayed spreading of an initial hairline suture line may sometimes be avoided by using subcutaneous sutures made from permanent, i.e., nonabsorbable materials such as clear nylon.

If the wound is very deep, it may be necessary to place more than one row of subcutaneous sutures. The deepest row should be placed independently of the skin in the final layer or (if only one layer is necessary) in such a way that the most superficial portion of the suture bites into the bottom portion of the dermis. In that way, the subcutaneous sutures, when properly placed, have already virtually closed the skin (Fig. 6–17). Such mechanics as the direction of passing the needle must be given close attention. It is easy to slide the needle in almost parallel to the skin surface, which results in an inverted suture line. One must consciously place the needle with a backhand motion in such a way that the deeper

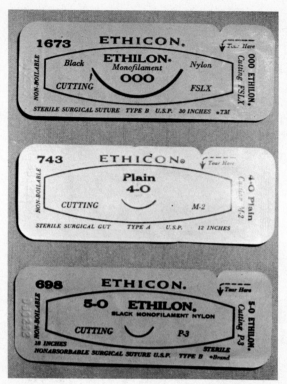

Figure 6–15. Commonly used suture material in plastic surgery. Note that the needle sizes for larger sutures are most often used in general surgery.

portion of the bite is wider than the bite at the surface in order to promote eversion of the skin edge (Fig. 6–18). The latter tends to produce a level skin edge when maturation of the scar is complete.

One is often asked how far apart sutures should be placed. The answer is in part dictated by the area one is working on. Sutures on an eyelid are placed closer together than those on the face or back. The distance is actually determined by the type of skin one is working with. The thinner the

skin and the finer the sutures, the closer the bite must be to the edges and the closer the sutures must be to each other. Regardless of their location, sutures should be placed so that (looking at the suture line in two dimensions) two adjacently placed sutures should form a perfect square, and (looking at it in three dimensions) all the tissues removed between two sutures should form a cube (Fig. 6–19).

When all these details have been considered, one has a wound that is already virtually closed. Skin sutures are usually nonabsorbable and, to some degree, depend on the surgeon's preference. The most commonly used skin sutures are artificial materials such as nylon or the natural fibers such as silk or cotton. Whether one places these as interrupted sutures or as a running suture is immaterial as long as the principles described in the remaining sections of this chapter are taken into consideration (Fig. 6–20). Small, interrupted, vertical mattress sutures can favorably counteract the natural tendency of some areas of skin (e.g., the nasolabial fold, the postauricular crease, or the palm) to become inverted.

SPLINTING OF THE WOUND

In order to promote healing and to avoid excessive motion of the area operated upon, splinting of the wound with strips of adhesive tape, a spray-on plastic dressing, or a single layer of gauze covered with collodion, is both effective and useful.

THE DRESSING

A dressing for a wound should, in the author's opinion, fulfill at least three criteria: (1) It should cover the wound; (2) it should splint the wound effectively; and (3) it should provide a mild degree

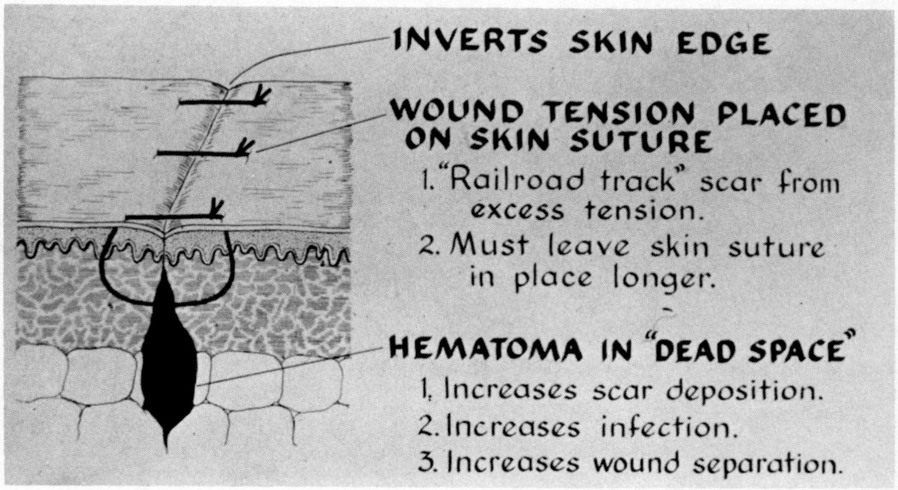

Figure 6–16. Possible surgical results from not using subcutaneous sutures.

INVERTS SKIN EDGE

WOUND TENSION PLACED ON SKIN SUTURE
1. "Railroad track" scar from excess tension.
2. Must leave skin suture in place longer.

HEMATOMA IN "DEAD SPACE"
1. Increases scar deposition.
2. Increases infection.
3. Increases wound separation.

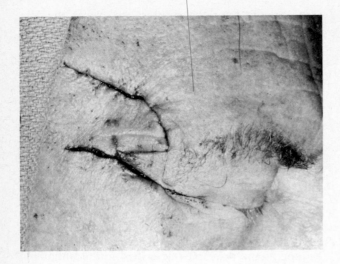

Figure 6–17. A wound closed with properly placed subcuticular sutures.

Figure 6–18. Correct and incorrect direction of needle passage.

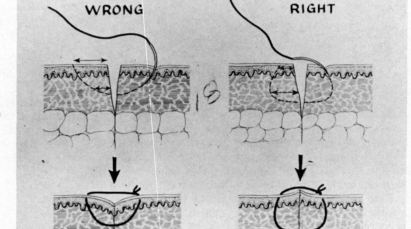

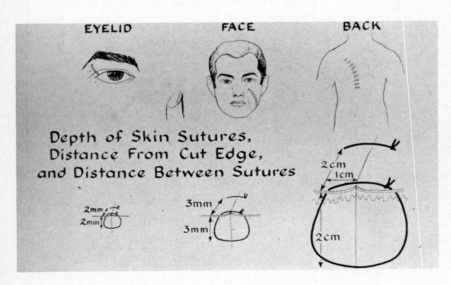

Figure 6–19. Appropriate placement of skin sutures for the eyelid, face, or back.

Figure 6–20. Common methods for placement of skin sutures in cutaneous surgery.

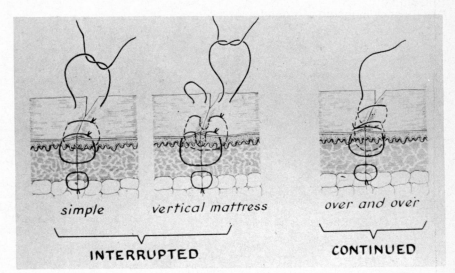

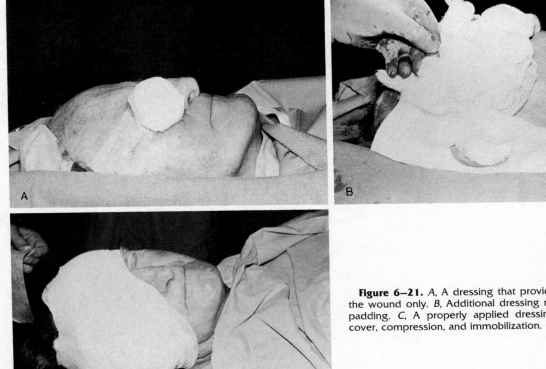

Figure 6–21. *A*, A dressing that provides coverage for the wound only. *B*, Additional dressing material provides padding. *C*, A properly applied dressing that provides cover, compression, and immobilization.

PROBLEM:
Discrepancy in length of wound edges

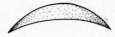

SOLUTION:

① Fudging*

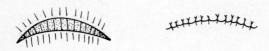

Figure 6–22.

Figure 6–22. Methods of solving discrepancy in the length of wound edges. (From Gorney M: Tissue Dynamics and Surgical Geometry, in Kernahan DA, Vistnes LM: Biological Aspects of Reconstructive Surgery. Boston, Little, Brown & Co, 1977. Reproduced with permission.)

② Shorten long side

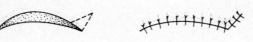

③ Lengthen short side

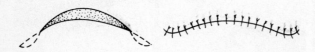

*Do not try fudging discrepancy
  of more than 10-20%

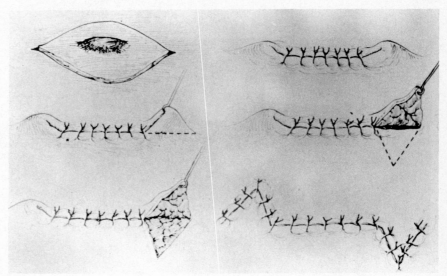

Figure 6–23. Possible solutions to the management of dog-ears.

of tissue compression to aid in hemostasis. A dressing with a piece of tape across the eye pad (Fig. 6–21A) fulfills only the first criterion. A dressing that achieves all three purposes for the same wound is seen in Figures 6–21B and C. A good padding in front of and behind the ear is comfortable for the patient, and fluffed-up gauze over the entire area operated upon is covered with a circumferential bandage.

EARLY REMOVAL OF SUTURES WITH CONTINUED SPLINTING

Proper placement of subcutaneous sutures, as discussed before, allows for earlier removal of sutures at three to five days, thus alleviating the telltale crosshatch markings. The skin has healed sufficiently by this time, and there should be no disruption of the wound. However, the hairline scar that everyone looks for is more apt to result if one of the splinting methods alluded to earlier is used. Ideally, this splinting should be continued for as long as collagen continues to be remodeled (about six weeks). But, for practical purposes, it is difficult to convince the patient to continue with the splinting for more than 10 to 14 days. Patients should be taught how to apply splinting material in case it comes off during washing or with natural oil or sweat production (particularly in warm weather).

SPECIAL PROBLEMS

Discrepancy in Length of Wound Edges

Discrepancies of less than 10% to 20% can be resolved by fudging, i.e., the discrepancy is carefully distributed evenly across the wound. Larger discrepancies can be solved by either shortening the long side or lengthening the short side (Fig. 6–22).

Dog-Ears

As mentioned earlier, dog-ears will result when the length-to-width ratio of a removed lesion is less than three to one. On rare occasions, it may be desirable to produce such a condition in order to distribute the scar over a different area. In that case, the dog-ear is picked up with a skin hook, with one side of it being incised as a continuation of the incision. The resulting flap is laid over the skin and excised either in continuation with the other suture line or by interrupting the suture line and removing a corresponding triangle of skin, which the created flap is fitted into (Fig. 6–23).

Wound Healing

The wound-healing process represents a complex interaction of soluble substances (chemical mediators), particulate structures (cells), and matrix proteins that are orchestrated to restore injured tissue to its functional state. Traditionally, wound repair has been divided into three phases: (1) inflammation (substrate phase), (2) proliferation (fibroblastic phase), and (3) maturation (remodeling phase). These phases are closely integrated and are regulated precisely by largely unknown control and signaling mechanisms. In this chapter, we will attempt to describe the salient features of each phase as well as present-day concepts regarding their orchestration.

THE WOUND-HEALING PROCESS

Inflammation

The immediate response to any type of tissue injury is the initiation of the inflammatory response. This is an exceedingly complex cascade of events in which biochemical mediators interact with specific cells to establish a functional matrix that provides the basis for continued repair.

Most cutaneous wounds result in hemorrhage and the release of proteolytic enzymes that can activate Hageman factor (Factor XII). Activated Hageman factor (XIIa) is a key substance that triggers several distinct systems that participate in inflammation: (1) the intrinsic coagulation system, (2) the kinin system, (3) the plasmin-fibrinogen system, and (4) the classic complement cascade.[1]

The major soluble mediators of inflammation consist of agents that modulate vascular permeability and cellular locomotion. Neutrophils, macrophages, platelets, fibroblasts, epithelial, and endothelial cells are vitally important participants in this sequence of events.

The factors that modulate vascular permeability include:

1. Polypeptides such as bradykinin and related substances as well as cationic proteases derived from lysosomal granules of neutrophils.
2. Vasoactive amines, including histamine derived from mast cells and serotonin, derived from platelets, basophils, and mast cells.
3. Acidic lipids produced from the unsaturated 20-carbon fatty acid, arachidonic acid.[2]

Arachidonic acid can be metabolized in at least two ways along either the cyclo-oxygenase pathway or the lipoxygenase pathway. Prostaglandins and thromboxanes are products of the cyclo-oxygenase pathway, whereas the 5-hydroxy-6,8,11,14-eicosatetraenoic acid (5-HETE) and the leukotrienes are products of the lipoxygenase pathway. The slow-reacting substance of anaphylaxis (SRS-A) consists of leukotrienes C4 and D4. The leukotrienes are particularly potent vasodilators and are among the most potent chemotactic substances known.

Enhanced vascular permeability occurs when microfilaments within endothelial and periendothelial cells contract. This results in an alteration of cell size thereby creating a fenestration between adjacent cells. Plasma proteins can penetrate these openings and reach the surrounding extravascular space. Tissue injury induces enhanced vascular permeability in a biphasic manner. First, an immediate permeability occurs within minutes that is transient and is mediated both by histamine and serotonin. Second, a delayed phase occurs over a three- to six-hour period that is independent of the immediate response and is probably mediated by bradykinin, prostaglandins, and leukotrienes.

Soluble substances that enhance chemotaxis can be classified structurally into three groups: (1) acidic lipids, (2) peptides, and (3) proteins. The 5-HETE are acidic lipids that are weak direct chemotactic mediators, whereas the leukotrienes are among the most potent chemotactic agents for polymorphonuclear leukocytes ever identified.[4] Peptides are another category of chemotactic factors derived from the activation of complement. Both C5a and C3a are cleavage products of the fifth and third components of complement respectively. They are liberated following tissue injury and are potent chemotactic agents. Proteins, particularly various proteases, are also present in damaged tissue where they can degrade various components.

Following tissue injury, red blood cells, platelets, and neutrophils are initially attracted to the site of the wound. Platelets are technically not cells but rather organelles derived from megakaryocytes, which are present in early clot formation. Their cytoplasm contains numerous granules that can release hydrolytic enzymes, serotonin, β-thromboglobulin, and platelet-derived growth factor (PDGF). PDGF is a cationic polypeptide indispensible for the growth of connective tissue cells in culture. This substance is chemotactic for polymorphonuclear leukocytes and monocytic leukocytes and is mitogenic for fibroblasts. Current evidence indicates that PDGF is vital for the initiation of the wound repair process.[5]

Within 12 hours, neutrophils enter the wound in large numbers in response to the chemotactic stimuli described above. They degranulate thereby releasing potent proteolytic enzymes such as collagenases that appear to be preferentially active against type I collagen.[6] They are also phagocytic and can ingest various structural components. This influx of polymorphonuclear leukocytes persists for 24 to 36 hours and provides an initial system that can reduce the risk of infection by destroying colonizing bacteria.

The most important and sustained cellular element to arrive at the wounded area is the macrophage. These marrow-derived phagocytic cells evolve from monocytes that enter the wound from the bloodstream. In addition to phagocytosis, these cells provide a number of substrates essential for wound repair. They also release chemotactic factors that attract additional macrophages and fibroblasts to the site of injury. Fibroblasts are critical for effective wound healing since they are responsible for collagen synthesis.[7]

In the first few days following injury, a fibrin latticework is formed. A key constituent of this matrix is an insoluble, high molecular weight glycoprotein known as fibronectin, which is elaborated by fibroblasts and endothelial cells and is found in the serum.[8] This pivotal substance plays an important role in the adhesion of cells to various surfaces. Fibronectin appears early in the fibrin latticework, is chemotactic for, and guides the migration of fibroblasts and epithelial cells into the wound.[9] Collagen is synthesized by fibroblasts and is also deposited in the fibronectin-fibrin matrix. Fibronectin is known to bind preferentially to type III collagen and to denatured collagen,[9, 10] both of which are prevalent in granulation tissue and in immature tissue. As wound healing progresses, type I collagen becomes predominant, and fibronectin disappears from the matrix.[11]

At the conclusion of the inflammatory phase, the soluble and particulate components essential for the repair process are in place. The predominant cellular constituents of the wound at this time are macrophages and fibroblasts. They elaborate materials that are critical for the second phase of wound healing, i.e., proliferation. A schematic representation of the wound-healing process is depicted in Figure 7–1.

Proliferation

The key element in this second phase of wound healing is the fibroblast, a cell that is richly endowed with mitochondria, endoplasmic reticula, and Golgi's vacuoles, which are essential for protein synthesis. The fibroblasts are motile and some possess myofibrils that assist later in wound contracture. Fibroblasts prefer a surface on which to attach and

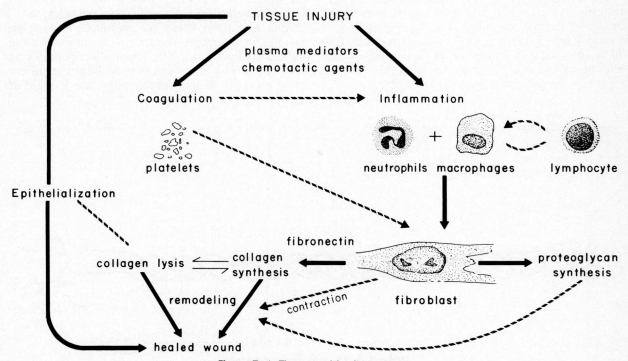

Figure 7–1. The wound-healing process.

migrate, and in wounds they adhere to fibrin and collagen and function most efficiently in a slightly hypoxic, acidic environment rich in ascorbate.[12]

Fibroblasts synthesize collagen, the principal structural protein of the body's connective tissue, as well as elastin and proteoglycans.

Collagen is not a single substance but a group of helical proteins synthesized by fibroblasts and secreted into the extracellular space, where additional glycosylation occurs (Fig. 7–2). Collagens possess the following characteristics:

1. They are composed of three separate peptide chains of approximately one thousand amino acids each (alpha chains). Glycine occurs in every third position, making a repeating structure of Glycine-X-Y. Thus, one third of the collagen chain is glycine and another third is proline or hydroxyproline. X and Y may be any amino acid, but either hydroxyproline or hydroxylysine is usually found in the Y position.

2. Each alpha chain is twisted into a right-handed helix, three of which lie parallel to one another. The entire structure is then twisted into a left-handed "superhelix." This provides for extraordinary rigidity in a compound that is 300Å long but only 15Å in width.

To date, at least nine structurally and genetically separate collagens have been identified.[14–18] Type I and type III collagens are essential in the wound repair process. Type I is the most abundant collagen found in adult skin and is located in the dermis. Two of its three alpha chains are identical (α-1) and a third is similar (α-2). Type III collagen, found primarily in embryonic and fetal tissue, is present initially in dermal wounds but is subsequently replaced by type I collagen as the wound matures. As will be seen, type IV collagen is present in basement membranes and may also play a role in the wound-healing process, especially epithelialization.

A review of the stepwise synthesis of collagen is essential for an understanding of the manner in which this protein becomes incorporated into the healed wound (Fig. 7–3).

Procollagen is the intracellular precursor of the extracellular tropocollagen. It is procollagen that is actually synthesized in and secreted by the fibroblast. The extracellular tropocollagen molecules spontaneously associate in a programmed manner to form collagen fibers.

Procollagen is synthesized by transcription and translation in the usual manner, but it is important to keep in mind that no transfer RNA exists for hydroxyproline or hydroxylysine. Two amino acids, proline and lysine, are added to the chain and then hydroxylated post-translationally by two specific enzymes, prolyl hydroxylase and lysyl hydroxylase. Cofactors include ferrous iron, α-ketoglutarate, and vitamin C. The role of vitamin C is critical for hydroxylation, and it appears that lactate enhances the activity of these enzymes. Deficiency of vitamin C diminishes collagen synthesis, and scurvy is the resulting clinical disorder.

Following alignment of the peptide chains, disulfide bonds are added at the terminal positions, and the helical configuration of the molecule is assumed. The procollagen molecule then moves from the endoplasmic reticulum to the Golgi apparatus, where galactose is attached and the procollagen molecule is secreted from the cell. The microtubular system is important in collagen transport, and colchicine, which inhibits microtubular transport, may diminish collagen secretion. Once in the extracellular space, the procollagen molecule possesses long terminal ends termed registration peptides, which enable the alpha chain to assemble in a parallel fashion at the proper distance to assume the superhelical configuration. The registration peptides are then split off by the action of procollagen aminoprotease and procollagen carboxypeptidase to yield the

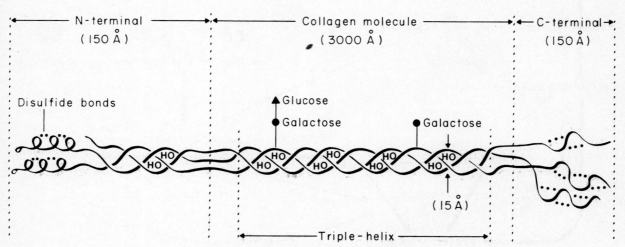

Figure 7–2. The structure of collagen.

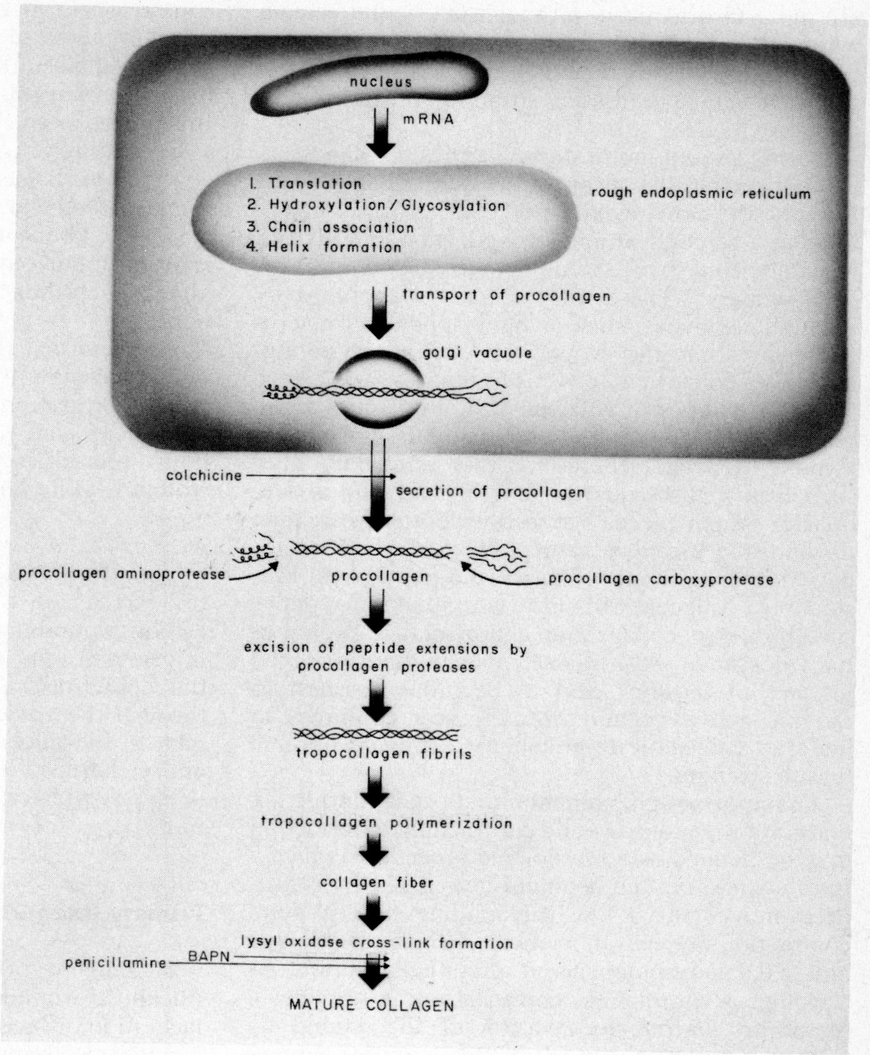

Figure 7–3. Sequence of events in collagen synthesis.

tropocollagen molecule. A deficiency of these enzymes in cattle and sheep results in dermatosparaxis, which is characterized by increased fragility of collagen[19] and diminished tensile strength of connective tissue.

Tropocollagen then aggregates to form fibrils. A key step at this stage is the formation of collagen cross-links, a process whereby aldehyde groups are introduced into the molecule. The enzyme responsible for this is lysyl oxidase. Inhibition of this enzyme results in lathyrism, in which there is generalized weakness of all connective tissue. A chemical called β-aminoproprionitrile is a specific inhibitor of lysyl oxidase, which is derived from the sweet pea. This compound causes diminished intermolecular cross-links thereby weakening the structure of collagen. Penicillamine also inhibits this enzyme by binding to the aldehyde groups and reducing cross-link formation. New collagen can be detected within two to three days of wounding and peaks at five to seven days. The efficiency of collagen synthesis is greatly influenced by both vascularity and oxygen supply. It is felt that an increased rate of collagen synthesis may persist for up to six months following injury, which is well into the third phase of wound repair, i.e., maturation.

Maturation

As the wound matures, continuous remodeling of the scar occurs. As the scar evolves, collagen fibers and fiber bundles become more densely packed, with loss of water and glycosaminoglycan from the wound. This permits closer approximation of the sites on the molecule that facilitate covalent cross-linking. The collagen thus becomes increasingly insoluble, which provides a major increase in tensile strength of the wound. Compared to the surrounding uninjured tissue, collagen fibers within a scar are quite disorganized, although fibers that remain within a scar are generally oriented along lines of tension. It is well documented that a cutaneous scar never regains the tensile strength of the skin it replaced.[19, 20]

During wound maturation, a delicate balance exists between collagen synthesis and collagen lysis. Initially, the newly synthesized collagen exists essentially as a gel, and wound strength is poor. Collagen is catabolized by proteolytic enzymes known as collagenases.[21] These enzymes are elaborated by inflammatory cells, such as neutrophils and macrophages, within the wound and by regenerating, migrating epidermal cells. Collagenases are specific for various types of collagen and always attack the collagen molecule at the same site. Following enzymatic cleavage, there are two remaining fiber segments, a three-quarter length piece and a one-quarter length piece. These polypeptides can then unwind and are very susceptible to further degradation by additional proteases and peptidases. Presumably, collagen with little cross-linking is more susceptible to collagenase action and is preferentially degraded. Also, those collagen fibers oriented in lines of tension seem to be more resistant to enzyme activity. Therefore, the scar continues to undergo enzymatic remodeling to provide optimal tensile strength.

An important phenomenon that occurs during the maturation phase is wound contraction. Contraction may be defined as a physiologic process by which a full-thickness wound is diminished in size by centripetal movement of the surrounding skin. Wound contraction involves movement of the entire dermis and takes place independent of epithelialization. As a wound is contracting, epithelialization provides a temporary barrier to invasion of the wound by microorganisms, but much of this migrated epithelium is lost in the fully contracted wound.

The amount of available skin surrounding a wound, and not the size of the wound itself, determines the extent to which a wound will contract. There is some evidence that contraction proceeds at a fairly uniform rate of 0.6 to 0.75 mm per day.[19] However, the shape of a wound may influence the rate: Circular wounds contract at a slower rate than rectangular or stellate ones.

A specialized cell called the "myofibroblast" is believed to be the key element in wound contraction. This cell has features both of fibroblasts (collagen synthesis) and smooth muscle cells (contractility). These cells are most highly concentrated in either a granulating wound or an arterial wound. They are scarce or absent in wounds healing by primary intention. The nuclei of these cells possess numerous indentations, and the cytoplasm possesses contractile myofibrils. They have desmosomes and tight intercellular junctions and attach to the underlying substrate.[22] They respond to smooth muscle

contractors (e.g., epinephine and serotonin) and can be inhibited by such compounds as prostaglandin E, and cytochalasin B.[23] It also appears that myofibroblasts contain microtubules that are vulnerable to such drugs as colchicine and vinblastine.

Interestingly, collagen is not essential for wound contraction. It has been shown that wound contraction proceeds normally in the scorbutic animal. Collagen fibers are not contractile and cannot shorten under physiologic conditions. A scar is relatively inelastic, because it contains few elastic fibers. Also, its collagen fibers are more dense than those in normal skin and tend to be oriented along lines of original tension.

The maturation phase of wound healing proceeds for at least one year, as the scar undergoes continuous remodeling. The approximate timing of wound-healing phases is shown in Figure 7–4.

TYPES OF WOUND HEALING

Skin wounds may be classified by the extent of injurious insult. A superficial wound involves only the epidermis; a partial-thickness wound extends through the epidermis and into the superficial dermis; a full-thickness wound extends through the entire dermis. Wounds heal by primary intention, delayed primary closure, or by secondary intention.[24]

Primary Intention

Healing by primary intention occurs when full-thickness wounds are approximated shortly after laceration or incision. The epidermis and dermis are coapted. Prerequisites for this type of healing are a clean wound (free of foreign bodies, nonviable tissue, or bacterial contamination) and an adequate blood supply to the margins.

Epithelialization and wound contraction have only small roles in wound healing by primary intention. Minimal epithelialization occurs within 24 hours, whereas increased collagen synthesis is detectable 24 hours after wounding and peaks at five to seven days. The strength of these wounds is provided by collagen cross-linking; epithelialization provides no strength for the closed wound. The strength of the primarily closed wound increases for many months, but the resultant scar never totally recovers the tensile strength of the surrounding normal skin.

Delayed Primary Closure

Delayed primary closure is advisable in contaminated skin wounds or in patients who are severely injured and must be stabilized before the manage-

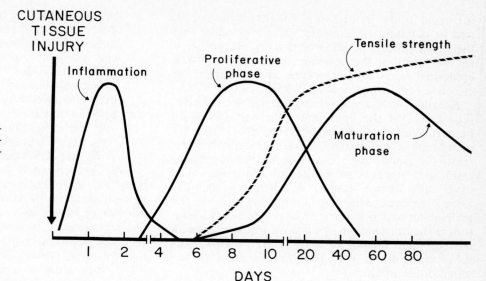

Figure 7–4. Approximate timing of the phases of wound healing and the development of tensile strength.

ment of cutaneous injuries. Delayed primary closure does not delay the development of tensile strength or the ultimate strength of the wound and substantially decreases the likelihood of infection.

Secondary Intention

Healing by secondary intention allows wounds to close without surgical intervention. All aspects of the wound-healing process are involved, with contraction being the most important phenomenon in closure. Collagen synthesis and epithelialization play valuable supportive roles. The advantages of healing by secondary intention include the simplicity of postoperative care. The wounds are relatively pain-free and rarely bleed or become infected. This method is particularly prudent in those cutaneous malignancies with a high risk of recurrence, especially in the midface, periorbital, and periauricular areas. Depending on the location, the cosmetic result is often quite excellent. Wounds on concave surfaces of the *n*ose, *e*ye, *e*ar, and *t*emple (NEET areas) often heal with imperceptible scars. Wounds on convex surfaces of the *n*ose, *o*ral lips, *c*heeks, and *c*hin (NOCH areas) heal with variable results and may be best managed by immediate surgical repair. Finally, wounds on the *f*orehead, *a*ntihelix, eye*l*ids, and the *r*emainder of the nose, lips, and cheeks (FAIR areas) often heal with flat hypopigmented scars, which are cosmetically satisfactory to most patients.[25]

NEO-ANGIOGENESIS

The wound-healing process requires a synchronized cascade of interdependent events to proceed normally. The nutritional supply to the tissue is interrupted at the moment of tissue injury, and yet formation of the surrounding connective tissue matrix requires additional energy. Cell replication and collagen synthesis cannot be initiated without oxygen, amino acids, glucose, trace metals, and vitamins. The new vascular system within a wound begins as bud-like structures once sufficient collagen gel is formed to support the vestiges of new blood vessels. These budding structures meet and fuse forming small loops that interconnect to expand the system. The advancing edge of granulation tissue is characteristically rich in such microvasculature. Many of these new vessels are short-lived because collagen synthesis gradually decreases and high oxygen tensions are no longer necessary. As the scar develops further, much of this new vasculature spontaneously involutes.[26]

In the primarily closed wound, this extensive neovascularization process is not required. Damage to tissue in such wounds is normally minimal, and the wound edges are readily united. Activation of coagulation occurring after wounding is followed by fibrinolysis with recannulation of certain damaged vessels. Some vessels may also re-anastomose across the wound edge, although the exact mechanism for this is unknown. Relatively few fibroblasts are needed to provide support for the moderately compromised microvascular system of the primarily closed wound, and the entire healing process proceeds with much less energy expenditure than that of other wounds.

The exact stimulus for angiogenesis in the wound-healing process is not known, but it appears to involve macrophages and perhaps platelets as well.[27]

EPIDERMAL WOUND REPAIR

The epidermis provides a continuous, intact barrier between the body and the environment. Following tissue injury, its structural integrity is destroyed, and to maintain homeostasis, it is imperative that the repair process be initiated quickly. Recent studies indicate that the structure and function of the epidermal basement membrane unit is critical for effective repair of skin wounds (Fig. 7–5).[28]

Keratinocytes are present within the various stratified layers of the epidermis, whereas only basal keratinocytes are in direct contact with the basement membrane zone matrix. Basal keratinocytes are relatively small, have a low cytoplasm-to-nuclear ratio, and are able to proliferate and divide. The basal cells contain keratin, but it is an immature form compared with the keratinizing cells in the malpighian and granular cell layers and in the stratum corneum. Once the cells have lost contact with the basement membrane zone (BMZ) matrix, they move vertically in a nonproliferative mode of terminal differentiation.[29]

The BMZ of human skin is divided into four components:

1. Plasma membrane of the basal keratinocyte.
2. Lamina lucida—an electron-lucent space of 30 to 50 mm that contains laminin, a large, noncollagenous, cysteine-rich glycoprotein synthesized by epidermal cells. In addition, the bullous pemphigoid antigen is located in this region.
3. Lamina densa—an electron-dense zone composed of type IV collagen that is specific for the basement membrane. Also located within or surrounding this area is a heparin-sulfate-proteogylcan complex, which is believed to function as a molecular sieve. In addition, the KF-1 antigen, (so named because it reacts with the KF-1 monoclonal antibody) has been identified in the lamina densa. Its exact function is

unknown, but it may help to stabilize the basement membrane zone.
4. Sublamina densa—the zone that contains anchoring fibrils, collagen fibers, and microfibrillar bundles. Also within this zone is the epidermolysis bullosa antigen (EBA), which has been identified on the basis of circulating antibodies in patients with this disease. Additionally, anchoring fibril antigens (AF-1 and AF-2) have been identified from their reactivity with AF-1 and AF-2 monoclonal antibodies.[28, 30]

Type V collagen is also associated with certain basement membranes as well as endothelial and smooth muscle cells. Its exact location and function are just beginning to be delineated.[30]

The basement membrane zone therefore separates the proliferating basal keratinocytes from dermal collagen, proteoglycans, fibronectin, and elastin. It may serve as a selective filter and regulate various growth and inhibitory factors that influence epidermal cell behavior.[31]

Following tissue injury, the epidermal cells begin a migratory process that will ultimately resurface the wound. This process is known as epiboly. Epibolin is a soluble substance that has been isolated and appears to mediate this response. The cells adjacent to the wound, both basilar and suprabasilar, become flattened, lose many of their junctional complexes, and develop pseudopodal extensions of their cytoplasm. They also develop phagolysosomes, a prominent rough endoplasmic reticulum, and the Golgi complexes.[32] Microfilaments can also be seen in the cytoplasm. These consist of the contractile protein actin, which undoubtedly assists in cellular locomotion. These disappear after the wound is healed.[33]

Epidermal cells migrate in sheets while maintain-

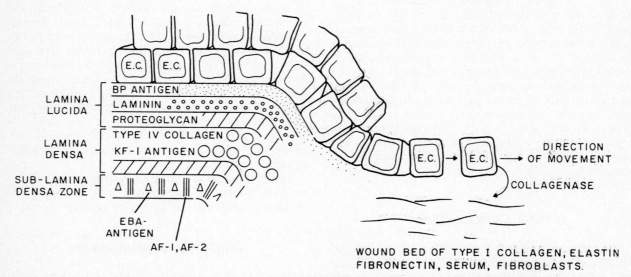

Figure 7–5. Hypothetical structure of the epidermal basement membrane unit. The early stages of epidermal cell migration after wounding is also shown.

ing their desmosomal attachments between cells intact. Their movement appears to occur by an ameboid action that requires the extension of broad lamellipodia. Another theory proposes a rolling and sliding movement of cells with some leapfrogging of one cell over another.[34] These cells continue to migrate until they come in contact with other sheets of epidermal cells migrating from the opposite side of the wound. When the wound is completely covered by epidermal cells, the process stops, the cells form additional desmosomal attachments and revert to their normal morphology.

It appears that epidermal migration may be influenced by electric potentials across the wound. In one study,[35] enhanced re-epithelialization could be achieved by delivering a weak electric current to a silver anode embedded in the skin wounds of laboratory animals. Interestingly, an increased rate of collagen synthesis was also observed in the dermis. It appears that the natural voltage gradient is more positive in the area close to the wound and becomes more negative further away from the wound. This concept of changing electric fields influencing wound healing may partly explain the enhancement of wound healing that occurs in a humid milieu.

When the basement membrane zone is injured, the epidermal cells come into direct contact with dermal elements such as fibronectin, proteoglycans, and type I and type III collagens. The exact signal for epidermal migration is not known; perhaps it involves loss of contact inhibition or loss of the basement membrane itself. Interestingly, it has been shown that migrating epidermal cells produce type V collagen. Also, these migrating cells continually produce a type IV collagenase, which theoretically aids in the migration process by dissolution of the preferential attraction that epidermal cells have for type IV collagen.[30] The migration takes place in the moist areas of fibrin deposition beneath the superficial crust. It has been shown that wound healing may be slowed if the damaged tissue dehydrates excessively, forcing the migration into a deeper plane. It is also known that epithelialization is enhanced by a humid atmosphere or by a hydrophobic dressing.[36] This concept is fundamental to the rational use of occlusive dressings discussed below.

Evidence is growing that the presence of soluble factors may influence epidermal migration as well as cell-matrix interactions. After wounding, epidermal cells are also exposed to serum that contains platelet-derived growth factor, a substance that is chemotactic for endothelial cells and fibroblasts.[5] As already mentioned, epibolin has been isolated from the serum and is known to enhance cell migration.[37] Human epidermal growth factor is a heat-stable polypeptide present in numerous body fluids.[38] Its actions include stimulation of mitosis in fibroblasts and epidermal cells, an increased replicative epithelial cell life span, and suppression of contact inhi-

bition in cell culture. The exact role, if any, of epidermal growth factor in human wound repair has not yet been defined.

Finally, it should be emphasized that skin sutures result in the formation of small wounds that also become epithelialized. These epithelialized suture tracts are normally removed by an intense inflammatory macrophage infiltrate. This is occasionally accompanied by a foreign body reaction that is mistaken for a "stitch abscess." Often, remnants of keratinocytes are trapped within the suture tract giving rise to small inclusion cysts. Such suture tracts may be minimized by using skin tapes instead of sutures or by removing the sutures at 48 to 72 hours and then using skin tapes.

FACTORS AFFECTING WOUND HEALING

Nutritional Factors

It is now known that normal wound healing is dependent upon specific nutritional requirements. These are summarized in Table 7–1.[39] Since more energy is required during the repair process, there is an increased consumption of carbohydrates, amino acids, and lipids. Protein deficiency impairs

TABLE 7–1. Nutritional Factors in Wound Healing

Nutrient	Role in Healing Process
Proteins	Essential for neo-angiogenesis, protoglycan and collagen synthesis, fibroblastic function, wound remodeling
Carbohydrates and fats	Supplies energy for cells; necessary for normal inflammation phase
Vitamin A	Essential for neo-angiogenesis; epithelialization; labilizing effect on lysosomal membranes
Vitamin C	Cofactor in hydroxylation of proline and lysine; necessary for normal fibroblastic function and resistance to infection
Vitamin E	Antioxidant; stabilizes cell membranes
Vitamin B complex	Cofactors of enzyme systems in protein, carbohydrate, fat metabolism
Iron	Divalent iron necessary for hydroxylation of lysine and proline in collagen synthesis
Copper	Contained in lysyl oxidase; necessary for the formation of collagen cross-linkages
Zinc	Associated with RNA and DNA polymerase; involved in vitamin A metabolism
Magnesium	Activates enzymes in protein synthesis and energy-producing cycles
Manganese	Activates enzymes in glycosylation of procollagen; required for proteoglycan synthesis

fibroblastic proliferation, neo-angiogenesis, proteoglycan and collagen synthesis, and wound remodeling. Compromised immune mechanisms lead to a higher risk of wound infection. Defective metabolism of carbohydrates and lipids results in decreased energy for cellular functions. Decreased availability of fatty acids may result in diminished prostaglandin and leukotriene synthesis.

Minerals and other trace elements are essential for the healing process. Calcium is a cofactor required by many enzyme systems, including tissue collagenases. Likewise, magnesium is essential for many enzymes, especially those related to energy-producing cycles. Iron is necessary for collagen synthesis. Specifically, divalent iron is a cofactor for the enzymes that hydroxylate lysine and proline. Copper is also essential for collagen synthesis because lysyl oxidase, the enzyme that promotes the conversion of lysyl and hydroxylysyl to their aldehydes in the final cross-linking process, requires this metal. Zinc is a ubiquitous element associated with a number of critical enzymes, such as RNA and DNA polymerase, and is involved in the metabolism of vitamin A. Manganese is also required for the activity of several enzymes, especially in the glycosylation of procollagen and the synthesis of proteoglycans.

Vitamins also play a significant role in the wound-repair processes.[40] Vitamin C is needed for hydroxyproline and hydroxylysine synthesis. The normal function of fibroblasts and leukocytes are impaired by a deficiency of vitamin C, and resistance to infection is diminished.[41] Vitamin A appears to be essential for normal epithelialization, for collagen synthesis, and for the cross-linking of collagen and wound closure. Vitamin A is believed to have a labilizing effect on lysosomal membranes. As will be seen, this is opposite to the stabilizing effect of glucocorticoids. Glucocorticoids can inhibit prolyl hydroxylase and thereby suppress wound healing, which can be restored by the administration of vitamin A. Presumably, this vitamin influences the inflammatory response and stimulates fibroblast activity and epithelialization.[42] The exact function of vitamin E in the repair process is unclear. It appears to stabilize cell membranes but also may protect vitamin A from oxidation because of its potent antioxidant properties.

Systemic Drugs

Numerous medications have stimulatory or suppressive effects that may alter the normal wound-healing process (Table 7–2).[43]

Corticosteroids inhibit the healing process because of anti-inflammatory, antiproliferative, immunosuppressive, and vasoconstrictive properties. More specifically, if they are given prior to injury,

TABLE 7–2. Systemic Drugs and Wound Healing

Agent	Effect
Glucocorticosteroids	Inhibitory
Diphenylhydantoin	Stimulatory
Anticoagulants	Inhibitory
Phenylbutazone	Inhibitory
Aspirin	Inhibitory
Colchicine	Inhibitory
Penicillamine	Inhibitory
Actinomycin D	Inhibitory
Bleomycin	Inhibitory
Carmustine	Inhibitory

the inflammatory phase will be suppressed. The depressive effects involve leukocytes, macrophages, lymphocytes, mast cells, and fibroblasts with resultant decreases in collagen synthesis, neovascularization, epithelialization, and contraction. Additionally, there is an increased susceptibility to infection because of the immunosuppressive effects of these compounds.

The type, timing, and dosage of steroids is critical. Steroids with the most potent anti-inflammatory properties have greatest detrimental effects on the wound-healing process. Low doses (10 mg/day) of prednisone have little or no effect; moderate doses (10 to 30 mg/day) of prednisone have a minimal influence; however, doses of 40 mg/day or more will substantially inhibit the process. The most profound effect is noted when steroids are administered prior to tissue injury. If they are delayed until 72 hours after wounding, the inflammatory phase of wound healing is intact, and there is less of a detrimental effect.[43]

Cytotoxic and immunosuppressive agents can theoretically suppress the wound-healing process.[44] Possible mechanisms include suppression of the inflammatory response, decrease in fibroblast proliferation, and fibroblast protein synthesis. Experimental studies have indicated that actinomycin, bleomycin, or carmustine would have the greatest detrimental effect, with carmustine being the most potent. Vincristine and methotrexate may exert a mild suppressive effect. Azathioprine, chlorambucil, nitrogen mustard, and cyclophosphamide are believed to have little influence on healing responses.

Nonsteroidal anti-inflammatory agents, such as phenylbutazone and aspirin, decrease wound strength. This effect may be secondary to their anti-inflammatory properties and to the antiplatelet activity of aspirin.

Phenytoin is known to have a significant effect on connective tissue, as evidenced by the gingival hyperplasia that accompanies its administration in some individuals. Some studies have suggested that this is due to enhancement of fibroblastic proliferation, but the principal action may relate to inhibiting the secretion or the synthesis of collagenase.[45]

Environmental Factors

A number of environmental factors may influence the wound-healing process. Pathogenic bacteria, such as *Staphylococcus aureus* and *Streptococcus pyogenes,* may invade the wound and stimulate an intense leukocytic response that can interfere with wound healing. It is generally agreed that systemic antibiotics are optimally effective when given prior to surgery for the prevention of wound infection.[46]

Oxygen tension is critical for normal wound healing, and there is evidence that the rate of wound healing may be limited by oxygen supply. Oxygen is required for cell replication, migration, and protein synthesis and is essential for hydroxylation of collagen. If arterial P_{O_2} is increased, there is a slight concomitant increase in collagen synthesis, but the majority of the oxygen is consumed by the tissue.[26] It has been shown that artificially high oxygen tensions, e.g., in hyperbaric oxygen chamber, enhance wound healing; whereas anything that interferes with the delivery of oxygen to the wound, e.g., hypovolemia secondary to hemorrhage or anemia, hinders efficient repair.

Environmental temperature also influences the wound-healing process. Warm temperatures of up to 30°C favor healing, but cooling of the skin to 12°C is detrimental to healing.[19]

Another important influence in the healing of superficial wounds is the maintenance of wound tissue hydration. Denuded dermis exposed to air with subsequent dehydration and crust formation creates a mechanical barrier to epidermal migration. The epidermis at the wound edge is also incorporated into the crust. With air exposure, epithelialization takes 2 to 3 days, but occlusion shortens the healing time to 18 to 24 hours.[36]

COMPLICATIONS OF CUTANEOUS WOUND HEALING

Complications of wound healing after trauma or surgery include hematoma formation, undesirable wound tension, infection, and hypertrophic scars or keloids. (The latter two are considered separately later in this chapter.) Additionally, wounds occurring in patients with diabetes mellitus present special problems.

Bleeding is one of the most common complications following trauma or surgery. Most bleeding after cutaneous surgery is from the deep dermal plexus. Proper hemostasis during the procedure and adequate approximation of the wound margins help prevent this complication. Delayed bleeding results in the formation of a hematoma—a space-occupying lesion that compromises repair, diminishes tensile strength, and may predispose a patient to wound dehiscence or infection.

Excessive tension at the wound margin can compromise blood supply and wound strength, decrease rates of repair and wound contraction, and increase the final width of the scar. If excessive tension is apparent, an alternate method of closure, such as flap, graft, or partial closure with delayed repair, should be considered.

Infections usually occur in cutaneous wounds that are primarily closed. Wounds allowed to heal by secondary intention rarely become infected. Surgical wounds may be classified as clean, clean-contaminated, or dirty. Clean wounds are those created in a strict aseptic environment in which contaminated organs have not been entered; less than two percent of such wounds become infected. Clean-contaminated wounds are those created with exposure to microflora; the infection rate is reported to be 5 to 10 percent. Contaminated wounds are those in which large bacterial populations are encountered during surgery; the infection rate is 20 to 40 percent.[46]

The usual postoperative wound infection becomes manifest after four to eight days and is characterized by pain, tenderness, swelling, redness, and increased temperatures. *Staphylococcus aureus* is among the common causative agents. If wound infection occurs within the first 48 hours, the causative agent is often β-hemolytic streptococci. In certain situations, it may be desirable to administer antibiotics prophylactically. Oral antibiotics should be administered at least 24 hours prior to surgery and generally need not be continued longer than 72 hours after surgery.[46]

Concomitant diseases, such as diabetes mellitus, can greatly complicate wound healing. In general, the wound repair process is delayed, and this is thought to be caused by microvascular disease that interferes with neovascularization, blood flow, and oxygen supply. Furthermore, polymorphonuclear leukocytes function abnormally in diabetic individuals, so there is a defective adherence to vascular membranes, decreased migration, phagocytosis, and bacterial killing.[26] In addition, insulin deficiency suppresses collagen deposition in wounds, even in the absence of diabetic microvascular disease.[43]

MODULATION OF THE WOUND-HEALING RESPONSE

With the knowledge gained from basic research in wound healing, attempts have been made to modulate the repair process. These efforts have concentrated on both the local application of agents, especially on superficial wounds, and systemic medications.

Most would agree that superficial wound healing is enhanced in a humid environment. Topically applied agents, such as corticosteroids, have been extensively studied for their effects on wound healing. Fluorinated steroids, such as triamcinolone acetonide, decrease the rate of re-epithelialization and reduce collagen synthesis. Hydrocortisone does not effect epidermal resurfacing, but does reduce collagen synthesis.[47]

Antibacterial ointments are often used on wounds. Neosporin contains polymyxin B sulfate, bacitracin zinc, and neomycin in a petrolatum base. It has been found to enhance epidermal healing, and it is believed that the bacitracin zinc is the component responsible for this response.[47] Neomycin may lead to allergic sensitization, especially if applied to partial- or full-thickness wounds. Silver sulfadiazine and benzoyl peroxide (10 to 20 percent solutions) both enhance epidermal resurfacing in wound healing.[48]

A unique agent used in the treatment of suppurative cutaneous wounds is dextranomer, a high molecular weight dextran derivative. This is manufactured as dry, insoluble, spherical beads, 0.1 to 0.3 mm in diameter. The beads are very hydrophilic because of their high hydroxyl group content. One gram of dextranomer can absorb four grams of fluid when saturated. The beads are sterilized by gamma radiation and act by absorption of wound exudate, which enhances wound healing by removing necrotic material, proteolytic enzymes, and bacterial toxins. Dextranomer causes a decrease in tissue pressure at the wound surface creating negative pressure that enhances migration of beneficial nutrients from the bloodstream. Thus, healthy granulation tissue proliferates and re-epithelialization proceeds normally. The advantages of this approach are that there are no systemic or local side effects. The beads are insoluble and do not decompose. The major limitation of this approach is the requirement for an exudative wound.

Systemic medications that have been used to modulate the repair process generally influence collagen synthesis. The effect of corticosteroids has been mentioned. The lathyrogenic substance beta-aminopropionitrile (BAPN), which inhibits the enzyme lysyl oxidase, interferes with covalent collagen cross-linking. Poorly cross-linked collagen is then more susceptible to tissue collagenase and may decrease the scar. Although this medication is highly toxic, it is currently being investigated clinically in humans.[50] Another lathyrogenic agent, penicillamine, is available for clinical usage. Penicillamine decreases the tensile strength of wounds by chelating cross-linking sites in the oxidative deamination of lysine.[26] However, the necessary dosage for significant clinical improvement is quite toxic.

Another agent that alters wound healing is colchicine. The mode of action is disruption of the microtubular system so that secretion of procollagen is blocked. Additionally, tissue collagenase is stimulated, as is the release of histamine-containing granules from mast cells.[51] Colchicine in combination with lathyrogenic agents has been used with limited success to treat keloids and hypertrophic scars.[52]

The complex structure of collagen and its intricate biosynthetic pathway with strict enzymatic and co-factor requirements make collagen an ideal target for agents that can modulate wound healing. One approach is the incorporation of proline analogues into the polypeptide chain. This results in an abnormal triple helical configuration, and normal collagen synthesis is interrupted. One such analogue, 3,4-dehydroproline, is an example of this type of agent.[53] Much research is needed in this field.

SPECIAL CONSIDERATIONS

Occlusive Wound Dressings

The advantages of wound healing in a humid environment have been known for more than two decades.[54, 55] Only recently have occlusive dressings been developed to maximize the advantages of humid wound healing. These dressings, which are either permeable or impermeable to oxygen, are listed in Table 7–3. Clinical studies have shown that wounds treated with occlusive dressings have less erythema, pain, swelling, and tenderness, and the cosmetic results of the scar are often superior.[56–58]

Occlusive dressings have been shown to enhance the wound repair process in both acute and chronic wounds.[59] Dermal wound healing as well as epidermal repair is improved.[57, 60] The beneficial effects are possibly due to improved epidermal migration on a moist wound matrix, increased partial pressure of oxygen, maintenance of electric potentials across the wound, improved availability of soluble growth factors, and protection from invasion of pathogenic bacteria.[61] Indeed, it was a fear of precipitating infections that initially delayed the popular use of these dressings. In practice, wound infections treated in this way have not been a problem. The

TABLE 7–3. Occlusive Wound Dressings

Dressing (Trade Name)	Composition
Vigilon	Polyethylene oxide hydrogel with polyurethane backing
Duoderm	Hydrocolloid particles (pectin and gelatin) in a hydrophobic polymer
Op-Site	Polyurethane film
Tegaderm	Polyurethane film
Epilock	Polyurethane film
Synthaderm	Polyurethane film
Bioclusive	Polyurethane film
Mediskin (+ silver)	Porcine collagen
Biobrane	Nylon-silicone composite with porcine collagen

number of bacteria is not as important as the pathogenicity of the organisms. It is entirely possible that residental microflora may exert a beneficial effect, although this is unknown.[62] Each individual dressing creates a specific wound environment, and it is advantageous to evaluate this environment and the bacterial barrier characteristics in vivo.[63]

Currently, there are several types of occlusive dressings: postoperative dressings; cutaneous ulcer dressings; dressings for traumatic, superficial, and partial-thickness wounds; postoperative dermabrasion dressings; and support dressings for grafts. In addition, the following skin conditions may benefit from this approach: blistering diseases, dermatitis factitia (both treatment and prevention), intravenous catheter care, chronic eczematous dermatitis, and decubitus ulcers.[56] As further knowledge of the wound-healing process is obtained, there will undoubtedly be newer occlusive dressings and more indications for their use.

Keloids and Hypertrophic Scars

Keloids and hypertrophic scars are abnormal collections of collagen resulting from an abnormal wound-healing response. Alibert first coined the French term *chéloïde* (from the Greek, *chēlē*, crab's claw) in the early 1800s.[64] By definition, hypertrophic scars result from injury or surgery, remain within the normal boundaries of the wound, and will gradually decrease in size. Keloids may occur spontaneously or after injury, may extend beyond the margins of the original wound by invading surrounding tissues, and will recur if removed.[65]

Clinically, keloids are dense fibrous lesions varying in size from a few millimeters to large lobular masses. They occur most often in patients between 10 and 30 years of age with equal sex distribution. They are more common in darker-skinned individuals but occur in all races.[66] Sites of predilection are on the upper back, shoulders, anterior chest, and upper arms—less frequently on the lower extremities, face, and neck.

Histologically, both keloids and hypertrophic scars exhibit abundant collagen deposition within the dermis. The arrangement of the collagen bundles is more random than in the mature scar, and they are loosely connected in layers with no orientation to the epithelial surface.[67] Myofibroblasts are present in actively growing keloids, and some composed entirely of myofibroblasts have been reported.[68] Collagen synthesis in keloids is greater than in hypertrophic scars, and synthesis in both is greater than that in normal scars or in unwounded skin.[69] Furthermore, the relative amount of type III collagen appears to be increased, and keloid collagen is more soluble than dermal collagen.[70] Interestingly, both keloids and hypertrophic scars contain an abundant number of mast cells. It is known that histamine stimulates cell growth in fibroblastic cultures,[71] and it is possible that the pruritus associated with these growths may be due to increased histamine levels.

In addition to increased collagen synthesis, proteoglycans and water are also increased in keloids and hypertrophic scars. Most of the glycoprotein is chondroitin-4-sulfate, which is present in greater amounts than in normal skin.[72] One study has suggested that the abundance of this glycoprotein may protect keloidal tissue from collagenase degradation.[73] Another mechanism of altered collagen degradation may contribute further to accumulation of fibrous tissue. Collagenase levels are normal or increased but may be inhibited by α_2-macroglobulin and α_1-antitrypsin, which have been shown to accumulate in keloids.[74]

The treatment of keloids is generally unsatisfactory and is detailed elsewhere.[67, 69] (See Chapter 48.) Recommended modalities include conventional surgery, cryosurgery, radiation therapy, intralesional corticosteroids, lathyrogenic agents, antimetabolites, and antihistamines. Of these, intralesional corticosteroids are the mainstay of therapy. The regression of a keloid is probably secondary to decreased collagen synthesis and the altering of collagen degradation by reduced tissue levels of α_2-macroglobulin and α_1-antitrypsin.[21] If used after surgical excision, corticosteroids lessen the recurrence rate by decreasing fibroblast migration and reducing the inflammatory reaction. Although a malignant change rarely occurs in a keloid or hypertrophic scar, a biopsy of all lesions unresponsive to treatment should be done to exclude dermatofibrosarcoma protuberans.[75]

Finally, laser surgery has been reported to be successful in treating keloids and hypertrophic scars. The initial clinical studies were performed with the argon laser at high-power densities and with the carbon dioxide laser at lower-power densities.[76] More recently, the neodymium-yttrium-aluminum-garnet (NdYAG) laser has proved to be efficacious in treating keloids and hypertrophic scars.[77]

LASERS AND WOUND HEALING

In the past decade, the use of biomedical laser systems has increased greatly. Both the argon and carbon dioxide lasers have been used in cutaneous surgery for a number of conditions.[78] Recently, tunable dye lasers and NdYAG lasers have been added to the therapeutic armamentarium.[77, 79]

The carbon dioxide laser has been the most extensively studied in terms of wound healing. Following impact, varying degrees of tissue damage occur. There is a central carbonized crater in which no cellular detail can be seen.[80] This is a V-shaped zone whose depth depends on the total energy applied.

Beneath and peripheral to this is a zone of coagulation necrosis with surrounding edema.[81] Peripheral to this, epidermal cells exhibit necrosis and loss of organelles.[82] The area of coagulation necrosis expands during the initial 48 hours following injury. This corresponds to a horizontal thermal gradient extending from the core of injury.[83] Epidermal regeneration begins, but the total healing time appears to be greater than with scalpel-cut wounds.[84] One recent study[85] suggests that this is due to a delay in onset of epidermal migration, although the rate of migration is similar to that in scalpel-cut wounds. Dermal wound healing proceeds slowly with extrusion of necrotic collagen and a decreased inflammatory and fibroblastic response.[86] Wound contraction, however, appears to be similar in laser-, scalpel-, and electrosurgery-induced wounds.[87] Studies assessing tensile strength following laser surgery are contradictory.[88, 89] The development of tensile strength may be slower in tissues treated by a CO_2 laser, but the ultimate tensile strength is at least comparable to that of scalpel-cut wounds.[90]

A recent study has shown that the NdYAG laser selectively suppresses collagen production in both fibroblast cultures and normal skin.[77] This cannot be explained entirely by thermal effects and appears to be the result of suppressed fibroblast function. These same authors also report laboratory evidence that low-energy lasers using helium-neon (HeNe) or gallium-arsenide (GaAs) stimulate collagen production in human skin and fibroblast cultures. This stimulatory effect was not confirmed when the helium-neon laser was used in a porcine wound model.[91] Undoubtedly, future studies and the development of new laser systems will enhance our knowledge of the wound-healing process.

WOUND TREATMENT UTILIZING TISSUE GROWN IN CULTURE

In recent years, it has been demonstrated that cultured epidermal autografts could be used to cover partial-thickness wounds.[92] This has tremendous potential usefulness in covering large areas of cutaneous tissue destroyed by trauma or burns. Cell culture techniques have been scaled up so that small pieces of epidermis can be expanded to 10,000 times their original surface areas in three to four weeks.[93] Recent studies have shown that culture epidermal autografts used in experimental animals resurfaced wounds significantly faster than a semiocclusive dressing.[94] These grafts had a thicker epidermis with well-formed rete ridges compared to healed control wounds. Using this technique, it is unlikely that the graft will contain Langerhans' cells, melanocytes, or Merkel's cells, nor are hair follicles or sweat glands likely to regenerate. Some investigations have reported a slight reduction in wound contraction with this technique.[95]

Exciting new research is being conducted to develop stronger materials composed of a collagen matrix and epidermal cells.[96] Further innovations include material with a dermal component composed of collagen, modified in vitro by fibroblasts, then seeded with epidermal cells.[97] These techniques significantly reduce wound contraction, suggesting that contraction is predominantly influenced by the connective tissue matrix. Further advances may lead to significant improvement in the ability to treat extensive areas of wounded skin in the future.

REFERENCES

1. Lambert WC, Cohen PJ, Klein KM, Lambert MW: Cellular and molecular mechanisms in wound healing: Selected concepts. In Eaglstein WH (ed): Clinics in Dermatology: Wound Healing, Vol 2, no 3. Philadelphia, JB Lippincott, 1984, pp 17–23
2. Ward PA: The acute inflammatory response and the role of complement. In Dineen P, Hildick-Smith B (eds): The Surgical Wound. Philadelphia, Lea & Febiger, 1980, pp 19–25
3. Camp RDR: Prostaglandins, hydroxy fatty acids, leukotrienes, and inflammation of the skin. Clin Exp Dermatol 7:435–444, 1982
4. Bickers DR, Elias PM, Marki R, et al: Dermatologic needs in drugs and instrumentation. J Am Acad Dermat 5:983–990, 1984
5. Seppa H, Grotendorst G, Seppa S: Platelet-derived growth factor is chemotactic for fibroblast. J Cell Biol 92:584–588, 1982
6. Horwitz AL, Hauce AJ, Crystal RG: Granulocyte collagenase: Selective digestion of type I relative to type III collagen. Proc Natl Acad Sci USA 74:897–901, 1977
7. Wohl SM: The role of monuclear cells in the wound repair process. In Dineen P, Hildick-Smith B (eds): The Surgical Wound. Philadelphia, Lea & Febiger, 1981, pp 63–74
8. Mosher DF, Furcht LT: Fibronectin: Review of its structure and possible functions. J Invest Dermatol 77:175–180, 1981
9. Repesh LA, Fitzgerald TJ, Furcht LT: Fibronectin involvement in granulation tissue and wound healing in rabbits. J Histochem Cytochem 30:351–358, 1981
10. Enguall E, Rooslahti E, Miller EJ: Affinity of fibronectin to collagens of different genetic types and to fibrinogen. J Exp Med 147:1584–1595, 1978
11. Kurkinen M, Vaheri A, Roberts PJ, et al: Sequential appearance of fibronectin and collagen in experimental granulation tissue. Lab Invest 43:47–51, 1980
12. Van Winkle W Jr: The fibroblast in wound healing. Surg Gynecol Obstet 124:369–386, 1967
13. Bornstein P, Byers PH: Collagen metabolism. In Current Concepts, Upjohn Co, 1980
14. Prockop DJ, Kivirikko KI, Tuderman L, Guzeman NA: The biosynthesis of collagen and its disorders. New Engl J Med 301:13–23, 77–85, 1979
15. Prockop DJ, Kivirikko KI: Hereditable disease of collagen. New Engl J Med 311:376–385, 1984.
16. Bentz H, Morris NP, Murray LW, et al: Isolation and partial characterization of a new human collagen with an extended triple-helical structural domain. Proc Natl Acad Sci USA 80:3168–3172, 1983
17. Sage H, Trueb B, Bornstein P: Biosynthetic and structural properties of endothelial cell type VIII collagen. J Biol Chem 258:13391–13401, 1983
18. Van der Rest M, Mayne R, Ninomiya Y, et al: The structure of type IX collagen. J Biol Chem 260:220–225, 1985
19. Peacock EE Jr: Wound Repair. Philadelphia. W. B. Saunders, 1984

20. Cohen IK, McCoy BJ, Diegelmann RF: An update on wound healing. Ann Plast Surg 3:264–272, 1979

21. Harper E: Collageneases. Ann Rev Biochem 49:1063–1078, 1980

22. Gabbiani G, Lelous M, Bailey AJ, et al: Collagen and myofibroblasts of granulation tissue: A chemical, ultrastructural and immunological study. Virchows Arch 21:133–145, 1976

23. Ryan GB, Cliff WJ, Gabbiani GB: Myofibroblasts in human granulation tissue. Human Path 5:55–67, 1974

24. Carrico TJ, Mehrhof AI Jr, Cohen IK: Biology of wound healing. Surg Clin N Amer 64:721–733, 1984

25. Zitelli, JA: Secondary intention healing: An alternative to surgical repair. In Eaglstein WH (ed): Clinics in Dermatology: Wound Healing, Vol 2, no 3. Philadelphia, JB Lippincott, 1984, pp 92–106

26. Hunt TK, Dunphy JE (eds): Fundamentals of Wound Management. New York, Appleton-Century-Croft, 1979

27. Hunt TK, Andrews WS, Halliday B, et al: Coagulation and macrophage stimulation of angiogenesis and wound healing. In Dineen P, Hildick-Smith G (eds): The Surgical Wound. Philadelphia, Lea & Febiger, 1981, pp 1–18

28. Katz SI: The epidermal basement membrane zone—structure, ontogeny, and role in disease. J Am Acad Dermatol 11:1025–1037, 1984

29. Boutwell RK: Factors promoting epidermal cell proliferation. In Dineen P, Hildick-Smith G (eds): The Surgical Wound. Philadelphia, Lea & Febiger, 1981, pp 90–96

30. Woodley DT, O'Keefe EJ, Prunieras M: Cutaneous healing: A model for cell matrix interactions. J Am Acad Dermatol 12:420–433, 1985

31. Martin GR, Kleinman HK, Gross-Muller V, et al: Regulation of tissue structure and repair by collagen and fibronectin. In Dineen P, Hildick-Smith G (eds): The Surgical Wound. Philadelphia, Lea & Febiger, 1981, pp 110–122

32. Odland G, Ross R: Human wound repair. I. Epidermal regeneration. J Cell Biol 39:135–151, 1968

33. Gabbiani G, Ryan GB: Development of a contractile apparatus in epithelial cells during epidermal and liver regeneration. J Submicr Cytol 6:143–157, 1974.

34. Krawczyk WS: Pattern of epidermal cell migration during wound healing. J Cell Biol 15:300–317, 1971

35. Alvarez DM, Mertz PM, Smerbeck BS, et al: The healing of superficial skin wounds is stimulated by external electric current. J Invest Dermatol 81:144–148, 1983

36. Rovee DT, Kurowsky CA, Lobun J, et al: Effect of local wound environment on epidermal healing. In Maibach HI, Rovee DT (eds): Epidermal Wound Healing. Chicago, Yearbook Publishers, 1972, pp 159–181

37. Stern KS: Epibolin: A protein of human plasma that supports epithelial cell movement. Proc Natl Acad Sci USA 78:6907–6911, 1981

38. King LE, Carpenter GF: Epidermal growth factor. In Goldsmith LA (ed): Biochemistry and Physiology of the Skin. New York, Oxford University Press, 1983, pp 269–281

39. Ruberg RL: Role of nutrition in wound healing. Surg Clin N Amer 64:705–714, 1984

40. Boucek RJ: Factors affecting wound healing. Otol Clin N Amer 17:243–264, 1984

41. Ringsdorf WM, Cheraskin E: Vitamin C and human wound healing. Oral Surg 231–236, 1984

42. Pollack S: Wound healing: A review. III. Nutritional factors affecting wound healing. J Dermatol Surg Oncol 5:615–619, 1979

43. Pollack S: Systemic drugs and nutritional aspects of wound healing. In Eaglstein WH (ed): Clinics in Dermatology: Wound Healing, Vol 2, no 3. Philadelphia, JB Lippincott, 1984, pp 68–80

44. Falcone RE, Nappi JF: Chemotherapy and wound healing. Surg Clin N Amer 64:779–794, 1984

45. Bauer EA, Cooper TW, Tucker DR: Diphenylhydantoin therapy of recessive dystrophic epidermolysis bullosa: Clinical trials and proposed mechanism of action. Clin Res 28:563–569, 1980

46. Adinolfi MF, Nichols RL: Postoperative cutaneous wound infections. In Eaglstein WH (ed): Clinics in Dermatology: Wound Healing, Vol 2, no 3, Philadelphia, JB Lippincott, 1984, pp 86–91

47. Eaglstein WH, Mertz PM, Alvarez DM: Effect of topically applied agents on wound healing. In Eaglstein WH (ed): Clinics in Dermatology: Wound Healing, Vol 2, no 3, Philadelphia, JB Lippincott, 1984, pp 112–115

48. Alvarez OM, Mertz PM, Eaglstein WH: Benzoyl peroxide and epidermal wound healing. Arch Dermatol 119:222–225, 1983

49. Parrish LC, Witkowski JA: Dextranomer in dermatologic conditions. Int J Dermatol 18:480–484, 1979

50. Peacock EE Jr: Control of wound healing and scar formation in surgical patients. Arch Surg 116:1325–1329, 1981

51. Chapil M, Peacock EE Jr, Carlson EC: Colchicine and wound healing. J Surg Res 28:49–56, 1980

52. Peacock EE Jr: Pharmacological control of surface scarring in human beings. Ann Surg 193:592–597, 1981

53. Salvador RA, Tsai I, Marcel RJ: The in vivo inhibition of collagen synthesis and the reduction of prolylhydroxylans activity by 3,4 dehydroproline. Arch Biochem Biophys 174:381–386, 1976

54. Winter CD: Formation of scab and the rate of epithelialization of superficial wounds in the skin of domestic pig. Nature 193:293–294, 1962

55. Hinman CC, Maibach, H, Winter GD: Effect of air exposure and occlusion on experimental skin wounds. Nature 200:377–378, 1963

56. Eaglstein WH: Experiences with biosynthetic dressings. J Am Acad Dermatol 12:434–440, 1985

57. Linsky CB, Rovee DT, Dow T: Effect of dressing on wound inflammation and scar tissue. In Dineen P, Hildick-Smith G (eds): The Surgical Wound. Philadelphia, Lea & Febiger, 1981, pp 191–206

58. Eaton AC: A controlled trial to evaluate and compare with sutureless skin closure technique (Op site skin closure) with conventional skin suturing and clipping in abdominal surgery. Br J Surg 67:857–860, 1980

59. Alper JC, Welch EA, Ginsberg J, Bogaars H, Maquire P: Moist wound healing under a vapor permeable membrane. J Am Acad Dermatol 8:347–353, 1983

60. Winter GD: Epidermal regeneration studied in the domestic pig. In Rovee DT, Maibach HJ (eds): Epidermal Wound Healing. Chicago, Yearbook Medical Publishers, 1972, pp 71–112

61. Eaglstein WH: Effect of occlusive dressings on wound healing. In Eaglstein WH (ed): Clinics in Dermatology. Wound Healing, Vol 2, no 3. Philadelphia, J. B. Lippincott, 1984, pp 107–111

62. Mertz PM, Marshall DA, Eaglstein WH: Occlusive wound dressings to prevent bacterial incision and wound infection. J Am Acad Dermatol 12:662–668, 1985

63. Vaghese M, Balin AK, Carter DM, Caldwell D: Local wound environment under synthetic dressings. J Invest Dermatol 82:395, 1984 (Abstract)

64. Alibert JLM: Quelques recherches sur la chéloïde. Mémoires de la Société Médicale d'Émulation, p 744, 1817

65. Peacock EE Jr, Madden JW, Trier WC: Biologic basis of treatment of keloid and hypertrophic scars. South Med J 63:755–760, 1970

66. Murray JC, Pollack SV, Pinnell SR: Keloids: A review. J Am Acad Dermat 4:461–470, 1981

67. Murray JC, Pollack SV, Pinnell SR: Keloids and hypertrophic scars. In Eaglstein WH (ed): Clinics in Dermatology: Wound Healing, Vol 2, no 3. Philadelphia, J. B. Lippincott, 1984, pp 121–133

68. James WD, Besancenez CD, Odom RB: The ultrastructure of a keloid. J Am Acad Dermatol 3:50–57, 1980

69. Cohen IK, McCoy BJ: Keloid: Biology and treatment. In

Dineen P, Hildick-Smith G (eds): The Surgical Wound. Philadelphia, Lea & Febiger, 1981, pp 123–131

70. Bailey AJ, Bazin S, Sims TJ, et al: Characterization of the collagen of human hypertrophic and normal scars. Biochem Biophys Acta 405:412–421, 1975

71. Russell JD, Russell SB, Trupin KM: The effect of histamine on the growth of cultured fibroblasts isolated from normal and keloid tissue. J Cell Physiol 93:389–393, 1977

72. Kischer CW, Shetlar MR: Collagen and mucophysaccharides in the hypertrophic scar. Connect Tissue Res 2:205–213, 1974

73. Linares HA, Larson DL: Proteogylcans and collagenase in hypertrophic scar formation. Plast Reconstr Surg 62:589–593, 1978

74. Diegelmann RF, Bryant CP, Cohen IK: Tissue alpha globulins in keloid formation. Plast Reconstr Surg 59:418–423, 1977

75. Manalan SS, Cohen IK, Theogaraj SD: Dermatofibrosarcoma protoberans or keloid—a warning. Plast Reconstr Surg 54:96–98, 1974

76. Henderson DL, Cromwill TA, Mes LG: Argon and carbon dioxide laser treatment of hypertrophic and keloid scars. Laser Surg Med 1:93–101, 1980

77. Abergel RP, Meeker CA, Lam TS: Control of connective tissue metabolism by lasers: Recent developments and future prospects. J Am Acad Dermatol 11:1142–1150, 1984

78. Arndt KA, Noe JM, Rosen S (eds): Cutaneous Laser Therapy: Principles and Methods. Boston, John Wiley and Sons, 1983

79. Anderson RR, Jaenicke KF, Parrish JA: Mechanisms of selective vascular changes caused by dye lasers. Lasers Surg Med 3:211–216, 1983

80. Rainoldi R, Candiani P, de Virgilis G, et al: Connective tissue regeneration after laser CO_2 therapy. Int Surg 68:167–170, 1983

81. Schenk P: Die Ultrastruktor von Haut- und Schleimhautgeweben nach CO_2-lasereinwirkung. Laryng Rhinol 58:770–776, 1979

82. Ben-Bassat M, Ben-Bassat M, Kaplan I: A study of the ultrastructural features of the cut margin of skin and mucous membrane specimens excised by carbon dioxide laser. J Surg Res 2:77–84, 1976

83. Mihashi S, Jako GJ, Incze J, et al: Laser surgery in otolaryngology: Interaction of CO_2 laser and soft tissue. Ann NY Acad Sci 263–294, 1983

84. Hall RR: The healing of tissue incised by a carbon dioxide laser. Br J Surg 59:222–225, 1971

85. Moreno RA, Hebda PA, Zitelli JA, et al: Epidermal cell outgrowth from CO_2 laser and scalpel-cut explants: Implications for wound healing. J Dermatol Surg Oncol 10:11; 863–868, 1984

86. Carney JM, Kamat BR, Stern RS, et al: Cutaneous tissue repair after focused CO_2 laser irradiation. Laser Surg Med 5:180–181, 1985 (Abstract)

87. Fry TL, Gerbe RW, Bostros SB, et al: Effects of laser, scalpel and electrosurgical excision on wound contracture and graft "take." Plast Reconstr Surg 65:729–731, 1980

88. Cochrane TP, Beacon JP, Creasey GA, et al: Wound healing after laser surgery: An experimental study. Br J Surg 67:740–743, 1980

89. Buell BR, Schuller DE: Comparison of tensile strength in CO_2 laser and scalpel skin incisions. Arch Otolaryngol 109:465–467, 1983

90. Finsterbush A, Rousso M, Asher H: Healing and tensile strength of carbon dioxide laser incisions and scalpel wounds in rabbits. Plast Reconstr Surg 70:360–362, 1982

91. Hunter JG, Leonard LG, Snider GR, et al: Effects of low energy laser on wound healing in a porcine model. Laser Surg Med 3:328–329, 1984 (Abstract)

92. Eisinger M, Monden M, Raaf JM, et al: Wound coverage by a sheet of epidermal cells grown in vitro from dispersing single cell proportions. Surgery 80:287–293, 1980

93. Gallico GG III, O'Connor NE, Compton CC, et al: Grafting of burns with cultured epithelium prepared from autologous cultured human epithelium. New Engl J Med 311:448–451, 1984

94. Alvarez OM, Biozes DG: Cultured epidermal autografts. In Eaglstein WH (ed): Clinics in Dermatology: Wound Healing, Vol 2, no 3. Philadelphia, JB Lippincott, 1984, pp 54–67

95. O'Connor NE, Mulliken JB, Banks-Schlegal S, et al: Grafting of burns with cultured epithelium prepared from autologous epidermal cells. Lancet 1:75–78, 1981

96. Burke JF, Yannas IV, Quinby WC: Successful use of a physiologically acceptable artificial skin in the treatment of extensive burn injury. Ann Surg 194:413–428, 1981

97. Bell E, Ehrlich HP, Battle DJ, et al: A living tissue formed in vitro and accepted as a full thickness skin equivalent. Science 211:1042–1054, 1981

JOHN H. DONOHUE, M.D. / THEODORE R. SCHROCK, M.D.

8

Emergencies in Outpatient Skin Surgery

Life-threatening complications of dermatologic surgery are rare. When they occur, however, they must be recognized and treated with speed and skill. The prevention and treatment of some emergencies that may arise during skin surgery are discussed in this chapter.

PREPARATION FOR SURGICAL EMERGENCIES

An essential step in the management of emergencies is preparation for their occurrence. Training of staff, availability of emergency equipment, and communication links with emergency services in the community must be planned long before the development of an intraoperative crisis.

Office employees and clinic personnel should be trained to administer basic cardiopulmonary resuscitation (CPR). Courses in these techniques are available in most communities. If the surgeon's office or clinic is covered by a hospital on-call resuscitation team, employees must be familiar with the phone number and other details of activating this service. When it is further removed from a medical center, each employee should be able to contact the local emergency medical service. Important phone numbers should be posted. Staff members should know how to reach other physicians in the same building who might be available to help in an emergency. The physician who operates in the office setting should be trained in the techniques of advanced cardiac life support. Instruction in advanced cardiac life support is readily available through the Red Cross or the American Heart Association.

Basic equipment and supplies for the management of emergencies must be available. These items should be checked periodically to assure that they are in good working order. Less equipment is required if a "code blue" team is immediately available.

The following items are needed for the treatment of office emergencies. An asterisk denotes items that are usually carried by members of hospital resuscitation teams.

1. Cardiac arrest board
2. Oxygen tank with adapter and tubing
3. Bag-valve mask for administering oxygen
4. Oral-pharyngeal airways* (or esophageal obturator)
5. Laryngoscope*
6. Endotracheal tubes*
7. Suction apparatus and tubing
8. Intravenous starter kit including:
   a. Several bags of intravenous solution (e.g., 5% dextrose in water)
   b. Intravenous administration sets, extension tubing, and stopcocks
   c. Various intravenous catheters for both peripheral and central line insertion
   d. Tourniquets, tape, and armboards
   e. Skin prep solution
9. Cardiac monitor and defibrillation unit
10. Emergency medications
    a. Aminophylline
    b. Atropine
    c. Bretylium tosylate
    d. Calcium chloride
    e. 50% Dextrose in water
    f. Diazepam (Valium)
    g. Diphenhydramine hydrochloride (Benadryl)
    h. Dobutamine hydrochloride
    i. Dopamine hydrochloride
    j. Epinephrine (1:1000 and 1:10,000 solutions)
    k. Hydrocortisone
    l. Isoproterenol
    m. Lidocaine
    n. Metaproterenol sulfate inhaler (Alupent)
    o. Morphine sulfate
    p. Naloxone hydrochloride (Narcan)
    q. Nitroglycerin (0.3 mg sublingual tablets)
    r. Sodium bicarbonate
    s. Sodium pentobarbital (Nembutal)
    t. Terbutaline sulfate
    u. Thiobarbital
11. Syringes, needles and solutions (e.g., sodium chloride and water) for injections

The final aspect of preparation for emergencies is making certain that all employees are aware of their respective roles, if a crisis develops. Rehearsals are helpful to define responsibilities and identify gaps that must be filled. Preparation will shorten the response time and improve the outcome of emergency events in outpatient surgery.

PREVENTION OF EMERGENCIES

Many emergencies can be prevented by obtaining the patient's medical history and performing a basic physical examination. A history of previous illness, especially of vital organ systems (cardiovascular, pulmonary, hepatic, and renal), should be elicited. Current care and medications for these conditions should be noted. Personal and family history of bleeding disorders should be obtained. Allergies and side effects of previous drug administration must be known.

Physical examination is directed toward the problem to be treated, but in addition, the patient's overall health is assessed. Signs of acute cardiovascular or pulmonary decompensation should be sought. Evidence of acute infection might require cancellation of an elective minor procedure. Laboratory tests are not needed routinely for minor outpatient surgical procedures, but studies should be requested to clarify suspected acute systemic disease.

Physician awareness of possible complications of surgical procedures helps prevent mishaps. For minor procedures, toxic effects of drugs are the principal concern. The maximum safe dose, adverse reactions, and cross reactions with other medications should be known to the operating physician.

TREATMENT OF SPECIFIC EMERGENCIES

Vasovagal Syncope

Even minor surgical procedures may cause intense emotional stress for the patient. Apprehension, pain, or other unpleasant experiences, such as the sight of blood, may result in excessive vagal stimulation. Fainting may occur in these circumstances, especially when the patient rises from a recumbent posture. Peripheral vasodilatation with inadequate increase in cardiac output results in cerebral hypoperfusion and loss of consciousness. The patient is usually pale and diaphoretic and has a slow, regular pulse rate and normal blood pressure. Loss of consciousness is transient and is not accompanied by uncontrolled movements or fecal and urinary incontinence, as seen in seizures. The greatest risk to the patient in this situation is injury resulting from a fall.

The incidence of syncopal episodes is minimized by preparative explanation of the procedure, the use of sedatives, and intraoperative reassurance. Surgical procedures should be done with the patient recumbent. Patients should be assisted to their feet slowly at the completion of the operation. Patients who look or feel ill at the end of a procedure should remain supine, have vital signs checked, and arise slowly when they feel improved.

When syncope occurs, those in attendance should try to prevent injury from a fall and return the patient to the supine position. Trendelenburg's position improves cerebral blood flow, and cold compresses on the head and face will help revive the patient. Vital signs should be noted. Complete restoration of mental status and cardiopulmonary function should occur quickly. Failure of either of these events to occur implies a different, more serious problem, such as stroke, seizure, or myocardial infarction.

Hemorrhage

Most patients with significant congenital or acquired bleeding abnormalities have had some symptoms or signs of unusual bleeding before undergoing minor surgery. Defects of vasoconstriction, platelet numbers or function, and the coagulation cascade can cause excessive operative hemorrhage. A history of spontaneous bleeding from multiple sites (e.g., mucosal surfaces), excessive bleeding from minor trauma, or the occurrence of petechiae or large ecchymoses should alert the physician to a probable bleeding disorder. A family history of similar problems suggests the presence of a congenital coagulation defect. Drugs, especially anticoagulants and platelet cyclo-oxygenase inhibitors (e.g., aminosalicylic acid), can cause excess hemorrhage during surgery. These medications may need to be stopped or reversed before an operation. Underlying disease states (e.g., liver disease or malabsorption of vitamin K) may also cause hemostatic abnormalities and should be screened for preoperatively if there is a history of abnormal bleeding.

The most common form of bleeding abnormality is thrombocytopenia, which can be detected by simple examination of a peripheral blood smear. If there is a suspicion of a bleeding diathesis, a platelet count, bleeding time, prothrombin time, and partial thromboplastin time comprise a good panel of tests to clarify the disorder. More specific studies may be required.

If the history fails to reveal any hint of coagulopathy, the most likely cause of bleeding during a procedure is inadequate control of blood vessels in the operative field. Pressure should be applied and hemostasis achieved with cautery or clamping and ligation. If close attention is paid to good surgical technique, blood loss should be minimal and the need for transfusion nonexistent.

Drug Toxicity

Local anesthetics are the most commonly used drugs in outpatient surgery, and most toxic drug reactions are caused by these agents. Toxicity is related to the total dose of drug and the rate of administration. Reactions are not always seen at the same serum drug level, even in the same patient. Systemic absorption must occur in order to cause toxicity. Individual characteristics of the particular drug, such as lipid solubility, ionization in serum, protein binding, biotransformation, and excretion patterns are factors in drug toxicity.

To avoid toxicity, the surgeon should use the smallest dose necessary for anesthesia. All local anesthetics have maximum recommended doses (see Table 8–1). Doses should be lower in children, the elderly, and patients with debilitating illness. Agents with amide linkage (including lidocaine, bupivacaine, etidocaine, and mepivacaine) are metabolized by the liver, so maximum tolerable doses are lower in patients with liver disease and congestive heart failure. A vasoconstricting agent, usually epinephrine in a 1:200,000 dilution, can be used to slow systemic absorption and prolong local action of anesthetic agents. Epinephrine should be avoided in patients with cardiovascular disease and hyperthyroidism, and it should not be used in distal extremities, the nose, or the penis because it may cause irreversible ischemia of these tissues. Cocaine has potent vasoconstrictive properties of its own and requires no such additive. Care must be taken to avoid direct intravascular administration of local anesthetics, since such a bolus may deliver a toxic dose instantaneously. The injection needle should be aspirated frequently while placing the local block.

If a dose of local anesthetic is excessive or is given too rapidly, early indications of toxicity may develop. Most of these symptoms and signs result from high concentrations in the central nervous system. Dizziness, tinnitus, nystagmus, diplopia, dysphoria, slurred speech, shivering, twitching, and tremors of the face and intrinsic muscles of the hands are among these early manifestations. Numbness of the tongue and circumoral area are frequent symptoms, but they may reflect local anesthetic action rather than toxicity. When a reaction occurs, the procedure should be halted, oxygen delivered by mask, and an intravenous infusion started. Barbiturates or diazepam increases the seizure threshold and should be given to prevent this complication. Doses of 1 to 2 mg/kg of thiopental or pentobarbital or 2.5 to 5.0 mg of diazepam up to a total dose of 0.1 to 0.2 mg/kg are recommended in this situation. Both of these medications inhibit respirations, and the patient's breathing should be checked frequently.

Progression of the toxic reaction to local anesthetics leads to grand mal seizures. Diazepam or barbiturates may be utilized to control the seizure activity. Diphenylhydantoin should not be given, since it may increase seizure activity in this situation. Seizures often last only one to two minutes, but more serious side effects may be masked during this period. Further development of toxicity leads to general depression of the CNS, in part manifested by cardiovascular collapse and respiratory arrest. Besides the effects on the circulation mediated by the blockade of autonomic nerve function, local anesthetics have direct relaxation effects on cardiac and vascular wall musculatures. With a fully developed toxic reaction from a local anesthetic, artificial support of circulation and respiration are needed (for treatment, see the section on cardiopulmonary arrest below).

If epinephrine has been used for vasoconstriction, signs of catecholamine toxicity may occur. Palpitations and headache are the most common symptoms; others include shortness of breath, fear, anxiety, nausea, and faintness. On examination, patients are often restless and have tachypnea, tachycardia, hypertension, pallor, tremors, and vomiting. Usually, the signs of epinephrine toxicity are clearly distinguished from other emergencies. In the vast majority of cases, no specific therapy is needed because the half-life of epinephrine in serum is short. Small doses of intravenous propranolol (0.5 to 1.0 mg, repeated as necessary every few minutes) can be administered with ECG monitoring, but this should be reserved for cases of severe hypertension and tachycardia in which there is danger of stroke or myocardial injury. Prevention of such side effects again depends on limiting the dose and rate of absorption of epinephrine into the systemic circulation. Epinephrine toxicity is minimized by the use of dilute epinephrine solutions (1:200,000), a maximum dose of 0.25 mg, and the avoidance of intravenous administration.

Drug Allergy and Anaphylaxis

Adverse immunologic reactions can occur with any drug, although certain compounds, such as proteins and substances that form haptens (e.g., penicillins), are more likely to be allergenic. Symptoms are frequently mild and involve only pruritus, a rash, or urticaria. More severe reactions may result in vomiting and diarrhea, angioneurotic edema,

TABLE 8–1. Maximum Doses of Local Anesthetics

Drug	Plain	With Epinephrine
Cocaine	200 mg	—
Procaine	Ineffective	1000 mg
Chloroprocaine	Ineffective	1000 mg
Tetracaine	100 mg	200 mg
Lidocaine	300 mg	500 mg
Mepivacaine	300 mg	500 mg
Prilocaine	600 mg	600 mg
Bupivacaine	175 mg	225 mg
Etidocaine	300 mg	400 mg

Doses are calculated for a 70 kg healthy patient. Doses should be altered according to age, weight, and condition of patient.

laryngeal edema, bronchospasm, hypotension, and cardiovascular collapse. Allergic reactions can be mediated by either cellular or humoral components of the immune system. The most feared form of allergic response is anaphylaxis, which is an immediate reaction (within seconds to several minutes) caused by the presence of IgE antibodies that react with the allergen. Airway obstruction and cardiovascular insufficiency need to be checked for and treated promptly in order to prevent permanent injury or death.

Although frequently implicated as allergens, local anesthetics rarely cause allergic reactions, except for dermatitis in people who come into contact with them frequently. Most of the documented cases of allergic response to local anesthetics have been caused by agents with ester linkage (e.g., procaine, chloroprocaine, tetracaine); the para-aminobenzoic group in these compounds may be responsible. Preservatives (e.g., methylparaben in multiple-use vials) are the most common source of allergy to local anesthetic solutions.

Allergic reactions to local anesthetics are best avoided by taking a history, preliminary skin testing (if necessary), single usage vials (no preservatives), and using amide rather than ester linkage agents. Cross-reactivity between anesthetics of amide or ester linkage will occur, making the use of a similar compound for a patient with an allergic history unwise and dangerous. Atopic patients may be at increased risk for developing allergic reactions and should be carefully watched after administration of any medication.

The prevention of allergic reactions to other medications includes similar measures, including a thorough history and investigation of previous drug reactions, skin testing (when necessary), and avoidance of substances likely to cause an allergy or anaphylaxis (e.g., proteins or drugs that will cross-react with known allergens). If known allergens must be used, desensitization should be attempted by an experienced physician or by premedication with steroids (prednisone 50 mg every six hours for three doses, the last dose one hour before the procedure) and antihistamines (diphenhydramine 50 mg intramuscularly one hour before the drug exposure) can be tried. Intravenous access should be available when administering a drug known to have caused an allergic response, and emergency drugs and a means of establishing a secure airway must be at hand, since premedication may not avoid an anaphylactic reaction.

Serious allergic reactions usually occur quickly after the administration of the offending substance. Anaphylactic reactions often start within 30 seconds after exposure and usually are fully manifested within 5 to 10 minutes, although this is dependent on the route of introduction and the speed of systemic absorption. Early warning symptoms of severe allergic response include generalized warmth and flushing with local or diffuse erythema, pruritus, and urticaria. These symptoms may be accompanied by a sense of impending doom; nausea and vomiting; tingling and edema (frequently involving the face, mouth, and tongue); tightness of the chest and throat; and palpitations.

As soon as a significant allergic reaction is suspected, the patient must be placed in a supine position with the head down. Epinephrine solution (0.2 to 0.5 ml of a 1:1000 dilution) should be administered subcutaneously and repeated as necessary every 5 to 15 minutes. If the offending drug was injected peripherally, a tourniquet may be used to slow further absorption, as may local injection of epinephrine. Intravenous access should be obtained at the first possible moment in case the allergic response progresses. Oxygen should be given by mask initially, and inhalant bronchodilators (isoproterenol, metaproterenol, or terbutaline) are used for moderate bronchospasm. Subcutaneous terbutaline (0.25 mg) or an intravenous bolus of aminophylline (5.6 mg/kg over 15 to 30 minutes) are reserved for more severe bronchial constriction. Antihistamines and corticosteroids have no immediate effect on the developing anaphylactic response and do not need to be given during the initial treatment. If signs of upper airway compromise develop, immediate endotracheal intubation should be performed. Delay may result in the need for an emergency cricothyroidotomy or tracheostomy to establish an airway. Hypotension due to cardiovascular collapse is treated with rapid fluid infusion and vasopressor agents (such as epinephrine or dopamine) if fluid alone is inadequate to maintain blood pressure. Should cardiac arrest occur, CPR is carried out as outlined below. Any patient suffering a severe allergic reaction must be admitted to a hospital as soon as transport can be achieved safely.

Asthma

With the stress of a surgical procedure, a person with asthma can become acutely symptomatic. The preoperative history should alert the physician to this condition. The lack of symptoms and signs other than bronchospasm differentiates asthma from allergic reactions to drugs. The attack can vary from mild wheezing to severe bronchospasm, and the treatment varies accordingly.

For a mild episode of bronchospasm, an inhalant bronchodilator, such as metaproterenol or terbutaline, should be tried first. These may be repeated if initially unsuccessful. If additional treatment is needed, subcutaneous epinephrine (0.2 to 0.5 ml of a 1:1000 solution) can be given every 15 to 30 minutes. This drug should be used cautiously when the patient also suffers from cardiac or hyperthyroid disease. The next step is intravenous aminophylline in a loading dose of 5.6 mg/kg over 15 to 30 minutes (decrease dosage between 50 and 75% of the total, if the patient is currently on a theophylline medication) followed by a continuous infusion of 0.6 mg/kg/hr for an adult (0.3 mg/kg/hr for chronically ill patients and 0.9 mg/kg/hr for smokers). Oxygen should be administered in all cases. In severe cases that fail to respond, corticosteroids may help, although benefit is not seen acutely and it is probably best to use steroids only after arrival at the hospital.

Myocardial Infarction

Patients with coronary artery disease can suffer myocardial ischemia or infarction during minor surgery. Severe substernal chest pain with shortness of breath, diaphoresis, and pallor should be managed by immediate termination of the operative procedure and initiation of therapeutic maneuvers. The goals of treatment are relief of symptoms, if possible, and prevention of complications if infarction is evolving.

Nitroglycerine (0.3 mg) is given sublingually, oxygen is administered by mask, vital signs are measured, and an intravenous line is started. An electrocardiogram monitor, preferably with the capability to obtain a 12-lead ECG should be attached to the patient. Failure to eliminate pain with two or three tablets given 5 to 10 minutes apart or failure of ischemic ECG changes to resolve should raise serious concern about a myocardial infarction. Intramuscular morphine sulfate in doses of 10 to 15 mg (or 1 to 4 mg of intravenous morphine) help provide pain relief, but it must be used cautiously, especially in the presence of hypotension. Increasing enthusiasm for prophylactic lidocaine to prevent arrhythmias has developed over recent years. A bolus of 75 to 100 mg of plain 1% lidocaine is given intravenously, and a 2 mg/min constant infusion (1 mg/min with congestive failure, hypotension, or liver disease) is begun. Because most prehospital deaths from myocardial infarction are caused by arrhythmias, the patient must be rapidly transported to a hospital where cardiac monitoring can be instituted. Treatment of shock and specific arrhythmias are discussed below.

Cardiogenic Shock

Shock is any situation where inadequate perfusion of vital organs occurs. The causes of this hypoperfusion include hypovolemia (usually from blood loss), sepsis, neurologic disturbances of vascular tone, anaphylaxis, and cardiac disturbances. In the setting of outpatient surgery, hypovolemic and septic shock are not likely to occur. Anaphylaxis and a form of neurogenic shock (vasovagal syncope) have already been discussed. Cardiogenic shock during minor operations is most likely the result of an acute decompensation of cardiac function, either an arrhythmia or an infarction.

Symptoms related to the underlying cause of cardiogenic shock may be apparent, e.g., palpitations often accompany arrhythmias, and ischemic chest pain is present with a myocardial infarction. Because of insufficient blood flow to the brain, the symptoms of cardiogenic shock may include restlessness, anxiety, and thirst in the early stages and then apathy, obtundation, and coma later. Peripheral perfusion is impaired, and vasoconstriction makes the patient appear pale. The extremities are cool and moist. Blood pressure is low, and the pulse is rapid, irregular, or both. Cardiogenic shock is easily differentiated from syncope in which the pulse is usually slow and the symptoms and signs resolve rapidly. A rapid pulse is present with epinephrine toxicity, but the blood pressure is normal or elevated.

The presence of arrhythmias is suspected from the pulse rate and rhythm, but it is confirmed by ECG monitoring. The treatment of specific arrhythmias is discussed under cardiac arrest. Shock due to myocardial infarction occurs when a large amount of myocardial function is lost; it denotes a poor prognosis, even with aggressive therapy. Congestive failure, manifested by signs of fluid overload will be apparent. Lack of adequate hemodynamic monitoring makes attempts at aggressive treatment in the prehospital setting potentially dangerous. Cautious use of morphine, extremity tourniquets, and a beta agonist, such as dobutamine (starting dose of 1 to 2 μg/kg/min) or dopamine (1 to 10 μg/kg/min) should be begun in an unstable patient while arranging for immediate transfer to a coronary care unit.

Cardiopulmonary Arrest

The most immediate threat to life is cessation of effective cardiac activity due to either asystole or arrhythmia (e.g., ventricular fibrillation). In both situations, the patient becomes unconscious within a few seconds. There is either a feeble or absent pulse and spontaneous respirations cease. A brief attempt should be made to arouse the patient, and a quick check for breathing and pulse precedes initiation of cardiopulmonary resuscitation. Immediate recognition of arrest and commencement of resuscitation are critical to prevent ischemic cerebral injury and to improve chances for survival. The goal of prehospital management of a patient suffering cardiac arrest is the restoration and maintenance of adequate ventilation and circulation. It is hoped that the patient can be stabilized sufficiently to reach a facility where more intensive therapy can be instituted.

The basic principles of CPR should be followed

when beginning treatment of a patient with a cardiac arrest. An assistant should call the hospital resuscitation team (if available) or the community emergency medical service immediately. An airway is established by tilting the head back and lifting the neck. If the resuscitator has experience with either the head-tilt-and-chin-lift or head-tilt-and-jaw-thrust techniques, these are generally regarded as superior to the head-tilt-and-neck-lift technique of opening the airway. If there are no spontaneous efforts at breathing with an open airway, four deep breaths are given by the mouth-to-mouth technique or with a firmly fitting mask and bag if available. Upon completing these ventilations, the carotid pulse should be checked. If no pulse is appreciated, CPR should be begun.

The patient must be placed on a firm surface (floor or back board) before beginning chest compressions. Position of the hands, degree of compression, number of compressions, and timing with respirations should follow the recommendations of the American Heart Association to assure maximal cardiac output and to avoid chest wall injury. During this time, the cardiac monitor and defibrillator unit should be set up and charged. An intravenous line is started, through which drugs can be delivered during the resuscitation. If someone present is familiar with the techniques and the equipment is available, a more secure airway should be obtained. Endotracheal intubation is the best way to accomplish this, but experience with the method is required. Suctioning of oral and gastric secretions may be needed for adequate visualization of the larynx. An esophageal obturator or a mask-valve-bag with an oropharyngeal tube are second choices for airway maintenance. None of these activities should interfere with providing ventilation and cardiac compressions for more than 30 seconds.

The ECG tracings in cardiac arrest show three distinct patterns: fibrillation, asystole, and electromechanical dissociation. If ventricular fibrillation is noted and countershock is available within two minutes of the onset of arrest, a shock of 200 to 300 joules should be tried to defibrillate the heart. Paddles should be placed so that the current traverses the heart, usually one to the right of the sternum just below the clavicle and the other lateral to the nipple in the left anterior axillary line. With a longer delay, 0.5 to 1.0 mg of epinephrine (5 to 10 ml of 1:10,000 solution) and sodium bicarbonate (one or two ampules of 44.6 mEq in 50 ml) are given before attempting defibrillation. Two discharges of 200 to 300 joules are tried, and the resultant rhythm is checked between the countershocks. A third shock of 360 joules is given if the first two are unsuccessful in converting the heart to an organized rhythm. Depending on the duration of arrest, additional doses of bicarbonate are administered in an effort to lower the fibrillation threshold.

When conversion to a supraventricular rhythm is achieved, a 75 to 100 mg lidocaine bolus and continuous infusion of 2 mg/min should be started. Recurrent fibrillations require further shocks, lidocaine, procainamide, and sometimes bretylium. Less energy for defibrillation is usually needed with recurrent fibrillations, and smaller electrical discharges reduce myocardial injury.

Ventricular asystole carries a worse prognosis than fibrillation and may occur primarily or after fibrillation or electromechanical dissociation. Asystole usually implies a severe metabolic disturbance, extensive injury of the heart, or both. Epinephrine and bicarbonate are given intravenously first; an ampule of calcium chloride (5 ml of a 10% solution) is administered next if there is no response to the first two drugs. Intravenous atropine in a dose of 0.5 to 1.0 mg is the next step in attempting to restore an electric complex. Intracardiac epinephrine or intravenous infusion of isoproterenol may restore myocardial activity. Additional bicarbonate is given at the rate of one ampule every 10 minutes, or as needed by pH determination, if arterial blood gases can be done. The insertion of a ventricular pacemaker only rarely restores an effective ventricular rhythm.

With electromechanical dissociation, the ECG shows organized electric activity, but there is no effective myocardial contraction. A breakdown in calcium ion transport in the myocardium may be responsible for this condition, which carries a grave prognosis. After starting basic resuscitation, intravenous epinephrine and bicarbonate are given followed by calcium chloride (the same doses previously mentioned for asystole). Intravenous isoproterenol or additional intravenous or intracardiac epinephrine may be of benefit. An additional ampule of sodium bicarbonate is given every 10 minutes or as arterial pH determination indicates need. Antishock garments may be of use. It is imperative to distinguish pericardial tamponade from electromechanical dissociation, since the former condition is readily treatable by aspiration of the pericardial sac and may mimic the latter.

Arrhythmias may occur primarily or subsequent to conversion from fibrillation, asystole, or electromechanical dissociation. Recognition of these arrhythmias and knowledge of their treatment is critical to maintain stable cardiac function until arrival at a hospital. Oxygen should be given by mask and intravenous access should be obtained. Additional steps in securing ventilation and circulation are instituted as needed.

1. Premature Ventricular Contractions. These are best treated with lidocaine that is given as an intravenous bolus of 75 to 100 mg and subsequent 2 mg/min constant infusion. Procainamide is required for those situations in which this arrhythmia fails to respond to lidocaine.

2. Bradycardia. Bradycardia may result from sinus, junctional, or atrioventricular block irregularities. When no hypotension or premature ventricular contractions are present, no treatment is needed for a pulse above 50. A rate below this or the presence of hypotension or premature ventricular contractions requires intravenous atropine (0.5 mg, with a dose repeated every five minutes as necessary). An intravenous infusion of isoproterenol at rates of 2 to 20 μg/min should be started when atropine is not working; the dose is titrated by heart rate and pressure response. Acute second- and third-degree atrioventricular blocks are best treated by inserting a temporary cardiac pacemaker as soon as possible.

3. Supraventricular Tachyarrhythmias. Supraventricular tachyarrhythmias result from excessive catecholamine levels or irregularity of cardiac automaticity or conduction. Treatment of these conditions without measurement of hemodynamic parameters, such as cardiac output, may be dangerous, but continuation of such arrhythmias may result in increased myocardial injury. If hypovolemia is suspected, a trial of fluid infusion is in order. Treatment with pressor agents, such as intravenous infusions of dopamine or dobutamine may increase cardiac output and lower heart rate, but both drugs may increase myocardial irritability and cause worse arrhythmias. Small doses of intravenous propranolol (0.5 to 1.0 mg) can be given cautiously, but this is usually best done in an intensive care situation. Countershock and intravenous loading with digoxin are also best reserved until the patient reaches the hospital.

4. Ventricular Tachycardia. Ventricular tachycardia is treated with lidocaine or procainamide infusion when an adequate blood pressure is present. When the patient is hypotensive or unresponsive, cardioversion should be performed and a constant lidocaine infusion started after a better rhythm is obtained.

Although immediate use of advanced cardiac life-support techniques at the site of arrest improves survival, the inability to convert the patient to a rhythm with good perfusion should not delay the transportation of the patient to the hospital. CPR should be continued with minimal (≤ 30-second) interruptions while transferring the patient to a stretcher and while moving. If a good cardiac activity and airway have been obtained, continued monitoring of vital signs and cardiac rhythm must be maintained while en route. The physician should remain with the patient until the receiving hospital is reached and care can be transferred to another doctor.

SUGGESTED READINGS

Colmer RW, Hirsh J, Marder VJ, Salzman EW: Approach to the bleeding patient, in Colman RW, Hirsh J (eds): Hemostasis and Thrombosis. Philadelphia, J. B. Lippincott, 1982, pp 694–700

Covino BG, Vassallo HG: Local Anesthetics' Mechanisms of Action and Clinical Use. New York, Grune and Stratton, 1976, pp 123–148

deJong RH: Local Anesthetics, ed 2. Springfield, Ill, Charles C Thomas, 1977, pp 247–275

Donegan JH: Cardiopulmonary resuscitation, in Miller RD (ed): Anesthesia. New York, Churchill Livingstone, 1981, pp 1493–1529

Durerman N, Pons P, Rosen P, Marlin R: Prehospital management of cardiac arrest, in Harwood AL (ed): Cardiopulmonary Resuscitation. Baltimore, Williams and Wilkins, 1982, pp 127–133

Matheu A, Battit GE, and DiPadua D: Anaphylactic and anaphylactoid reactions to anesthetic agents and other drugs used during anesthesia, in Matheu A, Kahn BD (eds): Immunologic Aspects of Anesthetic and Surgical Practice. New York, Grune and Stratton, 1975, pp 261–287

Parker CW: Systemic anaphylaxis, in Parker CW (ed): Clinical Immunology. Philadelphia, W. B. Saunders Co, 1980, pp 1208–1218

Raj PP, Winnie AP: Immediate reactions to local anesthetics, in Orkin FK, Cooperman LH (eds): Complications in Anesthesiology. Philadelphia, J. B. Lippincott Co, 1983, pp 51–74

Ritchie JM, Greene NM: Local anesthetics, in Gilman AG, Goodman LS, Gilman A (eds): The Pharmacological Basis of Therapeutics, ed 6. New York, Macmillan Publishing Co, 1980, pp 300–320

Schwartz SI: Hemostasis, surgical bleeding and transfusion, in Schwartz SI, et al (eds): Principles of Surgery, ed 4. New York, McGraw-Hill Book Co, 1984, pp 81–113

Shires GT, Canizaro PC, Carrico CJ: Shock, in Schwartz SI, et al (eds): Principles of Surgery, ed 4. New York, McGraw-Hill Book Co, 1984, pp 115–164

Standards and Guidelines for Cardiopulmonary Resuscitation (CPR) and Emergency Cardiac Care (ECC): JAMA 244, 453–509, 1980.

Stewart, RD: CPR in prehospital care, in Auerbach PS, Budassi SA (eds): Cardiac Arrest and CPR: Assessment, Planning and Intervention, ed 2. Rockville, MD, Aspen System Corporation, 1983, pp 225–232

Webb-Johnson DC, Andrews JL: Bronchodilator therapy. New Engl J Med 297:476–482 and 758–764, 1977

Wyngaarden JB, Smith LH Jr: Cecil Textbook of Medicine, ed 16. Philadelphia, W. B. Saunders Co, 1982

9

J. NILAS YOUNG, M.D. / DAVID J. DUGAN, M.D.

Techniques of Cardiopulmonary Resuscitation

The type of death under discussion is that which occurs unexpectedly. . . . The first one I recall was when I was a surgical intern in Baltimore. The patient could not be revived. . . . My belief is that surgeons should not turn these emergencies over to the fire department. We should take care of them ourselves.[1]

CLAUDE BECK, 1941

Cardiopulmonary arrest is described by Jude as "the total arrest of the circulation or ineffectual circulation of oxygenated blood for a period of four to six minutes so as not to sustain biological life."[2] The tissues most sensitive to oxygen deprivation are located in the central nervous system. Tissue injury is probably reversible for up to six minutes, but beyond this time, cell death occurs. It is thus extremely important that a rapid diagnosis of cardiopulmonary arrest be made followed by immediate resuscitative measures.

Causes of Cardiopulmonary Arrest

Hopefully, cardiopulmonary arrest will be a rare event during surgical procedures on the skin. When it occurs, it will most likely be in association with either drug reactions or in patients with coronary artery disease. The presence of coronary disease should be ascertained when any type of surgical procedure is contemplated. Patients with severe or progressive angina pectoris or those recently recovered from myocardial infarction are at an increased risk for cardiac arrest. The signs and symptoms preceding arrest in these patients are often those associated with angina pectoris or myocardial infarction, e.g., retrosternal pain that radiates to the neck or arms, shortness of breath, apprehension, perspiration, weakness, or fainting.

Cardiovascular collapse secondary to the use of drugs or local anesthetic agents can be caused by either an anaphylactic (allergic) reaction or the absorption of local anesthetic into the bloodstream. Severe reactions to local anesthetics are rarely allergic and are usually secondary to bloodstream absorption. The severity of the reaction occurring from a local anesthetic is dependent on the rate of absorption, which is increased in such areas as the

upper respiratory passages and the urethra. Therefore, using local anesthetics in these regions requires special care. Verbal contact with the patient while using a local anesthetic is often helpful in detecting the early symptoms of impending severe reactions.[3] Apprehension, bradycardia, pallor, perspiration, loss of consciousness, convulsions, or apnea may indicate circulatory arrest.

The two most common clinical patterns of anaphylaxis are profound shock or respiratory distress. The signs associated with an allergic reaction anaphylaxis usually include urticaria, edema, pruritus, wheezing, paresthesias, and loss of consciousness.

Recognition of Cardiopulmonary Arrest

The presence of cardiopulmonary arrest in an unconscious patient is best determined by evaluation of respiration and circulation. The chest should be observed for evidence of respiratory motion. If none is noted, the rescuer should place his ear next to the patient's mouth to determine if spontaneous breathing is occurring. The carotid artery provides a readily available central pulse and should be palpated to detect effective circulation (Fig. 9–1). Cyanosis or dilated pupils may also be present but this is a less reliable finding. Any patient who is unconscious without evidence of spontaneous breathing or a palpable pulse should be considered as having a cardiopulmonary arrest, and cardiopulmonary resuscitation (CPR) should be immediately administered.

Techniques of Cardiopulmonary Resuscitation (CPR)

CPR techniques are designed to support the cellular functions of the vital organs by providing

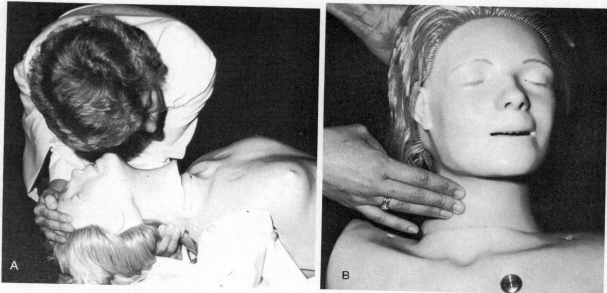

Figure 9–1. *A,* Detection of spontaneous breathing. *B,* Palpation of carotid pulse.

artificial circulation of oxygenated blood. In 1973, the National Conference of Standards for Cardiopulmonary Resuscitation and Emergency Cardiac Care established the essential guidelines for two levels of treatment—basic life support and advanced life support. Basic life support is emergency first aid to establish an open airway and to administer artificial ventilation and external cardiac compression, i.e., the ABCs of CPR (airway, breathing, and circulation). Advanced life support includes the use of drugs, electric defibrillation, and stabilization of the patient. The sequence of events in both basic and advanced phases are listed in Table 9–1. It should be stressed that although CPR involves many different aspects, the most important are the basic maneuvers of airway maintenance and cardiac compression.[4–6]

Basic Life Support

The patient should immediately be placed on his back on a hard surface. If emesis occurs, the patient

TABLE 9–1. Proper Sequence in Cardiopulmonary Resuscitation

1. Recognition—check respirations and carotid pulse.
2. Summon help.
3. Place patient on hard surface.
4. Establish open airway—tilt head, remove any foreign body and dentures from mouth.
5. Respirations—four quick breaths then ventilate at a rate of 12 times per minute.
6. External cardiac compression—60 strokes per minute.
7. Defibrillator, drugs, and supplemental oxygen, if available.
8. Transport to appropriate medical facility.

should be turned on his side toward the resuscitator. Striking the patient's back between the scapulae may help to dislodge aspirated material (Fig. 9–2).

In the supine position, unconscious patients have a closed airway because the head flexes on the cervical vertebral column, thus acutely angulating

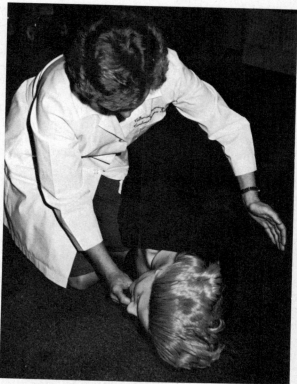

Figure 9–2. If emesis occurs, the victim is rolled towards the resuscitator. Striking between the scapulae may help to dislodge aspirated material.

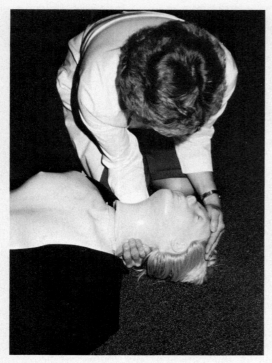

Figure 9–3. The head-tilt position.

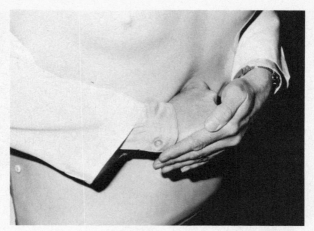

Figure 9–4. The abdominal thrust for upper airway obstruction.

the pharynx and closing the airway.[7] The airway must be opened by tilting the forehead backward with one hand, while simultaneously elevating the patient's neck with the other hand (Fig. 9–3). Any foreign body, aspirated material, or dentures in the mouth must be removed.

Although uncommon in the setting of a physician's office, respiratory embarrassment may occur because of upper airway obstruction by a foreign body, such as food. In addition to the previously mentioned interscapular blow, the abdominal thrust of the Heimlich maneuver may also be beneficial. This is performed by the rescuer placing the closed fist of one hand between the xiphoid process and umbilicus and then with his open hand pressing against the fist four times into the victim's abdomen with a quick inward and upward thrust. It is best performed by standing behind the victim, who is standing or sitting (Fig. 9–4). If the victim is unconscious, the manuever may be performed with the rescuer straddling the supine victim.

Ventilation may be performed by the mouth-to-mouth method, with a ventilating bag, or with an endotracheal tube. Although a properly placed, cuffed endotracheal tube provides the ideal approach to artificial ventilation, valuable time should not be lost by an inexperienced rescuer attempting to place an endotracheal tube or searching for equipment. A pharyngeal airway and a ventilating bag with supplemental oxygen are extremely useful and require little time or proficiency. If ventilatory

equipment is unavailable, simple mouth-to-mouth breathing is beneficial and capable of providing adequate respiratory support.

The mouth-to-mouth method is accomplished by maintaining the head-tilt position and pinching the victim's nose with the free hand. The resuscitator then takes a deep breath, and, sealing his mouth over the patient's mouth, forcefully blows into the patient's airway (Fig. 9–5). The rescuer then once again places his ear next to the patient's mouth to detect exhaled air, which, in association with good chest expansion, indicates good ventilation and an adequate airway. If the airway appears adequate, four quick breaths are delivered without allowing

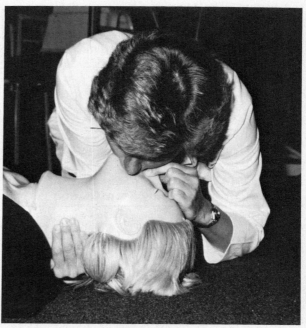

Figure 9–5. The technique of mouth-to-mouth ventilation. Note that the head-tilt position is maintained.

the patient to exhale fully. In exceptional circumstances, laryngeal edema or a foreign body may prevent a patent airway. In this situation, the performance of an emergency cricothyroidotomy by percutaneous puncture of the circothyroid membrane can provide a quick airway (Fig. 9–6).

The next step is to provide adequate circulation by external cardiac compression. This is accomplished by placing the heel of one hand just below the midpoint of the sternum, and then the heel of the second hand on top of the first (Fig. 9–7). In this position, the hands should overlie the midportion of the heart, which is approximately at the junction of the middle and lower thirds of the sternum. While performing external cardiac compression, the fingers should not touch the chest wall, since this can transmit enough pressure to the costal cartilages and ribs to fracture them. Pressure applied too low on the sternum may cause laceration of the liver by the xiphoid process.

With the resuscitator close to the victim's side and with his shoulders directly over the victim's sternum, the sternum is compressed 1½ to 2 inches. The

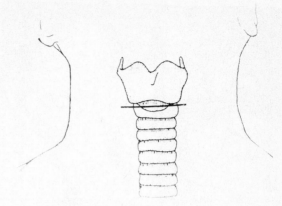

Figure 9–6. Incision for cricothyroidotomy.

compressions should be performed smoothly with only a slight pause at the depth of each compression to allow for ejection of blood from the heart. Cardiac compression should be carried out at a rate of approximately 60 strokes per minute.

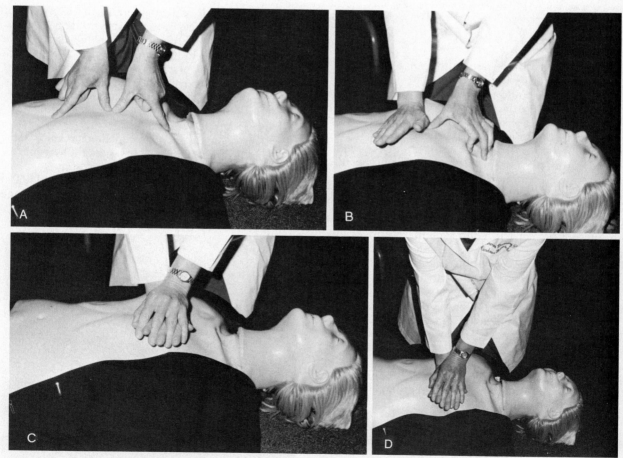

Figure 9–7. External cardiac compression. A, Locating the midpoint of the sternum. B, The heel of one hand is placed just below the midpoint of the sternum. C, Final position of the hands. D, The resuscitator is close to victim's side, and her arms are as straight as possible.

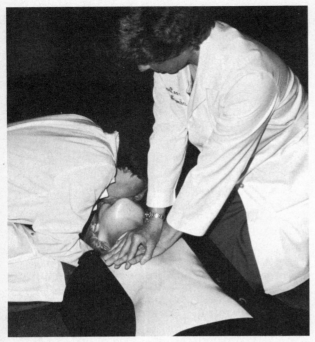

Figure 9–8. When two resuscitators are present, they should be positioned on opposite sides of the victim to allow for easy exchange of duties.

The situation differs depending on whether one or two resuscitators are present. With one resuscitator, a cycle should consist of two quick lung inflations followed by 15 cardiac compressions. To maintain 60 beats a minute, the compression rate will have to be approximately one every 0.75 seconds. With two persons performing the resuscitation, the cardiac compression rate should be one per second and ventilation should be 12 per minute. Counting aloud by the person doing cardiac compression (e.g., one thousand one, one thousand two) is helpful. It should be noted that no break in the rhythm of cardiac compression should occur. The resuscitators should be situated on opposite sides of the patient, since this allows easy exchange of positions without interruption (Fig. 9–8).

By external cardiac compression, a systolic blood pressure of more than 100 mm Hg can be achieved. Diastolic pressure, however, approaches zero, and there is a resultant mean pressure of approximately 40 to 50 mm Hg. Cerebral blood flow is usually 30 to 40% of normal and has been shown to remain adequate for periods of two to three hours when attained by external cardiac compression and ventilatory support alone.[8, 9]

Advanced Life Support

If possible, advanced life support measures should be incorporated into all resuscitative efforts. As mentioned earlier, these involve the use of an elec-tric defibrillator and drugs in association with basic life support methods.

The patient who suffers a cardiopulmonary arrest usually has abnormalities of cardiac rhythm, e.g., premature beats, bradycardia, and sustained ventricular or atrial tachycardias. In the acute setting, the precipitating causes are usually those of decreased myocardial perfusion and hypoxia. Sudden cardiac rhythm disturbances, particularly those of ventricular origin, remain the most important cause of sudden death. The incidence in the healthy population is unknown, but 90% of patients with myocardial infarction have ventricular arrhythmias to some extent.[10]

The presence of a defibrillator unit (Fig. 9–9) is useful in dealing with cardiac arrest. Within seconds, leads from the unit may be attached to the patient allowing visualization of the type of cardiac rhythm. According to electrocardiographic criteria, there are three main types of arrest. One is complete asystole with no apparent cardiac activity. The second is ventricular fibrillation. The third is cardiovascular collapse with ventricular complexes but no effective blood pressure, e.g., ventricular tachycardia or bradycardia (Fig. 9–10).

If a defibrillator is available and the presence of ventricular fibrillation or tachyarrhythmia is discernible, then immediate conversion of the arrhythmia may be obtained by a countershock. This is performed by placing one of the defibrillator paddles at the base of the heart in the right second intercostal space, and the other paddle near the cardiac apex below the left nipple (Fig. 9–11). Then, 400 watt-seconds are applied for a duration of 4 to 6 milliseconds. This sequence can be repeated as necessary. It is unlikely that there is any benefit to countershock when ventricular asystole is present.

Modern defibrillator units are small, portable, and usually simple to operate. Defibrillation can be done

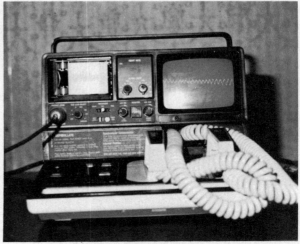

Figure 9–9. Portable defibrillator apparatus.

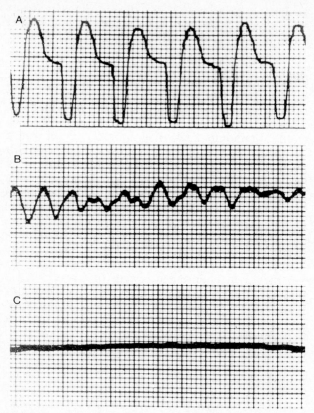

Figure 9–10. The three most common ECG patterns seen in circulatory arrest: *A,* Ventricular tachycardia. *B,* Ventricular fibrillation. *C,* Asystole.

quickly so that basic cardiopulmonary resuscitative measures are interrupted only briefly. Caution should be exercised in the use of the defibrillator paddles. A special coating gel should be applied evenly and thinly to the paddle surfaces. Failure to properly apply the gel can result in burns, and an excessive amount prevents proper electrical conduction. Special conductor pads may be used that eliminate the need for placing the paddles on the patient's skin.

Cardiovascular Drugs

Although the number of potentially beneficial cardiac drugs is large, most cardiac arrests are successfully managed by no more than three or four. Table 9–2 provides a list of commonly used drugs and their dosages.

The approach to the pharmacology of cardiopulmonary arrest should be based on the physiologic pathology present. Almost all patients who sustain cardiopulmonary arrest rapidly develop metabolic acidosis, which must be controlled to some extent for adequate cellular function. In addition, the response of the myocardium to drugs such as epinephrine is greatly reduced when acidosis is present. One of the most useful drugs that can be given initially is sodium bicarbonate. A safe dose is usually 50 mEq every 5 to 10 minutes. Excessive use results in alkalosis and myocardial depression.

Myocardial stimulants are used in the treatment of ventricular depression and asystole. Probably the most readily available and most effective of these is epinephrine given as 5 ml of a 1:10,000 solution. Epinephrine has the effect of a direct myocardial stimulant as well as producing peripheral vasoconstriction, thus elevating blood pressure and enhancing myocardial perfusion.[11] Additional drugs, such as dopamine and Isuprel, may also be beneficial cardiac stimulants. Atropine 0.5 mg is useful for

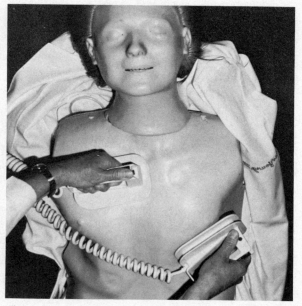

Figure 9–11. Defibrillator paddle positions: second right interspace and below left nipple.

TABLE 9–2. Drugs Used in Cardiopulmonary Resuscitation

Drug	Purpose	IV Dosage
Sodium bicarbonate	Reverses acidosis	50 mEq
Epinephrine	Cardiac stimulant	5 ml in a 1:10,000 solution
Isuprel	Cardiac stimulant	0.1–0.2 mg
Dopamine	Cardiac stimulant	400 mg in a 250 ml IV drip
Calcium chloride	Cardiac stimulant	10 ml in a 10% solution
Atropine	Sinus bradycardia	0.5–1.0 mg
Lidocaine	Ventricular irritability	100 mg bolus in an IV drip, 2–3 mg/min
Aminophylline	Bronchospasm	250 mg in a 250 cc IV drip
Diazepam (Valium)	Convulsions	5–10 mg

sinus bradycardia. Calcium chloride (10 ml of a 10% solution) may improve myocardial contractility.

The sequence of events for drug administration in a patient with cardiopulmonary arrest could be the following: 50 mEq of sodium bicarbonate and 5 ml of a 1:10,000 solution of epinephrine followed by 10 ml of a 10% calcium chloride solution. This sequence may be repeated every 5 to 10 minutes. Since medications should be given intravenously if possible, and because resuscitation cannot be halted for more than a few seconds at a time, it is almost always necessary for assistants to be available to carry on basic cardiopulmonary resuscitation while an intravenous route is established. If necessary, the medications may be injected directly into the heart by inserting an intracardiac needle in the left fourth intercostal space along the left sternal border.

The use of a myocardial depressant, such as lidocaine, may be necessary in the face of recurrent ventricular tachycardia or ventricular ectopic beats. Lidocaine is best given intravenously as a 100 mg bolus and then as an intravenous drip at a rate of 2 to 3 mg/min.

Therapy for drug reactions should include discontinuing the offending drug and the management of specific nervous system symptomatology, such as convulsions. Convulsions are usually treated with sedatives, such as phenobarbital or diazepam (Valium).

Anaphylactic reactions should be treated with 1 ml of a 1:10,000 solution of epinephrine given intravenously. For associated severe bronchospasm, aminophylline may be helpful.

Evaluation of Rescue Efforts

Every two to three minutes, the effectiveness of the resuscitative effort should be evaluated. The carotid pulse should be checked to determine if cardiac compression is producing an adequate result or if spontaneous cardiac activity has resumed. Dilated and nonreactive pupils indicate cerebral anoxia and cell damage. Pupils that are dilated but reactive imply inadequate cerebral oxygenation, although cellular death has probably not occurred. The decision to terminate CPR is the responsibility of the physician in charge. When the pupils have been dilated and nonreactive for more than 20 minutes, it is unlikely that the victim's central nervous system function can be fully restored.

Assistance and Transport

Although basic life support can be carried out by one resuscitator, assistants allow for advanced resuscitative measures to be provided. If possible, the patient should be transported immediately to a medical facility, but at no time during transport should cardiopulmonary resuscitation be interrupted for more than a few seconds.

Children and Infants

Children and infants require CPR methods adapted to their smaller body size (Fig. 9–12). The child's or infant's back is supported with an arm if necessary. An infant's head is best kept in a semitilt position, since extreme tilting of the supple neck tissues produces angulation of the airway. External cardiac compression is carried out using the tips of the index and middle fingers for infants or the heel of the hand for children. The ventricles in infants and children lie in a higher position, and compression should be at the midsternal level.[12] The sternum is depressed one inch in infants and approximately 1½ inches in children at a rate of 100 times per minute. For artificial ventilation, the rescuer's mouth covers both the nose and mouth of the child, and breathing is done at the rate of 25 to 30 times per minute.

Summary

This chapter has provided a review of emergency life support. The importance of well-coordinated resuscitative efforts has been emphasized. In general, the correct application of the basic techniques of airway maintenance and breathing and circulatory assistance is the main determinant of success. Hope-

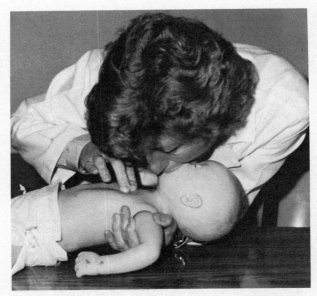

Figure 9–12. Infant resuscitation. The resuscitator's mouth covers the nose and mouth of the infant. Cardiac compression is done with fingertips; the back is supported by the resuscitator's hand and arm.

fully, all physicians will be interested in this crucial facet of medical care and provide themselves with frequent instruction and practice in this area.

REFERENCES

1. Beck CS: Resuscitation for cardiac standstill and ventricular fibrillation occurring during operation. Amer J Surg 54:273, 1941
2. Jude R: Classification of etiology, prevention and treatment of cardiac arrest, in Advances in Cardiopulmonary Resuscitation. New York, Springer-Verlag, 1977
3. Cullen SC, Larson CP: Essentials of Anesthetic Practice. Chicago, Year Book Medical Publishers, 1974
4. Gordon AS et al (American Heart Association Committee on Cardiopulmonary Resuscitation and Emergency Cardiac Care): Standards for cardiopulmonary resuscitation (CPR) and emergency cardiac care (ECC). JAMA 227:837, 1974
5. Standards and guidelines for CPR and emergency cardiac care. JAMA 244:453, 1980
6. Sanders AB, et al: The physiology of cardiopulmonary resuscitation. JAMA 252:3283, 1984
7. Shapter RK et al: Cardiopulmonary resuscitation: Basic life support. Clinical Symposium 26, No. 5, Ciba 1974
8. Oliver GC Jr. Effect of closed-chest cardiac massage on the aortic pulse during ventricular fibrillation. Lancet, 1303, June 13, 1964
9. Oldham HN: Cardiopulmonary Arrest and Resuscitation, in Gibbon's Surgery of the Chest. Philadelphia, W. B. Saunders Co, 1983
10. Watanabe Y, Dreifus L: Arrythmias—Mechanisms and pathogenesis, in Soderman WA, Soderman TM (eds): Pathologic Physiology: Mechanisms of Disease. Philadelphia, W. B. Saunders Co, 1974
11. Resnekov L: Vasoactive cardiac and supportive drugs, in Advances in Cardiopulmonary Resuscitation. New York, Springer-Verlag, 1977
12. Birch LH: Mechanical external cardiac compression and ventilation during cardiopulmonary resuscitation, in Advances in Cardiopulmonary Resuscitation. New York, Springer-Verlag, 1977

Cold Steel Surgery

2

10

MARVIN E. CHERNOSKY, M.D.

Scalpel and Scissors Surgery as Seen by the Dermatologist

This chapter deals with surgery in which the scalpel or scissors or both are the primary, but not the only, cutting instruments used. Other sharp or destructive instruments and modalities such as the razor blade, dermal curette, skin punch, chemical cauterants, electrosurgical equipment, and cryosurgical materals will be mentioned for certain procedures.

Local anesthesia and the doctor's surgical training, self-confidence, ability, personality, and time are factors limiting office skin surgery. Lack of time is often offered as an excuse by the dermatologist as the reason he or she does not perform more office surgery, but both the physician's and patient's time is saved by avoiding hospitalization. Advantages of office-performed surgery and lists of appropriate surgical equipment and materials are given in Chapter 2.

Appropriate immunization with hepatitis B vaccine should be taken by the dermatologist and all assistants.

OFFICE SURGICAL ASSISTANTS

Convenience and time savings result by consistently operating with the same personally trained assistant, nurse, or doctor. A well-informed person outside the surgical field is needed to provide equipment and supplies and to aid in certain procedures.

THE PREOPERATIVE PATIENT

Most patients undergoing office surgery do well during and after the operation because they are ambulatory and do not have acute systemic illnesses. Nevertheless, the physician must record a review of systems and make specific inquiries about bleeding tendencies, drug allergies (including to anesthetics), allergic contact dermatitis to medicines or adhesive tape, keloid formation, scarring tendencies, and what medications the patient is taking. Except for certain minor procedures, elective surgery should not be performed on patients receiving anticoagulants. Consultation with the prescribing physician usually results in an arrangement where the patient can be taken off the drug for a few days pre- and postoperatively. Aspirin is contraindicated from several days to three weeks before an operation because of its effect on platelet aggregation in blood clotting. Blood pressure should be recorded, but a general physical examination is not required in most instances. For most closed surgery (defined below) and fairly extensive procedures that are to be scheduled, a complete blood count, blood glucose level, SGPT assay, and VDRL and hepatitis-associated antigen tests should be ordered. If the history indicates an easy bruising or bleeding tendency, a prothrombin time and partial thromboplastin time are obtained. If the patient is chronically ill, less than one year old, or very elderly, appropriate consultation with the regular physician may be indicated. Before extensive procedures in some patients, I recommend multivitamins containing zinc.

FACTORS AFFECTING SUSCEPTIBILITY TO INFECTION

A number of well-studied factors affect a patient's susceptibility to postoperative infection. The following patient-related factors should be considered prior to surgery:
1. Damaged or diseased skin and callosities.
2. Diabetes.
3. Debilitation.
4. Hypogammaglobulinemia (congential or acquired).
5. Shock.
6. Severe malnutrition (as in alcoholism).
7. Long-term antibiotic therapy.
8. Corticosteroids.
9. Granulocytopenia due to nitrogen mustard, methotrexate, radiation, etc.
10. Emotional stress.
11. Environment—crowded home, staphylococcal or other bacterial carriers, and poor hygiene.

The following are doctor-related factors:
1. Instrument trauma—the unknowing or careless operator can produce unnecessary amounts of devitalized tissue by the crushing action of forceps or clamps. A sharp, single-prong skin hook should be used when possible.
2. Hematomas.

3. Air spaces—so-called "dead spaces" resulting from improper wound closure become filled with serosanguineous material, which offers an ideal place for the growth of microorganisms.
4. Foreign bodies—suture material, glove powder, or aberrant tissue within a wound provide a locus for microorganism growth.
5. Epinephrine in infiltration anesthesia—a possibility proposed by some surgeons, but not valid in my experience.
6. Indequate sterilization procedures.

SEDATION AND ANALGESIA

Preoperative sedation is used only occasionally. For scheduled surgery, night-before or preoperative sedation can be given by mouth, e.g., flurazepam hydrochloride (Dalmane) or diazepam (Valium). A combination of intramuscular and intravenous meperidine (Demerol) and promethazine hydrochloride (Phenergan) is given before more extensive surgery.

Drugs for postoperative pain control include acetaminophen (Tylenol), propoxyphene napsylate and acetaminophen (Darvocet-N), codeine, or meperidine (Demerol). These last two agents may cause nausea, which can be controlled by isopropamide iodide and prochlorperazine (Combid). Specific dosages of the above drugs have been avoided because they are given on a patient-weight basis, and their contraindications and side effects should be well known by the physician prescribing them. The patient must be warned about a possible overdose and advised not to take other self-prescribed medications.

ANESTHESIA

Local infiltration is generally used. Nerve blocks are not as reliable, and their effects develop more slowly. Care should be taken not to insert the anesthesia intravascularly. The smallest volume of anesthesia required to produce the desired effect should be used, and if any reaction occurs, injection should be terminated and appropriate corrective measures taken. The reader is referred to the two previous chapters concerning office emergencies.

Much has been written about the relative advantages, disadvantages, toxicities, and allergic indices of the many drugs used for local anesthesia, and no attempt to summarize these data will be made here. For most closed surgical procedures (defined below), I use 0.5% lidocaine with 1:200,000 epinephrine, which produces capillary constriction. For patients with contraindications and when performing open surgery or surgery in acral areas (e.g., the digits or penis), the epinephrine may be omitted.

Although lidocaine causes pain when injected, its speed of effect is valuable. The manufacturer states that 60 ml of the 0.5% solution without epinephrine is safe in an adult, but this amount has never been required for surgery I have performed. I have never observed a toxic reaction, and only on rare occasions has a possible allergic reaction occurred. Lidocaine does not cross-react with procaine, which has a higher index of sensitivity. For that occasional patient who claims he is allergic to all "-caine" anesthesia, I infiltrate 1% solution of diphenhydramine hydrochloride (Benadryl).

Localized cryoanesthesia is used when incising and draining infected lesions, even though it presents disadvantages such as pain, short duration, difficulty with localization to small areas (with sprays), and the possibility of pigmentary changes resulting from excess freezing. A spray, such as ethyl chloride and dichlorotetra-fluoroethane mixture (Fluoro-ethyl), or solid material (dry ice) can be used.

General anesthesia in a hospital is occasionally used for extensive procedures, such as surgery for hidradenitis suppurativa.

ANTIBIOTICS

Generally, antibiotics are not administered before or after surgery except for an inflamed and infected lesion, extensive closed surgery in cosmetically important contaminated areas near the nose or mouth, or surgery that is required in infected or potentially infected skin such as pustular acne. If antibiotics are given, they are started one day or more before surgery, if possible, and continued several days postoperatively. Certain topical antimicrobial agents are also used postoperatively, as described below.

OPEN SURGERY VERSUS CLOSED SURGERY

In open surgery, the tissue is incised or excised, sometimes cauterized chemically or electrically, or frozen and left open to heal secondarily. The operating tips of instruments are maintained in a sterile condition. Wearing gloves protects the operator from patients with certain types of pathologic conditions. I wear gloves where skin contact with potentially infected fluids and tissues is inevitable, e.g., operations involving a large number of lesions or large abscesses, surgery for rhinophyma or hidradenitis suppurativa, intraoral or genital surgery, and lip shaves. However, for punch biopsies or removal of a few small lesions, I do not routinely wear gloves, because skin contact with blood and tissue usually does not occur. Open surgery is often chosen because of its simplicity, time savings, and economy. Other indications for it include infected wounds, the presence of virus in certain papillomas (verruca vulgaris, or molluscum contagiosum), and the superficial nature of some lesions (seborrheic or actinic keratoses). The rapidity of performing most open surgical procedures allows them to be performed when the patient first presents himself.

Closed surgery produces wound healing by primary intention, because the wound is closed with sutures, tape, or staples in a sterile field utilizing drapes and gloves. Closed surgery may give superior cosmetic results.

Patients should be informed about what to expect. No operation is without some possible undesirable side effects. Consent forms are signed by the patient for some major procedures, especially those performed for cosmetic reasons.

OPEN SURGICAL PROCEDURES

No attempt will be made to mention all types of lesions that may require surgery, but certain conditions will be used to illustrate basic procedures. The skin site is prepared with 70% alcohol. If it is grossly contaminated, water and pHisoHex or Hibiclens followed by 70% alcohol or povidone-iodine (Betadine) solution or both are used. In such areas as the scalp, a small amount of hair may need to be shaved, and a postoperative bandage is not used.

If bandages (Telfa Pad) are applied postoperatively, they are removed later in the day and usually not replaced. The drying effect of air exposure inhibits bacterial growth, which is particularly important in moist hot environments. Some surgeons leave occlusive or partially occlusive dressings or antibacterial ointments on the wound to keep it moist, which, according to some studies, promotes faster epithelialization. For unbandaged wounds on normally dry areas, the patient is encouraged to keep them dry (although many do not), and the wounds usually heal well. For wounds in moist or closed areas (such as the eyelid border, oral commissure, or axilla and beneath a pendulous breast, genitalia, or intergluteal fold), warm water compresses (sometimes with Burow's solution) or hot sitz baths are used twice daily. Betadine solution or 70% alcohol or both are applied. In cases of extensive or deep open surgery, I request the patient to return in one week, because a significant percentage of such wounds will form a purulent exudate beneath the crust. At this stage, better healing occurs by removing the crust, cleaning the base with hydrogen peroxide, and applying 10% silver nitrate solution. Postoperative analgesics or sedation is not required for most open surgery.

Excisions Without Anesthesia

One of the simplest open surgery techniques is the removal without anesthesia of small lesions such as seborrheic keratoses or acrochordons. Large numbers can be snipped off with microscopic dissecting scissors or removed with a curette. Pressure for a few minutes produces hemostasis.

Callosities and Clavi

These lesions can be pared down by use of a sharp no. 10 or 15 Bard-Parker blade or a new double-edged razor blade held so its sharp edge is curved, allowing only the desired portion of skin to be cut. Practice results in competence in this bloodless procedure. Caustic materials, such as trichloroacetic acid, may then be applied, followed by a 40% salicylic acid plaster and repeated paring several days later.

Nevus Cell Nevi

Melanocytic nevi can be cut off with scissors or sliced off with a sharp scalpel at the skin surface and the base of the wound lightly electrodesiccated to produce hemostasis and hopefully to destroy any remaining nevus cells. This furnishes adequate material for histopathologic studies. Scalpel excision and primary wound closure should be used for very active appearing junctional or dysplastic nevi, for nevi with terminal hair, or for lesions in which a diagnosis of melanoma is seriously suspected.

Benign Tumors and Cysts

Small benign lesions, such as mucoceles, papillomas, pyogenic granulomas, hamartomas, and small epidermal inclusion cysts, can be removed with scissors followed by pressure hemostasis, Monsel's solution (ferric subsulfate), or electrodesiccation.

A larger cyst can be eliminated by scalpel excision and primary wound closure (discussed later) or by making a small linear incision into the lesion. Cystic contents are expressed by finger pressure, the wall is clamped with a hemostat, and gentle oscillating forces are applied. As the cyst loosens and begins to emerge from the opening, a second hemostat is applied to the cyst (Fig. 10–1), and this alternating technique is repeated until the wall is removed. Any remaining pieces of the cyst can be removed with a dermal curette. Pressure usually results in hemostasis, but pinpoint electrodesiccation or coagulation may be needed. Because the skin has not been excised, the wound edges usually approximate each other without the use of suture or tapes. If the area is infected, the wound should be irrigated with sterile saline solution and a drain placed for 24 to 48 hours. If, during the above procedure, the cyst cannot be removed with hemostats as described, dissection of tissue around the sac with scissors may be required.

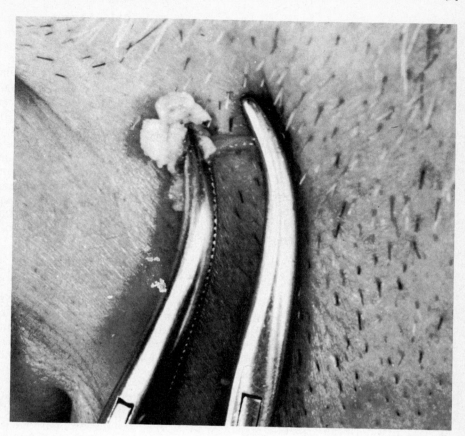

Figure 10–1. Cyst wall being delivered by oscillating forces applied to clamped hemostats.

Chalazia of the eyelids may point to the skin surface or eyelid border, but more often they are deep to the tarsal plate close to the palpebral conjunctiva. After dropping local anesthesia (Ophthane) into the eye, chalazion forceps are clamped around the mass, the eyelid is everted, a 2 mm punch incision is performed, tiny double-pointed Stortz scissors are used to cut out a plug, a 1 mm curette is used to clean out the cystic structure, and pressure is applied to obtain hemostasis. Antibiotic eye drops and hot compresses are used postoperatively.

Pyogenic Abscesses

The incision and draining of a purulent abscess is frequently inadequate because of the doctor's timidity or lack of proper anesthesia or both. Pathogenic microorganisms in the inflamed tissue may contraindicate local infiltration anesthesia. Local cryoanesthesia is often used, but its limitations have been discussed above. Parenteral sedation may be required. A no. 11 Bard-Parker scalpel blade is used to incise deep and long enough to permit adequate drainage. Material can be taken for bacterial cultures and sensitivity studies. A rubber drain or Nu-Gauze may be inserted for 24 hours and replaced several times if needed.

Verruca Vulgaris and Verruca Plantaris

The size of the wart may not at first be appreciated. Better visualization of its borders follows application of mineral oil or 70% alcohol to render the stratum corneum more translucent. Sometimes calloused overlying skin must be shaved off. To decrease the possibility of dissemination of virus, the needle used for infiltration anesthesia should not penetrate the wart. Scissors should be held in an inverted position with points curved downward to allow cutting around the wart in a direction roughly perpendicular to the skin surface. Taking advantage of a fulcrum principle, the Freer elevator is used to lift the wart from its base. If the correct cleavage plane has been attained, the underside of the wart appears convex, smooth, shiny, greyish-white, and avascular. Hemostasis and destruction of any remaining virus-infected cells are accomplished by light electrodesiccation and, if needed, Monsel's solution, sterile Gelfoam packing, and a pressure dressing. Electrodesiccation in certain areas should be avoided in order to avoid excessive scarring, but this may increase the recurrence rate. Many statements in the literature indicate that electrodesiccation is contraindicated on plantar surfaces because of painful postoperative scars. I do not find this to be the case, and for that rare occasion when a tender or hypertrophic scar develops, adequate treatment is available in the form of intralesional corticosteroids or x-ray therapy or both.

Dermal Curettage

The use of the sharp curette is detailed in another chapter. In addition to its use for various benign tumors, it is frequently used in the curettage and desiccation times-two procedure for basal and squamous cell cancers, which has a cure rate greater than 95%.[1] Recently, curettage followed by shave excision of the base with histologic control has been described,[2] but others believe that this more involved and expensive technique is unnecessary.[3, 4]

The Lip Shave

The lip shave is indicated when a large portion of the vermilion border is involved with leukoplakia. After infiltration anesthesia, a new no. 15 scalpel blade is used to shave off the lesion (Fig. 10–2A). Hemostasis is accomplished by bipolar electrocoagulation using a flat straight or hockey-stick active electrode and Monsel's solution. One end of the specimen is marked with dye so that the dermopathologist can orient the specimen. Any area shown to have malignant changes can be treated further. Figure 10–2B shows the postoperative results several months later.

Rhinophyma

Rhinophyma, a condition resulting from long-standing uncontrolled rosacea, is manifested by enlargement of follicular orifices, telangiectasia, papules, and diffuse cutaneous hypertrophy. Before surgical procedures are undertaken, medical treatment and advice to the patient should be given.

For active rosacea and early forms of rhinophyma, telangiectatic vessels can be destroyed with an epilating needle and fine electrodesiccating current. Acneiform rosacea papules can be incised and sutured. Localized areas of tissue hypertrophy can be treated with partial success by repeated intralesional injections of triamcinolone acetonide 3 to 10 mg/ml or by scapel excision utilizing appropriate skin flaps when required.

In some respects, rhinophyma resembles elephantiasis nostras verrucosis, a condition which has been attacked surgically.[5]

For the patient with mild rhinophyma involving most or all of the nasal surface (Fig. 10–3), two methods are advocated: (1) cryosurgery using sufficient liquid nitrogen spray to produce a bullous reaction or (2) dermoplaning under localized cryoanesthesia (Fluoro-ethyl). Details of dermabrasion are given in other chapters.

For the patient with advanced rhinophyma (Fig. 10–4A), a two-stage surgical approach is preferred. After preoperative sedation, the entire nose is infiltrated with 0.5% lidocaine without epinephrine. Some writers indicate that nerve blocks are sufficient, but I have not found this to be the case. A

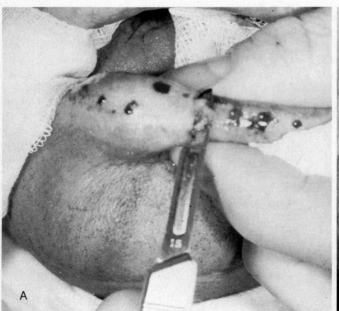
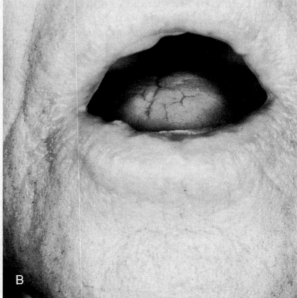

Figure 10–2. *A,* Leukoplakic skin is being shaved off the lip with a scalpel. *B,* Appearance of patient five months after the operation.

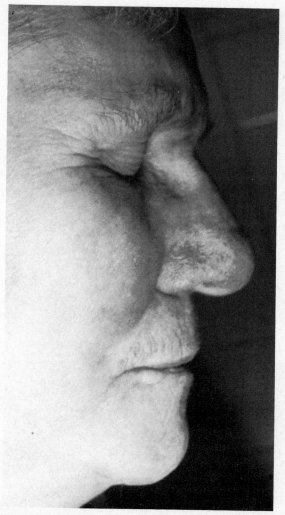

Figure 10–3. A patient with mild to moderate rhinophyma may be a candidate for dermoplaning or liquid nitrogen cryosurgery.

of the excess tissue with scalpel or razor blade, sometimes utilizing the insertion of long needles to guide and limit the depth of the excision. I find the excessive amount of bleeding with this procedure to be annoying, and in my experience, no better cosmetic results are obtained. Caustics, such as full-strength monochloroacetic acid, have been recommended to control hemorrhage, but these materials can cause as much scarring as electrosurgery, and extreme caution must be exercised when using them close to the eyes.

Excision and coverage with full-thickness skin grafts have been used, but in my opinion, this time-consuming procedure does not result in superior cosmetic appearance. New electric dermatomes for paring down tissue and ultra-high-speed equipment for dermoplaning are being evaluated for use on rhinophyma.

Hidradenitis Suppurativa

Axillae, breasts, genito-inguinocrural areas, perineum, and buttocks can be involved because hidradenitis suppurativa is based on occlusion and subsequent infection of apocrine glands. The early acute stage, sometimes called apocrinitis, consists of moderately tender, firm, sometimes erythematous dermal nodules, which may be misdiagnosed as inflamed epidermal inclusion cysts or furuncles. The nodules extend laterally and deeply and form multiple sinus tracts opening on the surface. At first, they contain a yellowish, translucent, gelatin-like, thick material, but they become pustular with ensuing bacterial infection. Scar formation results in further occlusion of glands and extension of the process.

For early stages of hidradenitis suppurativa, conservative treatment should be tried. The doctor should take the time to develop a good rapport with the patient and explain the recurring nature of the disease. A promise of a cure without recurrence should not be made. The patient should agree to return to the office when indicated and not to neglect the condition. Incision and drainage of lesions and bacterial cultures and sensitivity studies are carried out. Appropriate systemic antibiotics are given in full dosage for an extended period of time together with systemic steroids, provided there are no strict contraindications. Skin care includes the use of antibacterial cleansers such as Hibiclens or Safeguard and topical clindamycin in a nonocclusive base. The patient must be followed, but sometimes, from a combination of patient and doctor neglect or unrealistic promises of cures by each new doctor consulted, the condition progresses insidiously over a period of years and becomes a major problem. Aggressive surgery should not be delayed until patients can no longer move their arms because of

hockey-stick active electrode is used on a bipolar electrosection unit to excise slices of tissue. The nose is stabilized by inserting a finger in one naris or by grasping the columella between the thumb and forefinger. The electric current provides some hemostasis, but Monsel's solution and pressure may be required. Healing is complete in three to six weeks.

Some surface irregularities and scarring remain. Under local cryoanesthesia with Fluoro-ethyl, the surface of the nose is dermoplaned with a coarse diamond fraise. The result four months later is shown in Figure 10–4B. Hypopigmentation may remain postoperatively. The procedures not only correct the rhinophyma but usually prevent recurrence of active rosacea even though active disease might be manifest in other areas.

Some authors advocate a one-step paring down

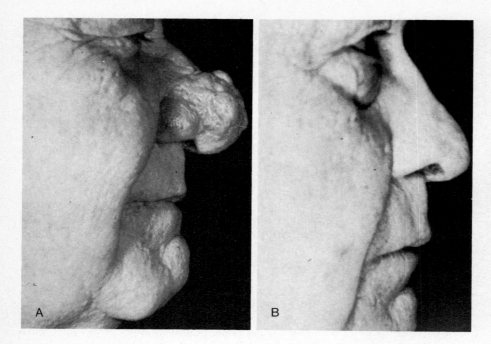

Figure 10—4. *A*, Preoperative appearance of a patient with advanced rhinophyma. *B*, Appearance after a two-stage surgical procedure.

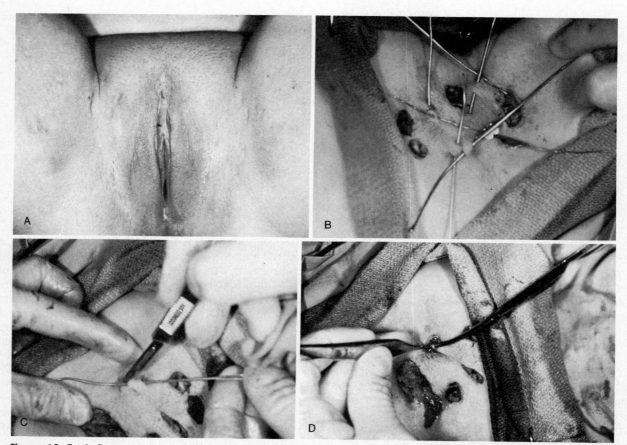

Figure 10—5. *A*, Preoperative condition of patient with long-standing hidradenitis suppurativa appears minimal because of suppression with systemic steroids, antibiotics, and topical treatment. *B*, Flexible lacrimal probes inserted into the sinus tracts; some cystic areas and tracts have already been removed. *C*, A scalpel is used to cut tissue over the probe. *D*, Edges of tissue overhanging the tract are grasped with toothed forceps and trimmed off with scissors.

Illustration continued on opposite page

pain, sit down without discomfort, perform sexual intercourse, or put up with the malodorous discharges that soil their clothing. Furthermore, longstanding, extensive hidradenitis suppurativa has been associated with cachexia, anemia,[6] and interstitial keratitis.[7]

If large areas of tissue are affected, the patient should have general anesthesia. Figure 10–5A shows a patient who had persistent hidradenitis suppurativa for years. Erythema, edema, and sinus drainage do not appear great because of suppression for many weeks with topical and systemic medications. Flexible lacrimal probes are inserted into the sinus tracts (Fig. 10–5B). A scalpel is used to cut through the superficial tissue to the probe (Fig. 10–5C). Redundant tissue overhanging the base of the tract is excised with surgical scissors (Fig. 10–5D). The contents and lining of the tract and cavities are removed with a sharp curette (Fig. 10–5E). The completely exposed area is then electrodesiccated or electrocoagulated (Fig. 10–5F) to promote he-

mostasis, destroy any remaining tract lining, and temporarily destroy nerve endings in the area for a relatively pain-free recovery. Bandages are not applied (Fig. 10–5G). On some patients several hundred tracts, blind pouches, cysts, and acneiform lesions have been removed during one operation.

The healing time of wounds depends upon their size and the overall systemic condition of the patient (Fig. 10–5H). After reepithelialization, the patient should reinstitute the antibacterial soap. Periodic observations are mandatory. If small lesions develop, they should be treated surgically under local anesthesia in the office.

In lieu of the above marsupialization procedure, small resectable lesions can be excised, drains placed, and the wound closed with sutures (as described below). Some surgeons advocate extensive excisions, such as the removal of all of the skin of the axillae and covering the area with a skin graft. This may result in sufficient loss of sweat glands that it causes a symptomatic dry intertrigo.

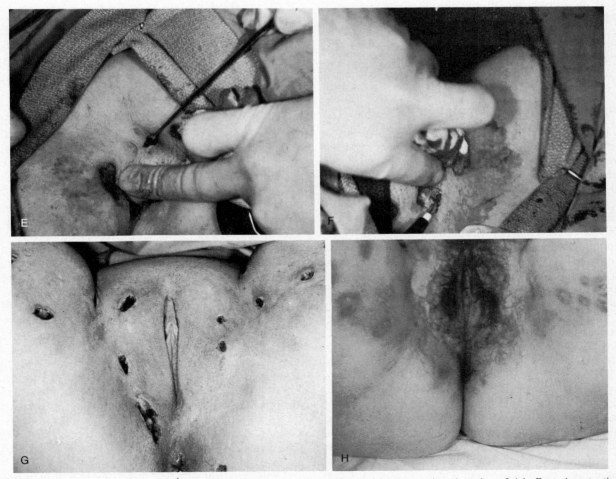

Figure 10–5 Continued. E, The tract lining is curetted. F, Electrocoagulation of the areas has three beneficial effects (see text). G, Postoperative appearance of patient. H, Patient three months after the operation. She remained symptom-free for two years without systemic medication or incision and drainage of additional lesions.

CLOSED SURGERY

There has recently been a growing interest in and greater utilization of dermatologic surgery, especially closed techniques performed in an office setting. This is witnessed by the growth of the American Society for Dermatologic Surgery to over 1490 members, publication of the *Journal of Dermatologic Surgery and Oncology,* more attention paid to this field by the American Board of Dermatology and the Association of Dermatology Professors, and the larger number of surgical educational programs being offered. Dermatologists are performing more closed surgery and are utilizing more complex techniques when required.

The reader is referred to material in the first portion of this chapter that applies to closed surgery. Closed procedures require a significant amount of time, and I perform such operations on Monday and Tuesday of each week so that early postoperative complications, if any, as well as suture removal will not occur during the weekend.

At the time of scheduling, certain laboratory tests are ordered (see above), and patients are requested to wash the operative site for several days with 4% chorhexidine skin cleanser (Hibiclens), avoiding the eyes and ears.

Preoperative Preparation of the Patient

Some patients undergoing closed surgery require preoperative sedation. The area of skin prepared for surgery must be adequate and large enough to allow for extending incision lines. Preoperative removal of hair by shaving or clipping has been contraindicated by some investigators because of an associated increase in postoperative infection.[8] They recommended no preparation or use of depilatory cream. But long hair interferes with operative techniques, and depilatories often cause primary irritation and occasionally allergic contact dermatitis. If shaving is performed, it should be done *immediately* before the surgery,[9] although short vellus hair, eyebrows, and sometimes pubic hair need not be removed. If the lesion is on the face, neck, or scalp, adjacent hair is taped down with Micropore Skin-Tone Surgical Tape or confined in a turban fashioned from a towel and clips. Skin contaminated with hair oil or other material is cleaned with ether. The site is then scrubbed with Hibiclens and water. The surface is dried with sterile gauze squares and painted with Betadine solution. Indistinct borders of surface lesions are marked with a pointed stick dipped in 2% gentian violet solution before infiltration anesthesia is administered.

Instruments and Materials for Closed Surgery

Prepared autoclaved packs contain the following:
1. Two sterile towels
2. One sterile eyesheet
3. Two sterile swabs
4. Sterile 2 × 2, 12-ply sponges
5. Two hemostats
6. One Hudson forceps
7. One Ochsner clamp with teeth

To this basic pack, the following dry-heat or factory-sterilized sharp instruments and materials are routinely added by using transfer forceps:
1. Bard-Parker handle, no. 15 scalpel blade
2. Curved, double-pointed, microscopic dissecting scissors
3. Olsen-Hegar needle holder and combined scissors with Ochsner diamond jaws
4. Suture scissors, 1 end blunt, 1 end pointed
5. Laschal Precision Suture Tome, Model 403, with a no. 15 slot
6. Skin hook
7. Suture materials
8. One 10 cc syringe
9. One 21-gauge needle
10. One 27- or 30-gauge needle

Additional special instruments such as probes, self-retaining retractors, tenotomy scissors, and Casteneri's rhytidectomy dissection scissors are added to the tray as required. A bipolar electrocoagulation unit with sterile electrodes or active electrode tip should be at hand. Usually, a mask is not worn unless the operator or assistant has a cough or suspects the onset of an upper respiratory tract infection. Sterile gloves are always employed when contact with blood or tissues is likely. Some doctors claim they do not need gloves and seldom have postoperative infections. One explanation lies in the fact that there is a wide variation in opinion as to what constitutes an infection. Some physicians simply ignore sizable amounts of edema, erythema, and wound drainage! Furthermore, surgeons who do not wear gloves are probably more likely not to use buried sutures, and this allows them to get by with less stringent aseptic techniques. The use of gloves to help protect the surgeon from hepatitis has recently been stressed.[10, 11] Sterile cloth towels and eyesheets made of 250-weave pima cotton are still preferred in my office because they do not tear or shred into the wound. Many types of disposable drapes are available, and I do use them at times.

The Incision

Consideration must be given to the direction of lines of incision. Among the influencing factors are

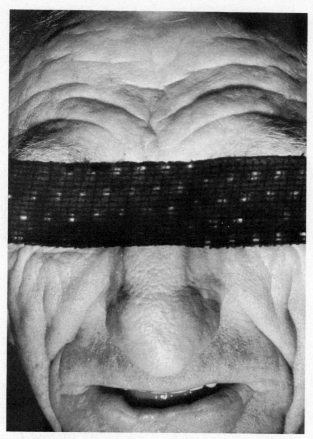

Figure 10–6. Wrinkle lines are helpful in determining the direction of surgical incision lines.

wrinkle lines of the skin that run perpendicular to the long axis of the major underlying musculature (Fig. 10–6). Note, for example, that wrinkle lines, or lines of expression, on the forehead run horizontally at right angles to the frontalis muscle. Incisions placed in such a manner that the scar (the suture line) is parallel to these lines will give the best cosmetic results. Wrinkle lines on the extremities run circumferentially. On the anterior trunk, they are directed horizontally except over the pectoral muscles in the male. Diagrams showing details have been published elsewhere.[12, 13]

Wrinkle lines vary, and in many people, especially the young, they are not clinically evident. They can be made visible by contracting appropriate underlying muscles such as when saying "cheese," grimacing, or hyperextending the shoulders, but these lines may not coincide exactly with those that will develop naturally with aging. Compression of the skin gently between thumb and forefinger held 2 or 3 cm apart results in regular folds of skin if the pressure is parallel to wrinkle lines and irregular folds if it is perpendicular to them. The patient should be in the sitting or standing position, a

neutral position, when determining incision lines. This is especially true for incisions on joints, face, and neck and for patients with sagging skin and subcutaneous tissues. If in doubt about the placement of incisions, one can excise the lesion in a circular configuration, undermine the edges, and then by using skin hooks pull the edges together in different directions to find the least resistance.

Langer's lines of skin tension, previously used as a guide for incisions, often run at angles to wrinkle lines; but when both types of lines coincide, excellent postoperative healing can be expected. Examples of such locations would be on the neck and just inferior to the eyes. In some instances, such as over the bony pretibial area, I find that a longitudinal suture line gives the best result, even though this direction is perpendicular to the wrinkle lines.

Factors other than wrinkle lines and Langer's lines must be considered. Figure 10–7 shows an acceptable postoperative scar on the right upper lip of a patient who had a lesion with a larger horizontal than vertical dimension. A small, horizontal, fusiform excision was made that, in this case, was perpendicular to wrinkle lines. Previous surgery in an area has to be considered because of residual, less-flexible scar tissue. Scars can be placed in areas hidden by eyeglasses, scalp hair, or a beard. Incisions should not cross major lines of expression or flexural creases.

When planning for excisions, care must be taken to try to prevent the loss or distortion of structures of cosmetic or functional importance, such as the eyebrow, eyelid border, lip, scalp border, sideburn, columella, sublingual frenulum, or fingernail. Procedures somewhat more complex than a fusiform excision may be required. In some areas where incisions are likely to extend deeply, anatomic di-

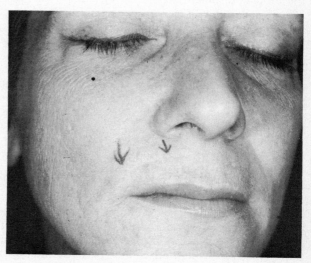

Figure 10–7. In this case, the suture line is perpendicular to the direction of wrinkle lines.

rection and location of major blood vessels, nerves, and other structures must be considered.

Some surgeons routinely mark the lines to be incised with gentian violet. A series of parallel lines perpendicular to what is believed to be the resulting suture line is then placed as a guide for suturing the wound edges. I do not use these markings except for certain procedures, such as on the eyebrows or lips.

An adequate length-to-width ratio should be planned for a fusiform defect. My experience indicates that a ratio greater than 2 or 3 to 1 will often suffice, but a 3 or 4 to 1 ratio may be preferable at times.

Sometimes, it is helpful for the surgeon and assistant to place tension on the skin to be incised. The scalpel blade should be held perpendicular to the skin surface. Often, the novice surgeon will have a tendency to slant the blade as it traverses an arcing line, resulting in beveled skin edges whose surfaces do not closely approximate when sutured. Incisions should be as deep at the ends as they are at the center. When clinical judgment indicates that pathologic tissue is deep and not attached to the integument, a single linear incision is used.

Hemostasis

The use of 1:200,000 epinephrine in the infiltrated anesthesia, when not contraindicated, helps prevent bleeding from small vessels. Larger vessels are clamped with small curved hemostats, which are touched with the sterilized tip of a bipolar electrocoagulator by an assistant not within the sterile field. Another efficient method is to grasp the bleeding vessels with the microbipolar forceps attached to the bipolar terminals of the Hyphecator. Less than 1% of severed vessels require ligation. To insure against slippage, a suture (white Dexon-S, Vicryl, Ethibond, or Mersilene with a round noncutting needle) can be placed close to the clamped end of the vessel and then tied around it. Because of the retraction of vessels, most hemostasis in scalp wounds is accomplished by placing large approximating sutures that encompass a large amount of tissue.

Dissection and Excision Beneath the Skin Level

These procedures are accomplished with the scalpel, curved scissors, and the spreading action of hemostats. After excision of pathologic tisue, skin flaps as well as wound edges may be undermined to prevent undue tension during closure. Where there is little subcutaneous fascia, blunt dissection can be performed with the finger or the piercing and

spreading action of a hemostat. The scalpel should not be used by an inexperienced operator or by anyone in a casual manner. Using a skin hook to hold the skin up and under direct vision, the surgeon should undermine the dermis at a level in the superficial subcutaneous fat. In the scalp, dissection should be below the galea aponeurotica. To fill in large deep defects, deeper undermining may be required.

Wound Closure

Wounds should be closed in anatomic layers to eliminate dead air spaces and to allow proper union during healing. Even though suture closure will provide some hemostasis, it should not be relied upon to do so except in certain areas such as the scalp.

Tension sutures bring tissue edges toward each other and reduce tension on the healing wound surfaces. Approximating sutures are used to properly align the interface of the cut tissues to produce primary healing. They should be placed close to the wound edges. Individually tied sutures are used most often in dermatologic surgery. Because continuous sutures are fixed only at each end of the wound, they can be inserted more quickly but may cause uneven approximation, predispose to multiple stitch infections, or allow complete wound dehiscence if any one portion breaks. Unnecessary strangulation of vascular supply occurs if sutures are tied too tightly.

The question always arises about how far apart or how many sutures should be used. One should use only as many sutures as needed. Figure 10–8 shows surface sutures closely spaced around the point of the chin and farther apart at the superior

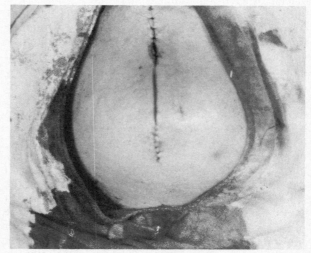

Figure 10–8. Wound closure by irregularly spaced sutures (see text).

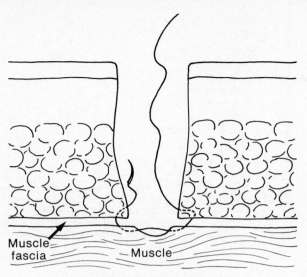

Figure 10–9. Muscle fascial suture.

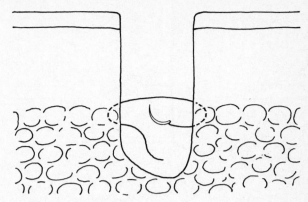

Figure 10–11. Superficial subdermal and subcutaneous suture placed so knot will be deep.

end. Subcutaneous sutures are causing near approximation in the center. I most often use the Olsen-Hegar needle holder and combination scissors to place sutures while holding the tissues with a sharp single-pronged skin hook.

Figure 10–9 illustrates a simple suture used to close muscle fascia deep within the wound. A round noncutting needle should be employed to avoid causing any additional hemorrhage. Figure 10–10 illustrates the placement of an interrupted subcutaneous suture used to approximate tissues and relieve tension from surface edges. If the suture is close to the surface, the knot should be placed in the deep loop as in Figure 10–11. The loop of this buried suture can be placed horizontally to the skin surface in a small wound that allows only one suture, the net effect being that of two buried sutures in relation to the long axis of the suture line (Fig. 10–12). Some writers have indicated that buried sutures

should seldom, if ever, be used in cutaneous surgery, but I disagree with this view. Because of wound healing rates and scar tensile strength, proper use of buried sutures is important.

Figure 10–11 shows the position of a superficial suture passing through the lower dermis so that the knot and suture ends will face away from the sur-

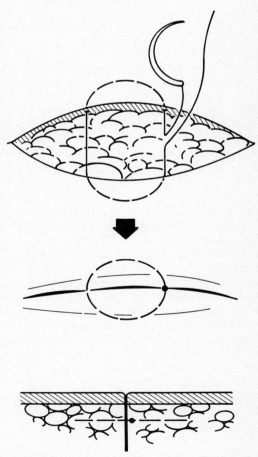

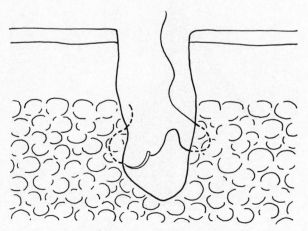

Figure 10–10. Subcutaneous suture.

Figure 10–12. Horizontally buried subcutaneous suture.

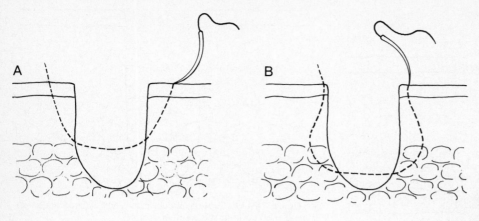

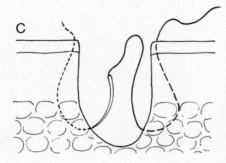

Figure 10–13. Near-far—far-near everting suture. *A,* Incorrect procedure. *B,* Correct procedure. *C,* Frequently, each edge of the wound must be handled separately.

face. This type of suture is used in areas where there is not enough subcutaneous fascia to suture together.

Figure 10–13 illustrates the near-far—far-near everting approximating suture. The "near" and the "far" refer to the distance from the cut wound edges. Encompassing greater masses of deep tissue produces desired eversion of the wound edges, which flatten out postoperatively. If stitches are inserted first at each end, placement of remaining sutures is facilitated by an assistant producing tension on the wound edges by holding the first stitches (Fig. 10–14).

Horizontal (Fig. 10–15A) and vertical (Fig. 10–15B) mattress sutures are used primarily as tension sutures and to produce eversion. They aid in hemostasis but should not routinely be relied upon to do so. Bolsters made from cutting single- or double-layered strips from the cardboard in the suture package can be placed between the skin surface and loops of mattress sutures to disseminate pressures. A half-buried, horizontal mattress suture is used to avoid piercing the surface of a pointed tip of the tissue. The suture remains buried in the tip of tissue opposite the knot by passing in and out of the cut vertical surfaces. The locking vertical mattress suture is designed to act as a combination tension and approximating suture. This is accomplished by passing the needle shown in Figure 10–15B through the

loop of suture on the opposite (left) side of the wound and then recrossing and tying the knot. An improved vertical mattress suture leaves no noticeable suture-produced cross marks on the skin.[14] The suture enters the skin surface at one edge, remains buried in the opposite edge, and is brought out as

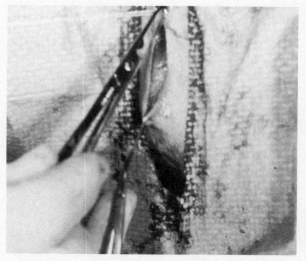

Figure 10–14. Longitudinal tension, placed on the wound edges by an assistant, aids in the placement of remaining sutures.

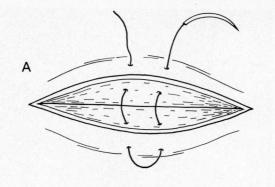

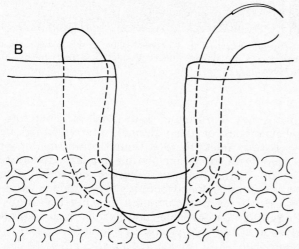

Figure 10–15. *A,* Horizontal mattress suture—used mainly as a retention suture when there is unavoidable tension on the edges. *B,* Vertical mattress suture—used as a retention suture and to evert wound edges.

close to the point of entrance as possible. Because the knot will bury itself, it is tied over a separate loop of suture, which facilitates removal later.

Intracuticular or subdermal continuous sutures do not produce "railroad tracks" because they pierce the skin surface only at each end (Fig. 10–16). This allows them to be left in for up to six or eight weeks

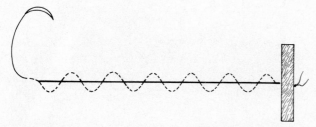

Figure 10–16. Intracuticular or subcutaneous continuous suture.

in areas where healing is slow (e.g., the lower extremities in the elderly) or to prevent wide scars in areas such as the upper trunk, arm, or shoulder (Fig. 10–17).

Although the suture needle is usually grasped by the needle holder at right angles, the suturing of this type of running stitch is facilitated by angling the needle point toward the wound edge being pierced. Figure 10–18A shows the needle angulating toward the skin edge opposite the operator, and Figure 10–18B shows the needle pointing back to the edge closest to the operator. If the wound is longer than 5 cm, the suture is brought to the surface at intervals to facilitate removal by cutting at these places. If the suture is placed below the dermis, additional surface-approximating sutures or tape splints may be required. When properly placed within the dermis, no additional sutures are needed.

Continuous surface sutures are not used commonly, except when stainless steel wire is inserted over joints where there is no strong subcutaneous fascia, or on the distal lower extremities of elderly patients where the dermis is thin and healing slow. Ends of the sutures are tied, or preferably anchored with crimped lead beads.

Protrusion of excess tissue near the ends of the wound, so-called dog-ears, should be avoided in fusiform excisions by an adequate length-to-width excision ratio, deep excision of enough tissue near the ends of the wound, adequate undermining of wound edges, and beginning the closure at the ends of the wound. Despite these precautions, dog-ears may occur in fusiform excisions and during more complex procedures. Figure 10–19 shows four methods of repair. The dotted lines indicate additional skin incisions or excisions.

Wound Healing in Relation to Sutures

Many studies indicate that a healed wound never becomes as strong as normal skin.[15–17] The mechanisms suggested to explain development of strength in a scar are: (1) an increase in the amount of collagen, (2) an increase in the extent of cross-linking of collagen, and (3) some type of interaction between collagen fibers and the ground substance. Forrest and Jackson demonstrated increased intermolecular covalent cross-linking in guinea pig scars but not in human scars, and therefore they suggested that long-term tensile strength cannot be correlated to this factor.[18]

Tensile strength studies have indicated that scar tissue recovers only 10 to 30% of its maximum strength at 14 days postoperatively. Furthermore, Forrester and colleagues claim that wound toughness or ability to resist rupture (energy absorption) is incompletely described by measurements of tensile strength.[16] When extension, or "give," is taken

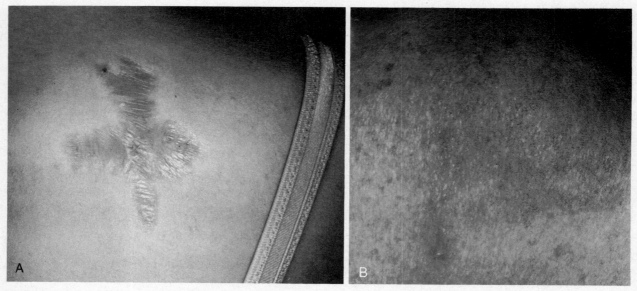

Figure 10–17. *A,* Three-month postoperative site on shoulder. Surgery performed in a hospital prior to this writer's initial examination. *B,* Three-month postoperative vertical suture line scar (see arrows) on shoulder utilizing buried 5-0 Mersilene suture and a running 4-0 Prolene intracuticular stitch that was left in place six weeks.

into account, the recovered energy absorption (compared to normal skin) is only approximately 8% at 10 days and 50% at 150 days postoperatively. Further evidence for ongoing activity in scars is provided by collagen kinetics using tritium-labeled proline.[17] This study showed a higher rate of synthesis and degradation in scar tissue than in normal skin for 90 days postoperatively.

These basic studies, plus the all-important clinical fact that one must prevent the spreading of a postoperative scar if possible, would indicate that some material is needed to bind wound edges together

that is not removed in 3 to 21 days. Therefore, subcutaneous or deep dermal sutures should be employed, unless there is wound contamination or a scarcity of fascia and dermis available to suture together. Gut sutures in or buried beneath the skin should be abandoned because they produce excessive tissue reaction compared to synthetic sutures. Present-day absorbable polyglycolic acid sutures (Dexon-S) and polyglactin 910 sutures (Vicryl) retain only 55% of original tensile strength at 14 days and 20% at 21 days after implantation. The newer polydioxanone (PDS) monofilament absorbable su-

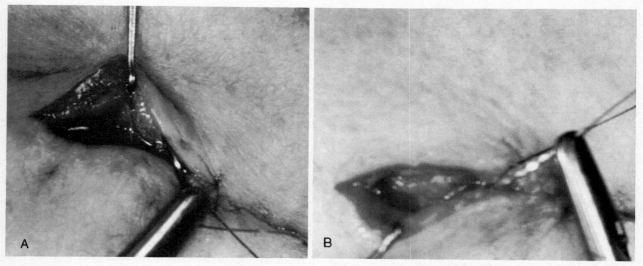

Figure 10–18. *A,* A needle pointing toward the wound edge to be sutured. *B,* Needle points toward the tissue to be sutured.

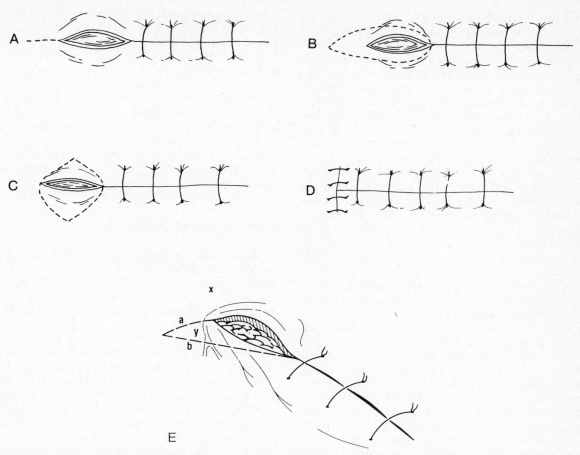

Figure 10–19. Four methods to repair dog-ears at the ends of wounds. *A,* First method. *B,* Second method. *C* and *D,* Third method. *E,* Fourth method; line "a" shows the extension of a suture line; tissue "y" is pulled over tissue "x" to determine the location of the second excision line "b"; closure of the wound results in a curved suture line.

tures do retain tensile strength longer (14% at 56 days), but one wonders if the retained tensile strength of these buried sutures is sufficient to consistently obtain the desired narrow suture line scar. For subcutaneous and subdermal tissues, I presently continue to use nonabsorbable sutures because they maintain most of their tensile strength when measured up to 24 months postoperatively,[19] and they evoke less tissue reaction than other sutures.[20–22]

Suture Materials

Proper choice of suture materials is related to wound healing factors, as previously outlined. Many writers have simply stated what they like to use without explaining their choice. Because a suture is traumatic and a foreign body, needles and materials should be the smallest size consonant with anatomic location, mobility of the area, and tension of the tissues. A curved, reverse cutting-edged, 3/8-inch eyeless needle with suture swaged to the end passes easily through skin and subcutaneous fascia without much trauma. The recently developed Precision Cosmetic Needle (Ethicon) with conventional cutting tip and square shank offers some improvement in strength, sharpness retention, and needle holdability. Needles with a round, tapered noncutting shank are used on deep muscle fascia and other areas where a cutting-edged needle may needlessly sever blood vessels.

White Vicryl or Dexon-S (4-0 or 5-0) is used on deep muscle fascia. On subcutaneous fascia and deep dermal surfaces, white 5-0 polyester fiber suture (Mersilene, Ethibond, Ticron) is used because: (1) its synthetic composition produces little tissue reaction and (2) it maintains tensile strength for an extended period of time. The polybutilate (on Ethibond) or silicone (on Ticron) coating lowers the friction coefficient, which allows the suture to pass through tissues easily and to tie without grabbing or sticking, but this characteristic does not allow much tension on the first double loop when instrument-tying a knot. When cutting the suture, ends should safely protrude about 2 mm away from the knot. The higher friction coefficient of Mersilene makes it better for instrument ties (with a needle holder), but it causes some resistance the first time the suture is pulled through tissue. This is greatly reduced after it becomes coated with tissue fluids. Skin surgeons should discipline themselves by using only as little buried suture as required. The multifilament braided nature of Mersilene produces a low memory (i.e., a tendency to stay tied), and therefore suture ends should be cut adjacent to the knot by sliding the scissors (held at 90 degrees) on the suture down until the knot is felt and rotating the scissors about 30 degrees before cutting. The Laschal Precision Suture Tome, described in Chapter 2, is easier to use and more efficient when cutting sutures adjacent to the knot.

Synthetic nonabsorbable, monofilament sutures are usually used on the skin because they produce the least tissue reaction. Nylon or Prolene (5-0 or 6-0) is used on the face, neck, breast, and some other areas with delicate skin, and in sizes 2-0, 3-0, or 4-0 on the trunk and extremities and in any location for intracuticular running or mattress type retention sutures. Stainless steel wire is employed as noted previously. Vicryl or Dexon-S (3-0, 4-0, or 5-0) is used as interrupted surface sutures on mucous membranes, vulva, penis, and perineum, because these areas invariably develop some postoperative tissue reaction, and absorbable sutures avoid painful and tedious removal. Soft, nonsticking, strong Ethibond (5-0 or 4-0) is used on areas such as the lip and eyelids. For small wounds, for some contaminated wounds, or when subcutaneous suturing affords near approximation, surface closure with tape (Steri-Strip or Clearon) is used.

In addition, I have had some experience with various clip or stapel instruments used for skin closure. Presently, I use the Auto-Suture (see Fig. 2–6), particularly to close 4 to 6 mm punch biopsy sites or excisions of small lesions where optimum cosmetic results are not required. Its timesaving features allow many procedures to be performed during a routine office visit. Partially used packets of staples are washed immediately and later sterilized by ethylene oxide at a nearby hospital. Several brands of disposable instruments have recently become available.

Tying Sutures

The square knot is used routinely. I often apply a third knot on top of the square knot, and sometimes a fourth knot when using a monofilament suture with high memory (i.e., an increased tendency to return to its untied state). A surgeon's knot, consisting of a double first loop, is used when the wound edge tension provokes a loosening of a knot before it can be completed. The first loop can be further "locked" to maintain tension temporarily by holding both ends of the suture tight and crossing over to bring one end next to the other before tying the second loop. Instrument ties are usually used in skin surgery to save time and suture material. If the combination needle holder and scissors is used, sutures can be cut rapidly without the need of an assistant. Hand ties are valuable when ligating a blood vessel or when there is considerable tension on skin edges.

When to Drain a Wound

Indications for placement of a drain in a wound include the following: (1) infected or potentially infected wounds, (2) foreign body (inclusion cyst material), (3) difficult to control capillary hemorrhage, and (4) areas subjected to excess movement (neck or axilla).

After suturing part of the edges closed, a drain can be placed by inserting a hemostat through the dependent end of the wound and pushing it underneath the sutures until the tip appears on the surface close to the opposite end. A drain (a sterilized rubber band or strip from a rubber glove) is grasped and pulled through the wound. The protruding lower end can be anchored with a single surface suture. Care must be taken when applying the balance of the sutures not to sew the drain into the depth of the wound. Drains are usually removed in 24 hours.

Wound Dressings

Postoperative dressings often are not used on such areas as the axilla, perineum, and mucocutaneous junctions. When small areas of hair are shaved, such as on the scalp or beard, a small neat-appearing dressing can be attached to the skin by the use of flexible collodion. In other areas, a sterile Telfa-Pad is placed against the closed wound, after which gauze squares and tape are applied. Appropriate thickness of dressings and application of tape should be employed to cause some pressure on the area to aid in immobilization and prevention of hemorrhage. For procedures on the extremities, especially distally, an elastic bandage may be applied over the tape. On occasion, for even better immobilization, I have used isoprene splints (Orthoplast) for a few days postoperatively. These splints are malleable when heated with warm water and become firm when cool. Except for minor procedures, I usually have the patient return in one day to check for any complications and to reduce the size of the bandage. Patients are instructed to change their own bandages periodically. Some surgeons apply an antibiotic ointment postoperatively.

A recent report[23] advocates the postoperative application of an opaque, nonsterile, semipermeable woven tape over the suture line for several days without changing it. This approach is based on the work of Rovee and coworkers who demonstrated: (1) faster epithelialization of occluded nonsutured incisions than of air-exposed ones and (2) a more level plane of epithelialization in occluded wounds than in air-exposed ones.[24] I wonder if their findings would be significant at the clinical level when applied to carefully approximated wound edges. Occlusive or partially occlusive materials produce increased microbial populations and stratum corneum maceration that should be considered, especially in climates with high ambient temperature and humidity. Op-Site (a transparent film occlusive to microorganisms but permeable to air and moisture vapor), Vigilon (hydrogel formulation of water and polyethylene oxide), and Duoderm (a flexible hydroactive dressing) have all proved to be effective in the healing of open wounds, but their routine use in approximated wounds is not well established.

Suture Removal and Skin Splinting

Sutures should be removed as soon as possible after taking into consideration the original tensions on the wound edges, anatomic site, mobility of the area, rate of wound healing, presence or absence of infection, and future plans for splinting the skin. In general, interrupted approximating sutures are removed from the face in three to four days, from the neck in five to seven days, from the scalp in seven days, from the trunk and upper extremities in 12 to 14 days, and from the lower extremities in 14 to 28 days. Wound healing on the distal lower extremities of the elderly is especially slow. Retention sutures may be left in place longer than approximating sutures. At times, only a portion of the sutures are removed. Continuous intracuticular or subcutaneous sutures may be left in place for several weeks.

Skin splints in the form of Micropore Skin-Tone Surgical Tape, Steri-Strips, or Clearon are applied when sutures are removed. On hairy areas such as the beard, hair may grow through a single layer of the paper tape instead of pushing it off. Patients should not change their own splints because they are likely to subject the wound to harmful stress. They are instructed to return for replacement when splints begin to loosen, not after they come off. The removing force on each end of the splint should be toward the suture line. Acetone or ether is used as a solvent. Skin splints are kept on two to six weeks

after suture removal, and their importance should not be underestimated.

Tissue Expanders

When primary skin closure utilizing various skin flap procedures is not possible, skin grafts may be required, although the resulting cosmetic appearance is often not desirable. Recent work by Argenta[25] and others on tissue expansion promises more primary closures without grafts. Inflatable tissue expanders are placed under normal skin adjacent to the lesion (see Chapter 54). Repeated inflation causes the skin to expand. This excess tissue is then used to primarily close the wound.

Specific Operative Procedures

For the remainder of this chapter, some specific procedures will be discussed to illustrate techniques previously described. No attempt will be made to outline all pathologic conditions and indications for closed surgery.

Fusiform Excision on the Eyelid

Figure 10–20 shows an adequate length-to-width ratio, undermined skin flaps, and wound edges held taut by tensions on sutures placed at the ends. Excellent cosmetic results can be obtained without buried sutures on the eyelids. Ethibond is used because its softness prevents the cut ends from sticking into the skin. Because of the difficulty of applying them and the nuisance to the patient, postoperative bandages are often omitted in eyelid surgery.

Vertical Fusiform Excision of the Eyebrow

Figure 10–21A shows a basal cell carcinoma and the proposed lines of excision. Note that the suture line is not parallel to the wrinkle lines. The dark crust within the lesion represents a previous 2 mm punch biopsy. For most suspected malignancies, a small incisional biopsy is performed, and at the return visit, a thorough explanation is given regarding the histologic diagnosis, possible methods of treatment, prognosis, need for future preventive measures, and necessary follow-up visits. A good rapport is thus developed with the patient. This lady chose closed surgery. Another person might have chosen the quicker, less troublesome, cheaper curettage and desiccation method and would not have been upset with a hairless, depressed white scar. The five-year cure rate for both methods is essentially the same.

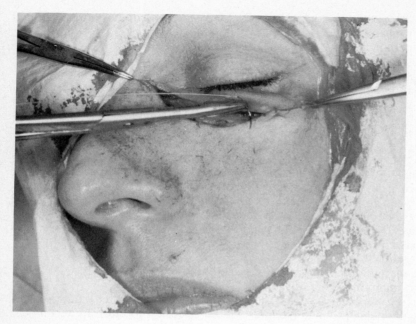

Figure 10–20. Fusiform wound on the eyelid.

Contrary to many statements in the literature citing the need for removing or destroying 4 to 10 mm of adjacent normal-appearing skin, I have obtained a high cure rate using 2 to 5 mm borders of normal skin in most small, moveable, well-defined and probably shallow basal or squamous cell carcinomas.[26, 27] This is consistent with the observations by others about the accuracy of visual assessment of basal cell carcinoma margins.[28] To accomplish this, one must mark very carefully the tumor margin prior to infiltration anesthesia, utilizing a sharp pointed stick dipped in gentian violet solution. Frequently, 4 to 6 power magnification is used. Figure 10–21B shows the postoperative results six months later. About 1/4 to 1/3 of the length of an eyebrow can be excised in this manner without causing excessive asymmetry.

Larger normal skin borders are required for sclerosing basal cell carcinoma, highly aggressive squamous cell carcinoma, and large lesions (over 20 mm).

Pigmented Lesions

Scalpel excision and primary closure of pigmented nevi often results in better cosmetic appearance than removal by scissors and electrodesiccation. For nevi with terminal hairs, care must be taken to excise deeply enough to include hair bulbs and papillae. Only 1 or 2 mm borders of normal skin are needed for intradermal nevi, but slightly larger ones are preferred for compound, junctional, and dysplastic nevi.

Before attempting excisional biopsy of a suspected melanoma, the reader is directed to published techniques related to specific types.[29] The writer believes that the office-based dermatologic surgeon should

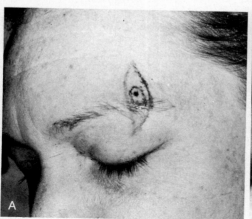
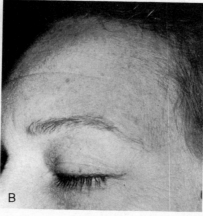

Figure 10–21. *A,* Biopsy-proven basal cell carcinoma in the eyebrow; incision lines are marked. *B,* The patient six months after surgery.

in most cases limit his definitive excisions of melanomas to a thickness of less than 0.76 mm.

Keloids and Hypertrophic Scars

If seen early, these expanding fibrotic tumors should be repeatedly injected with 10 mg/ml of triamcinolone at three- to six-week intervals. Preinjection cryosurgery using liquid nitrogen produces edema permitting easier introduction of the corticosteroid.[30] Older avascular keloids do not respond as well and may require excision. Intralesional steroids are used pre- and postoperatively. In addition, for tissues in certain locations in selected patients, an x-ray treatment with half-value layer of 1 to 2 mm aluminum, 400 roentgen (air dose at skin surface) can be given to the well-shielded suture line and may be repeated four weeks later. Careful observations and repeated intralesional application of triamcinolone up to one or two years postoperatively may be required. Figure 10–22 demonstrates such a case.

Excision with Unequal Wound Edges

Figure 10–23 shows a variation of the fusiform excision required to remove an irregularly shaped lesion. The wedge of tissue removed from the inferior edge makes it shorter than the superior edge. A similar triangle of tissue was excised from the superior edge to make it equal in length to the inferior one. If the difference in wound edges is not too great, one suture can be placed in the center of the wound, and then by equally bisecting the remaining segment with sutures, a smooth closure results.

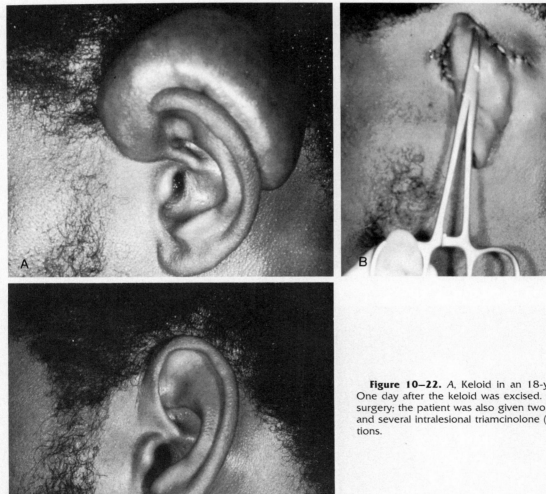

Figure 10–22. A, Keloid in an 18-year-old male. B, One day after the keloid was excised. C, Six years after surgery; the patient was also given two x-ray treatments and several intralesional triamcinolone (10 mg/ml) injections.

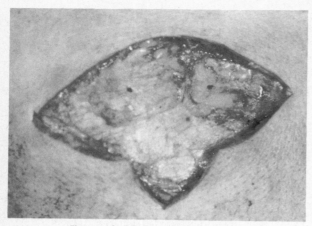

Figure 10–23. An irregular excision.

Chondrodermatitis Nodularis Chronica Helicis

This tender lesion, usually on the helix but sometimes on the antehelix of the ear, should first be treated conservatively with intralesional application of triamcinolone (10 mg/ml) at three- or four-week intervals. If this fails, a fusiform excision of skin (with a length-to-width ratio of 3 or 4 to 1) and a piece of underlying cartilage is performed with a scalpel (Fig. 10–24). If the overlying skin does not appear ischemic and atrophic, a single incision is made, and a wedge-shaped piece of underlying cartilage is excised. Very little deformity results.

Epidermal Inclusion and Sebaceous Cysts

These common masses are often ignored by both patient and physician. If they are in areas subjected to trauma, adjacent to important anatomic structures such as the ear canal or eye, draining malodorous material, becoming inflamed and tender, or in cosmetically important areas, removal should be performed before they grow to a large size.

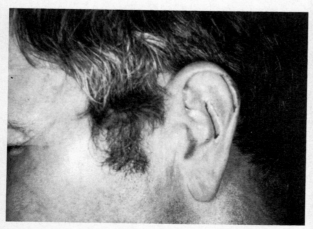

Figure 10–24. Incision lines for chondrodermatitis nodularis chronica helicis.

Infected, fluctuant cysts should be incised and drained and later excised. In the absence of infection, a routine fusiform excision of skin and cyst is carried out and the wound sutured. For small cysts, especially those where cosmetic results are not so important, a narrow fusiform excision can be made, the cyst is dissected out with scissors, and the wound taped or stapled together. If, during this procedure, the cyst wall is ruptured, it can be grasped with hemostats and gradually advanced to surface as previously described in the section on open surgery.

Triangle-to-T Excisions

Sometimes, the shape of the lesion, direction of wrinkle lines, and adjacent anatomic features require an excision that results in a T-shaped suture line. Figure 10–25A shows a biopsy-proven basal cell carcinoma on the upper lip and skin excision lines. After excision (Fig. 10–25B), the triangular-shaped skin flaps are undermined (Fig. 10–25C), and subdermally placed interrupted sutures result in near approximation (Fig. 10–25D). A corner stitch (half-buried horizontal mattress suture) with cardboard bolster is used together with interrupted surface sutures (Fig. 10–25E) to produce an excellent cosmetic result two months later (Fig. 10–25F). Figure 10–26 shows other uses for the triangle-to-T procedure.

O-to-Z Excision

Closure of a circular excision (O-shaped) results in a Z-shaped suture line that moves tissue along an axis approximately 90 degrees to the skin moved when closing a fusiform excision. To avoid pulling an eyebrow superiorly, an O-to-Z procedure is useful when excising a tumor adjacent to it (Fig. 10–27).

Figure 10–28A shows a biopsy-proven basal cell carcinoma outlined with proposed skin incisions. Incisions are made (Fig. 10–28B), flaps are undermined (Fig. 10–28C), skin edges are pulled together (Fig. 10–28D), and the wound is sutured (Fig. 10–28E). Three months after the operation (Fig. 10–28F), no disturbance of the eyebrow location is seen.

Excision With M-Plasty Closure

To reduce the length of a regular fusiform excision suture line, a single or double M-plasty (crown procedure) can be used (Fig. 10–29). Figure 10–30 shows an excision of the upper lip that avoids the vermilion border by this technique.

V-to-Y Tissue Movement

One method of pushing tissue in a given direction to release tension or to fill a void consists of making

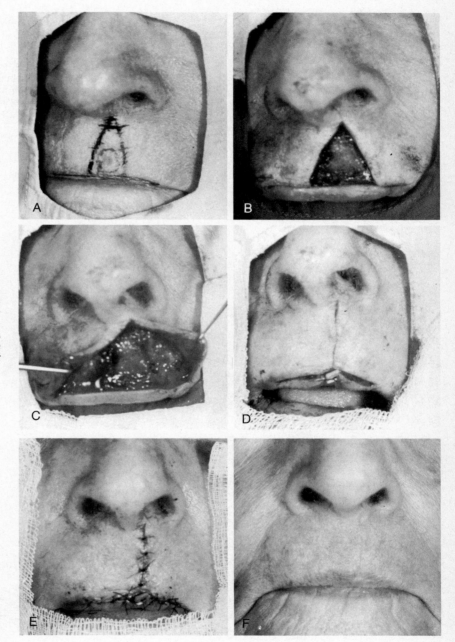

Figure 10–25. *A,* A basal cell carcinoma and the proposed excision lines. *B,* The triangular excision and horizontal skin flap incisions. *C,* The skin flaps are undermined. *D,* Subdermal and half-buried mattress corner sutures in place. *E,* The wound is approximated with surface sutures. *F,* Appearance two months after excision.

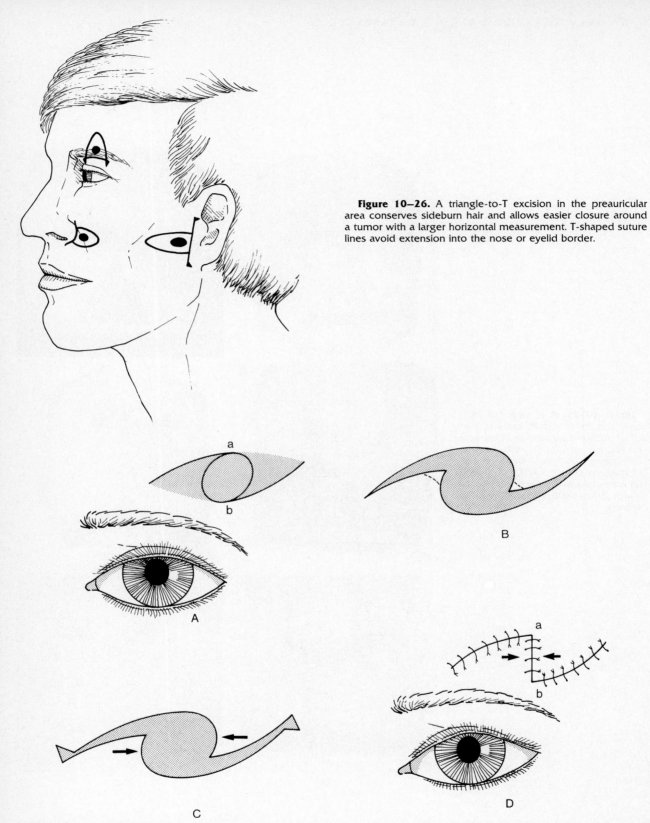

Figure 10–26. A triangle-to-T excision in the preauricular area conserves sideburn hair and allows easier closure around a tumor with a larger horizontal measurement. T-shaped suture lines avoid extension into the nose or eyelid border.

Figure 10–27. The O-to-Z excision. *A,* Circular lines of excision for a tumor next to the eyebrow and the medial and lateral curving skin incisions; the stippled areas away from the excision indicate the extent of undermined skin flaps. *B,* Sometimes the points of skin flaps are rounded off, as indicated, by dotted lines. *C,* Sometimes Burow's triangles are excised to prevent buckling of the skin; arrows point in the direction that the skin is pulled for closure. *D,* The wound is closed without disturbing the eyebrow position.

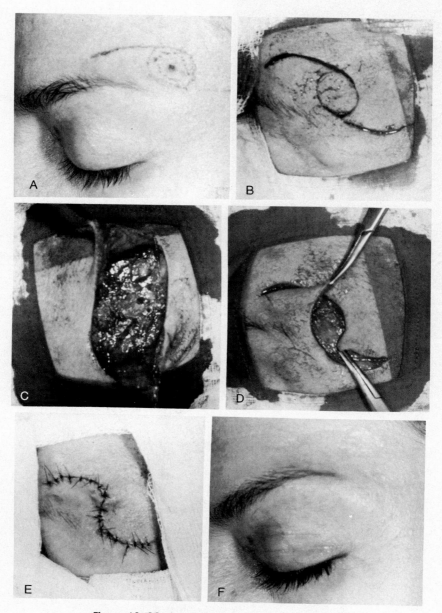

Figure 10–28. *A* to *F*, An O-to-Z excision of cancer.

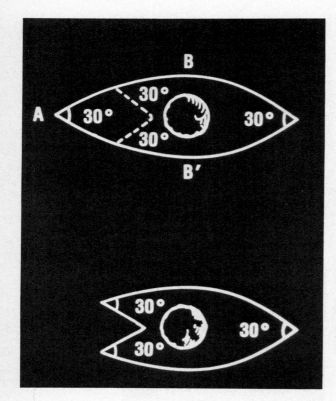

Figure 10–29. M-plasty is used to shorten the length of a regular fusiform excision.

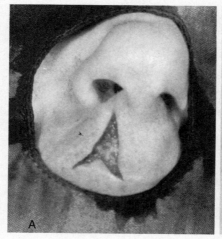
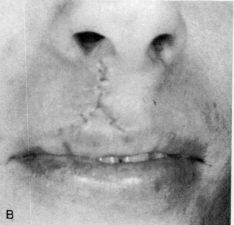

Figure 10–30. *A*, Tumor excised from the upper lip. *B*, Appearance three days later.

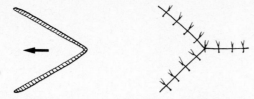

Figure 10–31. The closure of V-shaped incisions to produce Y-shaped suture lines results in tissue movement in the direction of the arrow.

V-shaped skin incisions, then undermining the skin, and suturing the wound together to produce Y-shaped suture lines (Fig. 10–31). This technique is utilized in the excision described below.

Fusiform Incisions with Double Island Sliding Grafts

Because the basal cell carcinoma (diagnosed by a punch biopsy) shown in Figure 10–32A is adjacent to the eyebrow, it cannot be excised by either a routine fusiform excision or an O-to-Z procedure because of its large horizontal dimension. Figure 10–32B shows the proposed incision lines, and Figure 10–32C shows the same area after tumor excision. The preserved skin at both ends is still attached to the subcutaneous fat layer and is gently pulled together and sutured (Fig. 10–32D). Half-buried horizontal mattress sutures with bolsters are placed at points 1 and 2, and the V-shaped defects at points 3 and 4 are sutured, resulting in Y-shaped suture lines. Figures 10–32E to G show the postoperative results. This operation could be described as a rectangular excision with double island sliding grafts and double V-to-Y closures. Unlike split- and full-thickness free grafts, these small island grafts are nourished by intact vessels beneath them. If not stretched by moving too great a distance, they will routinely heal with acceptable cosmetic results.

Double or Single Advancement Flaps

Figure 10–33A illustrates a biopsy-proven basal cell carcinoma in the lateral end of the left eyebrow with skin incision markings for excision and double advancement flap closure. Figure 10–33B shows the rectangular excision of the tumor, and Figure 10–33C shows the medial and lateral skin flaps. In this case, the medial flap is longer so that the eyebrow will be extended more laterally to partially compensate for the excised tissue. Undermining of these flaps should be just below the dermal hair papillae in order to preserve the eyebrow. The wound is closed (Fig. 10–33D), resulting in an acceptable cosmetic result two months later (Fig. 10–33E) that produces no noticeable asymmetry of the eyebrows in the frontal view (Fig. 10–33F).

Closure of Defect by Skin Rotation

Palpation of the skin around the biopsy-proven lentigo maligna shown in Figure 10–34A reveals the most redundant skin to be inferior to the lesion. A triangular excision with the long axis horizontally is closed by the rotation of a flap from the inferior to superior sides (Fig. 10–34B). Extensive undermining was required to prevent tension on the flaps. This is important because blood flow in skin flaps is inversely proportional to tension on the flap.[31] In order to prevent a dog-ear, a Burrow's triangle of tissue was excised medially (Fig. 10–34C). Figure 10–35D shows the patient four years later.

Triangle-to-Y Excision

Figure 10–35A shows a nevus sebaceus on the right anterior temporal scalp. The triangular-shaped lesion was excised (Fig. 10–35B). Several methods could be used to close this defect, but care should be taken to keep suture lines covered by scalp hair. After widely undermining skin edges, closure of the wound was possible by starting at each point of the triangle and proceeding toward the center (Fig. 10–35C and D).

Rhomboid Transposition Flap

The rhomboid transposition flap used to close excisional defects is often preferred because it:
1. Allows use of redundant adjacent tissue.
2. Allows the direction of a skin closure to be changed in order to avoid tension on nearby margins or structures such as the lip, eyelid, or eyebrow.
3. Results in patterned angulated suture lines that often give better cosmetic results than a long straight one.
4. Prevents suture lines from crossing joints.
5. Avoids tension at right angles to suture lines near joints.

The mechanics of this procedure have recently been reviewed[32] and are summarized in Figure 10–36. The skin lesion L is excised leaving a rhomboid-shaped defect (points A, B, C, and D). The skin flap (C, D, E, and F) and recipient defect (A, B, C, and D) are undermined in the areas of cross-hatching, or smaller areas if a smooth closure without tension can be accomplished. The flap is then rotated in the direction of the arrow so that points D, E, and F superimpose points B, A, and D, respectively. Flap rotation could be from the right side (B to D) or from the left or right side using A as a pivotal point instead of C.

Figures 10–37A to F illustrate the excision of a carcinoma of the left cheek and defect closure by a transposition flap.

Text continued on page 120

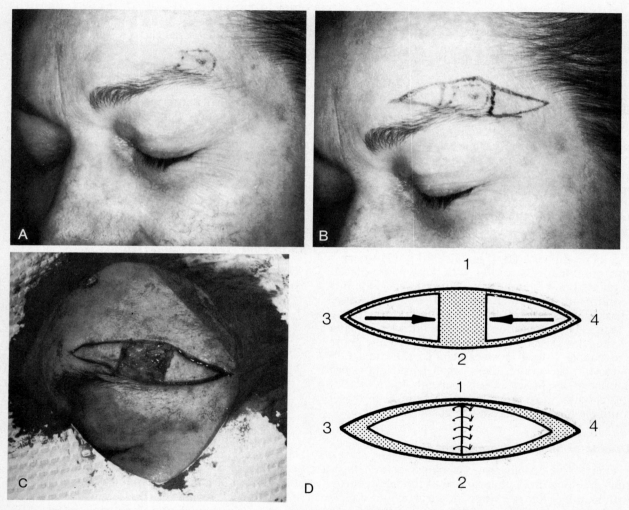

Figure 10–32. *A,* A biopsy-proven basal cell carcinoma. *B,* Proposed incision lines. *C,* The tumor is excised; the skin incisions at both ends of the fusiform design are carried into the subcutaneous fat layer. *D,* The movement of tissue to close the defect.

Illustration continued on opposite page

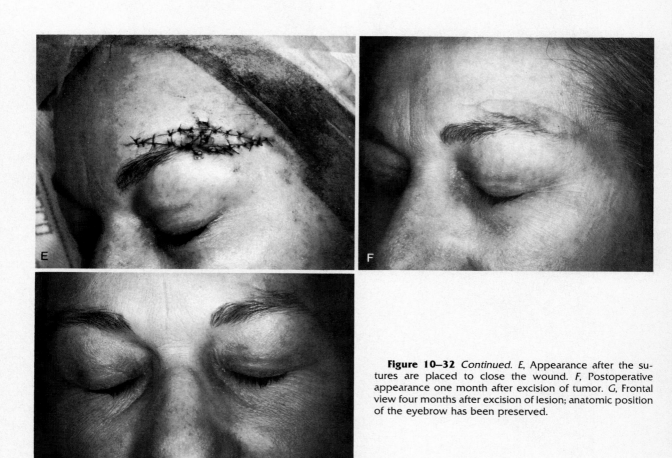

Figure 10–32 *Continued. E,* Appearance after the sutures are placed to close the wound. *F,* Postoperative appearance one month after excision of tumor. *G,* Frontal view four months after excision of lesion; anatomic position of the eyebrow has been preserved.

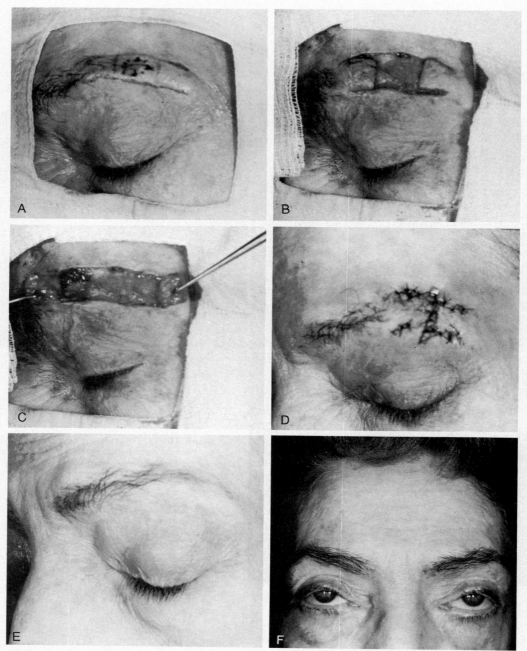

Figure 10–33. *A,* A biopsy-proven carcinoma at the end of the eyebrow. *B,* Excision and incisions are completed. *C,* Skin flaps are mobilized. *D,* The wound is sutured; note half-buried horizontal mattress corner sutures with bolsters. *E,* Appearance two months after the operation. *F,* The frontal view shows no noticeable eyebrow asymmetry.

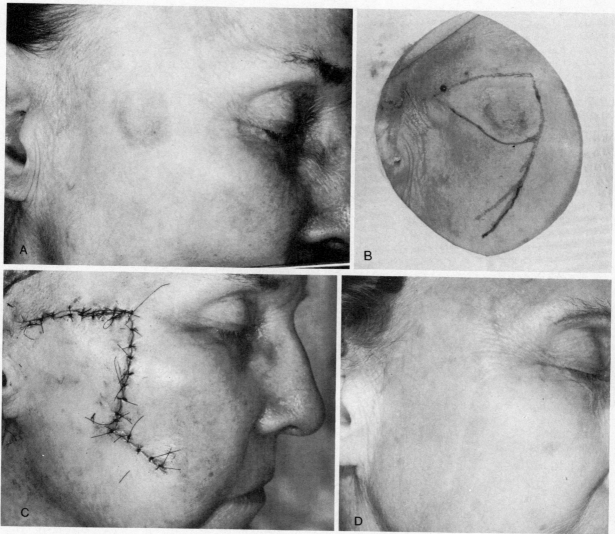

Figure 10–34. *A,* Most of the available loose skin is inferior to the lesion. *B,* After the excision, extensive undermining of the skin inferior to the lesion is carried out; in addition to these incisions, a triangle of tissue is removed from the medial side at the lower end of the flap incision to allow a smooth closure. *C,* The flap is rotated and sutured. *D,* Appearance four years later.

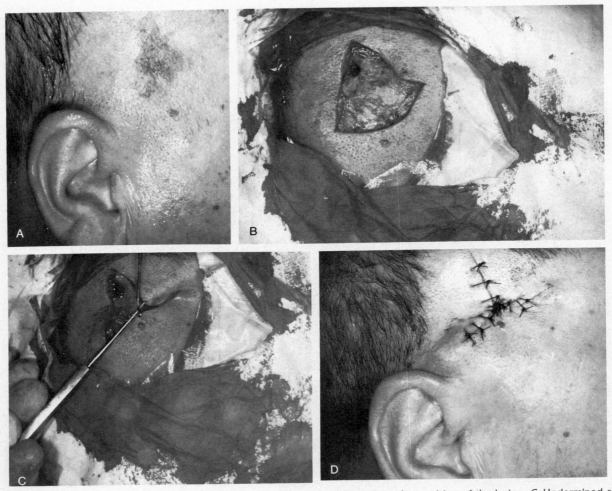

Figure 10–35. *A*, Nevus sebaceous on temporal scalp. *B*, The triangular defect after excision of the lesion. *C*, Undermined skin edges are pulled together for suturing. *D*, Sutures are in place.

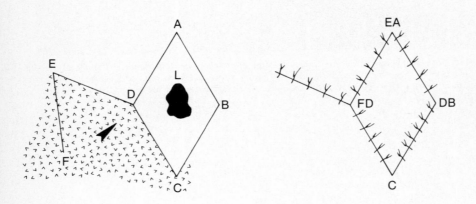

Figure 10–36. The rhomboid transposition flap; sometimes the skin flap (CDEF) does not have to be as large as the recipient site (ABCD).

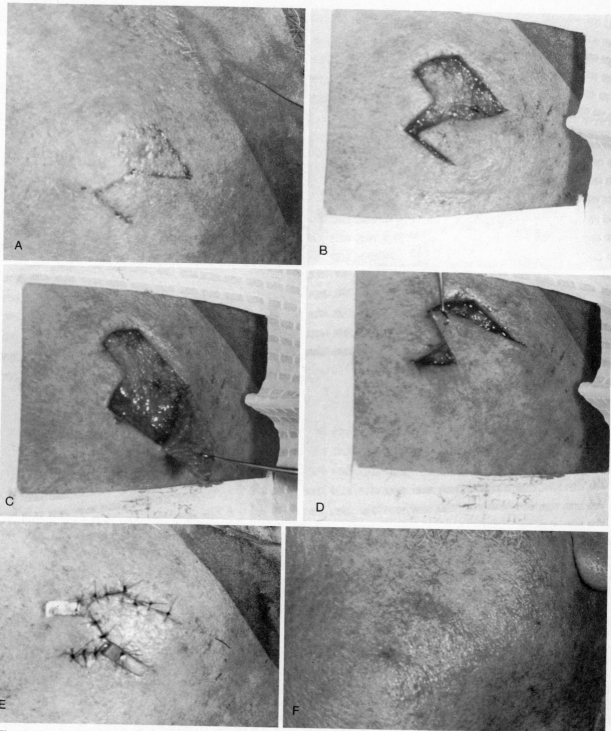

Figure 10–37. *A*, Biopsy-proven basal cell carcinoma of the left cheek with an outline of the proposed rhomboid excision and the inferolateral transposition of the skin flap. *B*, The carcinoma is excised and the skin flap borders are incised. *C*, The skin flap is undermined. *D*, The skin flap is transposed to cover the defect. *E*, The wound is sutured; note the use of half-buried horizontal mattress sutures (corner stitches) with cardboard bolsters. *F*, Suture lines are hardly visible after six months.

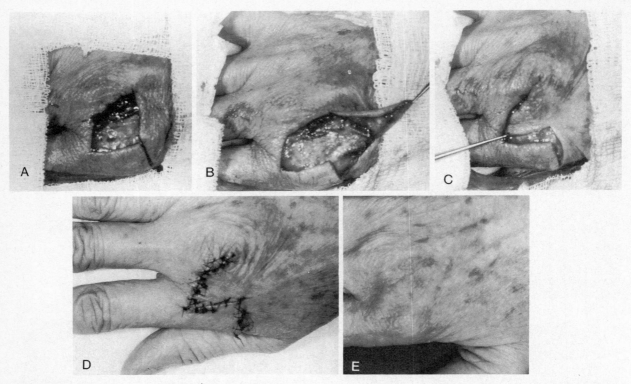

Figure 10–38. *A,* Rhomboid defect and skin flap over the metacarpal phalangeal joint. *B,* The skin flap is undermined. *C,* The skin flap is rotated and transposed to cover the wound. *D,* The wound is sutured. *E,* Four months after the closure of the defect; note the smooth tensionless closure without suture lines crossing over the joint.

Figure 10–38A shows the rhomboid defect and flap incision following the removal of a squamous cell carcinoma over the right second metacarpal-phalangeal joint. The flap is undermined (Fig. 10–38B), transposed (Fig. 10–38C), and sutured (Fig. 10–38D). The wound is hardly visible four months after the operation (Fig. 10–38E).

Vermilionectomy

A vermilionectomy is indicated at times when dealing with precancerous and cancerous conditions of the lip. The patient shown in Figure 10–39A has widespread leukoplakia on the lower lip and superficial, biopsy-proven squamous cell carcinoma to the right of the midline. Figure 10–39B shows the completed excision with a single suture at each end of the wound grasped with a hemostat to be held by an assistant to help immobilize the lip. The labial mucosa is undermined with tenotomy scissors while being held with the sharp single-pronged skin hook (Fig. 10–39C). Wound edges are aligned carefully by placing a single midline suture (Fig. 10–39D), and closure is completed (Fig. 10–39E). Ends of a soft Ethibond suture will not stick to or irritate adjacent tissues. A dye mark or suture is placed at one end of the excised tissue to maintain anatomic orientation, a requirement for the pathologist to be able to assure adequate excision.[33]

Fusiform Excision With Z-Plasty Closure

A chronic labial fissure or other small lesion can be removed by a narrow fusiform excision and Z-plasty closure, as indicated in Figure 10–40. Skin flaps X and Y are undermined and transposed so that point B of flap X goes to point D, and point A of flap Y goes to point C. This results in a smooth closure, because the distance between A and B is increased and the suture line becomes directed horizontally. This change of direction of the skin tension and suture lines is useful to repair scar contractions and to move tissue at other times when needed. The Z-plasty has also been used when extensive axillary excisions are required to control hyperhidrosis.[34]

V-Excision of the Lip

Figure 10–41A shows a deep biopsy-proven squamous cell carcinoma of the upper lip outlined with gentian violet. Unfolded sponges in the corner of the mouth and a suction apparatus are used to keep the field clear of blood and saliva. With an assistant tightly holding one lip edge and the operator the other, a V-shaped wedge is excised (Fig. 10–41B). Note that the length of excision on the mucous membrane is not as great as on the skin surface. The severed ends of the superior labial artery must be carefully isolated, clamped, and ligated with

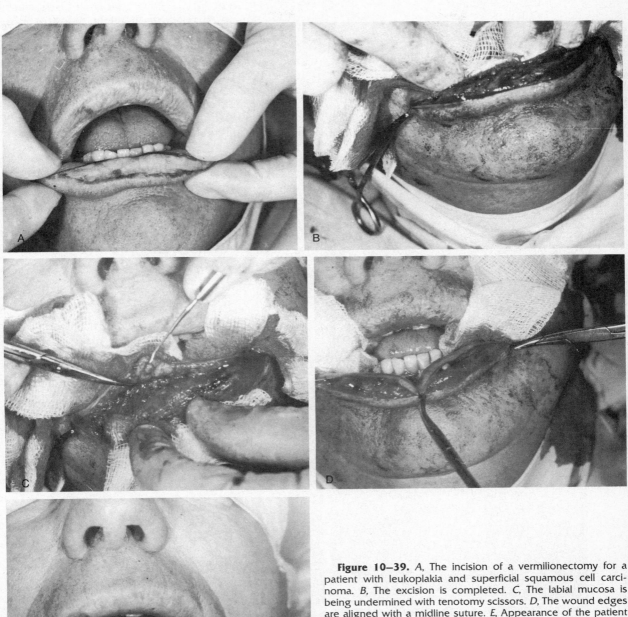

Figure 10–39. *A,* The incision of a vermilionectomy for a patient with leukoplakia and superficial squamous cell carcinoma. *B,* The excision is completed. *C,* The labial mucosa is being undermined with tenotomy scissors. *D,* The wound edges are aligned with a midline suture. *E,* Appearance of the patient immediately after the vermilionectomy.

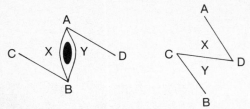

Figure 10–40. Fusiform excision and Z-plasty closure.

sutures. Bipolar electrocoagulation is used on small vessels.

Suturing begins by the use of interrupted 5-0 Vicryl or Dexon-S on labial mucous membranes,

after which this type of suture is used on deep muscle fascia. Properly placed 5-0 Mersilene sutures (with ends cut adjacent to knots as previously described) on subcutaneous fascia result in near approximation of surface edges, which are then closed with interrupted 6-0 monofilament nylon or Ethibond sutures (Fig. 10–41C). Figure 10–41D shows the patient 24 hours later. Note the mild hematoma and edema commonly observed after surgery on the upper lip. An appropriate cosmetic result is obtained six months later (Fig. 10–41E).

Figure 10–42A shows another patient with a biopsy-proven squamous cell carcinoma of the mid-lower lip, and Figure 10–42B shows the same patient

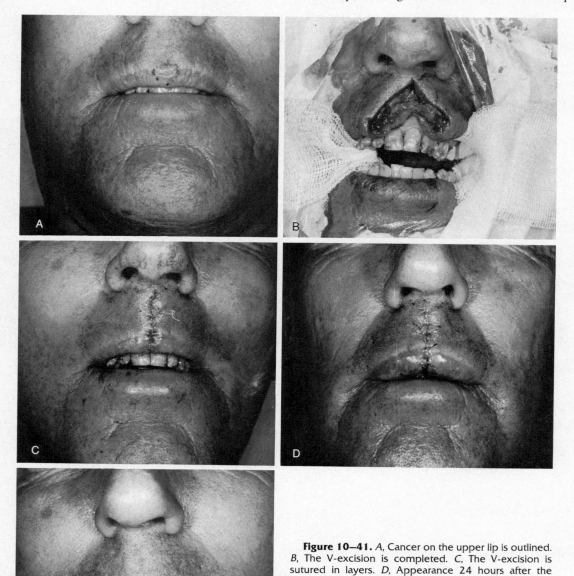

Figure 10–41. *A*, Cancer on the upper lip is outlined. *B*, The V-excision is completed. *C*, The V-excision is sutured in layers. *D*, Appearance 24 hours after the operation. *E*, Appearance six months after the operation.

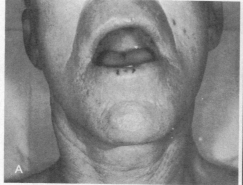
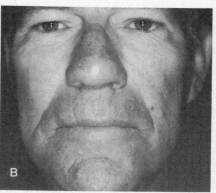

Figure 10–42. *A*, A biopsy-proven, indurated squamous cell carcinoma at the midline of the lower lip. *B*, Postoperative appearance after a V-excision.

several months after V-excision. If at all possible, the V-excision on the lower lip should be directed inferolaterally to avoid crossing the major horizontal crease line of the chin. This is illustrated by another patient in Figure 10–43.

V-Excision of the Pinna

V-excisions as previously described are applicable for other structures such as the ala nasi and ear. Figure 10–44A pictures a punch-biopsy–proven squamous cell carcinoma with proposed lines of excision. With the operator and assistant firmly holding the ear in place, a triangle of tissue is cut out using slow movements of the scalpel through the entire helix (Fig. 10–44B). When accomplishing hemostasis, cartilage should not be damaged with the electrocautery. Edges of skin are approximated with interrupted monofilament nylon sutures that do not pass into cartilage (Fig. 10–44C). Three months later, the ear (Fig. 10–44D) compares favorably with the opposite (nonoperated) ear (Fig. 10–44E).

Earlobe Surgery

Surgical treatment of certain earlobe tumors and traumatic lacerations may require special considerations. Because of the small confinements of the lobe, buried sutures and electrocoagulation of vessels should be avoided. Pressure for a short time usually controls bleeding. Although the earlobe is appendiceal, epinephrine can usually be included with lidocaine (Xylocaine) anesthesia unless exposure to low ambient temperatures is expected. When possible, tumor excision should be through the posterior surface. Laceration repair from an earring and restoration of the pierced lobe can be accomplished in a one-step procedure by sewing a stainless steel ear post in place at the same time.[35]

Nail Surgery

Fingernails and toenails can be safely and quickly removed for various appropriate reasons. Local infiltration anesthesia (without epinephrine) is used after thorough skin preparation. A small curved hemostat or curved surgical scissors are used to free the nail from paronychial tissues, eponychium, and subungual bed. The nail plate is then grasped with Ochsner forceps and extracted. Proximal and lateral nail sulci should be probed or gently curetted to ensure that no pieces of nail remain. Hemostasis is usually accomplished by a simple pressure dressing, although Monsel's solution may be required. After the first 24 hours postoperatively, I usually start patients on soaks of Alibour's or Burow's solution.

Ingrown toenails can be disabling. Hot soaks for

Figure 10–43. A V-excision of the lower lip; note the suture line is at an inferolateral angle to avoid crossing the horizontal chin crease.

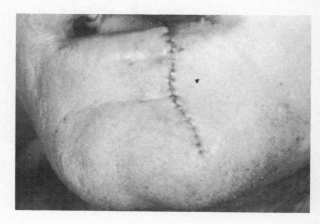

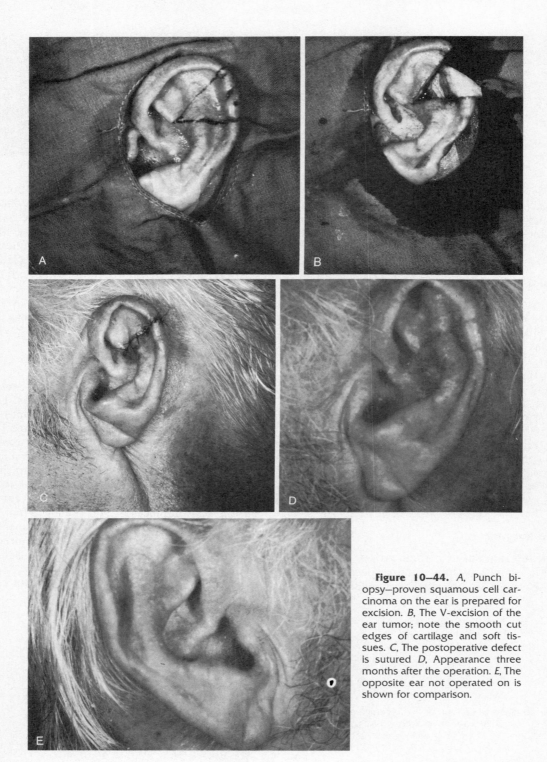

Figure 10–44. *A,* Punch biopsy–proven squamous cell carcinoma on the ear is prepared for excision. *B,* The V-excision of the ear tumor; note the smooth cut edges of cartilage and soft tissues. *C,* The postoperative defect is sutured *D,* Appearance three months after the operation. *E,* The opposite ear not operated on is shown for comparison.

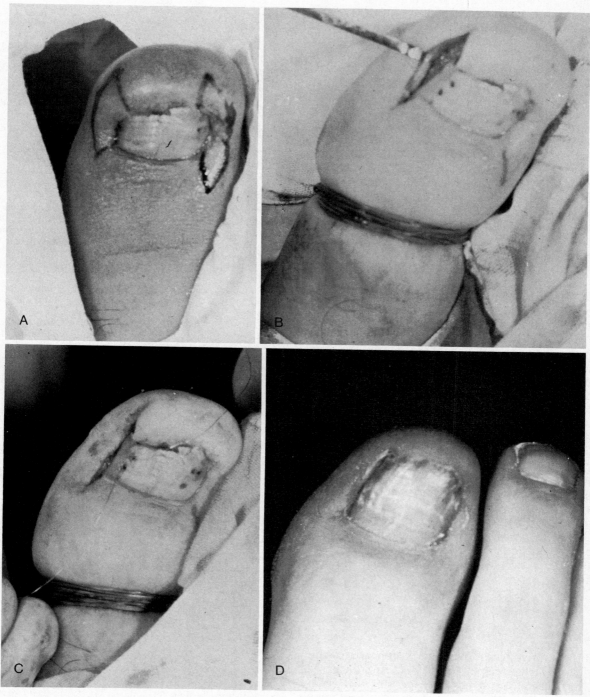

Figure 10–45. *A,* Incision lines for medial and lateral ingrown toenail edges. *B,* One fusiform excision has been made. *C,* A horizontal mattress suture brings the lateral wound edge beneath the nail plate. *D,* Postoperative appearance of toe.

inflammation and systemic antibiotics for infection should be administered when indicated. Unless the condition is too advanced, I attempt conservative therapy. A longitudinal groove that thins the nail plate to a fraction of its original thickness is placed 2 or 3 mm from the lateral ingrowing edge. The Moto-Drill with a no. 11 dental burr is used. This thinning makes the plate flexible, and a podiatric probe curette is used to lift the edge and clean debris from the groove. Any erosion and granulation tissue is cauterized with silver nitrate. Compacted wisps of cotton, made by rolling fibers between the thumb and forefinger, are dipped in a 70% alcohol solution and packed beneath the ingrown edge. This packing is changed at intervals until the nail grows out over the soft tissue. Patients are instructed not to wear tight shoes or to cut off the nail corners.

If the nail has ingrown too far to allow this conservative method, other surgery must be undertaken. I do not favor cutting the nail plate in most instances because the regenerating plate will again impinge upon soft tissues and ingrow. Occasionally, the edge of the nail plate is removed together with the corresponding proximal nail matrix resulting in a narrower nail plate. A rubber band tourniquet is applied. Two longitudinal skin incisions allow the proximal nail fold to be lifted up in order to expose the matrix. A sharp curette used down to the bone removes the necessary part of the matrix. An alternate procedure utilizing curettage and phenol to destroy the matrix without lifting up the proximal nail fold has recently been described.[36]

In most cases, attention should be given to the removal of excessive paronychial tissue (Fig. 10–45A). After applying a rubber band tourniquet, fusiform excisions of any tissue that extends into the subungual bed are carried out (Fig. 10–45B). Using a no. 3 dental burr, two holes are made in the plate, close to the excised area. A large single horizontal mattress suture (2-0 or 3-0 Prolene) is then placed starting downward through one of the holes in the nail. The lateral wound edge is thus pulled beneath the edge of the nail (Fig. 10–45C). Figure 10–45D shows the same toe several months after the operation.

SUMMARY

Preoperative, operative, and postoperative material for selected scalpel and scissors surgery as seen by the dermatologist has been presented. Because of many factors (the decreased use of x-ray therapy for skin cancer being only one), dermatologic surgery in the past few years has been utilized more and has become more varied and complex. I hope the revisions and additions in this chapter since the last edition of *Skin Surgery* accurately reflect most of the changes.

REFERENCES

1. Chernosky ME: Treatment for early squamous cell and basal cell carcinomas: Preliminary study of 3,817 primary skin cancers. Southern Medical Journal 71:802–803, 806, July, 1978
2. Brooks NA: Curettage and shave excision. J Am Acad Dermatol 10:279–284, 1984
3. Spiller WF, Spiller RF: Treatment of basal cell epithelioma by curettage and electrodesiccation. J Am Acad Dermatol 11:808–814, 1984
4. Knox JM: Treatment of skin cancer (Letter to the Editor). J Am Acad Dermatol 12:3, 589, March 1985
5. Chernosky ME, Derbes VJ: Elephantiasis nostras of the abdominal wall. Arch Derm 94:757–762, Dec 1966
6. Tennant FS, Bergeron JR, Stone OJ, et al: Anemia associated with hidradenitis suppurativa. Arch Dermatol 98:138–140, 1968
7. Bergeron JR, Stone OJ: Interstitial keratitis associated with hidradenitis suppurativa. Arch Dermatol 95:473–475, 1967
8. Alexander JW, Fischer JE, Boyajian M, et al: The influence of hair-removal methods on wound infections. Arch. Surg 118:347–352, 1983
9. (editorial) Preoperative depilation. Lancet 1:13311, June 1983
10. Smith JG, Chalker DK: Viral hepatitis: A hazard for dermatologists. Seminars in Dermatology 3:2, 136–139, June 1984
11. Leyden JJ, Smith JG, Chalker DK, et al: Serologic survey for markers of hepatitis B infection in dermatologists. J Am Acad Dermatol 12:4, 676–680, April 1985
12. Kraissl CJ: Selection of appropriate lines for elective surgical incisions. Plast Reconstruct Surg 8:1–28, 1951
13. Baer RL, Kopf AW: Dermatologic office surgery. Year Book of Dermatology. Chicago, Year Book Medical Publishers Inc, 1963–1964 series, pp 7–47
14. Castrow FF, Canavati F: An improved mattress suture. J Derm Surg 2:237–239, June 1976
15. Dunphy JE, Jackson DS: Practical application of experimental studies in the care of the primarily closed wound. Am J Surg 104:273–282, 1962
16. Forrester JC, Zederfeldt BH, Hayes TL, et al: Tape closed and sutured wounds: A comparison by tensiometry and scanning electron microscopy. Br J Surg 57:729–737, 1970
17. Forrester JC: Mechanical, biochemical, and architectural features of surgical scars. Biol Med Phys 14:1–34, 1973
18. Forrest L, Jackson DS: Intermolecular crosslinking of collagen in human and guinea pig scar tissue. Biochim Biophys Acta 229:681–689, 1971
19. Postlethwait RW: Long-term comparative study of nonabsorbable sutures. Ann Surg 171:892–897, 1970
20. Herrmann JB, Kelly RJ, Higgins GA: Polyglycolic acid sutures. Arch Surg 100:486–490, 1970
21. Madsen ET: An experimental and clinical evaluation of surgical suture material II. Surg Gynecol Obstet 97:439, 1953
22. Postlethwait RW, et al: Wound healing II. an evaluation of surgical suture material. Surg Gynecol Obstet 108:555, 1959
23. Harris DR: Healing of the surgical wound. J Am Acad Dermatol 1:197–207, Sept 1979
24. Rovee DT, et al: Effect of local wound environment on epidermal healing. In Maibach HI, Rovee DT (eds): Epidermal Wound Healing. Chicago, Year Book Medical Publishers Inc, 1972
25. Argenta LC, Marks MW, Pasyk KA: Advances in tissue expansion. Clinics in Plastic Surgery, 12:2 April 1985
26. Chernosky ME: Treatment for early squamous cell and basal

cell carcinoma. In Neoplasms of the Skin and Malignant Melanoma. Chicago, Year Book Medical Publishers Inc, 1976

27. Chernosky ME: Squamous cell and basal cell carcinomas: Preliminary study of 3,817 primary skin cancers. Southern Medical Journal 71:802–803, 806, July 1978

28. Epstein E: How accurate is the visual assessment of basal carcinoma margins? Br J Dermatol 89:37–43, 1973

29. Castrow FF, Chernosky ME: Scalpel excision of primary cutaneous malignant melanomas without metastasis. J Dermatol Surg Oncol 5(2):109–111, Feb 1979

30. Ceilley RI, Babin RW: The combined use of cryosurgery and intralesional injections of suspensions of fluorinated adrenocorticosteroids for reducing keloids and hypertrophic scars. J Dermatol Surg Oncol 5(1):54–56, Jan, 1979

31. Larrabee WF Jr, Holloway GA Jr, Sutton D: Wound tension and blood flow in skin flaps. Ann Otol Rhinol Laryngol 93:112–115, 1984

32. Monheit GD: The rhomboid transposition flap re-evaluated. J Dermatol Surg Oncol 6:6, June 1980

33. Freeman RG: Handling of pathologic specimens for gross and microscopic examination in dermatologic surgery. J Dermatol Surg Oncol 8:8, Aug 1982

34. Hill TG: Radical excision and reconstruction of axillary skin. J Dermatol Surg Oncol 9:4, April 1983

35. Chernosky ME: One-step procedure for earlobe surgical repair and ear post replacement (Letter to the Editor). J Am Acad Dermatol 12:721–723, April 1985

36. Seigle RJ, Swanson NA: Nail Surgery: A review. J Dermatol Surg Oncol 8(8):659–666, 1982

11

ERVIN EPSTEIN, M.D.

Shave Surgery

Superior cosmetic results may be obtained by shaving off certain benign lesions even with the skin. This maneuver requires some experience to obtain all of its potential benefits. Cicatrization is rare because of the superficial nature of the excision, although hypertrophic scarring may develop in such notorious areas as the chest and feet. The therapeutic results are excellent in most nonmalignant tumors, especially with intradermal nevi.

Indications

The main use of shave surgery is in the removal of intradermal nevi. These lesions are usually elevated, soft, dome-shaped, flesh-colored to light brown, and often contain hair. In Orientals, Indians, and blacks, they may be a dark blue or black in color. Flat black nevi may also be removed by this procedure. In such cases, the shaving is carried below the surface of the skin, but only to a shallow level. If histopathologic examination should reveal the presence of a melanoma, one can return and excise the entire area without any adverse effect on the prognosis. Elevated pedunculated fibromas and warts may be eradicated in the same manner. Bleeding is controlled with the electrodesiccating current, trichloroacetic acid, or both.

Technique

The lesion is elevated by the injection of a local anesthetic. The assistant holds the skin taut. The operator selects the proper size scalpel (with a no. 10 or 15 blade) and slices the lesion off level with the adjacent normal cutaneous surface. Identical results can be obtained by using a sharp shaving blade held in a hemostat. It may be necessary to smooth the edges with small surgical scissors. If the lesion is pedunculated, the base may be snipped off with the scissors.

Bleeding is controlled by the application of trichloroacetic acid, which must be then washed off with rubbing alcohol. If the acid is left on too long, scarring may result. The base is then electrodesiccated lightly to produce an eschar and to further control any bleeding or oozing.

The wound is not dressed except for sprinkling some talcum powder onto the surface. The patient is instructed to leave the treated area alone—no dressings, no medication—and to keep it dry. The crust is shed in 10 to 14 days in most instances.

Complications

Complications are encountered very rarely. The superficial nature of the excision makes secondary infection very uncommon. Eczematization is avoided by withholding topical applications, including antibiotics and antiseptics. As stated previously, scarring is not to be expected.

Results

As a rule, the cosmetic results are excellent unless the excision is too superficial or too deep. In the former case, one can return and extend the removal to a deeper level that is even with the normal skin. These excisions usually heal without any trace and the eventual cosmetic results surpass those produced by excision and suturing or by any other approach. Recurrences are uncommon despite the fact that, in intradermal nevi, the nevus cells are not completely removed. Occasionally, a black macule may develop in a portion of the skin from which the nevus was excised. Histopathologic examination reveals only pigmentation. Although this darkening may be permanent, it is not hazardous.

LOUIS C. ARGENTA, M.D. / REED O. DINGMAN, M.D.

12

Skin Grafting

To transplant or to graft can be defined as removing a group of living cells from one area of the body (donor site) and transferring them to another area of the body (recipient site) where they can multiply and produce new living cells. The rapid development of grafting has required new and more specific terms to be coined. Autograft denotes that the graft is transferred from one area to another within the same individual. Allograft is exchanged between two individuals of the same species. Xenograft designates the transplant of tissue between individuals of different species. Isograft is usually a form of allograft between two individuals from a very highly inbred strain of animals. Brephoplasty indicates the grafting of embryonic tissue between two individuals.

Usually, if certain technical points are followed and complications do not intervene, autografts of skin are successful. Skin allografts, usually from cadaveric donors, have been used in humans as a temporary cover for large defects. These grafts are almost invariably rejected after the host appears to have briefly accepted them. The immunologic process of rejection occurs between the allograft and the host, resulting in the separation of the graft. Xenografts, especially from pigs, have been extensively used to temporarily cover large areas, especially following major burns. These grafts are never accepted but merely form a barrier to protect the host from the environment. They are usually removed after several days and replaced with a new xenograft until the patient becomes stabile enough to permit autografting.

BACKGROUND

Although skin grafting evolved primarily in the early nineteenth century, several primitive attempts occurred. In India as early as the fifth century A.D., Sushruta described the reattachment of skin segments after slapping the wound to produce hyperemia. It has since been shown that grafts with an increased blood supply are usually more successful.

Baronio[2] in 1804 described an itinerant ointment salesman who detached a portion of his forearm skin and replaced it after applying his ointment. Eight days later, the merchant displayed his arm with the skin reattached.

Bunger[3] in 1823 presented the first clinical report of a successful free skin graft. He removed skin from the lateral surface of the upper thigh and grafted it to a nasal defect. Interestingly, Bunger's procedure included slapping of the donor area before excision of the graft, as Sushruta had advised.

Reverdin[4] was one of the principal pioneers in skin grafting. He used a small stylette to take small transplants of skin in the donor area, which were removed very superficially and transferred to the recipient area. This produced a recipient site with a large number of small islands, and the defect was closed by epithelialization. Ollier[5] stressed the importance of including dermis in the graft and was able to take larger pieces of skin of up to 8 cm^2. He also emphasized the importance of immobilizing the graft with bandages to insure a "take." Thiersch[6] in 1874 evolved a method of removing large, very thin "dermo-epidermic grafts in large sheets to cover large wounds."

The true forerunner of today's split-thickness skin graft evolved from the work of Blair and Brown[7] in 1929. These authors took thicker grafts than the original Thiersch graft and were able to apply them to a wide variety of clinical uses. The introduction of the dermatome by Padgett[8] in 1939 greatly facilitated the widespread use of these grafts.

SPLIT-THICKNESS SKIN GRAFTS

The thickness of the human skin varies greatly with the region of the body and an individual's age and sex. Southwood[9] measured skin from a wide group of patients and demonstrated that its thickness varies from 17/1000 to 150/1000 of an inch. The thickness is greatest on the soles and palms. The eyelids and postauricular area are the thinnest. The dermis is usually from 15 to 20 times thicker than the epidermis depending on the site. The adult skin is approximately 3.5 times thicker than a newborn's, but by the age of five, skin thicknesses are usually the same as in adults.[10] Skin from females is generally thinner than in males, especially in the dermal layer.[11]

All split-thickness skin grafts contain the epidermis and a portion of the dermis. The thickness of the graft determines the relative amount of dermis included. Split-thickness skin grafts are classified according to the amount of dermis taken in the graft. These subdivisions are: thin grafts (Thiersch), generally less than 10/1000 of an inch; intermediate grafts, usually 12/1000 to 18/1000 of an inch; and

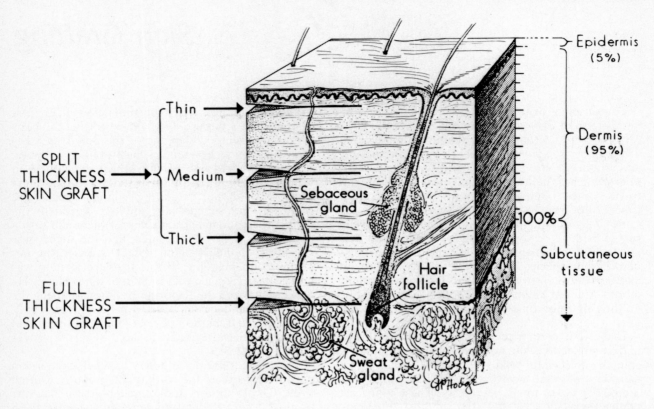

Figure 12–1. Various depths of split- and full-thickness skin grafts. All split-thickness skin grafts leave some dermis; full-thickness grafts remove the entire dermis and most adnexal structures, leaving no potential for regeneration.

thick grafts, generally from 18/1000 to 28/1000 of an inch. A thin graft is translucent, and a thick graft is opaque (Fig. 12–1).

Clinical Applications of Skin Grafts

When faced with a specific defect, the surgeon must decide whether the wound is best covered by a split-thickness skin graft, a full-thickness skin graft, a composite graft, a skin flap, a myocutaneous flap, or a free flap. In general, skin grafts can be used to close any wound in the body that has sufficient blood supply to nourish the graft. The production of granulation tissue in an open wound is a good indication that adequate blood supply exists. Areas with notoriously poor blood supply that will not support a graft include bone denuded of its periosteum, tendons denuded of peritenon, nerves denuded of perineurium, or cartilage denuded of perichondrium. Coverage of such wounds is best obtained with flaps that carry their own blood supply.

Skin grafts may be used as a permanent or temporary cover for a wound. In cases where the patient's general condition precludes larger opera-

tive procedures, a split-thickness skin graft can be applied to an open wound, thus facilitating the control of infection. When the patient's general condition warrants and if local infection has been controlled, the split-thickness skin graft can be removed and a full-thickness graft or flap applied to provide more acceptable and stable coverage.

Split-thickness skin grafts have been applied directly to lung, pericardium, and other vital structures.[12] These organs accept the graft, but their removal at a later date can prove to be very difficult. These organs are best covered by flaps. Provided that there is adequate underlying soft tissue, a split-thickness graft can be stable over an extremely long period of time. If applied over hard surfaces, such as the skull with only a minimal amount of pericranium, the glabrous nature of the skin graft results in easy breakdown of the wound. Likewise, skin graft areas persistently exposed to trauma such as the hands and feet are apt to break down, and grafting in these areas is generally not recommended.

Split-thickness skin grafts may be applied to the flexor surfaces of the body, where they are especially prone to develop contractures producing less-than-optimal results. Prolonged splinting in extension over these surfaces, especially of the neck, is indi-

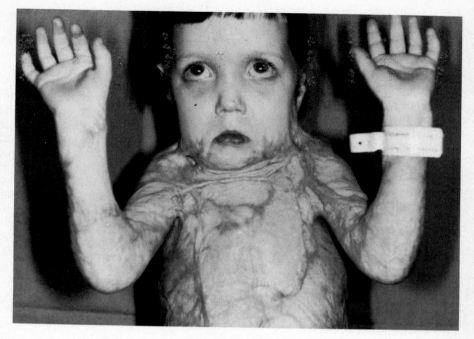

Figure 12–2. Severe contracture occurring in a three-year-old girl after skin grafting for burns. Note the severe immobilizing scar of the flexor surfaces of the neck and elbows. The use of long-term stent and pressure dressings have made such deformities unusual today.

cated if contracture is to be avoided (Fig. 12–2). Usually within six to eight months, most contracture has occurred and splinting can be relieved. Unfortunately, uninterrupted splinting, which is carried on to minimize contracture, may result in significant joint stiffness, particularly in the hand, wrists, and elbows of the elderly. Splints should be removed on a regular basis and the patient put through a regimen of active and passive range-of-motion exercises at least twice a day.

Split-thickness skin grafts may be used for replacement of mucosa in the mouth, nose, and vagina. On these surfaces, significant contracture of the graft may occur and splinting is necessary. Intraoral prostheses should be worn for four to six months to minimize contracture. When a split-thickness skin graft has been used for vaginal reconstruction, splinting must be used for a prolonged period of time, especially if the patient is sexually inactive. Most vaginal grafts are therefore not recommended until the patient is old enough to dilate herself or to be sexually active.

Although some change does occur in the skin when placed in the mouth or vagina, a significant amount of keratinization continues, and a true transformation to mucosa does not occur. Placement of skin in the conjunctiva of the eyelids is not recommended.

Donor Site

The skin is not uniform but has considerable variation in hair-bearing quality, thickness, vascu-larity, color, and texture from one area of the body to another. The most important aspect of taking split-thickness skin grafts, however, is the variance in color. Ideally, the split-thickness skin graft should be taken from an area adjacent to the wound so that color and texture match as close as possible to the denuded area. Unfortunately, in such areas as the face and arms, the scarring produced by taking the graft is unacceptable and other sites must be sought.

Small amounts of split-thickness skin to cover areas of the face may be taken from the postauricular area or anywhere in the neck above the clavicle. The taking of large grafts, however, results in unacceptable scarring.

The scalp is an excellent source of skin that is a good color and texture match to facial skin. This skin is best taken after careful shaving with a free hand knife. The infiltration of the scalp of a large amount of 0.5% lidocaine (Xylocaine) with 1:200,000 epinephrine will produce a surface more amenable to harvesting. When grafts are of thin to moderate thickness (10/1000 to 12/1000 of an inch), very little hair growth is noted in the grafted skin.[13] Regrowth of hair on the scalp will be essentially normal provided that full-thickness grafts are not taken.

Although skin can be harvested from anywhere on the extremities, buttocks, or abdomen, the permanent change that occurs in the donor site dictates that the graft be taken from an area that can be hidden by a bathing suit. Today's bathing suits can make this a formidable challenge. If normal skin is available, the outline of underwear briefs is marked on the patient preoperatively. A split-thickness skin graft is then harvested from the buttock so that the scar will be hidden beneath the underwear or bathing suit. Harvesting grafts from the frequently exposed abdomen is a practice which should be condemned except in cases where large amounts of skin are necessary, such as for burn victims.

Unfortunately, a split-thickness skin graft taken from the thighs, abdomen, and buttocks frequently assumes a yellowish, slightly discolored, or brownish appearance when it is placed elsewhere on the body. Thinner grafts tend to become darker than thicker ones.[14]

Skin Graft Bed

If the skin graft is to survive, the recipient bed must have an adequate vascular supply, and the graft must be brought into contact with it. The relative vascularity of recipient beds varies considerably. Bone with the periosteum removed, cartilage with the perichondrium removed, and tendons with the peritenon removed are essentially avascular on their surface and, as such, will not nourish a skin graft. Dermis, fascia, muscle, and most viable tissues have a good blood supply that permits vascularization of the graft. Recipient beds, which have a more limited blood supply, require a longer period for successful vascularization of the graft. These beds also require longer immobilization of the graft and more care than those with greater vascularity. Tissue that has been exposed to large doses of radiation or sites adjacent to areas of chemotherapeutic agent extravasation generally have a poor blood supply and are less-than-optimal sites for the placement of grafts. Fat has a poor blood supply and does not make a good recipient bed. Wounds that have been left exposed to the environment will develop a highly vascular bed termed granulation tissue, which is, by definition, infected. The longer standing the granulation bed is, the poorer a recipient site it makes.

Evaluation of the Recipient Site

Two types of wounds generally require split-thickness skin graft. The first are acute wounds resulting from the extirpation of lesions, after the rotation of flaps, or after the loss of skin secondary to trauma. The second type is a chronic wound that has been exposed for several days and has formed granulation tissue.

The bleeding evident in an acute wound attests to adequate blood supply and the bed's adaptability to accept a skin graft. Similarly, the presence of granulation tissue in a chronic wound attests to an adequate blood supply. Wounds in which bone is exposed acutely or chronically reveal a nonbleeding area, which therefore will not accept a graft.

The second most important factor in determining the take of a skin graft is the quantitative and qualitative bacteriology of the wound. Since a person usually lives in symbiosis with bacteria, all open wounds are immediately colonized by endogenous flora. Exogenous flora may exist if the wound has been contaminated from external sources. Unusual flora may occur when exposure to animals occurs, such as in farm injuries. Usually, the flora that colonizes chronic open wounds is endogenous and secondary to the direct split of bacteria from the wound edges or from the patient's own blood-borne contamination.

Numerous studies have documented that wounds containing less than 10^5 bacteria per gram of tissue can usually be considered as noninfected and will accept a skin graft. Wounds with greater than 10^5 bacteria per gram of tissue are, by definition, infected, and the take of a skin graft is statistically very unfavorable.

Robson and Krizek have developed a rapid slide technique that has been used clinically for several years. The technique requires a small amount of tissue taken with a punch biopsy or scalpel and a quantitative assay of this material.[15, 16] The entire procedure takes about 30 minutes.

If less than 10^5 bacteria are present, the graft can be applied directly. If more than 10^5 bacteria are present, then steps must be taken to decrease the bacterial count. Mechanical débridement of all necrotic and foreign material is mandatory, since even the smallest foreign bodies potentiates the growth of bacteria. Exuberant granulation tissue should be removed surgically. Electrocautery or an epinephrine-containing solution applied to the granulating bed will usually achieve hemostasis.

Usually, systemic antibiotics are ineffective in decreasing the bacterial count in a granulating wound. Topical antibiotics, especially silver sulfadiazine (Silvadene) and neomycin, decrease bacterial growth in open wounds. Biologic dressings, including amnion, allografts, or xenografts, may be placed over infected wounds and changed at 24-hour intervals to reduce significantly the number of bacteria.[15]

The Technique of Taking Split-Thickness Grafts

Any sharp blade can be used to take a split-thickness skin graft. Several devices have been developed that greatly facilitate the taking of grafts and allow for safe, rapid, and uniform procedures. Small split-thickness skin grafts can be taken with a Weck blade or an ordinary safety razor blade. Larger knives include the Humby knife, the Blair knife, and the Ferris-Smith knife. The Humby knife controls the thickness of the graft to be taken with shims. More modern knives are fitted with an adjustable roller that has the advantage of insuring that the blade depth will not change significantly while cutting a skin graft. A Goulian knife is a modification of a Weck straight blade with a blade protector. Preset protectors determine the thickness of the graft.

All of these knives function best when skin is taken from a relatively fixed area such as the buttock, arm or leg. Areas with considerable flaccidity, such as the abdomen, are not as easily removed. With practice, however, considerable expertise can be developed so that extremely long and wide grafts can be taken with ease from almost any donor site.

The Drum Dermatome

There are three types of drum dermatomes in use today: the Padgett, the Reese, and the Schuchardt dermatomes. All three can take large grafts (up to 4 × 16 inches) of precise thickness.

The basic ingredient in these devices is a drum that is coated with glue (Fig. 12–3). As the drum is rolled across the skin, the skin adheres to the drum and is held in position. A knife blade is manipulated back and forth across the drum on a piston and precisely cuts a graft of predetermined thickness. Various glues have been developed for these dermatomes.

The drum dermatome can be used on almost any surface. Grafts are more easily taken in a circumferential direction around the thigh or abdomen rather than longitudinally. These devices allow the surgeon to take grafts of unusual shapes. Using a template from the recipient site, glue is applied only to a similar area on the drum, so as the drum is rotated, only that portion of skin is removed.

Air-Driven and Electric Dermatomes

These dermatomes include the Brown, Padgett, Stryker, and Castroviejo designs. Power-driven dermatomes greatly facilitate the taking of extensive grafts in a short period of time. The simplicity of these devices makes it possible for inexperienced surgeons to achieve success with minimal practice (Fig. 12–4). The graft thickness is controlled by calibration knobs on either side of the instrument. Tension is applied on the donor site, and a lubricant (usually oil) is applied. The dermatome is then pushed uniformly across the skin surface removing as much skin as necessary. The savings in operative time of these devices quickly offsets the initial expense. The Castroviejo dermatome was designed for taking split-thickness grafts of mucosa from the mouth and lips. This is a very small device designed for a specific purpose; it facilitates the taking of grafts in constricted areas.

As soon as the graft has been removed, it should be applied immediately to the recipient site without washing or soaking in solutions of any kind. If it is necessary to delay the use of a graft, the raw surfaces should be folded together and the graft placed on a

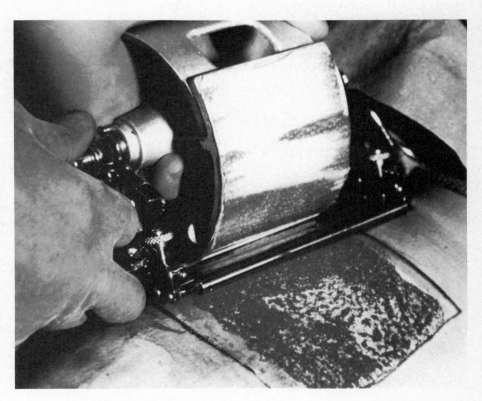

Figure 12–3. The Padgett Dermatome. Adhesive is applied to both the dermatome and skin; rotation of the dermatome drum with one hand while the other moves the blade back and forth results in uniform grafts of precise thicknesses.

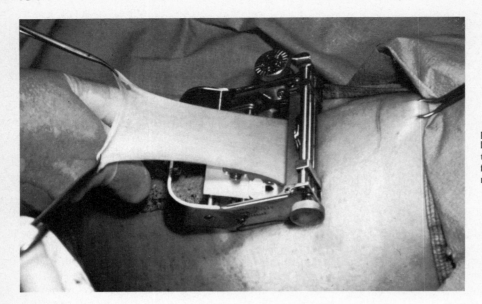

Figure 12–4. The Browne air-powered dermatome can take very large pieces of skin at uniform thicknesses. Such dermatomes are faster and easier to use than the more complicated drum devices.

sterile sponge moistened with saline solution. Grafts should not be soaked in other solutions. Grafts left on a side table while hemostasis is insured quickly dry out and compromise the final result.

When a limited area is to be grafted or an optimal cosmetic result is desired, the skin should be applied as a continuous sheet. When hemostasis is incomplete or where the wound has been open for a period of time, multiple holes should be cut in the graft with a 10-gauge needle or a No.11 knife blade to allow fluids to escape. When large areas must be covered from a limited donor site, as in the case of burns, grafts can be meshed. Multiple mechanical and manual devices are available that produce multiple uniform slits in the graft, usually about 2 mm apart (Fig. 12–5). When tension is applied to the

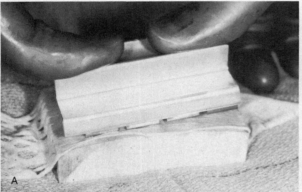

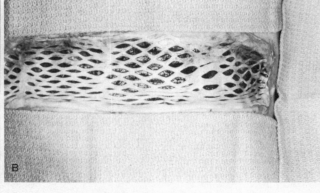

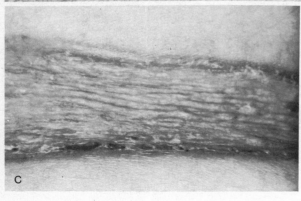

Figure 12–5. *A,* A simple skin-graft meshing device; multiple blades in an aluminum holder rapidly mesh skin grafts and permit coverage of very large areas. *B,* A meshed skin graft in place. Multiple fenestrations are helpful in grafting contaminated or weeping wounds and can also almost double the surface area of a graft when a minimal amount of donor area is available. The small fenestrations heal by secondary epithelialization. *C,* The same skin graft three months later; all of the fenestrations have healed together by secondary intention. While useful for the trunk and extremities, mesh grafts frequently have an uneven surface and do not give optimal results in the facial area.

graft, multiple openings appear. Such devices will allow the graft to be expanded up to three times its previous surface area.

Fixation of the Graft

When thin split-thickness skin grafts are applied to an appropriate recipient site, there is almost immediate fixation of the skin graft. It is important to fix the graft as firmly as possible in order for it to have an optimal chance of taking. Sutures are the most common method used for fixation. Either absorbable or nonabsorbable sutures can be employed. Fine chromic sutures allow fixation of the graft for several days and eliminate the need for suture removal. Surgical staples are quite effective but must be removed within five to seven days to avoid scarring.

Surgical adhesive tape positioned radially across the graft can be helpful. Surgical adhesives have found relatively little use, since most surgeons tend to fix the graft irregularly or to separate it from the bed. Tie-over fiber dressings that minimize motion are an effective and desirable method of fixing grafts to the recipient area (Fig. 12–6). They are useful in the facial area and neck where motion could disrupt the graft. Tie-over fiber dressings are constructed in the following manner. If the graft is sutured about its circumference, 4-0 black silk or nylon sutures are left approximately six to eight inches in length. Sutures are placed at intervals around the wound. A nonadherent gauze is applied directly to the skin graft. Over this is placed a bolus of either saline-soaked cotton or a more porous synthetic fiber. The bolus is held by an assistant while the operator ties sutures from the opposite side over the bolus. Such dressings provide fixation of the graft with uniform, firm pressure.

As long as no obvious signs of infection occur, the tie-over dressing can be left in place for approximately five days. If any signs of infection occur (e.g., odor or erythema), the graft should be removed and the wound treated in an open fashion. A delay of 24 hours after seroma or hematoma occurs almost uniformly dooms the graft to failure. Translucency of the graft or any other sign of nonadherence requires lancing it, preferably with a No. 11 knife blade. The fluid beneath it is then removed by pressure with sterile cotton-tipped applicators.

Barring infection or seroma, most grafts are adherent within eight hours after placement. They continue to gain greater adherence during the next several days.[17]

Physiology of the Graft Take

For several hours after a graft is placed over the recipient site, it is nourished and survives by "plasmatic circulation," or the absorption of plasma-like fluid from the recipient area.[18] This fluid is absorbed into the capillary network of endothelial-lined spaces of the graft dermis. At the same time, a fibrin network forms between the graft and the recipient bed to secure the graft in place. If the graft becomes progressively affixed to the site channels connecting existing blood vessels, the recipient area with those in the graft are established. Thin grafts develop a viable pink color within 12 to 15 hours, whereas a thicker graft may appear cyanotic for several days. New capillaries grow from the recipient area into the graft.[19, 20] These new vascular channels grow into existing vessels of the skin graft to re-establish circulation.

Concurrent with the development of blood vessels, new lymph vessels develop for lymphatic drain-

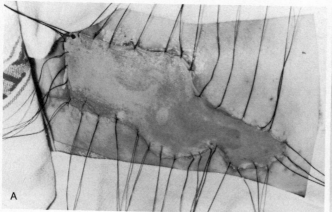
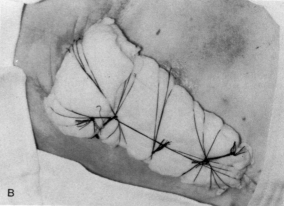

Figure 12–6. *A,* A split-thickness skin graft sutured to the neck. Since this is a cosmetic area, no fenestrations are made in the graft, which is fixed circumferentially with 5-0 silk sutures. *B,* A typical stint device. Fiber-filled cotton is placed over a nonadhesive gauze that has been applied to the neck graft; the sutures are tied together to maintain a uniform pressure for five to seven days.

age, which is usually established by the fourth or fifth postoperative day. This ingrowth depends upon absolute uninterrupted contact of the graft to the recipient site. The thin fibrous network that holds the graft to the bed serves as an adhesive material to prevent slippage. Ideally, the graft should be placed in the recipient site under the same physiologic tension as the donor area. This allows for less interference with the development of new circulation.

Postoperative Management of Skin Grafts

All skin grafts contract, but thin grafts contract more than thicker ones. The degree of contracture depends upon the recipient bed and the physiologic reaction of the patient to repair. The application of splints is helpful to avoid contracture. In the facial area, postoperative splinting is difficult. On the arms and legs, however, splinting with supportive dressings or casts may be necessary for as long as six weeks. The neck, oral mucosa, nasal lining, and vagina are particularly prone to contracture and may require even more prolonged periods of time.

The prolonged application of uniform pressure to a skin graft minimizes eccentric contractures. Jobst elastic dressings can be applied to almost any surface and are relatively comfortable for the patient. Their long-term effect has been gratifying, but they must be applied to the skin graft as early as possible and be worn as much as possible to achieve optimal results.

Care of the Donor Site

Donor sites for split-thickness skin grafts heal by re-epithelialization of the remaining structures. New cells develop from intact epithelium adjacent to hair follicles, sebaceous glands, and sweat glands and migrate across the denuded area until epithelialization is completed. Donor sites from which thick grafts have been removed heal more slowly than those from which thin grafts have been taken.

Donor sites may be left exposed to the air so that a thin protective crust is formed. Such crusts are spontaneously sloughed after epitheliazation has been completed, which takes from five to 10 days. Such treatment of a donor site, however, is quite painful and prone to infection.

The use of petrolatum gauze and other impregnated gauzes has given way over the past several years to synthetic occlusive membranes. Such membranes have the distinct benefit of almost totally alleviating pain at the donor site.

Once the skin graft has been harvested, a gauze soaked with a 1:400,000 epinephrine solution is applied to the donor site. In three to five minutes, hemostasis has occurred and the gauze is removed.

A bio-occlusive dressing such as Op-Site is applied to cover the wound. This dressing is left intact for eight to 10 days after which it may be soaked off in the tub or shower. Epitheliazation usually occurs by this time and discomfort is minimal.

Late Changes in the Grafted Skin

Usually, skin grafts from the neck and the post-auricular and facial areas retain their natural pink color and have a relatively normal appearance when used to repair facial defects. Grafts taken from below the clavicle may develop a yellowish or brown appearance. Such grafts, when used in the facial area, become conspicuous because of their poor color match. Thin split-thickness grafts may become darker over time than thick grafts, making them less desirable.

Hyperpigmentation of a skin graft can be distressing to the patient and is probably due to the stimulation of melanophores from exposure to sunlight (Fig. 12–7). Patients should be advised to strictly avoid sun exposure on split-thickness grafted areas

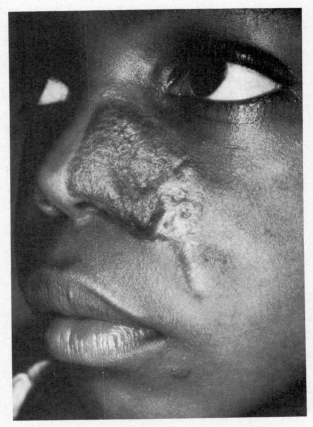

Figure 12–7. A hypertrophic and hyperpigmented scar on a black patient who underwent split-thickness skin grafting for a nasal defect. Skin grafts in blacks frequently become both hyperpigmented and, despite the application of pressure dressings, hypertrophied.

for a reasonable period of time. Sunscreens should be worn over the facial grafts for at least six months. Occasionally, dermabrasion of a hyperpigmented graft can decrease the amount of pigmentation.

It is unusual for split-thickness grafts to retain the ability to grow hair and for sebaceous or sweat glands to continue functioning. Such functions occur occasionally with deep split-thickness skin grafts. Because of the lack of sebaceous function, grafted areas are frequently dry and crusty in the early postoperative period. Skin lubricants or topical ointments, such as bacitracin, are helpful in preventing excessive breakdown.

Nerves grow gradually into areas where split-thickness skin grafts have been applied. Although the degree of sensation is seldom as good as before the grafting, some return of sensation can be expected. Sensation in thin grafts returns more quickly than in thick ones; it may be noted as early as five weeks postoperatively and usually is completed after two years.

The cosmetic appearance of a split-thickness graft improves over time. Discrepancy in thickness between the graft and normal skin, which may be disturbing to the patient in the early postoperative period, eventually diminishes. The development of underlying fat and scar tissue smooths out the area. The application of uniform and constant pressure to such grafts is helpful.

Skin grafts placed in children seem to grow in proportion to the development of the child.

FULL-THICKNESS SKIN GRAFTS

A full-thickness skin graft (Wolfe graft) contains the entire thickness of the dermis as well as the epidermis. Full-thickness grafts more closely resemble normal skin in color, texture, and hair growth; therefore, they are desirable in closing defects of the facial area when immediately adjacent skin is insufficient or unsuitable. As previously mentioned, grafts taken from a highly vascular area have a greater tendency to survive than those taken from less vascular areas.

Donor Sites for Full-Thickness Skin Grafts

The amount of a full-thickness graft that can be taken is limited by the ability to close the donor site primarily. If large areas of full-thickness grafts are needed, then the donor site must be closed with a split-thickness graft taken from another site.

The postauricular surface of the ear and mastoid area are excellent sources of full-thickness grafts that match facial skin. Grafts as large as 2×3 cm can be removed and the site closed primarily. Although the retroauricular sulcus can be decreased significantly, the general contour of the ear is not

distorted. If larger grafts are needed, then a split-thickness graft must be applied.

The supraclavicular region can provide a larger area for full-thickness grafts. Its color and texture match facial skin almost as well as that taken from the postauricular area. Enough skin can be removed from this region to cover the nose, cheek, or upper eyelid. Scars produced in this area, however, can be quite objectionable, particularly in women.

When smaller amounts of skin are needed, the preauricular area is almost an ideal source. Hair taken with such grafts will survive and grow in another area of the face. The age and general looseness of the skin will determine how much of this tissue can be removed.

The upper eyelid can be taken from elderly patients if some redundancy of tissue occurs. In most patients, however, only a narrow ellipse can be removed without deforming the eyelid.

The inguinal crease is an ideal source for large full-thickness grafts. The surgeon must be careful that pubic hair is not taken because it will be transplanted to another site. If some hair grows in the graft, it can be removed by electrolysis.

Taking Full-Thickness Skin Grafts

Since the amount of tissue that can be taken is relatively restricted, it is important that an exact template of the recipient area be prepared (Fig. 12–8). This can be done with transparent materials that can be sterilized and do not stretch. A cloth towel or aluminum sheet can be used. Transparent exposed x-ray film is ideal. An outline of the defect is made and cut to appropriate shape and then placed over the donor area. Since only a minimal amount of shrinkage occurs with full-thickness grafts, the graft should be taken only slightly larger than the defect.

After transferring the template design to the skin, a full-thickness graft is removed with the scalpel. An injection of lidocaine (Xylocaine) with epinephrine minimizes blood loss and accentuates the separation of the dermis from underlying fat. The skin is incised into the dermis, and the graft is retracted with a skin hook and then excised through the layer of fat.

After the graft has been removed, the epidermal surfaces are placed downward and a small pair of scissors is used to take as much fat as possible from the back of the graft. Fat on the undersurface acts as a barrier against vascularization of the graft.

Hemostasis of the recipient site must be absolute, or vascularization of the full-thickness graft will fail. The graft should be placed in the recipient area under normal physiologic tension without stretching it and without leaving undue laxity, which interferes with vascularization. The graft is accurately fixed to the recipient area with circumferential sutures to

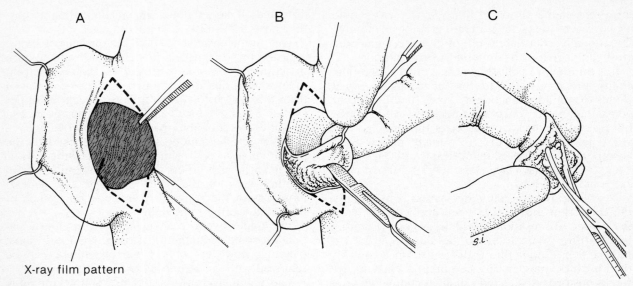

A   B   C

X-ray film pattern

Figure 12–8. The technique for taking full-thickness grafts from behind the ear. *A*, The pattern of the defect on x-ray paper is transposed to the donor site. *B*, A full thickness of skin and subcutaneous tissue is taken, and the donor site is closed primarily. *C*, All fat should be removed with fine scissors to maximize the "take" of the graft.

prevent motion. Any motion will seriously affect full-thickness grafts, because it disrupts the fibrin bond between the graft and the recipient area. Since a longer time is necessary for full-thickness grafts to take, they should not be placed in infected areas or in long-standing wounds. If the full-thickness graft is desirable but cannot be used because of infection in an open wound, the wound is first covered with a split-thickness graft. After this has taken and the area is clear of infection, the skin graft can be excised and replaced with a full-thickness graft for cosmesis.

Postoperatively, full-thickness grafts will assume the color that they had at their initial donor area (Fig. 12–9). Grafts taken from the face and above the clavicle will therefore be more reddened than those taken from the inguinal area or abdomen. Sensation will return to full-thickness grafts more slowly than to split-thickness grafts. Partial function of the sebaceous and the sweat glands may be retained in a full-thickness graft. Hair follicles incorporated in a full-thickness graft will frequently go into a telogen phase lasting from one to two months after transplantation. Such hair, however,

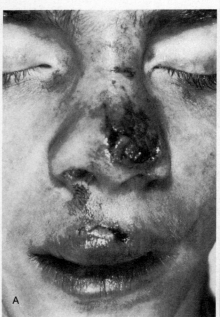
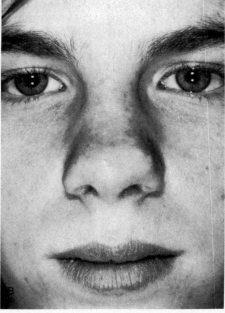

Figure 12–9. *A*, A seven-year-old boy with a full-thickness avulsion injury of the nose with minimal loss of subcutaneous tissue. *B*, The same patient two years after treatment with a full-thickness graft from the postauricular area; note the excellent contour and color match.

will usually grow back after the full-thickness graft takes.

REFERENCES

1. Converse JM: Reconstructive Plastic Surgery (Ed 2) 7 vols. Philadelphia, W. B. Saunders Co, 1964
2. Baronio G: Degli innesti animali. Milan, Stamperia e Fonderia del Genio, 1804
3. Gnudi MT, Webster JP: The Life and Times of Gaspar Tagliacozzi. 1545–1599. New York, Reichner, 1950
4. Reverdin M: Greffes épidermiques; expérience faite dans le service de M. le docteur Guyon, à l'hôpital Necker. Bull. Soc. Impériale Chir., 10:2, 1870
5. Ollier L: Greffes cutanées ou autoplastiques. Bill. Acad. Méd., 1:243, 1872
6. Thiersch C: Über die deineren anatomischen Veranderungen bei Aufheilung von Haut auf Granulationen. Arch Klin Chir 17:318, 1874
7. Blair VP, Brown JB: Use and uses of large split thickness grafts of intermediate thickness. Surg Gynec Obstet 49:82, 1929
8. Padgett EC: Calibrated intermediate skin grafts. Surg Gynecol Obstet 69:799, 1939
9. Southwood WF: The thickness of the skin. Plast Reconstr Surg 15:423, 1955
10. Kazanceva ND: Growth characteristics of skin thickness in children and its significance on free skin grafts. Acta Chir Plast (Prague) 11:71, 1969
11. Grabb WC, Smith JW: Plastic Surgery. Boston, Little, Brown & Co, 1979
12. Dingman RO, Argenta LC: Reconstruction of the chest wall. Ann Thor Surg 32:202–208, 1981
13. Crawford BS: An unusual skin donor site. Brit J Plast Surg 17:311, 1964
14. Ponten B: Grafted skin—observations on innervation and other qualities. Acta Chir Scand Suppl 257, 1960
15. Krizek TJ, Robson MC: Evolution of quantitative bacteriology in wound management. Am J Surg 130:579, 1975
16. Robson MC, Krizek TJ, Heggars JP: Biology of surgical infections. In Current Problems in Surgery, Ravitch MM (ed). Chicago: Yearbook Medical Publishers Inc, 1973
17. Polk HC: Adherence of thin skin grafts. Surg Forum 17:487, 1966
18. Clemmesen T: Experimental studies on the healing of free skin autografts. Dan Med Bull Suppl 14, 2:1, 1967
19. Smahel J: The healing of skin grafts. Clin Plast Surg 4:409, 1977
20. Smahel J, Clodius L: The blood vessel system of free human skin grafts. Plast Reconstr Surg 47:61–66, 1971

13

ALFRED S. KETCHAM, M.D., F.A.C.S. / FREDERICK L. MOFFAT, M.D., F.R.C.S.(C)

Cancer of the Skin and the Surgical Oncologist

The best opportunity to cure a patient of cancer is
afforded the first physician who treats the disease.
—ALFRED S. KETCHAM

Cancer of the skin is an exceedingly common clinical problem that is managed competently for the most part by surgeons in this country. With the exception of melanoma, skin cancers are relatively indolent tumors that metastasize or invade major structures late in their course. They cause negligible morbidity and mortality when diagnosed promptly and treated appropriately. However, the cure rate in the United States for cutaneous cancers other than melanoma is currently only 70% to 85%. We suggest that, if all patients afflicted with these malignancies received optimum therapy when medical attention is first sought, more than 98% would be cured. With this in mind, it is appropriate that a chapter in this book be devoted to a review of the principles of surgical management of malignant neoplasia of the skin.

The conventional and best primary treatment of most skin tumors is wide surgical excision. The extent of resection required is dictated in part by the site of origin and histologic type of the lesion being treated. The gross and histologic extent of the primary tumor and the presence or absence of invasion into vital structures or the spread to regional lymph nodes are also major determinants of the extent of surgery necessary for adequate treatment. Appropriate primary surgical excision of skin malignancies should eliminate the rather distressing therapeutic problems posed by patients presenting with local recurrence in the face of previous "conservative" surgery, "shave" excision, topical chemical treatment, cryotherapy, fulguration, curettage, or injudicious radiotherapy.

When wide surgical excision is undertaken as definitive primary therapy, the cancer must be excised en bloc with adequate peripheral and deep margins of uninvolved tissue. While preservation of sufficient regional tissue for cosmetically and functionally acceptable wound closure is a significant consideration (especially for lesions of the face, hands, or digits), total excision of the cancer with histologically tumor-free margins is of paramount importance. The patient is better served at the outset by an adequate wide resection than by a "cosmetic" excision; the latter may result in local persistence or recurrence of tumor for which a major ablative procedure will be necessary.

Treatment efficacy is also compromised by lax follow-up of patients with a past history of skin cancer. The postoperative monitoring of a patient who has had a small skin cancer excised is not infrequently undertaken in a cavalier manner. Such a patient is at risk of presenting with extensive recurrent or metachronous skin cancer that is amenable only to disfiguring or disabling surgical treatment. Even when such patients are followed conscientiously, nodularity in a surgical scar may mistakenly be attributed to a foreign-body reaction or early ulceration to defective wound healing. Only a high index of suspicion for recurrent neoplasia will prompt early biopsy of such seemingly innocuous changes in an attempt to detect recurrence at a time when it can be easily treated.

BIOPSY TECHNIQUES

Anesthesia

In general, local anesthesia is best achieved by infiltration of a 1% or 2% lidocaine solution around the tumor. A small caliber needle is used to inject the anesthetic, and infiltration is carried out slowly in order to minimize patient discomfort. Epinephrine-containing anesthetic may be used unless the patient has atherosclerotic heart disease, or the lesion in question is situated on an appendage perfused by an end artery (i.e., a digit, the nose, the ear, or the penis). Lidocaine should not be injected directly into skin tumors because of the theoretical risk of dislodging and disseminating tumor cells into the dermal lymphatics or blood vessels. A "ring" block or proximal infiltration may be used for a cancer on a digit or the ear.

Punch Biopsy

In general, needle aspiration or trocar needle biopsy techniques are of little use in the diagnosis of skin cancer.[2] Shave biopsies are not recommended because they may not provide the pathologist with a satisfactory specimen for accurate diagnosis and assessment of the depth of invasion. On the other hand, punch biopsies are often performed to obtain a tissue diagnosis in patients with suspicious skin lesions. This technique is easy to use and lends itself well to office practice. Bleeding may be controlled with pressure or silver nitrate cauterization; suture closure of a punch biopsy wound is generally unnecessary.

A few words of caution regarding punch biopsies are warranted. The punch biopsy instrument must be sharp to prevent undue patient discomfort or excessive distortion and crushing of the biopsy specimen. Disposable punch biopsy instruments serve adequately, but become dull quickly. The operator must be sure to label specimens carefully and to identify what part of the lesion each is from when multiple punch biopsies of a large tumor are taken. Because only a limited portion of tissue is removed, the biopsy should be taken from the most worrisome part of a tumor; for instance, the thickest portion of a pigmented lesion should be biopsied. Furthermore, the biopsy should include the full thickness of epidermis and dermis for optimal histologic assessment. Biopsies taken from the base of an ulcerated lesion will show only necrosis unless a full-thickness specimen is obtained. Finally, it cannot be stated too strongly that a punch biopsy must never be regarded as definitive therapy for skin cancer, even when the entire tumor is included in the specimen. There is no place for "punch therapy" in the treatment of neoplasms of the skin.

Incisional Biopsy

Surgeons are reluctant to cut through a neoplastic skin lesion because of the theoretical risks of causing tumor cell implantation deep within the operative wound or of promoting tumor dissemination. While it is indeed preferable to perform excisional biopsy where possible, experience has shown that incisional biopsy techniques are safe and seldom complicate subsequent definitive therapy if the incision is oriented appropriately.

Incisional biopsies are best taken with a no. 11 or 15 scalpel. A strip of tissue is removed, its long axis oriented radially with respect to the lesion. The biopsy specimen samples the central and peripheral areas of the tumor as well as adjacent normal skin. The biopsy should include all layers of the skin so that the pathologist can assess the extent of vertical tumor growth. For obvious reasons, this technique is in no way therapeutic.

Excisional Biopsy

This technique involves removal of the entire lesion, leaving a defect which often must be closed with sutures. The tumor is not violated and the pathologist can give a very accurate appraisal of the tumor's histology, invasiveness, and peripheral extent of growth. This technique is preferable to an incisional or punch biopsy, if feasible.

When excising a skin lesion for biopsy, careful consideration should be given to the orientation of the resulting scar. The incision should be placed so that subsequent definitive surgical resection of the area is curative and produces a satisfactory cosmetic and functional result. Again, a simple excisional biopsy should seldom be considered adequate local treatment by itself.

SURGICAL TREATMENT OF SKIN TUMORS

While the principles of surgical treatment vary somewhat with the site and histologic type of skin cancer, there are some general rules that apply to all skin malignancies. If these are followed, local recurrence should seldom be a complication of treatment for most skin cancers.[3]

Specimen Margins and the Pathologist's Role

The issue of what constitutes an adequate margin of excision is very contentious. The definitive surgical resection must encompass the biopsy incision and tract and include the margins of uninvolved tissue adjacent to the tumor. Generally, basal cell carcinomas can be cured by en bloc excision with normal tissue margins of 5 mm at all points peripheral and deep to the lesion. Squamous cell carcinomas should be excised with margins of 10 mm. These guidelines are not applicable to large, neglected neoplasms; such lesions require excision of wider margins of uninvolved tissue for a curative result.

Special consideration must be given to lesions of the face, hands, and digits in the interests of cosmesis and function. Skin tumors overlying joints or located on the nose or ear not infrequently invade underlying cartilage, ligaments, or bone; adequate treatment requires en bloc removal of portions of these structures with immediate reconstruction. It is most important to establish intraoperatively by frozen section examination that the margins of resection are free of disease. These complicated lesions are best managed by individuals with expertise in surgical oncology and reconstructive surgery.

Malignant melanoma is the most dangerous and capricious of the common skin tumors and therefore must be considered separately. This tumor not uncommonly recurs as satellite nodules in surgical scars, in adjacent uninvolved skin, or under skin grafts. Where possible, peripheral margins of 2 to 5 cm should be removed with the lesion. The deep margin of resection should extend at least to the underlying fascia. Controversy exists as to whether the fascia should be taken with the specimen. It is the authors' opinion that the deep fascia should be removed, especially if the melanoma is ulcerated or deeply invasive.

It is apparent from the foregoing discussion that the pathologist performs an indispensable service in the surgical management of skin tumors. Ideally, the pathologist should see the lesion before and during surgery; realistically, he or she should at least be invited into the operating room to be shown how the specimen relates spatially to the surgical wound. In this regard, we recommend a small sterile specimen board, the edges of which have been labeled superior, inferior, left, and right. The specimen is properly oriented on the board, pinned in place and submitted to the pathologist. This technique has the added advantage of preventing postoperative tissue shrinkage that might lead the pathologist to conclude erroneously that insufficient margins of normal tissue have been excised.[4] Alternatively, the edges of the specimen can be marked with sutures, using one suture for the superior edge, two for the inferior edge, and so on. Detailed records of the significance of these sutures should be made on the patient's chart and on the pathology requisition.

Some wounds are best evaluated for adequacy of margins by re-excising 1 to 2 mm of the wound edge after tumor removal but before wound closure. These separately taken margins are then labeled and sent for frozen section interpretation.

Prior to closure of the operative wound, the pathologist must assess the specimen margins by frozen section microscopic examination to confirm that no disease has been left behind. If a margin is close to or involved by cancer, it is a simple matter to re-excise that margin and do another frozen section examination. If the operative wound has been closed without confirmation of tumor-free margins and cancer is found in the margins on subsequent examination of the permanent tissue sections, it may be impossible to determine where the residual tumor is. When undermining of wound edges and suture closure of the wound have been done, residual tumor cells may inadvertently have been spread a considerable distance from the original positive margin; radical re-excision of the wound may then have to be undertaken. Such a patient pays a formidable price for inadequate confirmation of tumor-free margins at the time of the initial procedure.

Occasionally, examination of the permanent sections several days after surgery reveals a positive or close margin that was missed intraoperatively despite what was thought to be a thorough frozen section assessment. If the lesion is not a melanoma and the patient is intelligent and compliant, the surgeon may elect to follow the wound closely. Any suspicious nodularity or other changes should be biopsied without delay and radical re-excision undertaken if tumor persistence is confirmed.

Technical Considerations

Removal of a skin cancer en bloc with adjacent normal tissue is essential for a curative result. It is equally important that the surgeon take some technical precautions in closing or reconstructing the skin defect to prevent inadvertent implantation of tumor cells. Once the lesion is removed and the margins of resection are reported to be free of tumor, the surgical team should change gloves and use new instruments for the remainder of the procedure. The occurrence of tumor implantation when the wound edges are being undermined and sutured is thereby minimized. The presence of viable tumor cells in washings from the gloves and surgical instruments used to resect a cancer has been documented; the potential for disease recurrence due to wound contamination by surgical personnel is very real.[5]

If it is anticipated that a skin graft will be required for wound closure, the graft should be taken and the donor area dressed before the cancer is excised. When the necessity for a graft becomes apparent only after the primary tumor has been removed, the surgical team should use new gowns and gloves, prepare and drape the donor site separately, take the graft with fresh instruments, and then dress the donor site before proceeding further.

A case is cited to illustrate the phenomenon of iatrogenic tumor cell implantation. A 54-year-old white female presented with a squamous cell carcinoma of the skin of the bridge of the nose. The lesion was excised only to recur two and four years later. On removing the second recurrence, it became apparent intraoperatively that a skin graft would be required for wound closure; a full-thickness graft was taken from the postauricular area with the same instruments used to excise the tumor. Within two years, the tumor had recurred in the nasal skin graft and involved the underlying bone. She had also developed an ulcer in the postauricular donor site, which, on biopsy, proved to be squamous cell carcinoma. The histologic characteristics of the original skin tumor, the three local recurrences, and the postauricular lesion were identical. Five years after appropriate treatment, the patient was free of any new primary tumors. It is most unlikely that this woman had metachronous skin primaries; rather it can safely be concluded that her postauricular cancer was implanted by the surgeon during her third operation as a result of tumor cell transplantation.

Regional Lymphadenectomy

In addition to treating the primary skin cancer, one must not forget that concomitant regional lymphadenectomy may be indicated in some instances. Removal of clinically negative regional lymph nodes at the time of resection for primary skin cancer is the subject of much debate. However, therapeutic regional node dissection must be undertaken in skin cancer patients with clinically evident nodal metastases. Lymphadenectomy should be performed in continuity with resection of the primary tumor whenever technically and cosmetically possible. If the practitioner is not competent to undertake excision of the primary tumor and regional lymph nodes in a patient requiring such a procedure, a surgeon with the necessary expertise should be consulted.

SKIN TUMORS BY HISTOLOGIC TYPE AND SITE

Basal Cell Carcinoma

This is the most indolent of all skin malignancies and can be cured by any of several therapeutic modalities.[6, 7] Metastases from basal cell cancers are extremely rare.[8] However, these tumors are locally invasive and, if neglected or inadequately treated, can develop into disabling or even life-threatening lesions.[9] Basal cell carcinomas must be treated by adequate wide excision.

In general, basal cell carcinomas should be excised with normal tissue margins of at least 5 mm. For uncomplicated small lesions, this can ordinarily be accomplished under local anesthesia in an outpatient setting. We believe that conventional surgical excision is preferable to other forms of local therapy. Only one visit is required for adequate treatment, and the resulting scar is barely noticeable if Langer's skin lines are respected. Other modalities, such as radiation or Mohs' chemosurgery, give favorable results, but multiple outpatient visits are usually necessary. These treatments are therefore costly, and patient compliance is a potential problem.

Basal cell carcinomas are commonly multifocal, especially on sun-exposed areas of the body.[10] In excising a basal cell cancer, the surgeon may unknowingly cut through a small adjacent tumor thereby leaving a "positive margin" in the specimen. Such unfortunate occurrences may be avoided by careful preoperative inspection of the surrounding skin with a magnifying glass. The importance of accurate labeling of the edges of the operative specimen is, again, apparent.

Basal cell tumors arising near the orbit or on the nose, ear, or dorsum of the hand or foot require special consideration. Such lesions must be totally excised, but care must be taken to ensure a good functional and cosmetic result. This may necessitate the use of skin flaps or other tissue transfers for which special surgical training is required. Extensive and neglected basal cell cancers that invade underlying structures are often only amenable to major surgical procedures outside the province of most general surgeons. These patients are best treated at the outset by a surgical team with the requisite expertise.

Squamous Cell Carcinoma

In terms of biologic behavior, skin cancers with a mixed basal and squamous cell histologic appearance are indistinguishable from pure squamous cell carcinomas. All of these tumors are locally destructive (Fig. 13–1) and can metastasize widely. It is imperative that the initial surgical treatment be curative. Inadequate resection of the primary tumor is attended by a local recurrence rate of 50% and an ultimate mortality rate of 20%.

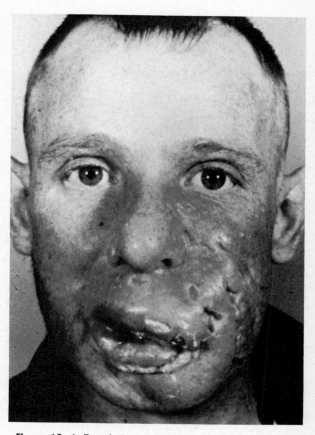

Figure 13–1. Deeply invasive squamous cell carcinoma misdiagnosed as a fungal infection and treated as such for two years before a biopsy was done. Radical surgical resection was necessary, followed by multiple reconstructive procedures. The patient was disease-free 15 years after appropriate treatment.

Squamous cell cancers of the skin should be widely excised taking 1 cm margins of surrounding skin and subcutaneous tissue whenever possible. The margins of resection must be checked intraoperatively by frozen section examination to ascertain whether any tumor cells remain in the operative wound. If periosteum, galea, muscle, tendon, or cartilage are involved by the tumor, then even multiple frozen sections may be misleading in determining the extent of invasion. In such cases, the surgeon must rely on his clinical judgment in deciding how much tissue must be removed.

Keratoacanthomas and subungual squamous cell carcinomas are difficult to diagnose both clinically and histologically.[11, 12] Keratoacanthomas are benign lesions, despite their rapid growth pattern and capacity to erode underlying bone. They closely resemble squamous cell carcinoma histologically. If diagnosed correctly by biopsy, they can be watched; with time, keratoacanthomas may regress completely.[13] Subungual carcinomas are slow growing and metastasize late in their course, but amputation at least one joint proximal to the tumor is usually required for cure. These lesions are not infrequently observed by medical practitioners for variable periods of time before the diagnosis is considered and then confirmed.

Radiation-Induced Skin Cancer

The now discredited use of ionizing radiation to treat acne or benign keratoses in adolescents and young adults has given rise to a population of middle-aged patients who have diffuse or multifocal precancerous and malignant changes in the irradiated skin.[14, 15] It is neither necessary nor practical to excise all affected skin and undertake reconstructive surgery. Close and careful followup, excisional biopsy when indicated, and wide resection of confirmed cancer will result in good long-term control.[16] It must be emphasized that a biopsy should be performed for any and all suspicious changes in previously irradiated skin without delay.

Surgical excision of cancer arising in heavily irradiated skin is often complicated by delayed healing due to radiation-induced hypovascularity. Neither primary wound closure nor split-thickness skin grafts will suffice in many instances; skin pedicles or myocutaneous flaps must be transferred into the surgical defect for satisfactory healing. Occasionally, major amputation may be necessary for adequate control of cancer arising in skin severely damaged by ionizing radiation. The consequences of not carrying out appropriate surgery primarily in this clinical setting are illustrated by the following case.

A 57-year-old rural surgeon who had used fluoroscopy extensively for 20 years presented with premalignant changes in the skin of both hands.

Over the next eight years, multiple conservative excisions of ulcerating lesions on both hands were undertaken, followed by partial amputations of several digits and, finally, amputation of one hand. He died two years later of pulmonary metastases after first undergoing axillary node dissection and then forequarter amputation for regional recurrence. It is quite likely that a more radical approach initially might have spared this patient's life and perhaps partial function of one or both hands. Such patients are rarely well served by conservative therapy undertaken to preserve important parts of the body.[17]

Atypical fibroxanthoma of the skin is a spindle cell variant of squamous cell carcinoma. These lesions tend to occur in radiation-damaged skin. The treatment of choice is adequate surgical excision, which provides an excellent cure rate.[18, 19]

Carcinoma Arising in Cutaneous Scars

It has long been recognized that carcinomas may develop in chronic fistulae, wounds, sinuses, ulcers, keloids, burns, and chronic osteomyelitis.[20, 21] Frostbite has also been implicated as a cause of skin malignancy.[22] A classical example of cutaneous "scar cancer" is the squamous cell carcinoma arising in skin that has been burned in the remote past, the so-called Marjolin's ulcer. One early report suggested that 18% of all skin tumors of the scalp, trunk, and proximal extremities arise in scar tissue and that 38% of all skin malignancies on the hand arise from old wounds.[23]

The treatment of these skin cancers is radical excision, removing all cicatricial tissue en bloc with the tumor. The underlying fascia should also be excised. The surgical wound may be closed with a skin or composite tissue flap or with a split-thickness skin graft. The advantage of the former method of closure is that cutaneous or myocutaneous flaps withstand the trauma, irritation, and stress of weight-bearing much better than a split-thickness skin graft. However, local recurrence is more likely to be diagnosed early when the wound has been covered with only a split-thickness skin graft.

Malignant Melanoma

Of the common primary tumors of the skin, melanoma is the least predictable and the most life-threatening. Irrespective of the extent of invasion (as measured by Breslow's tumor thickness or Clark's histologic level), it is imperative that primary melanomas be widely excised with adequate peripheral margins of 2 cm or more, incorporating the underlying fascia in the deep margin of resection. In general, local recurrence is a distressingly frequent consequence of overly conservative resection.[24] Unfortunately, local recurrence, satellitosis, or both may occur even after radical resection (Fig. 13–2).

As a general rule, the extent of tissue resected with the primary tumor should preclude primary closure of the wound except in areas such as the torso. Wide undermining of the surrounding skin to permit primary closure may be unwise, because this theoretically increases the risk of local tumor implantation. The use of Z-plasties and local skin flaps remains controversial for the same reason.[25, 26] Furthermore, thick tissue flaps may mask local recurrence and thereby delay appropriate treatment.

Some surgeons treat patients who have head and neck melanomas by conservative resection and primary closure of the wound. This is an acceptable practice only if the patient is intelligent and willing to be followed closely. Such a patient should be fully informed of the increased risk of local recurrence inherent in such a treatment plan before undergoing surgery. Melanomas arising in the head and neck tend to be aggressive tumors.[27]

Digital and subungual melanomas are treated best by amputation at least one joint proximal to the lesion (Fig. 13–3).[28]

Patients who present with clinically evident re-

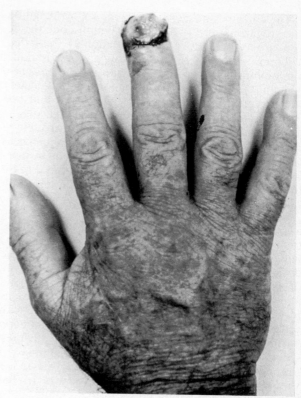

Figure 13–3. A subungual melanoma of the finger that should be managed by a digital amputation; in the case of the long finger, a ray amputation would likely give the best functional result.

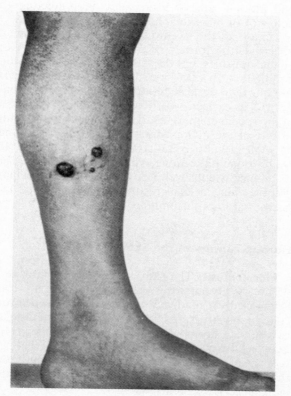

Figure 13–2. A nodular melanoma invading through the papillary dermis, with local satellitosis. This was managed by en bloc wide resection with 3 cm margins of normal skin. A simultaneous prophylactic superficial inguinal node dissection revealed no nodal metastases.

gional lymph node metastases in addition to the primary tumor should undergo simultaneous resection of the primary and regional lymphatics, preferably in continuity if feasible. When suspicious regional lymphadenopathy is present or develops subsequent to successful treatment of the primary tumor, fine needle aspiration or biopsy should be undertaken to confirm or rule out metastatic disease. If regional metastases are confirmed, lymphadenectomy should be performed after a full metastatic workup has been done.

A number of retrospective studies and two prospective trials have addressed the question of elective regional lymphadenectomy at the time of resection of the primary lesion in patients with clinically negative nodes.[29–39] As of this writing, the various points of contention on this subject are still unsettled. At issue are the criteria by which patients with Stage I melanoma, who are at high risk for regional nodal micrometastases but who are unlikely to have systemic disease, can be discerned. The major concern of many surgeons is that the morbidity of regional lymphadenectomy cannot be justified in patients with early Stage I disease who are unlikely to have occult nodal disease, or in those whose melanomas are probably already widely disseminated.

The current data suggest that the following guidelines regarding elective regional lymph node dissection are reasonable.[38] Thin melanomas (less than 0.76 mm thick) are rarely associated with nodal micrometastases or distant spread of disease, whereas thick lesions (4 mm or more) are associated with a very high incidence of both nodal and systemic occult melanoma. Prophylactic nodal dissection should be avoided in these circumstances. However, melanomas of 0.76 to 3.9 mm in thickness have an increasing risk of nodal micrometastases (up to 60%) but a low risk of disseminated disease (less than 20%); patients with these lesions are candidates for elective node dissection.

Overall, Stage I melanomas on an extremity have a lower probability of occult regional nodal spread than melanomas situated elsewhere. Trunk lesions have a high risk of regional spread but it can be difficult to predict which nodal basin is harboring disease in individual patients. Patients with head and neck melanomas and those with trunk lesions in whom lymphoscintigraphy suggests that the skin around the primary tumor drains to one lymph node basin should be considered for elective regional lymphadenectomy. In patients with melanomas of the head and neck, the radical neck dissection should include the parotid gland because of the intraparenchymal lymph nodes in that gland.

Melanomas in males are somewhat more aggressive than those in females; elective lymph node dissection should be more seriously entertained in men with superficial lesions than in women with comparable tumors. The gross appearance of the lesion has some importance in determining whether elective node dissection is indicated. Ulcerated melanomas are more often associated with nodal micrometastases than are nonulcerated lesions. Lentigo maligna (Hutchinson's freckle) is almost never associated with nodal disease, whereas nodular or acral lentiginous melanomas frequently are.

Finally, the position of the primary tumor relative to the regional nodes may have some bearing on the decision to do elective lymphadenectomy. Melanomas overlying the neck, parotid glands, axillae, or groins are ideally situated for en bloc removal of the primary tumor and the lymphatics. One is more inclined to perform lymphadenectomy in these circumstances than when the primary lesion and the regional nodes are far removed from one another, other factors being equal.

In recent years the dysplastic nevus syndrome has come to light as a strong predictor of melanoma in affected individuals.[40–43] This syndrome follows both familial and sporadic epidemiologic patterns. Dysplastic nevi tend to be larger than truly benign moles and have irregular borders, variegated color, and erratic growth patterns. They may occur on unexposed areas of the body. Affected persons do not necessarily have large numbers of moles but do have a very high risk for developing invasive melanoma in their dysplastic nevi. The recognition of this syndrome has underscored again the importance of maintaining a high index of suspicion with respect to apparently innocuous pigmented lesions. A biopsy of moles should be performed whenever the slightest doubt exists concerning their biologic behavior.

Adnexal Tumors of the Skin

Tumors of the skin adnexa are rare; few studies involving significant numbers of patients have been done.[44] The skin adnexa originate from the same ectodermal cell line as epidermal cells, and as a result, the histology of adnexal tumors is similar to that of other skin neoplasms.[13] Most of these lesions present as discrete nodules that, having been present for many years, suddenly increase in size. They are from a few millimeters to several centimeters in diameter.[45] There is no known etiology for most of these tumors. Their biologic behavior is quite variable; however, it should be noted that local recurrence rates for even low-grade adnexal neoplasms are as high as 40%, and distant spread may occur in 6% to 10% of patients. Histologic appearance and grading are of little value in predicting the behavior of individual adnexal skin tumors.

Tumors of the sweat glands are either eccrine or apocrine, the former occurring more often on the palms and soles and the latter in the axillary, pubic, perianal, and scrotal skin. The axillae are a frequent site of origin of these lesions.[46] These tumors should be widely excised with frozen section examination of the specimen margins. If the tumor is in proximity to one of the major lymph node basins, there may be some benefit to undertaking immediate en bloc lymph node dissection, even when these nodes are not clinically enlarged. Long-term follow-up is mandatory; delayed local recurrence and regional metastases are not uncommon.

Fibrous Tumors of the Skin

Fibromatosis. The skin is occasionally the site of origin for fibromatoses. These conditions are characterized by a tendency to recur locally and invade contiguous structures.[47–51] They do not metastasize as a rule. A fibromatosis generally becomes increasingly aggressive with each recurrence. Treatment consists of wide local excision with or without radiotherapy. Chemotherapy may be used in combination with surgery for recurrences.

Desmoid Tumors. Desmoids are fibromatous tumors that classically arise in the abdominal wall musculature but may also occur in the skin.[50–52] Wide local excision is the treatment of choice, but the surgeon must be cognizant of the fact that these tumors may arise in the underlying fascia or muscle and involve the skin secondarily. Cutting through a desmoid results in a locally recurrent tumor that behaves more aggressively. Only rarely are desmoids responsive to hormones, steroids, or x-ray treatment.[53–55]

Keloids. Although keloids are not neoplastic lesions, total excision is mandatory in treating these abnormal scars surgically. Recurrence is a frequent and distressing outcome. The concomitant use of steroids or low-dose radiotherapy is occasionally helpful.

Pseudosarcomatous Fasciitis. This fibrous skin tumor tends to invade skin and subcutaneous tissue precipitously.[56] If widely and totally excised with margins of normal tissue, local recurrence is uncommon.

Dermatofibrosarcoma Protuberans. This low-grade dermal sarcoma may occasionally metastasize.[57–61] It tends to occur in patients aged 20 to 40 years. The lesion presents as solitary or multiple, hard, erythematous cutaneous nodules. The local recurrence rate following excision is as high as 80%. The lesion invades adjacent normal tissue by developing microscopic stellate projections of neoplastic cells. Radical excision with generous margins of deep fascia and muscle and skin margins of at least 4 to 6 cm is essential.

Tumors of the Scalp

Less than 2% of epithelial malignancies occur in the scalp.[62] The most common primary cancer of the scalp is melanoma followed, in descending order of frequency, by basal cell and squamous cell carcinomas, fibrosarcoma, rhabdomyosarcoma, angiosarcoma, leiomyosarcoma, liposarcoma, lymphoma, adenocarcinoma, adenocystic basal cell cancer, and leukemic infiltrates.

The so-called turban tumor (Fig. 13–4) is a dermal cylindroma of the scalp.[63] This lesion probably arises from eccrine sweat glands. Multiple lesions are common, and the marked vascularity has persuaded some practitioners to recommend electrocoagulation as the preferred method of treatment. Dermal cylindromas do not metastasize, but local recurrence is a problem. Wide local excision is the standard treatment.

Surgical excision is the treatment of choice for most scalp neoplasms. If the lesion is only minimally invasive, a wedge resection down to the subaponeurotic space may suffice. Primary closure of the resulting defect is usually possible. However, the scalp is nonelastic and very vascular; the surgeon must be prepared for bleeding and difficult wound closure problems following either major or minor scalp resections. If the excision has included the galea and periosteum, the wound should be covered by a full-thickness flap from the scalp, shoulder, or chest. Split-thickness skin grafts do not take on bone denuded of periosteum.

Radiotherapy is seldom the preferred method of treatment for scalp neoplasms. The close proximity of bone and the tough fibrous characteristics of the scalp make radiotherapy difficult to administer without incurring serious local complications. Electrocautery and cryotherapy are useful for only a few scalp lesions.

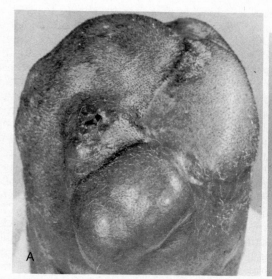
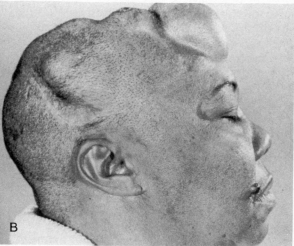

Figure 13–4. The turban tumor. *A* and *B*, The propensity for local recurrence is illustrated in this lady in whom the cylindroma is once again in evidence despite multiple excisions and closures with rotational scalp flaps.

Tumors of the External Ear

Tumors of the ear arise from both epithelial and mesothelial tissues; neoplasms originating in skin, muscle, and cartilage all occur here. Basal cell and squamous cell cancers are most frequently encountered, followed by melanomas and, rarely, sarcomas. The external ear is rarely involved by tumors arising in the mastoid air cells or parotid gland, although it may be included in the surgical resection of these lesions.

Benign tumors of the ear are easily managed by local resection when they are recognized early in their course. Malignant lesions must be treated by full-thickness wedge resection of the external ear including the underlying cartilage. Invasion of the cartilage by basal cell or squamous cell carcinomas is a very common occurrence. Meticulous closure of the resulting defect in the ear produces an excellent cosmetic result.

When the tumor is extensive or invades the external auditory canal (Fig. 13–5), resection of the entire ear may be necessary. Surgical reconstruction should be undertaken only by an experienced plastic surgeon. In general, a skillfully designed prosthesis gives a better cosmetic result than surgical reconstruction following removal of the external ear.

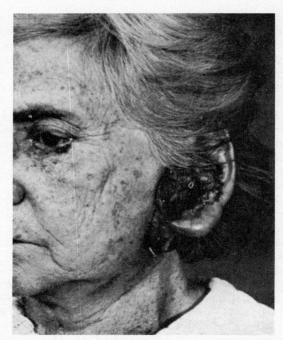

Figure 13–6. A carcinoma of the lower lip that was neglected by the patient for three years. Radical excision, superficial parotid lobectomy and radical neck dissection were undertaken. Despite the presence of metastatic disease in the preauricular, submental and submandibular lymph nodes, the patient was free of disease nine years later.

Cancer of the Lip

Cancer of the lower lip is approximately 20 times as common as cancer of the upper lip. The lip is a common site of origin for cancer in the head and neck; carcinomas of the lip account for 25% to 30% of all tumors of the oral cavity.[64, 65]

The most common histologic type of lip cancer is squamous cell carcinoma, which tends to spread laterally across the surface but can also infiltrate deeply into the lip muscle. Nodal metastases from the lower lip are seen in 10% of the cases and are found most often in the submental and submandibular lymph nodes. Cancers of the upper lip spread to the regional nodes in 20% of cases; these lesions metastasize more often to the preauricular and parotid lymph nodes than to the submandibular glands.

The treatment of primary lip cancer consists of either surgery or radiotherapy. Overall, the efficacy of these methods of treatment is comparable. For optimal cosmesis and function, however, small cancers (involving less than one third of the lip) are preferably excised, although a better result is obtained with radical radiotherapy for more extensive lesions. When lip cancers are treated surgically, intraoperative frozen section examinations must be done to confirm that the margins are free of tumor.

Surgical removal of early lip cancers is done by the V-excision technique. Primary closure is then performed, taking care to obtain realignment of the vermilion border to avoid a "step" deformity in the lip. For more extensive lesions, a flap from the opposite lip can be rotated on a labial arterial pedicle, as in the Estlander or the Abbé procedures.[66] Cancers involving the labial commissures require meticulous closure with rotational flaps (Fig. 13–6).

Some practitioners have employed chemical dessication, electrocautery, or lip shaves to treat early lip cancers and have justified these methods by the belief that labial cancer is not deeply invasive in its early stages. While these procedures undoubtedly have a place in the management of minimal disease or premalignant changes (carcinoma in situ or leukoplakia), it is important to remember that lip cancer is a lethal disease. Some series report five-year survival rates of only 70% for carcinoma of the lip. It is imperative that the initial treatment of these tumors be curative; this is generally possible only by resorting to wide surgical resection or radical radiation.

Prophylactic radical neck dissection is not necessary for early low-grade cancers of the lip. These patients should be followed carefully and neck dissection undertaken if submental, submandibular, or jugular nodal metastases develop. The authors perform prophylactic suprahyoid dissection or, occasionally, radical neck dissection when the primary lesion is extensive, when there has been rapid growth of the primary tumor, and when the primary

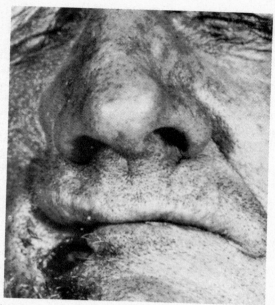

Figure 13–6. A carcinoma of the lower lip that was neglected by the patient for three years. Radical excision, superficial parotid lobectomy and radical neck dissection were undertaken. Despite the presence of metastatic disease in the preauricular, submental and submandibular lymph nodes, the patient was free of disease nine years later.

tumor has a high-grade histologic appearance. Patients with cancers of the upper lip undergo ipsilateral superficial parotid lobectomy and radical neck dissection only when there is palpable neck disease or when the primary lesion is advanced. Lymph node biopsy is generally not required to confirm the presence of cervical metastases. The decision to do a neck dissection can be made on the basis of fine needle aspiration cytology or clinical judgment alone.

Secondary Tumors of the Skin

Cutaneous metastases from tumors elsewhere in the body are uncommon but not rare (Fig. 13–7). The most common tumor to metastasize hematogenously to the skin is carcinoma of the breast, followed by gastrointestinal cancers, melanoma, and lung carcinomas.[67, 68] Tumors occurring in a surgical scar following resection of a visceral cancer are generally considered to be iatrogenic.[69] Experimentally, cancers have also been shown to metastasize to sites of trauma or remotely placed surgical wounds ("scar oncotaxis"), although this phenomenon has not yet been shown to occur clinically.

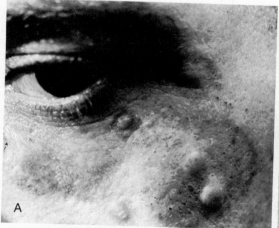

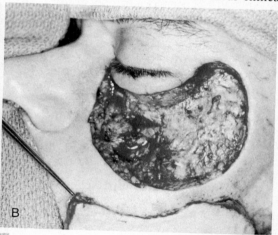

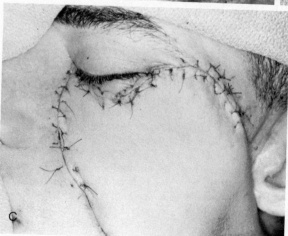

Figure 13–7. *A,* Malar cutaneous metastases that developed two years following radiotherapy for a preauricualr "fullness" that was never biopsied. Biopsy of the malar lesions revealed metastatic parotid cancer. *B,* The cutaneous metastases were removed en bloc. *C,* A deltopectoral flap was used for reconstruction. Unfortunately, the patient subsequently developed a massive preauricular recurrence and multiple pulmonary metastases.

The treatment of true cutaneous metastases from visceral cancer is predicated on the extent of tumor spread in the individual patient and on what palliative treatment is available. If chemotherapy is used, the medical oncologist might prefer to preserve a cutaneous metastasis as an "indicator" lesion in order to follow the tumor's response to treatment. In other circumstances, cutaneous secondaries may be widely excised.

Tumors recurring in an operative wound should be widely excised. Many patients with wound implants have been cured by aggressive excision of their recurrent disease.

Melanoma metastasizes to the skin in one of two ways: It may spread locally, giving rise to satellitosis, or distantly (i.e., by in-transit metastasis). In either circumstance, radical excision offers the only realistic chance of cure or palliation.

Cutaneous Manifestations of Visceral Malignancies

A number of dermatologic conditions strongly suggest underlying malignant neoplasia.[70] There are also certain skin conditions that are parts of clinical syndromes in which cancers predictably occur, such as the previously discussed dysplastic nevus syndrome. It is important that surgeons, the major providers of therapy for solid tumors, be familiar with these skin conditions.

Paget's Disease. Occurring in the skin of the breast or the perineum, Paget's disease presents as an eczematous eruption. The diagnosis is made by biopsy, but treatment is directed toward the inciting neoplasm of the breast or vulva. Total excision of the skin lesion and the underlying tumor is mandatory for a satisfactory result.

Arsenical Keratosis. This precancerous condition is sometimes associated with the development of bronchogenic carcinoma, bladder cancer, or carcinoma of the renal pelvis. Because these cancers are all amenable to curative surgery, it is important to consider the possibility of these neoplasms being present in patients with arsenical keratoses.

Bowen's Disease. About 80% of patients with Bowen's disease also have or will develop other epithelial cancers.[71] Both types of tumors, once identified, should be treated independently and aggressively.

Multiple Nevoid Basal Cell Carcinoma. Syndromes of multiple nevoid basal cell carcinomas tend to be familial. They occur in association with skeletal anomalies, cerebellar medulloblastomas, ovarian neoplasms, and fibrosarcomas. The underlying visceral lesion should be widely resected whenever possible.

Gardner's Syndrome. The cutaneous manifestations of Gardner's syndrome include soft tissue, epidermal, and myoepithelial inclusion cysts. Hypertrophic scarring following removal of the skin lesions is suggestive of this syndrome.[72] The most significant lesions in Gardner's syndrome are the adenomatous polyps that occur throughout the small and large bowel. These polyps may be profuse and have a high probability of undergoing malignant degeneration. Prophylactic subtotal colectomy with close endoscopic follow-up of the rectal stump or panproctocolectomy are recommended for this condition. The development of the continent ileostomy and pelvic pouch has made these major prophylactic procedures more acceptable to patients with polyposis syndromes. If a bowel cancer has already developed in a patient with Gardner's syndrome, this lesion should be treated in the standard manner.

Von Recklinghausen's Disease. Patients with von Recklinghausen's disease have a definite predisposition to malignant degeneration of their neurofibromas or the development of other visceral cancers. About 16% of these patients will develop tumors such as fibrosarcomas or pheochromocytomas. Recognition of von Recklinghausen's disease should prompt a practitioner to maintain close surveillance of the patient for visceral neoplasms. These tumors should be treated aggressively in the usual manner when they occur.

Acanthosis Nigricans. This disorder in adults may be the harbinger of bronchogenic carcinoma or adenocarcinoma of the stomach, breast, uterus, or ovary. Definitive treatment of the inciting neoplasm will cause acanthosis nigricans to remit, and local recurrence or distant spread of the cancer may be heralded by the reappearance of the skin lesion.

Dermatomyositis. One of the so-called collagen diseases, dermatomyositis has a peculiar association with visceral neoplasia. Afflicted patients have a fivefold greater risk of developing cancer than the general population. Even when the patient is debilitated by dermatomyositis, visceral cancer should be treated as aggressively as it is in patients who do not have such chronic illnesses.

SUMMARY

It is apparent from the foregoing discussion that skin cancers must be treated properly when they are first brought to the medical practitioner's attention. This usually means wide surgical excision with adequate margins of uninvolved tissue. Regional lymph node dissection should also be undertaken, preferably en bloc with the primary lesion, when lymph node metastases are evident or for tumors in which elective removal of clinically negative lymph nodes is indicated. Surgeons should be cognizant of clinical situations in which special surgical expertise is required and be prepared to refer these cases to appropriate specialists if they have not had the requisite training or experience. Surgeons and other medical practitioners should also be aware of dermatologic syndromes associated with local or visceral neoplasia.

REFERENCES

1. Ketcham AS: A surgeon's approach to the patient with advanced cancer. In Schoenberg B, Carr AC, Peretz D, et al (eds): Psychosocial Aspects of Terminal Care. New York, Columbia University Press, 1972, pp 88–97
2. Chu EW, Hoye R: The clinician and the cytopathologist evaluate fine needle aspiration cytology. Acta Cytol (Baltimore) 17:5, 1973
3. Glass RL, Perez-Mesa CM: Management of inadequately excised epidermoid carcinoma. Arch Surg 108:50–51, 1974
4. Beirne GA, Beirne CG: Observation on the critical margin of complete excision of carcinoma of the skin. Arch Dermatol 80:344–345, 1959
5. Fisher JC, Ketcham AS, Hume RB, et al: Significance of cancer cells in operative wounds. Am J Surg 114:514–519, 1967
6. Hayes H: Basal cell carcinoma: The East Grinstead experience. Plast Reconstr Surg 30:273–280, 1962
7. Phelan JT, Milgrom H, Stoll H, et al: The use of Mohs' chemosurgery technique in the management of superficial cancers. Surg Gynecol Obstet 114:25–30, 1962
8. Wermuth BM, Fajardo LF: Metastatic basal cell carcinoma. A review. Arch Pathol 90:458–462, 1970
9. Cornelius CE: Bone: A site of metastatic basal cell carcinoma. Arch Surg 104:848–850, 1972
10. Litzow TJ, Perry HO, Soderstrom CW: Morpheaform basal cell carcinoma. Am J Surg 116:499–512, 1969
11. Shapiro L, Baraf CS: Subungual epidermoid carcinoma and keratoacanthoma. Cancer 25:141–152, 1970
12. Erich JB, Trucker AL: Deforming xanthomatous tumors of the face: Report of case. Ann Surg 155:477–480, 1962
13. Rosai J: Skin tumors and tumor-like conditions. In Rosai J (ed): Ackerman's Surgical Pathology (Ed 6). St. Louis, C V Mosby Co, 1981, pp 81–152
14. Pack GT, Davis J: Radiation cancer of the skin. Radiology 84:436–441, 1965
15. Lenz M: Radiotherapy of epithelioma of the skin. Arch Dermatol Syph 53:588–596, 1946
16. Conway J, Hugo NE: Radiation dermatitis and malignancy. Plast Reconstr Surg 38:255–268, 1966
17. Martin H, Strong E, Spiro RH: Radiation-induced skin cancer of the head and neck. Cancer 25:61–71, 1970
18. Danese CA, Grishman E, Oh C, et al: Malignant vascular tumors of the lymphedematous extremity. Ann Surg 166:245–253, 1967
19. Hudson AW, Winkelmann RK: Atypical fibroxanthoma of the skin: A reappraisal of 19 cases in which the original diagnosis was spindle-cell squamous carcinoma. Cancer 29:413–422, 1972
20. Arons JS, Lynch JB, Lewis SR, et al: Scar tissue carcinoma: Part I. A clinical study with special reference to burn scar carcinoma. Ann Surg 161:170–188, 1965
21. Arons MS, Rodin AE, Lynch JB, et al: Scar tissue carcinoma: Part II. An experimental study with special reference to burn scar carcinoma. Ann Surg 163:445–460, 1965
22. DiPirro E, Conway H: Carcinoma after frostbite: A case report. Plast Reconstr Surg 38:541–543, 1966
23. Longacre JJ: Scar Tissue: Its use and abuse. Springfield, Ill., Charles C Thomas, 1972
24. Ketcham AS, Lawrence W, Pilch YH, et al: Symposium on melanoma. Contemp Surg 2:87–113, 1973
25. Ballantyne AJ: Malignant melanoma of the skin of the head and neck. Am J Surg 120:425–431, 1970
26. Conley JJ, Pack GT: Melanoma of the head and neck. Surg Gynecol Obstet 116:15–28, 1963
27. Catlin D: Cutaneous melanoma of the head and neck. Am J Surg 112:512–521, 1966
28. Das Gupta T, Brasfield R: Subungual melanoma. Ann Surg 161:545–662, 1965
29. Goldsmith HS, Shah JP, Kim DH: Prognostic significance of lymph node dissection in the treatment of malignant melanoma. Cancer 26:606–609, 1970. See also Shah JP, Goldsmith HS: Incontinuity versus discontinuous lymph node dissection for malignant melanoma. Cancer 26:610–614, 1970
30. Fortner JG, Das Gupta T, McNeer G: Primary malignant melanoma on the trunk. Ann Surg 161:161–168, 1965
31. McGovern VJ: The classification of melanoma and its relationship with prognosis. Pathology 2:85–98, 1970
32. Dellon AL, Ketcham AS: Surgical treatment of stage I melanoma. Arch Surg 106:738–739, 1973
33. Fortner JG, Woodruff J, Schottenfeld D, et al: Biostatistical basis of elective node dissection for malignant melanoma. Ann Surg 186:101–103, 1977
34. Kapelanski DP, Block GE, Kaufman M: Characteristics of the primary lesion of malignant melanoma as a guide to prognosis and therapy. Ann Surg 189:225–235, 1979
35. Veronesi U, Adamus J, Bandiera C, et al: Inefficacy of immediate node dissection in stage I melanoma of the limbs. New Engl J Med 297:627–630, 1977
36. Sim FH, Taylor WF, Ivins JC, et al: A prospective randomized study of the efficacy of routine elective lymphadenectomy in management of malignant melanoma: Preliminary results. Cancer 41:948–956, 1978
37. Cohen MH, Ketcham AS, Felix EL, et al: Prognostic factors in patients undergoing lymphadenectomy for malignant melanoma. Ann Surg 186:635–642, 1977
38. Balch CM, Cascinelli N, Milton GW, et al (eds): Cutaneous melanoma: Clinical management and treatment results worldwide. Philadelphia, J. B. Lippincott Co, 1985, pp 131–157
39. Ketcham AS, Lawrence W Jr, Pilch GH, et al: Symposium on melanoma. Contemp Surg 2:87, 1973
40. Reimer RR, Clark WH, Greene MH, et al: Precursor lesions in familial melanoma. A new genetic preneoplastic syndrome. JAMA 239:744–746, 1978
41. Clark WH, Reimer RR, Greene M, et al: Origin of familial malignant melanomas from heritable melanocytic lesions. "The B-K mole syndrome." Arch Dermatol 114:732–738, 1978
42. Sagebiel RW: Histopathology of borderline and early malignant melanomas. Am J Pathol 3:543–552, 1979
43. Elden DE, Goldman LJ, Goldman SC, et al: Dysplastic nevus syndrome: A phenotypic association of sporadic cutaneous melanoma. Cancer 46:1787–1794, 1980
44. Futrell JW, Kruger GR, Morton DL, et al: Carcinoma of sweat glands in adolescents. Am J Surg 123:594–597, 1972
45. Futrell JW, Krueger GR, Chretien PB, et al: Multiple primary sweat gland carcinomas. Cancer 28:686–691, 1971
46. Miller RE, White JJ: Sebaceous gland carcinoma. Am J Surg 114:958–961, 1967
47. Das Gupta TK, Brasfield RD: Benign and malignant tumors and tumor-like conditions of fibrous tissue. Am Cancer Soc 19:202–210, 1969
48. Petri WH: Aggressive fibromatosis of the mandible. J Oral Maxillofac Surg 40:663–667, 1982
49. Ajagbe HA, Daramola JO: Fibro-osseous lesions of the jaw: A review of 133 cases from Nigeria. J Nat Med Assoc 75:593–598, 1983
50. Naylor EW, Gardner EJ, Richards RC: Desmoid tumors and mesenteric fibromatosis in Gardner's syndrome. Report of kindred 109. Arch Surg 114:1181–1185, 1979
51. Waddell WR: Treatment of intra-abdominal and abdominal wall desmoid tumors with drugs that affect the metabolism of cyclic 3'5'-adenosine monophosphate. Ann Surg 181:299–302, 1975

52. Masson JK, Soule EH: Desmoid tumors of the head and neck. Am J Surg 112:615–622, 1966

53. Cole NM, Guiss LW: Extra-abdominal desmoid tumors. Arch Surg 98:530–533, 1969

54. Brasfield RD, Das Gupta TK: Desmoid tumors of the anterior abdominal wall. Surgery 65:241–246, 1969

55. Das Gupta TK, Brasfield RD, O'Hara J: Extra-abdominal desmoids: A clinicopathological study. Ann Surg 170:109, 1969

56. Toker C: Pseudo-sarcomatous fasciitis: Further observations indicating the aggressive capabilities of this lesion, and justifying the inclusion of this entity within the category of the fibromatoses. Ann Surg 174:994–1001, 1971

57. Stout AP: Juvenile fibromatosis. Cancer 7:953–978, 1954

58. McPeak CJ, Cruz T, Nicastri AD: Uncommon sarcoma shows potential for metastasis. Ann Surg 166:803–816, 1967

59. Harry RD, Kruger RL, McLaughlin CW: Elastofibroma dorsi. Am J Surg 125:773–774, 1973

60. Taylor HB, Helwig EB: Metastatic tumors of the skin. Cancer 15:717–725, 1962

61. Adams JT, Saltzstein SL: Metastasizing dermatofibrosarcoma protuberans. Report of two cases. Am Surg 29:879–886, 1963

62. Conley JJ: Malignant tumors of the scalp. Plast Reconstr Surg 33:1–15 and 163–170, 1964

63. Whiffen JD: Dermal cylindroma. Plast Reconstr Surg 31:70–73, 1963

64. Binder SC, Cady B, Catlin D: Epidermoid carcinoma of the skin of the nose. Am J Surg 116:506–512, 1968

65. Bennett JE, Moore TS, Vellios F, et al: Surgical treatment of skin cancer of the nose. Am J Surg 117:382–387, 1969

66. Wise RA, Baker HW: Surgery of the head and neck (Ed 3). Chicago, Year Book Medical Publishers Inc, 1968, pp 142–155

67. Reingold JM: Cutaneous metastases from internal carcinomas. Cancer 19:162–168, 1966

68. Brownstein M, Helwig EB: Metastatic tumors of the skin. Cancer 29:1298–1307, 1972

69. Dunham LJ: Cancer in man at site of prior benign lesion of skin or mucous membrane. A review. Cancer Res 32:1359–1374, 1972

70. Goltz RW: Cutaneous clues to visceral cancer. Hosp Med 5:33–45, 1969

71. Graham JG, Helwig EB: Bowen's disease and its relationship to systemic cancer. Arch Dermatol 80:133–159, 1959

72. Gardner EJ, Richard RC: Multiple cutaneous and subcutaneous lesions occurring simultaneously with hereditary polyposis and osteomatosis. Am J Human Genet 5:139–147, 1953

R. K. WINKELMANN, M.D., PH.D.

14

Skin Biopsy

The biopsy is a useful diagnostic surgical procedure for skin disease, skin tumors, and systemic disease. It can be performed readily with minimal risk to the patient and with maximum effectiveness in diagnosis. There is no area of skin or mucous membrane that cannot be examined. Skin, nails, tongue, genital skin, and mucosa are equally amenable to the office biopsy procedure. The physician can perform adequate biopsies easily in the office or treatment room with minimal assistance and risk.

A biopsy is taken to provide a surgical sample for analysis by microscopic and laboratory methods. While the problems of cutaneous biopsy are small compared with the biopsy of a visceral organ such as the liver or kidney, basic principles govern the clinical judgment of selecting tissue for biopsy and the surgical procedures involved. The fundamental problem involves safely excising enough tissue for diagnosis with minimal risk to the patient. All the organization and selection of procedure is made to ensure such a result.

The physician must decide, first, the location of the lesion and what surgical method should be used to study it. The most satisfactory result will be one in which a large sample of tissue is excised so that a full range of the pathology may be observed. It is important to include normal skin for reference. A recent review of a series of erythema nodosum biopsies emphasized that only 25% of punch biopsies had provided enough tissue for diagnosis of this disease. It requires considerable skill and perhaps some luck to obtain a diagnosis of an inflammatory lesion of the face when the sampling is done with only a 2 or 3 mm Keyes' punch. If the patient requires a biopsy, then the procedure should acquire enough tissue for the pathologic diagnosis. Cosmetic considerations are important but only after the primary purpose of the biopsy is accomplished.

The nature of the disease will determine the area to be sampled and the size of the biopsy. Tumors, inflammatory dermatoses, ulcers, and wheals must be dealt with individually. No general rule applies except to take enough tissue. The purpose of the biopsy is to obtain a sample of the pathologic condition—the larger the sample, the better the opportunity for an accurate diagnosis.

TUMORS

It is always best to remove a tumor in toto. It is possible to use a punch biopsy to enclose a junctional nevus for removal; however, it is frequently easier to excise the superficial nevus with curved iris scissors or a sharp scalpel. The least damage to an unknown tumor, the better; so excision for diagnosis with a rim of normal tissue is preferable. When a tumor is so large that it is not possible to excise it in toto, then it should be removed in its firmest area by a wedge or section that moves from normal skin to the center of the lesion, carrying through the depth of the entire skin and subcutaneous tissue. Excising an exophytic nodule may not provide a true picture of a tumor because the tissue is often altered or metaplastic in such areas and has undergone necrosis or hemorrhage. When the biopsy of an ulcerative tumor is to be performed, the edge of the ulcer extending from normal skin into the necrotic base of the tumor should be excised deeply into the subcutaneous and fascial tissues. The biopsy of the base of a necrotic tumor ulcer is often a useless procedure.

When clinical judgment indicates that the lesion is malignant and invading deep tissue, one should reflect on why the biopsy is being performed. It is often best to plan definitive treatment for such a lesion at the same time that the biopsy is done. This means a surgical procedure for definitive therapy, one that includes a biopsy to confirm the diagnosis by frozen section during surgery. There can be no quarrel with an excision of a melanoma on the extremities between tourniquets in the office or hospital operating room with definitive tissue diagnosis during the procedure. Because only half the lesions clinically suspected of being melanoma actually are, some selectivity is necessary in deciding which lesions should be removed with all precautions. Most recently, clinical criteria for melanoma have increased the diagnosis for true melanoma dramatically; however, suspect lesions will always require the conservative physician to handle such lesions carefully.

INFLAMMATORY LESIONS

It is always best to perform a biopsy on a mature lesion of an inflammatory process. It is undesirable to obtain an early undeveloped lesion or an involuting or secondarily traumatized, infected, or treated lesion for this purpose. The skill of the clinician is important for accurately selecting representative areas. In most instances, it is wise to pick a reasonably sized lesion (1 to 2 cm in diameter). Larger lesions are more likely to be undergoing involution or may demonstrate the effects of trauma or therapy. If a large lesion is selected, the edge of the lesion is preferable because the active border may indicate the true pathologic process and, at the same time, give comparison with normal and older, central lesional skin. A biopsy of a crust is not as helpful as a sample of the inflammation that produced it.

A biopsy of vesicles and blisters should be done when they are new and small in size. Older and larger blisters frequently show re-epithelialization of a bulla base that can occur within 24 to 48 hours and distort the pathologic picture. Similarly, the varying degrees of inflammation or infection in older blisters may handicap the pathologist. It is imperative that early blister lesions be removed for immunofluorescence studies. Frequently, the surrounding erythematous skin or normal skin may give the most accurate immunofluorescent results, as in dermatitis herpetiformis. The blister may be too inflammatory with masses of leukocytes, fibrin, and dermal and epidermal necrosis. If only such a blister is available for biopsy, the edge of this larger blister may be the best site for selection. At times, trauma may produce a Nikolsky sign, and the biopsy of such a bulla often best represents the pathologic condition. Only rarely does the denuded blister base provide positive information. Suprabasalar acantholysis can be present in pemphigus, Darier's disease, or familial benign chronic pemphigus.

Most biopsies of purpuric lesions must be small in order to show a definitive pathologic process. Larger purpuric lesions frequently show only hemorrhage or tissue necrosis. Hyalinized necrotic tissue is the end result of most cutaneous abscesses, infarctions, and burns. There is a uniformity of such pathologic processes, so a central biopsy of the lesion may offer an opportunity to find a central thrombosed vessel in such a lesion.

Granulomatous noduloulcerative lesions vary so much in histologic patterns that no specific guide can be given that will be successful for all lesions. A small well-developed lesion can be excised in toto, or the active edges of the lesion may yield a diagnostic specimen when a full-thickness biopsy into the subcutaneous tissue is taken. Erythematous areas in scars may turn out to be sarcoidosis, lupus vulgaris, or leprosy. A biopsy of atrophic, scarring, or evolutionary granulomas (such as necrobiosis lipoidica, granuloma annulare, rheumatoid nodules, or the Churg-Strauss granuloma) should be done in the inflammatory stage or area and away from sclerosis and atrophy. Biopsies of morphea and scleroderma should include subcutaneous tissue to demonstrate the lymphocytic panniculitis present in some lesions. A biopsy of all forms of panniculitis must be carried out by the surgical excision technique in order to provide a large area of normal and involved subcutaneous tissue.

BIOPSY METHODS

Physicians should choose the technique that suits their requirements and skills. Tissue for biopsy may be removed by surgical excision, curettage, punch, electrocutting technique, or chemosurgery. Surgical excision is the preferred method, because it rapidly and neatly provides tissue and good control. Other methods may be used, but the sampling possibilities and pathologic process results are usually compromised.

Surgical Excision

Although outlined in greater detail later, three surgical methods for biopsy are commonly available. The most frequently used is scalpel excision. An elliptic excision of a lesion or portion of tissue through all of the skin layers is optimal. The incision should follow Langer's lines. Suture placement should approximate the skin edges and should not exert undue tension on them. Pathologic tissue tolerates pressure and tension poorly. Mattress sutures or through-and-through sutures 1 cm away from the wound edge are often necessary. Only minimal suturing should be done to decrease the trauma to pathologic skin. Subcuticular or similar approaches to skin closure are excessive and often cause trouble. Occasionally, only skin tapes will be adequate.

Surgical excision using a pair of iris or curved scissors may be all that is required for a small and superficial lesion. With the scissor points, dermal dissection can be performed around the lesion. This technique always provides dermal tissue and a rim of normal tissue. With care, full-thickness dermis can be maintained throughout the scissor excision. This is a satisfactory procedure for superficial nevi, keratoses, verrucae, and such exophytic lesions as papillomas. With light electrodesiccation or cautery, the remaining dermal bed will shrink the excised area to half its original size, and it can then heal readily by secondary intention. This is a preferred superficial surgical biopsy method.

A second procedure for superficial biopsies is the shave technique—an easy means to provide diagnostic tissue in most instances. The scalpel or razor blade slices horizontally through the epidermis and superficial dermis and removes the surface lesion. Unfortunately, the scalpel used in this way does not have the mobility and utility of the pointed scissors. It is possible to obtain only the crust or stratum corneum of some lesions by this method. Frequently, only traces of papillary dermis are found in such biopsies. Therefore, although the extent and margins of the lesion are known, its depth is not studied adequately. Holding the razor blade at a slight curve may give a good dermal sample. This modality provides an easy cosmetic and therapeutic surgical approach to superficial skin lesions, but care must be taken to provide a satisfactory sample for pathology. It is used frequently for papillomas and keratoses. It should not be used routinely for pigmented or epithelial malignancies.

The Punch Biopsy

The development of the punch biopsy instrument has significantly improved the development of dermatology by providing an easy way to take a biopsy of full-thickness skin for diagnosis or therapy. The ease of biopsy, the uniformity of the specimen obtained, and the ready healing of the operative site, have made this method a favorite in most dermatologic offices. The amount of time saved in using this biopsy method as opposed to a surgical excision has often been a factor in its use.

Keyes' hand punches are routinely available from 1 to 8 mm in diameter as well as in larger sizes. A similar range of punch sizes may be purchased for use with a hand-held rotary surgical planing instrument; disposable plastic punches are also manufactured (Fig. 14–1). The metal punches must be sharp-

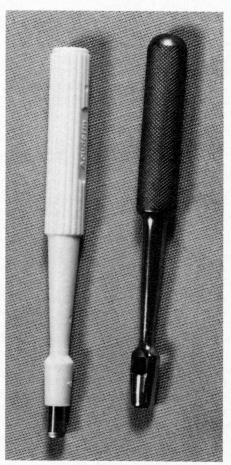

Figure 14–1. The standard 5 mm Keyes punch and the disposable plastic punch.

ened about once a year. Note that, with sharpening, the length of the punch will diminish, so older punches may not be adequate for deep biopsies.

After anesthesia, the punch may be held against the skin lesion to be biopsied and twirled, while firm vertical pressure drives the punch into the tissue. The column of epidermis and dermis will hang loosely on a pedicle of connective tissue in the circular hole in the dermis created by the punch. Gently, the tissue may be raised by atraumatic forceps or by a skin hook, and the base snipped off by the scissors. It must be emphasized that in cutting the sample free, the deepest possible line of excision must be used. Dermal punch biopsies that are too superficial occur frequently with small-diameter punches. To avoid this, the punch must penetrate cleanly through the dermis so that only subcutaneous tissue holds the biopsy in place. Then the tissue can be lifted high enough from the biopsy hole to cut it free at a deep level. In most instances, a superficial punch biopsy is either a wasted attempt or only a partial success at obtaining pathologic tissue.

When the lesion is in the deep dermis and subcutaneous tissue, the punch biopsy may also fail. At times, the punch cannot reach the level of the pathologic condition. Then, the double punch biopsy method must be used. The first punch biopsy must be cut free and then the hand punch reinserted into the biopsy hole. Holding the subcutaneous tissue firmly from the sides with one hand, the biopsy is again rotated to produce a second core of deeper tissue. This method is particularly useful for subcutaneous metastatic lesions. Of course, a larger punch size increases the size and depth of the sample and of the volume of pathologic material available for study. A surgical excision should be considered in such instances.

Because the punch biopsy hole is round, it heals more slowly by secondary intention than oval or linear wounds. In areas where the skin is freely movable and expansile, an oval punch biopsy hole, which heals more neatly, can be created by spreading the skin under tension between two fingers along the lines of Langer. This produces a slightly oval punch biopsy hole. This technique will not work in areas where the skin is more firmly fixed, such as the scalp, hands, and feet.

To properly obtain a biopsy of the scalp follicles, the punch biopsy should be tilted 15 to 20 degrees along the axis of hair growth. Remember, the dermal papilla of a growing scalp hair is in the subcutaneous tissue, so a 5 to 6 mm punch biopsy is the minimum practical size. The rotary punch biopsy has been used for the nail bed and works well if the punch is sharp. Biopsy of the cheek and mucous membranes with a hand punch is easy and effective and usually provides a good sample of deeper tissue more readily than a scalpel or scissor excision.

Once the biopsy is removed, pressure with sterile

gauze for a few minutes will frequently provide all the hemostasis necessary for small punch biopsies. Additional hemostasis may be accomplished by fibrin foam or other hemostatic agents packed in the lesion. It is also possible to use Monsel's solution, aluminum chloride, or electrodesiccation, if convenient. On occasion, when the punch penetrates a large vein or artery, a single stitch may be necessary. Many dermatologists routinely suture punch biopsies. A single 4-0 silk suture in a small punch biopsy on the face may help healing, if the biopsy is superficial. A large mattress suture of 3-0 silk may be helpful in eliminating the dead space in an 8 mm punch biopsy cavity. In pathologic material, necrotic or infected tissue may cause inflammation so that stitches may need to be removed early.

Curettage Biopsy

For many years, electrodesiccation and curettage have been standard therapy for cutaneous tumors. The successful statistics related to basal cell carcinoma show that it is a reasonable and safe method. In addition, the use of light electrodesiccation can provide hemostasis as well as desiccation and destruction of skin tumors. The physician who uses curettage for biopsy often places many small fragments of tissue in the bottle of fixative and believes that this is sufficient for pathologic study. The disorientation of the tissue, the fragmentation and traumatic changes in the tissue, often leads the pathologist to despair about giving rational answers as to what the basic lesion was and how completely it was removed.

Some of these objections can be overcome by using a larger ring curette or a small bone curette. If these instruments are kept sharp, a single firm stroke down and through a lesion, such as a basal cell carcinoma, will usually scoop out the tumor intact, or a massive portion of it, for a biopsy. Under these circumstances, there is no point in placing small fragments of tissue in the fixative. Another easy method is to use a small pair of curved, pointed scissors to take a biopsy before desiccation and repeated curettage. Often, a major mass of superficial cutaneous tumor can be removed surgically before seeking out the firm fibrous tissue bed of normal dermis with the curette.

Electrocautery Biopsy

The cutting current of electrosurgical instruments can be used to produce a biopsy. Although the edges of the tissue show electrical and thermal injury, the central portion of a large lesion can be used for pathologic studies. A pointed needle may be used to outline and to cut through the tissue.

The loop attachment is often easier to use with the current on a high electrocutting setting. A firm downward and through stroke can move the loop rapidly into, under, and through a cutaneous lesion, removing a large portion for microscopic study. It is particularly easy to do this with protuberant lesions, such as papillomas or seborrheic keratoses.

Anesthesia

The biopsy requires rapid onset, short-lived anesthetic agents. Infiltration of the skin provides immediate anesthesia and, as the infiltrate is cleared by the lymphatics, the anesthetic effect fades within one hour. Lidocaine (Xylocaine) is the agent of choice because of the low incidence of sensitization and cross-reactivity. Diphenhydramine (Benadryl) solution may be used by local injection for patients with sensitivity to the anesthetic. If neither of these drugs are desirable, regional block of a cutaneous nerve is possible.

Only on rare occasions is freezing the surface epidermis with Freon or ethyl chloride all that is necessary to do a punch biopsy.

Anesthetic agents should be infiltrated slowly into the tissue. Rapid intradermal infiltration under pressure may produce edematous and vascular artifacts. In block anesthesia, the anesthetic agent is injected into four sides of the field, but not directly into the tissue for biopsy. This requires more time to perform and for the skin to become anesthetized. For granulomatous infections, it is particularly desirable because mycobacterial cultures may be inhibited by "-caine" anesthetics.

After the Biopsy

Stitches may be removed at appropriate intervals after the biopsy depending on the depth of the biopsy, the purpose of the stitch, and the nature of the condition diagnosed. Mattress sutures and sutures in punch biopsies should be left in place 5 to 7 days or longer, if reasonable. Cosmetic stitches on the face may be removed in 72 hours.

The punch biopsy may be dressed daily with Telfa or gauze dressing; isopropyl alcohol may be used as a disinfectant. If a hemostatic material such as fibrin foam is used, the biopsy should be checked at 24 hours to remove this material and to apply another dressing to the lesion. The patient should be instructed to expect some slight drainage from the lesion. It is useful to indicate that the lesion will heal best if kept dry and at rest. It is wise to emphasize that dressings are useful to keep out debris and absorb drainage, but that with moisture and heat, healing may be retarded and infection promoted. Lesions on the scalp and mucous membranes frequently require little or no care, except protection from physical damage.

THE SPECIMEN

The purpose of the biopsy is to obtain tissue for study, and so the planning of what to study and how to accomplish it must be finished before the biopsy procedure is started. Fixatives must be prepared and ready, and the special procedures ordered at the time of biopsy.

While the biopsy may appear to be dense tough tissue, it still must be handled carefully with atraumatic instruments. When it is removed from the body, it is sensible to place it on gauze moistened with saline solution or on Telfa in a closed petri dish, if there are still some judgments to be made about future studies.

Frozen Section

The ready availability of the modern cryostat makes a frozen section a common procedure. It is an office procedure for some dermatologists and is replacing the delayed Mohs' method of tissue evaluation to check the edges of tissue for residual tumor. With a small investment in instruments and in training for a technician, all office surgery can be monitored for completeness during the procedure. A record of a permanent, as well as frozen, hematoxylin and eosin section can be available.

If the frozen section is available at another location, the biopsy may be rapidly transported safely by wrapping it in gauze moistened by a sterile physiologic salt solution. A petri dish with the edge taped makes a handy container.

Fixation

Fixation of tissue will depend somewhat on the laboratory that the physician uses. Staining procedures are standardized according to the fixation, so it is wise to use the fixative recommended by the particular laboratory. It is not wise to change laboratories without checking to see what differences in routine fixatives may exist. Buffered 10% formalin is a routine fixative, because it is simple and its tendency to acidify can be neutralized effectively. It permits tissue shrinkage in the warm paraffin. Many tissue components are washed out in the fluid phase. Because it is such a poor nuclear fixative, other methods of fixation such as Zenker's, Helly's, or Bouin's solutions may be preferred by an individual pathologist.

It is important to have a large volume of fixative for the biopsy. The standard tonsil bottle with a minimum of 30 ml of fixative is appropriate for a punch biopsy up to 8 mm in diameter. Larger punch biopsies or excision biopsies are optimally treated with larger volumes of fixative. It is best that the small mailing vials of fixative often provided should not be used for anything but small samples of tissue. This is unfortunate, because it does seem to imply that a smaller piece of tissue is adequate when, in fact, the limitations of size are obvious. One should not mail the piece of tissue in an equal volume of fixative solution. The more fixative solution the better. One should also be sure that the vial is adequately sealed.

Before the tissue is placed in the fixative solution, it should be pressed firmly on a stiff piece of paper or light cardboard in order to avoid some shrinkage during fixation. The tendency for the dermal connective tissue to contract and produce a curved specimen with a bowed epidermis can be avoided. Such shrinkage is neglible with small biopsies.

It is often advisable to bisect a large specimen prior to fixation. The surfaces *not* to be cut are marked with India ink (Fig. 14–2). This indicates the remaining cut surface for pathologic examination. In addition, a surface marker of indelible ink (e.g., silver nitrate) can be used to mark the other surfaces for the technician. Bisecting a scalp biopsy along the plane of hair follicles will ensure longitudinal cuts of the appendages. Bisection also helps to orient the tissue at right angles to the skin surface so that oblique or angled sections are not cut. The easiest way to bisect a specimen for these purposes is to place the sample, epidermis facedown, on a cork or wooden board. After orientation of the specimen, a single-edged razor blade or scalpel can then be used to bisect the specimen cutting first through the subcutaneous tissue; each half may be put in a separate fixative bottle. If a question arises about the volume of fixative, only one half needs to be embedded and cut. Both halves are often mounted side by side and cut together in some laboratories. The tumor may be bisected twice so that the edges may be checked for completeness of excision. A section parallel to the surface from the bottom of the specimen is also necessary (Fig. 14–3). A large irregular tumor such as a melanoma may need serial sampling, as in Figure 14–4.

Hematoxylin and esoin sections following paraffin embedding are usually the only studies required for common skin tumors. In addition, some laboratories routinely perform elastic fiber or Giemsa's stains. A combination of Giemsa's stain and aldehyde fuchsin (for elastin) is an excellent second routine study to perform. It divides the epidermis into proliferative and differentiating layers and indicates the pattern of collagens and elastin. It specifically shows the mast cell and emphasizes the red blood cells and eosinophils.

Cutting and staining skin sections is not as easy

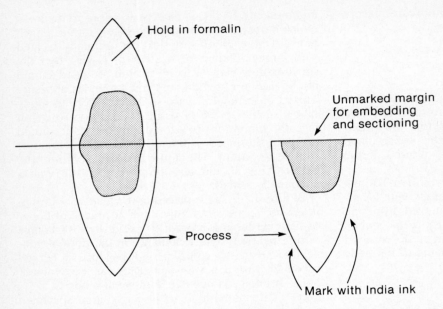

Figure 14—2. Method of processing an excisional biopsy for histologic diagnosis. (From Peters MS, Winkelmann RK: The biopsy. *Dermatologic Clinics* 2:209–217, 1984.)

as handling a uniform tissue with massive amounts of parenchyma and minimal amounts of stroma, such as kidney or liver tissue. Accordingly, some pathology laboratories regularly produce poor to bad sections of skin. It is possible to cut and stain skin just as well as any other tissue, but this requires some effort and training. Do not be content with bad sections. Inform the pathologist that the performance of his tissue laboratory is not up to an appropriate standard. If the problem is not corrected, change laboratories. Only good technique can provide an adequate basis for pathologic interpretation.

SPECIAL STUDIES

Frequently, a specific diagnosis indicates that it will be useful to have special stains performed on a given piece of tissue. Where possible, these should be anticipated and ordered at the time the tissue is

cut originally. Table 14–1 lists these procedures and the clinical indications that might call for them.

For fat stains, the fixed tissue must be sectioned on a freezing microtome. This, of course, cannot be done on tissue that has been embedded in paraffin. Accordingly, the procedure must be ordered and the laboratory informed that frozen sections are necessary for a fat stain. Many histochemical procedures are done on fresh frozen tissue or on frozen tissue with a short-duration fixation. There are only a few histochemical procedures that are more than curiosities. In routine pathologic study with an office cryostat, it is possible to do phosphorylase, respiratory enzymes, acid phosphatase, cholinesterase, and peptidase assays. Although these tests increase the understanding of the pathology, they are usually not necessary for diagnosis.

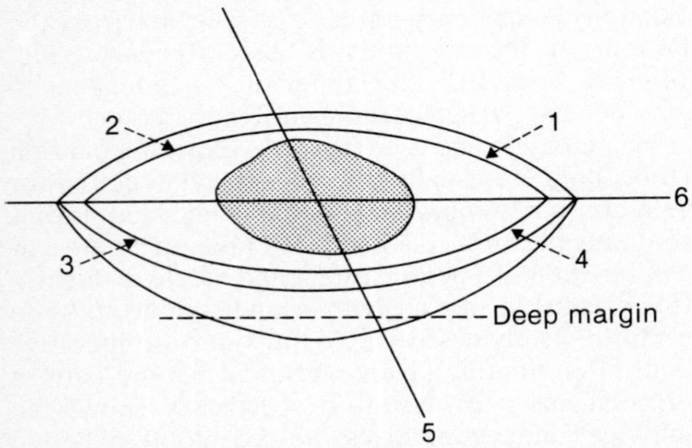

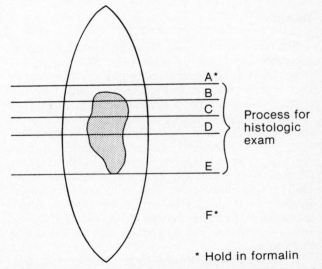

Figure 14—3. Technique for checking the margins of a basal cell carcinoma removed by an elliptical excision. (From Peters MS, Winkelmann RK: The biopsy. *Dermatologic Clinics* 2:209–217, 1984.)

Figure 14—4. Technique for handling the excisional biopsy of a suspected melanoma. (From Peters MS, Winkelmann RK: The biopsy. *Dermatologic Clinics* 2:209–217, 1984.)

TABLE 14–1. Special Histopathology Stains

Indication	Method
Elastin	Orcein Aldehyde fuchsin
Connective tissue	Mallory's or Masson trichrome Movat's pentachrome
Reticulin	Silver (foot's) Periodic acid–Schiff
Mast cells	Toluidine blue Giemsa's Acridine orange
Melanocytes and melanin	Silver nitrate (Becker's)
Nerve	Protein-silver (Bodian's)
Mucopolysaccharides	Alcian blue Colloidal iron (Hale's)
Glycogen	Periodic acid–Schiff and with diastase
Lipid	Frozen section—Sudan or oil red O, Sudan black B Paraffin section—acid hematein (Baker)
Amyloid	Congo red—polarize Periodic acid–Schiff Methyl violet Thioflavine T
Calcium	Silver (von Kossa's)
Iron	Perl's potassium ferrocyanide
Fungus	Periodic acid–Schiff Acridine orange Methenamine silver (Gomori's)
Bacteria	Gram's Giemsa's
Spirochete	Silver (Levaditi's)
Acid-fast bacteria	Ziehl-Neelsen Auramine-rhodamine

Electron Microscopy

Fixation for electron microscopy (EM) is accomplished by use of buffered glutaraldehyde solution. This should be made or provided fresh each week. When the specimen reaches the laboratory, additional osmium or other fixation is added. The solutions vary according to the individual laboratory, though the principles remain the same, and it is necessary to follow the procedure of the laboratory that processes the tissue in order to obtain the best results.

Optimum fixation is obtained by rapid excision of the biopsy and immediate immersion in a meniscus of glutaraldehyde fixative on a cutting block. With a scalpel or razor blade, the tissue of interest should be diced into 1 mm cubes. Eight to 10 cubes of tissue can then be lifted from the smaller volume of fixative to the fixation vial for rapid transport to the laboratory. If every effort is made to get the specimens quickly to the EM preparation laboratory, then the remainder of the fixation and embedding procedures will not distort the tissue.

One may expect thick sections stained in toluidine blue or Giemsa's to be returned from the EM preparation laboratory. They will cut several sections from each small block for viewing so that a decision can be made as to which tissue should be cut for thin sections and EM viewing. These thick sections are now used routinely for pathologic study of the kidney and are becoming common in dermatopathology. General dermatopathology may use them routinely in time because they can reveal much more than just the melanosomes and Langerhans' granules for which EM is commonly used. The ability to demonstrate virus particles in dermatologic conditions is a major indication for electron microscopy.

Microbiologic Specimens

After the excision of tissue, the specimen should be kept moist and transported rapidly to the laboratory. The tissue provides its own transport medium. The biopsy should be wrapped in sterile gauze, moistened with sterile physiologic saline solution, and placed in a sterile container.

Immunofluorescence

The biopsy specimen should be snap-frozen in liquid nitrogen. It is convenient to wrap the specimen in aluminum foil for freezing. After freezing, it may be placed in a test tube and labeled. The test tube can then be sent to the laboratory in an insulated flask or cup containing liquid nitrogen. It may be packed in dry ice for a short trip, but this is less desirable. It should be stored in a $-70°C$ freezer. The freezing compartments of office refrigerators or freezers are usually from $-5°$ to $-20°C$ and are not acceptable. Transport media for immunofluorescence produce variable results. Because a negative result cannot be surely ascribed to the disease but may be due to the transport medium, it is not a recommended procedure. If it is important to do immunofluorescence, it is important to do it correctly. Indications for immunofluorescence of skin biopsies are shown in Table 14–2.

Touch Imprint Preparations

After a biopsy is made, the cellular infiltration may be assessed by touch imprint or dermogram. The biopsy is placed on dry gauze and gently blotted to remove blood cells and clots. The skin biopsy is bisected and the cut surface so exposed is placed on a glass slide and then on an adjacent spot and with gentle pressure streaked the length of the slide. This

TABLE 14–2. Direct Immunofluorescence

Pathology	Biopsy Site	Results
Pemphigus	Perilesional	Intercellular substance with IgG
Pemphigoid	Perilesional	Basement membrane zone with linear IgG ± complement
Herpes gestationis	Perilesional	Basement membrane zone with linear complement; also IgG
Dermatitis herpetiformis	Normal skin	Dermal papillae with IgA
Lupus erythematosus	Lesional and normal skin	IgM, IgG, IgA, and complement along the basement membrane zone
Leukocytoblastic vasculitis	Early lesions	Immunoglobulin, mainly IgM, and complement in vessels
Henoch-Schönlein purpura	Early lesions	IgA in vessels

is repeated for a total of three parallel spots and streaks. A specimen will give standard blood cell morphology when stained with Wright's or Giemsa's stain after air drying. The parent tissue used may now be fixed and studied pathologically, but it should be noted that distortion is common. It is a good practice to take another adjacent biopsy for the routine histology.

Clusters of lymphoreticular cells are observed in benign and malignant lymphoid tumors of the skin. Malignant tumor cells can be identified on such preparations. Sézary's cells may be obtained from touch preparations of Sézary's erythroderma. The histiocytes of histocytosis X show a typical hyalin histiocytic morphology. It is possible to obtain cells with organisms by this means in leprosy and Donovanosis (granuloma inguinale). The cells of malignant melanoma, basal cell carcinoma, and squamous cell carcinoma can be studied and identified by this method, although routine histology is adequate.

Monoclonal Antibody Studies

Monoclonal antibodies are available for many cell constituents. Factor VIII is shown in endothelial cells and therefore can mark vascular tumors. S-100 protein antibody stains nerve, Langerhans' cell, histiocytosis X, and nerve and pigment tumors. Antibodies to vimentin, laminin, keratin peptides, actin and myosin, collagen I and IV; and special antibodies to pemphigoid antigen, Merkel's cell, and keratohyaline can be used to classify skin changes and tumors. Carcinoembryonic antigen is found in some cases of Paget's disease. Monoclonal studies are generally performed on frozen tissue, though in some cases the antigen resists fixation and paraffin embedding. The most frequent use of monoclonal antibodies is to define lymphoid cell populations in the skin. An outline of commonly used antibodies is listed in Table 14–3.

ADMINISTRATIVE PROCEDURES

Each office should keep a biopsy book in which biopsies are identified by the patient's name, address, clinical practice number, and date of biopsy. Depending on the number of biopsies, the numbering may be sequential from the beginning of the practice or may start again each year with the addition of identifying numbers for the year of biopsy.

The biopsy book should also contain demographic information about the patient such as age, date of birth, address, and telephone number. A relative's name and address is an additional piece of information that often proves useful. Clinical information about the disease may be given in shorthand form as diagnosis, duration, and location of disease and location of biopsy. The routine and special studies ordered should also be included. This information may be spread across one page or, depending on the type of ledger, may require two pages. The material on subsequent patients can be kept in columns for ready access to the day's biopsies. With adequate biopsy material, a page can be devoted to each day.

All this material should be sent to the pathologist. If the pathologist does not provide a small accession slip with the bottle of fixative, then this information should be typed on a form or index card and sent with the biopsy to the laboratory.

All dermatologists know that dermatopathology requires inspection of the gross tissue or the dermatologic eruption. Therefore, the clinician must provide a similar advantage to the dermatopathologist who will primarily be looking at the histopathologic picture. By providing more clinical information and the differential diagnosis to the pathologist,

TABLE 14–3. Monoclonal Antibodies

Antibodies	Cells
leu 1	Peripheral T cells
leu 2a, OKT 8	Suppressor/cytotoxic T cells
leu 3a	Inducer/helper T cells
HLA-DR, OK1a	B cells, activated T cells, and some monocytes
OKT 6	Common T cells and Langerhans' cells
OKM 1	Monocytes and null cells
B-1	B cells

the best possible microscopic and clinical correlation is possible.

Most pathologists will return a slide or the block or both. These should be filed by date, name, and patient number. An index file should be kept so that cross-indexing may be possible. Slides can be filed away according to diagnosis or according to date of biopsy. For administrative purposes, it is easier and often best to file by date of biopsy, but for study purposes, filing slides by diagnosis offers tremendous advantages. The ledger book provides the date of biopsy, and the diagnostic slide file can arrange the slides according to date of accession so that ready access by name, diagnosis, and date of biopsy is provided. Good records make pathology a working part of the practice and provide an opportunity for continued review and study of the practice experience.

Electrosurgery

3

15

Electrosurgery

GEORGE L. POPKIN, M.D.

Electrosurgery has been used by dermatologists for well over 60 years, and a large amount of practical experience has accumulated over this time. The indications, advantages, disadvantages, and limitations of electrosurgery are well recognized by now.

The advantages of electrosurgery, although well-known to dermatologists, are less appreciated by other physicians. This method of treatment is not time-consuming and is ideally suited to office and clinical practice of dermatology. It requires few instruments, and patient acceptance is high. When used in properly selected cases, it yields acceptable to excellent cosmetic results in both benign and malignant lesions. As with every modality of therapy, the cumulative experience and acquired skill of the operator influence the results obtained.

DEFINITION

Electrosurgery is a modality that utilizes controlled electric currents to produce selective destruction of tissues. These currents may be generated by spark gap, radio tube, transistorized, or battery-operated electrosurgical equipment.

EQUIPMENT

Equipment for electrosurgery ranges from relatively inexpensive to high-priced machines found in hospital operating rooms. Generally speaking, less expensive equipment (with exceptions noted below), suffices for most conditions requiring extirpation by dermatologists.

In the lower price range are the Birtcher Hyfrecator (Fig. 15–1), the Sybron Coagulator (Fig. 15–2), the Burton Electricator (Fig. 15–3), and the Cameron-Miller Technicator (Fig. 15–4). These spark gap units are capable of delivering a satisfactory current for electrodesiccation, but they lack bipolar cutting currents.

In the higher price range are the Cameron-Miller (Fig. 15–5), the Birtcher Blendtome (Fig. 15–6), and the Sybron Bovie Bantam (Fig. 15–7). These machines provide, in addition to a spark gap electrodesiccative current, bipolar cutting and coagulating currents produced either by spark gap or radio tube high frequency currents or by a combination

of both. There are also machines that use transistorized circuits (Figs. 15–5 and 15–8) and that produce electrodesiccating, cutting and coagulating currents.

Physics of Electrosurgical Equipment

The value of high-frequency electrosurgical machines lies in conversion of office line current and voltage into usable and controlled currents suitable for the destruction of certain lesions.

When high-frequency currents of proper magnitude and frequency are generated and passed through tissue, heating is produced by the intrinsic resistance of tissue to the passage of such electromagnetic energy. If that energy is dispersed between two large indifferent electrodes, as it is in equipment

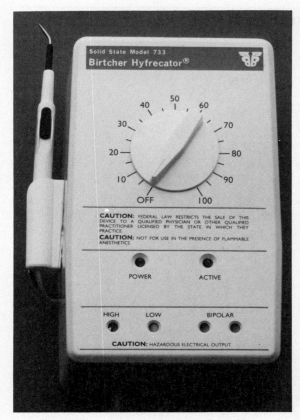

Figure 15–1. Courtesy of Birtcher Corporation.

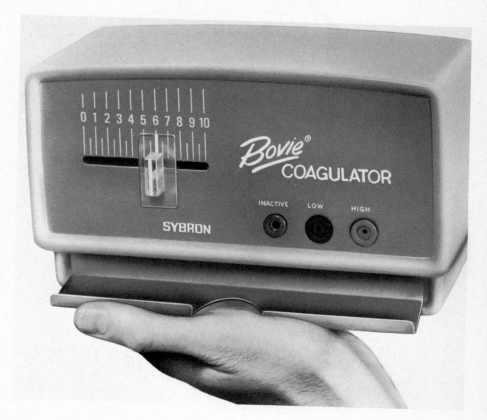

Figure 15–2. Courtesy of Sybron Corporation.

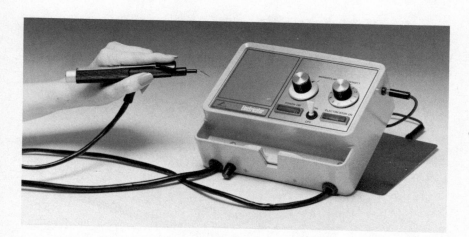

Figure 15–3. Courtesy of Burton Corporation.

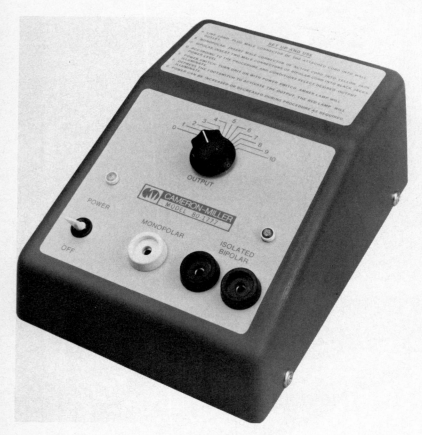

Figure 15–4. Courtesy of Cameron-Miller, Inc.

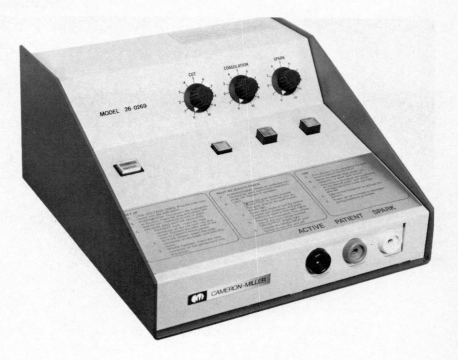

Figure 15–5. Courtesy of Cameron-Miller, Inc.

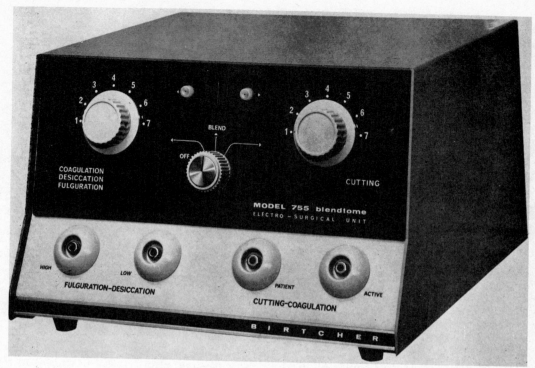

Figure 15–6. Courtesy of Birtcher Corporation.

Figure 15–7. Courtesy of Sybron Corporation.

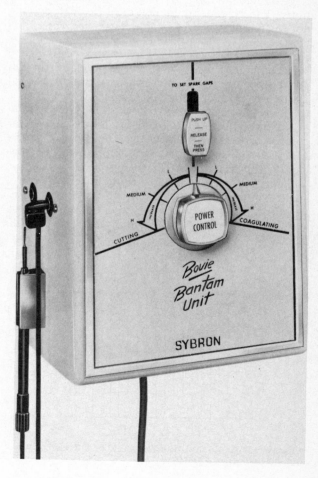

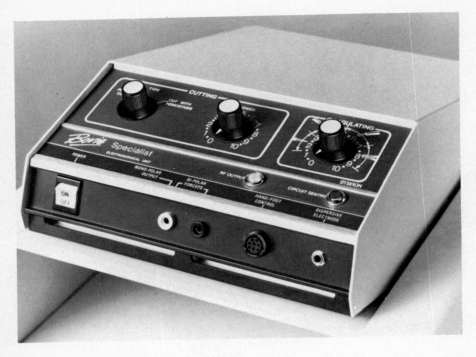

Figure 15–8. Courtesy of Sybron Corporation.

for medical diathermy (Fig. 15–9), regulatable heat is generated and can be used for indicated conditions. The current frequency must be high enough not to stimulate nerves or muscle tissue.

In a similar fashion, if one of the electrodes is reduced to a fine point, energy is applied to a very small volume of tissue and results in its destruction around the electrode tip. This is termed surgical diathermy (Fig. 15–10).

The term electrodesiccation describes destruction of skin growths by Oudin current, i.e., a monopolar current derived from a spark gap machine (Fig. 15–11A), or the equivalent current produced by machines with transistorized circuits.

Figure 15–12 diagrams the circuit of a typical spark gap apparatus. Line voltage is stepped up to several thousand volts by means of a transformer. When the voltage is sufficient both to charge the capacitors and also to break down the air resistance between the spark gaps, the capacitors discharge their voltage. Current then flows through the high-frequency circuit and into a transformer with variable coupling to the output. Recharging and discharging of the capacitors give rise to a series of highly damped, oscillating wave trains (Fig. 15–11A) that produce the desired high-frequency current.

A blocking capacitor prevents inadvertent transmission of low-frequency voltage to the patient and safeguards against shock from the line current. Volt-

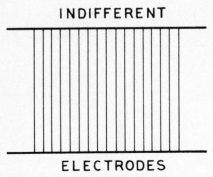

Figure 15–9. Medical diathermy—indifferent electrodes at top and bottom.

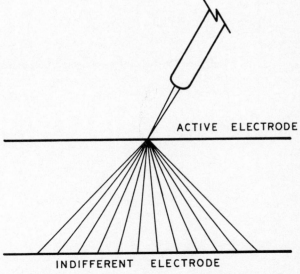

Figure 15–10. Surgical diathermy—indifferent electrode at bottom.

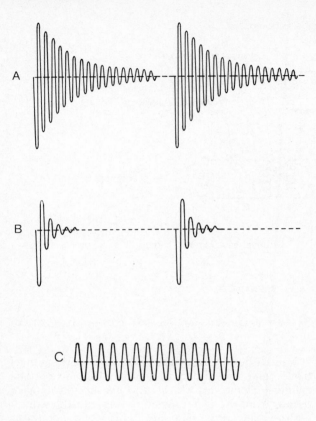

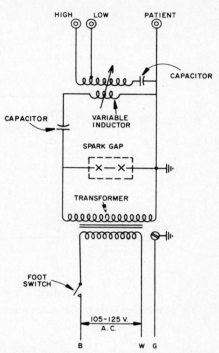

Figure 15—12. Schematic circuit of a spark gap apparatus. (Courtesy of Sybron Corporation.)

Figure 15—11. Wave forms: *A,* damped; *B,* moderately damped; *C,* undamped; and *D,* blended damped and undamped currents.

age to the patient is increased by means of an Oudin step-up transformer. The patient acts as a ground in monopolar equipment. Electrons are then dispersed into the patient's body as well as into surrounding objects.

In the simplified triode vacuum tube circuit (Fig. 15–13), there are three divisions, as in the spark gap design—the power source, the oscillating circuit, and the patient's circuit.

Input energy from alternating current line voltage is rectified and supplied as positive direct current high voltage to the plate (anode) of a triode vacuum tube. Low voltage is supplied by the transformer to heat the filament (cathode). The driving force to move electrons to the anode comes from the high voltage on the plate. The grid is interposed between the plate and filament. When the grid is positively charged, it neutralizes a space charge of electrons between the cathode and the plate resulting in an increased density and flow of electrons to the plate. When the grid is negatively charged, the flow of electrons ceases.

A tuned oscillatory circuit is connected between the grid and filament and develops high-frequency alternating current. Unlike the spark gap circuit, where the amplitude of the oscillations falls rapidly to zero because it generates highly damped current (see Fig. 15–11A), the vacuum tube circuit feeds back a portion of its output energy by inductive coupling from the plate to the oscillatory circuit. This energy is supplied at the proper time of the cycle and prevents the amplitude of the oscillations from dying down, producing a high-frequency undamped current (Fig. 15–11C). This additional energy input has been likened to someone giving a person on a swing a push to keep the swing from stopping.

By inductive coupling, this high-frequency undamped alternating current is induced in the patient's circuit. With the use of an active electrode (either a wire or a blade) and an indifferent or dispersive electrode, a cutting current is produced.

Monopolar electrodesiccation produces an output current in the range of 500 to 750 mA at a voltage in excess of 2000 volts. The bipolar cutting current is usually in the range of 200 to 700 mA at a lower voltage (less than 2000 volts). Bipolar electrocoagulation is produced by a high-frequency current at a low voltage (typically 1500 volts) with a current output between 300 to 600 mA.

Bipolar cutting current is produced with spark gap machines by increasing the frequency of the successive wave trains, i.e., they are moved more

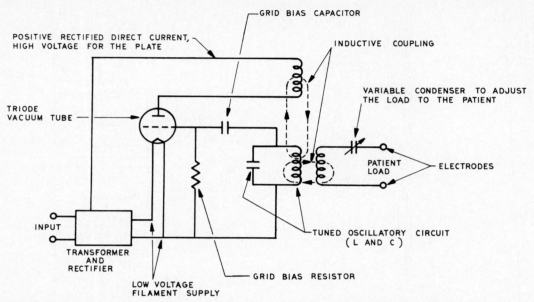

Figure 15–13. Schematic circuit triode vacuum tube. (Modified from Elliot JA: Electrosurgery. *Archives of Dermatology,* 94:340, 1966.)

closely together (Fig. 15–11B). This type of moderately damped current more closely simulates the pure undamped cutting current (Fig. 15–11C) produced by the radio tube apparatus.

In the battery-operated electrolysis unit used for epilation (Fig. 15–14), power is provided by a 22.5-volt B battery. This is linked in series with a milliammeter, a variable resistor, and two electrodes (an active and a dispersive electrode).

A low-voltage, low-amperage galvanic current produces ionization in the patient's tissues. At the positive pole (anode), acids, such as hydrochloric acid, are produced with the release of oxygen and the migration of iron ions into the skin. The acids cause vasodilation, coagulation of tissue protein, and pain. At the negative pole (cathode), sodium hydroxide is formed with liberation of hydrogen. The hydroxides cause liquefaction of the tissues with minimal pain.

This cathode terminal is always the working electrode, and the anode is a large dispersive metal cylindric electrode, which prevents the tattooing of tissues from the iron ions migrating into the skin.

Both the spark gap and radio tube apparatus generate finely controlled currents suitable for epilation and other purposes, such as the destruction of telangiectases. In the case of the spark gap unit, extra resistance is introduced into the circuit to provide the finely controlled currents suitable for epilation.

For the reader who is interested in further information on the physics of electrosurgery the author suggests two articles — one by R. Jackson[1] and the other by J. A. Elliot.[2] The material in this section on physics has been largely drawn from their work and modified with the assistance of J. R. Popkin-Clurman. J. W. Martin (Cameron-Miller, Inc.) supplied information on current ranges and Figure 15–

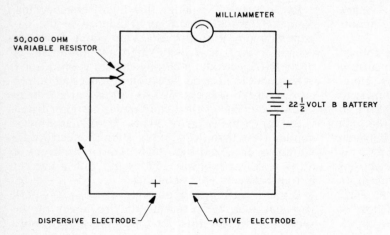

Figure 15–14. Schematic circuit for a battery-operated electrolysis unit. (Modified from Jackson R: Basic principles of electrosurgery. *Canadian Journal of Surgery,* 13:354–361, 1970.)

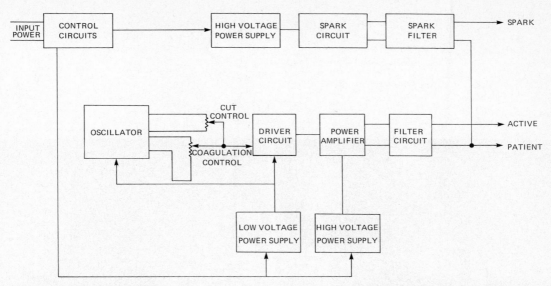

Figure 15–15. Circuitry diagram of a transistorized apparatus, such as the Cameron-Miller 26–0268 unit.

15, which shows the circuitry in a transistorized apparatus.

TREATMENT FOR BENIGN LESIONS

The removal of benign lesions should be done with minimal destruction of surrounding normal tissue. However, when treating malignant lesions, the primary aim is complete removal or destruction of malignant growth. The cosmetic end result, while important, must be a secondary consideration. Physicians know that patients often do not return for follow-ups. For this reason, malignant lesions should be treated with the understanding that there may not be a second chance to eradicate the malignancy.

Warts and seborrheic keratoses provide good examples of benign lesions handled well by electrosurgery (Figs. 15–16 to 15–20). Ordinarily, local anesthesia is used. An electrodesiccating spark of medium intensity is applied to soften the hyperkeratotic surface of the wart. Small curved scissors incise the junction between the wart and normal skin. The curette scrapes off the softened electrodesiccated tissue. By constricting the skin between the index finger and the thumb or by spreading the skin between these two fingers when the lesion is on a flat surface (Fig. 15–16E), sufficient hemostasis is obtained, permitting surgery to be carried out in a relatively bloodless field. Following complete wart removal, a spark of lower intensity is used to secure hemostasis.

An alternate method for surgical removal of a wart is also suggested. After local anesthesia is produced, scissors are used, as previously described, to incise the border of the wart and normal skin. With the curette, the wart is scraped from its bed.

Preliminary hemostasis is produced by finger pressure and styptics, such as 35% aluminum chloride in 50% isopropyl alcohol or Monsel's solution, are applied. If any pinpoint bleeders are not coagulated by these styptics, light electrodesiccation can be used to control bleeding.

When electrodesiccation is attempted in a field welling up with blood, the effective heat of the spark is dissipated by the cooler blood. This is avoided if pressure hemostasis is performed before applying the electrodesiccating spark.

Not all warts should be managed routinely by electrodesiccation. Flat warts of the face may leave small depressions or scars or both when treated by curettage and electrodesiccation. These lesions may respond to many types of therapy including suggestion. If it becomes necessary to treat verruca plana of the face by surgical methods, one should first treat a small inconspicuous test area using curettage only. My preference is for liquid nitrogen therapy for flat warts using superficial freezing of short duration. Because the knee and elbow also tend to scar very easily, liquid nitrogen therapy may be preferable in these locations. However, it should be noted that the skin of some patients will develop scarring from procedures producing minimal injury to the dermis.

In some instances, scarring follows treatment of plantar warts. In the author's experience, this is less likely to occur when the wart is removed with a minimal destruction of subjacent and surrounding tissue by the methods described above. To help reduce the frequency of plantar wart recurrences, attention should be paid to such coexistent problems as faulty weight bearing, hyperhidrosis, shoes that do not fit correctly, and abnormalities in underlying bones of the feet.

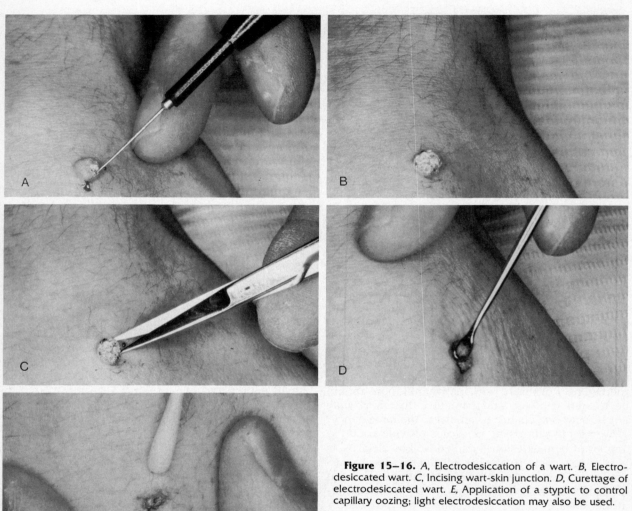

Figure 15–16. *A,* Electrodesiccation of a wart. *B,* Electro-desiccated wart. *C,* Incising wart-skin junction. *D,* Curettage of electrodesiccated wart. *E,* Application of a styptic to control capillary oozing; light electrodesiccation may also be used.

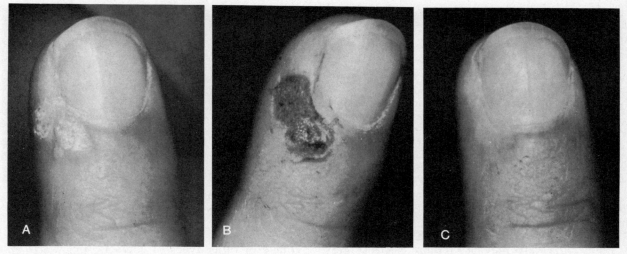

Figure 15–17. *A,* Periungual wart. *B,* Appearance after completing curettage and electrodesiccation. *C,* Healed result three months after treatment.

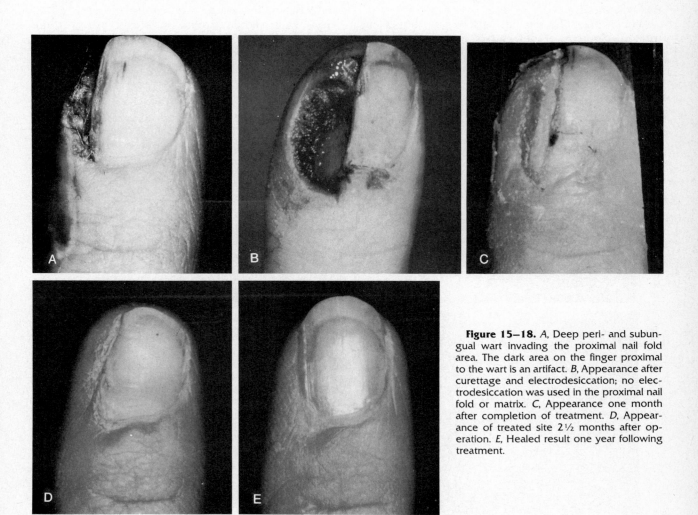

Figure 15–18. *A,* Deep peri- and subungual wart invading the proximal nail fold area. The dark area on the finger proximal to the wart is an artifact. *B,* Appearance after curettage and electrodesiccation; no electrodesiccation was used in the proximal nail fold or matrix. *C,* Appearance one month after completion of treatment. *D,* Appearance of treated site 2½ months after operation. *E,* Healed result one year following treatment.

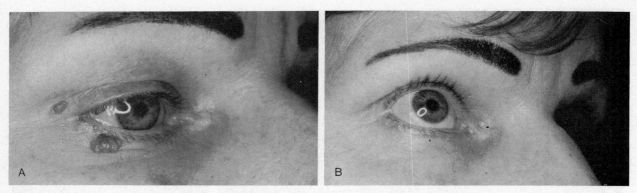

Figure 15–19. *A*, Seborrheic keratoses involving eyelids. *B*, Appearance one month after treatment by electrodesiccation and curettage.

Anogenital warts may also require electrosurgery after podophyllin or other local chemical cauterants fail. Depending upon the patient's pain threshold and the degree of involvement, careful local anesthesia may suffice for this electrosurgery. Rarely, general anesthesia in a hospital may be needed for this treatment.

When present, vaginal discharge should be treated. Sources of new warts in sexual contacts should be investigated. Patients vary greatly in their susceptibility to acquire warts through sexual inter-

course or other types of contact. Anal warts may require anoscopy and proctoscopy to determine whether warts coexist in the anal canal or rectum. Because anal warts and some acuminate genital warts are very vascular, the author prefers to use bipolar electrocoagulating current to treat them.

Occasionally, warts will require biopsies. Situations that should arouse suspicion are wartlike growths that are not typical even when located on fingers, under nails, or in the periungual fold. Squamous cell carcinoma of the fingernail bed and peri-

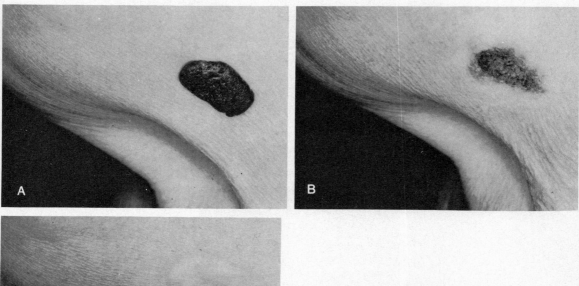

Figure 15–20. *A*, Seborrheic keratosis located on the neck of an elderly woman. *B*, Appearance of wound after electrodesiccation and curettage. *C*, Seven months after treatment showing difference in pigmentation compared with untreated surrounding skin.

ungual areas is not common but should be considered when lesions are not typical or are extremely persistent. Wartlike lesions of the anogenital areas may also cause diagnostic confusion. Bowen's disease and bowenoid papulosis in these areas may mimic warts.

Rarely, true warts invade the proximal nailfold and result in nail dystrophy, which may be permanent (Fig. 15–17C). The author's preference for treatment of warts in these locations is to use curettage alone. Should the wart recur, curettage plus electrodesiccation may be performed at the next treatment.

Skin tags may be scissor-excised to the base followed by application of a styptic. They may also be electrodesiccated with a spark of fine intensity. When they are electrodesiccated, small scissors may be used to remove them at skin level, or they may be left to fall off spontaneously.

For hemangiomas, a scissor-type biopsy can be performed followed by curettage and electrodesiccation (Fig. 15–21).

The majority of pigmented nevi are amenable to office therapy (Figs. 15–22 and 15–23). The dermatologist by history, clinical inspection, and judgment should ascertain whether the nevus shows any changes that suggest the possibility of melanoma. If such a suspicion exists, conservative total excisional biopsy is desirable when possible. If the lesion is too large or if the excision would require extensive surgery or the loss of a portion of a digit, a partial excisional biopsy is indicated prior to definitive therapy.

Occasionally, pigment will persist following treatment of benign nevi by electrodesiccation and curettage. In very few cases, the nevus will regrow above the skin surface and require further treatment. Should patients desire total removal of nevi, conservative surgical excision should suffice.

If the lesion appears to be a benign intradermal or compound nevus elevated above the surface of the skin, a "shave type" biopsy may safely be performed to just above the skin level with a scalpel or small curved scissors (with the concave side toward the skin surface). The remainder of the nevus may then be lightly electrodesiccated to skin level. If the nevus has hair within it and the patient wishes to have this hair removed, epilation should

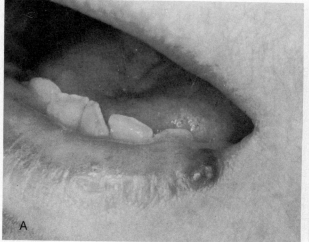

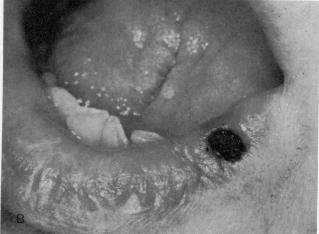

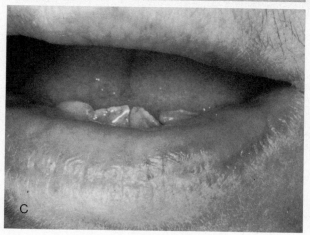

Figure 15–21. *A,* Benign hemangioma before treatment. *B,* Appearance following scissor-type biopsy, curettage, and electrodesiccation. *C,* Healed result one month after treatment.

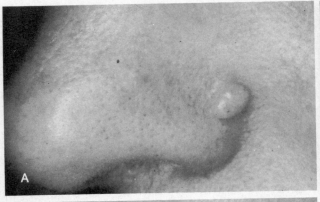

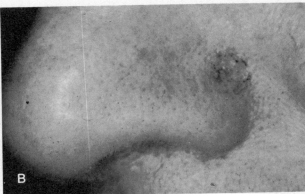

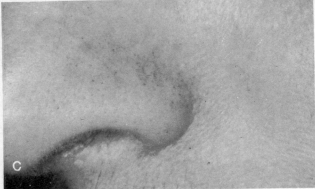

Figure 15–22. *A*, Intradermal nevus on the nose. *B*, Appearance after "shave type" biopsy and electrodesiccation; the same result may be obtained by bipolar cutting current. *C*, Healed site two months after treatment.

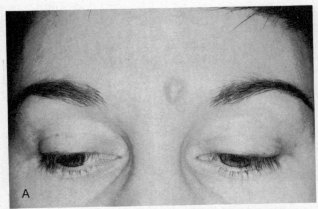

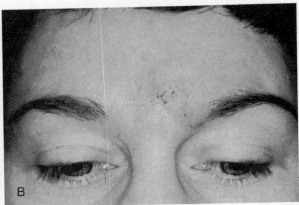

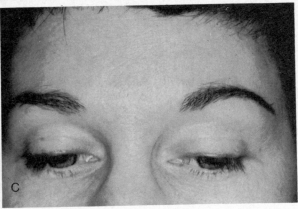

Figure 15–23. *A*, Intradermal nevus on the forehead. *B*, Appearance after "shave type" biopsy and treatment by a spark gap bipolar cutting current. *C*, Appearance six months later.

be performed prior to electrodesiccation, since the epilation may destroy some of the nevus.

Experience with epilation of hairs in a pigmented nevus followed by a shave type biopsy and electro-desiccation at a later date leaves much to be desired because of the frequent persistence of hair in the nevus following epilation. It may be less time-consuming and less costly in the long run to the patient to remove the hairy pigmented nevus initially by conservative surgical excision and suture closure.

When pigment persists following electrodesiccation of the nevus, liquid nitrogen cryotherapy may be beneficial. Complete blanching of all pigment may not be possible. However, application of liquid nitrogen for 10 to 15 seconds with moderate pressure at monthly intervals usually diminishes pigment intensity. Pigment intensity may also diminish spontaneously over a period of time.

TREATMENT FOR PREMALIGNANT AND MALIGNANT LESIONS

The use of curettage and electrodesiccation for actinic keratoses will be considered briefly, since newer methods of treatment, such as fluorouracil and liquid nitrogen, are available. These treatments are simple to use and usually yield excellent results. However, for isolated keratoses or those that are thicker than usual, curettage and electrodesiccation still remain an excellent method of treatment. A biopsy should be done in thickened or indurated actinic keratoses to make certain that a squamous cell carcinoma has not supervened.

Most actinic keratoses can be eradicated by vigorous curettage and minimal electrodesiccation. Occasionally, a keratosis will recur and be confirmed by a biopsy. These lesions will require heavier electrodesiccation. In a similar fashion, arsenic keratoses may be treated by electrodesiccation and curettage. However, this type of treatment is more difficult for the patient when there are many arsenic keratoses on the palms and soles.

Curettage and electrodesiccation find widespread use for treating basal cell carcinoma, squamous cell carcinoma and Bowen's disease (Figs. 15–24 to 15–27). In the case of basal cell carcinoma, the carcinomatous tissue, together with the underlying fibroblastic stroma (rich in mucopolysaccharides), is much softer in consistency than the surrounding normal epidermis and subjacent healthy dermis. This enables the surgeon to separate the diseased soft tissue from the firm, surrounding normal epidermis and dermis by curettage. There have been reports of a high incidence of recurrence of Bowen's disease when treated by this method.[3] The author's personal experience is at variance with these findings, although the case selection may very well be different.

Salasche,[4] Edens and coworkers,[5] and Sughe d'Aubermont and Bennett[6] performed microscopic examination on sites of basal cell carcinoma immediately following treatment by curettage and electrodesiccation. They noted tumor persistance rates of 30%, 37%, and 33.3%, respectively. Salasche's study pertained to basal cell carcinomas of the nose and nasolabial folds. Spiller and Spiller[7] and Knox and colleagues[8] in carefully selected lesions of basal cell carcinoma up to 2 cm in size that had been treated by curettage and electrodesiccation achieved a cure rate of 97%. Spiller and Spiller noted that lesions of the nose and nasolabial folds and lesions larger than 2 cm were more likely to recur after treatment with this modality.

Such high cure rates for basal cell carcinoma treated in this manner (as reported by Spiller and Spiller and Knox and colleagues) indicate that other factors may explain the discrepancy between their findings and those of Salasche, Eden and coworkers, Sughe d'Aubermont, and other experienced dermatologists who carefully employ this method of treatment for selected lesions of basal cell carcinoma. It is postulated that immune mechanisms[9] and the inflammatory aspects of wound healing following treatment[4, 7] by curettage and electrodesiccation may play a role in the further removal by

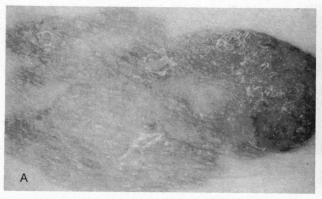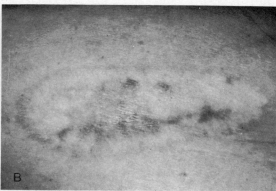

Figure 15–24. A, Large plaque of Bowen's disease located on the abdomen of an elderly patient. B, Appearance eight months after curettage and electrodesiccation to destroy the lesion.

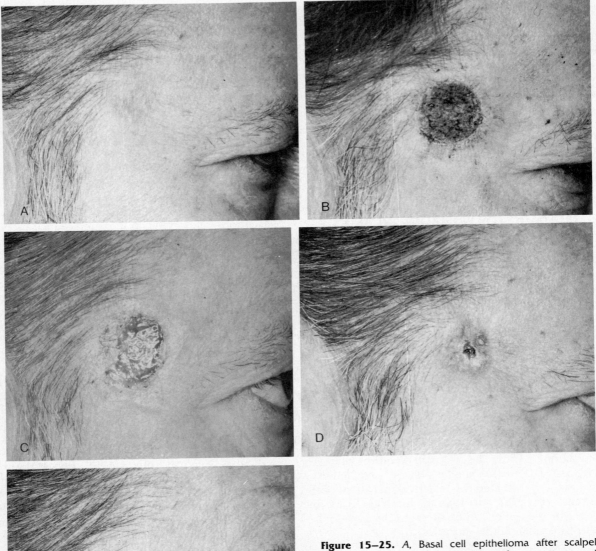

Figure 15–25. *A*, Basal cell epithelioma after scalpel "shave type" biopsy. *B*, Appearance after curettage and electrodesiccation, showing the extent of treatment. *C*, Appearance 2½ weeks after treatment, showing healthy granulation tissue at the operated site. *D*, Appearance five weeks after curettage and electrodesiccation. *E*, Appearance eight months after treatment.

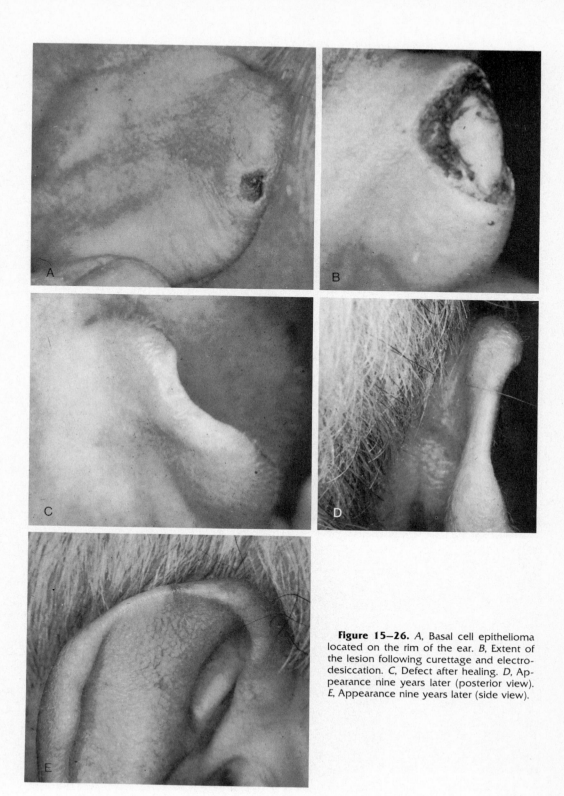

Figure 15–26. *A*, Basal cell epithelioma located on the rim of the ear. *B*, Extent of the lesion following curettage and electrodesiccation. *C*, Defect after healing. *D*, Appearance nine years later (posterior view). *E*, Appearance nine years later (side view).

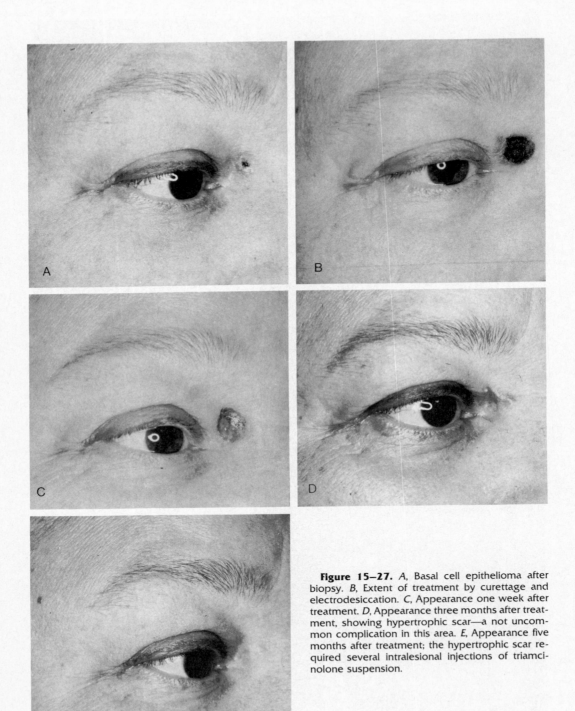

Figure 15–27. *A,* Basal cell epithelioma after biopsy. *B,* Extent of treatment by curettage and electrodesiccation. *C,* Appearance one week after treatment. *D,* Appearance three months after treatment, showing hypertrophic scar—a not uncommon complication in this area. *E,* Appearance five months after treatment; the hypertrophic scar required several intralesional injections of triamcinolone suspension.

the body of basal cell carcinoma tissue that may be persistent immediately after curettage and electrodesiccation.

Elderly patients with sun-damaged skin may present some problems for treatment by curettage and electrodesiccation. Firm scraping action by the curette may tear the thin atrophic epidermis and also penetrate the thin dermis, resulting in false information about the extent of the lesion.

The morphea type of basal cell carcinoma, basal cell carcinoma that recurs in scars, or basal cell carcinoma that has a strong fibrotic or scarring tendency are best treated by other modalities. Because of the intimate admixture of basal cell tissue and fibrotic tissue, the physician is unable to secure the necessary information from the feel of the curette, since there is little "mushy" tissue to separate.

Basal cell carcinomas located in certain anatomic areas are better treated by other methods. These include lesions involving the ala and tip of the nose, the lip vermilion-skin junction, the eyelid margins (except for very small lesions), and the canthi. Eradication of lesions in these areas may result in significant cosmetic or functional defects or both. X-ray therapy, unless contraindicated, is more appropriate, although work with liquid nitrogen cryosurgery shows much promise. Lesions that invade deeply and may be fixed to periosteum or perichondrium or that invade bone or cartilage are best treated by other techniques. Excessively large and complicated lesions of basal cell carcinomas are probably better treated by other modalities — except large lesions of superficial basal cell carcinoma, which may be treated successfully by curettage alone or by curettage and electrodesiccation. Such lesions may be seen with a tumor extending up to several centimeters in size.

Alternate methods of treatment for the superficial type of basal cell carcinomas include cryosurgery with liquid nitrogen and grenz ray therapy. One suggested schedule for grenz ray therapy is 500 roentgens (of the thickest HVL for grenz rays) three times a week for a total of 5000 roentgens.

For some recurrent or complicated lesions, Mohs' chemosurgery or excisional surgery should be considered. Menn and colleagues[10] have shown that recurrence rates of basal cell carcinoma are high when retreated by methods other than Mohs' chemosurgery. Reymann[11, 12] and McDaniel[13] have used curettage alone for treatment of basal cell carcinoma. While cosmetic results in general tend to be better with this technique, cure rates are likely to be consistently higher with the combination technique of curettage followed by electrodesiccation. Eradication of the lesion during the first treatment session should be the aim of the dermatologist.

TREATMENT FOR SKIN MALIGNANCIES

After securing local anesthesia, the skin around the lesion is fixed firmly between the thumb and index finger. This maneuver also achieves a degree of pressure hemostasis. The curette is then drawn across multiple diameters of the lesion with a firm scraping motion until all soft tissue has been removed.

Continued pressure hemostasis with the index finger and thumb is maintained, and a cotton applicator moistened with 35% aluminum chloride in 50% isopropyl alcohol or other suitable styptic is applied to the curetted site. Isolated bleeders that are not coagulated by this styptic may then be electrodesiccated.

The next step in treatment is careful electrodesiccation using a spark of medium intensity applied to the entire curetted tumor base. This electrodesiccation includes a peripheral rim of apparently normal tissue and is repeated two or more times. If any soft pockets are encountered, a curette with a small diameter tip should be used to eradicate them.

Oozing and redness around the treated area are noted in seven to 10 days; crusts will form later. Healing time is dependent upon the extent and depth of involvement and the anatomic location. Lesions of the face tend to heal more rapidly than other areas; those on the legs are the slowest to heal. Occasionally, an inflammatory halo develops around the treated area, which may indicate low-grade pyoderma under the crust. The crust should be removed and appropriate topical measures instituted. If granulation tissue develops in excess of normal amounts, topical silver nitrate therapy (5% to 10%) is instituted at weekly intervals until more normal healing ensues.

When selected lesions of Bowen's disease (e.g., intraepidermal squamous cell carcinoma) and squamous cell carcinoma of the skin are treated in a similar fashion, the author's experience indicates that high cure rates are achieved.

Hypertrophic scars (Figs. 15–27E and 15–28A) are not uncommon complications when destruction of the lesion has resulted in the loss of full-thickness skin. Ordinarily, such scars will improve spontaneously over several months. Monthly intralesional injections of triamcinolone acetonide (the concentration adjusted for the lesion) assists in the resolution of the hypertrophic scar.

In the author's experience, true keloids are seldom seen following curettage and electrodesiccation of basal cell carcinomas. When they do occur, they are likely to be found over the deltoid and presternal areas and on the upper back or the neck below the mandible. Treatment of true keloids is at present unsatisfactory. Intralesional steroid therapy (5 to 40 mg/ml of triamcinolone) at monthly intervals may be helpful. However, it may be necessary to continue this treatment over a long period of time. If the keloid has thickened, it may be shaved down to just above the surface of the skin and then injected with intralesional steroids. X-ray therapy or cryotherapy combined with intralesional steroids may be necessary to treat some keloids.

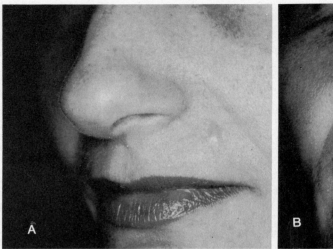
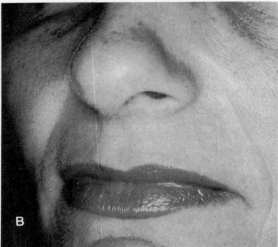

Figure 15–28. *A,* Hypertrophic scar following curettage and electrodesiccation of basal cell epithelioma. *B,* Healed result after treatment by intralesional triamcinolone injections.

OTHER USES FOR ELECTROSURGERY

The bipolar electrocoagulating current is useful for treating bleeders encountered in excisional surgery. The current is adjusted to a medium setting. The patient must be in firm contact with the dispersive electrode. A sterilized pair of stainless steel jeweler's forceps may be used to grasp the bleeding vessel. The active electrode is touched to the forceps, resulting in point electrocoagulation. Alternatively, bipolar electrocoagulating current can be applied across the tips of the forceps used to grasp the bleeding vessel. These forceps are connected to an isolated source of bipolar coagulation current.

On some of the spark gap machines, bipolar coagulation current (with extra resistance introduced into the circuit) provides a serviceable epilating current. Bipolar cutting currents are produced by the spark gap, radio tube, and transistorized apparatus. The undamped, radio tube, high-frequency alternating currents yield an effect on the tissue of cutting with minimal coagulation. The bipolar cutting current derived from the spark gap machine produces a cutting effect with more coagulation. However, in practice, the speed with which the active electrode is drawn through the skin determines to some extent how much coagulation takes place during the cutting procedure. This same principle is operative for cutting currents obtained from the spark gap, radio tube, and transistorized electrosurgical units.

The bipolar cutting current is useful in removing the excess tissue found in rhinophyma, trichoepithelioma, and keloids. It may also be used to treat large intradermal nevi in which some degree of sculpting may be needed, e.g., one occupying the nasal fold and originating from the adjacent ala nasae. While electrodesiccation and curettage give similar results, the sculpting effect is more easily achieved with the bipolar cutting current.

Bipolar cutting current is also useful in rhinophyma and enables the practitioner to remove the hypertrophic lobulations with minimal bleeding and with good visual control of the depth of tissue removal. The patient's nose may be anesthetized by means of a bilateral infraorbital nerve block. In addition, nerve filaments from the infratrochlear nerve must be blocked by a fan-type infiltration at the root of the nose. The tip and sides of the nose derive additional innervation from the external nasal nerves. These must be blocked because they emerge at the junction of the cartilaginous and bony portions of the sides of the nose.

If it is difficult to produce an infraorbital block, the branches of the infraorbital nerves supplying the alae nasi and rim of the external nares may be anesthetized by injecting anesthetic solution in a plane just above the maxilla in the nasal sulcus

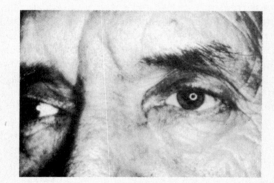

Figure 15–29. Skin fold following treatment of a basal cell epithelioma by curettage and electrodesiccation.

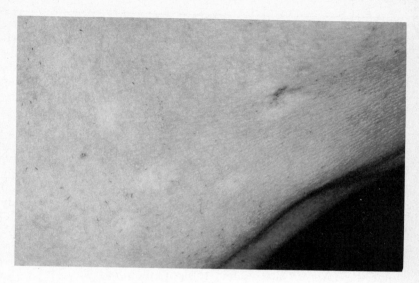

Figure 15–30. Hypopigmentation of the neck following treatment of a verruca in the bearded area of a 65-year-old patient. Hypopigmentation is often seen in older patients whose skin has some degree of actinic damage.

lateral to the alae nasi and toward the midline at the same depth under the external nares.

The main problem in external nasal anesthesia is caused by the vascularity of the area that results in the loss of anesthesia and necessitates reinjection.

After suitable anesthesia has been secured, the hypertrophic lobules are removed by a combination of cutting and superficial shaving. It is advisable to have the patient sit up periodically during this procedure. The sides of the nose may be inspected to ensure that reasonable symmetry is being maintained.

An alternate and similarly effective method is to remove the rhinophymatous tissue in circumscribed areas. A reasonable amount of tissue may be removed under local infiltration anesthesia at each office visit.

Dermabrasion and scalpel surgery may also be used to sculpt the external surface of the nose. The chief advantage of the bipolar cutting current lies in its ability to seal the blood vessels as the operation proceeds. Occasionally, a more vigorous bleeder will be encountered. This complication is handled by switching to the bipolar coagulating current and touching the active electrode to the bleeding vessel.

The author has had some experience with the "discing" method of treating selected skin malignancies of the face and neck in older patients. In this simple technique, the scalpel or bipolar cutting current is used to remove the carcinoma down to, and including some of, the superficial layer of subcutaneous fat. The specimen is suitably marked with a suture for orientation and sent to the pathologist for examination of the adequacy of the excised margins. Bleeding vessels may be electrodesiccated or electrocoagulated. The wound is then left to granulate and epithelialize. The patient changes dressings on a daily basis until a firm crust forms on the wound.

Zitelli[14] has published an excellent review of healing by secondary intention that will assist those practitioners who plan to use the discing method for treating selected skin malignancies.

REFERENCES

1. Jackson R: Basic principles of electrosurgery. Can J Surg 13:354–361, October, 1970
2. Elliot JA: Electrosurgery, its use in dermatology with a review of its development and technologic aspects. Arch Dermatol 94:340, 1966
3. Graham JH, Helwig EB: Precancerous skin lesions and systemic cancer. In Tumors of the Skin. Chicago, Yearbook Medical Publishers Inc, 1964
4. Salasche SJ: Curettage and electrodesiccation in the treatment of midfacial basal cell epithelioma. J Amer Acad of Dermatol 8:496–503, 1983
5. Edens BL, Bartlow GA, Haghighi P, Astarita RW and Davidson TM: Effectiveness of Curettage and Electrodesiccation in the Removal of Basal Cell Carcinoma. J Amer Acad of Dermatol 9:323–388, 1983
6. Sughe d'Aubermont PC, Bennett, RG: Failure of curettage and electrodesiccation for removal of basal cell carcinoma. Arch Dermatol 120:1456–1460, 1984
7. Spiller NF, Spiller RF: Treatment of basal cell carcinoma by curettage and electrodesiccation. J Amer Acad of Dermatol 11:808–814, 1984
8. Knox JM, Freeman RG, Duncan WC, et al: Treatment of skin cancer. Southern Medical Journal 60:241–246, 1967
9. Dobson RL, Thiers BH: Yearbook of Dermatology. Chicago, Yearbook Medical Publishers Inc, 1981, p 106
10. Menn H, Robins P, Kopf AW, et al: The recurrent basal cell epithelioma. Arch Dermatol 103:628–631, 1971
11. Reymann F: Treatment of basal cell carcinoma of the skin with curettage. Arch Dermatol 108:528–531, 1973
12. Reymann F: Basal cell carcinomas of the skin, treatment with curettage. Arch Dermatol 111:877–879, 1975
13. McDaniel WF: Therapy for basal cell epitheliomas by curettage only. Arch Dermatol 119:901–903, 1983
14. Zitelli JA: Wound healing by secondary intention. J Amer Acad of Dermatol 9:407–415, 1983

16

SCHOCH, JR., M.D.
EUGENE P.

Endothermy Excision

Epstein[1] has reviewed the rapidly growing interest in dermatologic surgery and the response of organized teaching programs to this need. Much of this enthusiasm has been expressed in the emphasis on cosmetic surgery. Some dermatologists are skilled in plastic surgical techniques, such as sliding grafts and Y- and Z-plasties. Others transplant hair and plane faces. The vast majority of practicing dermatologists, however, are content to apply their surgical knowledge and skills to the ablation of benign or malignant skin tumors. Scalpel surgery has been previously described in this book. This chapter will address one aspect of electrosurgery, the special variant of endothermy or cutting current excision.

CHARACTERISTICS OF ELECTROSURGICAL CURRENTS

In 1893, d'Arsonval[2] described tissue heating effects of radio-frequency currents. Ward[3] in 1925 demonstrated that damped oscillations produced by a spark gap apparatus caused *coagulation* of tissue and that undamped pure sinusoidal current produced a *cutting* effect. These two basic principles apply today in modern electrosurgical techniques: (1) electrodesiccation (fulguration) and (2) coagulation and cutting (electrosectioning). Electrodesiccation is the process of producing dehydration of a tissue by the contact or near contact of an electrode through which a simple monopolar damped sinusoidal current is passed. This type of current is generated by a spark gap apparatus, e.g., the Birtcher Hyfrecator. The uses of this technique have been described in Chapter 15.

Electrocoagulation and cutting currents employ a bipolar setup by which a very small active electrode concentrates the current and produces rapid heating at the point of application. A large dispersive electrode (indifferent or ground plate) in broad contact with the skin is used to minimize the current density and heating at the other end of the body circuit. Samuel Ayres, Jr.,[4] has reviewed the physics and current characterization in the third edition of this book.

Endothermy or excisional electrosurgical generators employ a bipolar, undamped sinusoidal current in the frequency range of 1 to 2 MHz. This is produced usually by a vacuum tube or solid-state oscillator, but some spark gap machines are capable of generating a cutting current. Tissue cutting is not the result of a hot cautery tip (electrocautery) but rather is due to the dissolution of molecular structure by the electric arc in the immediate path of the electrode.[5] Some electrosurgical units produce coagulation, cutting, and a combination current with both characteristics.

The various modes of current have distinctive biologic effects that can be utilized for specific surgical purposes. The pure cutting current causes the least tissue damage during cleavage and most closely resembles scalpel excision. There is little or no hemostasis in such cutting, and the wound may be sutured to heal in the primary manner if desired. The coagulating current is used to control hemorrhage by direct coagulation of small vessels or by applying the electrode to the tip of a hemostat that has been clamped on a larger vessel. The blended current (part cutting and part coagulating current) produces more hemostasis during the actual cutting but also produces more tissue destruction because of coagulation.

INDICATIONS

Although numerous benign growths can be managed by electrosurgery,[6] other methods, such as cryosurgery or scalpel excision, may be preferable in selected cases. Excisional electrosurgery (endothermy) is primarily a procedure for removing cutaneous malignancies.

Recurrent basal cell carcinomas are good candidates for endothermy (Fig. 16–1A). Morphea-like basal cell carcinomas and those arising in areas of radiodermatitis or scars are well managed by this technique. In addition, squamous cell carcinomas of almost any cutaneous area and of the lip respond well. Of course, the presence of metastases requires additional surgical management. Malignant melanomas may be removed by this method. Modern-day criteria as to which melanomas can be treated by wide local excision alone include lentigo maligna and superficial spreading melanoma, levels I and II, which are less than 0.76 mm thick without palpable lymph nodes.[7] Many authorities also employ this modality in nodular melanoma.

PROCEDURE

The diagnosis of a neoplasm is usually made or confirmed by a biopsy of a portion of the lesion. If the tumor is small, a total excisional biopsy may be more appropriate.

The operative field is prepared in the usual manner. The skin is scrubbed with an antibacterial soap, and a topical noninflammable antiseptic is applied.

A local anesthetic such as 1% or 2% lidocaine with or without epinephrine (1:100,000) is infiltrated around and beneath the lesion. If the area is on a peripheral digit or if the patient has a cardiovascular contraindication to the use of epinephrine, plain lidocaine should be injected.

The indifferent electrode, usually a large stainless steel plate, is carefully placed in smooth, even contact with the patient's skin at a remote point. The active electrode is usually a needle but may be a flat blade, loop, or another shape according to the surgeon's preference. The machine is set for cutting operation. The lesion to be excised is marked out with sterile ink or by means of light electrodesiccation. The size of seemingly normal tissue border may vary for 0.5 to 3.0 cm or more depending on the nature of the tumor and the surgeon's judgment. The outline is generally a circle or oval but may be elliptical if suturing is anticipated.

The energized needle is stroked along the pattern line cutting through the skin. One edge of the island of tissue is held with a pair of rat-tooth or Allis forceps, and the cut is extended down to a depth beneath the tumor mass. This is usually in subcutaneous fat, but in deep growths, it may extend down to fascia, muscle, or periosteum. The disc is then lifted so that it may be dissected away from the underlying supportive tissue. This dissection plane is parallel to the surface. As the electrode advances, the tissue splits effortlessly.

Hemostasis is achieved by electrocoagulation of bleeding points by direct application of the electrode (with a coagulation setting, not a cutting one) or by energizing the tip of a hemostat clamped on a vessel. Very large vessels are isolated and ligated at each border of the cavity. The operative site should then be dry. The base is painted with 1% aqueous gentian violet solution then dusted with polymyxin B-bacitracin-neomycin (Neosporin) powder and absorbable gelatin sterile powder (Gelfoam). One layer of fine mesh gauze and several bulky gauze pads are applied and secured with Elastoplast. This dressing is left undisturbed for three to five days, when it is removed in the office. If there is no hemorrhage, the wound is left open to the air and Neosporin powder is applied twice daily. The immediate postoperative appearance of the wound is shown in Figure 16–1B, and the appearance three months later in Figure 16–1C.

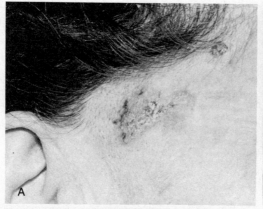

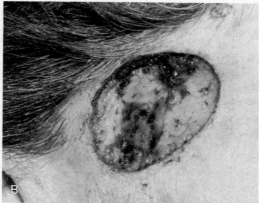

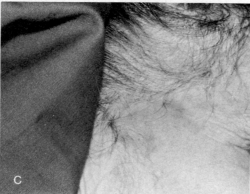

Figure 16–1. *A,* Recurrent basal cell carcinoma of the skin on the temple. *B,* Wound resulting from electrosurgical excision immediately after surgery. *C,* Scar resulting three months after surgery. (From *The Journal of Dermatologic Surgery,* 2:241, 1976. Copyright 1976, *The Journal of Dermatologic Surgery and Oncology,* Inc.)

ADVANTAGES

Endothermy excision is an office procedure requiring a minimum of equipment and assistance. Usually, less normal tissue is sacrificed because the disc includes only the tumor and a smaller peripheral zone of normal tissue than with elliptical scalpel surgery. Although there is not the microscopic control as with Mohs' chemosurgery (fixed or fresh techniques or both), the entire disc from endothermy excision is submitted for histopathologic study. Should there be encroachment on any border by malignancy, the excision may be enlarged the following day. The wound is usually allowed to granulate and heal by secondary intention. The resulting scars are usually acceptable and durable (Fig. 16–1C).

DISADVANTAGES

Occasionally, hemorrhage may occur several days postoperatively from the sloughing of coagulated vascular tissue or from trauma to the granulating bed. Simple pressure usually controls the small bleeders, but sometimes larger vessels must be ligated. Healing is slow and there may be hypertrophic scarring. Granulation tissue may be exuberant during healing of large wounds, which encourages more scar formation. Should excessive scars develop, intralesional corticosteroid injections or superficial x-ray therapy or both are useful. Usually, three or four doses of x-rays, 300 rad each (HVL 1.0 mm of aluminum), given every two weeks will suffice.

SPECIAL PRECAUTIONS

Excisional electrosurgery in general does present some special problems.[8] Radio frequency output may interfere with other electrical instruments in the area. Modern shielding and design of apparatus minimize this problem.

High-frequency burns may occur if the dispersive electrode is in contact with a small surface, such as a bony prominence creating a localized high current density. Also, if the wire connection from the machine to the dispersive electrode is broken, alternate grounding pathways develop, which produce burns at the exit site.

Explosions and fire arising from electrosurgical use in an environment containing explosive anesthesia (e.g. operating room areas and gas-filled hollow organs) are unlikely since few dermatologic electrosurgical procedures are performed under such circumstances. Modern operation room protocol and anesthesiologists also preclude such a possibility. Fire from flammable local antiseptics used in patient preparation may occur. Surgeons should avoid the use of alcohol, ether, and similar skin cleansers before electrosurgery.

Finally, implanted cardiac pacemakers may be disrupted by high-frequency currents flowing through the body. The demand type of pacemakers are especially susceptible. Patients with such devices probably should be treated by alternative methods.

CONCLUSION

Dermatologists are constantly losing ground to other medical disciplines. The management of cutaneous malignancies should remain primarily within the domain of dermatologists. The methods of treatment should be versatile. Each case of skin cancer should be individualized, and the patient should be offered the particular advantages of scalpel surgery, electrosurgery, cryosurgery, or radiotherapy or a combination of these.

REFERENCES

1. Epstein E: Skin surgery today. Dermatol Digest, no. 11, 1976
2. d'Arsonval MA: Production des courants de haute fréquence et de grande intensité; leurs effets physiologiques. C R Soc Biol 45:122–124, 1893
3. Ward GE: Value of electrothermic methods in the treatment of malignancy. JAMA 84:660–666, 1925
4. Ayres S Jr: Endothermy and electrocoagulation. In Epstein, E (ed): Skin Surgery, ed 3. Springfield, Ill, Charles C Thomas, Publisher, 1970, pp 251–260
5. Battig CG: Electrosurgical burn injuries and their prevention. JAMA 204:1025–1029, 1968
6. Elliott JA: Electrosurgery. Arch Dermatol 94:340–350, 1966
7. Kopf AW, et al: Malignant Melanoma. New York, Masson Publishing USA Inc, 1979, pp 179–180
8. National Fire Protection Association: High frequency electrical equipment in hospitals. No. 76 CM, 190

17

ERVIN EPSTEIN, M.D.

Cautery Excision

Along with the rest of the world, surgery has made great strides during the past thirty years. Not only has the scope of the specialty been extended and morbidity and mortality decreased by better anesthesia and supportive care, but operative techniques have been improved tremendously. Since early surgeons did not have the training of present-day operators, they were forced to rely upon cruder approaches and instruments. During that era, the use of actual cautery was important in the performance of radical surgery, including mastectomy, thoracotomy, and ruthlessly destructive operations for advanced malignancy.

Dr. James Percy, the inventor of the Percy cautery, had much to do with the erstwhile popularity of this form of surgery. Percy, who specialized in oncologic surgery, was one of the first surgeons in this field. He had his own service at the Los Angeles County Hospital for many years complete with his own resident, rotating interns, a ward, an operating room, and an inexhaustible supply of patients suffering from inoperable cancer. He operated on these individuals every Thursday starting at eight in the morning and ending at ten in the evening. Even when he was in his seventies, it was not unusual for him to be operating and lecturing to an audience of physicians from all over the world.

He was a competent showman and so attracted a large number of observers into his amphitheater. Since the main portion of his practice consisted of patients with inoperable malignancies, many died on the table, but a few were saved because he was able to perform more radical removals than his more conservative colleagues. He believed that the cautery bearing his name attained a degree of heat that prevented the patient from feeling pain. Therefore, he performed most of his surgery, including major procedures within body cavities, without anesthesia! Since there is considerable radiation of heat from the cautery, a very stoic patient was needed for such an approach. Patients had such confidence in this master that they gladly submitted to the operation, despite the fact that Percy never minimized the risks inherent in the ultraradical surgery. The opportunity of watching this man in action influenced my earlier dermatologic surgery to a significant extent.

In the 1930s, we encountered many more extensive skin cancers than we do today. Possibly, this is due to the publicity that cancer has received from the media and cancer societies. Regardless of the reason, there has been a diminution in the size and extent of such neoplasms encountered in private practice. For instance, I remember vividly one of my earlier patients, a hard-headed individual who had diagnosed the lump on his shoulder as a "boil." One night, when his wife and daughter left him alone while they attended a movie, he attempted to incise the alleged boil with a pair of scissors. Being a man of great determination, he managed to deeply lacerate the lesion. Unfortunately, instead of pus, blood poured out of the self-inflicted wound. The bleeding continued at a reduced rate until the following morning, when he came into the office. Despite the fact that the mass was at least double the size of a regulation baseball, the patient was placed on a table in the office, and the sarcoma was excised under local anesthesia with a Percy cautery. The patient lived for several years, succumbing eventually to pulmonary and other metastases. The surgical wound healed eventually with only moderate scarring and with no evidence of local recurrence during the remainder of his life. It is doubtful that one could perform surgery of this extent under local anesthesia outside of a hospital with any other modality.

Another extensive, though comparatively simple, operation that can be done with a cutting cautery is the excision of the skin and subcutaneous tissue for the eradication of hidradenitis suppurativa. When this can be done in the office without general anesthesia, the surgery is considerably simplified. It is in this simplification that the advantages of cautery surgery are most noticeable.

DEFINITION

Cauterization refers to the destruction or removal of tissue by heat or chemicals. Surgical cauterization concerns only the use of heat; the destruction may be accomplished by a number of heated instruments shaped like a loop, a blade, a needle, or a ball or in other configurations. For all practical purposes, the cautery has proven to be of greatest value in the excision of malignant tumors. Other indications include certain precancerous dermatoses, such as leukoplakia and erythroplasia of Queyrat, and localized granulomas, such as deep fungus infections and tuberculosis. Other methods have proven to be more applicable in most infections, disseminated granulomas, and benign neoplasms. Only the blade type of cautery will be considered in this chapter since it is concerned with "cautery excision."

EQUIPMENT

The equipment needed to perform cautery surgery is inexpensive. There are many types and brands on the market, but in this discussion, I will confine myself to the Post and the Percy cauteries. It should be emphasized that these are hot cauteries, which exert their action through thermal elevation. Also, the intent of cauterization in this section is excision—not destruction—of a mucocutaneous lesion, usually a neoplasm.

Basically, the two cauteries vary only in size. The Post cautery is the smaller of the two and so is more applicable for work on the skin. The instrument consists of a six-inch long handle with a light on top that theoretically should illuminate the operative field. Actually, the lamp is too weak to accomplish anything except notifying the operator that the cautery is turned on. A cutting blade is attached to the end of the handle by a small bolt and nut, which must be applied tightly or the current will not flow to the blade. The equipment is activated by elevating a sleeve to the top of the handle.

The blade is said to be made of silver and is supplied in various shapes and sizes, including straight and curved blades, needles, and rods. When the cautery is plugged into a wall socket with the blade firmly attached and the sleeve raised, the blade quickly becomes hot. This cautery is manufactured by the Post Electric Company of Andover, New Jersey. Recently, Post has upgraded their cautery by introducing a new set of controls allowing for more accurate setting of the current produced. However, the handle and blades are unchanged.

The Percy cautery is much larger and more austere, without a light, a sleeve and other amenities. Actually, it resembles an old-fashioned soldering iron and has a variety of interchangeable tips. It is merely plugged into a socket, and after a moment or two, it is ready to operate.

TECHNIQUE

Preoperative preparation is minimal. Only the most apprehensive patient requires sedation or tranquilizers.

The skin need not be cleansed or sterilized. The superheated cautery attends to both tasks adequately as it sears the tissues. Of course, one should use rubbing alcohol or another antiseptic before injecting a local anesthetic; however, alcohol is inflammable and it must evaporate before using the hot cautery on the skin.

It is not amiss to warn the patient about the pungent odor of burning flesh. Few individuals develop a fondness for this aroma, especially when they realize that their own tissues are being singed. The smoke may be dissipated by forcibly exhaling.

Drapes are not necessary, and in fact, if one is fastidious and insists on their use, the edges must be far enough away from the operative field so that the inflammable cloth or plastic does not contribute to an untoward event, such as a conflagration, which can be embarrassing.

Anesthesia is not an important phase of the procedure. If necessary, one could operate on a stoic patient without any anesthetic agent at all. On the other hand, the injection of a local anesthetic has much to recommend it. Procaine, lidocaine, or whatever the operator prefers can be inserted intradermally and subcutaneously along the proposed incision line. This will eradicate the *pain* of the burning, but the patient should be warned that this will not prevent feeling some heat radiation from the cautery. The surgeon must remember that if the surrounding unanesthetized skin is inadvertently touched with the hot tip, the patient will complain loudly and bitterly.

General anesthesia may be employed, if desired. Intravenous preparations are preferred for this purpose. If inhalation anesthesia is utilized, one of the inflammable or explosive gaseous mixtures must not be administered.

Now for the operation itself (Fig. 17–1). One can judge when the cautery is ready for use when a square of absorbent cotton can be cut through without undue pressure. In excising a lesion, one makes an incision in the skin with the tip of the cutting blade. The incision should extend all the way around the tumor and be of sufficient depth so that one can cut under the neoplasm. After the growth has been surrounded by a charred ditch, one corner is elevated by a skin hook or toothed forceps. Then the blade is rotated from the vertical position to a horizontal one, and the lesion is removed by undercutting it completely. Although one cannot readily identify all of the microscopic prolongations, the amount of peripheral and deep normal tissue that should be sacrificed can be judged by the experienced operator. A margin of 0.5 to 1 cm is adequate in most instances. This should be greater for a melanoma or a sarcoma. When the specimen has been removed, one can cut through it and identify the type and extent of the lesion: dead white if it is an epithelioma, jet black if it is melanoma, and purulent if it is hidradenitis suppurativa or a deep mycosis such as coccidioidomycosis. If the extent of the excision does not appear to be adequate, especially in depth, one can excise additional tissue during the primary operation.

As a rule, hemostasis is complete. In fact, the comparatively low temperature of circulating blood allows one to dissect blood vessels with this technique. It is astounding how a cancer that is adherent to the wall of a large blood vessel can be excised without damaging the vein or artery. However, it must be admitted that this is not always successful. I will never forget the time that a surgeon opened the subclavian artery with a Percy cautery. The blood splattered the ceiling, and the patient was exsanguinated within a few moments. Small bleeders, even spurters, can be caught with hemostats and cauterized or tied. Most small excisions, such as those a dermatologist would tackle, can be performed in a bloodless field without the use of hemostats. This is a major advantage.

No attempt is made to obtain primary closure of the defect. Even in a small wound, this would be unwise because of the discharge that follows the operation. The burned tissue, of which a certain amount remains in vivo, is sloughed, commencing about the third day after the operation and continuing for seven to 10 days. Since the material resembles pus, an inexperienced surgeon may fear that the wound is infected and institute local or systemic antibiotic therapy. One postoperative patient who changed physicians in midstream was told that the wound was infected and was treated for an infection, and then sued the original surgeon for malpractice. One must remember that the purulent-appearing discharge is normal and does not indicate the presence of an infection.

Basically, a nonadherent dry dressing should be used. Telfa or ordinary gauze with a tiny amount of boric acid ointment (Borofax) or petrolatum on it to prevent the bandage from sticking to the wound is satisfactory. One should use as little adhesive tape as possible and try to apply it in different directions with each changing—horizontal, vertical, or in the form of an X—since the wound will take about one month to heal. In this length of time, if one applies the tape over the exact same area, skin irritation will probably occur. The first dressing is left in place for two to four days. After the aforementioned discharge starts to soil the gauze, the bandage is changed daily until the discharge ceases. As the granulation tissue becomes exuberant and extends

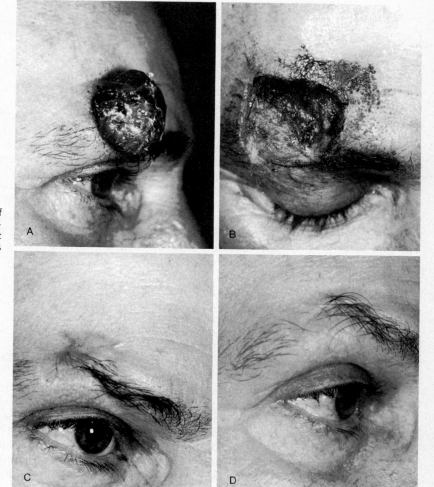

Figure 17–1. *A,* Melanoma. *B,* Extent of cautery excision (note the conservative sacrifice of normal tissue). *C,* Cosmetic result six weeks after surgery. *D,* Result six years after surgery.

above skin level it is treated twice a week with a silver nitrate or copper sulfate stick to reduce it to the desired level. Healing proceeds from both the base of the wound and from the sides. In most cases, healing is complete in about four weeks. It is apt to be delayed in very large wounds or wounds on the scalp and the feet. If a membranous bone is exposed, as on the forehead or scalp, the defect may not heal unless the surface of the bone is roughened with a curette.

The period of morbidity may be shortened by applying a graft to the healthy granulation tissue. However, this additional procedure is not essential.

Scarring is unpredictable. In many instances, a circular cicatrix contracts and forms a linear scar resembling that following an excision and suturing operation. Commonly, it remains in a coin-shaped form becoming white and atrophic. Occasionally, a hypertrophic scar develops, specially on the feet or on the chest and breast. All in all, the cosmetic results are equal to or surpass those obtained by other electrosurgical approaches.

ADVANTAGES OF CAUTERY SURGERY

With refinements of surgery in general, the use of hot cautery has declined in popularity. The question might be asked why this modality should be perpetuated or what advantages, if any, are inherent in this approach. When we examine this method, we find a number of important features that suggest it should not become extinct.

Cautery surgery is simple and does not require extensive training to perform. Naturally, the experienced operator does superior work, but even the novice can obtain respectable results. An extensive setup is not necessary, and the equipment is inexpensive. A sterile field is not a prime requisite as it is in cold steel surgery.

Hemostasis is adequate and usually complete. There is little need to catch and tie bleeders. Most bleeding points can be eliminated by touching them with the hot blade. Flowing blood in large blood vessels tends to cool the cautery, so these structures are seldom damaged, although they may be opened with disastrous results. With experience and care, one can dissect neoplastic tissue off major blood vessels. Bleeding seldom obscures the operative field.

While the cosmetic results may leave something to be desired, the sequelae compare favorably with those following other electrosurgical modalities. If electrodesiccation and curettage is as extensive as the cautery excision, the scar is less disfiguring with the latter procedure. The tendency of these cicatrices to contract and form linear scars usually results in a satisfactory postoperative appearance. The lip usually regenerates very well after a partial or total

cautery excision. Surgical scars tend to improve with time, while those following x-radiation become more marked, which means that the eventual appearance of most cautery excisions is superior to the atrophy and telangiectasia following cancericidal doses of ionizing radiation. In the removal of cutaneous malignancies, the operator has the advantage of a built-in safety factor. Most recurrences of skin cancers result from the inadequate sacrifice of grossly normal tissue surrounding the tumor. After the completion of a cautery excision, several millimeters of charred tissue sloughs off from the sides and the bottom of the wound. Therefore, the cautery may compensate to some extent for surgical timidity. Also, since there is no necessity to close the wound, one can be more radical than when an excision and repair procedure is contemplated. Healing is accomplished by the formation of granulation tissue, which becomes covered with epithelium mainly from the periphery of the wound. Skin grafting is unnecessary but can be utilized, if desired.

The cautery cuts more slowly than the scalpel or the endothermy knife. However, the elimination of many steps, such as the clamping and tying of blood vessels, the need for undercutting the adjacent skin, and wound closure or skin grafting or both, makes cautery excision a rapid method of removing cutaneous tumors. While there is less bleeding during cautery surgery than endothermy, cautery takes more time.

DISADVANTAGES OF CAUTERY SURGERY

Slow healing is the main limitation of cautery surgery. An average-sized epithelioma requires four to five weeks for complete recovery. This may extend into a period of months if the excision is extensive. Healing on the breast, scalp, and leg is particularly sluggish. However, the rate of recovery can be accelerated by skin grafting or Elastoplast dressings.

The cosmetic results are erratic. As stated previously, the scars are often comparatively inconspicuous, but in some cases, they become hypertrophic or contractile resulting in an unsatisfactory appearance.

THERAPEUTIC RESULTS

All therapeutic accomplishments necessarily vary with the skill of the operator and the selection of cases. Therefore, published series offer no proof of the superiority of one approach over another in the treatment of cancer. Even comparisons of series of patients treated by different methods by the same operator do not establish superiority or inferiority of a particular form of treatment, because an individual's skill and training is not the same with each method he or she may employ.

Remembering the old adage, "There never was a skin cancer that could not have been cured at one time with a hot nail," one must realize that the use of an actual cautery for excision of a cutaneous malignancy is effective. In the hands of an expert, it is a valuable tool in the fight against cancer.

The ordinary small basal cell or squamous cell epitheliomas encountered in dermatologic practice can be removed easily and completely by cautery excision. Large neoplasms of these types can be excised if they are confined to the skin, accessible mucous membranes (such as the lips), and subcutaneous tissue. If the lesions invade the orbit, bones, or lymph nodes, other methods should be employed. However, if desired, the primary tumor may be removed by cautery excision prior to lymph node dissection or enucleation of the eyeball. Only the most advanced epitheliomas of the skin and lips are not amenable to this treatment. In the hands of an experienced operator, simple cautery excision offers an excellent prognosis in these neoplasms.

The basic outlook in melanomas and sarcomas is different. Because of early metastases, any local therapy may prove to be only of temporary benefit. The rapid and extensive local spread of sarcomas poses another technical problem. However, the removal of these primary tumors can be accomplished as well by cautery as by any other modality. Cautery allows for the removal of large areas of surrounding normal skin. One does not have to consider technical problems, such as closure, that often act as a deterent to adequate removal. In a study of 28 patients with sarcoma involving the skin, this approach proved to be as successful as amputation and with much less disability. Since these tumors occur often in younger age groups, disability becomes an important consideration.

Precancerous lesions may also be removed with a cutting cautery. In some instances, the lesions are superficial and more easily destroyed by less destructive approaches. This is particularly true of actinic and seborrheic keratoses. However, it is very valuable in leukoplakia, erythroplasia of Queyrat, and other extensive and more penetrating processes.

Malignancy of the skin constitutes the prime indication for cautery excision. Better cosmetic results can be obtained in most benign neoplasms by other approaches. However, if such a lesion is extensive and poses great technical difficulties in its excision or destruction, removal by a cutting cautery might well be the treatment of choice. It should be remembered that the cosmetic results following cautery removal are unpredictable and sometimes unsatisfactory. This factor is of importance only in benign lesions. In the case of a malignant new growth, the unsightly scar can be improved later by excision and grafting, by intralesional injection of steroids, or by abrasive approaches. The same is true in the treatment of localized granulomas where prompt surgical removal may eradicate a focus and prevent dissemination of the infection.

In summary, we can say that actual cautery surgery is seldom used in dermatology today. However, because it offers certain advantages, it might be wise to reconsider the tendency to push it into oblivion.

18

KIRK A. BARBER, M.D. / ROBERT JACKSON, M.D.

Electrolysis

DEFINITION

Electrosurgical epilation (electrolysis) includes all methods of hair removal using either alternating or direct (galvanic) electric currents. Electrosurgical epilation is a safe and permanent method of hair removal.

HISTORICAL BACKGROUND

The idea of using an electric current to remove hair was first reported in 1875 by an American ophthalmologist, Dr. Charles E. Michel, who used it for the elimination of ingrowing eyelashes.[1, 2] In 1879, Dr. W. A. Hardaway discussed the treatment of hirsutism with this method.[3] Galvanic (direct) current introduced by a fine needle was used to produce dissolution of the hair root. By the mid-1920s high-frequency alternating currents (diathermy) were in use to produce epilation by an electrical injury to the hair papilla.[4-6] Today, methods using galvanic current have now been largely replaced by the alternating current methods, which have been greatly refined.

INDICATIONS

Patients presenting themselves for treatment of hirsutism have already decided that they consider themselves abnormally hairy. The physician should then determine whether there is an underlying organic disorder producing the excessive hair growth. The differential diagnosis of hirsutism is not the purpose of this chapter, and the reader is referred to any of the major dermatologic textbooks for further information on this subject.

Electrolysis may be indicated in the following situations:

1. Excessive facial hair of the beard, mustache, outer ear, and nose
2. Isolated large dark terminal hair scattered on the breasts, nipples, chin, or elsewhere
3. Terminal hairs on facial moles that are to be removed by the shave biopsy technique
4. Terminal hairs extending beyond the "bikini" area
5. Hair that persists in a hair-bearing skin graft used to cover a defect in a non–hair-bearing area
6. Terminal hairs from the neck that frequently become ingrown.

As a general rule, hair follicles showing inflammatory changes should not be epilated.

Before recommending electrolysis, the physician should decide how much hair is excessive. Some families and races have excessive hair. The physician should be aware of trichomania[7] where the patient's problem is due to a poor self-image—not excessive facial hair. Removal of a small amount of hair is not likely to restore emotional balance—the problem will just reappear in a different form.

Also, considering the cost and time involved in extensive electrolysis, the physician should discuss alternatives with the patient: shaving, removal by wax, chemical epilation, bleaching with alkaline hydrogen peroxide, and the use of a pumice stone.

Today, dermatologists rarely perform electrosurgical epilation. Professional electrologists have attained a high degree of expertise and are easily found in most major cities. The purpose of this chapter is to inform the reader of the theory, methods, techniques, and complications of electrosurgical epilation.

BASIC PRINCIPLES OF ELECTROLYSIS

The regulation of growth and differentiation of the epidermis and its appendages is determined by dermal factors.[8-10] Embryologically, the hair is first seen as an accumulation of epidermal basal cells forming the hair germ at three to five months of gestation. As the germ descends into the dermis, there appears an accumulation of mesenchymal cells directly below it. This group of cells will be encompassed by the descending epidermal cells and will become the dermal papillae of the mature follicle. The surrounding epidermal cells will form the hair matrix. The lower portion of the follicle will be encased by a connective tissue sheath composed of cells similar to those of the dermal papillae and distinct from those of the upper follicle sheath.

The dermal papilla is thought to regulate the induction and organization of the hair matrix. The volume of the hair matrix, and subsequent size of hair produced, is directly proportional to the size of the dermal papilla; the mitotic index at a given level of the matrix is inversely proportional to the distance from the base of the papilla.[11]

Controversy exists as to which portion of the hair follicle must be destroyed in order to produce permanent epilation. Early animal work, which was supported by indirect human studies, suggested that one must destroy the upper third of the hair follicle.[12-14] If this was not done, the hair was thought to regenerate from the dermal connective tissue sheath and the inner and outer root sheaths.[15, 16]

Human studies utilizing histologic observations of hair follicles after epilation suggest that the lower portion of the follicle must be destroyed and that the infundibulum and sebaceous glands regenerate themselves.[17, 18] These authors consider the destruction of the hair papilla necessary for permanent epilation.

It is thought that the tissue is destroyed by a combination of coagulation necrosis from the heat generated by the high-frequency waves and the resulting inflammatory reaction about the tissue.

ELECTROSURGICAL EPILATION

Galvanic Current

This low-voltage, low-amperage current produces chemical ionization in the tissues to which it is applied.[19] Epilation devices that use galvanic (direct) current have largely been replaced by those using high-frequency alternating current as the preferred method of electrosurgical epilation. The galvanic current method is as effective, and probably safer and less painful, but it is considerably slower.

Machines specifically designed for professional electrologists often incorporate both damped and undamped alternating currents either for separate or blended use. A galvanic current may also be added. Small hand-held galvanic current units have been devised for self-epilation (Perma-Tweez). A clinical study by Sternberg suggests that these units are an acceptable method of epilation if performed properly.[20] However, the Dermatologists Group Committee of the British Medical Association condemned these instruments as unsafe.[21] The difficulty in accurate placement of the needle in the follicle by the patient with the significant chance of pitted scarring was their main objection.

High-Frequency Alternating Current

Conventional electrosurgical machines of both the spark gap and vacuum tube design (see Chapter 15) can be adjusted to produce a mild epilating current. Monoterminal epilation is possible, and special epilating needles are available for most units. These fine needles are either stainless steel or platinum and may have a rounded point to help prevent penetration of the follicular wall. Each machine should be calibrated prior to use to produce a minimal spark that will only impart a mild sensation of heat when tested on the wet thumbnail of the operator.

Technical advances have produced equipment specifically designed for epilation. These machines utilize a higher frequency (shorter wavelength) than standard electrosurgical equipment. Solid-state circuitry has been incorporated into many of the newer models along with the availability of both damped and undamped alternating currents. Automatic power and time controls are standard features on most units. This allows the operator to preset the current intensity and the duration of application so that, when the circuit is closed, a finite amount of current is delivered. Manual operation is also possible. Most manufacturers will provide information regarding the initial current settings recommended for a particular machine.

Recently, another electrosurgical technique has been advocated for permanent hair removal. This method also utilizes high-frequency alternating current, but the active terminal is not a platinum wire but instead a tweezer device. The tweezer grasps the hair close to the skin surface, and a slight tension is applied in the direction of the hair growth. Once the hair has been "treated," it will slip out painlessly, and there is little chance of scarring.

A simplified theoretical explanation of this new technique is as follows: The hair with a dielectric potential of three (water has a dielectric potential of 80) is used as an insulator; the tweezer and dermal papilla serve as electrical plates in the creation of a capacitor. Resistance is present within this system at the matrix-papilla interface, and therefore, heat is generated resulting in coagulation of the papilla.

Independent dermatologists, dermatopathologists, and electrical engineers have certified that this technique causes necrosis through the generation of heat in the papilla and hair matrix.[22] The *permanence* of the hair removal is presently being disputed, and clinical studies are needed to document this before it can be widely advocated.[23]

TECHNIQUE

Electrosurgical epilation by any method is tedious, so both operator and patient should make themselves comfortable. Some patients will require mild sedation, and others may request a topical anesthetic. The patient should wash with soap and water prior to the visit, and a 70% alcohol solution, witch hazel, or other cleansing lotion is applied and allowed to dry completely before the treatment. Good lighting and some method of magnification is also required. Several types of magnifying lenses with lights are available, or some operators prefer magnifying attachments for eyeglasses.

Once the patient is comfortable and the area to be treated is lighted and magnified, the actual epilation can be started. The skin is placed under tension, and the direction of the hair to be epilated is discerned. The needle is inserted in this direction into the follicle along the hair shaft to a depth calculated to be close to the dermal papilla or until a slight resistance is felt. No pain should be experienced. The correct current is then applied.

Determining the correct current depends on the area being treated, the size and character of the hair, and the individual patient. It is important that the current be sufficient to destroy the lower portion of the follicle and papilla. However, as the current is increased, more pain is appreciated and the chances of scarring increase.

The effect of the current is determined by the intensity multiplied by time. With high-frequency epilation, the amount of pain is related more to the duration of the application than to the intensity, so many operators use multiple short bursts of current to reach the desired amount. The wire needle should *never* be moved while the current is being applied because this results in increased pain and, if close to the skin surface, may cause undesirable scarring.

A pair of fine forceps is used to remove the hair once it has been treated. The hair should slide from the follicle without resistance; if it does not, more current should be applied.

The number of hairs that may be treated at one time is usually limited by the tolerance of the patient. A skilled operator can usually remove 200 hairs in an hour. In order to lessen the chances of scarring, the hairs should be approximately 4 mm apart. A predetermined current suitable for a specific type of hair in a certain location of a particular individual may be selected by using the automatic controls. This allows the operator to treat similar types of hair with the same current settings and to be more efficient. A thinning technique is used for large areas of coarse hair. The coarsest hairs are treated first and, with repeated treatments, a gradual thinning is produced. The removal rate also depends on the amount of follicular distortion and scarring produced by previous skin disease or treatments.

RESULTS

Regrowth is to be expected and should not discourage the patient or the operator. Estimates place the average amount of regrowth at approximately 15% to 25%. The major factors influencing these figures are: (1) inadequate current allowing regeneration of a dermal papilla, (2) distorted follicles that do not allow proper application of the current, and (3) the phase in the hair cycle at the time of treatment (early anagen hairs will not be seen and therefore not treated, and telogen hairs will not allow access to the papilla).

Peereboom-Wynia[24] has documented the permanence and safety of electrosurgical epilation when comparing galvanic current and high-frequency diathermy in the removal of beard hair from hirsute women. Both methods reduced the hair density by approximately 60% to 80%. Hairs that regrew after high-frequency diathermy were generally of smaller diameter than before treatment, and there was a relative increase in the percentage of dysplastic and dystrophic hairs. Theoretically, these smaller hairs are easier to treat.

It should be remembered that the basic transformation of vellus to terminal hair on the face due to such factors as age, estrogen or androgen levels, and race, will continue to occur. This means that five or 10 years after the removal of many large facial hairs, new ones require removal.

COMPLICATIONS

In the hands of a competent operator, serious complications resulting from treatment are uncommon. All patients will experience some pain at the time of treatment and varying degrees of erythema and edema after the treatment. These will resolve in approximately three to seven days. Pin-point bleeding points may be present if the follicular wall is penetrated. If the current has been incorrectly placed or overdone, then superficial erosions and crusting will occur, and the chances of scarring and, rarely, secondary bacterial infection are increased.

The possibility of postinflammatory hyper- or hypopigmentation should be considered also, particularly in dark-skinned patients. Multiple pitted follicular scars are the result of improper treatment and are avoidable. Hypertrophic scarring and keloid formation are rare. A small test area should be treated and reassessed in three to six months if one is concerned about the possibility of adverse scar formation. An adequately sterilized needle for each patient is a necessity. Most electrologists use 70% alcohol; however, it is highly flammable. Chernosky[25] points out the possibility of hepatitis transmission and recommends dry heat sterilization.

Many different products are promoted for use before and after epilation, and one should always be aware of the possibility of the patient developing allergic contact dermatitis. If significant inflammatory reaction and crusting are produced, a hydrocortisone-antibiotic cream should be used.

Electrosurgical epilation requires technical skill and patience, because it is often a long and frustrating experience for both operator and patient. The goals and the possible length of treatment, the probability of regrowth, the chances of complications, and the cost should be discussed with the patient before commencing a course of therapy. Constant reassurances to the patient are necessary, and often a pretreatment photograph is of help.

Electrologists have the ability to perform a necessary and needed service to the community, but they also have the potential of doing great harm. In the United States and Canada, there are no standard licensing requirements, and only a few areas require certification of competence.[26, 27] Many competent professional electrologists realize the potential problems in maintaining standards, and organizations of electrologists* have been formed and are actively seeking solutions. If physicians wish to perform electrolysis, they must have the time, patience, and superb eyesight required. If not, it becomes the responsibility of individual physicians to recommend competent electrologists to their patients.

---

*Directory of Professional Electrologists, 30 East Fortieth Street, Suite 505, New York, NY, 10016. International Guild of Professional Electrologists, 3425 Kingsbridge Avenue, Suite 102, Riverdale, NY, 10463.

REFERENCES

1. Michel CE: Trichiasis and distichiasis. St. Louis Clin Rec 2:145–148, 1875
2. Blackwell G: Dr. Michel, inventor of electrolysis. Electrolysis Digest 22:23–42, 1975 (April)
3. Hardaway WA: The treatment of hirsuties. Arch Derm 4:337–340, 1879
4. Lerner C: The treatment of hypertrichosis by electrocoagulation. NY State J Med 42:879–882, 1942
5. Niedelman M: Epilation, fifteen-year comparative evaluation of electrolysis and electrocoagulation. Arch Phys Med 26:290–296, 1945
6. Ellis FA: Electrolysis versus high frequency currents in the treatment of hypertrichosis. Arch Derm Syph 56:291–305, 1947
7. Darier J: A Textbook of Dermatology. Philadelphia, Lea & Febiger, 1920, p 406
8. Spearman RIC: The structure and function of the fully developed follicle. In Jarrett A (ed): The Physiology and Pathophysiology of the Skin. New York, Academic Press, 1977
9. Kollar ES: The induction of hair follicles by embryonic dermal papilla. J Invest Derm 55:374–378, 1970
10. Oliver RF: Vibrissae dermal papillar influence on epidermal tissues. Br J Derm 81 (Suppl 3):55–65, 1969
11. Van Scott, et al: Determinants of rate and kinetics of cell division in scalp hair. J Invest Derm 41:269–273, 1963
12. Oliver RF: Whisker growth after removal of the dermal papilla and lengths of follicle in the hooded rat. J Embryol Exp Morph 15:331–347, 1966
13. Oliver RF: Ectopic regeneration of whiskers in the hooded rat from implanted lengths of vibrissa follicle wall. J Embryol Exp Morph 17:27–34, 1967
14. Inaba M, et al: Regeneration of axillary hair and related phenomena after removal of deep dermal and subcutaneous tissue by a special "shaving" technique. J Dermatol Surg Oncol 4:921–925, 1978
15. Oliver RF: Histological studies of whisker regeneration in the hooded rat. J Embryol Exp Morph 16:231–244, 1966
16. Inaba M, et al: Histological study of the regeneration of axillar hair after removal with subcutaneous tissue shaver. J Invest Derm 72:224–231, 1979
17. McKinstry CT, et al: Epilation by electrocoagulation: Factors that result in regrowth of hair. J Dermatol Surg Oncol 5:407–411, 1979
18. Kligman AM, Peters L: Histologic changes of human hair follicles after electrolysis: A comparison of two methods. Cutis 34:169–176, 1984
19. Jackson R: Basic principles of electrosurgery. Can J Surg 13:354–361, 1970
20. Sternberg, TH: Clinical Study of Perma-Tweez Self Use Electrolysis. Los Angeles, General Medical Company, 1972
21. Caldwell I: Electronic pencil (letter). Br Med J 2:591–592, 1972
22. Affidavits available from Depratron Inc., Abington, PA
23. Crumay HM: Epilation. In Goldschmitt H (ed): Physical Modalities in Dermatological Therapy. Berlin, Springer-Verlag, 1978, pp 197–199
24. Peereboom-Wynia JDR: The effect of electrical epilation on the beard hair of women with idiopathic hirsutism. Arch Derm Res 254:15–22, 1975
25. Chernosky ME: Permanent removal of superfluous hair. Texas Med 67:72–78, 1971
26. Mahoney, MG: Electrolysis: A dark horse referral. Cutis 18:213–214, 1976
27. Wagner RF, Tomich JM, and Grande PJ: Electrolysis and thermolysis for permanent hair removal. JAAD 12:441–449, 1985 (March)

Special Procedures

19

SAMUEL AYRES, III, M.D.

Hair Transplantation

THE PUNCH GRAFT METHOD FOR MALE PATTERN BALDNESS

Biological Considerations—Concept, Rationale, and Fallacies

The multiple punch scalp autograft technique of Orentreich for male pattern baldness utilizes the now well-recognized fact, particularly stressed by Montagna and by Orentreich, that the propensity of certain scalp hair follicles in the adult male to become progressively transformed into vellus hair follicles, i.e., miniaturized (Fig. 19–1), rather than producing coarse hairs throughout life, is a gene-determined inherent quality of these particular follicles in men having this hereditary predisposition. Histologically, the bald scalp contains as many hair follicles as the nonbalding fringe. The miniaturization of the follicles is associated with a shortening of the anagen phase and/or a prolongation of the telogen phase.

The fact that individual coarse hairs (a few or many) may continue to grow in areas subject to a marked degree of male pattern baldness and the fact that the basic pattern has many "variations on the theme" and degrees of intensity illustrate the individualistic behavior of the hair follicles even within the overall pattern.

Male pattern baldness is triggered by a *normal adult male androgen level*, but only if the man is genetically predisposed, i.e., if the genes for male pattern baldness have been inherited from either the paternal or maternal side of the family or both. If the tendency is present in the heredity of both parents, then the individual may exhibit it to a more severe degree than any of his forebears. Furthermore, only those follicles that are genetically susceptible are responsive to the androgen stimulus.

Burton and colleagues found that male pattern baldness was *neither* associated with an increase in plasma testosterone nor related to other markers of masculinity—such as the sebum excretion rate; body hair density; or bone, skin, and muscle thickness—thus, conclusively demonstrating that male pattern baldness, occurring in an adult male, is *not* an expression of virility or of *excess* androgen production (reassuring as this popular fallacy may be to some bald men). Rather, the genetically susceptible follicles show increased 5α-reductase activity. This converts the *normal* male level of testosterone

or androstenedione in the cytoplasm of these follicles (reflecting the circulating level) to dihydrotestosterone, which is more active metabolically. This conversion occurs at an increased rate compared to genetically nonbalding follicles.

According to Price, the dihydrotestosterone is quickly bound to a specific cytoplasmic androgen receptor protein to form the steroid-receptor complex. This complex transports the dihydrotestosterone to the cell nucleus where it is bound to chromatin, and where it initiates the translation and transcription of genetic information.

Age is the third factor in male pattern baldness (or androgenetic alopecia) in addition to heredity and normal adult male androgen production. Therefore, Orentreich has suggested the term "andro-chronogenetic" to cover all three. According to a study of white men by Norwood, approximately one third show some cosmetically significant degree of recession, thinning, or more pronounced baldness by their mid-thirties, half by age 50, and two thirds by their mid-sixties. As a general rule, the earlier the onset of hair loss, the more severe it will become, and the later the onset, the milder. The general expectation is that male pattern baldness tends to progress with increasing age, but obviously the exact pattern, degree, and pace of hair loss varies greatly in different individuals.

Smith and Wells have suggested that male-type alopecia in both men and women is caused by a multifactorial genetic mechanism with a partially dominant gene. Orentreich believes that, just as in men, the three factors of heredity, age, and androgen production are responsible for female pattern baldness and that the normal androgen level in women (roughly two thirds that of men) is sufficient to trigger hair loss in those women who are genetically predisposed. In addition, he states that some 150 androgenic pharmaceuticals, including some oral contraceptives and wheat germ oil, can be sources of exogenous androgens.

Montagna, and previously, Hamilton, has emphasized that all persons, male and female, have hairlines practically down to the eyebrows at about the sixth fetal month and that the subsequent retreat of the hairline to that of the newborn infant and subsequently to that of the older child, etc., is microscopically exactly analogous to the process that occurs in male pattern baldness, viz., a progressive shrinking down of each new "generation" of follicles

198

in the area in question producing progressively finer and finer hairs until finally only vellus hairs are found. Therefore, the baldest scalp has the same sort of vellus hairs that are found on that man's (or any person's) forehead.

Montagna has also observed that frontal baldness occurs to a substantial degree in the mature adults, compared to the young animals, which have hair down to their eyebrows, of our fellow primates, the stump-tail macaque, the orangutan, and, to some degree, the chimpanzee.

Thus, male pattern baldness is a gene-determined pattern of scalp hair growth and is *completely unrelated* to such alleged causes as nervous tension, seborrhea, seborrheic dermatitis, "plugged follicles," poor scalp circulation, scalp muscle tension, a too tight galea aponeurotica, the wearing or non-wearing of hats, or shampooing too frequently or too infrequently.

Although 5α-reductase blockers, such as progesterone and spironolactone, administered topically and/or intradermally, which Orentreich advocates, may theoretically slow down the progression of male

pattern baldness, the author knows of no *controlled* observations in which increased hair growth actually occurred to a cosmetically significant degree, and Tromovitch and coworkers concur. Even such drastic measures as castration or the systemic administration of high doses of estrogen, at the most, slow down or perhaps stop the progression of male pattern baldness, but they do not cause hair to regrow in cosmetically significant amounts. It is thus unrealistic to expect this to occur with progesterone or other antiandrogens.

The relatively recent use of topical minoxidil, a potent and potentially toxic oral antihypertensive with vasodilating properties, has apparently resulted in some increased hair growth in some men with moderately thin hair due to male pattern baldness. However, when its use is stopped, hair loss recurs. This also happens in some patients even despite continued use. It has produced no significant growth on scalps that are extensively bald or have only vellus hairs, according to De Villez. A recent report by Franz shows no significant absorption from limited topical use, but that issue remains unresolved.

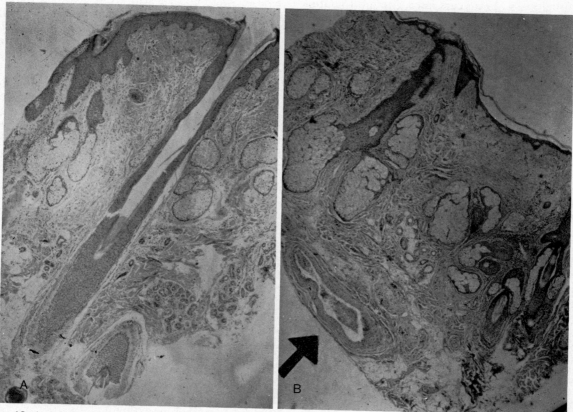

Figure 19–1. *A,* Histologic section from the coarse hair-bearing (donor) area of the scalp of a patient with marked male pattern baldness, showing large hair follicle (and a portion of another) extending through the dermis and into the subcutaneous fat. The thickness of the section occupies the entire photomicrograph. *B,* Histologic section from the bald scalp of the same patient and at the same magnification showing three markedly attenuated follicles with prominent sebaceous glands. Note the much narrower diameter of hair shaft sections and that the full thickness section of skin including subcutaneous fat is substantially thinner than in A (cf. Fig. 19–52). The large blood vessel in subcutaneous fat (at arrow) clearly demonstrates that there is no lack of adequate blood supply to the bald scalp.

Its mechanism of action is at present not understood. Its value in dealing with male pattern baldness to a cosmetically significant degree is probably marginal at best and will certainly require several more years for adequate evaluation, as emphasized by Weiss and West.

Orentreich states that a normal, nonbalding male or female scalp (containing around 100,000 hairs) sheds about 100 hairs a day. At any given time, about 10% to 15% are in telogen (resting phase) for three months and 85% to 90% are in anagen (growing phase) for three to five years. However, the number of hairs shed daily may vary from zero to over 200 in a cyclic fashion, with the greatest loss in November and the least in June in the northern latitudes. This emphasizes the pitfalls inherent in evaluating medications or processes alleged to retard or stop hair loss in male (or female) pattern baldness.

Orentreich in a classic experiment clearly demonstrated this individualistic behavior of scalp follicles by transplanting a single punch graft from the posterior scalp to the anterior border of the receding frontal hairline in a man with progressive male pattern baldness. Two years later, the graft continued to grow coarse hair with undiminished vigor as though it were in its original site, despite the further recession of the frontal hairline by one to two centimeters. On the other hand, the graft that had been transplanted from the bald scalp to the posterior hairy scalp remained bald. These observations, which conclusively demonstrate the phenomenon of *donor dominance in male pattern baldness*, have been confirmed many thousands of times over a much longer period of observation. Thus the basis for having confidence in the permanence of this technique is provided by Orentreich's 30-year experience, the author's 25-year experience, and that of many others (Fig. 19–2).

Naturally, the permanence is contingent upon obtaining grafts from the temporoparietal and occipital fringe—areas not subject to male pattern baldness—and, inasmuch as the exact extent and pattern varies in different individuals, the grafts must be obtained from within the clearly "safe" area in a patient whose baldness is relatively early or still progressing.

SELECTION OF PATIENTS AND CONTRAINDICATIONS

As in other forms of cosmetic surgery, it is essential that the prospective patient have a thorough understanding not only of the procedure and of the limitations inherent in hair transplantation in general, but also of how this applies to him specifically so that he will have realistic expectations. Not all individuals with male pattern baldness are suitable candidates for hair transplantation. If the area of baldness is very large and the donor supply is very limited, it may be impossible to achieve an aesthetically acceptable result. This is especially true if the hair is dark and straight and the skin is light, which produces an unaesthetic tufted appearance due to color contrast, when adequate filling in between grafts is impossible to achieve. On the other hand, if the skin and hair are close to the same color value (a natural camouflage effect), even a relatively limited amount of grafting (compared with the size of the bald area) may give an acceptable result, provided that a good strategy is utilized in placing the grafts and aided by styling (Fig. 19–3). Patients with very curly to kinky hair achieve better coverage with a comparable amount of grafting than those with relatively straight hair (Fig. 19–4).

In any event, there is often a compromise between what would constitute relatively definitive coverage for moderately extensive baldness (say, 600 or more 4.0 mm grafts) and what is available (perhaps only about 300 or 400 grafts). A patient with a very narrow and/or sparse fringe (donor area) and a correspondingly very large bald area, or someone whose fringe may be wider but in which the lower half to two thirds is sparse to very sparse may have a potential of only 150 to 200 grafts. This is perhaps only one third, one fourth, or even a much smaller fraction of the amount required for relatively definitive coverage. The unfavorable supply-demand ratio makes such a patient a borderline candidate at best and, depending upon his hair and skin color, perhaps an unsuitable candidate. (See the section on scalp reduction.) Of course, some patients have potential donor areas of such poor density (regardless of width) that they are clearly not candidates for hair transplantation under any circumstances (Fig. 19–5).

If the patient is young with minimal recession or thinning, but with a potential, based on family history, for much greater hair loss in the future, grafting should be deferred until it is more clearly indicated. Even then, the hairline should not be placed too low, both for aesthetic reasons and to conserve the available donor supply for more effective use later when it is really needed. In summary, borderline, poor, or unsuitable candidates for hair transplantation are, relatively speaking, either too bald or not bald enough, and ideal candidates have both a favorable supply-demand ratio and hair and skin colors that do not sharply contrast. People with light blond, silver, or salt-and-pepper gray hair have the potential for especially good cosmetic results (Figs. 19–2, 19–3, and 19–6).

The patient should be cautioned before starting the procedure that it is very difficult and, in some instances, impossible to provide a completely natural-looking frontal hairline with grafting. Some surgical scarring, however minimal, is inevitable on

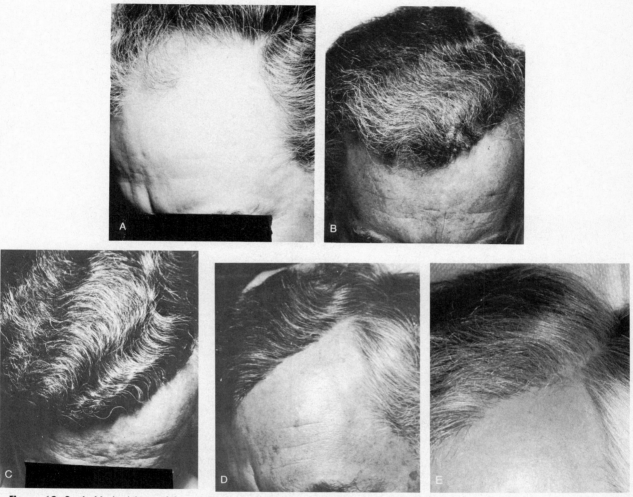

Figure 19–2. *A*, Marked loss of frontal hair caused by male pattern baldness in a 49-year-old patient. *B*, Appearance seven months after beginning the multiple punch scalp grafting procedure. Note the frizziness of the grafted hair, which is characteristic of early growth and presumably a consequence of telogen defluvium, induced by temporary ischemia of the grafts (see Fig. 19–22B). *C*, Appearance after 15 months; patient received 295 grafts over a period of nine months. *D*, Appearance after four years and nine months; an additional 21 grafts had been placed along and just behind the left frontal hairline and at the apex 1½ years after the start of the procedure. Note that the frizziness seen at seven months had largely disappeared by 15 months, and that the grafted hair texture now appears completely normal for this individual. *E*, Appearance 20 years after beginning the hair transplantation; the patient returned for grafting in his progressively thinning crown (not shown), but grafted hair in the frontal scalp continues to grow vigorously.

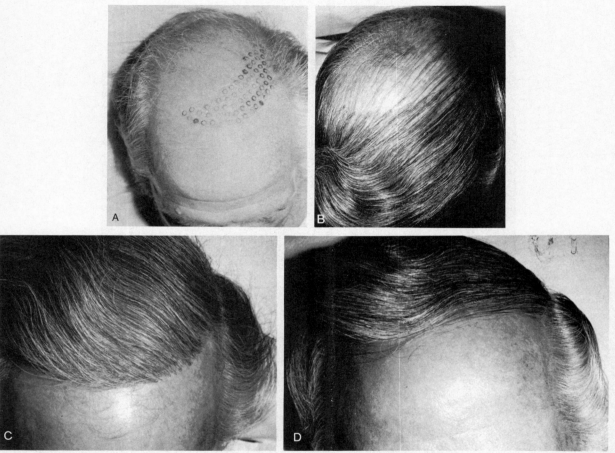

Figure 19–3. *A*, Patient, 55 years old, with very extensive male pattern baldness, poor crown mobility, and a silver-gray fringe of fair to sparse density shown marked for the first session of 65 (4.0 mm) grafts placed in 3.5 mm holes. Note the pronounced asymmetry with a ledge extending along the fringe of the parting side and the creation of a moderately receded left temporal hairline. At subsequent sessions grafting was extended further posteriorly and to the right, but a greater number of grafts with the best density were placed to the left and center. *B*, Appearance 17 months later after the patient received a total of 433 (4.0 mm) grafts in six sessions within one year. A large area of the crown (at top of figure) remains bald, and the hair is styled forward and across. An additional 80 grafts followed, including filling in along the posterior margin adjacent to the bald crown to achieve a more natural blending. *C*, Same as B with the hair combed back, showing the grafted hairline terminating at the part, on patient's left, with a moderate temporal gulf. No hairline refinement (see the section, "Filling in with Minute Grafts, Especially for Hairline Refinement") had been done at the time, but natural camouflage provided by the gray hair makes it less necessary, even with the hairline exposed. *D*, Same as B and C with hair styled forward and across. Patient is parting hair slightly lower than in C, combing a little of the upper fringe hair on the left across and into the grafted hair, thus enhancing the coverage and causing the styled hairline to be lower than the more conservative (slightly receded) grafted hairline shown in C. This is useful to obscure a hairline that has not been refined, especially when a marked color contrast between the hair and skin exists and/or when hypopigmentation of the grafts occurs (not present here).

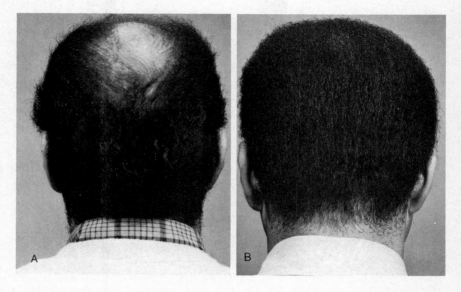

Figure 19–4. *A,* Patient, 29 years old, with extensive male pattern baldness and light skin; the black frizzy hair has a fringe of good width and density. Note the lowest extent of crown baldness (cf. Fig. 19–27). *B,* Appearance 27 months after the start of extensive punch grafting. Good coverage is enhanced by frizzy hair texture and styling. The grafted hair has continued to grow for 22 years, despite the progressive thinning of original hair in a narrow zone that is adjacent to the permanent fringe hair on the lower posterior and lateral area of the crown.

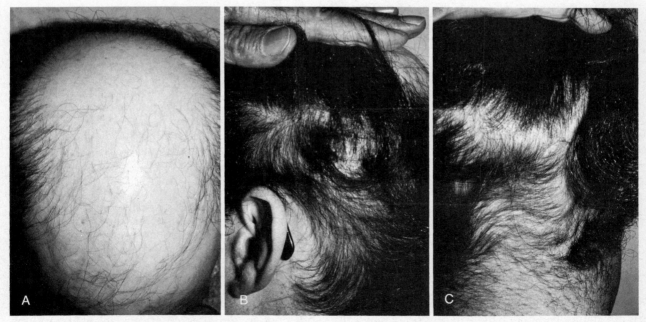

Figure 19–5. *A, B,* and *C,* Patient, 38 years old, with very extensive male pattern baldness, fair to moderate crown mobility, and a relatively narrow fringe (especially posteriorly) of sparse to very sparse density. Because of the unfavorable supply-demand ratio compounded by his black straight hair and light skin (poor camouflage), the patient, who already wore a conventional hairpiece, was considered by the author not to be a candidate for punch grafting. He also shows a light nevus flammeus (barely visible in the black-and-white photograph) in the extremely sparse suboccipital-nuchal area (*C*) and relatively mild scars in the anterior and posterior bald scalp from previous suture loop placements for attaching a hairpiece that had subsequently been removed (*A*).

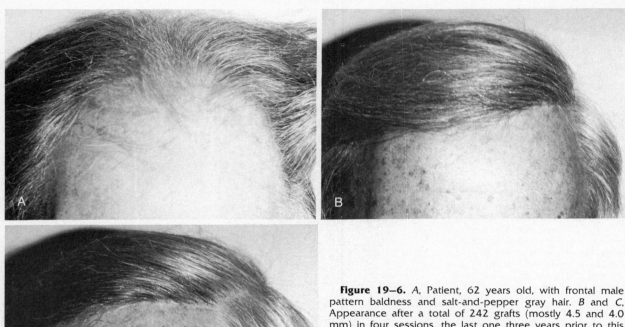

Figure 19–6. *A,* Patient, 62 years old, with frontal male pattern baldness and salt-and-pepper gray hair. *B* and *C,* Appearance after a total of 242 grafts (mostly 4.5 and 4.0 mm) in four sessions, the last one three years prior to this photograph. Hairline refinement on left to mask mild hypopigmentation at hairline would enhance result. Note proper forward angling of grafted hairs.

close inspection. As noted above, good results in patients with dark hair and light skin are the most difficult, especially at and immediately behind the hairline. The use of minute grafts for hairline refinement can minimize, but may not entirely prevent, some degree of artificiality if the hairline is completely exposed.

Hypopigmentation of the grafts is especially prevalent in patients who have red hair and ruddy, or nontanning skin, which has been heavily sun-exposed for many years (Fig. 19–7). This is due to the grafts having been obtained from the sun-protected fringe area of the scalp, placed adjacent to the sun-exposed skin of the bald scalp or forehead. These patients may never get good skin color matching, despite graduated sun exposure, whereas those with medium, olive, or dark skin may eventually achieve a good match (Fig. 19–8). However, even when the grafts themselves match the adjacent skin quite well, some degree of hypopigmented scar line along the anterior border of the grafts is quite common (Fig. 19–6). This is not preventable, but it should be anticipated and the patient made aware of it *before* the grafting is begun. The most practical solution besides hairline refinement (or possibly tattooing, as advocated by Berger) is styling the hair in a

forward or forward and across manner to avoid unduly exposing the frontal hairline (Fig. 19–3).

Excessive acceleration of hair loss in a recipient area of only slight thinning may result from prematurely grafting in such an area. Thus, grafting should be avoided in an area of only minimal thinning, especially if the *donor* hair is relatively sparse, because the loss of hair caused by grafting in such an area will almost certainly result in no net gain and more likely a net loss of hair in the recipient area, for several months or perhaps until hair growth from two or three sessions has occurred. In other words, things may get worse before they get better. This is due to two causes: (1) the purely mechanical loss of whatever hairs occupy the sites where the recipient holes are cut and (2) the frequent induction of premature telogen defluvium in at least some and perhaps many of the *residual* hairs in the area adjacent to the sites of graft placement resulting from the trauma of the surgery. Although these lost telogen hairs are generally replaced after about three months, they tend to return as still finer hairs than before the defluvium. This follows the natural history of male pattern baldness in which successive "generations" of hairs are progressively finer and shorter, which are produced by successively smaller

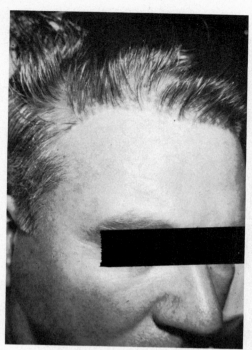

Figure 19–7. Patient, 46 years old, with red hair and fair, ruddy, sun-exposed skin as he appeared when first seen by the author. Extensive grafting (three sessions) had been performed by another operator about one year previously. Note hypopigmentation and cobblestoning of virtually all of the grafts, a low temporal hairline (cf. Figs. 19–83 to 19–88), and a poor yield of hairs in many of the grafts.

tion of residual hair growth or else adjacent follicles will be destroyed, resulting in numerous unsightly bald spots in place of mere thinning. If the yield of hairs per graft is poor (because of improper technique or taking grafts from a donor area of poor density or both), the net result will be a worse rather than an improved cosmetic appearance. Thus, the author basically agrees with Unger on the issue of performing grafting in *relatively* early hair loss, provided that the potential extent of the future loss is taken into account, that an adequate donor supply is available, and that a careful technique is used.

Norwood has correlated certain criteria with ultimate hair growth and found a predictive value for better growth in those patients who have loose (mobile) thick scalps, a good donor site hair density that yields grafts of good quality, and no excessive scarring in the grafts. The converse correlated with poor hair growth (Fig. 19–9). On the other hand, he found no correlation between hair growth and depth of follicles within grafts, amount of bleeding, difficulty of planting grafts, coarseness or fineness of hair, sizes of grafts (3.5, 4.0, or 4.5 mm), and the number of grafts planted at each session (however, see the section, "Number of Grafts per Session").

Unfortunately, excessive scarring, *unless already present elsewhere preoperatively*, is only of value retrospectively in accounting for poor hair growth and could only be predicted by routinely performing a limited number of grafts and then waiting four months for results before proceeding with larger numbers, as suggested by Norwood. Although logical, the author does not find this practical or necessary as a *routine* measure, but it is certainly prudent to do so when patients give a history or show evidence of hypertrophic or keloidal scarring anywhere on the body. This is particularly appro-

follicles. This is in contrast to the transplanted hairs in the grafts that return in three months as coarse as before the defluvium.

Unger has properly emphasized that, if grafting is done in patients with relatively mild thinning, the *recipient site* holes must be cut parallel to the direc-

Figure 19–8. *A*, Patient, 37 years old, with black hair, medium skin color of good tanning capacity, and extensive male pattern baldness, who also had a wide fringe of good density. *B*, Appearance after 17 months. A total of 605 (4.0 mm) grafts were placed in 3.5 mm holes over an 11-month period in all bald areas. Note the good color matching of grafts with adjacent skin at the hairline, despite the fact that subsequent hairline refinement had not been done prior to this photograph.

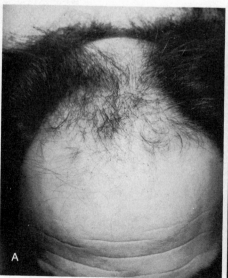
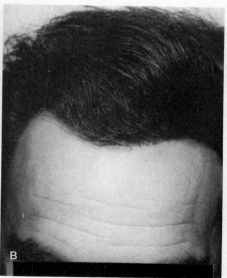

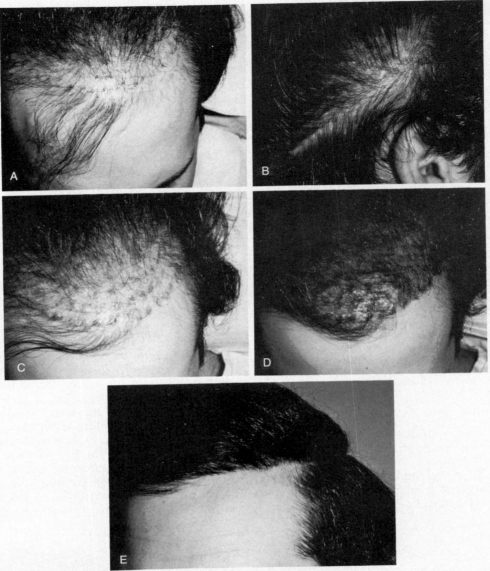

Figure 19–9. *A* and *B*, A 27-year-old man, as he appeared when first seen by the author, who two years previously had had four rows of grafts placed in the anterior scalp by another operator for recession and moderate, though extensive, thinning caused by male pattern baldness. This was followed 15 months later by punch excision of the first two rows by a second operator at the patient's request, leaving relatively large depressed (not hypertrophic) scars with some residual hairs. The yield in the remaining two rows was fair to sparse. The donor area had fair density in the upper portion and was sparse to very sparse in the lower portion, where some previous donor site scars were located. The latter, which had apparently healed without closure, were not hypertrophic and there was no history or evidence of hypertrophic scarring elsewhere on the body. The patient requested excision of all scars and remaining grafts in the anterior scalp, but this was not deemed practical and resumption of punch grafting was advised. *C*, Appearance 2¼ months later after placing 68 (4.0 mm) grafts in 3.5 mm recipient holes that followed the original grafted hairline. Patient had persistent recipient site bleeding with graft elevation at the time of surgery, which responded to manual pressure. The pressure dressing was left on for 2 days, and when observed on the third postoperative day, there was no graft elevation. However, shown here is moderate cobblestoning of some of the grafts, especially on patient's right side and center. A second session of 76 grafts followed, again with persistent graft elevation from bleeding perioperatively, but no elevation after the second and seventh postoperative days. *D*, Appearance 2¼ months after C showing satisfactory early hair growth from the first session 4½ months before with considerable spontaneous improvement in cobblestoning. A third session of 73 grafts followed, with less bleeding and temporary graft elevation. *E*, Same patient 25 months after A following two additional sessions of 66 and 50 grafts, including considerable hairline refinement with small to minute grafts during the fifth session (6 months before), there is a satisfactory cosmetic result with an exposed hairline.

Legend continued on opposite page.

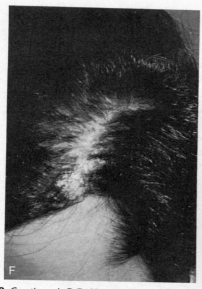

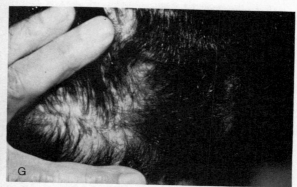

Figure 19–9 *Continued. F,* Deliberate exposure of heavily grafted area behind hairline, showing relatively poor yield of hairs in many of the grafts with moderate hypertrophic scarring. *G,* Many of the donor sites, both the earlier ones allowed to heal without closure and later ones closed by interdigitation (in the medium low midposterior fringe) show relatively persistent moderate hypertrophic scarring. Conclusion: This patient apparently has a hypertrophic diathesis, not apparent when he was first seen by the author, that resulted in a generally disappointing yield of hairs per graft, yet a quite acceptable cosmetic result.

priate when contemplating remedial hair transplantation on a patient, many of whose grafts placed by a previous operator show a poor or even negligible yield of hairs, with or without the presence of scarring, especially if the grafts were harvested from a donor area of reasonably good density (Fig. 19–10).

One should, of course, inquire about a history of intolerance to medications, especially local anesthetics, (however, the incidence of true allergy to lidocaine is apparently extremely low). Relative or absolute contraindications to elective cosmetic surgery (which may require appropriate laboratory tests when indicated) include a hemorrhagic diathesis or the patient's use of anticoagulants, severe or uncontrolled diabetes, a cardiovascular condition or medication interdicting the use of epinephrine in the local anesthetic (e.g., propranolol, according to Foster and Aston), hepatitis B, unusual scarring, or anything else that would constitute a significant risk to one's general or cutaneous health in view of the fact that a purely cosmetic surgical procedure is contemplated.

Psoriasis, unless severe, would not be an absolute contraindication, since any isomorphic response induced by the grafting would presumably be responsive to appropriate treatment. However, the patient should be warned of this, and only a relatively limited amount of grafting should be done initially. Seborrheic dermatitis should be controlled as well as possible prior to grafting, although this is mainly a matter of convenience and does not adversely affect the end result. Folliculitis of the scalp should

be controlled by systemic antibiotic administration, if necessary.

There is no upper age limit, assuming that the patient's general health is satisfactory. The procedure works as well on a patient in his seventies as in his twenties or thirties.

DONOR AND RECIPIENT PUNCH SIZES FOR BASIC COVERAGE

For *basic coverage* the author generally uses 4.0 mm (or 4.25 mm) grafts placed in 3.5 or 3.25 mm recipient holes, depending on which results in a better fit. The grafts are usually placed about the same distance apart in all directions as the diameter of the recipient holes. The use of 4.5 mm grafts placed in 3.75 or 4.0 mm holes is also acceptable, especially when the donor area is relatively sparse. For very flaccid scalps (despite heavy infiltration with normal saline), 4.25 or 4.5 mm grafts placed in holes 1.0 or 1.25 mm smaller may be appropriate. Sometimes, especially in patients with dark straight hair and relatively light skin, in whom the avoidance of artificiality is the most difficult, some or all of the recipient holes in the first row of the anterior hairline can be 3.0 mm, into which 3.5, 3.75, or even 4.0 mm grafts are placed—which size, again, depending on proper fit. Thus, the graft is usually 0.5 mm larger than the recipient hole, allowing for slight shrinkage of the graft and slight expansion of the hole, but in some patients 0.75, 1.0, or even 1.25 mm difference, or infrequently, only 0.25 mm, gives

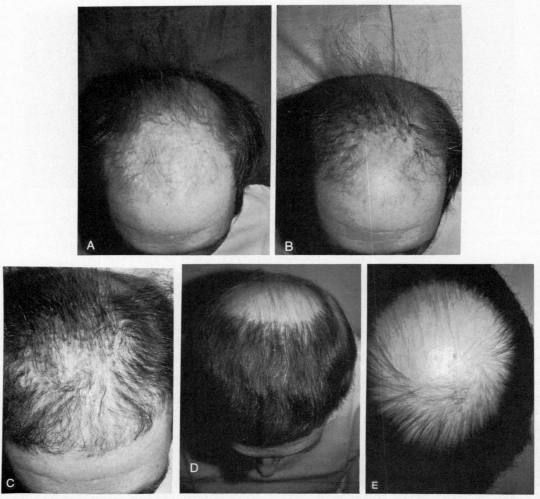

Figure 19–10. *A,* Patient, 38 years old, with extensive male pattern baldness, as he appeared when first seen by the author. About six years before, 100 grafts in two sessions had been placed in the anterolateral and midscalp areas by another operator. Most graft sites are devoid of hair with only depigmented scars, others have two to four hairs, and a couple have six or eight. Donor site scars indicated that the grafts were taken from the upper donor areas, which had the best available density (fair to moderate); the lower donor areas were fair to very sparse. *B,* Appearance 6½ months after placing 32 (4.0 mm) grafts into 3.5 mm recipient holes. The yield is good in most of the grafts, although sparse in some. *C,* Appearance 22 months after A, showing results of an additional 209 grafts in four sessions and a good yield of hairs per graft (commensurate with donor site density). This suggests that the very poor yield obtained by the previous operator was due to faulty technique rather than intrinsic factors. *D* and *E,* Appearance after two more sessions (three years after A) showing results of a total of 348 grafts. With hair combed straight forward (patient's preference), the incompletely filled-in anterior hairline leaves the crown bald because donor supply was inadequate for definitive coverage of all areas. Patient was not interested in reduction despite moderate crown mobility. Subsequently, 76 more grafts were placed and refinement of the posterior border of grafted area adjacent to the bald crown was achieved. (Patient's face is at bottom of figure in A to D and at the top in E.)

the best fit. If, due to these variations, too large a space between recipient holes has been left at a first session, this can be at least partially compensated for at the next session by appropriate corrections of graft and recipient hole sizes.

The author does not use grafts larger than 4.5 mm, as these tend to result in a more artificial appearance, particularly at the hairline and especially if they are not thoroughly filled in at subsequent sessions. If there is a marked contrast in color between hair and skin, this further aggravates the aesthetic problem. Large grafts are also more prone to elevation, resulting in a cobblestone appearance, and may have few or no hairs in their centers, presumably due to ischemia (Fig. 19–11). Nevertheless, Stough, unlike the author and most others, uses 5.0 mm grafts placed about 1.0 mm apart at the first session to form the basic frontal hairline.

RECIPIENT SITE PLANNING

Anticipating Future Hair Loss

The ratio of available donor supply to actual (or, in a young man, *potential*) baldness must be considered and proper strategy used in distributing the grafts by concentrating them in certain areas, such as anteriorly. The emphasis should be on the parting side, sometimes creating an asymmetric ledge on that side, extending posteriorly into the midscalp and the anterior crown adjacent to the fringe, or alternatively (especially if scalp reduction is not appropriate or desired), concentrating on the crown and perhaps midscalp, with, in either case, appropriate styling for maximum cosmetic impact, rather than scattering them relatively sparsely over a large bald area (Figs. 19–3, 19–12, and 19–13). However, scalp reduction in suitable candidates can substantially improve this supply-demand ratio. In any event, future hair loss should be anticipated and planned for, based on the patient's age, family history, and even subtle evidence of thinning; and a sufficient donor supply should be preserved for future use, even if reduction is to be used, in patients with progressively thinning hair (Fig. 19–14).

Thus, hair transplantation is frequently a long-term proposition, with perhaps a limited amount of grafting being done in a receded frontal-temporal area initially, with additional sessions performed over a period of five, ten, or even twenty years at suitable intervals as required, in patients with relatively early hair loss when first seen, but with progressive hair loss due to male pattern baldness (Figs. 19–2 and 19–14 to 19–16).

The Frontal Hairline

It is essential to give sufficient attention to the aesthetics of a proper frontal hairline by careful planning using a marking dye prior to surgery. If in doubt, it is preferable to create initially a hairline higher than the patient desires with considerable temporal recession or gulf, and thus to retain the option of possibly lowering it later. It is simple enough to lower a grafted hairline and obviously much more difficult to correct one that has been placed too low. Patients often have completely unrealistic notions of what their hairlines should be, and the operator should not necessarily give the patient whatever he wants, if it is not aesthetically

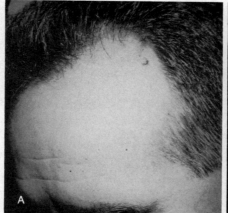 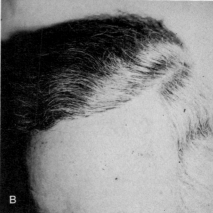

Figure 19–11. *A*, Patient, 35 years old, who had a limited number of grafts placed in the receded temples by another operator. There was very sparse yield and one very large graft (about 8 mm) placed relatively low on the left temple, which gave a ring-like appearance with hairs growing only around most of the periphery (the central portion was completely bald). This is one of the problems inherent in using excessively large grafts. The graft exchange technique was then used piecemeal to replace the large graft that was placed too low. Conservative temporal hairlines were created with 63 (4.0 mm) grafts in four sessions, which blended into the thinned and receded apex. Previously grafted hairs were preserved wherever possible when placing new grafts. The patient returned six years later with considerable progressive thinning in the anterior scalp, including the apex, the midscalp, and crown, for which an additional 272 grafts were placed in all these areas in four sessions over a five-year period. There were 120 (4.5 mm) grafts placed in 4.0 mm holes and the rest were 4.0 mm grafts in 3.5 mm holes. *B*, Appearance 12 years after A. Note that the patient's hair has turned gray, enhancing the cosmetic result. Proper placement of the grafts has resulted in a moderate forward angling of the grafted hair. Another 70 grafts were placed later to fill in small gaps in the frontal hairline and other scalp areas.

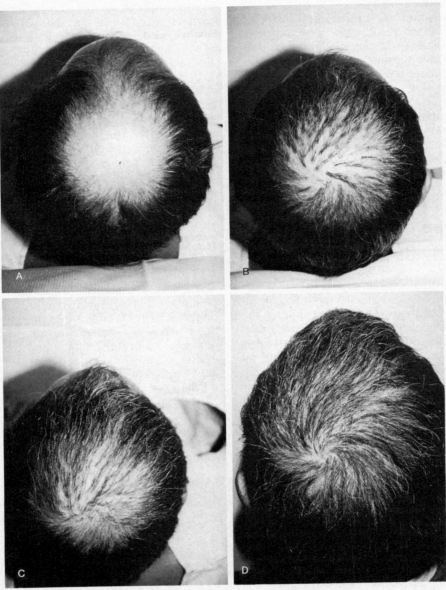

Figure 19–12. *A,* Patient, 49 years of age, with extensive crown and frontal baldness who was seen prior to the availability of crown reduction and who requested coverage of the crown with forward styling of hair. *B,* Appearance six months after 92 (4.5 mm) grafts were placed in 4.0 mm recipient holes in the crown and oriented to establish the beginning of a whorl pattern. A session of 101 (4.5 mm) grafts followed, which filled in the area and advanced the coverage anteriorly. The patient wore a clip-on hairpiece until the coverage was adequate. *C,* Appearance 15 months later; a session of 104 (4.5 mm) grafts followed. *D,* Appearance six years later; completion of the whorl pattern is evident. Patient is styling hair forward and keeping it rather short, but has no difficulty covering donor site scars, which healed without closure. Patient received a total of 446 grafts in 5 sessions to the crown, midscalp, and midanterior scalp. Graft sizes of 4.5, 4.0, 3.5, and 3.0 were placed respectively in 4.0, 3.5, 3.0, and 2.5 or 2.0 recipient holes. The smaller sizes were used in the later sessions to refine the center of the whorl and included peripheral trimming of the grafts, as required, to fit the circular and ovoid holes remaining among the grafts from earlier sessions.

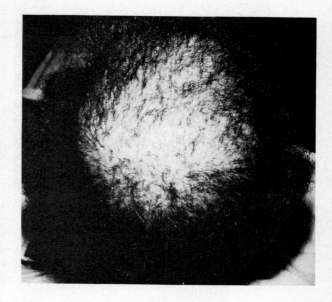

Figure 19–13. When first seen by the author, this 39-year-old patient showed poor distribution of grafts (anterior scalp is at top of photograph). The patient had 540 grafts in eight sessions by another operator over a period of nine months; the sessions had ended two years previously. His donor area was of moderate density in the upper portion and very sparse in the lower. There were donor site scars in all portions; the yield of grafts varied from good to sparse or nil. There was a greater concentration of grafts anteriorly than elsewhere (even here the coverage was sparse), but the many grafts scattered over the large bald top and crown produced an unattractive tufted appearance that ineffectively covered his baldness. Although his brown hair was curly to kinky, there was insufficient coverage to achieve any cosmetic benefit in this area.

acceptable. Of course, it should *never* be placed lower than the patient requests. In fact, some patients prefer to start grafting considerably above the eventual hairline, either to help avoid detection that grafting is being done or to temporize on a decision about the definitive hairline or both. The neophyte operator can avoid some of the serious errors in aesthetic judgment all too commonly seen by initially following this course and by refusing to restore his patient's hairline to match the photograph in his high school year book (Fig. 19–7).

Based on the aesthetic rule that the face can be divided approximately into thirds, i.e., one third from the point of the chin to the nasocolumellar angle, one third from the latter to the glabella, and one third for the forehead (from the glabella to the apex of the frontal hairline), the author usually allows at least the upper third, and frequently slightly to somewhat more for the forehead to be on the safe side—but never less than a third. Usually, a gently curving hairline—anteriorly convex and varying slightly with facial configuration, and *within certain limits*, patient preference—is created, with an acute angle at the temporal gulfs on each side of the forehead, especially on the parting side. A slight blunting of the temporal gulf is permissible on the nonparting side. The part is ideally situated on a vertical line extending approximately from the junction of the middle and lateral thirds of the eyebrow or the outer canthus of the eye (as seen from directly in front), although it may have to be more laterally placed, depending on the width of the bald area and the present or anticipated eventual height of the lateral fringe. The lateral end of the frontal hairline should ideally terminate at the part, or possibly medial to it, but not lateral to it, which would cause the hair to be parted later through

grafted hair. This does not look natural unless a considerable amount of refinement is done, both at and for a considerable distance behind the hairline. However, an ill-defined orientation, rather than a sharp parting of the hair, may be a satisfactory solution in some men.

After the proposed hairline is marked with gentian violet or other dye, it should be observed from the front and both sides to be certain that adequate temporal gulfs have been created, that it is not straight across, and especially that it is not slanted downward at the temples. It is essential that the patient also see this (Fig. 19–17). What *might* be an acceptable hairline on a man in his early twenties may look inappropriately juvenile when he is in his forties, fifties, or sixties. Planning a hairline is an extremely important step and *must not* be a casual, offhand decision.

Following the outline of the partially erased dye-marked hairline, the author then uses a dull manual punch of appropriate size (see the section "Donor and Recipient Punch Sizes for Basic Coverage") that is wet in 1% or 2% gentian violet (which is soluble in alcohol but relatively insoluble in blood or normal saline), contained in an ink stamp pad, to mark the individual prospective recipient hole sites after the area has been cleansed with an appropriate skin antiseptic. Thus, the location of the sites and the number of grafts to be obtained at that session are determined (Figs. 19–17 and 19–18).

One advantage of using a dull punch as a marking instrument, which creates a hollow circle with the gentian violet rather than making a solid dye mark with a cotton-tipped applicator, is the ability to see the number and caliber of residual hairs inside the circle if it is in an area of thin but not completely bald scalp (e.g., in a transitional area from bald or

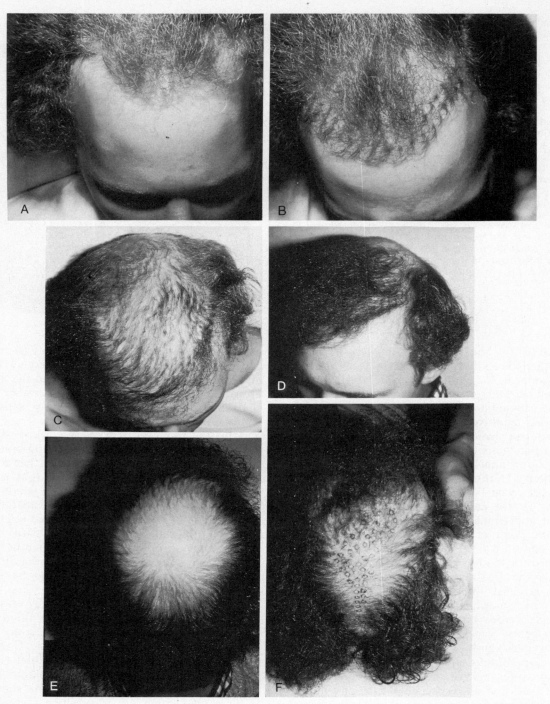

Figure 19–14. *A*, Patient, 20 years old, with rapid progressive thinning of anterior scalp and midscalp, some thinning of the crown, and a family history of marked male pattern baldness in a maternal uncle and of temporal recession in his father. The author first advised the patient 1½ years before to defer grafting for mild recession of the temples and minimal thinning along the hairline. *B*, Appearance four months later after 36 (4.5 mm) grafts were placed in 4.0 mm holes to establish a conservative (relatively high) anterior hairline, with a partial second row in the temples. Note the further hair loss; probably some was due to natural progression and some was accelerated by the grafting. An additional 36 grafts were then placed. *C*, Appearance two years later; rapid progression of balding had continued in all areas, including the crown. Four months before this photograph, 82 (4.5 mm) grafts were placed to fill in and extend into the midscalp, especially on the left (parting) side. Subsequently, 87 (4.5 mm) grafts were placed in the midanterior scalp and midscalp that extended further posteriorly and emphasized the left side. Another 64 grafts were placed in the anterior and midanterior scalp 4½ months later, for a total of 305 grafts. *D* and *E*, Nine months after C, there was fairly good coverage of the anterior scalp and midscalp aided by naturally curly to frizzy hair and forward and across styling that left the crown exposed (top of figure in both E and F show frontal area). *F*, Same patient, 16 months after D and E, following four scalp reductions by Drs. T. G. Mayer and R. W. Fleming, showing placement of 68 (4.0 mm) grafts into 3.5 mm holes in the residual bald crown, including reduction scars and into previously grafted anterior and midanterior scalp, filling in.

212

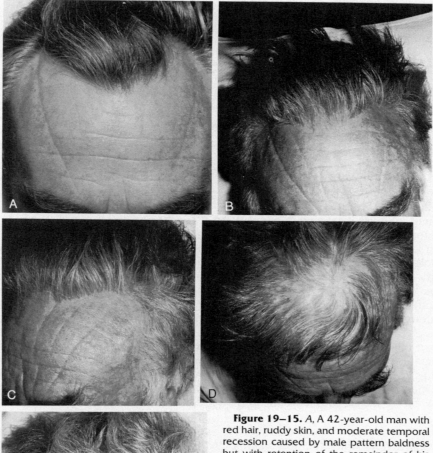

Figure 19–15. *A*, A 42-year-old man with red hair, ruddy skin, and moderate temporal recession caused by male pattern baldness but with retention of the remainder of his hair, including the apex. *B* to *D*, Appearance 16 years later after receiving 112 (4.0 mm) grafts in the receded temples during four sessions over a seven-month period. Grafted hair (now gray) has continued to grow vigorously—whereas the apex, lateral temples (B and C) and midanterior scalp (D—forehead is at bottom of photograph) have continued to lose hair. Patient parts hair on the right. Deep furrows in the forehead and scalp are an inherent characteristic of this individual and are intensified by heavily sun-exposed skin. Persistent growth of grafted hair, despite gradual loss of adjacent hair, validates Orentreich's concept of donor dominance in male pattern baldness. B and C show minimal, mildly hypopigmented, scalloped scars along the anterior border of the grafts. Color matching of the grafts and adjacent skin is quite good considering the patient's type of skin. *E*, Appearance 7½ months later, showing the result of two sessions in the apex and lateral temples. Additional grafting in these areas and a bald area behind the apex (D) followed. Hairline refinement would enhance the result.

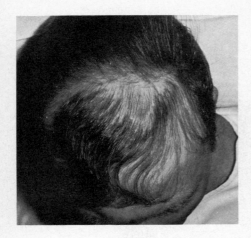

Figure 19–16. A 57-year-old man on whom the author had performed punch grafting in the frontal scalp mostly within the first two years, beginning 20 years earlier. Persistent growth of grafted hair, despite gradual loss in the midscalp, demonstrates donor dominance in male pattern baldness. Additional grafting followed.

markedly thinned receded temples to a retained apex forelock of relatively good density). Thus, the operator can decide whether the hairs to be lost in creating the recipient hole are excessive in quantity and/or quality compared to the anticipated number in the graft to be placed there. If the sacrifice is excessive, the circle of dye can be eliminated or moved to a slightly different location. In addition, a dot of green ink can be placed in the center of each circle to facilitate counting, especially if the grafts are distributed in a way that makes counting difficult, such as a circular area over the crown, or if one is using two or more different sizes of marking punches in anticipation of cutting corresponding recipient holes (Figs. 19–19 and 19–20). The green ink dots also help identify circles that might become partially erased by blood or saline during the procedure.

It is preferable to plan on placing the grafts *slightly* less than one recipient hole diameter apart along the first row of the anterior hairline (i.e., between 3.0 and 3.25 mm apart if 3.25 or 3.5 mm holes are planned for the placement of 4.0 mm grafts). This avoids possible excessive space between grafts in the first row when filling it in at a subsequent session. For areas behind the first row, grafts are usually placed approximately one recipient hole diameter apart in each row (about 3.25 to 3.5 mm for 4.0 mm grafts). The rows are placed a similar distance apart in anticipation of filling in the spaces at subsequent sessions (Figs. 19–17 to 19–20).

If one places grafts much closer together than this, it will necessitate using smaller grafts at a subsequent session; more importantly, if a large amount of grafting is performed at a session, placing the grafts too close together greatly increases the likelihood of ischemia and hence a poor yield of hairs per graft or even necrosis of grafts. (See the section, "Number of Grafts per Session.")

Thus, four sessions are required to achieve *basic*

coverage in any one area, assuming that the grafts are placed approximately one recipient hole diameter apart in all directions at each session.

Because younger men sometimes insist on parting their hair at or near the midline rather than the more conventional lateral temple location, the author has attempted to accede to their request in some instances. No attempt should be made to create an actual part by slanting grafts at diverging angles, as this will result in an artificially broad and cosmetically unacceptable part line. However, by repeated placement of minute grafts to fill in any small spaces remaining after the four basic sessions have been completed (with hairs oriented forward at about 60 degrees), a refinement at and for a considerable distance behind the hairline can be achieved in this area by creating a sufficiently dense effect to be cosmetically acceptable. As with hairline refinement, the greater the color contrast between hair and scalp, the more filling in is required to achieve a natural effect (Fig. 19–21).

Because of the subtle gradation of hair texture and density at the anterior border of the temporal "points" at the lateral aspects of the forehead, it is usually best to avoid grafting in this area. Otherwise, an unnaturally sharp-appearing hair margin is very apt to result, particularly with dark hair and light skin. The use of grafts with fine and/or relatively sparse hair, especially if it is gray or blond, and refinement with minute grafts, *might* produce an acceptable result. As Norwood has emphasized, the grafts must be inserted at a very acute angle pointing down. Styling this hair forward may still be necessary, however, to avoid an unaesthetic appearance.

The author has had a few occasions to create a feminine hairline in male transsexuals who had some temporal recession. Here, one deliberately, but conservatively, lowers and rounds the lateral frontal temporal hairline, thus blunting the temporal gulfs, in contrast to the usual mature masculine hairline.

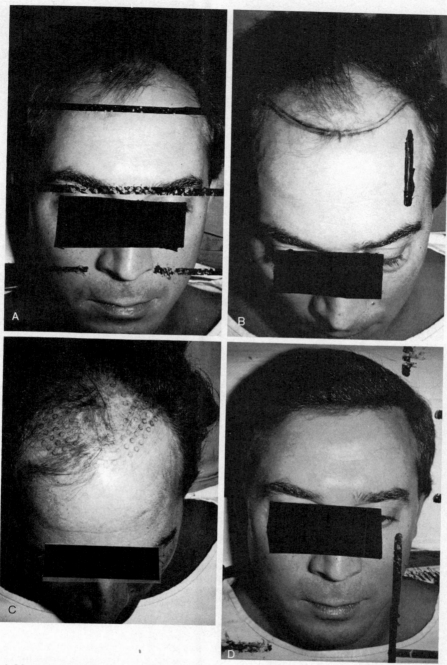

Figure 19–17. *A*, A 33-year-old man with pronounced frontal baldness (also shown in Figs. 19–59, 19–70, and 19–80). The face has been divided horizontally into thirds. *B*, A conservative, gently curving, anteriorly convex, frontal hairline is marked (two slightly different alternatives) that terminates at the part line on the patient's left and creates an adequate temporal gulf. (Compare with D and also with Figure 19–81A for a lateral view in a similar patient.) *C*, The 100 (3.5 mm) recipient sites for 4.0 mm grafts are marked with gentian violet. Spacing is considerably further apart than 3.5 mm in the midanterior scalp behind the first four rows (cf. Fig. 19–18). *D*, Appearance after completing the hair transplantation. Face is divided into thirds, as in A; distance from the glabella to the *apex* of the hairline is *at least* one third of the face. Note that the patient's *grafted* hairline terminates on his left at the part line, which is vertically above the outer canthus of the eye (also indicated in B).

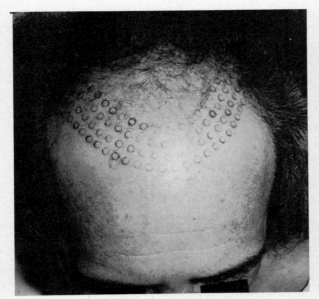

Figure 19–18.

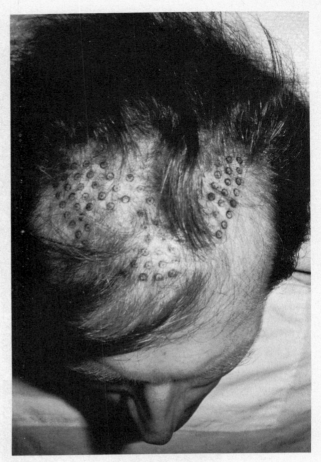

Figure 19–20.

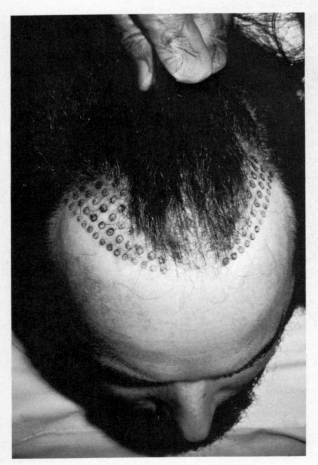

Figure 19–19.

Figure 19–18. A 35-year-old patient with extensive frontal male pattern baldness. The 100 (3.5 mm) recipient sites for 4.0 mm grafts were marked with gentian violet using a dull punch and were placed approximately 3.5 mm apart in all directions, except for the first row where they are slightly closer together. Note that four rows have been marked, and no grafts are to be placed in the midanterior bald area during this session. When viewed from the front, the termination of the first row laterally on the left (parting) side is almost vertically above the outer canthus of the eye, which creates a proper temporal gulf (cf. Fig. 19–60).

Figure 19–19. A 31-year-old patient with moderate temporal recession due to male pattern baldness and long straight black hair, showing 3.0 mm gentian violet marks for the first row and 3.5 mm for the other prospective recipient sites, into which 31 (3.5 mm) and 47 (4.0 mm) grafts, respectively, were subsequently placed. Green ink dots in the center of each circle facilitate counting. Grafting in thinning apex was deferred because of concern about temporary appearance, as patient parts hair in center.

Figure 19–20. A 58-year-old patient with extensive frontal hair loss caused by male pattern baldness but with areas of retained frontal hair of fairly good density. Prospective recipient sites (3.5 mm) for 68 (4.0 mm) grafts have been marked to avoid areas of retained hair (cf. Fig. 19–74).

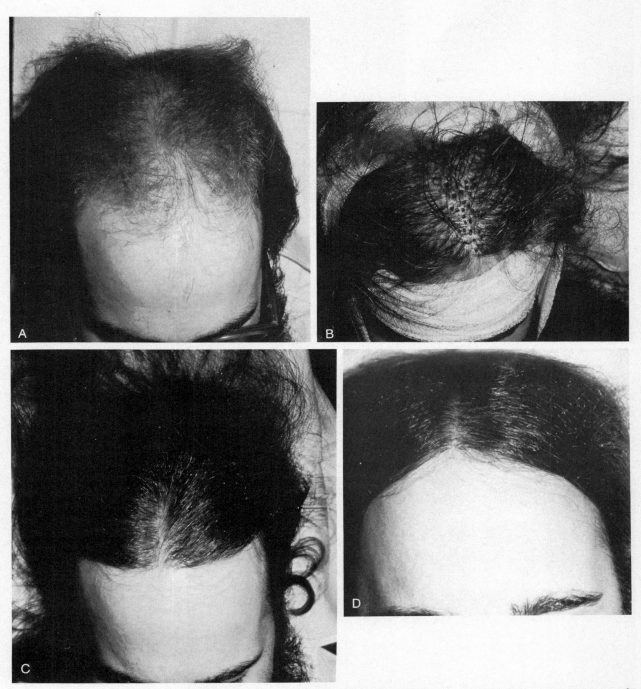

Figure 19–21. *A*, A 30-year-old man with extensive and marked thinning caused by male pattern baldness. *B*, Appearance after extensive punch grafting of frontal scalp showing a refinement session in the center of the scalp where he wants to part his hair, with minute circular and ovoid recipient holes (3.0, 2.5, 2.0 and 1.5 mm) placed in the remaining spaces. *C* and *D*, Appearance after B, plus a similar session seven months prior to these photographs. A further refinement session followed.

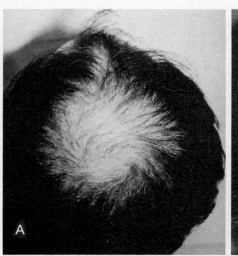

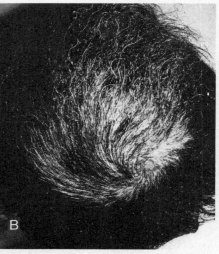

Figure 19–22. *A,* A 38-year-old patient with a very thin to nearly bald crown caused by male pattern baldness. He also has marked frontal recession and thinning with moderate thinning of the midscalp and a wide fringe of good density. Subsequently, 85 (4.0 mm) grafts were placed in 3.5 mm recipient holes on the crown. *B,* Appearance 11 months later after receiving 79 additional grafts on the crown 2½ months after the first session and 78 grafts in the frontal area four months after that. He shows surprisingly good coverage for only two sessions on the crown. Note that the natural whorl pattern of the crown has been re-created, following a pattern of sparse residual hair shown in A, and that the kinkiness of the ends of long hairs growing anteriorly represent earlier growth following telogen defluvium, whereas portions of hairs closer to the scalp (later growth) are relatively straight (see Fig. 19–2B to D).

The same principle applies to women who have a temporal recession due to female pattern baldness, a point emphasized by Norwood.

The Crown (Vertex)

For the most definitive result, the author prefers to simulate the natural whorl or spiral configuration of hair growth on the crown, if discernible, by observing the orientation of any residual, even vellus, hairs or, if not, then arbitrarily placing it to be most compatible with the direction of hair growth and/or styling in the anterior scalp (Figs. 19–12, 19–22, and 19–23). This applies whether it is done as the sole procedure or as the completion of a combined approach preceded by reduction of the crown (and frequently midscalp). However, if the bald crown is relatively large (especially if the frontal scalp is also bald) and/or if the donor supply is limited (especially if reduction is not appropriate but perhaps even following reduction), and if there are still not enough grafts to create an adequately filled in whorl, then it may be preferable to concentrate the grafts adjacent to the fringe along the parting side with grafts spaced progressively more

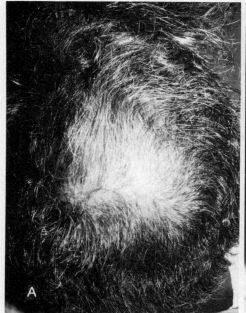

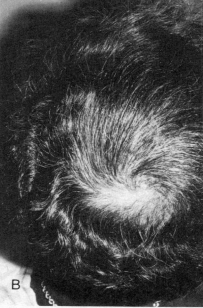

Figure 19–23. *A,* A 58-year-old man with relatively pronounced thinning caused by male pattern baldness in a limited area of the crown with milder peripheral thinning. Frontal thinning and recession were also present. *B,* Appearance two years later after four sessions during which a total of 207 (4.0 mm) grafts were placed in 3.5 mm holes over 13 months. Grafting was also done in the anterior scalp. Note the creation of a natural crown whorl pattern. There was additional grafting after this photograph.

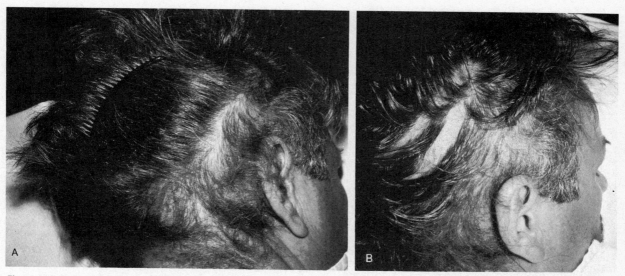

Figure 19–24. *A*, The right posterolateral fringe area of a 39-year-old man with moderately extensive male pattern baldness, showing marked contrast between the good density of the upper portion and the extremely sparse lower portion. *B*, Hairs have been clipped short in two rows in the upper and midposterolateal area of good density, avoiding the extremely sparse lower lateral and posterolateal area, in preparation for taking grafts followed by interdigitated closure (see Fig. 19–31).

widely apart over the rest of the bald crown. Considerable dependence upon styling may be necessary to accomplish reasonable coverage, especially in the case of straight hair. On the other hand, *relatively* widely spaced and evenly distributed grafts *may* give adequate coverage if the hair is curly or frizzy, especially if there is not too great a color contrast between hair and scalp.

DONOR SITE PLANNING

Donor areas having the best available density should be selected for those grafts to be placed in the most critical locations—such as on the side of the scalp on which the hair is parted or from which it is oriented, especially for the first few rows, or in the center of the whorl of the crown.

When a large amount of grafting is required, the donor supply can be conserved by using the grafts of *relatively* sparser, but still acceptable, density in less critical locations, such as the midscalp, the anterior area on the lateral aspect of the side *opposite* the parting side, or the periphery of the crown. When this is done, it should be stressed to the patient in advance that not all of his grafts will have as good a yield as the best ones. Similarly, grafts can be spaced more widely apart and/or less complete filling in with repeated sessions can be done in the less critical areas, thus preserving a sufficient supply of grafts of good quality, so that the maximum impact can be created in the areas where it is most needed.

It should be stressed that many patients have a marked difference in density in different portions of

the donor area or fringe. Frequently, the best density occurs *relatively* high with much sparser growth in the lower third or half (Fig. 19–24). Obviously, grafts taken from areas of very poor density will have a very poor yield, regardless of technique. Furthermore, sparse areas low on the fringe may tend to get even sparser with time so that grafts taken from here cannot be expected to continue to grow hair of even fair density and quality in some patients. Thus, aside from poor technique in taking and preparing grafts, one of the most frequently seen errors is taking grafts from too low an area on the fringe in order to avoid taking them from too high an area.

Norwood has pointed out that the short sparse curly hair seen low in the lateral scalp above and adjacent to the ears in some young men, which is apparently referred to by barbers as "whisker hair" because of the resemblance, is not only unsuitable for grafting because of its poor density (with the prospect of becoming even sparser with time) but is also believed to be an indicator of future extensive male pattern baldness (Fig. 19–25).

Naturally, grafts must not be taken from too high an area on the posterior or lateral fringe either, i.e., areas which may be subject to future hair loss in a patient whose baldness is still progressing. Grafts also should not be taken from above (medial to) the part line (actual or intended) or so close below (lateral to) it that donor site scars would be exposed. Thus, one can take grafts higher up laterally on the side opposite that on which the patient parts his hair.

By wetting the hair, a future line of demarcation between the "safe" fringe and progressively balding

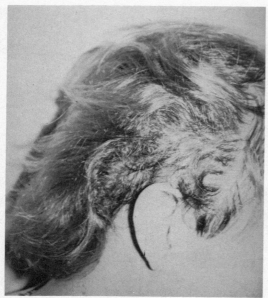

Figure 19–25. A 23-year-old man with mild thinning and recession (not shown) caused by male pattern baldness demonstrating "whisker hair"—very sparse, short, dark (in a blond individual), curly hair adjacent to the ear—an extremely poor source of donor material.

areas may often be more readily seen in patients with relatively early to moderate thinning over the crown and midscalp (Fig. 19–26). In any event, a reasonable margin of safety should be allowed for along the upper margin of the fringe by "assuming the worst" in case of doubt.

The author has observed that in many men the lowest extent of crown baldness in the *midline*

posteriorly is approximately a finger's breadth above a horizontal line connecting the tops of the ears, as seen from behind. This can vary considerably (frequently higher, rarely much lower) but is of some value in determining *roughly* the upper limit of the "safe area" in the *midline posteriorly* (but *not* posterolaterally or laterally where the natural arciform curve must be followed) in patients with early baldness (Figs. 19–4A, and 19–27).

In many individuals, grafts obtained from the moderately low, *but not too low*, midposterior donor area contain slightly to somewhat finer caliber hairs compared to those coarser hairs higher up in the posterior, posterolateral, or lateral scalp; yet they are not of too sparse density, as are those commonly seen slightly lower down. If these finer hairs are used in the first (and perhaps second) rows of the frontal hairline, a more natural and less stark effect may be achieved, particularly in patients with black hair and relatively light skin. This is less important in light blond or gray-haired individuals. In fact, the latter are usually grayer on the sides of the fringe, especially anterolaterally, and darker in the midposterior aspect (usually the last area to turn gray). In this situation, the camouflaging effect of placing the grayer hair on the frontal hairline may well be preferable to using the slightly finer but darker hair from the midposterior scalp (Fig. 19–28).

Because many individuals have a nevus flammeus involving varying portions of the nuchal, suboccipital and occipital areas (Fig. 19–5C), grafts taken from these areas should preferably not be placed in or near the frontal hairline or center of the whorl of the crown, although Unger has noted that they tend to become lighter after being transplanted. An

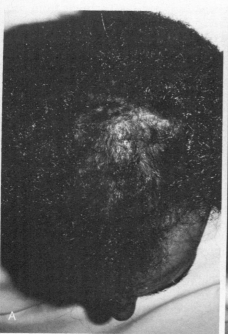
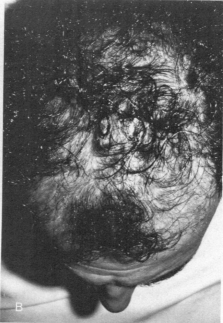

Figure 19–26. *A,* A 47-year-old man with extensive thinning caused by male pattern baldness. *B,* Wet hair shows more clearly the line of demarcation between the balding area and "safe" fringe hair available for obtaining grafts, which will produce permanent hair. Difference in lighting between the two photographs exaggerates somewhat the contrast between them.

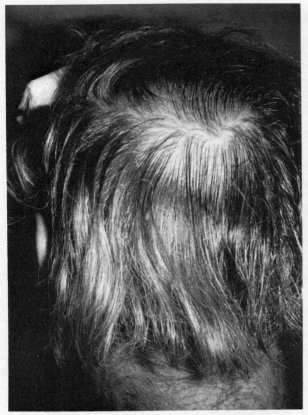

Figure 19–27. A 49-year-old man with moderate thinning of the crown caused by male pattern baldness, demonstrating that the line of demarcation between balding and "safe" fringe hair in the *midline posteriorly* is frequently about a finger's breadth above a horizontal line joining the tops of the ears, as viewed from behind, made more evident by wetting the hair. The upper row of just completed donor sites (closed by interdigitation) is barely visible through the combed-over hair somewhat below this point.

exception might be a patient with fair or ruddy skin in whom hypopigmented grafts would be anticipated and in whom grafts taken from an area of nevus flammeus (if not too intensely erythematous) might help mask hypopigmentation.

THE PUNCH GRAFTING PROCEDURE

Preoperative Care and Medication

It is essential during the initial consultation or, if need be, subsequently for the patient to achieve a basic understanding of the nature of male pattern baldness and of the rationale and essential details of the hair transplantation procedure, especially the need for repeated sessions. The limitations, especially as to hairlines, must be made clear so that the patient does not have unrealistic expectations, particularly if he is a less-than-ideal candidate. He should be given a reasonable estimate of the number of grafts likely to be needed, taking into account future hair loss, as well as some idea of his likely donor supply, both in quality and quantity, so he has a concept of what his supply-demand ratio is.

The patient should be instructed to avoid products containing aspirin for 10 to 14 days preoperatively and perhaps antihistamines for a few days, to avoid interference with normal blood coagulation. However, the author has performed grafting on a number of occasions when these instructions were ignored without significant blood-clotting problems. Alcohol should be avoided on the day of surgery as well as heavy exercise, which may increase bleeding. The patient should shampoo the hair the night before or day of the surgery.

Preoperatively, a mild to moderate tranquilizer and/or an analgesic (avoiding aspirin) may be given, especially for apprehensive patients and for long sessions. The author also gives the patient 500 mg of erythromycin, cephalexin, or other suitable oral antibiotic, which is continued, one gram daily, for two to several days postoperatively.

TECHNIQUE—DONOR SITE

Patient Position and Preparation

The patient should be on an adjustable operating table in the prone position for taking grafts from the donor area, and supine with varying degrees of head elevation for placing them in the recipient sites. If sitting upright in a chair, some patients may experience syncope. The author concurs in Alt's recommendations that the patient's head be placed in a headrest (Prōn-Pillō, for example) facing straight down rather than turning the head to one side when obtaining the grafts from the posterior fringe, and that the patient lie completely on his side with the side of the head supported by a pillow when harvesting grafts from the lateral fringe. This prevents distortion of the skin resulting from twisting the neck, which would prevent cutting the grafts exactly parallel to the direction of the hair follicles.

Relatively narrow strips of hair, appropriately curved to the arciform configuration of the donor area, are clipped short with small curved scissors, preferably with blunt points, leaving the hairs just long enough (0.5 to 1 mm) to indicate: (1) the direction of the hair shafts and hence of the follicles beneath the surface when cutting the grafts and (2) the direction of intended hair growth when placing them. In addition, areas of good and of poor density are often seen more clearly after the hair has been clipped. If left too long, inadvertent traction on the hairs postoperatively could result in grafts being pulled out. Two or more horizontal rows are clipped; the number, distance between them, and the length are determined by the number of grafts to be taken at that session. The hair is left long

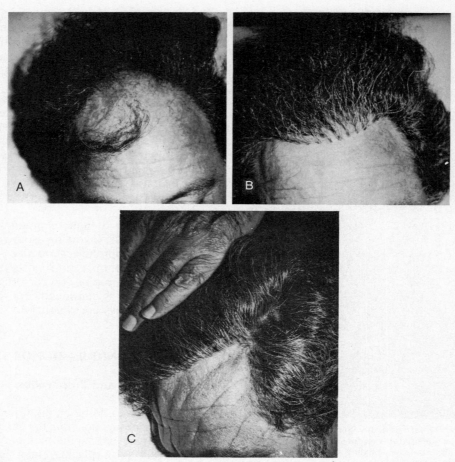

Figure 19–28. *A*, A 48-year-old patient with marked frontal-temporal recession and thinning, together with moderate midscalp and considerable crown thinning caused by male pattern baldness. Subsequently, 60 (4.5 mm) grafts were placed in 4.0 mm holes in the frontal-temporal area, with five rows on the left and three on the right (patient parts his hair on the left). The best density grafts were placed on the left, and grafts from the lateral fringe that contained more white hairs were placed in the first row, especially on the left. *B*, Appearance 13½ months later. Note the predominance of white hairs in the first row of grafts. For his next session 72 similar grafts were placed in alternate rows (i.e., beginning new second, fourth, etc., rows). *C*, Appearance three years after the first session. At his third session of 70 similar grafts (one year before), the remaining spaces in the first and alternate rows were filled in. Some of the 4.5 mm grafts were trimmed and fitted into 3.0 mm ovoid holes in the first row. Photograph shows the result of three sessions with the left frontal hairline exposed and with remaining spaces in alternate rows covered by hair in the solidly grafted first row. Note the aesthetic enhancement from using grafts that contained a maximum number of white hairs in the first row of this patient with predominantly black hair.

between the rows for better temporary coverage (Fig. 19–24B). Not wearing the hair too short over the donor areas facilitates this.

The donor areas are cleansed with alcohol and/or other skin antiseptics such as chlorhexidine.

Local Anesthesia and Normal Saline Infiltration

For the donor area, the author generally uses 1% lidocaine with 1:100,000 epinephrine (unless contraindicated by cardiovascular status or propranolol medication, as stressed by Foster and Aston) as a local anesthetic, injected *intradermally*, gently and slowly. A control syringe and a one-inch 30-gauge needle are used with a field block technique supple-

mented by intradermal infiltration throughout the area. Dermal jet injection or nerve block are alternative techniques. Immediately before cutting every few grafts, the area to be cut is heavily infiltrated *intradermally* with injectable normal saline in order to achieve maximum turgor, which helps to obtain well-cut grafts (Fig. 19–29). This is especially important in patients with flaccid scalps but is helpful in all.

Cutting and Removing the Grafts

After anesthetizing the donor area, the circular punch grafts are taken in horizontal rows where the hair has been clipped short. Each graft is about 1.5 to 2.0 mm from the adjacent one in the horizontal

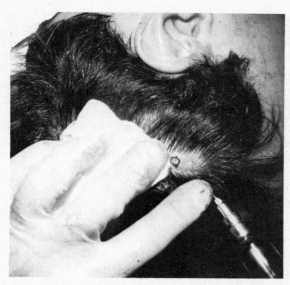

Figure 19–29. Injecting normal saline intradermally immediately before cutting every few grafts in order to obtain good turgor and thus a well-cut graft. This figure and Figures 19–33 to 19–35 illustrating donor site techniques are oriented so that the operative field is viewed as it would be by the operator, who is positioned at the patient's head, the top of which is at the bottom of the figure.

thus providing the patient with a nontender side of his head to sleep on following each session.

At later sessions, grafts can be obtained from between the rows as required, thus permitting a high yield of grafts from a given donor area (Fig. 19–30B). Of course, sufficient space must eventually be left between each individual donor site in all directions or unduly large bare areas will be created, especially when interdigitating closure is *not* done because of contiguous donor site scars with little or no hair remaining between them for coverage (Figs. 19–31 and 19–32).

The author has for many years used the power punch exclusively for cutting the grafts in the *donor* area, but uses power and/or manual punches to cut the *recipient* site holes. Power punches offer the advantage of slightly greater operative speed, less operator fatigue, and greater patient acceptance (in the donor areas) than the manually operated ones and, provided that the punches are extremely sharp *and do not rotate eccentrically*, an accurately cut graft and, hence, a good yield of hairs can be obtained. Alt has actually shown power-cut grafts to be superior to those cut manually. A rather small, light (5½ ounces) hand-held motor of adequate power (the Bell International Hand Engine) has proved to be most satisfactory in the experience of a number of operators including the author. Of course, care must be taken to avoid entangling and thus pulling out long hairs in either the donor or recipient areas.

The extreme importance of using an exquisitely sharp punch, whether power or manual, to cut the grafts cannot be overemphasized. The author and others have long preferred the Australian-made (or more recently, the U.S.-made Australian type) car-

direction, but each row is separated from the one above or below it by 6 or 7 mm if no donor site closure is planned (Fig. 19–30A). The rows should be substantially farther apart (1.0 to 1.5 or 2.0 *cm*) when the interdigitating closure technique is used (Figs. 19–24B, 19–41D, and 19–44). Alternate sides of the lateral, posterolateral, and/or posterior scalp can be utilized at subsequent sessions, if feasible,

Figure 19–30. *A*, Right posterolateral donor area after removal without closure of 100 (4.0 mm) grafts. The grafts with the hairs cut short were removed 1.5 to 2.0 mm apart in the horizontal direction, in six rows, each row 6 to 7 mm apart. At the second session grafts were taken from the left side, and at the third session they were taken from between these rows on the right. Note the good density in the upper and midposterolateral scalp with an ample margin of safety below the bald crown. Hairs are much sparser in the lower scalp and well below the bottom row of grafts. *B*, Donor area on the left side 1½ years later after removing a total of 400 (4.0 mm) grafts in four sessions of 100 grafts each alternating sides. The normal scars resulting from healing without closure are visible only when deliberately exposed, provided the hair is not cut too short.

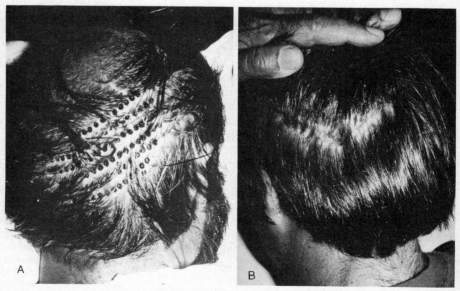

The fourth session (the second one taken from the left side) was seven months previously. Ample residual donor site hair remains despite relatively heavy, but not excessive, harvesting.

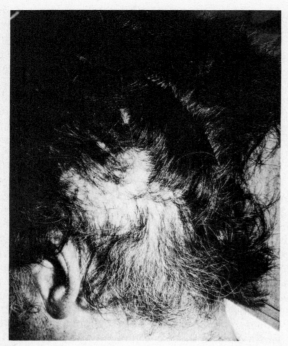

Figure 19–31. A 44-year-old man as he appeared when first seen by the author, showing excessive harvesting of the donor area. He had received about 250 to 300 (4.5 and 5.0 mm) grafts by another operator during a period ranging from 3 years to seven months before. The recipient area (not shown) had a generally sparse yield of hairs per graft. The donor area demonstrated a good density in the middle and upper portions and sparse to very sparse density in the lower portion, from which a substantial number of grafts were taken. Subsequent grafting by the author (avoiding sparse donor sites) resulted in a good yield per graft (see Fig. 19–24).

bon steel punches, which are harder than the generally used stainless steel ones and are therefore capable of acquiring and maintaining (with resharpening) a far superior edge. (Whether power or manual, extreme sharpness of punches is of less critical importance in cutting *recipient* site holes.)

The rheostat of the power unit is set at about 5000 rpm, first having observed the punch rotating at the slowest speed in order to avoid using one that wobbles or vibrates owing to a bent or eccentrically placed mandril, which destroys follicles at the periphery of the graft. Sometimes, inserting the mandril into the chuck at various depths will correct the problem. A somewhat dull punch may be less easily detected by the operator when using a power unit because much more effort is required to cut with a dull punch manually. Therefore, *extremely sharp* punches to cut the grafts are especially critical when using a power unit. The ability to shave off easily a hair from the operator's forearm with a punch's cutting edge is a good measure of its sharpness.

If a power punch is used, the entire depth of the cut should be angled parallel to the direction of the hair shafts. The hairs point inferiorly, so the punch

should be directed superiorly and at the same angle (Fig. 19–33). The punch should be either rotating prior to contact with the skin or barely touching it at the proper angle. The skin should be held taut by the operator's other hand. If the power is cut off by the foot switch before removing the punch from each donor site, spattering of the patient and operator with blood can largely be prevented.

Hemostasis is best achieved by removing the graft and suturing closed any donor site hole with any heavy (especially arterial) bleeding as it occurs and by direct and persistent manual pressure with gauze squares on those with milder bleeding by the patient and/or assistant.

If a manual punch is used to cut the donor sites, it is held perpendicular to the surface until the skin is just barely cut in order to prevent it from slipping and creating too ovoid an outline. Then, in a continuous motion while fully rotating the punch, or pressing on it lightly while exerting either a very slight twist or a slight to moderate twisting back and forth motion, the angle is changed to correspond to the same angle at which the hairs emerge from the surface. The cut is made through the dermis and well into the subcutaneous fat and parallel to the hair shafts. As with the power punch, if the angle of the cut varies significantly from that of the hair

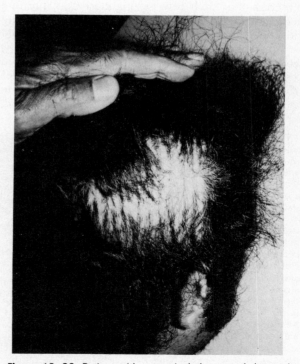

Figure 19–32. Patient with excessively harvested donor site as he appeared when first seen by the author. Very little hair remains in this portion of his right lateral and posterolateral scalp making coverage very difficult even when his hair is combed over the area. He had received 500 punch grafts in five sessions two months apart beginning 1½ years before by another operator.

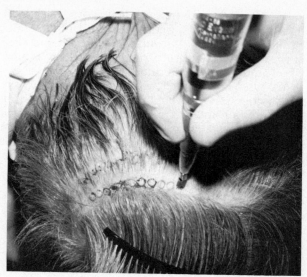

Figure 19–33. Using a 4.0 mm Australian carbon steel punch powered by Bell International Hand Engine, the operator cuts grafts at the same angle as clipped hair shafts emerge from the skin. Each cut is separated from the adjacent one in the same row by about 1.5 to 2.0 mm. Although not shown, digital pressure should be made immediately above and below donor sites, both during saline infiltration and cutting of grafts, to maintain maximum skin tautness, as advised by Alt. A curved comb holds hair out of the operative field. The patient is in a prone position (facedown) and using a headrest. (See text for proper positioning of the patient's head and body to avoid distortion when cutting grafts.) Lower row has just been closed by interdigitation.

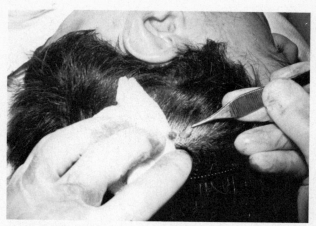

Figure 19–34. Checking a graft that has just been cut to be certain it was cut parallel to the hair shafts in all directions and sufficiently below the level of the follicular bulbs before additional grafts are cut. The patient is lying on his side with his head on a pillow for harvesting grafts in this lateral donor area.

shafts beneath the surface, follicles will be needlessly cut across tangentially, hence reducing the yield, sometimes drastically. The Stough modification of the Orentreich manual punch has a relatively thick and gently tapered conical handle with circular grooves, which is convenient for grasping while exerting a twisting back and forth motion. Orentreich preferred a continuous rotation when using his narrower knurled handle design.

Whether a power or manual punch is used, all aspects of the edges of the grafts should be carefully inspected as they are cut (initially and at least every few cuts thereafter) by pulling them outward gently with rat-tooth Adson forceps, or cutting them free for inspection. This will ensure that the cut has been sharp, parallel to the hair shafts (neither too nearly vertical nor too acute but at the same angle), and to a sufficient depth (about 5 mm or more). The cut should extend deeply into the subcutaneous fat into which the follicular bulbs extend and thus be clearly beneath them, especially on the superior side of the tangential cut, in order to avoid damage to the bulbs when the grafts are subsequently cut free (Fig. 19–34).

Each graft is gently grasped at the cut edge of the epidermal surface with narrow pointed 1 × 2 rat-tooth Adson forceps, in order to avoid traumatizing

the follicles by squeezing the graft with the forceps. It is then pulled outward and cut loose at the base with curved iris scissors (preferably having a gentle S-curve shape), taking care not to cut across any follicular bulbs (Fig. 19–35) by making certain that the cut with the punch has been deep enough. A convenient number of grafts can be cut but left attached, and then each, or perhaps every second or third, graft can be inspected either before or after it has been cut free. In either case, the grafts should be cylindrical, not conical or otherwise distorted, and any indicated corrections should be made for an improper angle and/or depth of cut, a dull or eccentrically rotating punch, etc., before harvesting subsequent grafts. Using a coarse-toothed straight comb and/or forceps to lift them gently from the site, the grafts are placed in a Petri dish and covered with sterile normal saline (Fig. 19–36).

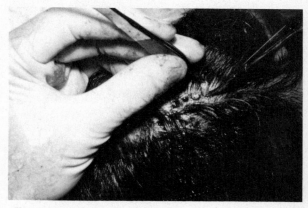

Figure 19–35. A graft is being cut free at a safe depth (well beneath the follicular bulbs) with S-curved iris scissors while being grasped gently at the epidermal edge and pulled outward with narrow-nosed, rat-tooth Adson forceps.

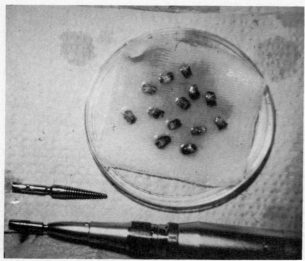

Figure 19–36. Several grafts have been placed in normal saline solution in a Petri dish. Intact hair shafts and a cylindrical (not conical) shape indicate they have been cut correctly. Also shown are a power punch and a Stough manual punch (4.0 mm).

The grafts will survive for at least several hours as long as they are kept wet. Excessive heat from a hot light and excessive evaporation of the normal saline resulting in a hypertonic solution must also be avoided. Grafts can be segregated into different Petri dishes or portions of them according to size of grafts, density and/or caliber of hairs, and the proportion of white hairs for appropriate placement later (Fig. 19–37).

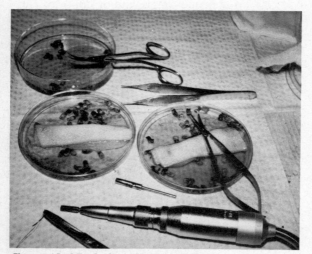

Figure 19–37. Grafts being kept in normal saline solution (until placed in recipient holes) are shown in two Petri dishes at the bottom of the photograph. They have been segregated according to density, caliber of hairs, and graft size. The other Petri dish with normal saline solution contains bald plugs from the recipient site, which will be discarded. Also shown are 1 × 2 rat-tooth Adson forceps, S-curved iris scissors, small spring-handle scissors (for trimming grafts), a punch with a narrow mandril (for insertion into the chuck of a power unit), and the handpiece (with a punch inserted) of the Bell International Hand Engine.

It is important to remove any short hair shaft fragments that adhere to the cut surface of the grafts because they would, of course, act as foreign bodies in the wound. (For graft trimming, see the section "Technique—Recipient Site.")

Alt has demonstrated with excellent ultra-close-up photographs the importance of a number of factors responsible for producing a nearly perfect graft, i.e., a somewhat tangential cylinder but with straight sides; not conical, with no epidermal lip or otherwise distorted, and with no damage to or loss of peripheral hair follicles (Figs. 19–38 and 19–39). His careful observations have corroborated the opinions held by this author and others for many years as well as adding new insights.

Of great importance is the use of extremely sharp punches of carbon steel, as previously emphasized. Normal saline infiltration should be used routinely to produce good turgor and thus a clean cut without compression and resulting distortion. This is especially important in patients with flaccid scalps. However, Alt has stressed the importance of heavily infiltrating only small areas, then cutting a few grafts at a time because the turgor is lost quickly. He advises adjacent digital pressure during infiltration and cutting in order to aid in maintaining turgor and immobilization. Too rapid advancement of the punch into the skin and the increased pressure required with a dull punch and with the manual as opposed to the power punch causes compression of the skin with resultant distortion and follicle damage, as demonstrated photographically by Alt. Pinski has summarized most of the requisites long stressed by the author and others for obtaining the "perfect plug."

With proper technique, the average 4.0 mm graft obtained from an area of moderate density usually contains about 15 to 17 hairs, although, as previously stressed (see the section, "Donor Site Planning"), the inherent follicle density may vary markedly in different portions of the donor area in the same patient (Fig. 19–24) as well as between different individuals (Fig. 19–5), and the grafts may contain only eight or 10, or even fewer hairs from sparse areas, or as many as 20 or 25 hairs, sometime more, from areas of good density. Larger or smaller grafts would naturally vary accordingly in their yield. Of course, poor technique or judgment can substantially or even drastically reduce the yield of hairs in grafts obtained from even a donor area of good density (Figs. 19–10 and 19–40).

Interdigitated Donor Site Closure

The author's previous policy was not to close the donor sites (except where required for hemostasis) because the scars resulting from healing without closure often tend to be somewhat (and sometimes substantially) smaller than the donor site holes,

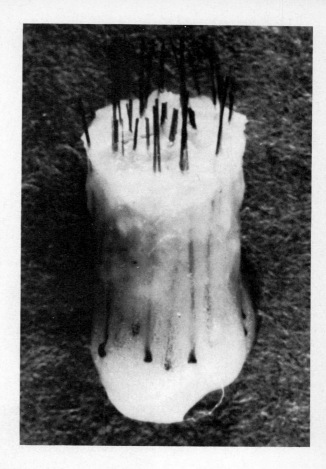

Figure 19–38. An ideal graft cut with an extremely sharp, power-driven, Australian-made, carbon steel punch and aided by normal saline infiltration to produce adequate skin firmness. Follicles at the periphery are intact, with no transection of bulbs from the hair shafts. The sides of the graft are straight with a smooth, glistening surface. (Courtesy of Thomas H. Alt, Sr., M.D.)

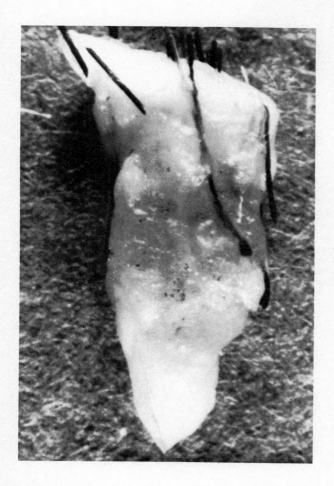

Figure 19–39. Graft cut with a dull punch and without saline infiltration requires excessive downward pressure, resulting in compression of the soft subcutaneous fat, which causes splaying of the bulbs, creating a cone effect and transection of the bulbs. It also causes a depression of the epidermis, resulting in an oval lip of skin with transected hairs. A dull punch cuts an irregular surface that does not reflect light at the same angle, causing a dull, rather than a glistening, surface. (Courtesy of Thomas H. Alt, Sr., M.D.)

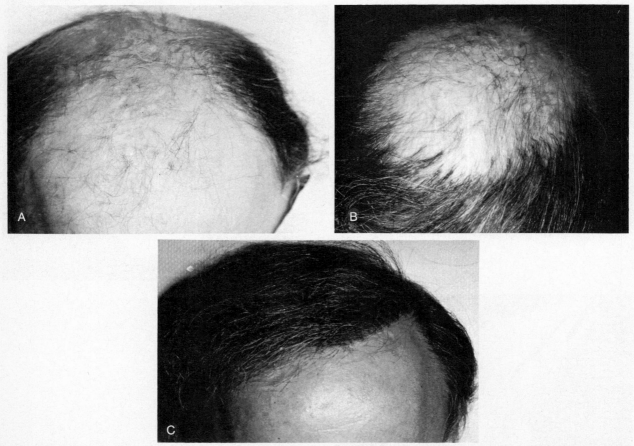

Figure 19–40. *A,* A 52-year-old man with extensive male pattern baldness and a fringe of moderate density in the upper portion and very sparse in the lower as he appeared when first seen by the author. Ten years before he had between 100 and 200 grafts placed on the anterior scalp, midscalp, and crown by another operator. The yield was good on only a few, fair on a moderate number, and sparse to nil on many. There was also considerable hypopigmentation and atrophic scarring. The donor site scars were normal (i.e., not hypertrophic) and were in areas of adequate density. *B,* Appearance 16 months later after a total of 185 (4.0 mm) grafts were placed in 3.5 and 3.75 mm holes during three sessions in the anterior scalp. Excellent yield of hairs per graft is apparent in scattered grafts along posterior border of grafted area, adjacent to bald crown. Face is at bottom of photograph. *C,* Appearance 14 months later after two additional sessions of 64 and 62 grafts, including some smaller sizes in and near the hairline, which still needs further refinement. An additional 57 grafts followed, including the use of grafts with finer and/or sparser hairs to create a more natural blending into the bald crown.

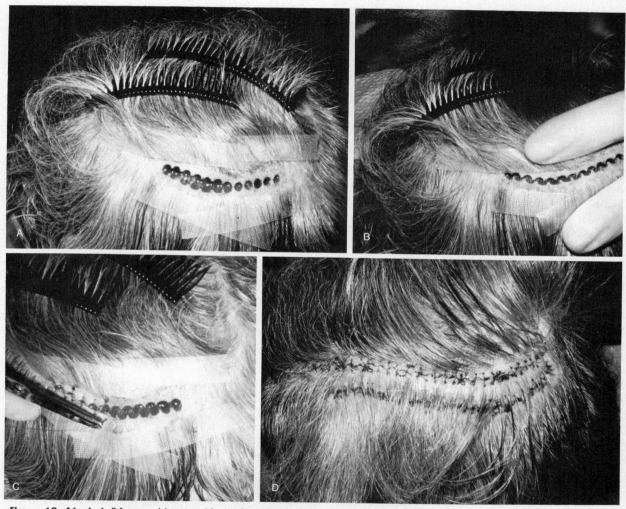

Figure 19–41. *A,* A 54-year-old man with moderately extensive male pattern baldness, showing preparation for interdigitated closure of a single row of donor sites. A portion of the bridges connecting the 4.0 mm holes have been cut with iris scissors parallel to the hair shafts and follicles. Patient is in a prone position with the head supported in a neutral position (facedown) for work on the posterior and left posterolateral donor area. Top of the patient's head is at the top of the figure in A to D. *B,* Demonstrating interdigitation of tips to arcs. *C,* Sutured closure of tips to arcs using a continuous running suture with occasional interrupted sutures for security and hemostasis. *D,* Completed closure of 65 donor site holes in two single rows. This was the second session on the patient's left side and grafts were obtained from areas between the rows shown in Figure 19–43A.

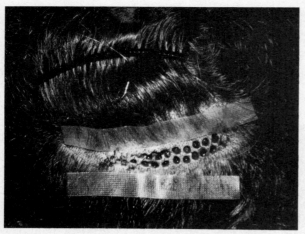

Figure 19—42. A 44-year-old man with moderate male pattern baldness showing interdigitating closure in progress of a double row of 4.0 mm donor sites. Patient's head has the same orientation as in Figure 19—41.

whereas the scars following *conventional* sutured closure tend to spread. On numerous occasions, the author's comparison of donor site scars resulting from previous closure of the holes and of those resulting from leaving them open showed that the scars are virtually indistinguishable.

However, the relatively recently described technique (Carreirao and Lessa, Pierce, and Unger) of cutting the skin bridges separating the donor site holes (angling the incision parallel to the hair follicles to avoid damage) and then suturing them closed by interdigitating the resulting tips to arcs, generally produces a relatively narrow wavy or zigzag linear scar, which is usually significantly less apparent than the scars following either of the above procedures. The author uses single or double rows of holes for the interdigitated closure (Figs. 19—41 and 19—42), whereas some operators use triple rows. This procedure helps prevent excessive thinning of the residual donor area hair after extensive graft removal

and/or allows more grafts to be harvested, thus in effect extending the donor supply by reducing the total amount of scarring relative to the amount of hair remaining (Figs. 19—30 to 19—32 and 19—43 to 19—45).

In an analogous procedure that the author has found useful, relatively large, confluent, and/or numerous donor site scars resulting from previous healing without closure or conventional sutured closure can be removed with a punch and an interdigitated closure done, resulting in substantial narrowing of the scars (Fig. 19—46). The periphery of such excised scar plugs may at times provide a few intact hair follicles that can serve as a source for minute grafts for hairline refinement.

Another technique used by some operators (e.g., Morrison, Nordstrom, and Hill) is to take two or three rows of grafts as close together as possible, both vertically and horizontally, then to totally excise the remaining skin (utilizing this as a source of additional small grafts), to extensively undermine the borders as in a scalp reduction, and to suture it closed. This procedure can also be modified to achieve total harvesting of limited donor areas that have previously been heavily or even excessively harvested, thus increasing the donor supply without undue donor site exposure. However, extensive donor area excision with undermining in effect constitutes a "fringe reduction" and would appear to be somewhat at cross-purposes to a bald crown or midscalp reduction, if the latter has already been done or is contemplated. This opinion is also expressed by Unger.

TECHNIQUE—RECIPIENT SITE

Local Anesthesia

The frontal scalp (especially the midline) generally requires a higher concentration of local anes-

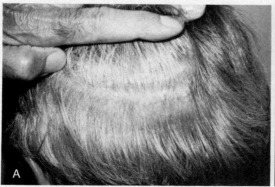
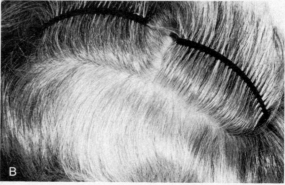

Figure 19—43. *A*, The donor area of the same patient as in Figure 19—41 three weeks after the first interdigitated closure on the left side showing normally erythematous, narrow zigzag linear scars, which represent the posterior and posterolateral aspect of the lower of two long closure lines similar to those in Figure 19—41D. *B*, Appearance five months after interdigitated closure. Scar is virtually invisible, even with hair parted precisely on the scar line (posterolateral aspect of the upper of two long closure lines). Compare with Figure 19—30.

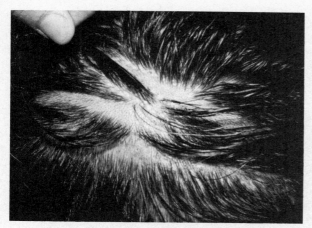

Figure 19—44. A 43-year-old man with extensive male pattern baldness, showing left lateral and posterolateral donor area 3½ and 6½ months after interdigitated closures and immediately before a third harvesting of grafts from the left side. Four rows of hypopigmented, relatively narrow, zigzag linear scars are visible only because the adjacent hair between the scars has been clipped short in preparation for taking additional grafts (cf. Fig. 19—30).

thetic than other areas of the scalp; the author uses 2% lidocaine with 1:100,000 epinephrine as a field block, which is supplemented by 1% lidocaine with 1:100,000 epinephrine infiltrated further posteriorly.

Cutting Recipient Holes

Using either a manual or power punch or both (see below), the recipient holes are cut following the outlines created by the gentian violet markings, and using the same technique with the punch as in cutting the grafts from the donor sites. One must be sure to cut them to a sufficient depth to ensure a good fit of the graft and flush with the surface. Initially, however, it is wise to cut only one or two holes, to remove the bald plug, and to try temporarily placing one or more grafts as a test to be certain that the size ratio (e.g., a 4.0 mm graft placed in a 3.5 mm hole) results in a proper fit. If not, a correction can be made in the recipient hole size (e.g., 3.25 mm if 3.5 mm is too ample for a 4.0 mm graft) before cutting any more holes. The fit should be neither too tight, resulting in excessive compression and probably graft elevation (cobblestoning), nor too loose, resulting in an excessively wide scar around the periphery of the graft, a yield of fewer hairs than the hole could accommodate, a graft that might come out too easily during the early postoperative period, and/or a graft depressed below the adjacent surface. Thus, if most or all of the recipient holes were cut and then found to be too large for the grafts that had already been obtained, no correction could be made, whereas if the holes were found to be too small, they could, of course, be enlarged. In patients with flaccid scalps, regardless of the temporarily increased turgor created in the *donor* sites by normal saline infiltration in order to be able to cut better quality grafts, there is a greater shrinkage of the graphs than in patients with better inherent turgor. In such cases, the author prefers to place a 4.25 or 4.5 mm graft into a 3.5 or 3.25 mm recipient hole, whichever combination results in a proper fit.

When cutting each punch of skin, which will eventually be discarded, from the bald or thinning recipient site, careful attention should be paid to slanting the punches at an angle of approximately 60 degrees and orienting them in the same direction as the normal hair growth in any given area (guided

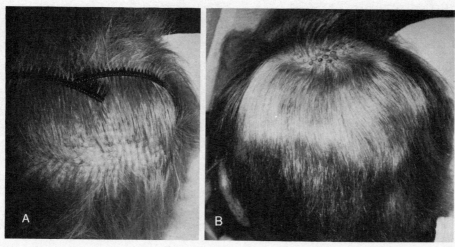

Figure 19—45. *A,* A 41-year-old man, showing normal donor site scars (no closure) in a heavily, but not excessively, harvested donor area that is deliberately exposed. Photograph was taken at the same time as Figure 19—82C and D during which a total of 675 grafts (mostly 4.5 mm) had been harvested. (Cf. Figs. 19—30 to 19—32.) *B,* Same patient can adequately cover his wide donor area when hair is dry and combed normally but perhaps only marginally when it is wet. Coverage is aided by camouflage provided by bleached blond hair. Crown shows recipient site gentian violet markings preparatory to further filling in.

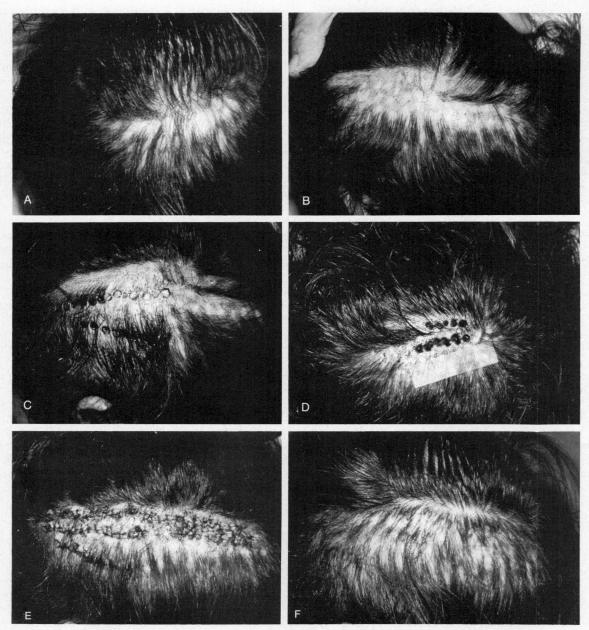

Figure 19–46. *A* and *B,* A 27-year-old man who had had 200 to 300 grafts placed by two previous operators (five years and four years before first being seen by the author) because of moderately extensive male pattern baldness. The result was a marginally low hairline and many sparse to very sparse grafts (not shown). The donor area shows many excessively large and confluent donor site scars. *C,* Same patient showing a 4.5 mm punch excision of 14 large scars in progress, together with hair-bearing punch grafts (4.0, 3.5, 3.0, and 2.5 mm) for remedial and hairline refinement in the anterior scalp. In addition, three minute grafts of three to six hairs each were obtained from the periphery of some of the excised scars and also used for hairline refinement. *D,* A different patient with similar but smaller donor site scars after punch excision of scars and cutting of skin bridges preparatory to interdigitated closure, as was done to patient in C. *E,* Same patient as in C at the completion of interdigitated closure. *F,* Same patient as in E 4 weeks after the operation showing marked improvement in excised scars but with much more scar excision still to be done.

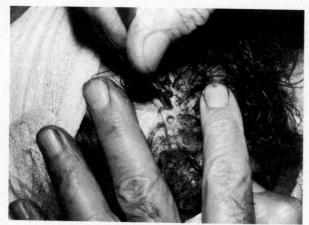

Figure 19–47. Cutting 3.5 mm recipient site holes for 4.0 mm grafts using a power punch in the patient's left frontal hairline and following gentian violet markings. Punch handle is angled about 60 degrees anteriorly from the skin surface in the direction of normal hair growth in the frontal area so that the cutting edge of the punch is directed at a corresponding angle posteriorly. Manual punch technique is similar. Operator's left hand is holding long grafted hairs from the first session many months before out of the way to prevent entanglement by the rotating punch. Because this is the patient's second session, recipient holes are cut and grafts are placed in staggered or offset positions creating new rows between the original first, second, and third rows and so on (see Fig. 19–54).

by residual hairs, if any). That is, the cutting edge of the punch is usually directed posteriorly to slightly posteromedially in varying degrees on the frontal scalp and midscalp, so that the direction of the short cut hairs in the grafts and hence of the eventual hair growth will be pointing, respectively, in an anterior to slightly anterolateral orientation (Figs. 19–47 and 19–48). It is usually, though not invariably, directed in a spiral fashion over the crown so that the eventual direction of hair growth will follow the normal whorl pattern (Figs. 19–12, 19–22, and 19–23). Without proper orientation of the holes and corresponding placement of the grafts, the subse-

quent growth of hair in the grafts will be at artificial angles and directions. This produces an unnatural and unattractive appearance (Fig. 19–49) and also makes it impossible to fill in the area adequately at subsequent sessions. The proper placing and angling of the recipient holes, especially at the frontal hairline, requires meticulous attention to detail so that the eventual hair growth will be aesthetically acceptable.

Tromovitch prefers to have the hairs emerge from the skin at a much more acute angle than the author does, producing a "shingling" effect. If the donor supply is very limited in relation to the area of baldness, then this probably will give better coverage, especially in patients with dark straight hair and light skin, if only two instead of four or more sessions per area are planned. However, for the most natural-appearing hairline, especially if it is likely to be exposed, the author prefers to simulate nature as closely as possible. Sometimes a *very subtle* (not extreme) left-to-right or right-to-left orientation in the frontal scalp, in order to facilitate the eventual styling or combing of the grafted hair, can be achieved by appropriate angling of the recipient site holes and corresponding placement of the grafts. However, even if the patient plans to comb his hair straight back, the recipient holes should be cut and the grafts placed so that the eventual direction of hair growth will slant about 60 degrees *forward* (the usual orientation) *not* backward.

An exception to the crown whorl pattern would be cases in which only a limited coverage is possible. Grafts would be placed primarily or even entirely on either the left or right lateral crown and/or midscalp extending medially from the area adjacent to the fringe, and the resulting hair would be combed across to cover the remainder of the crown. In this case, a fairly definite left-to-right or right-to-left orientation would be appropriate.

When using the power punch, the manual punch is frequently also employed by the author and ori-

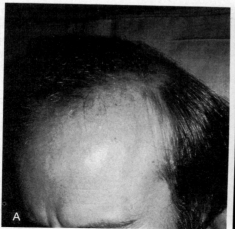 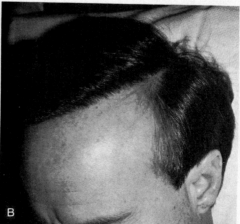

Figure 19–48. *A,* A 37-year-old man with marked thinning and recession caused by extensive male pattern baldness. (Same patient as in Fig. 19–30.) *B,* Appearance one year after the completion of extensive grafting over a three-year period. Note the forward angle (approximately 60 degrees) of hair growth.

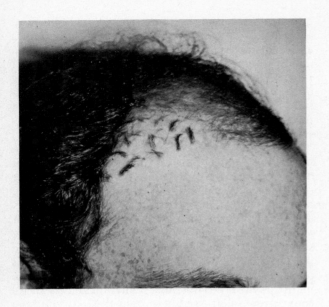

Figure 19–49. A 20-year-old man with frontal-temporal recession and thinning caused by male pattern baldness as he appeared when first seen by the author. He had 50 punch grafts placed in the receded temples by another operator 20 months previously, which resulted in a too low temporal hairline—an outcome based on a decision that the patient says was made without his knowledge or participation prior to surgery. Grafts were also too widely spaced, and there was poor yield in some, moderate cobblestoning, and grafts with hairs pointing in every direction, including laterally, medially, and posteriorly (see Fig. 19–86).

ented vertically to complete the angled cut made by the power punch, thus cutting sufficiently through the galea in the posterior portion of each hole (e.g., in the anterior scalp) to achieve adequate depth of the recipient site hole without excessive contact of the power punch with the pericranium and the resultant grinding sensation and sound, which is unpleasant to the patient (Fig. 19–50). Alternatively, the angled cut with the power punch can be changed to a vertical cut at the completion of the cut for the same reason. With the power punch, considerable care is required to avoid entangling and pulling out any long hair in the area, such as growth resulting from earlier grafting sessions or residual hair (Fig. 19–47). In these circumstances, some operators use manual punches only. Although, as a convenience to the operator, some routinely cut any long hair in the recipient area short (whether it is residual hair or growth from grafts placed earlier), the author prefers to work around these hairs, even though it is more time-consuming, out of consideration for the patient.

The author prefers to cut all or at least most of the recipient sites, then to cut a dozen or so bald plugs loose at their bases with curved iris scissors (cutting deeply enough to ensure a good fit when the grafts are placed) while grasping and pulling them outward with rat-tooth Adson forceps (Fig. 19–51), followed by placing a corresponding number of properly trimmed grafts and so on (see below).

Graft and Recipient Hole Trimming and Graft Placement

In order to prevent graft elevation (cobblestoning) one must compensate for the fact that the bald scalp is generally somewhat thinner [frequently about 20% thinner in baldness of long standing (Figs. 19–1 and 19–52)] than the coarse-hair–bearing scalp; however, this is a *consequence and not a cause* of male pattern baldness. *Excess* subcutaneous fat and galea aponeurotica, if any, are trimmed from the bottoms of the grafts with small curved scissors, preferably spring-handled, or with iris scissors taking great pains to avoid cutting off or traumatizing the bulbs of the deepest follicles, which extend into the fat, by not cutting too close to them. A gentle pulling away motion while cutting with the scissors helps to minimize the danger. Handling of the grafts while trimming should be gentle; one should avoid undue trauma by grasping them at the epidermal edge, preferably by using narrow pointed rat-tooth forceps (Fig. 19–53).

Overly zealous or careless trimming is an important cause of a poor yield of hairs and must be avoided. White hairs are especially vulnerable because of the difficulty of seeing them. It is much better to do little or even no trimming of the fat than to trim excessively close to the follicular bulbs and papillae. The author, who personally performs all phases of the transplantation procedure, generally custom trims each graft to fit a specific recipient hole immediately prior to placing it rather than having all grafts routinely trimmed of fat by an aide, as is commonly done (Fig. 19–54). Of course, if it becomes apparent that some or perhaps many or most of the grafts require removal of large amounts of subcutaneous fat in order to ensure a good fit, the author will trim a number of them, then place those that have been prepared, with additional individual trimming if required, and so on. *Peripheral trimming of grafts can also be done when indicated in order to fit a graft properly into a hole that may*

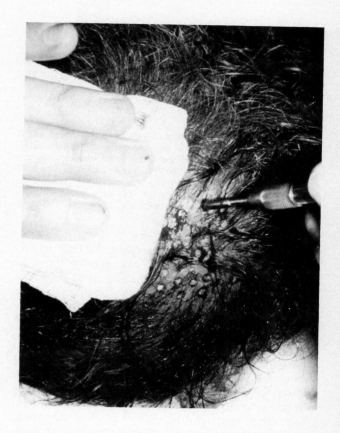

Figure 19–50. Manually deepening 3.5 mm recipient holes in the anterior crown, which have already been cut with a power punch. In this instance, a handle into which the power punch mandril had been inserted is being used as an alternative to the conventional manual punch (see Fig. 19–36). The punch is held and rotated slightly in a nearly vertical position in order to cut through the galea in the posterior portion of the bottom of the hole, which had been cut at a 60 degree angle (see text). Patient is maintaining manual pressure for hemostasis.

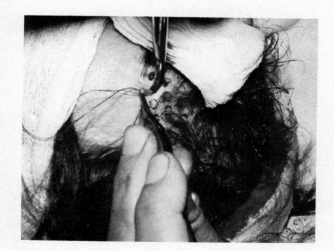

Figure 19–51. Cutting a bald plug free at the base with S-curved iris scissors while the plug is grasped with rat-tooth Adson forceps and pulled outward.

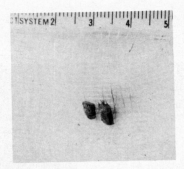

Figure 19–52. Plug of bald scalp skin from a recipient site is shown on the left and a coarse hair-bearing graft from the same patient's donor site (prior to being trimmed of subcutaneous fat) on the right, illustrating the difference in thickness. The bald specimen measures approximately 4.5 mm in thickness (i.e., depth), and the coarse hair-bearing specimen 5.0 mm. Both include the subcutaneous fat and were cut with 3.5 mm punches.

be too small, e.g., when enlarging the hole would damage adjacent follicles. It can also be done to enable a graft to fit into a smaller ovoid recipient hole (see section on "Subsequent Sessions") or to correct for an imperfectly cut, but usable, graft. Naturally, only those portions of the periphery *not* containing intact hair follicles are removed (Fig. 19–55).

The grafts after being judiciously trimmed free of *excess* subcutaneous fat, *but only to the extent required for a proper fit,* are carefully and gently placed using Adson forceps into the recipient holes, from which any clotted blood is first removed, rotating and pressing on them until they fit flush with the surface. Their short-clipped hairs should be pointed in the proper direction (generally forward in the anterior scalp), which has been determined by the direction in which the recipient site hole was cut (Figs. 19–56 and 19–57). Thus, both recipient site holes and hair-bearing grafts are in the approximate shape of tangential cylinders (Figs. 19–35, 19–36, 19–38, 19–47, and 19–52).

If a graft does not fit well (or anticipating that likelihood after initial experience) despite the removal of any clotted blood from the recipient hole and remains elevated above the surface, either additional galea must be removed from the bottom of the recipient hole (Fig. 19–58) or additional subcutaneous fat must be removed from the bottom of the graft (if this is possible without endangering the follicular bulbs) or both. The recipient hole can also be enlarged and/or a non–hair-bearing portion of the graft can be trimmed peripherally in order to achieve a proper fit. Care should be taken that adjacent long hairs, if any, in the recipient area are not inadvertently trapped beneath the grafts by lifting the hairs with Adson forceps. If any are, the graft trapping the hairs will abruptly pop out and require correct replacement.

Manual pressure is maintained, sometimes aided by a temporary pressure dressing, until the grafts appear to be secure (Fig. 19–58), and then any final correction of positioning of the grafts is made, followed by additional pressure before the final dressing is applied. This may entail repeated, time-consuming, and frustrating efforts before achieving the important goal of having all grafts absolutely flush with the skin surface, correctly oriented as to angle and direction, and free of bleeding (Figs. 19–59, and 19–60A). Persistent manual pressure exerted after placement of the graft is usually sufficient to stop even stubborn bleeding, but on rare occasions, heavy arterial bleeding will require suturing to close the prospective recipient site hole. Care should be taken that good hemostasis has been achieved in both donor and recipient areas before applying the final pressure dressing in order to help prevent distressing postoperative bleeding, which may also result in graft elevation.

Although it is true that there is a reduced vascular supply to the bald scalp as compared to the hairy scalp (in terms of the minute blood vessels of the subepidermal capillary plexuses), this is, as Montagna has emphasized, the apparent *result* of the reduced metabolic needs because of the greatly reduced size of the follicles and is *not* the *cause* of male pattern baldness. In any event, the large- and medium-sized blood vessels are present in entirely normal numbers (Fig. 19–1B), and anyone performing scalp surgery is frequently reminded during the

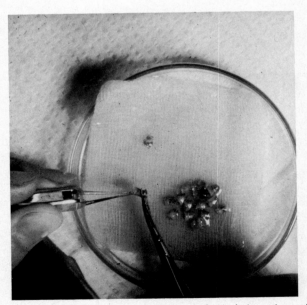

Figure 19–53. *Excess* subcutaneous fat is being trimmed from the deepest portion of the grafts with great care in order to avoid damage to follicular bulbs, using small rat-tooth Adson forceps and small curved spring-handle scissors. Adson forceps and iris scissors could also be used. Trimming should be only to the *minimum extent necessary* to achieve a good fit.

Figure 19–54. Custom trimming using 1 × 2 rat-tooth Adson forceps and small spring-handle scissors. Each graft should have removed only the minimal amount of subcutaneous fat actually necessary, if any, in order to achieve a satisfactory fit into a particular recipient hole. As much fat and galea as possible should first be removed from the bottom of the hole if the initial fit is not satisfactory. This technique is generally used by the author because it minimizes the likelihood of damaging the follicular bulbs.

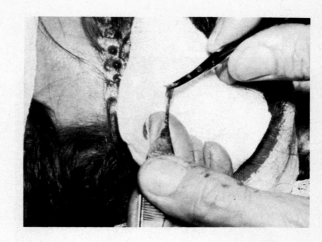

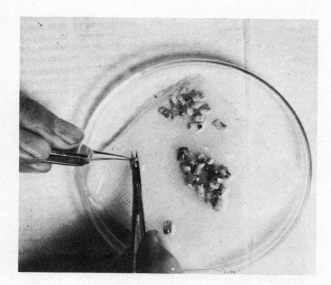

Figure 19–55. Trimming a 4.0 mm graft in order for it to fit in a 3.0 mm or 3.0 mm by 2.5 mm, or even a 2.5 mm recipient hole using fine-pointed rat-tooth forceps for handling and small curved spring-handle scissors. Only those portions of the periphery of the graft *not* containing intact hair follicles are carefully trimmed away to fit a specific recipient hole.

Figure 19–56. Placing grafts, properly oriented, in recipient site holes. Correct placement is aided by noting the direction of growth of the short-cut hairs in the grafts as well as by the slant of the grafts in relation to the slant of the recipient holes.

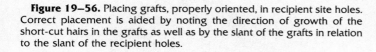

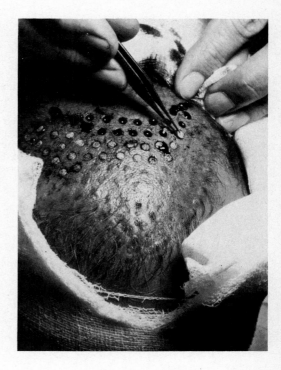

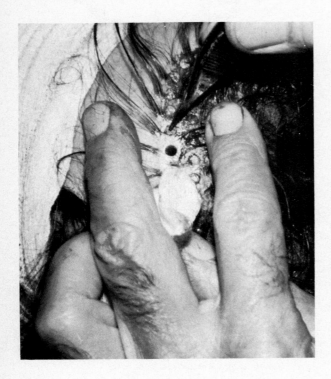

Figure 19–57. Pressing gently on the grafts to ensure that they are flush with the surface.

Figure 19–58. A fragment of galea at the bottom of a recipient hole in the left anterior scalp (which had not been adequately removed when the bald plug was cut free to create the hole) is grasped with Adson forceps and removed with S-curved iris scissors. Patient is making pressure for hemostasis and to keep secure those grafts already placed on the right side. Recipient sites on the left side have been cut, but bald plugs mostly remain attached. Moderately heavy bleeding is occurring at one recipient site on the left.

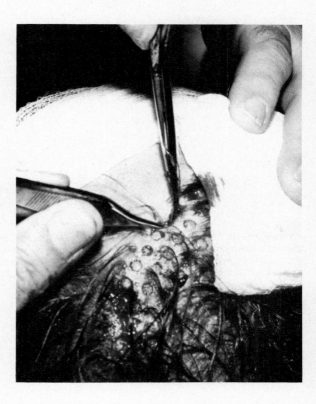

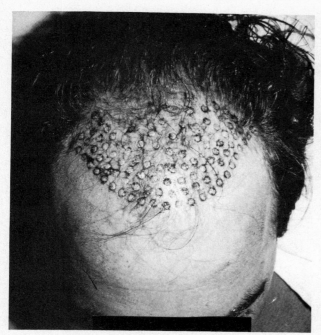

Figure 19–59. Same patient as in Figures 19–17, 19–70, and 19–80, immediately after placing 100 (4.0 mm) grafts into 3.5 recipient holes. Note the wider spacing behind the anterior four rows.

course of the surgery that the bald scalp as well as the coarse-hair–bearing scalp is exceedingly well supplied with blood (Fig. 19–58).

The author then applies a pressure dressing, firmly but not too tightly, in order to hold the grafts securely in place until fibrin clots have formed and to minimize and, if necessary, to absorb any bleeding. The dressing consists of the following elements, which incorporate both donor and recipient sites, and is generally left on overnight, occasionally longer. The layer next to the skin is a relatively nonadherent, porous, and fluid-absorbing dressing left dry or with a thin application of an antibiotic ointment. Next, four layers of gauze squares are applied; adjacent groups are taped together and both layers are secured to the forehead with transparent tape. Next, a wrap-around crimped gauze bandage is applied with tape holding it together and extending onto the sides of the neck, cheeks, and forehead to prevent upward displacement during the night (Fig. 19–60). If the crown has been grafted, the author prefers a dressing that also goes over the crown and under the chin for greater security. For appearance only, a loosely knit seaman's watch cap may be worn over the dressing.

Postoperative Care and Complications

Pain and discomfort following the procedure are usually relatively mild, although some patients may have moderate to considerable pain for a day or so. Moderate analgesia without aspirin and bedtime sedation may be desirable for one to several days postoperatively, especially following extensive grafting.

There is, of course, some tenderness of the operative sites, primarily in the donor areas, which may last to some degree for about three weeks or sometimes longer, but it is generally mild. Following interdigitated donor site closure, a majority of patients who have had a chance to compare find less discomfort than when donor sites are left open or are closed without interdigitation. Not suturing too tightly, of course, helps minimize discomfort. Occasionally, localized areas of pain and more marked tenderness occur in a portion of the donor site, especially where sutures have been placed tightly for hemostasis. More rarely, there is radiating pain requiring moderate analgesia. Increased sensitivity to touch and/or some degree of tenderness in the donor area may infrequently persist for weeks to months, especially when allowed to heal without closure.

A persistent neuroma at a painful and tender donor site present for many months was diagnosed clinically and confirmed microscopically in a patient who had very large donor site scars following punch grafting without closure, which was performed by another operator and seen by the author. Excision alleviated the symptoms.

Tenderness and swelling of the posterior cervical and suboccipital lymph nodes sometimes occur for a few days or longer, and itching, at times quite pronounced, may occasionally occur in the donor areas, mainly when closure is not done. Numbness of varying degrees is commonly noted, sometimes with later paresthesia, especially over the midanterior to the top of the scalp. This may last for several months to a year or two, sometimes longer (with perhaps indefinite partial numbness in occasional patients), following repeated extensive grafting procedures, especially anteriorly, because cutaneous sensory nerves in both recipient and donor areas have been cut. Sensation gradually returns to the grafts themselves.

Heavy physical exertion or bending over should be avoided for several days to a week or more following surgery in order to minimize the likelihood of postoperative bleeding, with the attendant hazard of graft elevation or possibly losing grafts. Moderate exercise is usually permissible after about four days. The patient should be instructed how to achieve hemostasis by making steady manual pressure with gauze squares on any bleeding site that might occur after removal of the pressure dressing.

When grafting is done over the frontal area, especially if extensive, it is quite common to have edema, sometimes marked, beginning over the forehead about the second postoperative day and ex-

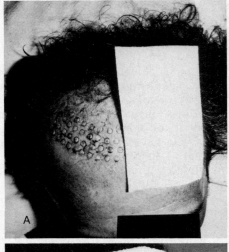

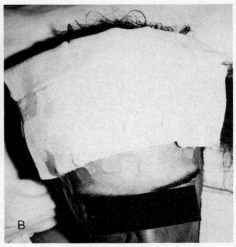

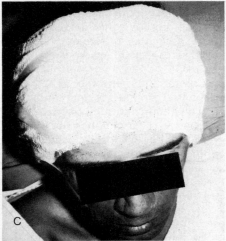

Figure 19–60. *A,* Same patient as in Figure 19–18 immediately after placing 100 (4.0 mm) grafts in 3.5 mm recipient holes, showing the first layer of an overnight (or longer) pressure dressing that will encompass the recipient and donor areas. A relatively nonadherent dressing has been applied to half of the recipient area, which can be left dry or covered lightly with an antibiotic ointment. *B,* Four thicknesses of gauze squares have been placed; both layers of the dressing were secured to the forehead with transparent tape. The same layers of dressing were then applied to the donor areas. *C,* A crimped gauze bandage roll has been applied and also secured by tape to the sides of the neck, cheeks, and forehead. If desired, a knit cap (not shown) may be worn over the bandage for appearance only.

tending later to the bridge of the nose and the eyelids, lasting from several days to a week or possibly longer. Sleeping with the head moderately elevated probably helps to diminish the tendency to edema as well as the likelihood of postoperative bleeding. Gently massaging the lower forehead from the center toward the temples may somewhat reduce the progression of edema to the eyelids once it has developed on the forehead. The use of ice packs may also help reduce edema, especially of the eyelids, to a degree. Rarely, periorbital ecchymosis may develop either spontaneously in conjunction with marked edema or apparently as a result of premature excessive exertion.

Unless contraindicated, a corticosteroid given orally or parenterally in adequate dosage (initially high then tapering), preferably beginning after the surgery and continuing for five to seven days postoperatively, usually prevents or at least greatly diminishes edema. The author routinely gives erythromycin (or cephalexin), one gram per day orally beginning at the time of surgery and continuing for

two to four days or, if a corticosteroid is given, for a matching number of days.

The pressure dressings are generally removed on the first postoperative day, although they may be left on for two or three days if more convenient or if persistent graft elevation and/or bleeding at the time of surgery has been a problem. If the dressings tend to adhere to the operative site because of clotted blood, the outer surface may be moistened with water and allowed to soak through briefly, after which they can usually be carefully peeled off by avoiding upward traction. *Very gentle* cleansing with a mild shampoo and water to remove dried blood from the scalp and hair can be done at this time or in a few days, taking great care to avoid displacing the grafts. Partial or even complete extrusion of one or more grafts from the recipient holes, with resulting desiccation, sometimes occurs after the dressing has been applied despite every effort to prevent it. It may result from persistent or recurrent bleeding beneath the graft, from the graft being either too large or too small for a proper fit, or from an

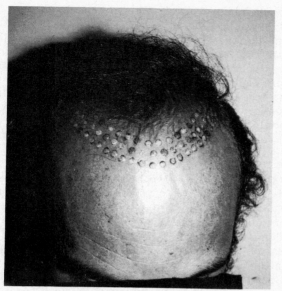

Figure 19—61. A patient on the third postoperative day with a slight erythema of the grafted area. The grafts vary from pale to erythematous to dark reddish purple in a few—the latter being slightly elevated due to clotted blood beneath them.

an antibiotic ointment applied or left alone. Fortunately, the normal scalp has an excellent healing capacity and great localized tissue resistance to significant bacterial infection, an infrequent problem in the author's experience. Deep pus formation beneath one or several grafts requiring incision and drainage and systemic antibiotic administration has occurred infrequently in the past. Cellulitis is a rare complication, which the author has not personally observed.

A case of severe *Pseudomonas aeruginosa* infection has been reported to the author in a personal communication. The patient responded to parenteral gentamicin administration together with removal of the infected grafts. The source of the infection was not determined.

Since the author began about 12 years ago using routine erythromycin prophylaxis against possible staphylococcal or streptococcal infection, even the benign superficial or occasional isolated deep pus formation in the recipient site has been virtually nonexistent.

After the crusts come off, the grafts are erythematous and gradually fade over a period of weeks to months (Fig. 19–63). A few or even many or all of them are sometimes slightly elevated above the surrounding surface at first, producing a mild cobblestone appearance, despite great care having been taken to ensure a placement as flush with the skin surface as possible, which is probably due to edema. Usually, these flatten out spontaneously, largely or completely, during the next several weeks or months.

Marked cobblestoning that persists is in most cases due to an improper fit of the graft in the recipient hole. Either the hole is too small or too shallow or both in relation to the size and/or thick-

excessive number of grafts (usually small or minute ones) being placed relatively close together when hairline refinement is done. An attempt should be made as soon as possible to correct any graft that is significantly elevated (unless it has become desiccated) or is improperly oriented.

After the initial pallor of the first couple of postoperative days (some of the grafts may be dark red to purple because of clotted blood beneath them as in Figure 19–61), the new grafts become pink then dark as minimal, moderate, or thick crusts develop during the next several days. The crusts are usually ready to be removed or come off with gentle washing between two and three weeks (Fig. 19–62). An antibiotic ointment (not cream) can be applied sparingly by the patient once or twice daily after a few days, or even sooner, in order to help prevent excessively thick crusts from developing and to facilitate their removal later. Some patients find this too messy and prefer daily gentle shampooing or simply leaving the area alone. The ultimate cosmetic result does not seem to be affected either way.

The grafts should be moderately secure after a week to 10 days and completely so after three weeks. It is, of course, possible to lose a graft by accidental trauma to the area or by careless combing, shampooing, or picking at the crusts during the first week or so.

Without the use of routine prophylactic systemic antibiotic administration, superficial follicular or nonfollicular pustules often occur in the graft sites during the first few days or so following grafting. They may be incised and drained as indicated and

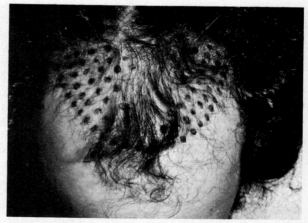

Figure 19—62. A patient on his tenth postoperative day showing normal crust formation following placement of 73 (4.25 mm) grafts in 3.5 mm holes at his second session. Grafts in alternate rows, including immediately anterior to this session's first row, placed two months before are practically invisible and have no hair growth yet because of telogen defluvium.

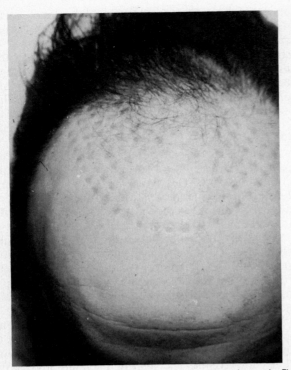

Figure 19–63. Appearance of a patient (also shown in Fig. 19–71) six weeks after a session of 112 (4.0 mm) grafts. Grafts are essentially flush with the surface, still somewhat erythematous, and devoid of hairs from telogen defluvium.

ness of the graft (Figs. 19–7 and 19–64). Persistent recipient site bleeding resulting in marked graft elevation will also cause cobblestoning if not corrected in the first few days. Cobblestoning can be leveled, at least substantially, by light electrodesiccation, repeatedly if required. Electrodesiccation avoids cutting off any hairs that may have grown in the grafts compared to scalpel shaving or dermabrasion, which are otherwise acceptable alternatives.

There are relatively infrequent instances when a hypertrophic diathesis apparently results in cobblestoning or even thickened scar-like elevations of the grafts, which may also be depigmented and have a poor yield of hairs, despite careful technique (Fig. 19–9). This same propensity may cause hypertrophic donor site scars, temporary or persistent, especially if the donor sites are not closed. It may also occur to some degree even with interdigitated closure and either with or without involvement of the grafts (Fig. 19–9).

When the donor sites are left open (i.e., allowed to heal *without* interdigitated closure), crusts form after a few days as well as in the recipient sites and are usually fairly thick (Fig. 19–65). They generally come off in two to three weeks leaving scars that are usually atrophic and erythematous at first, then gradually become hypopigmented (in relatively

light-skinned patients) in about three months or so. They tend to shrink to some extent, but there is considerable variation in size. In an occasional patient, the scars are quite small and inconspicuous even when searched for; whereas in most, they are only slightly smaller or about the same diameter as the holes that resulted from removal of the grafts. In most cases, the scars are readily covered by a moderate length haircut unless searched for, although a short crew-cut through which the scalp would be visible would necessarily expose them (Fig. 19–30B).

In patients who have had very heavy harvesting of grafts, donor site scars may be marginally visible, especially in those with dark hair and light skin and particularly if the hair is wet, mussed up, or somewhat short (Figs. 19–31 and 19–32). In contrast, the scars following *interdigitated closure* are usually a narrow wavy or zigzag line, at other times a bit wider, but in most instances much smaller than those resulting from healing without closure or from routine noninterdigitated closure. This permits better coverage of the donor area and/or the ability to obtain more grafts without undue exposure (Figs. 19–43 and 19–44). In patients with very *elastic* (as opposed to *mobile*) scalps, especially after repeated scalp reductions, even interdigitated closure scars may be relatively wide, especially on the upper lateral fringe area where the greatest stretching forces have been exerted by the reductions.

Although the closely clipped hairs in the grafts usually *appear* to be growing postoperatively, the follicles in most instances go into what has been presumed to be the telogen or resting phase as a

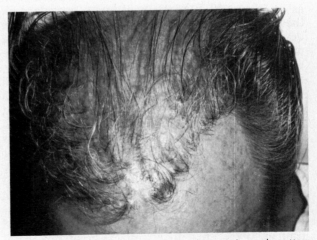

Figure 19–64. A 56-year-old man with extensive male pattern baldness as he appeared when first seen by the author. He had received 75 grafts in one session by another operator six months previously. Pronounced cobblestoning was present in many of the grafts, and those in the first row had been placed 1 mm or so apart. The yield varied from moderate to very sparse. Most of the grafts appeared to be at least 4.5 mm and possibly 5.0 mm.

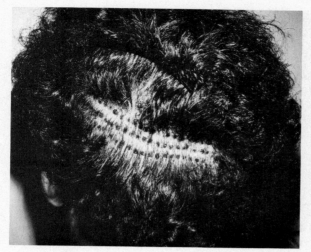

Figure 19–65. Donor area of a patient two weeks after the operation, showing normal crust formation when donor site holes are allowed to heal without closure.

the procedure and that topical application of minoxidil postoperatively shorten the three-month resting phase and/or cause fewer follicles to enter this phase are unsubstantiated by this author and others.

The beginning of new hair growth (anagen phase) may occur in a uniform manner with approximately all of the follicles beginning to grow vigorously at the same time, or it may be more uneven with some follicles proceeding ahead of others. The initial growth may be relatively fine and thus difficult to see when the hair is blond or white, followed by a normal coarseness in a few weeks. Frequently, the initial growth is of a frizzy or kinky texture for a number of months, even in a normally straight- or wavy-haired person. This is usually followed by restoration to an essentially normal growth characteristic for that individual after a period of several months to a year or longer, depending in part on how long the new hair is allowed to grow before the distal (earliest growth) portions are cut (Figs. 19–2 and 19–22). Sometimes, the change in texture may persist indefinitely in a few or even many or most hairs, at least to some degree.

Quite apart from this commonly seen and generally temporary phenomenon, in those cases where grafting is done in thinning rather than completely bald areas, the transplanted hair frequently appears coarse in comparison with the adjacent relatively

result of the trauma of the surgery (and especially because of the hypoxia induced by separation from their blood supply). The hair shafts, which were mostly below the skin surface at the time of surgery, are actually being extruded by the temporarily resting follicles. (Gloor claims that this is an anagen defluvium, rather than telogen as it is commonly designated, but to avoid confusion, it will be referred to here as telogen defluvium.) By about the third to fourth postoperative week, the hairs either fall out or may be readily plucked without resistance (Fig. 19–66). They frequently adhere to the underside of the crusts and come out with them when the latter are removed. Plucking any retained telogen hair shafts that persist after six weeks helps prevent their acting as foreign bodies with resultant delayed inflammation (with or without pustule formation) and probably also prevents their mechanical interference with new hair growth when it is due to occur. Not uncommonly, a few hairs in a number of the grafts and/or most or all in a few grafts do not fall out but continue to grow. Sometimes many, or rarely most or perhaps all, of the follicles do not go into telogen, but this, in the author's experience, is inconsistent and unpredictable, varying widely even in the same patient following different grafting sessions regardless of the length of session or other variables.

An interval of usually three months (although it can be two to four or occasionally more months) from the time of surgery (or a little over two months from the time the hairs become loose and fall out) is required before the resting follicles enter the new anagen phase and for the new hairs to start growing, after which they grow at the normal rate of approximately 1 cm per month. Claims that chilling the normal saline in which the grafts are stored during

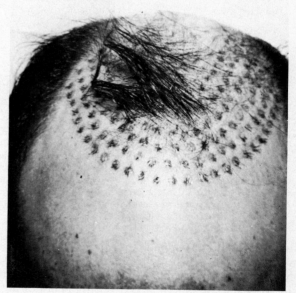

Figure 19–66. Appearance of grafts in a patient three weeks after the operation. Hair shafts have been extruded to a considerable length as follicles have gone into telogen and can now be readily plucked out. They also fall out spontaneously or as a result of shampooing. Direction and angle of hairs (about 60 degrees) in the grafts indicates that subsequent permanent hair growth will be properly oriented, i.e., the hair shafts are pointing anteriorly to anterolaterally. Grafts show moderate erythema and are flat or slightly elevated at this stage.

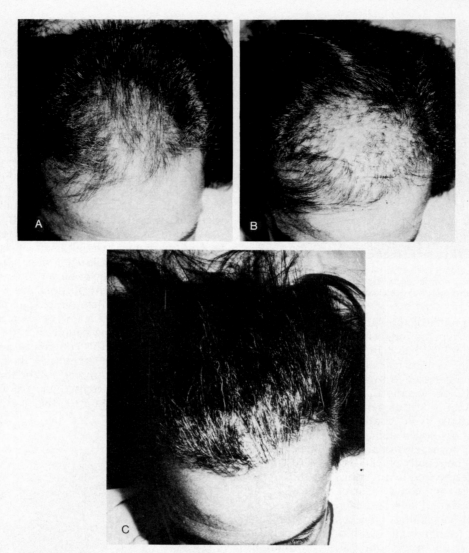

Figure 19–67. *A*, Patient in his midthirties with marked thinning of the anterior and midanterior scalp before grafting. *B*, Same patient showing telogen defluvium of residual thinning hair in the midanterior scalp caused by the trauma of placing 83 (4.0 mm) grafts in 3.5 mm recipient holes in this area five weeks previously. There is also the loss of residual hairs formerly occupying recipient sites when the holes were created. The result is considerable acceleration of hair loss in this area, an example of things getting worse before they get better. There are numerous erythematous "naked" grafts, mainly in the midanterior area from five weeks earlier, and hair-bearing grafts, mainly in the anterior area from an earlier session of 84 grafts nearly four months before this photograph was taken. *C*, Same patient seven months later. An additional 75 grafts were placed about 5½ months previously, and 92 grafts, including some smaller sizes, were done after this photograph.

fine and short hair remaining in the frontal area, which is characteristic of that found in progressive male pattern baldness. Blond hair is generally considerably darker as well as coarser in the donor area compared to the finer, lighter, and frequently sun-bleached thinning frontal hair in the same individual. Temporary or persistent actual darkening of light- to medium-colored grafted hair has been reported and has occasionally been seen by the author. Therefore, patients with recession at the temples but with retention of the hair at the apex should especially be warned that there may be at least a temporary and perhaps a lasting difference in texture and/or color between the transplanted and the adjacent residual hair.

At three to four weeks, a defluvium of varying degrees involving any *residual thinning* hair within and adjacent to the grafted area, sometimes also occurs, together with the usual temporary loss of the grafted hairs, in both cases apparently due to the induction of telogen in these follicles from the trauma of the surgery (Fig. 19–67). See the section, "Patient Selection and Contraindications" for a discussion of the consequences.

Although the trauma involved in placing additional grafts adjacent to previously placed grafts that have started to grow new hair does not regularly induce a new telogen phase, this does occur, at least to some degree (at times, to a considerable extent), when a large amount of grafting is done at a session. In any event, the defluvium is, of course, only temporary, and regrowth usually commences approximately three months from the last grafting session, although with one patient in the author's practice many months elapsed before growth resumed (Fig. 19–68). A grafting session performed during the telogen defluvium period of grafts placed at an earlier session usually does not cause a delay in the onset of new growth in the earlier grafts. Telogen defluvium sometimes occurs for about three months in the donor area adjacent to sites of graft harvesting, mainly when grafts are taken very close together in all directions, when excessively tight suturing is done, or when double or triple rows are removed with interdigitated closure.

When the transplanted follicles have completed their normal anagen (growing) phase after three to five years, they usually go into their telogen (resting) phase in a more or less random fashion in the same manner as the normal nonbalding scalp in which approximately 10% to 15% of its follicles are in telogen at any one time. However, occasionally, a substantial number, or perhaps most or all, of the follicles that had gone into telogen together as a result of a particular grafting session or sessions will again go into telogen simultaneously three to five years later. Thus, if a large amount of grafting has been done within a relatively brief period, there may be significant temporary defluvium until the new anagen phase begins again in three months. Although this phenomenon is not common and is, of course, only temporary, it could be a cause for considerable concern to both patient and physician if the mechanism involved is not understood. Orentreich has called attention to this, and it has also been observed by the author.

If there is sufficient available hair, it can be styled to cover the dark crusts at the graft sites as much as possible, aided by a hair spray. A hairpiece can be worn after the pressure dressing has been re-

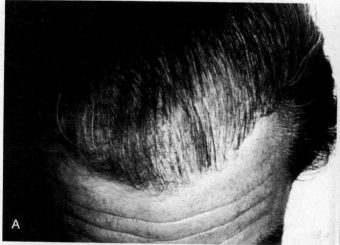

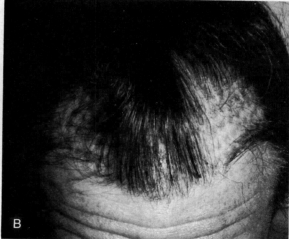

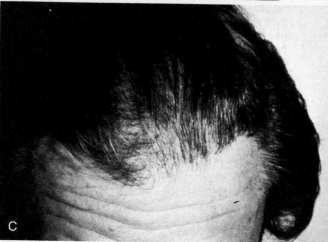

Figure 19–68. *A*, A 46-year-old man, who had some punch grafting in the receded temples performed by another operator 12 years before, with a fair to poor yield in many of the grafts and a somewhat low placement of the temporal hairline. Eight years previously, the author had placed 69 (4.0 mm) grafts in the same area, including a few in the progressively thinning apex. Following this photograph, 83 (4.0 mm) grafts were placed in the temple areas. *B*, Same patient two months later. In addition to the normal telogen defluvium of the recently transplanted hair revealing the erythematous "naked" grafts, a marked loss of hair has occurred in the old grafts as well, especially behind the grafted hairline. There was no regrowth of hair four months after A and only a little after five months. *C*, Same patient 17 months after B showing substantial regrowth but with some progressive thinning of the hair originally retained in the apex.

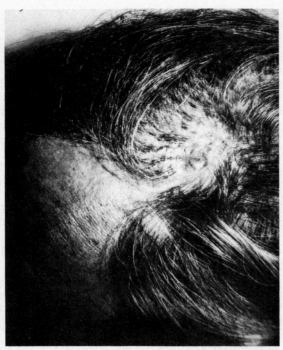

Figure 19–69. An apparent venous aneurysm in the left frontal-temporal recipient area at a graft site in a 45-year-old man about three weeks after a session of 58 grafts. At that time, the spaces remaining after extensive previous grafting were filled in with grafts ranging from 4.5 to 2.5 mm and placed in holes ranging from 4.0 to 1.5 mm, respectively. Also visible adjacent to the aneurysm are grafts in their "naked" (telogen) phase with a surrounding zone of temporary telogen defluvium of previously placed grafts. The lesion subsided spontaneously in about six weeks with no significant residual defect.

moved. Of course, if adhesive is used to secure it to the scalp, it should not be applied to an area that had been grafted within three weeks. Alternatively, the hairpiece can be attached with clips to the fringe hair.

Occasionally, an epidermal or hair-containing cyst or a granulomatous reaction to incarcerated hairs may occur in the recipient area, apparently caused by a graft that has inadvertently been placed in the recipient hole in a grossly incorrect orientation (sideways or upside down) or as a result of one graft having been placed on top of another in the same hole. Hairs that are clearly not growing out of the skin in a normal fashion but in a tight cluster and/or associated with giant comedones are the result of long hairs already growing in or adjacent to the recipient site having been trapped under a graft when it was placed (see the section, "Technique—Recipient Site").

A relatively uncommon occurrence is the development of a small- to moderate-sized arterial or venous aneurysm or pseudoaneurysm at a donor or recipient site two to six or more weeks postoperatively (Fig. 19–69). It usually subsides spontaneously over a period of several weeks, although sometimes

erosion of the thin wall with considerable bleeding can occur, requiring ligation.

The infrequent occurrence of a true arteriovenous fistula (as opposed to an aneurysm) in either the donor or recipient area that requires excision has been reported, but this has not occurred in the author's practice. A rare complication recently reported is the occurrence of multiple pyogenic granuloma-like lesions in the recipient area.

SUBSEQUENT SESSIONS

Basic Coverage—Placement and Time Intervals

Assuming grafts are placed one recipient-site width apart in all directions at each session (e.g., 3.5 or 3.25 mm for 4.0 mm grafts), four sessions in any one area are required in order to achieve *basic* full coverage (Fig. 19–70), although in less critical areas one may have to settle for perhaps only two or three sessions and/or space grafts more widely apart in order to conserve the supply of grafts. At such subsequent sessions following the initial one, at intervals of preferably two or more months in the same area, grafts are usually placed in staggered or offset positions thus starting (at the second session) new second, fourth, and sixth rows, for example. The original second row of grafts therefore becomes the eventual third row, the original third row becomes the fifth, and so on (Figs. 19–47, 19–51, 19–54, 19–57, 19–58, 19–71, and 19–72). At the third session, the remaining spaces in the first and now third and fifth rows are filled in deliberately creating *subtle* irregularities in the first row to avoid an excessively sharp hairline (Figs. 19–73 and 19–74). (Even at the first session, a *slight, but not excessive*, irregularity of the first row may be created.) At the fourth session, the remaining spaces in the second, fourth, and sixth rows are filled in (Fig. 19–75). The same basic formula applies to filling in the whorl pattern on the crown, except that usually a spiral pattern is followed (Fig. 19–12).

Although it takes longer to complete the grafting, if four or more months are allowed to elapse between each session (i.e., three months of telogen defluvium and a month or more of growth), then the exact location of hair growth from each session can be seen before proceeding with the next session, and therefore appropriate size and shape modifications in the recipient site holes and consequently of the graft sizes can be made. Thus, a space originally planned for placing a 4.0 mm graft into a 3.5 mm hole (at a second, third, or fourth session, for example) may actually require a 4.5 mm graft placed in a 4.0 mm circular hole or in an ovoid or pear-shaped 3.0 × 4.0 mm hole (created by overlapping circular cuts with a 3.0 mm punch or various com-

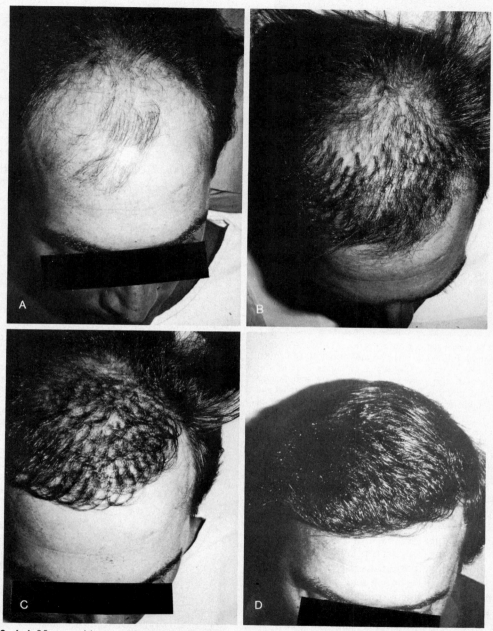

Figure 19–70. *A*, A 33-year-old man with pronounced frontal baldness. (Same patient as in Figs. 19–17, 19–59, and 19–80.) *B*, Appearance six months after 100 (4.0 mm) grafts were placed in 3.5 mm holes representing about three months of hair growth. Note the good yield of hairs per graft, which is more apparent posteriorly where the grafts were placed more widely apart. *C*, Same patient showing the result of two sessions five months after 94 similar grafts were placed in alternate rows. *D*, Same patient 2½ years after A. A total of 394 grafts in four sessions were placed over 15½ months to accomplish *basic* coverage. Hair is styled forward and across. Coverage shown is from grafted hair only. For hairline refinement on this patient, see Figures 19–17D and 19–80.

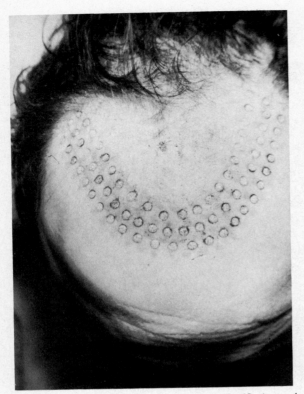

Figure 19–71. Same patient as in Figure 19–63 six weeks after first session, immediately after an additional 70 (4.0 mm) grafts were placed in rows staggered or offset behind the original first, second, and third rows, thus giving a balanced distribution of the grafts within the grafted area. Eight weeks would be preferable as a *minimal* interval for this amount of grafting.

binations of 3.5, 3.0, and 2.5 mm punches) in order to fill the space adequately without encroaching on adjacent previously grafted hairs (Fig. 19–75). It also permits the operator to see the hair shafts of previously placed grafts so that follicles at the periphery will not be sacrificed when new recipient site holes are cut (Figs. 19–47 and 19–75). In addition, both patient and operator can visualize the coverage being achieved and thus use the remaining donor supply where it is most needed. Thus, one may elect not to fill in as completely on the side opposite the part because the hairs from grafts on the parting side, with proper styling, in effect do double duty, helping to cover the opposite side as well as areas behind the first several rows.

If preferred by the patient, the first and other odd-numbered rows can be filled in at the second session, starting the new second row and so on at the third session. After the completion of four sessions, the result will be the same, but the temporary effect as hair growth occurs is a striped appearance that is more unnatural, especially with marked hair-skin color contrast. If grafting is being done as rapidly as possible (at two-month intervals)

rather than waiting for hair growth to occur before each subsequent session, then the staggered row approach has the advantage of allowing hair growth to occur in the first row before returning to fill it in at the third session (Figs. 19–73 and 19–74).

Number of Grafts per Session and Intervals Between Sessions—Safety Factors

Within certain limits, the author prefers to place a relatively large number of grafts during a session thus minimizing the total number of individual sessions. Depending upon the size of the area to be grafted, the supply of donor material, and the patient's desires, sessions of 40 to 75 grafts (4.0 or 4.25 mm) are common in the author's practice. Up to about 100 grafts can be placed at a single session if desired, especially if they are divided between two areas separated by a considerable distance (5 to 8 cm), such as the anterior scalp and crown or, alternatively, if a number of grafts are spaced substantially more than a recipient-site width apart.

To prevent ischemia and consequently a poor yield of hairs per graft or even graft necrosis (Fig. 19–76) with resultant atrophic or possibly hypertrophic scarring, an excessively large number of grafts (especially larger sizes) should not be placed at a single session. The grafts should not be placed too close together, and sessions for filling in between previously placed grafts should not be repeated after too short a time interval, especially if the total number of grafts at a session is large. Thus, if the number of grafts at a session is about 50 to 75, assuming they are placed about a recipient-site width apart in all directions, *at least* two months should elapse between sessions in the *same area*. The time period should preferably be longer (i.e., three

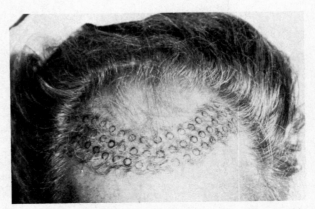

Figure 19–72. Same patient as in Figure 19–6 four months after 51 (4.5 mm) grafts were placed in 4.0 mm holes in four rows showing one month of growth. Sites marked for second session (three rows) are staggered or offset between the original four rows of grafts, thus creating new second, fourth, and sixth rows.

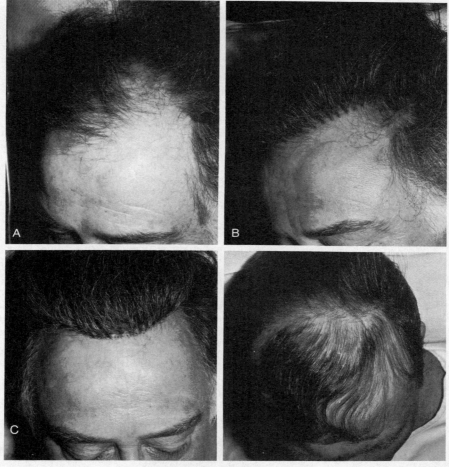

Figure 19–73. *A,* A 64-year-old man with extensive frontal-temporal recession and thinning caused by male pattern baldness. Grafting in a pattern similar to that used in the patient in Figure 19–17C followed. *B,* Same patient 13 months after his first and six months after his second session with a total of 206 (4.0 mm) grafts placed in 3.5 mm holes. Alternate spaces in each row remain to be filled in; therefore, half of his *basic* coverage in areas shown has been achieved. *C,* Same patient marked for his third session of mostly 3.5 mm holes. Eighty grafts (seventy-eight 4.0 mm and two 4.5 mm) were used to fill in the remaining gaps in the first, third, and fifth rows, especially on the left (parting) side. They were more widely spaced in the posterior area. The alternate spaces in the second, fourth, and sixth rows will require filling in to complete his *basic* coverage in the areas shown. Compare B and C with Figures 19–17B, C, and D; 19–80D; and 19–81A and B; and note similar lateral termination of the hairline with the creation of a temporal gulf.

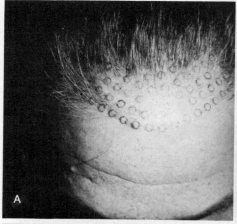

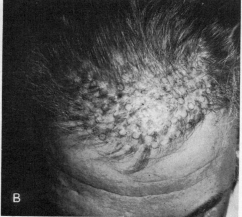

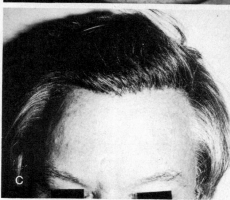

Figure 19–74. *A,* A 42-year-old man with blond hair and frontal recession and thinning caused by male pattern baldness marked for 4.0 mm recipient sites (for 4.5 mm grafts) in bald and noticeably thinned areas. (Cf. Figs. 19–19 and 19–20.) *B,* Same patient four months after the first session and two months after the second session. At the second session grafts were placed in rows staggered between the original rows, e.g., starting new second, fourth, sixth, etc. rows between those that became the first, third, fifth, etc. rows (the latter consist of grafts placed at the first session and now have hair growth). The two-month-old grafts of the second session are still "naked" and moderately erythematous. Note considerable telogen defluvium of the first session grafts in the center behind the original first two rows. (Cf. Figs. 19–67 and 19–68.) Recipient sites (4.0 mm) in the remaining spaces of the first, third, fifth, etc. rows (in which hairs are growing) have been marked. Apparent lack of circular markings in the first three spaces of the first row to the patient's right of the apex is an artifact caused by light application of gentian violet. *C,* Same patient five years after the start of grafting. At his fourth session, eight months after his first, the remaining spaces in the alternate even-numbered rows were filled in. At his fifth session four years after beginning, hairline refinement with smaller size grafts was done.

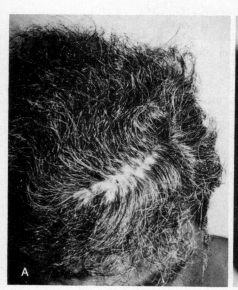

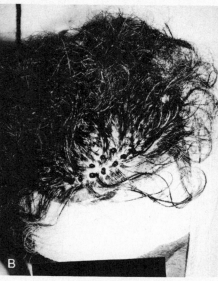

Figure 19–75. *A,* Same patient as in Figure 19–28 three years after his first session and one year after his third, with alternate spaces between grafts in the second and fourth rows deliberately exposed. *B,* Same patient and time as A, showing fourth session in progress at which 60 (4.5 mm) grafts were subsequently placed in the remaining spaces in the second, fourth, etc. rows. Most were placed in 4.0 mm circular holes, but some were fitted into ovoid and pear-shaped holes made by overlapping cuts with 3.5 and 3.0 mm punches; others were trimmed peripherally to fit 3.0 mm circular holes. Shown here are the recipient holes in the second and fourth rows *before* the grafts were placed. (See Fig. 19–96D.)

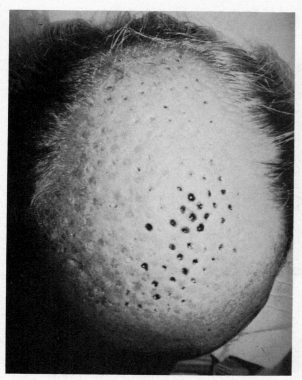

Figure 19—76. Necrosis of about 17 grafts caused by ischemia (shown after débridement) in the left-central midanterior scalp and midscalp of a 40-year-old man with extensive male pattern baldness. The photo was taken 2½ weeks after his second session consisting of 150 (4.5 mm) grafts placed in 4.25 and 4.0 mm holes over all aspects of the bald scalp but more widely spaced on the patient's right side. This followed a similar first session of 140 grafts by eight weeks. The patient, who had a wide donor area of good density (shown in Fig. 19—45), eventually achieved very satisfactory coverage (see Fig. 19—82). Nevertheless, the combination of relatively large grafts and recipient hole sizes; quite a large number of grafts at each session placed over the entire bald scalp; the spacing of the grafts that, in this case, proved to be too close together in the area of critical blood supply; and the interval of eight weeks, which would have been adequate under a different set of circumstances, all combined to create a relatively limited area of circulatory embarrassment resulting in graft devitalization and sloughing and healing with atrophic scars. The lost grafts were replaced at a subsequent session and the end result was not significantly compromised.

months) after the first two sessions, especially as the number approaches 100 or if 4.5 mm grafts are used. For a smaller number of grafts (40 or less) and/or smaller sizes, the intervals could be about six weeks.

Again, to avoid ischemia, the *posterior* margin of several rows of grafts placed in the frontal area should ideally be posteriorly concave, i.e., a crescentic outline (Figs. 19–18, 19–60A, and 19–71), rather than also placing grafts in the midanterior scalp to midscalp at the same session with resultant roughly semilunar outline (Fig. 19–63). However, depending upon the total number, a limited number of grafts could be placed more widely apart in the midscalp with safety (Figs. 19–17C and 19–59).

Filling in with Minute Grafts, Especially for Hairline Refinement

Because there will inevitably be some small spaces remaining after the four basic sessions in an area are completed, one can place grafts of appropriate size (2.5 to 4.0 mm) after waiting four to five months or more after the fourth session (thus allowing all the hairs that are going to grow to do so). These must be held gently with delicate rat-tooth forceps while being trimmed around the periphery with fine spring-handle scissors (avoiding intact follicles) and then placed into smaller-sized circular, ovoid, or irregularly shaped *recipient* holes (1.5 to 3.0 mm in diameter, respectively), which have been created in the remaining spaces. Ovoid or other shapes are achieved by overlapping circular cuts, thereby getting the optimum number of hairs into the space available without sacrificing adjacent previously grafted hairs. Thus, a 3.5 or 4.0 mm graft may be fitted (trimming peripherally as needed) into a 2.5 or 3.0 mm circular hole, a 3.0 mm graft into a 2.0 or 2.5 mm hole, and a 2.5 mm graft into a 1.5 or 2.0 mm hole. Similarly, a 3.0 or 2.5 mm graft, for example, can be placed into an ovoid hole created by two slightly overlapping circular cuts made by 2.0 or 1.5 mm punches or by a combination of the two sizes with or without peripheral trimming of the graft. Also, a 1.5 or 2.0 mm circular hole can be extended at one point by a small incision made with a no. 11 scalpel blade and/or a 16-gauge angiocath in order to accommodate a 2.5 mm graft.

It is particularly important to do this, in order to achieve relatively solid coverage at, immediately behind, and extending several rows behind the hairline and/or in the center of the whorl of the crown, especially when there is a marked color contrast (dark straight hair and light skin) (Figs. 19–12 and 19–77 to 19–80).

Variations of this hairline refinement technique include the following: (1) cutting 4.0 mm grafts longitudinally into smaller grafts containing two to four follicles each, trimming off excess fat and dermis plus the epidermis and inserting them into small scalpel stab incisions at or near the hairline (Nordstrom); (2) creating tiny two- or three-hair grafts by a longitudinal scalpel and scissors excision from the periphery of 4 mm grafts, then removing the epidermis and inserting them into randomly placed holes made by a 16-gauge angiocath a millimeter or more anterior to the previously grafted hairline (Marritt); and (3) gently removing single hairs from the periphery of 4.0 mm grafts with jeweler's forceps and inserting each hair into similarly placed holes created by an 18-gauge needle, using an electrocautery tip (without current) to dilate the hole immediately before insertion (Unger).

Thus, minute grafts of one, two, or three hairs

Text continued on page 257

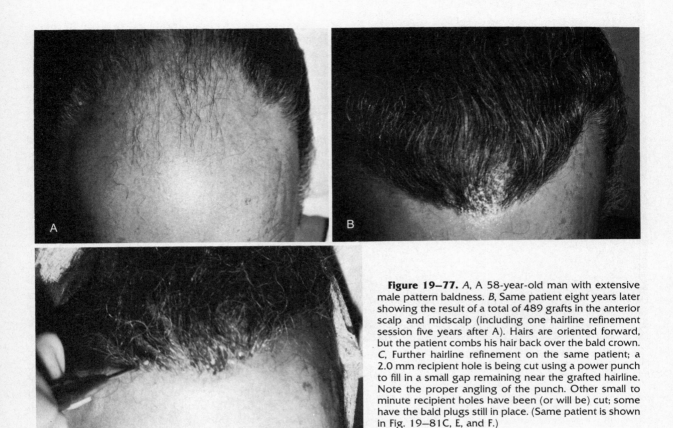

Figure 19–77. *A*, A 58-year-old man with extensive male pattern baldness. *B*, Same patient eight years later showing the result of a total of 489 grafts in the anterior scalp and midscalp (including one hairline refinement session five years after A). Hairs are oriented forward, but the patient combs his hair back over the bald crown. *C*, Further hairline refinement on the same patient; a 2.0 mm recipient hole is being cut using a power punch to fill in a small gap remaining near the grafted hairline. Note the proper angling of the punch. Other small to minute recipient holes have been (or will be) cut; some have the bald plugs still in place. (Same patient is shown in Fig. 19–81C, E, and F.)

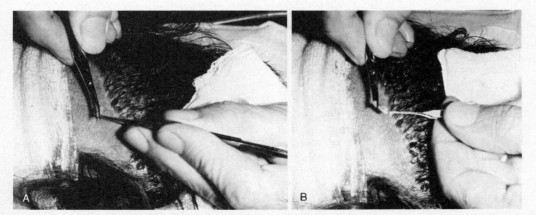

Figure 19–78. *A*, Hairline refinement: peripheral trimming of a 2.5 mm graft before placing it in a 2.0 or 1.5 mm recipient hole, using fine-pointed rat-tooth forceps and spring-handled scissors. *B*, Trimming excess subcutaneous fat from the bottom of 2.5 mm graft.

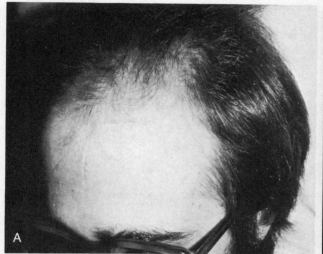

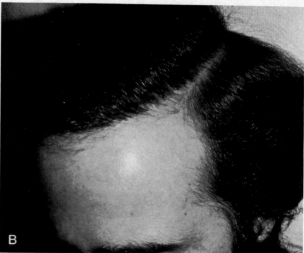

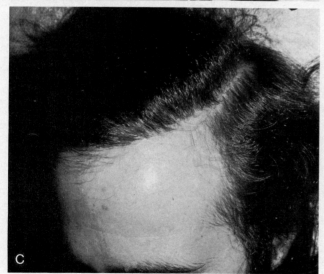

Figure 19–79. *A*, A 30-year-old man with marked and extensive thinning and recession caused by male pattern baldness. (Same patient as in Fig. 19–21.) *B*, Appearance two years and seven months later showing the result of four basic sessions with a total of 335 (4.0 mm) grafts placed in 3.5 mm holes. The first hairline refinement session followed with 59 grafts (4.0, 3.5, 3.0 and 2.5 mm) trimmed peripherally as indicated to fit into 3.5, 3.0, 2.5, and 2.0 or 1.5 mm holes, respectively. Ovoid combinations of these sizes and no. 11 scalpel incisions were used to extend the smallest size holes. The extreme left lateral hairline was extended slightly into the progressively thinning area adjacent to the fringe. *C*, Appearance 10 months later. The second hairline refinement session, which included the midanterior scalp and midscalp and emphasized the left side, followed and is shown in D, E, and F.

Illustration continued on following page

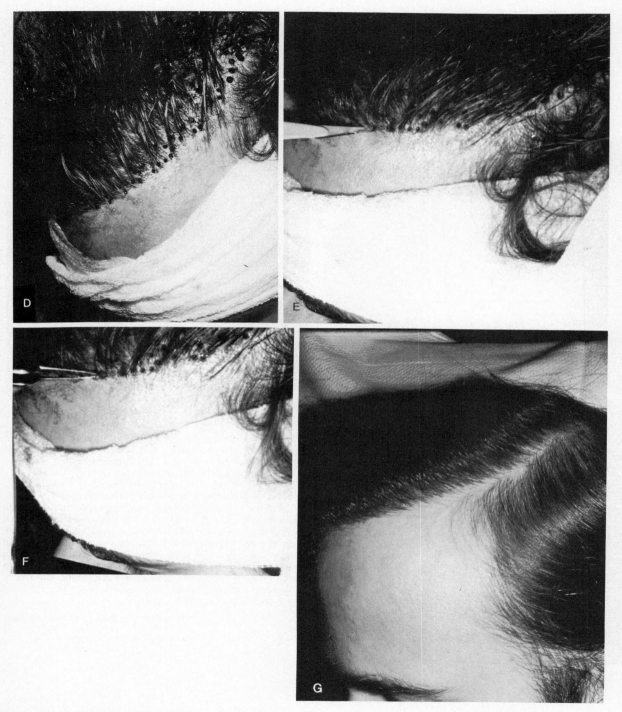

Figure 19–79 *Continued. D*, Recipient holes have been cut (3.25, 3.0, 2.5, 2.0, and 1.5 mm), including many 2.0 and 1.5 mm holes at and immediately behind the previously grafted hairline where minute spaces remained. *E*, Slight extension of a 1.5 mm hole at the hairline with a minute incision with a no. 11 scalpel blade. *F*, Placing a 2.5 mm graft that has been trimmed peripherally to fit the 1.5 mm hole in E (see Fig. 19–78A). It is grasped gently at the epidermal edge with small rat-tooth forceps. *G*, Same patient 20 months later, showing the results of the second refinement session on and behind the hairline. The photograph shows maximum exposure of the grafted hairline with lateral extension into the fringe, including a small zone of continued thinning adjacent to the upper border of the fringe. Patient is now wearing his hair parted in the center (see Fig. 19–21C and D).

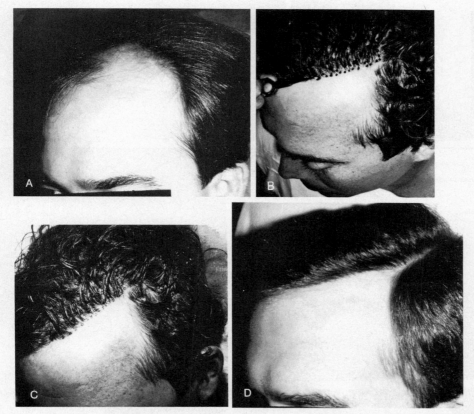

Figure 19–80. *A*, Same patient as in Figures 19–17, 19–59, and 19–70. (The old diagonal scar near the temple hairline from a previous suture loop placement for a hairpiece attachment is visible.) *B*, Same patient at his second hairline refinement session, showing mostly 2.0 and 1.5 mm recipient holes at and immediately behind the hairline. Some 1.5 and 2.0 mm holes were slightly enlarged by minute incisions with a no. 11 scalpel blade. Further behind the hairline are 3.5, 3.0, and 2.5 mm holes into which 4.0, 3.5, and 3.0 mm grafts were placed. A number of the holes are ovoid or irregular and were created by the overlapping cuts of two or more smaller sized punches in order to fill in properly the remaining minute, odd-shaped bald spaces without destroying hairs from the grafts placed at earlier sessions. Also shown is the placement of a 2.5 mm graft (peripherally trimmed as in Fig. 19–78A) into a 2.0 mm hole using fine rat-tooth forceps. (Shadow causes the hole, which is the same size as adjacent ones, to appear larger.) *C*, Same patient immediately after completing the placement of 2.5 mm grafts into 2.0 and 1.5 mm holes along and just behind the hairline. Larger sizes were used further behind the hairline. *D*, Same patient 15 months later, showing the result of the second hairline refinement session. The hairline appears quite natural despite the combination of dark straight hair and relatively light skin. Note the moderate forward angle of hair growth and moderate temporal gulf with the grafted hairline terminating at the part line. (A portion of the old hypopigmented linear suture loop scar is still barely visible there.) If desired by the patient, a *slight* lowering of the lateral portion of this conservative hairline would be acceptable.

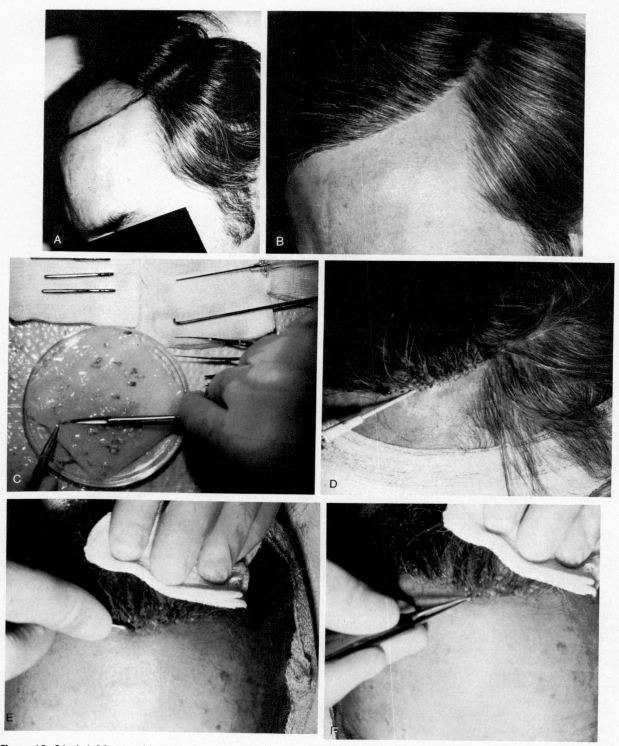

Figure 19–81. *A,* A 38-year-old man with extensive male pattern baldness after three scalp reductions and before the first anterior grafting session with preoperative hairline marked, viewed from the patient's left (parting) side. (Same patient as in Fig. 19–94; compare with Fig. 19–17B for anterior view of hairline marked with gentian violet in a similar patient.) *B,* Appearance after four basic grafting sessions in the anterior scalp (note creation of proper temporal gulf), plus grafting in the residual midscalp and crown areas, consisting mostly of 4.0 mm grafts placed in 3.5 mm holes. Minimal hypopigmented scarring along the anterior border of hairline grafts is present. (Cf. Fig. 19–6C.) *C,* Hairline refinement (same patient as in Fig. 19–77), showing creation of a one-, two-, or three-hair graft being trimmed from the periphery of a 2.5 or 3.0 mm graft (a 4.0 mm graft could also be used) with fine straight iris scissors.

Legend continued on opposite page

may be placed into a hypopigmented or scarred anterior border resulting from previous grafting (Fig. 19–81). With any of these techniques, two or more sessions are usually required for optimum refinement, preferably at intervals of 4½ or more months to allow for hair growth before proceeding. However, inserting grafts of 1, 2, or 3 hairs closely *anterior* to the grafted hairline, as distinguished from filling in small residual gaps *between* grafts at or behind the hairline, can be begun prior to the completion of basic coverage. This can be done along with the placing of regular-sized grafts, but at the end of the session in order to avoid their accidental loss.

Total Number of Grafts and Elapsed Time

The total number of grafts performed naturally depends upon both the extent of the baldness and the adequacy of the donor supply. A mild recession might require about 150 grafts, a moderately extensive frontal to midscalp baldness, 250 to 350 or more grafts (Figs. 19–2, 19–6, and 19–70), and extensive baldness, especially when involving the crown (without reduction), 500 to 600 or considerably more grafts, *if* the donor supply permits it (Figs. 19–3, 19–8, 19–12, and 19–82). Most men with male pattern baldness have enough hair in the posterior and lateral fringe to provide *at least* 300 grafts (4.0 mm) unless the donor area is very narrow and/or sparse, perhaps providing at best 150 to 200 grafts. On the other hand, some have enough for 600 or more (Figs. 19–8 and 19–82) while many are in the 400- to 500-graft range. When the supply of grafts is limited in relation to the size of the bald area, it is essential to plan the overall strategy carefully, *including scalp reduction when appropriate*, in order to place the grafts where they will do the most good and obtain maximum coverage when aided by combing or styling the hair. As stated earlier, curly or kinky hair (natural or "permed") has greater covering capacity per graft than straight hair.

It is advantageous to allow five, six, or more months to elapse after a second and/or a third session in patients with extensive baldness and relatively limited donor supply in order to evaluate the coverage being achieved and thus to utilize the remaining donor supply as effectively as possible by placing the grafts in subsequent sessions where they will achieve maximum cosmetic benefit.

Because of the time factors involved—three months of telogen, a minimum of two months between extensive grafting sessions in the same area, the need for *at least four sessions for basic full coverage in any one area*, especially with dark straight hair and light skin, (and probably a total of five, six, or more sessions if refinement with minute grafts for optimum coverage in critical areas is done), and the time required for the hair to grow to sufficient length—it is usually at least seven months to a year or more from the time grafting is started until significant cosmetic benefit is obtained and perhaps a year and a half *or more* for the final result.

CORRECTION OF UNAESTHETIC HAIRLINES

As stressed earlier (see the section, "The Frontal Hairline"), the creation of an excessively low frontal hairline, especially at the temples, must be avoided, as well as a low and sharply pointed apex with resultant biconcave or "Mephistophelean" hairline (Figs. 19–83 to 19–85). The author on numerous occasions has had to remove grafts that were placed too low on the forehead, especially at the temples, by other operators when apparently insufficient attention had been paid to aesthetic considerations.

Such low-placed hair-bearing grafts may be punched out and exchanged for bald grafts obtained from higher up (if still available). In this situation, both types of grafts are of necessity the same size. This must, of course, be done in stages if the low-placed grafts are close together. Alternatives to graft exchange are plucking, epilation, excision and suturing (which may give the best result if not too many grafts are involved), or removal of low-placed grafts, then cutting off their follicular bulbs from the undersides and replacing them. The end result

---

Figure 19–81 *Continued.* It is held by the epidermal edge with jeweler's forceps and the epidermis is then trimmed off. In addition to the 2.5 and 3.0 mm grafts, covered with normal saline on a gauze square in a Petri dish, there are a number of these tiny one-, two-, or three-hair grafts (which have already been trimmed from some of the larger grafts) located directly above the graft being trimmed. Also shown are 2.5, 2.0, and 1.5 mm power punches, a 16-gauge angiocath, an electrocautery tip, and small rat-tooth forceps. *D,* Same patient as in A and B, showing hairline refinement session at which 17 minute holes are being made with a 16-gauge angiocath immediately anterior to the grafted hairline. This was preceded by placing 4.0 and 3.5 mm grafts (minus one or two hairs) in ovoid and irregularly shaped holes made with 3.0 and 2.5 mm punches, combined with a no. 11 scalpel blade and/or 16-gauge angiocath extensions, in the small spaces remaining in the second row immediately behind the first row of earlier 4.0 mm hairline grafts. Placement of 17 one-, two-, and occasionally three-hair grafts in the 16-gauge angiocath holes followed. *E,* Dilating a 16-gauge angiocath hole with an electrocautery tip (without current) immediately before inserting a one- or two-hair graft. (Same patient as in Figs. 19–77 and 19–81C.) *F,* Same patient as in E who is having a one-, two-, or three-hair graft, which is held gently with jeweler's forceps, inserted into a 16-gauge angiocath hole immediately after dilating it with electrocautery tip.

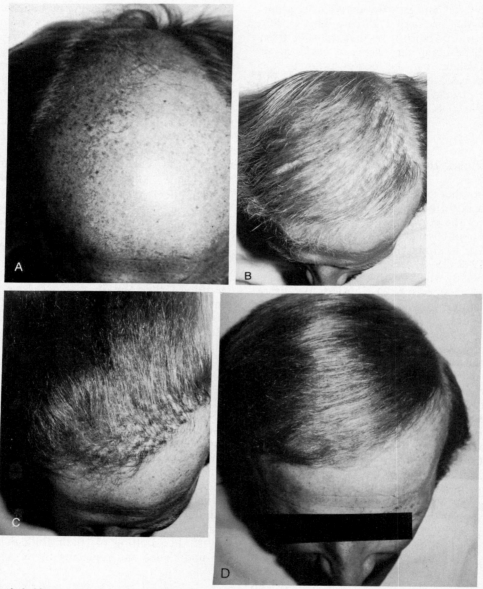

Figure 19–82. *A,* A 40-year-old man with extensive male pattern baldness and a wide fringe of generally good density, prior to the availability of scalp reduction. (Same patient as in Figs. 19–45 and 19–76.) *B,* Same patient, three months after the fifth session (12½ months after the first), showing growth from a total of 441 (4.5 mm) grafts (net) in four sessions. *C,* Same patient seven months after the sixth session (19½ months after the first), showing growth from a total of 675 grafts (mostly 4.5 mm) minus 17 grafts lost from necrosis for a net of 658. Immediately following this photograph, 100 grafts, eighty 4.5 mm and twenty 3.5 mm, were placed during the seventh session. Photograph shows that the patient is getting satisfactory coverage even with deliberate maximal exposure of the frontal hair. *D,* Same time as C, shows the enhanced cosmetic result achieved by forward and across styling that is enhanced by the camouflage of having light (bleached) blond hair and by parting the hair so that some of the uppermost left fringe is combed into the grafted hair. A year and a half later, 100 grafts (4.0, 3.5, and 3.0 mm) were placed, especially for left hairline and center of crown refinement, for a final total of 864 grafts net.

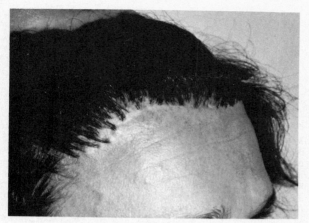

Figure 19–83. A 37-year-old man as he appeared when first (and last) seen by the author. He showed no significant degree of male pattern baldness but only a slight thinning immediately behind the grafts. He stated that although he had always had a high forehead, he had little actual thinning or recession before receiving a total of about 150 grafts in six sessions by two different operators beginning 6 years previously. The patient said that he had selected the present hairline himself and that the second operator had lowered it at the temples at his request. Shown is an excessively low, rounded temporal hairline with much depigmented atrophic and hypertrophic scarring and cobblestoning. The yield is moderate to fair to poor with many spaces, some quite wide, remaining between the grafts. Although this appears to be a particularly egregious example of the poor aesthetic judgment by an operator acceding to the patient's request (regardless of what he thought he wanted), the patient was concerned only about filling in the grafted areas to make it look more natural. He did not return.

may be improved by dermabrasion, but some scarring, usually with a degree of hypopigmentation, is inevitable. However, the result is generally still far superior to a bizarre appearing hairline (Figs. 19–86 and 19–87). A low temporal hairline can also be raised somewhat by scalp reduction, when appropriate, and a generally low hairline can be raised to some degree by a coronal incision forehead lift. Corrective measures may involve replacing all or substantial portions of many or most of the previously placed grafts when the yield is sparse to very sparse, especially when associated with depigmented scarring (Fig. 19–88).

GRAFTING IN BLACK PATIENTS

Hair transplantation in black patients can be effective, although the inherent density of the donor area is usually relatively sparse and often very sparse. However, this is at least partially compensated for by the excellent covering capacity of kinky hair as well as by the natural camouflage provided by dark hair and dark skin. Because of the spiral configuration of the follicles, there is, however, a greater loss of follicles at the periphery of the graft as it is cut than with relatively straight hair. There-

fore, using 4.25 or 4.5 mm grafts would be appropriate. Pierce, who has a large experience in performing hair transplantation on black patients, has indicated that keloid formation has not been a problem. However, as stated earlier, if any particular individual of any race gives a history of or shows evidence of keloid or hypertrophic scar formation, it would seem wise to perform only a small number of grafts (which would then serve as a test of both donor and recipient sites) followed by three or more months' observation before proceeding with more extensive grafting. In fact, the presence of true keloids, as opposed to hypertrophic scars, would very likely constitute an absolute contraindication or at least call for the greatest caution.

CONCLUSIONS

The punch-grafting technique of hair transplantation has stood the test of time, confirming Orentreich's premise of donor dominance in male pattern baldness as the rationale for the procedure. The patient can thus be reassured with a very high degree of confidence, based on extensive experience over more than 25 years of observation, that the grafted hair will be retained indefinitely in its new location, *provided* that it is obtained from scalp donor areas

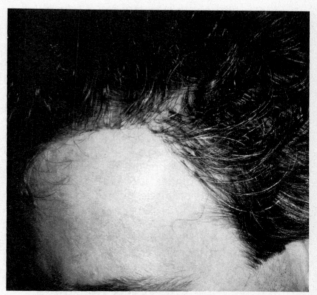

Figure 19–84. A 35-year-old man, as he appeared when first seen by the author after having a total of 105 grafts in three sessions, starting at age 23, by another operator. The patient stated that another physician had refused to do hair transplantation when the patient was 21 years old and that he had minimal temporal recession when grafting was started at the patient's insistence. The low rounded temporal hairline might have been acceptable (when completed) for a woman, but will become, if not corrected or hidden by hair styling, increasingly inappropriate as this patient becomes older.

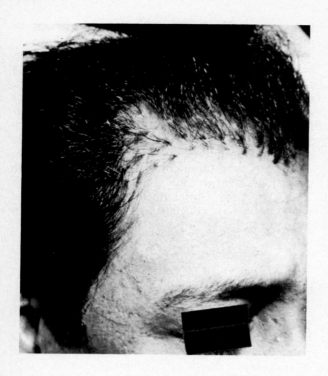

Figure 19–85. A 32-year-old man as he appeared when first seen by the author after having 60 punch grafts 1 ½ years before by another operator. This excessively sharp apex and low, rounded temporal hairline illustrates a biconcave or "Mephistophelean" hairline. The spaces between the grafts had not been filled in, which accentuated the tufted appearance made even more evident because of the patient's black hair. In addition, the grafts are generally spaced more than a graft (or recipient site) width apart in all directions, and the yield varies from excellent in a few to fair or sparse in most.

not genetically "programmed" to develop male pattern baldness. Of course, the patient actually has no more hair than before the procedure—in fact, perhaps somewhat less, depending upon the quality of the operative technique. However, the hair has been redistributed by permanently "borrowing" it from areas that can spare it and placing it where most needed to create a very effective illusion (if done properly) of having more hair. It can be combed, brushed, shampooed, or even pulled as well as dyed, tinted, bleached, permed, or straightened, and otherwise treated just as though it had been there all the time.

In properly selected patients, if performed with good aesthetic judgment and meticulous attention to detail (aided when appropriate by scalp reduction), punch grafting continues to be a highly effective procedure for the cosmetic improvement of male pattern baldness and certain other types of permanent hair loss. Its morale-boosting effect, resulting from an improved self-image, at least equals that after any other type of cosmetic surgery.

OTHER INDICATIONS FOR THE PUNCH GRAFT METHOD

Female Pattern Baldness

Those women (and occasionally men) who have extensive *diffuse* thinning of the scalp hair, in whom there is little or no area of essentially normal density to serve as a donor site, are obviously not amenable

to this procedure. However, some women with marked thinning in the frontal-temporal region or midscalp and crown (frequently with preservation of a frontal hairline margin) but retaining relatively normal hair density in the posterior (and sometimes lateral) scalp may benefit from grafting just as men with marked thinning due to male pattern baldness (Fig. 19–89). Naturally, the same criteria of donor supply vis-à-vis the size of the area of thinning are equally applicable. Frequently, there is only a very limited area of normal density in the midposterior scalp with sparse hair on the posterolateral and lateral fringe areas, so that the donor supply is grossly inadequate for the area of thinning. Because the more sharply defined patterned hair loss (and corresponding fringe area retention) commonly seen in men is rarely present in women, one cannot have the same degree of confidence in the permanence of the procedure in women as in men, although it is a reasonable assumption that an analogous mechanism is involved. However, placing grafts of fair to poor density (which may become even sparser in the future) in a large area of moderate to considerable thinning may result in an actual net loss of hair because of the resulting acceleration of hair loss frequently seen in the recipient area (see the section, "Selection of Patients").

Scars and Other Alopecias

Other scalp conditions that may lend themselves to punch grafting are: permanent localized alopecia

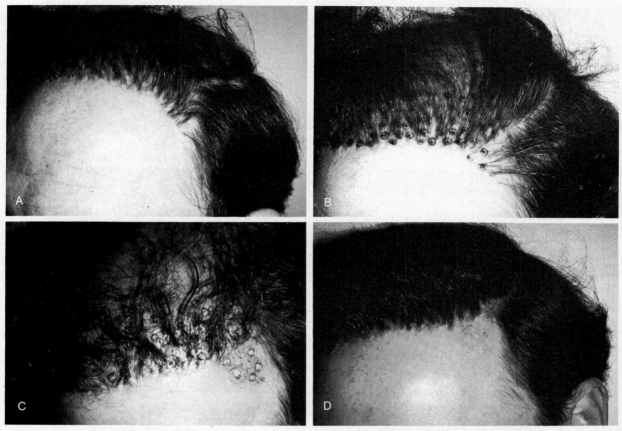

Figure 19–86. *A,* A 34-year-old man with extensive male pattern baldness as he appeared when first seen by the author. He had 85 grafts in two sessions (mostly 5.0 mm) placed seven years before and another 85 grafts in two sessions (also 5.0 mm) one year before. The temporal hairline is excessively low bilaterally. The grafts are oriented so that the hairs are pointing posteriorly in most of the grafts instead of pointing anteriorly as they should. The yield is highly variable, from good to fair to sparse to very sparse. There is hypopigmentation and scarring. *B,* Same patient at his first remedial grafting session, with preoperative recipient sites marked (mostly 3.5 mm for placement of 69 (4.0 mm) grafts). Sites of three low-placed, hair-bearing temporal grafts have also been marked, and their hairs have been cut short before exchanging them for bald grafts from recipient sites higher up. *C,* Appearance two months later. The second grafting session (of 69 (4.0 mm) grafts) is in progress and at the same time five additional bald plugs having been exchanged for five more low-placed hair-bearing grafts in the left temple. *D,* Appearance nine months later. The restoration of a proper temporal gulf has been largely accomplished, although some scarring is inevitable. Additional low-placed temporal grafts must still be removed and exchanged, including at least one adjacent to present hairline. Additional filling in with 4.0 mm grafts at and behind the hairline followed and hairline refinement with smaller grafts was begun. Because of the posteriorly slanting orientation of most of the original grafts on this patient, it was necessary to place fill-in grafts at the same angle in order to avoid the destruction of adjacent, previously grafted follicles, instead of the preferred, more natural-appearing, anterior angling.

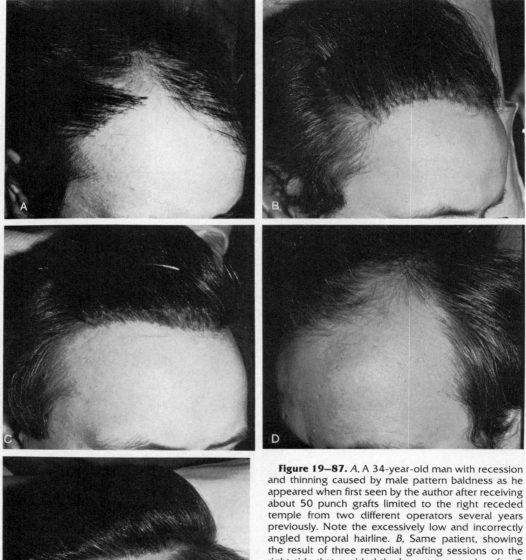

Figure 19–87. *A,* A 34-year-old man with recession and thinning caused by male pattern baldness as he appeared when first seen by the author after receiving about 50 punch grafts limited to the right receded temple from two different operators several years previously. Note the excessively low and incorrectly angled temporal hairline. *B,* Same patient, showing the result of three remedial grafting sessions on the right side that avoided the lowest temporal grafts. *C,* Same patient, showing the result of further grafting plus excision and suturing of the four lowest grafts on the right temple. Some of the previously placed grafts with sparse yield and some scarring (see A and B) were left intact immediately below the reconstructed hairline, which is usually not exposed because the patient combs his hair forward and across from the left (parting) side. *D,* Same patient, left side, as he appeared when first seen by the author. *E,* Same patient showing the result of extensive grafting on the left side and center, including one hairline refinement session. Note the creation of a proper temporal gulf with the grafted hairline terminating at the part and correct forward angling of grafted hairs (compare with A).

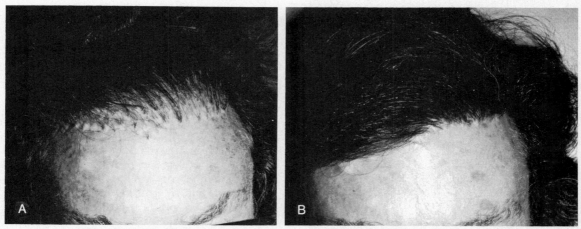

Figure 19–88. *A,* A 51-year-old man with fair, ruddy, and heavily sun-exposed skin as he appeared when first seen by the author after receiving about 80 to 100 grafts in two sessions about 1½ years before by another operator. All of the grafts are completely depigmented. Note also the depigmented areas on the right forehead, sites of past superficial removal of (presumably) actinic keratoses. Most of the grafts show a yield from sparse to nil and considerable scarring and cobblestoning. Donor area has moderate to fair density in the upper portion and sparse to very sparse density in the lower portion. *Donor* site scars, which are not hypertrophic, are mainly in the areas of moderate density, some from sparse areas. Patient states that he originally had a coronal incision brow (forehead) lift that resulted in a hairline (which was not significantly balding) being "too high." He then had punch grafting, which patient considered "a mess." *B,* Same patient 1½ years later showing the result of 222 grafts, mostly 4.0 mm, placed in 3.5 mm holes during three sessions. The hairline is exposed on the left side, but covered by styling on the right. A fourth session followed, including a substantial number of smaller sized grafts for hairline refinement—especially desirable because of the marked depigmented scarring resulting from the grafting done previously. Note the excellent yield and lack of scarring from the grafts placed in the last three sessions. A few grafts were also placed each time in the temporal portions of the relatively wide linear coronal incision scars (not shown). Conclusion: For the most part, the poor yield of hairs in many to most of the grafts placed by the previous operator was apparently caused by faulty technique. Poor selection of donor sites for some of the grafts also contributed to a minor extent, but in view of the result from remedial grafting, there was no scarring diathesis.

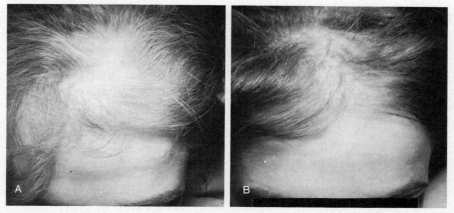

Figure 19–89. *A,* A 41-year-old woman with female pattern baldness characterized by marked frontal thinning over a limited area (of many years' duration) but with fairly good retention of the frontal hairline, moderate thinning of much of the scalp, and relatively good density in the lower posterior scalp. Patient has a rather strong family history of male pattern baldness (her father had moderate thinning; her maternal grandfather and uncle had marked male pattern baldness, but her mother and sister did not have thinning). *B,* Same patient 22 months after 15 grafts and 18 months after 25 grafts were placed in the thin frontal area. After 3½ years the grafts continued to grow hair, but the thinning process also continued in adjacent areas.

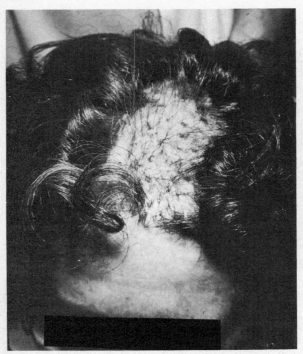

Figure 19–90. A 58-year-old woman with a large markedly atrophic thermal burn scar of the anterior scalp of many years' duration, showing the result of placing a total of 59 (4.0 mm) grafts, beginning 4½ years previously, throughout the scarred area. The yield is good in the grafts at periphery of the scars, especially along the frontal hairline but relatively sparse to very sparse in those more centrally placed, presumably because of poor vascularity. Additional grafting is obviously needed and should progress in stages from the periphery toward the center of the scar.

due to burns; radiation, surgical, laceration, or avulsion scars; and scars resulting from *burned-out* (*not* active) scarring diseases such as kerion, chronic discoid lupus erythematosus, and Romberg's disease (facial hemiatrophy or scleroderma en coup de sabre). With such atrophic scarring, especially if extensive, the poor vascularity in contrast to that in male pattern baldness presumably accounts for the observations by this author and others that, although the grafts take, the yield in terms of number of hairs per graft is relatively poor and sometimes very poor, especially in central portions of the scar, whereas it may be adequate at the periphery. Therefore, unless test grafting indicates otherwise, grafting should proceed stepwise from the periphery toward the center so that the better vascular supply at the periphery can supply the initial grafts. Their improved vascularity, in turn, can supply those grafts placed more centrally and so on (Figs. 19–90 and 19–91).

Additional indications include non–hair-bearing grafts used to repair trauma to the scalp, permanent traction alopecia, absence or marked thinning of the hair of the lateral temples and sideburns (with or without scarring) following a face lift (Fig. 19–92) or occurring as an inherent trait, and localized congenital alopecia (Fig. 19–93). Partial or complete loss of eyebrows, including loss from trauma and from Hansen's disease, may also be amenable.

With thin, atrophic scars or split-thickness grafts, it is necessary either to cut the recipient holes at a very acute angle or alternatively to cut them vertically, after which the grafts may be inserted nearly horizontally into a recipient pocket created by undermining (Fig. 19–91). For sideburns and low lateral temple areas, the grafts should be placed at an acute angle so that hair growth will be sharply downward (Fig. 19–92) and, for eyebrows, sharply laterally. Of course, eyebrows created from scalp hair will require trimming at regular intervals.

Although punch grafting has been reported to have been successfully used in a persistent site of alopecia areata, the very nature of this condition with its unpredictable recurrences and spontaneous regrowths would make this condition, in general, a rather dubious indication, in the author's opinion.

OTHER SURGICAL TECHNIQUES FOR MALE PATTERN BALDNESS

Scalp Reduction—A Valuable Adjunct to Hair Transplantation

The relatively recently (1977) developed scalp reduction procedure in which portions of the bald crown (and frequently midscalp) are excised with extensive undermining in the subgaleal plane, is, when properly performed, a highly useful adjunct to hair transplantation in patients with adequate scalp mobility. By reducing the size of the bald area, sometimes dramatically, the available donor supply is thereby extended, enabling it to be concentrated in the frontal scalp and providing more definitive coverage in individuals with moderately extensive male pattern baldness. These patients would formerly have been considered to be poor or borderline candidates for grafting because of an unfavorable ratio of donor supply to area of baldness.

Various excision patterns are used—midline ellipse, single- or double-Y, etc. (see Chapter 20, "Scalp Reductions")—in which up to 4 cm, sometimes more, may be excised at one procedure. This may be done two, three, or more times with a significantly large amount of bald skin eventually removed. Punch grafting can then be used to cover the remaining bald area, including the resultant excision scars, to the extent that the remaining donor supply allows. Reduction can precede (Fig. 19–94), follow (Fig. 19–95), or be done in alternation with punch grafting sessions in the frontal scalp.

If hair transplantation of the frontal hairline precedes reduction, the latter may result in an elevation

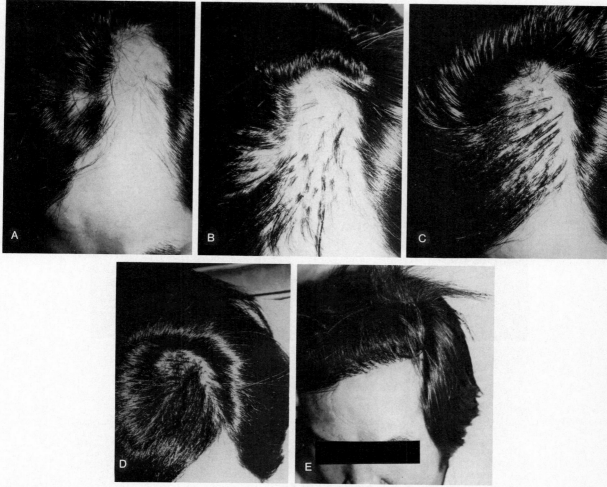

Figure 19–91. *A,* A 25-year-old man with facial hemiatrophy present since early childhood. Markedly atrophic skin in a vertical linear pattern involves the left frontal scalp and midscalp and extends down across the forehead and on the left side of the nose. Multiple medical grade silicone injections into the forehead area had been done by another physician with apparently considerable cosmetic improvement. After a test of 10 grafts placed near the hairline was successful, 30 (4.5 mm) grafts were placed in 4.0 mm holes throughout the scarred area. Where the skin was very thin, it was necessary to place grafts at an acute angle into the shallow undermined holes, but graft elevation was still unavoidable. *B,* Appearance five months after the session of thirty grafts showing good to moderate yield in most grafts but sparser growth from the posteriorly placed grafts. Forty grafts were then placed. *C,* Appearance six months later. The posterior portion continues to lag with sparser yield of grafts. Overall yield is good, however, and 40 more grafts were then placed. *D,* Appearance six months after an additional session of 75 grafts. *E,* Appearance three years after beginning (aside from test) showing the result of two further sessions of 82 and 80 grafts for a total of 357. Following this photograph 31 grafts were placed at and near the hairline. The majority of all the grafts used were 4.5 mm, but the later sessions included 4.0, 3.5, and 3.0 mm grafts trimmed and fitted into recipient holes of appropriately smaller sizes and shapes (including ovoid) at and immediately behind the hairline. Any gaps between grafts are especially noticeable in a patient with black straight hair and relatively light skin when the hairline is deliberately exposed.

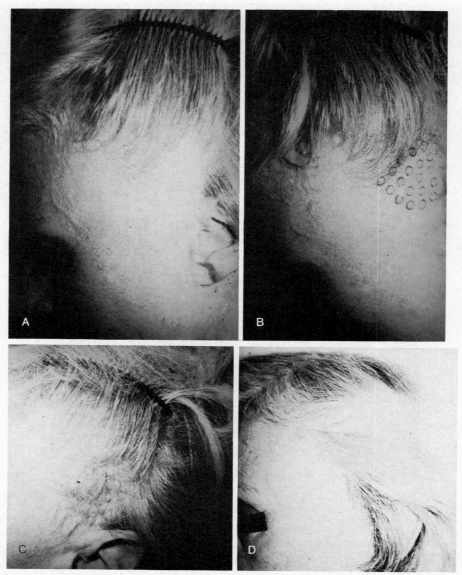

Figure 19–92. *A*, A woman, about 50 years of age, with loss of sideburns and temporal scalp hair above and anterior to the ears following a face lift. The incision scar is at posterior margin of the bald area and extends down immediately anterior to the ear. *B*, Same patient immediately after placing 19 (4.5 mm) grafts into 4.0 mm recipient holes in the area of alopecia, keeping the anterior and inferior margins of the grafted area relatively high. The grafts are angled so that hair growth will be directed rather sharply inferiorly. *C*, Growth is starting from the first session grafts and "naked" erythematous grafts from the second session are visible. *D*, Appearance two years after beginning grafting (four sessions). Note the correct downward direction of hair growth.

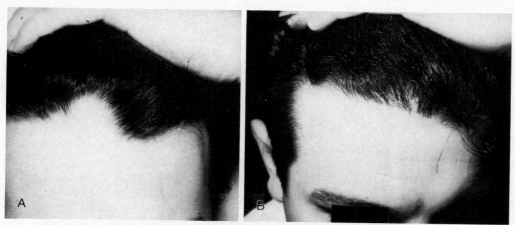

Figure 19–93. *A,* A 23-year-old man with a localized area of alopecia at the right frontal hairline present since birth. Of incidental interest is that his hair at the frontal hairline in this area slants posteriorly and posterolaterally, an uncommon orientation, in contrast to the usual anterior direction of hair growth. *B,* Appearance one year after beginning punch grafting. A total of only 33 grafts were placed in four sessions, mainly 4.0 mm grafts in 3.5 mm holes with several trimmed peripherally to fit 3.0 mm circular and smaller ovoid holes. Additional grafting is clearly needed to fill in the remaining small gaps evident when the hairline is critically exposed, as in this photograph. Hairline refinement is especially desirable here because of the color contrast between skin and hair and because the grafts had to be oriented with hairs slanting posteriorly in order to align them with his existing hair.

of the temporal hairline creating more recession than originally planned. This may be anticipated by: (1) initially creating a temporal hairline *slightly* lower than desired in anticipation of its being subsequently elevated by the reduction(s); (2) minimizing temporal hairline elevation by proper design of the reduction pattern (using an anterior-Y component as well as a posterior, i.e., a double-Y design); (3) lowering the temporal hairline by placing additional punch grafts to correct excessive elevation, if required, after reduction has been completed; or (4) a combination of these elements. Conversely, a previously grafted temporal hairline that is somewhat too low may be elevated moderately and thus made more aesthetically acceptable by a midline ellipse reduction pattern extending fairly far anteriorly.

Repeated reduction procedures may cause some thinning of the hair in the lateral and anterolateral fringe, especially the upper portion, which might cause a significant lowering of hair density and hence of hair yield in grafts obtained from those areas in patients with only fair to marginal density to begin with. In such cases, grafts should be taken from these areas either before or perhaps after only one reduction rather than after two or three. In patients with good or moderate density in the lateral fringe and in the posterior and posterolateral donor areas, where less stretching is likely to occur even from repeated reductions, the degree of thinning produced is probably not significant.

The trauma of the surgery may induce a three-month telogen defluvium adjacent to the excision following scalp reduction, so that, when multiple reductions are done, the upper margins of the lateral fringe are approached with successive reductions.

Especially in patients with an ill-defined transition between the thinning crown and fringe hair, it is, therefore, important to wait four or more months, if the advisibility of another reduction procedure is doubtful.

Patients, who have had a limited number of punch grafts placed on the crown and/or midscalp in the past as well as a substantial number placed anteriorly and who have only a limited donor supply remaining, may greatly benefit from retransplanting crown and midscalp grafts to suitable areas, such as the frontal scalp, for filling in and thus achieving a more definitive coverage. Careful attention must be paid to proper angle and depth when cutting and removing the grafts in order to avoid sacrificing follicles. Then reductions can be performed subsequently using the remaining donor supply for coverage of the residual bald areas and scars remaining after reduction (Fig. 19–96). Retransplantation and reduction can also be combined in a single procedure.

In some patients who have previously had a large amount of grafting over the crown but who have experienced progressive thinning in areas that are peripheral to the crown grafts, reductions can be done in the posterior and lateral crown and/or midscalp, thus, conserving the donor supply. In some of these patients, a prior retransplantation of a limited number of somewhat scattered grafts on the periphery of a more densely grafted central crown area may make it possible to perform a much more efficient reduction of the peripheral bald or markedly thinned crown than would otherwise be possible.

A recent innovation by Unger is the creation of rows consisting of several 4.5 or 5.0 mm punch holes, 2 to 3 mm apart in each row, in bald sites

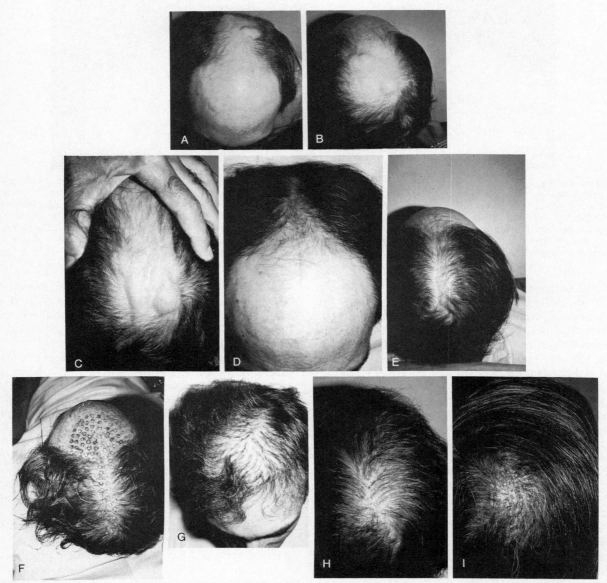

Figure 19–94. *A* and *B,* A 38-year-old man with extensive male pattern baldness. Multiple large recurrent epidermal or sebaceous cysts are present. Donor area varies from moderate density in the upper fringe to sparse in the lower and especially lower lateral region. *C,* Same patient demonstrating marked scalp laxity or mobility. *D* and *E,* Appearance after three scalp reductions using a midline ellipse with a posterior-Y pattern and removal of cysts (performed by Drs. T. G. Mayer and R. W. Fleming). Note the marked reduction in size of bald crown and much less, though significant, reduction of midscalp. *F,* Same patient showing placement of 92 (4.0 mm) grafts in 3.5 mm holes in the midscalp (more widely spaced on right) and the residual bald crown adjacent to and within the reduction scar. Photo was taken five weeks after placing 89 (4.0 mm) grafts that established four rows in the anterior scalp (six weeks after the third reduction). *G* and *H,* Appearance 8½ months after beginning grafting showing the results of one additional similar session in each area. H shows a developing whorl pattern in the residual crown. (Frontal area is at top of the photograph in H and I.) *I,* Appearance four months after 40 additional grafts were placed in the crown (i.e., only one month of hair growth from this session). The whorl pattern continues to be manifested. (See Fig. 19–81A and B for anterolateral views of the same patient, showing the result of four grafting sessions in the anterior scalp.)

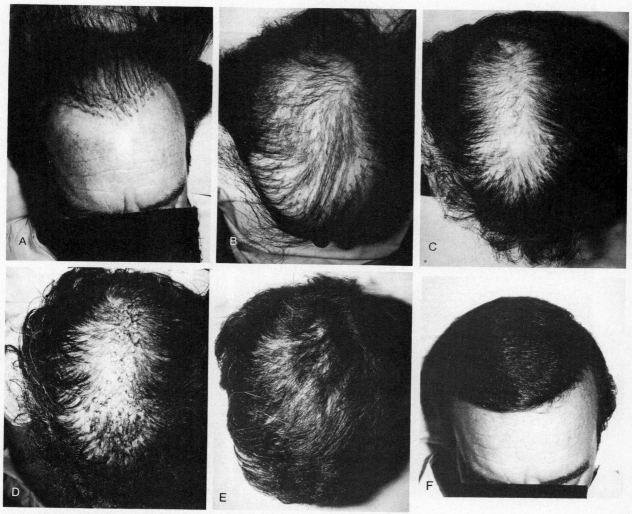

Figure 19–95. *A* and *B*, A 46-year-old man with extensive male pattern baldness as he appeared when first seen by the author. About 60 grafts in three rows had been placed three years before by another operator with moderate to fair yield in some and sparse to very sparse yield in many grafts. The crown had good mobility. The author then placed 229 (4.0 mm) grafts into 3.5 mm recipient holes in the frontal area during three sessions over 5½ months. (Frontal area is at bottom of the photograph in B to E.) *C*, Appearance 15 months after beginning frontal grafting and two months after a third scalp reduction (an anterior- and posterior-Y pattern performed by Drs. T. G. Mayer and R. W. Fleming). Note the good yield of hairs per graft and the substantial reduction in size of bald crown and midscalp. *D*, Appearance immediately after 88 (4.0 mm) grafts were placed by the author into 3.5 mm holes mainly in the residual bald crown and midscalp, including the reduction scar, with some placed behind left hairline. Seven months later 71 (4.0 mm) grafts were placed in 3.5 mm holes in the crown and midscalp. *E*, Appearance 5½ months later showing coverage achieved with grafted hair *only*. (There is *no* styling of left fringe hair across top of scalp to enhance coverage in E or F.) An additional 62 grafts to the crown, midscalp, and frontal scalp followed as well as hairline refinement with small to minute grafts. *F*, Appearance five months later showing the results of a total of 450 grafts by the author. A similar session of 78 grafts followed.

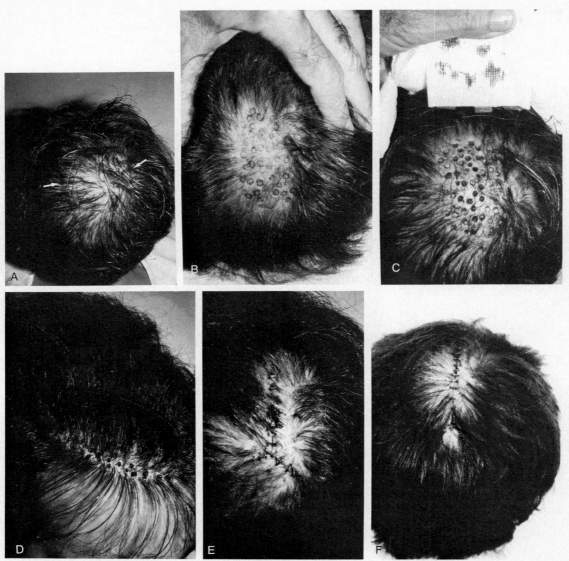

Figure 19–96. *A,* A 26-year-old man who had a total of 360 grafts placed in the anterior scalp and crown by another operator one to two years previously. The anterior scalp (not shown) was in need of hairline refinement, which was begun, but the patient was especially concerned about progressive thinning over the crown in view of his limited remaining donor supply. The problem in both areas was intensified by his having dark, straight hair and light skin. The photograph shows a moderately thin crown caused by male pattern baldness with a considerable number of the previous operator's punch grafts of variable yield. (Frontal area is at top of the photograph in A to F.) Prospective eventual reduction pattern has been indicated by arrows. *B,* Same patient with hair clipped short and 61 grafts within 4 cm wide area on crown marked for retransplantation. Limited scalp mobility is being demonstrated, compared to the marked mobility in Figure 19–94C. *C,* Same patient after punch excision of 61 grafts (most 4.0 mm, some 3.5 mm, and a few 3.0 mm) and followed by retransplanting 55 (six were not usable) to the anterior scalp. Bald plugs obtained from the creation of some of the recipient holes have been placed in donor holes closest to prospective reduction incision lines (and elsewhere for hemostasis). *D,* The same patient's recipient sites immediately behind the right and central anterior grafted hairline (patient parts hair on his right) where the author performed a hairline refinement session six months before. Retransplanted grafts were trimmed peripherally as required to fit the circular and ovoid holes made by 3.5, 3.0, 2.5, 2.0, and 1.5 mm punches. (See Figs. 19–75, 19–77, 19–79, and 19–80.) *E,* Appearance one day after a double-Y pattern scalp reduction was performed by Drs. R. W. Fleming and T. G. Mayer and 19 days after the retransplantation was performed by the author. All of the punch excision sites on the crown (except two or three) were included in the reduction excision. *F,* Appearance one day after the second reduction (four months after the first) and 17 days after a second retransplantation session at which 22 out of 29 removed crown grafts were usable and placed in the right anterior scalp near the hairline, as before. When the patient was seen eight months later, it was decided that further retransplantation and reduction were not indicated because of the tightness of his scalp, but rather additional punch grafting in the markedly reduced area of residual crown thinning, where some of the original grafts remain, was performed. (Courtesy of Drs. R. W. Fleming and T. G. Mayer.)

remaining between rows of grafts in areas previously partially transplanted. The skin bridges are then cut, and an interdigitated closure is done without undermining as in the donor area. This *mini reduction* or punch reduction results in previously placed grafts being brought closer together to produce better coverage without additional grafting, and thus it conserves a limited donor supply for use in more critical areas. It can be done concomitantly with punch grafting at a different site (Fig. 19–97).

The author has also used it either concomitantly with grafting or as an independent procedure: (1) to achieve additional benefit even after repeated conventional reductions when the remaining donor supply is severely limited, provided that the residual bald or thinning crown is not too tight (Fig. 19–98); (2) in patients who are suitable for but reluctant to have conventional reductions; (3) in lieu of retransplanting large numbers of crown grafts followed by conventional reductions in cases where a substantial amount of bald skin still remains between the grafts; and (4) to perform, in effect, a mini Z-plasty on linear scars following reduction in the posterior crown, including the midline and/or posterior branches of a Y-excision, provided there is not already considerable tension on the scar in which case it will spread again. As in punch grafting, the author has observed that a three-month telogen defluvium may occur in previously placed grafts adjacent to the mini reductions.

Because of the distorted proportions between the residual crown and the fringe after multiple scalp reductions, the ability to create a whorl pattern by punch grafting may be severely limited, but it can be attempted in some cases (Fig. 19–94). Because of the divergent directions of hair growth in the opposing fringes (depending upon the reduction pattern used), the angling of recipient holes and hence of eventual hair growth may have to be modified as required in order to avoid destruction of follicular bulbs. Grafts should be placed in the reduction scar as well as in residual bald or thinning crown remaining after reduction. Because of these aesthetic considerations, maximum reduction of the crown is not necessarily desirable, even if achievable, if it prevents the proper placement of grafts in these locations in order to achieve the most natural appearance possible. Fleming and Mayer prefer a conventional Z-plasty to correct this distortion.

Fusiform and Square Grafts

One variant of the punch graft technique is the use of fusiform grafts in place of circular or ovoid (when trimmed) grafts. Nataf excises fusiform grafts, 25 to 30 mm in length by 4 to 5 mm in width and inserts them into incisions in the recipient sites and closes the donor sites with sutures. He may later excise bald skin remaining between the rows of grafts. Although he claims that it is possible to attain more hairs per square centimeter than with punch grafts, he does not discuss the use of small peripherally trimmed punch grafts for achieving optimal density in aesthetically critical areas, such as the hairline and adjacent areas, as described by the author in this chapter.

Another variant is the removal of a strip of donor skin, which is cut into sections, so that each resulting graft is square or rectangular instead of circular thus producing a more even frontal hairline than is possible with circular punches. However, the author does not consider that to be an advantage but rather a disadvantage and prefers the *subtle* irregularity obtainable with circular punches, including minute grafts, when used properly.

Strip Grafts

The use of free strip grafts has long been advocated by some, but it is apparently difficult to create the slight irregularities and thus the more natural effects possible with properly performed punch grafting. In a number of examples of the strip graft technique observed by the author, there was a rather marked tendency toward elevation of the grafts, and only the central third of the width of the grafts was bearing hair (both lateral thirds were devoid of hair). This is evidently due to the technical difficulty in adequately controlling the angle of cutting when a long scalpel incision is made, thus resulting in two thirds of the width of the graft being without viable hair follicles (however, see Chapter 22, "The Strip Scalp Graft," for refinement of technique). In other instances, there were a number of sizable areas in the strip grafts totally devoid of hair that required punch grafts to fill them in (Fig. 19–99). However, with careful technique and good aesthetic judgment, strip grafts may be a feasible alternative to punch grafting in some instances, although this author does not use them. Some operators have combined punch grafts with strip grafts.

Flaps

Flaps, whether delayed rotation (Juri type), nondelayed bitemporal, or other types—*if* done with proper attention to aesthetic considerations and with surgical skill—can be an acceptable alternative to punch grafting in some patients with male pattern baldness. Because telogen defluvium does not usually occur (although it may occur in the distal portion of a flap), the patient receives "instant hair," at least in a limited area. Flaps involve considerably more radical surgery than punch grafting and consequently a substantially higher risk of untoward

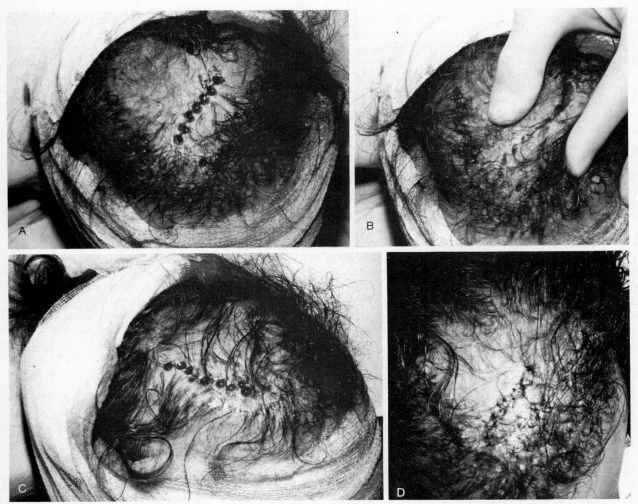

Figure 19–97. *A,* Mini or punch reduction being performed on a 40-year-old man with extensive male pattern baldness and limited remaining donor supply. Patient's forehead is at the bottom of all the photographs. He had 200 grafts placed in the anterior scalp by another operator 17 years previously, which resulted in a highly variable yield of many sparse to very sparse grafts. Five months before the author had placed 71 (4.0 mm) grafts, most in 3.5 mm holes mainly on the left (parting) side and on the central anterior and midanterior scalp, that resulted in a good yield of hairs per graft. Between and adjacent to previously placed grafts in the central bald midanterior scalp is a row of 7 (4.5 mm) holes resulting from punch removal of bald plugs of skin at about 2 mm intervals. The skin bridges separating the holes were then cut. Fifty-one recipient site holes (mostly 3.5 mm for 4.25 mm grafts) between previous grafts in the anterior scalp (mainly left and center with some on the right) were also cut, but bald plugs are still mostly in place, pending completion of the mini reduction. *B,* Demonstrating interdigitation before the sutured closure. *C,* A somewhat irregular row of nine punch excisions of bald skin between old grafts in the right anterior scalp, consisting mostly of 4.5 mm with some circular and ovoid (overlapping) 3.5 mm holes placed to avoid damaging existing hairs that are shown prior to cutting skin bridges. *D,* Appearance after completing two interdigitated closures (using 4-0 Prolene interrupted sutures) totaling 16 punch excisions of bald skin shown in A, B, and C (mini or punch reductions), thereby conserving the patient's limited remaining donor supply for use in the most critical areas—his left and central anterior scalp. Narrow zigzag scars resulted at the mini reduction sites when the patient was seen six months later, at which time 68 grafts (mostly 4.25 mm) were placed.

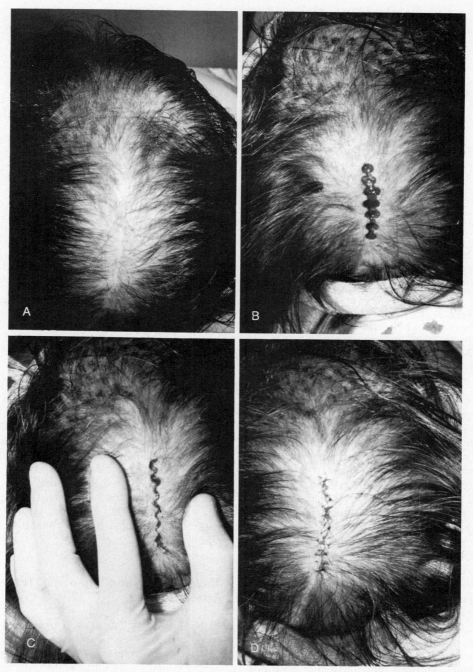

Figure 19–98. *A,* A 48-year-old man with extensive male pattern baldness who had previous punch grafting by another operator in the anterior scalp and, more recently, remedial grafting and hairline revision by the author. He also had two scalp reductions, and the residual bald scalp is now too tight to warrant further conventional reduction 8½ months after the second one. Because of his limited remaining donor supply, the author previously performed a mini reduction in the midanterior scalp (a total of ten 4.5 mm bald plug excisions in four rows) concomitantly with anterior punch grafting, which resulted in narrow zigzag scars. Patient's frontal area is at the top of all the photographs. *B,* Same patient beginning the mini or punch reduction with seven 4.5 mm punch excisions (later extended to eight) in the bald midcrown and the midline reduction scar with connecting skin bridges cut. *C,* Same patient demonstrating interdigitation prior to closure. *D,* Same patient with closure completed and the resulting modest additional scalp reduction. Also shown in B, C, and D are gentian violet markings for the recipient sites of 52 (4.0 mm) grafts that were subsequently placed in mostly 3.25 mm holes in the anterior scalp and midscalp. When the patient was seen four months later, there was some spreading of the mini reduction scar in the crown, the area where the scalp was the tightest. Therefore, punch grafting was begun in that area, as no further attempt at reduction was deemed advisable there.

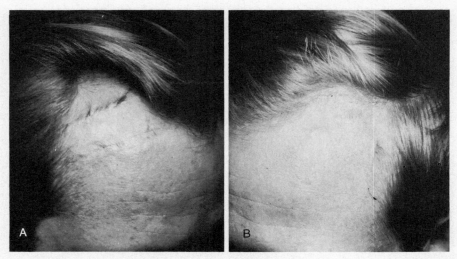

Figure 19—99. *A* and *B*, A 26-year-old man as he appeared when first seen by the author after having strip grafts placed in the frontal-temporal areas by another operator. Note the poor yield in relation to the width of the grafts, which are largely "naked" and also quite elevated. Hairs are oriented in opposite directions in the two grafts on the patient's right. Most important is the placement and especially the incorrect angling of these grafts, the lower one being much too low on the forehead at its lateral end, thus creating an aesthetically unacceptable hairline, even if it were successful in other respects. The vertically oriented strip grafts should not have been placed medial to the left temporal "point" in B. At least the lateral portion (and preferably all) of the lower graft on the patient's right should be excised. Then multiple punch grafting could create a *conservative* lowering of the original receded temporal hairline.

results, even major disasters, with very extensive loss of hair-bearing scalp caused by flap and/or donor site necrosis, in cases seen by the author.

Most flap procedures result in the hair being oriented posteriorly instead of the normal anterior direction of growth achieved by properly performed punch grafting. Excessive blunting of the temporal gulf is commonly seen, sometimes with extremely low temporal hairlines (Fig. 19–100) and is, to a degree, inherent in the procedure resulting from the attachment of the base of the flap(s) to the vascular supply. However, as with punch grafting, a sense of aesthetics is essential, and a properly designed flap can at least avoid the all too frequently seen unattractively low to bizarre temporal hairline. However, if a patient wants a somewhat more pronounced temporal gulf or recession (as many do), this would be technically impossible to achieve with flaps, whereas total flexibility in hairline design is possible with punch grafting. Flaps also frequently have excessively straight and artificial hairlines, often with broad scars made more conspicuous by the posterior direction of hair growth. However, with proper technique and aided by effective hair styling, many of these objections can be satisfactorily overcome. When required, punch grafting hairline refinement techniques can be used to improve unsatisfactory flap hairlines, including scars resulting from the nonsurvival of the distal portions of flaps, in the same way that it is used to correct poorly performed hair transplantation procedures.

By their very nature, flaps do not permit a more gradual approach, which is often an advantage rather than a disadvantage of the more slowly achieved results of punch grafting. Thus, the latter can be used to gradually fill in areas of only moderate thinning, to achieve a gradual and subtle lowering of a receded hairline, to fill in receded temples while avoiding a retained apex, or to fill in a residual bald crown and midscalp following reduction. Thus, flaps are essentially an all-or-nothing approach to male pattern baldness. In summary, there is a place for both punch grafting and flaps, and in either case, aesthetic considerations, good surgical judgment, and technical competence are essential.

"Galeoplasty" and Superficial Temporal Artery Ligation

"Galeoplasty" used as a primary procedure (*not* to be confused with multiple galeotomies or relaxing galeal incisions performed as a reasonable, albeit controversial, adjunct to scalp reduction—see Chapter 20) is based on the fallacious notion that male pattern baldness is due to interference in an adequate blood supply to the affected area of the scalp because of an excessive tightness of the galea. It is supposedly caused by excessive muscle tension that produces an abnormal degree of traction by the muscles at their attachments to the galea. However, despite the overwhelming evidence that male pattern baldness is clearly not due to these factors, there has nevertheless been an attempted revival of this illogical procedure. Its current advocates acknowledge that the alleged benefits, if any, are only temporary and furthermore sometimes employ grafts or flaps in addition, thus raising a serious question as to their rationale in using this operative procedure at all.

Another operation still being advocated is the ligation of the superficial temporal vessels, based on the opposite (and equally fallacious) notion that male pattern baldness is caused (at least in some cases) by too great a blood supply, which supposedly increases seborrhea and, in turn, hair loss. The advocates of both of these diametrically opposed "theories" and the operative procedures based on them totally ignore the overwhelming evidence that genetic predetermination of follicular growth behavior with resultant *donor dominance* is the key to understanding male pattern baldness and the rationale of the punch graft method (see section on "Biological Considerations—Concept, Rationale, and Fallacies").

PROSTHETIC DEVICES FOR MALE PATTERN BALDNESS (OTHER THAN CONVENTIONAL TOUPEES AND HAIRPIECES)

Weaving and Variations

Hair weaving is a technique in which human hairs are sewn together with nylon threads at their proximal ends to form hanks or wiglets, then several of these are woven into a network of tight braids. These braids, which are closely adherent to the scalp, have been created on the thinning scalp by weaving nylon threads into the residual scalp hair or into the fringe hair at the periphery of the bald scalp. As the patient's hair grows, it becomes necessary to reweave or reattach the braids of hair close to the scalp about every two months for as long as the device is used. Because of the constant mechanical traction produced, a traction alopecia may result, which has been observed by the author and by others. This may be temporary or permanent, depending upon how long the trauma has been imposed, but presumably, it could be avoided if excessively tight attachment and resulting traction are not permitted.

A more sophisticated variation involves inserting strands of natural matched hair with the same pattern and direction of natural hair growth into a light filamentous matrix that has been previously fitted to the bald area. A nylon thread is then attached to the bases of the fringe hairs without excessive tension, and the matrix containing the strands of hair is attached with other nylon filaments to the thread. This, of course, still requires periodic reattachment as the fringe hairs grow.

Suture Loops

A procedure that has had some popularity in recent years consists of placing multiple discrete loops of Teflon-coated stainless steel wire or nylon suture material in the scalp around the periphery of the bald area anteriorly and within the fringe adjacent to the bald scalp laterally and posteriorly. A thin netting is attached to the loops and then hanks or wiglets of human hair are attached to the netting, thus creating a more or less permanently attached hairpiece. Although the author does not know the degree to which this procedure finds long-term acceptance by the majority of recipients, he has performed hair transplantation on a considerable number of patients who subsequently had the suture loops removed. Others came in with the device in

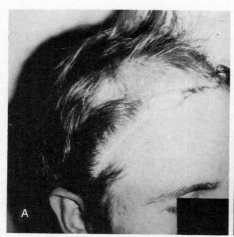 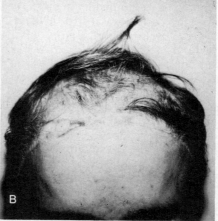

Figure 19–100. *A* and *B*, A 26-year-old man as he appeared when first seen by the author two months after having bitemporal rotation flaps. Note the extremely low temporal hairline with scars extending into the temporal "points" at the lateral aspect of the forehead. Hairs in the flaps are of good density but point in a posterior direction, which is the reverse of the patient's normal orientation. A slough in the central portion of the right flap has occurred plus temporary defluvium of the more medial portions of both flaps. Because of the patient's youth, the degree of present hair loss, and prospects for eventual extensive male pattern baldness (his considerable thinning and family history), the selection of this low temporal hairline, anteriorly concave (instead of convex), was especially unfortunate.

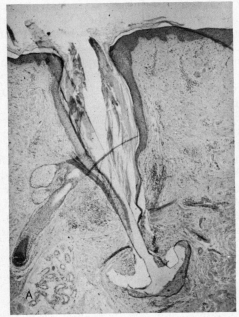
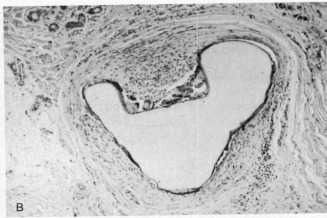

Figure 19–101. *A*, Photomicrograph of a biopsy specimen from the bald scalp of a 38-year-old man five months after the insertion of nylon filaments through individual vellus pilosebaceous openings. A nylon filament can be seen with a markedly dilated and keratin-filled pilosebaceous opening, through which the filament had been inserted and to the wall of which a vellus hair follicle and sebaceous gland are attached. The filament penetrates completely through this pilosebaceous unit, which is surrounded by a considerable amount of chronic inflammatory reaction, and extends into the lower dermis, where its arrowhead-shaped tip resides. The resulting cavity is *not* lined by epidermis. Clinically, the pilosebaceous openings appeared as large pits around the bases of the nylon filaments, which had been cut very close to the surface of the skin in order to prevent their being pulled out by traction against them, as occurred in the longer ones. *B*, Higher power photomicrograph of arrowhead-shaped tip of a nylon filament deep in the dermis, also 5 months after insertion, showing foreign body giant cells, chronic inflammation, and marked fibrosis surrounding it.

place but were dissatisfied with it and wanted grafting performed, which was subsequently done after removing the loops.

The most common complaints were constant discomfort from a pulling sensation or feeling of mechanical tension in the scalp, which the patients found extremely annoying, and difficulty in properly cleansing the scalp. One patient described this feeling as though he were "wearing a wet mop" after shampooing his scalp.

They all showed considerable chronic inflammation; there was usually evidence of low-grade infection or active purulent discharge (a case of septicemia has come to the author's attention) and sometimes a hypertrophic response of the skin around the openings as well. These findings were hardly surprising in view of the constant mechanical traction and the fact that the loops were creating a sinus tract deep in the dermis and subcutaneous tissues communicating with the surface. This is closely analogous to the situation in which synthetic implants were used (see subsections on "Synthetic Implants"). Considerable scarring accompanied healing after their removal (Figs. 19–5A, 19–80A and 19–80D), and there was resultant localized permanent hair loss in the fringe areas adjacent to

the area of male pattern baldness where some of the loops had previously been placed. However, this was subsequently corrected by means of the grafting.

This procedure is, in effect, simply another technique of attaching a hairpiece in lieu of the more conventional use of adhesive tapes or other types of adhesive material applied to the bald area or the use of clips to attach it to the hair in the fringe area. In addition to the likelihood of the suture loops eventually working through to the skin surface because of chronic inflammation, infection, and mechanical traction, there is also the unpleasant possibility of a sudden forceful pulling on the hairpiece that would cause considerable trauma to the scalp.

Tunnel Grafts

So-called tunnel grafts—utilizing skin grafts from behind the ears to create two epidermal-lined subcutaneous tunnels, one in the frontal area and one in the crown of the bald scalp, to which a hairpiece is then attached—has the advantage over suture loops of not creating a sinus tract. These tunnels can also be accidentally torn open by sudden forceful traction on the hairpiece, which, of course, could be repaired. This technique appears to be a physiologically sound means of attaching a hairpiece in a fairly secure manner.

Synthetic Implants—Unsuccessful Experimental Results

For the sake of completeness only, the author's experience with another technique before and during the early phase of his interest in punch grafting (1961) should be related.

A limited attempt was made to insert nylon filaments simulating hairs, with barbed or arrowhead-shaped tips into the bald scalp follicles, utilizing a modified hollow needle for insertion. However, because of the markedly reduced size and depth of the vellus follicles compared with the coarse-hair–bearing follicles, the filaments penetrated through the walls of the sebaceous ducts with which these vellus follicles are associated, and the tips were demonstrated microscopically to reside deep in the dermis or subcutaneous fat.

Most of the filaments came out within several weeks to several months, depending upon the shape and diameter of the barbed tips, the depth of insertion, and the length of the filaments. Far greater traction was exerted upon filaments left long than on those clipped short.

Histologic examination (Fig. 19–101) at seven weeks and five months after insertion showed a pronounced foreign body reaction and fibrosis. There was no evidence that the epidermal cells of the follicle walls of the vellus pilosebaceous units were attempting to line the sinus tracts created by the filaments. Thus, there was direct communication between the surface and the deep dermis or subcutaneous fat.

Therefore, inserting the filaments through the pilosebaceous openings was irrelevant, and the filaments were just as much outside the pilosebaceous units and in the deep dermal and subcutaneous tissues as if nylon sutures had been placed deep in the skin and the ends left long.

The attempted nylon filament implantation technique was a brief and extremely limited clinical experiment on volunteers who had given informed consent. The results were unsatisfactory, and it is definitely *not* advocated.

Synthetic Implants—Disastrous Results of Fraudulent Exploitation

During the period 1978 to 1980, there occurred a widely advertised commercial effort in a number of American cities to implant modacrylic fibers or natural hairs singly or in tufts, by inserting them, ostensibly under medical supervision, into the bald scalp by means of various mechanical devices, in some cases knotting the artificial hairs deep in the skin or subcutaneous tissue. A large number of very unfortunate results were seen. The "lucky" individuals were those in which the filaments simply pulled out in a few weeks, although not necessarily without some atrophic scarring. Others were much less fortunate, as the deeply imbedded, knotted filaments produced destructive bacterial infections (including *Staphylococcus, Klebsiella, Proteus,* and *Pseudomonas aeruginosa*) resulting in severe and extensive atrophic scarring. In addition to appropriate systemic and topical antibacterial therapy, it was necessary to remove often several hundred deeply knotted filaments painstakingly one at a time. Fortunately for other potential victims, the perpetrators are no longer in business.

SUGGESTED READINGS

Alt TH: Scalp reduction as an adjunct to hair transplantation. Cosmet Surg 1:1–9, 1981

Alt TH Sr: Evaluation of donor harvesting techniques in hair transplantation. J Dermatol Surg Oncol 10:799–806, 1984

Altchek DD, Pearlstein HH: Granulomatous reaction to autologous hairs incarcerated during hair transplantation. J Dermatol Surg Oncol 4:928–929, 1978

Auerbach R, Pearlstein H: Hair replacement. Cutis, 20:445, 1977

Ayres S III: Conservative surgical management of male pattern baldness. Arch Derm 90:492–499, 1964

Ayres S III: Baldness fallacy (Letters to the Editor). Medical World News 6:95, 1965

Ayres S III: Hair transplantation—The Orentreich technique for male pattern baldness, in Epstein E (ed): Skin Surgery, ed 3. Springfield, Ill, Charles C Thomas Publisher, 1970, pp 453–508

Ayres S III: Prevention and correction of unaesthetic results of hair transplantation for male pattern baldness. Cutis, 19:117–121, 1977

Ayres S III: Hair transplantation—The punch method for male pattern baldness, in Epstein E, Epstein E Jr (eds): Skin Surgery, ed 4. Springfield, Ill, Charles C Thomas Publisher, 1977, pp 327–388

Ayres S III: Hair transplantation—The punch method for male pattern baldness, in Epstein E, Epstein E Jr (eds): Skin Surgery, vol 1, ed 5. Springfield, Ill, Charles C Thomas Publisher, 1982, pp 437–529

Ayres S III: Hair transplantation for male pattern baldness: Aesthetic considerations and current status. Head and Neck Surgery 7:272–285, 1985

Ayres S III: Determining boundaries of the "safe" donor area in hair transplantation, in Robins P (ed): Surgical Gems, vol. 1, New York, Clinicom Publishing Co, 1986

Baran, R: New instruments for use in hair transplant techniques. J Dermatol Surg 1:47–48, 1975

Barros d'Sa AA, Heard CE: Arteriovenous fistula after hair transplantation. Br Med J, 1:340–341, 1978

Bendl BJ: Troubles with power punches in hair transplantations. J Dermatol Surg Oncol 3:594, 1977

Bendl BJ: The tunnel graft procedure for attachment of a hairpiece. Cutis 18:559, 1976

Blanchard G, Blanchard B: Obliteration of alopecia by hairlifting: A new concept and technique. J Natl Med Assoc 69:639–641, 1977

Borges AF: Prevention of cobblestoning in hair transplantation. J Dermatol Surg Oncol 4:168, 1978

Burton JL, Benhalim MM, Meyrick G, et al: Male pattern alopecia and masculinity. Br J Dermatol 100:567–571, 1979

Carreirao S, Lessa S: New technique for closing punch graft donor sites. Plast Reconstr Surg 61:455, 1978

Coiffman F: Use of square scalp grafts for male pattern baldness. Plast Reconstr Surg 60:228, 1977

De Villez RL: Topical minoxidil therapy in hereditary androgenetic alopecia. Arch Dermatol 121:197–202, 1985

Devine JW Jr: Square scalp grafts, combined with strip grafts for the treatment of male pattern baldness. Plast Reconstr Surg 62:716–721, 1978

Dick LA, Kurtin SB: Suture implantation for the correction of male pattern alopecia. Cutis 9:49–50, 1972

Farber GA, Burks JW, Salinger C: Hair transplants for male pattern baldness: Long-term subjective evaluation. Southern Med J 65:1380–1383, 1972

Fleming RW, Mayer TG: Short vs long flaps in the treatment of male pattern baldness. Arch Otolaryngol 107:403–408, 1981

Fleming RW, Mayer TG: Scalp flaps in the treatment of male pattern baldness, in Norwood, OT, Shiell, RC (eds): Hair Transplant Surgery. Springfield, Ill, Charles C Thomas Publisher, 1984, pp 278–314

Fleming RW, Mayer TG: Scalp flaps—Reconstruction of the unfavorable result in hair replacement surgery. Head and Neck Surgery 7:315–331, 1985

Foster CA, Aston SJ: Propranolol-epinephrine interaction: A potential disaster. Plast Reconstr Surg 72:74–78, 1983

Franz TJ: Percutaneous absorption of minoxidil in man. Arch Dermatol 121:203–206, 1985

Ginsburg JE: Hair transplants for male pattern baldness—Special clinical and mathematic considerations. Cutis 6:1113–1120, 1970

Gloor M: Secondary damage to hair follicles in full thickness skin autografts. Arch Dermatol Forsch 249:277, 1974

Goldman PM: Punch grafting the crown and vertex. J Dermatol Surg Oncol 11:138–141, 1985

Hagerman RD: Speed regulation of the power punch in hair transplantation. Cutis 8:333–335, 1971

Hagerman RD, Wilson JW: The skin biopsy punch: Evaluation and modification. Cutis 6:1139–1143, 1970

Hamilton JB: Male hormone stimulation is prerequisite and an incitant in common baldness. Am J Anatomy 71:451–479, 1942

Hamilton JB: Patterned loss of hair in man: Types and incidence. Ann NY Acad Sci 53:708–728, 1951

Hanke CW, Bergfeld WF: Fiber implantation for pattern baldness. JAMA 241:146–148, 1979

Hill TC: Closure of the donor site in hair transplantation by a cluster technique. J Dermatol Surg Oncol 6:190–191, 1980

Johnson WC, Baker GK: Use of steel pins in hair transplantation. J Dermatol Surg Oncol 3:220, 1977

Juri S: Use of parieto-occipital flaps in the surgical treatment of baldness. Plast Reconst Surg 55:456–460, 1975

Kabaker S: Flap procedures in hair replacement surgery, in Epstein E, Epstein E Jr (eds): Skin Surgery, vol 1, ed 5. Springfield, Ill, Charles C Thomas Publisher, pp 546–563

LePaw MI: Complication of implantation of synthetic fibers into scalp for "hair" replacement. J Dermatol Surg Oncol 5:201–204, 1979

LePaw MI: Therapy and histopathology of complications from synthetic fiber implants for hair replacement. J Am Acad Derm 3:195–204, 1980

Lewis LA, Resnik SS: Strip and punch grafting for alopecia of the eyebrow. J Dermatol Surg Oncol 5:557–558, 1979

Maloney JM, Lentora J, Yarborough J: Plasma concentration of lidocaine during hair transplantation. J Dermatol Surg Oncol 8:950–954, 1982

Marritt E: Single hair transplantation for refinement of the hairline: A practical solution. J Dermatol Surg Oncol 10:962–966, 1984

Mayer TG, Fleming RW: Short flaps—their use and abuse in the treatment of male pattern baldness. Ann Plast Surg 8:296–304, 1982

Mayer TG, Fleming RW: Hairline aesthetics and styling in hair replacement surgery. Head and Neck Surgery 7:286–302, 1985

Monell CM, Berman WE: The success or failure of the hair transplant. Arch Otolaryngol 97:265–268, 1973

Monell CM: Repair of sequelae from artificial fiber hair implants with hair-bearing punch grafting. Head and Neck Surgery 7:332–335, 1985

Montagna W: Structure and Function of Skin. New York: Academic Press Inc, 1958

Montagna W, Ellis RA: Biology of Hair Growth. New York: Academic Press Inc, 1958

Montagna W: Phylogenetic significance of skin of man. Arch Derm 88:1–19, 1963

Montagna W, Machida H, Perkins A: The skin of primates, XXVIII. The stump-tail macaque (Macaca speciosa). Am J Phys Anthrop 24:71–86, 1966

Montagna W, Uno H: Baldness in Nonhuman Primates. J Soc Cosmetic Chemists 19:173–185, 1968

Morrison ID: An improved method of suturing the donor site in hair transplant surgery. Plast Reconstr Surg 67:378, 1981

Nataf J: Special techniques of hair transplantation by fusiform grafts and flaps of many types. J Dermatol Surg Oncol 5:620–624, 1979

Nordstrom REA: Hair transplantation. The use of hairbearing compound grafts for correction of alopecia due to chronic discoid lupus erythematosis, traumatic alopecia and male pattern baldness. Scand J Plastic Reconstr Surg (suppl) 14:3–37, 1976

Nordstrom REA: Eyebrow reconstruction by punch hair transplantation. Plast Reconstr Surg 60:74–76, 1977

Nordstrom REA: Synchronous balding of scalp and hair-bearing grafts of scalp transplanted to the skin of the arm in male pattern baldness. Acta Dermatovener (Stockholm) 59:266–268, 1978/1979

Nordstrom REA: Punch hair grafting under split-skin grafts on scalps. Plast Reconstr Surg 64:9–12, 1979

Nordstrom REA: "Micrografts" for improvement of the frontal hairline after hair transplantation. Aesthetic Plastic Surgery 5:97–101, 1981

Nordstrom REA: Reconstruction of the temporal hairline. Aesthetic Plastic Surgery 5:103–106, 1981

Nordstrom REA: Hyperpigmentation of transplanted terminal hairs after punch hair grafting. J Dermatol Surg Oncol 8:787–789, 1982

Nordstrom REA: Methods to improve old results of punch hair grafting. Plast Reconstr Surg 72:803–809, 1983

Nordstrom REA: Change of direction of hair growth. J Dermatol Surg Oncol 9:156–158, 1983

Nordstrom REA: "Stretch-back" in scalp reductions for male pattern baldness. Plast Reconstr Surg 73:422–426, 1984

Nordstrom REA: Scalp kinetics in multiple excisions for correction of male pattern baldness. J Dermatol Surg Oncol 10:991–995, 1984

Nordstrom REA, Holsti LR: Hair transplantation in alopecia due to radiation. Plast Reconstr Surg 72:454–458, 1983

Nordstrom REA, Totterman SMS: Iatrogenic false aneurysms following punch hair grafting. Plast Reconstr Surg 64:563–565, 1979

Nordstrom REA, Wahlstrom T: Hair growth in subcutaneously buried composite hair-bearing skin grafts. Scand J Plastic Reconstr Surg 16:91–93, 1982

Norwood OT: Arteriovenous fistula resulting from hair transplant surgery. Cutis 8:263–264, 1971

Norwood OT: Hair Transplant Surgery. Springfield, Ill, Charles C Thomas Publisher, 1973

Norwood OT: Advantages of the electric power driven punch in hair transplants. J Dermatol Surg 1:39–40, 1975

Norwood OT: Male pattern baldness: Classification and incidence. South Med J 68:1359–1365, 1975

Norwood OT: Infection with hair transplant surgery. Cutis 23:642–645, 1979

Norwood OT: Whisker hair. Arch Dermatol 115:930–931, 1979

Norwood OT: Whisker hair—an update. Cutis 27:651–652, 1981

Norwood OT: Predicting hair growth for hair transplantations. J Dermatol Surg Oncol 7:477–480, 1981

Norwood OT: Transplanting temporal points, sideburns, and feminine hairlines. J Dermatol Surg Oncol 10:958–961, 1984

Norwood OT, Shiell RC: Hair Transplant Surgery, ed 2. Springfield, Ill, Charles C Thomas Publisher, 1984

Orentreich DS, Orentreich N: Hair transplantation. J Dermatol Surg Oncol 11:319–324, 1985

Orentreich N: Autografts in alopecias and other selected dermatological conditions. Ann NY Acad Sci 83:463–479, 1959

Orentreich N: Scalp hair replacement in man, in Advances in Biology of Skin: Hair Growth, vol 9. New York, Pergamon Press, 1969, pp 99–108

Orentreich N: Hair transplants: Long term results and new advances. Arch Otolaryng 92:576–582, 1970

Orentreich N: Hair transplantation: The punch graft technique, in Symposium on Cosmetic Surgery. Surg Clin N Am 51:511–518, 1971

Orentreich N: Hair transplantation. NY State J Med 72:578–582, 1972

Orentreich N: Hair transplants, in Maddin WS: Current Dermatologic Management, ed 2. St. Louis: C V Mosby Co, 1975, pp 26–32

Orentreich N: Medical treatment of baldness. Ann Plast Surg 1:116–118, 1978

Orentreich N, Orentreich DS: "Cross-stitch" suture techniques for hair transplantation. J Dermatol Surg Oncol 10:970–971, 1984

Pearlstein HH, Orentreich N, Berger RA, Auerbach R: Hair weaving—Another approach to the management of male pattern alopecia. Cutis 4:975–978, 1968

Pearlstein HH, Auerbach R: Gangrene and pyoderma of the scalp—An unusual complication of hair autograft technique. Cutis 8:133–136, 1971

Pierce HE: The uniqueness of hair transplantation in black patients. J Dermatol Surg Oncol 3:533–535, 1977

Pierce HE: An improved method of closure of donor sites in hair transplantation. J Dermatol Surg Oncol 5:475–476, 1979

Pinski JB: How to obtain the "perfect" plug. J Dermatol Surg Oncol 19:953–956, 1984

Price VH: Testosterone metabolism in the skin: A review of its function in androgenetic alopecia, acne vulgaris and idiopathic hirsutism including recent studies with antiandrogens. Arch Dermatol 111:1496–1502, 1975

Rabineau P: Surgical treatment of baldness using Juri's flap technique: Advantages and disadvantages compared with Orentreich's free graft technique. Cutis 25:511–515, 1980

Resnik SS: Surgical refinements of the hairline in hair transplant surgery. Head and Neck Surgery 7:312–314, 1985

Sarnoff DS, Goldberg DJ, Greenspon AH, Albom MJ: Multiple pyogenic granuloma-like lesions following hair transplantation. J Dermatol Surg Oncol 11:32–34, 1985

Schwartz RS, Downham TF II: Dangers of synthetic fiber implantation for baldness. Cutis 25:491–492, 1980

Sebben JE: A method of obtaining satisfactory anesthesia in the frontal portion of the scalp preliminary to hair transplantation. J Dermatol Surg Oncol 5:177, 1979

Selmanowitz VJ, Orentreich N: Hair transplantation in blacks. J Natl Med Assoc 65:471, 1973

Seltzer P: Reconstructive surgery of hair transplantation by improved motorized technique. Int Surg 51:354, 1969

Shuman R: Replacement of scalp hair by attachment to suture implants. J Dermatol Surg 2:333–334, 1976

Smith MA, Wells RS: Male-type alopecia, alopecia areata and normal hair in women. Arch Derm 89:95, 1964

Souder DE, Bercaw BL: Arteriovenous fistula secondary to hair transplantation. New Engl J Med 283:473–474, 1970

Stough, DB III, Berger RA, Orentreich N: Surgical improvement of cicatricial alopecia of diverse etiology. Arch Derm 97:331–334, 1968

Stough DB III: Punch scalp autografts for bald spots. Plast Reconstr Surg 42:450–453, 1968

Stough DB III: Some special aspects of hair transplantation. J Dermatol Surg Oncol 3:2, 1977

Stough DB III: Hair transplantation, in Epstein E, Epstein E Jr (eds): Techniques of Skin Surgery. Philadelphia, Lea & Febiger, 1979

Stough DB III: Esthetic consideration in hair transplantation. Cutis 16:747, 1975

Stough, DB III: Complications of hair transplantation. Cutis 6:645–651, 1970

Sturm H: The benefit of donor-site closure in hair transplantation. J Dermatol Surg Oncol 10:987–990, 1984

Takashima I, Montagna W: Studies of common baldness of the stump-tailed macaque (Macaca speciosa): VI. The effect of testosterone on common baldness. Arch Derm 103:527–534, 1971

Tezel J: Miniature drill expedites hair transplantation. Cutis, 6:461, 1970

Tromovitch TA, Kay D, Stegman SJ: Hair transplants. Cutis, 15:383, 1975

Tromovitch TA, Glogau RG, and Stegman SJ: Medical treatment of male pattern alopecia (androgenic alopecia). Head and Neck Surgery 7:336–339, 1985

Unger MJ, Unger WP: Management of alopecia of the scalp by a combination of excisions and transplantation. J Dermatol Surg Oncol 4:670–672, 1978

Unger MJ, Unger WP: Midline alopecia reduction combined with hair transplantation. Head and Neck Surgery 7:303–311, 1985

Unger WP: Alternatives in hair replacement. Cutis 19:623–628, 1977

Unger WP: A study of some innovations in hair transplanting. J Dermatol Surg Oncol 3:536–538, 1977

Unger WP: Timing of sessions in hair transplantation. Cutis 20:214–216, 1978

Unger WP: Planning in hair transplantation. J Dermatol Surg Oncol 5:536–541, 1979

Unger WP: Hair Transplantation. New York, Marcel Dekker Inc, 1979

Unger WP: Concomitant mini reductions in punch hair transplanting. J Dermatol Surg Oncol 9:388–392, 1983

Unger WP, Unger MJ: Alopecia reduction, in Epstein E, Epstein E Jr (eds): Skin Surgery, vol 1, ed 5. Springfield, Ill, Charles C Thomas Publisher, 1982, pp 530–545

Unger WP: A new method of donor site harvesting. J Dermatol Surg Oncol 10:524–529, 1984

Unger WP: Punch transplantation in "early" androgenetic alopecia. J Dermatol Surg Oncol 10:945–952, 1984

Unger WP: "MMunigrafts", in Robins P (ed): Surgical Gems, vol 1. New York, Clinicom Publishing Co, 1986

Uno H, Allegra F, Adachi K, Montagna W: Studies of common baldness in the stump-tailed macaque (Macaca speciosa): I. Distribution of the hair follicles. J Invest Derm 49:288–296, 1967

Vanderveen EE, et al: Topical minoxidil for hair regrowth. J Am Acad Dermatol 11:416–421, 1984

Vallis CF: Surgical treatment of the receding hairline. Plast Reconstr Surg 33:247–252, 1964

Vallis CP: Hair transplantation for male pattern baldness. Surg Clin N Am 51:519–531, 1971

Vallis CP: Hair Transplantation for the Treatment of Male Pattern Baldness. Springfield, Ill, Charles C Thomas Publisher, 1982

Vallis CP: The strip graft method in hair transplantation, in Epstein E, Epstein E Jr (eds): Skin Surgery, vol 1, ed 5. Springfield, Ill, Charles C Thomas Publisher, 1982, pp 564–579

Watson PE, Little WD Jr, Fields JP: Treatment of eyebrow loss with punch hair transplants. Cutis 6:176–178, 1970

Weiss VC, West DP: Topical minoxidil therapy and hair regrowth. Arch Dermatol 121:191–192, 1985

Weissman A, et al: Antiandrogenic effects of topically applied spironolactone on the hamster flank organ. Arch Dermatol 121:57–62, 1985

20

MARTIN G. UNGER, M.D. / WALTER P. UNGER, M.D.

Scalp Reduction

HISTORY

For many years, plastic surgeons have utilized advancement or rotation flaps or both to reconstruct scalp defects after areas of malignancy or cicatricial alopecia have been excised.[35, 36] In cases with larger defects, serial excisions have been successfully employed to remove areas that could not be excised in a single operation.[3] Although the field of scalp surgery progressed with the development and design of transposition flaps, it was not until the mid-1970s that the same techniques became incorporated into the treatment of male pattern baldness.

In the spring of 1976, the authors began excising areas of male pattern baldness in order to improve the ratio of donor sites to recipient sites in patients being treated with the Orentreich punch graft technique of hair transplantation.[4] The concept occurred to the authors as they were reviewing photographs for use in an upcoming text and happened on one showing the "before" of an area of cicatricial alopecia that was treated with excision rather than punch grafting; the "after" photograph showed its almost complete removal. The "before" photograph could have easily been mistaken for an area of alopecia in the crown, and the authors decided to try it on this next patient with vertex male pattern baldness. After completion of the first 60 cases, we decided to publish a paper on what was clearly an important new concept for the treatment of this condition. This paper was published in September 1978 in Journal of Dermatological Surgery and Oncology.[2] It has been credited with "the introduction of scalp surgery to a large segment of the surgical community."[5]

The authors were not alone in recognizing this concept. The Blanchard brothers apparently had the same idea at approximately the same time, and in fact, the publication of their paper preceded the authors' by nearly one year.[6] Subsequently, the authors have also learned that Sparkuhl and Kim had been using the same approach for several years but had neglected to publish the results.[7] At the International Hair Transplant Symposium at Lucerne, Switzerland, in February 1978, presentations on this subject were made by Sparkuhl as well as Stough and Webster.[8]

A large series on scalp reduction was published by Bosley and colleagues in February 1979.[9] In December 1980, Alt published his first paper, em-phasizing that larger areas of alopecia could be removed provided that extensive undermining, increased tension on closure, and galeotomies were utilized.[10] Significant contributions to this field have also been made by Norwood and Shiell,[11] Fleming and coworkers,[12] Nordstrom,[13] and Marzola[14] as well as others who have publicized and continued to modify and refine the procedure.

Although the term "hair lifting" and "alopecia reduction" have been used to describe this operation, the term "scalp reduction," first used by Sparkuhl in 1978,[7] has gained widespread acceptance for this procedure. Incorporation of one or more scalp reduction operations with the punch graft technique of hair transplantation has become increasingly utilized over the years, and it is carried out today on the majority of patients having extensive hair transplantation.

USEFULNESS OF SCALP REDUCTION

By combining the surgical reduction of an area of alopecia with punch graft hair transplantation, several useful benefits can be achieved.

1. If the same number of donor grafts is utilized, the reduced area of alopecia can be covered more densely.
2. A greater proportion of the original bald area can be covered with the same number of punch grafts if the density of the punch grafts remains the same.
3. In younger patients with less fully developed male pattern baldness, a reduction of the area of most advanced baldness can act as a stopgap before a final decision is made to proceed with punch transplanting; it also effectively conserves a significant donor area for future use.
4. In some cases, where the ratio of donor to recipient sites may initially be inadequate for hair transplantation, reduction of the area of alopecia may result in a satisfactory ratio for treatment.
5. When the remaining number of donor grafts is very limited and a portion of the bald crown is still present, this area can be surgically reduced or removed entirely.
6. Scalp reduction may be employed to elevate the superior border of the lateral fringe of normal hair on the parting side,[16] and thus, the part can be moved to a cosmetically more pleasing and more medial position.

7. Scalp reduction can be useful for correction of previously unsatisfactory punch transplantation in the following situations:
   a. Areas of poor graft survival, improper hair direction, or too sparse a dispersion of grafts can be surgically excised. If desired, satisfactory grafts can be removed from the area before or after it is excised and implanted for a second time into the remaining transplanted area.
   b. When male pattern baldness progresses, a hairless gap remains between the previous punch graft transplants and the narrower lateral or occipital area fringe or both, which can be surgically removed.

PATIENT SELECTION

As with any operative procedure, certain clinical factors must be taken into account, such as the general health of the patient, the degree of alopecia, the laxity of the scalp, the ultimate objective or goal of the patient, the age of the patient, and the psychological ability to accept the scalp reduction procedure.

General Health

Scalp reduction surgery is an elective cosmetic procedure. In this regard, the physician should ensure that the general health of the patient is satisfactory before the surgery is undertaken. As with any elective operation, the patient should have a general history taken and physical examination before the procedure. Coexisting medical conditions, such as hypertension, diabetes, and thyroid disease, should be controlled as well as possible. If a blood dyscrasia is present, all factors relating to that patient would have to be considered before a decision is made about whether the risks of elective surgery are justified. Special consideration also has to be given to patients with a history of hepatitis. The type and communicability of the hepatitis and whether the surgeon and staff have been vaccinated are important factors.

Degree of Alopecia

This operation is most useful in individuals with alopecia, classes 3 to 6, according to the classification of Norwood[17] and Hamilton.[18] It is important when classifying a patient to take into account the potential for future hair loss. In general, the larger the area of alopecia, the more useful scalp reductions are and the more important it is to include the prognosis for additional loss in your overall planning.

Scalp Laxity

The patients who benefit most from scalp reduction are, as expected, those whose scalps have the greatest degree of laxity. This is not to say, however, that this procedure cannot be done on anyone who does not have substantial scalp laxity. It is not unusual at the time of surgery to obtain results as good as or better than average on patients who preoperatively have only borderline scalp laxity. The degree of undermining and whether one is going to carry out galeotomies are also important additional factors to be taken into account.

A few patients have so little scalp laxity that scalp reduction is pointless. Fortunately, they represent a small minority. Another small group of individuals seem to benefit very little from even repeated scalp reductions. About the same area of alopecia quickly returns after each procedure and is accompanied by progressive thinning of the bald skin. This latter phenomenon suggests that most of the new laxity is primarily due to stretching of the alopecia site rather than the laxity of the entire scalp increasing, which occurs in most patients. Accurate before and after measurements should identify members of this small group and will prevent nonproductive repeated scalp reductions.

Objectives

A patient who is certain of his present and future objectives and who has adequate donor grafts to accomplish this end has little use for a scalp reduction. When making an estimate of the available donor grafts, however, the age of the individual and possible future advancement of male pattern baldness should be considered.

Scalp reductions are most valuable in those who intend to employ all or virtually all available donor grafts for as large and dense a coverage as possible. Patients whose ultimate objectives are not yet fully established should also consider scalp reduction. In such cases, the individual retains the option of more extensive or denser punch transplanting in the future.

Age

The older the patient, the more accurate is the estimate of the ultimate extent of male pattern baldness. When the end stage is certain, the need and number of scalp reductions can be fully appreciated. In younger individuals, it is wise to incorporate scalp reductions because the full extent of baldness will only be known at some future time.

Psychological Factors

Not all patients can psychologically accept having a portion of their scalp excised. Others are frightened by often unfounded rumors about punch graft transplantation and are hardly able to cope with yet another "unknown" procedure. For both reasons, scalp reduction in the authors' offices is usually carried out after one or two transplanting sessions have been performed. In this way, patients learn firsthand whether their fears are founded with regard to transplanting and can evaluate how well they would be able to tolerate a scalp reduction. Other pros and cons of doing scalp reductions before punch graft transplantation will be discussed later.

If the patient can accept the idea of the operation but not the actual procedure while awake, a general anesthetic can be used. In addition, a general anesthetic can also be used with patients who require higher concentrations of local anesthetic. Fortunately, the patients in each of these groups represent a small minority, and the added risks of a general anesthetic are best avoided if possible.

TIMING OF SCALP REDUCTION AND HAIR TRANSPLANTATION PROCEDURES

Most Common Sequence

Usually, two punch graft procedures, spaced six weeks apart, are performed on the anterior scalp using a U-shaped pattern. In addition, an "island" of grafts may or may not be placed posteriorly and is separated from the anterior portion of the U by a gap of alopecia 4 to 6 cm wide.[19] Alternately, the U-shaped area may be extended posteriorly on one (usually the left) or both sides. A three- to four-month interval is left between the second and third transplantation sessions as well as the third and fourth sessions. With most reduction patterns, the authors prefer to delay excision for six weeks after any punch transplanting and to use the same interval before any further transplanting is performed in the same general area. Thus, the first scalp reduction is most often carried out six weeks after the second and subsequent transplanting sessions. Midline and Y-shaped reductions, on the other hand, may be done as soon as two days before a transplant session, because these patterns do not compromise the blood supply to the anterior grafting in a U-pattern.

Scalp Reduction Before or During Hair Transplantation

There are advantages and disadvantages to doing scalp reductions before instead of during punch-grafting sessions. Alopecia reductions before transplanting have the following advantages:
1. Undermining is easier to carry out in areas that have not been punch-grafted.
2. Punch-grafting patterns do not have to take into account future ideal patterns of scalp reductions.
3. Estimates of how much skin can be removed by scalp reductions, and therefore how large an area can reasonably be attempted with the available number of donor grafts, are made more easily if scalp reductions are done first.
4. No special care is needed to avoid injury to previously transplanted grafts.

It should be noted that transplanting hair prior to scalp reduction does not affect appreciably the amount of tissue that can be removed in subsequent scalp reductions, providing the area of transplantation is undermined during the reduction operation.

Disadvantages of scalp reduction before transplantation include the following:
1. If scalp reductions are done first, the patient must wait longer before he sees hair growing on previously bald sites. The more reductions done, the longer this delay becomes.
2. Each scalp reduction results in some stretching of the scalp tissue in both the bald and hair-bearing areas. The latter supplies the donor punch grafts for later transplantation. Stretching of the hair-bearing skin causes a lower density of hair per unit surface area, fewer hairs per graft, and correspondingly less satisfactory results from transplanting such grafts.
3. As noted earlier, it is usually psychologically preferable to start with the better-known punch graft procedure.

There is no absolute answer to the question of whether to perform scalp reductions before or during transplant sessions. With most patients, the previously described sequence of operations is carried out. However, exceptions are made in specific instances—most often in younger individuals who are concerned about vertex alopecia but who also want to increase the possibility that they will have sufficient donor grafts left to transplant the anterior aspect of their scalp if hair loss occurs there later. In these cases, usually one or more scalp reductions are carried out prior to any hair transplantation.

In addition, a scalp reduction may be performed in a younger person in the central scalp region to intentionally delay the start of hair transplantation. The reason for this delay might be to allow the physician to make certain that the patient will become a good candidate for punch transplanting or, alternatively, to allow the patient some time to prepare psychologically or financially for hair transplantation. This interval may also result in a psychological accommodation of the patient to male pattern baldness so that transplantation may no longer be necessary, and in this case, only a fine scalp reduction scar would remain.

"Early" Scalp Reductions

Some controversy surrounds the question of whether one should perform a scalp reduction through an area of hair-bearing skin that is in the early stages of androgenic alopecia. No single answer is satisfactory for all individuals. In general, however, the presence of hair in an area that can be removed by a scalp reduction is not an absolute contraindication. Other factors must also be taken into account:

1. The patient's desire to complete the entire hair replacement and scalp reduction program as quickly as possible.
2. The patient's preference to carry out all operations on hair-bearing skin to avoid the embarrassment that might be produced later by similar operations when the scalp would have no hair left to camouflage the procedures.
3. The desirability of moving the part to a more medial position.
4. The patient's willingness to accept a temporary telogen effluvium, which may occur after a scalp reduction, in an area of hair-bearing skin. Telogen effluvium is an inconvenience that may, in fact, be tolerated better in the early stages of male pattern baldness when remaining and more lateral hair can still camouflage the region.

Some physicians believe that early scalp reductions might hasten the rate of hair loss in any given area. This has not occurred in any of the several thousand patients on whom the authors have operated. It is possible that other physicians who use significantly more tension in closing their wounds might cause a permanent hair loss on either side of the incision line, similar to that which occurs in some patients after a facelift operation because of considerable tension at and near the suture line. Obviously, the best solution to this problem is prevention by avoiding excessive tension, and by doing so, there is no exacerbation of the rate of hair loss, in the authors' opinion.

PATTERNS OF SCALP REDUCTION

In our original paper, six basic patterns of scalp reductions were described as examples of the many possible variations. The sagittal midline ellipse was incorporated in the original "star" pattern (Fig. 20–1), and the lateral crescent shape has been described by Alt.[5, 10, 15] In recent years, Marzola has described a pattern that consists of an incision anterior to the temple hair as well as along the margin of the lateral fringe.[14] From the beginning, it has been stressed and should be emphasized again that, even after performing several thousand operations, no one pattern is optimal for all patients. With each individual, the operation should be tailored to the patients' area of alopecia or pattern of previous hair transplantation.[1]

Sagittal Midline Ellipse

This pattern of excision has enjoyed widespread popularity over the years for the following reasons:[20]
1. It is effective in removing large areas of alopecia due to lateral mobility of the scalp.
2. It is the safest and technically the easiest pattern of excision to perform for the beginner.
3. There is no postoperative anesthesia or hypoesthesia of the scalp.
4. For the more experienced practitioner, this pattern can be used most easily concomitant with punch grafting.

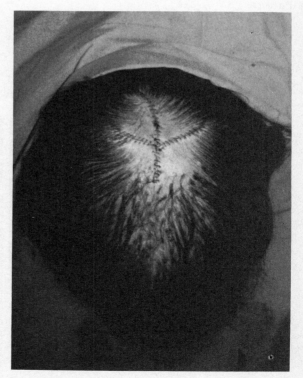

Figure 20–1. Modified "star" pattern. Note that the occipital end of the vertical component is curved to the patient's right to minimize the distortion of the hair direction.

In comparison to other designs, the principal disadvantages of this pattern are:

1. A central scar through the crown region almost always necessitates hair transplantation of that area.
2. In comparison to some patterns, e.g., the U-shaped pattern, less scalp tissue is removed anteriorly.
3. The most serious problem with this pattern is that repeated reductions produce a change in hair direction on each side of the scar that is difficult to camouflage. The bald area is also distorted by being slightly elongated. Nordstrom has described one method to improve this change in hair direction.[13] Because of this alteration in hair direction, the saggital midline ellipse also does not lend itself to the creation of a whorl pattern in the crown.
4. When the pattern is extended into the occipital region, an axe-like scar can be produced there. The best solution of this problem is prevention, which can be achieved by using an alternate pattern such as a Y-pattern, by stopping the excision at the margin of the occipital fringe, or by curving the end of the scar in the occipital region to one side. (Fig. 20–2).

Y-Pattern

This excision design has gained increasing popularity over the past few years. The principal advantages over the midline pattern are as follows:

1. A larger area can be excised with the Y-pattern as compared with a midline operation, given the same area of alopecia. This is true for two reasons: First, the laxity of the scalp is usually greatest in the crown region, and second, the increased total length of the incision allows more scalp tissue to be removed in that area. This holds true even with the double convex contour of the cranium.
2. Y-shaped scalp reduction allows the greatest area of alopecia to be removed if one is not transplanting the crown or crown and vertex regions and if no scar is left in those areas. For example, by positioning the lateral arms of the pattern to follow the anterior margin of the crown area, one can reduce the area of alopecia anterior to the crown, without creating a scar in the crown region itself. This is particularly useful when the patient is uncertain about the total area to be transplanted, when there is a paucity of donor area, or when the crown transplantation is significantly delayed.
3. In many patients, the Y-pattern scalp reduction conforms to the area of alopecia much better. This is particularly true of patients who have pear-shaped bald areas or persistent hair extending anteriorly from the occipital region.
4. Hair direction in the crown region is preserved much better by a Y-shaped scalp reduction (Fig. 20–3). This is a significant advantage and almost a necessity if a whorl pattern is planned for the crown region. Maintaining the normal hair direction is also particularly important in younger patients who are balding more rapidly in the crown and vertex than in the frontal area. By carrying out a reduction, transplantation of the crown can often be delayed several years and the donor area saved for the frontal region.

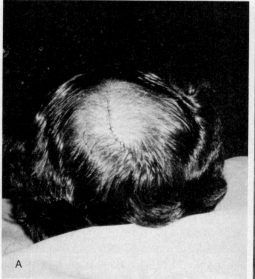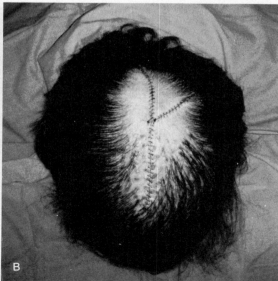

Figure 20–2. *A,* Posterior view of a modified sagittal midline ellipse. The occipital end of the incision is curved to prevent the distortion of the hair direction. *B,* Y-pattern variation. Note that the occipital end of the incision is curved as in A.

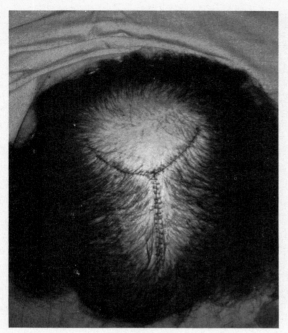

Figure 20–3. Y-pattern variation with the lateral components forming a semicircle around the crown.

has been reported,[10, 15] not a single case has occurred in the authors' experience with over 1500 cases using the Y-pattern. This specific topic was discussed at the Sixth National Symposium on Hair Replacement Surgery,[12] and the conclusion was that tip necrosis is extremely rare and virtually totally avoidable.

3. If the lateral components are initially placed at the anterior margin of the crown and then a Y-shaped reduction for the crown itself is desired, a fairly complicated situation develops. The second reduction can be carried out, if a one-inch bridge of tissue can be left between the two lateral component scars on each side of the midline and if at least three months have passed since the last excision. If these conditions cannot be met, a midline scalp reduction of the crown is indicated, even though the area removed will be smaller. This situation occurred only once in the authors' practice when a young man changed his mind about having a crown transplantation. Obviously, this type of problem cannot occur if only midline scalp reductions are repeated.

4. There is more interruption of the neurovascular supply of the scalp with a Y-shaped scalp reduction. Because each of the three flaps created with a Y has an excellent nerve and blood supply, this is not clinically important.

5. Because the total length of the incisions is longer with the Y-shaped scalp reduction, more time and effort is required for closure.

5. With the Y-shaped scalp reduction, a greater number of pattern variations are possible. The Y-shape can involve the entire dorsum or any other desired area. The vertical component may be short or almost the entire length of the area of alopecia. The lateral components may be short or long, straight or curved, and angled as most appropriate.

6. The Y-shaped scalp reduction allows an elevation of the occipital region impossible with a midline operation. By detaching the galea from the nuchal ridge of the occipital bone, an even greater advancement of the occipital hair can be achieved.

7. When large areas of scalp are removed with midline scalp reductions, a certain redundancy of tissue or dog-ears form posteriorly with closure of the wound. The Y-shaped incision allows the posterior dog-eared tissue to be dispersed over two areas instead of one.

8. With the Y-pattern scalp reduction no axe-like scar is produced in the occipital region.

The principal disadvantages of the Y-pattern are:

1. Technically, the Y-shaped scalp reduction is more difficult than the midline incision. Six wound edges must be approximated with the former, as opposed to two with the latter. Nonetheless, if one deals with each component of the Y-excision at a time, the complexity is dramatically reduced.[21] Basically, each component is treated similarly to a midline ellipse.

2. Although necrosis of the tip of the posterior flap

Y-Pattern Variations

By varying the length of the vertical component, the pattern can encompass the area desired, such as the anterior third or two thirds of the area of alopecia. When the vertical component is very long and the lateral arms short, the pattern resembles a rocket. Other variations include changing the angle at which the lateral arms meet the anterior element (a 45-degree angle is the most common, although the usual range is 30 to 90 degrees, asymmetric angles on each side, a midline excision with one lateral arm (Fig. 20–2B), and creating straight or curved lateral components (anteriorly or posteriorly). By curving posteriorly directed arms to form a semicircle around the crown (Fig. 20–3), a very useful pattern is created. With this variation, the vertical component is first reduced in size; the galea is closed; and then the posterior semicircle is reduced. This pattern is particularly useful to reduce the size of the crown when transplantation to that area is doubtful or significantly delayed.

Although the vertical component is usually placed in the midline, it can be positioned to either side and the lateral arms made of unequal length (Fig. 20–4). This is most useful for patients who have had

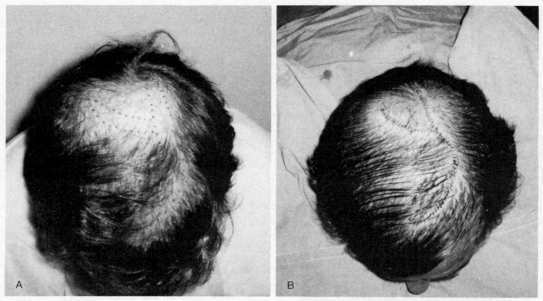

Figure 20—4. Y-pattern variation. Before (*A*) and after (*B*). The vertical component is positioned to the left of the midline.

previous punch grafting on one side up to the midline but none on the opposite side and the crown.

The lateral components of the Y are usually directed posteriorly. However, they can be positioned anteriorly (Fig. 20–5) or both anteriorly and posteriorly.[21] By positioning the arms forward toward each temple, the anterior transplanted U-shaped area can be preserved unchanged while the remaining area of alopecia is reduced in size. One's imagination is the only restriction to the number of variations of the Y-pattern possible.

The Lateral Patterns

In these patterns, part or all of the scar is placed at the periphery of the bald area. Included in this group are the S-, J- and C-types described by Unger and Unger[2, 19] as well as the lateral crescent-shaped pattern described by Alt.[10, 15] The principal advantages of these patterns are as follows:

1. The resultant scar is positioned at a more cosmetically favorable area (the periphery of the bald area).
2. As with the Y-pattern, there is no elongation of

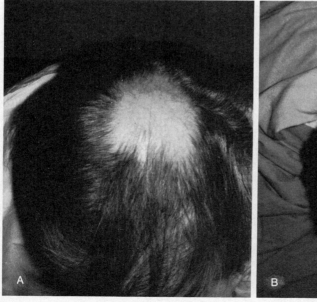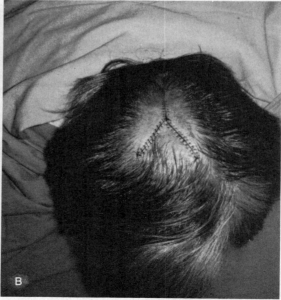

Figure 20—5. Y-pattern variation with anteriorly directed lateral components. *A*, Before—note the pear-shaped appearance of the area of alopecia. *B*, After.

the original area of alopecia or significant distortion of the hair direction.

3. Elevation of hair occurs in the occipital region. This is a distinct advantage over the midline pattern but not as effective as the elevation of the occipital region with the Y-pattern.

4. Because of the lateral position of the scar, undermining and galeotomies in the hair-bearing region on the side of the incision are technically easier to perform than with the midline or Y-pattern. Related to this advantage is the usefulness of this pattern to elevate the lateral fringe to a more medial position or, alternatively, to excise an area of alopecia between a previously transplanted zone and a receding lateral fringe.

5. This pattern preserves the possibility of creating a whorl pattern in the crown region that is intermediate in degree and significantly better than the midline pattern but less satisfactory than the Y-pattern.

The disadvantages of lateral patterns are:

1. Technically, the operation is slightly more difficult than the midline pattern.

2. Usually, some hypoesthesia or anesthesia is caused by transection of neurovascular bundles. This is nearly always of a temporary nature and located within the area of baldness itself.

3. One side of the scalp is elevated more than the other until surgery is carried out on the contralateral side. Usually, this is not significant if the hair is combed over the area of alopecia.

4. Similarly, if an intermediate zone of diminished hair growth exists between the dense lateral fringe and a sparse more central region, excision of the intermediate zone would cause an asymmetric appearance if the hair is not combed over the area of alopecia.

5. After a lateral pattern has been carried out on each side, the circulation in the remaining central scalp might be significantly impaired and consequently result in less successful growth from grafts placed within that region.

6. Because the total length of the incision is midway between that of a midline and a Y-pattern, the bald area removed is more than a midline excision, but less than a Y-pattern of the entire dorsum of the scalp.

The Marzola modification of the lateral pattern[14] in general has the same advantages and disadvantages as just previously noted. Because the incision extends along the anterior margin of the temple hair, an added advantage is created by allowing the lateral portion of the scalp to be rotated anteriorly as well as medially. However, the disadvantage of this operation is a scar at the anterior margin of the temple hair. Because of this scar, the authors have not utilized this pattern, but Marzola has obtained impressive results with this design.

U-Pattern

Since first described in 1978, the original pattern has been modified so that more tissue is removed along the lateral components on each side and less is removed anteriorly (Fig. 20–6).[22] The overall effect ensures that the anterior hairline is not moved superiorly to any significant degree while simultaneously taking greater advantage of the lateral mobility of the scalp. As the transplanted U is usually fixed to the periosteum by punch grafts, care is taken not to undermine the anterior area to further ensure minimal change in the distance from the nose to the hairline.

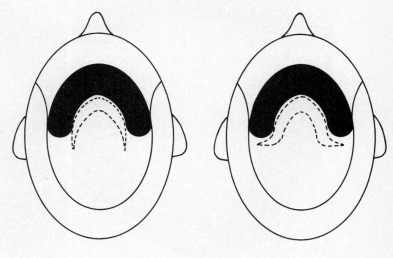

Figure 20–6. *A*, The original U pattern of uniform width. Dark U-shaped area of anterior hair transplantation is shown. *B*, A modified U pattern with a narrower anterior region and wider lateral components, which curve behind the transplanted area.

A   B

The principal advantages of this design are:
1. The scar is located immediately posterior to the anterior U-shaped area of punch transplantation (Fig. 20–7).
2. The lateral hairline areas can be raised for correction of previously faulty location.
3. Because of the length of the incision, a considerable area can be removed.

On the other hand, the most significant disadvantage of this design is the postoperative anesthesia present in the U-shaped flap created.

Miscellaneous Patterns

This group includes the T-pattern (Figs. 20–8), the I-pattern, the transverse or horizontal ellipse, and the crescent-shaped ellipse of the crown. The I-pattern, although one of the first described, has rarely been used. Usually, some alternate design is more suitable and conforms to the shape of the area of alopecia in a more natural fashion. The other patterns are still regularly used on selected patients.

Combined Patterns

Although usually only one pattern is used, the authors have employed in rare cases two patterns during the same procedure. On one occasion, the principal author carried out a U-shaped pattern in the anterior half of the dorsum of the scalp and a sagittal midline ellipse pattern in the posterior half. The purpose of this combination was to maximize the amount of tissue that could be removed from the anterior half of the area of alopecia. In one other case, a patient after punch graft transplants applied hot compresses that destroyed tissue in the midline area. In addition, this same patient had a remaining area of alopecia along the posterior and right side of the crown between the grafts and his lateral fringe. In this case, the lateral pattern was used to remove the gap in the crown region, and then it was combined with a sagittal midline ellipse to excise the area destroyed by the hot compresses.

The possibility of combining patterns is included in this chapter for completeness. In general, it should only be carried out in extreme situations and only by a surgeon who has had years of experience with scalp reductions. It should be pointed out that, in each of the two cases previously noted, one reduction pattern was carried out and completely closed before the other pattern was initiated.

Summary

In general, pattern selection varies with each patient. If the reduction involves the entire dorsum of the scalp, a Y-shaped pattern will be used if the area of alopecia is pear-shaped in nature or if there is a persistence of hair extending anteriorly from the occipital area. Alternately, if the bald area is an elongated oval, a midline sagittal ellipse or one of the lateral patterns can be used with equal success. For specific purposes, such as raising the hairline on one side, a lateral type of pattern is always used. When hair transplantation is going to be confined

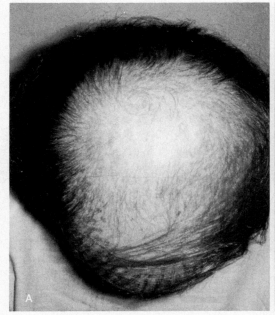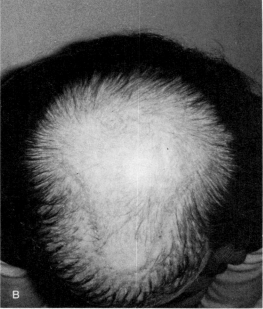

Figure 20–7. U pattern extending two thirds of the way posteriorly: Before (*A*) and after (*B*).

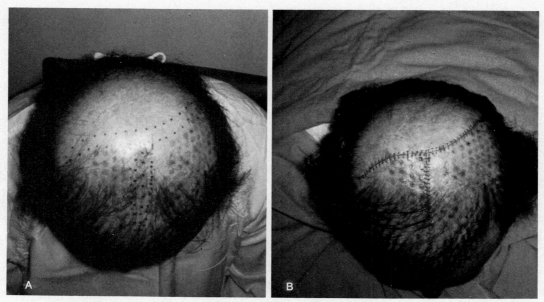

Figure 20–8. T-pattern variation with vertical component directed anteriorly: Before (*A*) and after (*B*).

to the anterior half of the dorsum of the scalp, a Y-shaped or U-shaped pattern is usually performed. With the crown and vertex areas, the Y-pattern is usually the procedure of choice, although the T-pattern, the horizontal ellipse, and the crescent-shaped ellipse are still frequently used if they conform best to the shape of the area of alopecia.

PREOPERATIVE INFORMATION

In the consultation prior to surgery, the authors initially discuss what the purpose of the scalp reduction is with regard to the particular patient. Specifically, the goal is reviewed—whether it is to achieve a greater density in a limited area, to provide coverage of a larger area with the same density, to preserve donor site grafts for the future, or to convert an unsatisfactory candidate for hair transplantation into a satisfactory one. The patient is told that the operation will remove as much tissue as the laxity of the scalp will allow. In explaining this, it is often useful to refer to the removal of extra "skin" in the bald area rather than referring to the scalp. Somehow, the word "skin" seems to be more psychologically acceptable to most patients. The reduction pattern to be used is then described to the patient. A diagram often proves useful.

It is important to describe the nature and location of the incisions and resultant scars as accurately as possible. If one is going to employ prophylactic antibiotics, the patient should be informed of this and given appropriate instructions. It is the authors' practice to prescribe erythromycin, 250 mg four times a day, which is started two hours *before* surgery. If one is going to use corticosteroids to minimize postoperative edema, this should also be reviewed. The authors use 5 mg tablets of prednisone. The daily dosage is as follows: Day 1, 30 mg; Day 2, 25 mg; Day 3, 20 mg; Day 4, 15 mg; Day 5, 10 mg; Days 6 and 7, 5 mg.

If diazepam or other medication is to be used, the patient is informed of this as well. In addition, when diazepam is used on the day of surgery, the patient is given a test of 10 mg which he takes during the evening about one week before the surgery in order to rule out idiosyncratic reactions to the drug. Patients must specifically be informed not to drive after taking this medication, both after the test dose and on the day of surgery. The expected postoperative course is fully explained as well as the possible side effects, such as a mild tightness of the scalp for one to four weeks, telogen effluvium developing adjacent to the incision in some patients who have hair remaining in the area of surgery, and the fact that a small seroma might occur creating a small temporary bump at each end of the incision.

Postoperative discomfort and edema in most patients is comparable to that experienced by them after punch graft transplantation. A minority find it worse or better. With the U- and J-shaped patterns, there is always some temporary postoperative hypoesthesia or anesthesia of the tissue within the arms of the U or J. If decreased sensation is usually expected following the particular pattern used, this should always be told to the patient prior to surgery.

For medicolegal reasons, one must also discuss possible complications. It is important that once the patient has been informed of them that they be put in the proper perspective. Usually, the best way of doing this is to relate in a reassuring fashion that only certain complications have occurred in one's own practice. In the hands of a competent physician, extremely few complications are encountered.

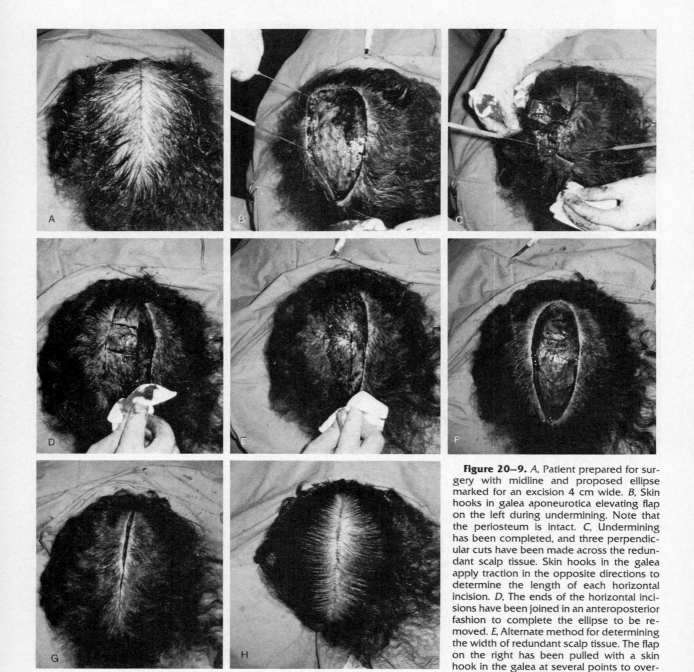

Figure 20—9. *A,* Patient prepared for surgery with midline and proposed ellipse marked for an excision 4 cm wide. *B,* Skin hooks in galea aponeurotica elevating flap on the left during undermining. Note that the periosteum is intact. *C,* Undermining has been completed, and three perpendicular cuts have been made across the redundant scalp tissue. Skin hooks in the galea apply traction in the opposite directions to determine the length of each horizontal incision. *D,* The ends of the horizontal incisions have been joined in an anteroposterior fashion to complete the ellipse to be removed. *E,* Alternate method for determining the width of redundant scalp tissue. The flap on the right has been pulled with a skin hook in the galea at several points to overlap the other flap. The staining of blood from the underside has marked the ellipse to be removed on the surface of the flap on the left. *F,* The resulting defect after an ellipse 4.2 cm wide has been removed. *G,* The galea aponeurotica has been closed with interrupted 2-0 Dexon sutures. *H,* Closure of the skin has been completed using a running 4-0 chromic catgut suture. Compare this end result with A. (Courtesy of *Head and Neck Surgery.*)

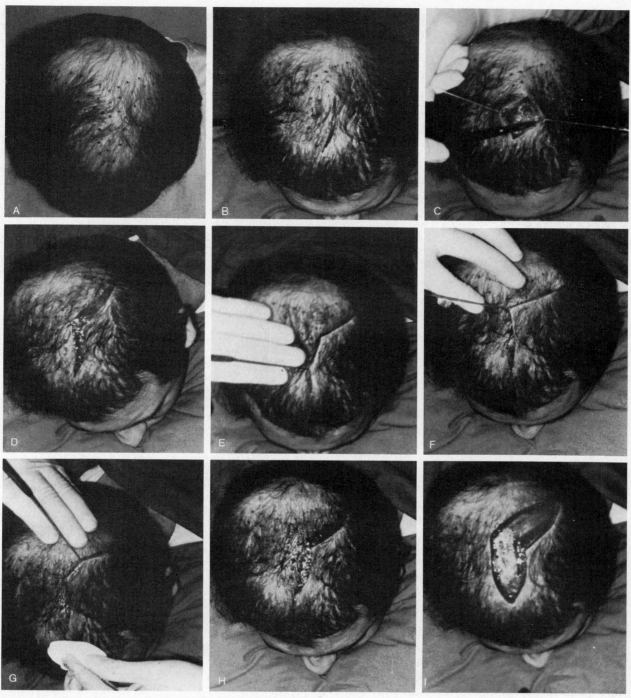

Figure 20–10. *A,* Preoperative markings for "Y" pattern. The midline and central dots for the lateral components are marked first. *B,* Initial incision along one side of the vertical component. *C,* Skin hooks separate the wound edges for undermining in a nontraumatic fashion. *D,* Second incision along the anterior margin of the lateral component. *E,* Overlapping of vertical component flaps. *F,* Overlapping of flaps at junction of the "Y." Elevated flap is first overlapped laterally and then posteriorly. *G,* Overlapping of lateral component flaps. *H,* The staining of blood on the underlying flaps marks the redundant tissue to be removed. This corresponds well to the preoperative markings. *I,* The extra tissue has been removed from the vertical component and the lateral component of the patient's left side. *J,* The flaps of the opposite lateral component are overlapped to mark redundant tissue. *K,* Defect which results after all redundant tissue has been removed. *L,* Galeal sutures have closed the lateral component on the patient's right side. *M,* Closure of the galea aponeurotica has been completed with interrupted 2-0 Dexon sutures. *N,* The skin edges have been closed with 4-0 chromic catgut sutures. The anterior two thirds of the original area of alopecia has been reduced in size. Compare this end result with *A.* (Courtesy of the *Journal of Dermatologic Surgey and Oncology.*)

Illustration continued on following page

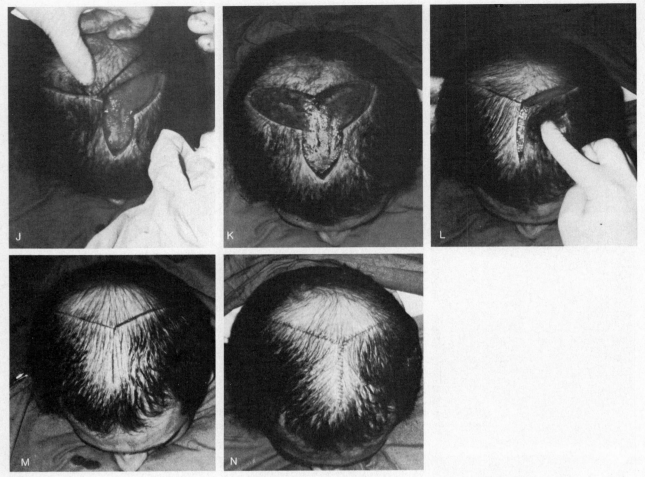

Figure 20–10 *Continued*

SURGICAL TECHNIQUE

Preoperative Preparation

This surgery has always been performed by the authors as an outpatient procedure. The patient arrives one hour before the scheduled time, removes all his clothing except underwear, and is given a hospital gown. While resting in bed, he is given either 15 mg of diazepam orally 30 minutes before surgery or 10 mg of diazepam intravenously immediately before it. Meperidine (Demerol), 50 mg intramuscularly 30 minutes before the operation, is optional with each patient. Photographs are taken and the pattern is marked on the area of alopecia. With the midline reduction, a series of dots are initially marked directly in the midline with a marker, such as the Micropoint Super Marker,* and then the proposed ellipse is added symmetrically (Fig. 20–9) on each side of the marks. With most patients, the accuracy of these markings increases

proportionately with the surgeon's experience in judging scalp laxity. For the beginner, the paper by Bosley and colleagues is helpful.[23] It is wise to terminate the posterior end of the ellipse within the area of alopecia in order to avoid a change in hair direction posteriorly. Alternately, as described earlier, the posterior end of the ellipse can be curved slightly to one side. (Fig. 20–2).

With the Y-shaped pattern, initially a series of dots is marked directly in the midline for the desired length. A mark is then made at the most posterior point along the lateral fringe on each side in a symmetric fashion. Another series of dots is then marked from the lateral side to the midline on one side so that the lateral line and midline markings meet at the desired angle. Markings are then made on the opposite side in a symmetric fashion. The proposed area for excision is then marked symmetrically on each side of the midline and two lateral lines previously marked (Fig. 20–10).

Similarly, with the S-, T- and I-patterns, the center of the proposed area to be excised is marked, and then the proposed area is outlined on each side.

With all lateral patterns (except the S), and the

*Micropoint Super Marker, Micropoint Inc., Sunnyvale, California

U-pattern, the marking technique is slightly different. Initially, a marking is made either along the periphery of the bald area for the desired length or immediately behind the U-shaped region of transplantation anteriorly. A judgment is then made about the width that can be excised, after which the proposed area for removal is marked and suitable tapering is carried out at each end.

Anesthesia

As in the past, a general anesthetic is used only for those patients who cannot psychologically accept being awake during the operation or for those who are extremely difficult to anesthetize with local anesthesia. Because a greater concentration of local anesthesia is required, the risk of toxicity increases proportionately. As noted previously, such patients represent a small minority. If a general anesthetic is used, local anesthetic with epinephrine should still be used along the proposed excision lines in order to minimize blood loss.

The procedure is almost always carried out with local anesthesia. Although 1% lidocaine with epinephrine 1:100,000 was initially used for local anesthesia, now 2% lidocaine with epinephrine 1:100,000 is often used. This provides a more intense anesthesia to the area involved, and because the volume required is usually 20 cc or less, the safety margin for any toxic reaction is still extremely good. A 30-gauge needle is used.

Field block anesthesia is produced by injecting in a circle around the circumference of the head inferior to the expected extent of undermining. Following this, local anesthetic is instilled for hemostasis along the proposed lines of the area to be excised. As an alternative, one can instill the local anesthetic into the incision lines only and use additional anesthetic, if required, during the undermining portion of the operation. The authors personally prefer the former technique, but occasionally use the latter.

Surgery

The operation is carried out under sterile surgical conditions. The patient is usually placed in a prone position with a bulky pillow under the chin for comfort. This positioning gives the greatest exposure to all areas of the scalp; however, care must be taken to avoid any blood running down onto the facial region. On the rare occasion when a general anesthetic is employed, the patient is usually positioned on his side.

After the surgeon has donned gloves and gown, the surgical area is cleansed with a chlorhexadine solution (Hibitane), and sterile drapes are applied. With the exception of the Y- and T-patterns, one initiates the operation by incising along the entire length on one side. This incision is carried out down to and through the galea aponeurotica, and the scalpel blade should be angled in order to avoid severing any adjacent hair follicles. If previous hair transplantation grafts are in the area, a 2 mm margin of safety is normally utilized. Surgical skin hooks are then used to separate the wound edges in a nontraumatic fashion, after which curved Mayo scissors are employed to undermine the loose connective tissue between the periosteum and the galea aponeurotica for 10 cm or more on either side (Fig. 20–9B). This dissection is relatively bloodless except in the vertex region where two or more perforators are often transected. The perforators as well as any other bleeding vessels are cauterized to obtain hemostasis.

There are two useful methods of determining the amount of redundant scalp tissue present. For the novice, the best way is to overlap the tissues by placing the portion of the flap to be removed on top of the other flap. Following this, a series of perpendicular incisions are made through the top flap, stopping at the point where the tissues will meet (Fig. 20–9C). Then, by joining the perpendicular cuts, the redundant tissue is effectively removed (Fig. 20–9D). Alternately, for more experienced surgeons, a skin hook attached to the galea can be used to pull one flap on top of the other. The staining of the blood on the underlying flap can be used as a marker for the amount of tissue to be removed (Fig. 20–9E). Once the redundant tissue has been discarded, hemostasis is again accomplished with cauterization to maintain as dry a field as possible (Fig. 20–9F).

For the Y- and T-patterns, the technique is similar but slightly different. Initially, one incises along one side of the midline component of the area to be excised (Fig. 20–10B). Following this, skin hooks are used, and extensive undermining is carried out (Fig. 20–10C). The second incision is then made at the anterior margin of the lateral component on the same side (Fig. 20–10D). After hemostasis has been controlled, additional undermining is usually carried out. The amount of redundant skin tissue present is then determined along the midline and lateral component on the same side (Figs. 20–10E to H). After using the blood on the underlying flap as a marker, the redundant tissue is removed (Fig. 20–10I). Hemostasis is again achieved with cautery. With the remaining lateral component, an incision is made along one side. Further undermining is performed, and then the redundant tissue is similarly measured and removed (Figs. 20–10J and K).

Closure of the reduction is always carried out in two layers. The galea aponeurotica is sutured using interrupted 2–0 Dexon or Vicryl sutures placed approximately 1.5 cm apart (Fig 20–9G). With the Y- and T-patterns, the lateral components are usually closed first and then the midline element (Figs. 20–10 L and M). The most medial suture with each lateral component is placed very close to the junction where the three flaps meet, whereas with the vertical component the most posterior suture is 0.5 cm from this junction.

During closure of the galea aponeurotica, it is imperative to have the patient refrain from talking, because this causes separation of the galeal edges from the contraction of the temporalis muscle on each side. Another important consideration is the strength of the galeal tissue itself. As previously reported,[12, 20, 24] six cases to date have been confirmed in which the galea aponeurotica has a soft, almost cheese-like, consistency rather than its normal strong fibrous nature. In view of this, it should be emphasized that the strength of the galea should be tested with a skin hook prior to any scalp tissue being removed. If the skin hook pulls through the galea as if it were butter, then no tissue should be removed, and closure is carried out immediately. If one has made the mistake of not testing for this and has already removed scalp tissue, the only solutions are closure with very large bites of galea, or interrupted retention sutures through the entire thickness of scalp tissue.

Once the galea has been closed, the skin edges are approximated with a running 4–0 chromic catgut suture (Fig. 20–9H). In patterns where three flaps meet at a junction, a single interrupted corner stitch is used, and then each component is closed with a running suture (Fig. 20–10N).

It is not necessary to apply a pressure dressing at the completion of surgery. Instead, three or four layers of gauze are placed over the area and then a piece of six-inch stocking modified to form a cap, is applied to hold the gauze in place (Fig. 20–11). In view of the simplicity of this dressing, the patient is instructed to remove it himself the next morning and then comb any hair present over the incision to hide it as effectively as possible.

AREAS OF CONTROVERSY

Tension of Galeal Closure

In the authors' view, the proper tension for closure of the galea occurs if the galeal edges just meet when the fingers are used to approximate the flaps toward each other. If one is questioning whether or not to remove additional tissue, the authors feel it is best to be conservative. Although one always wants to give patients the most benefit, elective cosmetic surgery is being performed, and it is in the best interest of both doctor and patient to err on the side of safety. Alt, among others, has advocated substantially more tension on galeal closure in order to maximize cosmetic gains.[5, 15] Obviously, each

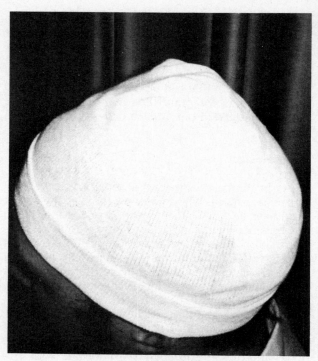

Figure 20–11. Postoperative dressing of gauze and stocking modified to form a cap.

surgeon will have to make his or her own decision about what the proper tension is for closure of this layer.

Interrupted Sutures Versus Continuous Suture Closure

There is some controversy about whether the galea should be closed with interrupted sutures or a continuous suture. The authors have always advocated interrupted sutures, because it is an accepted surgical principle that closure with interrupted sutures is always stronger than a continuous suture of the same material. This becomes even more important if tension for closure of the galea is increased.

Extent of Undermining

Although the area of undermining usually extends 10 cm or more on each side of the initial incision, the authors as a general rule do not dissect down to the attachment of the ears laterally or posteriorly separate the insertion of the occipital muscle from the nuchal ridge, except with certain uncommon reduction patterns referred to earlier. Although this more extensive undermining will enable additional scalp tissue to be removed, it results in increased bleeding during the operative procedure as well as a greater likelihood of postoperative hematoma, edema, and pain.

Galeotomies

The routine use of galeotomies for scalp reductions is still controversial. Although this technique allows an increased amount of scalp tissue to be removed, the practice similarily results in more bleeding during the operation and a greater risk of postoperative hematoma. In addition, the possibility of damaging the circulation to the overlying scalp tissue is markedly increased. Although there is unanimous agreement that galeotomies, if used, should be performed in the areas that are permanently hair-bearing rather than in areas of alopecia, it is also acknowledged that if that area is used as a donor area in the future, the number of hairs per graft will likely be diminished.

In the authors' experience, it has not been necessary or advisable to carry out parallel galeal incisions or both parallel and vertical incisions (scoring) of the galea except in rare cases. The two exceptions to this general rule are as follows: (1) when one has been slightly too aggressive and feels the tension on closure will be greater than ideal, and (2) when one wants to raise the hairline on the part side. In the last few years, even strong proponents of routine galeal scoring have begun to advocate a less aggressive approach. Alt, for example, no longer routinely scores the galea.[25]

Stretch-Back

The authors' objective in carrying out scalp reductions is to remove the redundant scalp tissue present. As related earlier, the ideal tension for closure of the galea occurs if the edges of the galea just meet when bimanual pressure is applied. The degree of stretch-back postoperatively in the authors' practice has been minimal and not clinically significant. It is logical that, if increased tension is utilized on closure of the galea, the amount of stretching of the scalp and resultant stretch-back would increase proportionately. Although Nordstrom has reported up to 50% stretch-back occurring postoperatively,[26, 27] the authors personally feel that this problem can be minimized by closing the galea without excessive tension. To date, Nordstrom is the only physician to have carried out a scientific study in this area. Although the number of patients he has studied is limited, he deserves recognition for focusing the authors' attention on this area. Obviously, further studies are required before this controversy can be resolved.

Intervals Between Scalp Reduction

Although some physicians advocate an interval of only four weeks between scalp reductions,[23] the authors recommend a minimum of eight weeks between operations and extend this to 12 weeks, if clinically indicated.

"Shaw Knife" and Carbon Dioxide Laser

In recent years, some physicians have employed either a Shaw knife (a hot knife) or a CO_2 laser in scalp reductions after incising of the epidermis and dermis initially with a standard scalpel. These instruments cauterize blood vessels as they cut through the tissue. With the Shaw knife, the blade is heated by electrocautery, whereas the CO_2 laser is used in the focused cutting mode to photocoagulate blood vessels. As expected, using either of these devices results in minimal operative bleeding and blood loss and a shorter operating time. A secondary benefit is the decreased likelihood of postoperative bleeding and hematoma formation.

The disadvantages of the Shaw scalpel are the cost of purchase and thermal tissue damage that may impede healing and adversely affect the quality of the scar. With the CO_2 laser, there is significantly less thermal tissue damage, and wound healing is less likely to be impaired. On the other hand, the purchase cost of the laser is far greater, and special training is required for its proper use. Fire and eye damage are potential dangers that must be avoided with the laser.

At the present time almost all doctors use the standard scalpel for reductions and epinephrine to decrease bleeding. Although there is less bleeding with the Shaw knife and CO_2 laser, either insufficient knowledge of their application in this field or their disadvantages have so far prevented their widespread use. Their role in scalp reduction surgery will be further clarified in the future.

CONCOMITANT SCALP REDUCTION AND PUNCH GRAFT TRANSPLANTATION

With certain patients who either have to travel a great distance for each procedure or are limited in the amount of time they can be away from work yet wish to progress as quickly as possible, a procedure combining both scalp reduction and punch graft hair transplantation can be performed. Usually, the scalp reduction operation is completed first followed by punch graft transplantation.

The ring block anesthesia is designed to encompass the area of reduction as well as the transplant recipient area. Most often, a saggital midline ellipse is surgically excised and a U-shaped area is transplanted anteriorly. Sometimes, a crescent of the crown or Y-shaped pattern has been used in combination with transplantation to the anterior region. On one occasion, a lateral pattern was carried out on the right side while transplantation was carried out to a ledge along the left side of the midscalp and crown regions. The primary consideration for the combined procedure is blood supply. If there is any question about whether the blood supply to either region will be compromised, it is wiser to carry out each procedure separately.

As noted earlier, concomitant scalp reductions are also used during repair sessions on patients who have had poor results with previous transplants. Worthwhile grafts are removed from the area to be excised and retransplanted in order to thicken the remaining areas.

Another type of combined procedures involves standard hair transplantation and mini reductions.[20, 28] Although it is acknowledged that repeated mini reductions may eventually save one standard type of reduction, one of the authors (M. G. Unger) does not routinely employ them. If the galea is not closed in a mini reduction, there is a significantly increased risk of bleeding and postoperative spreading of the scar. On the other hand, if one does close the mini reduction in two layers, the amount of time required is almost the same as that required for a standard type of reduction, and the latter procedure would have significantly more beneficial results.

The other author (W. P. Unger) uses mini reductions routinely in the midline during nearly all punch graft transplant operations, providing the excision lines are not close enough to the punch grafts being transplanted to distort the shape of the recipient sites. If one or two lines of holes are punched out and sutured closed in a single layer (after any intervening tissue has been removed), the resultant scar should be no worse than that seen when a similar maneuver in the donor area is carried out. Usually, 20 to 30 grafts can be "saved" during each transplant session by this simple procedure. However, if elliptical mini reductions are attempted, it cannot be emphasized enough that two-layer closure is necessary to avoid scars that are wide enough to have made the reduction futile.

Both authors use mini reductions in some individuals with poor punch graft transplant results. Sites that can be punched out and sutured closed are treated in this fashion in order to remove bald areas without consuming any of the limited remaining supply of donor grafts. These grafts are then used in sparse areas that are more cosmetically important or that are not amenable to excision. The main advantages of mini reductions in repair cases are that the configuration of the reduction can be whatever that of the defect is, e.g., S-, T-, L-, or I-shaped, and the punch used in boring out the bare sites may vary from 3 to 5 mm at different points along the pattern—depending on the size of the defect at that point. "Bridges" between the holes are cut and interdigitated prior to suturing (Fig. 20–12).

Tissue Expanders

The concept of tissue expansion prior to excision is credited to Radovan. Initially, the procedure was utilized for the expansion of chest tissue as part of

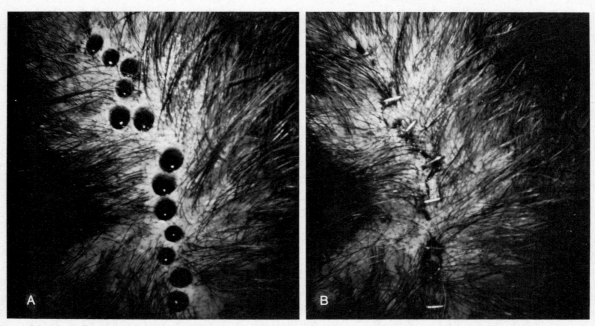

Figure 20–12. *A*, Thirteen holes, whose size was entirely dictated by the size of the hairless gaps, were bored out in a line whose configuration was also determined solely by the requirements of the site. *B*, The "bridges" between the holes were cut and the defect interdigitated before closure with stainless steel staples shown above. The staples will be removed in 10 days. Essentially 13 grafts were "saved" for use elsewhere. Three similar maneuvers at other sites in this patient were carried out concomitantly for a total "saving" of 48 grafts.

postmastectomy reconstruction. Following this, the technique was applied to the treatment of lesions of the limbs including giant nevi and tattoos.[29] In recent years, several physicians have applied the principles of tissue expansion to scalp surgery.[33, 34]

To date, tissue expansion of the scalp is most frequently being carried out to successfully remove large areas of cicatricial alopecia or post-traumatic defects. Recently, the use of one or more tissue expanders has been applied to the treatment of male pattern baldness.

With the first patient of the principal author, two custom-made banana-shaped expanders were placed along each side of the lateral scalp in the hair-bearing region, and after the first week, each device was expanded twice weekly. After six weeks, a scalp reduction operation was performed during which the two expanders were removed and virtually all of the area of alopecia, which measured 10 cm in width, was excised.

During the six months following that first patient, each new patient for scalp reduction was given the choice of one scalp reduction with tissue expanders, or alternately two or three standard reductions. Without exception, all patients elected to have the standard reductions performed. Despite this initial reluctance, since then several other patients have had tissue expansion reductions. In two cases, for the first time, previous punch graft donor area was expanded. Further details will be related in a publication now in press.[37]

By incorporating tissue expanders, an enlargement and a deformity of the scalp area is created, which has been compared to hydrocephalus, for at least several weeks. On the other hand, with standard reductions, there is minimal deformity, and the patient is usually able to return to work the following day. The author's conclusion is that, at the present time, scalp tissue expansion is a needed and valuable tool for correcting extensive abnormal regions of the scalp, but it has not yet been widely accepted for normal male pattern baldness because of the deformity created before the improvement is gained.

COMPLICATIONS

In the authors' experience (over 3000 operations), remarkably few complications have occurred. By far, the commonest complication has been a superficial catgut reaction. During the first year of carrying out scalp reductions, the skin sutures were left to dissolve, and 20% of the patients had these reactions. This consisted of either erythema or small pustules where the sutures penetrated the skin along the suture line. Treatment consisted of removing the sutures, after which the problem resolved in a few days without any long-term consequences. A 4–0 chromic catgut suture has continued to be used because of its closeness to normal skin color, but it

has since been removed after five to seven days. This has virtually eliminated the problem.

The next most common complication has been a deep catgut reaction. Initially, healing occurred beautifully, but then, after two to four weeks, a small opening would develop at one or more sites where 2–0 chromic catgut sutures had been used for galeal closure. If left untreated, often two or more openings coalesced (Fig. 20–13). This reaction occurred in 10% of the patients (12 patients) during the short time that the authors used catgut for the galea. Since that time, 2–0 Dexon has produced only three such cases, and none has occurred to date with 2–0 Vicryl sutures, although this material has been used much less frequently than Dexon. Treatment consists of suture removal and suitable daily cleansing until the openings are closed.

Temporary postoperative facial edema has occurred in approximately 20% of the authors' patients. The incidence of postoperative edema is far higher in those individuals who refuse or who medically cannot receive systemic steroids. Twelve patients have had wider scars than the usual fine line, and 10 patients have had a grooving or indentation of the scar itself. In all 10 cases, patients had a much thicker scalp depth than usual, yet this complication did not occur in the vast majority of other patients with similarly thick scalp tissues. Three patients had superficial necrosis of the skin edge, and a postoperative infection (*Staphylococcus aureus*) occurred in two patients despite prophylactic antibiotics. No other complications have been seen in our practice.

Postoperative bleeding, hematoma (especially

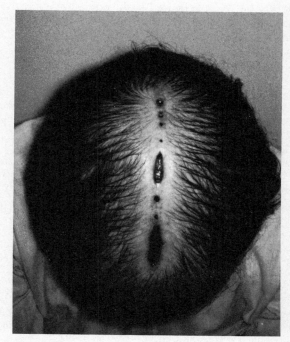

Figure 20–13. A severe "deep catcut reaction." Openings of suture sites have coalesced anteriorly and in the central region.

after galeotomies), wound dehiscence, flap necrosis, and permanent hair loss are all potential complications of scalp reductions.[30] One case of osteomyelitis of the skull has been reported.[31]

Norwood and coworkers have concluded that the incidence of complications decreases very significantly with increasing experience.[32] The authors' findings indicate that scalp reductions, in general, are safe and relatively complication-free when performed as recommended in this chapter.

CONCLUSION

The utilization of scalp reductions in combination with punch graft transplantation has now been carried out for over a decade. Modifications and improvements over the years have contributed significantly to the results, and the concept of scalp reduction itself has now gained widespread acceptance.

Attempts to remove the maximum amount of skin in each patient could conceivably lead to severe complications, such as wound dehiscence or permanent hair loss, and therefore it is always wiser to take a little bit less than a little bit more. When this is carried out by a competent physician, the likelihood of any complications is far less than with most cosmetic surgery procedures, and the resulting improvement in appearance and patient gratification is extremely rewarding.

Although our expertise and knowledge of scalp surgery have increased over the years, there are still several areas of controversy remaining. The ideal interval between repeated scalp reductions and the process of stretch-back are both important issues demanding further scientific study.

REFERENCES

1. Unger MG, Unger WP: Alopecia reduction, in Epstein E, Epstein E Jr: (eds): Skin Surgery, vol 1, ed. 5. Springfield, Ill, Charles C Thomas, 1982, pp 530–545
2. Unger MG, Unger WP: Management of alopecia of the scalp by a combination of excisions and transplantations. J Dermatol Surg Oncol 4:670–672, 1978
3. McGregor IA: Fundamental Techniques of Plastic Surgery and Their Surgical Applications. New York, Churchill Livingstone Inc, 1975
4. Orentreich N: Autographs in alopecia and other elected dermatological conditions. Ann NY Acad Sci 83:463–477, 1959
5. Alt TH: History of scalp reductions and paramedian method, in Norwood OT: Hair Transplant Surgery, ed. 2. Springfield, Ill, Charles C Thomas, 1984, pp 221–244
6. Blanchard G, Blanchard B: Obliteration of alopecia by hair-lifting: A new concept and technique. J Nat Med Assoc 69:639–641, 1977.
7. Sparkuhl K: Scalp reduction: Serial excision of the scalp with flap advancement. The International Hair Transplant Symposium, Lucerne, Switzerland, February 4, 1978
8. Stough DB, Webster RC: Esthetics and refinements in hair transplantation. The International Hair Transplant Symposium, Lucerne, Switzerland, February 4, 1978.
9. Bosley LL, Hope CR, Montroy RE: Male pattern reduction (MPR) for surgical reduction of male pattern baldness. Curr Ther Res 25:281–287, 1979.
10. Alt TH: Scalp reduction as an adjunct to hair transplantation, review of relevant literature, presentation of an improved technique. J Dermatol Surg Oncol 6:1011–1018, 1980.
11. Norwood OT, Shiell RC: Scalp reductions, in Norwood OT: Hair Transplant Surgery, ed. 2. Springfield, Ill, Charles C Thomas, 1984, pp 163–200
12. Fleming RW, Kabaker SS, Marritt M, Mayer TG: Panel discussion, The Sixth National Symposium on Hair Replacement Surgery, Palm Springs, Calif, March 29, 1984
13. Nordstrom REA: Change of direction of hair growth. J Dermatol Surg Oncol 9:156–158, 1983
14. Marzola M: An Alternative Hair Replacement Method, in Norwood OT: Hair Transplant Surgery, ed. 2. Springfield, Ill, Charles C Thomas, 1984, pp 315–324
15. Alt TH: Scalp reduction. Cosmet Surg 1:1–19, 1981
16. Unger WP, Unger MG: Alopecia reduction, in: Epstein E (ed.): Controversies in Dermatological Surgery. Philadelphia, W. B. Saunders Co., 1984, pp 329–336
17. Norwood OT: Hair Transplant Surgery. Springfield, Ill, Charles C Thomas, 1973
18. Hamilton JB: Patterned loss of hair in man: Types and incidence. Ann NY Acad Sci 53:708–728, 1951
19. Unger MG, Unger WP: Alopecia reductions, in Unger WP: Hair Transplantation, A Text. New York, Marcel Dekker Inc, 1979, pp 102–108
20. Unger MG, Unger WP: Midline alopecia reduction combined with hair transplantation. Head Neck Surg 7:303–311, 1985
21. Unger MG: The Y shaped pattern of alopecia reduction and its variations. J Dermatol Surg Oncol, 10:980–986, 1984
22. Unger MG: Scalp reductions. Facial Plastic Surgery, 2:253–258, 1985
23. Bosley LL, Hope CR, Montroy RE, Staub P: Reduction of male pattern baldness in multiple stages: A retrospective study. J Dermatol Surg Oncol 6:498–503, 1982
24. Unger MG, Kabaker S: Panel discussion, The International Advanced Hair Replacement Symposium, Birmingham, Ala, February 3, 1982
25. Alt TH: Personal communications, June 1984
26. Nordstrom REA, "Stretch-back" in scalp reductions for male pattern baldness. Plast Reconstr Surg 73:422–426, 1984
27. Nordstrom REA: Scalp kinetics in multiple excisions for correction of male pattern baldness. J Dermatol Surg Oncol 10:991–995, 1984
28. Unger WP: Concomitant mini reductions in punch hair transplanting. J Dermatol Surg Oncol 9:388–892, 1983
29. Radovan C: Personal communications, February 1984
30. Norwood OT, Shiell RD, Morrison ID: Complications of scalp reductions. J Dermatol Surg Oncol 9:828–835, 1983
31. Jones WJ: Osteomyelitis of the skull following scalp reduction and hair plug transplantation. Ann Plast Surg 5:480–482, 1980
32. Norwood OT, Shiell RD, Morrison ID: Complications and Problems of Scalp Reductions, in Norwood OT: Hair Transplant Surgery, ed. 2. Springfield, Ill, Charles C Thomas, 1984, pp 201–220
33. Manders EK, Graham WP 3rd, Shenden MJ, Davis TS: Skin Expansion to eliminate large scalp defects. Ann Plast Surg 12:305, 1984
34. Manders EK, Graham WP 3rd: Alopecia reduction by scalp expansion. J Dermatol Surg Oncol 10:967–969, 1984
35. Onizuka T, Ohmori S: Treatment of alopecia cicatricans using an artery flap. Plast Reconstr Surg 35:338, 1965
36. Huang TT, Larson DL, Lewis SR: Burn alopecia. Plast Reconstr Surg 60:763, 1977
37. Unger MG, Unger WP: Scalp reductions, in Unger WP: Hair Transplantation, ed 2. New York, Marcel Dekker Inc, in press.

21

SHELDON S. KABAKER, M.D.

Flap Procedures in Hair Replacement Surgery

A complete review of the techniques available for surgical hair replacement must include the scalp flap procedures wherein unipedicle hair-bearing scalp flaps can be used to create complete hairlines or half hairlines that are of great density and aesthetically acceptable. Although not all hair transplant surgeons perform them, scalp flap procedures should be understood by any physician involved with hair transplantation. The large delayed flaps devised by José Juri[1] of Argentina, the nondelayed flaps described by Elliott[2] and others, and the scalp reduction operation have all become important procedures in hair replacement surgery. Recent experiences with tissue expansion[3, 4] make this new procedure the treatment of choice in many cases of cicatricial alopecia. Tissue expansion also has some limited application in the treatment of male pattern baldness.

The reader should be aware that, while these operations involve the basic principles of flap surgery described elsewhere in this book, there are factors specific to the human scalp that have become apparent to this author through a 10-year experience with scalp flap procedures.[5, 6] Some previously little appreciated factors of scalp anatomy are of great importance in flap surgery, and their influence on procedures will be discussed later in this chapter.

ANATOMIC CONSIDERATIONS

The human scalp consists of a thick skin containing a tight pattern of hair follicles, glands, fat, fibrous tissue, lymphatic channels, and a vascular system. There is an abundance of interconnections of the blood supply that courses through the dermis and the subcutaneous layers of the scalp skin.[7] The only area of the scalp that is somewhat deficient in vascularity is in the saggital midline.

The vascular system consists of an abundance of anastomosing arteries and arterioles feeding the plentiful capillaries of the deep dermal layers. Five pairs of major arteries nourish the scalp. The paired supraorbital and supratrochlear vessels are branches of the ophthalmic artery; the paired superficial temporal arteries, postauricular arteries, and occipital arteries are derived from the external carotid system.

Beneath the vascular components of the scalp is the fibrous, tough galea aponeurotica, which anteriorly fuses with the frontalis muscle and posteriorly with the occipital muscle. Beneath the galea is a loose, fibroareolar layer overlying the pericranium. This loose fascial space allows for the sliding phenomenon utilized in moving scalp tissue (Fig. 21–1). The plane of separation and movement is not as distinct posteriorly as anteriorly where the galea is present.

Bald scalp is usually 30% to 60% thinner than hair-bearing scalp. The aging and balding scalp is less vascular than the youthful one. Scalp thickness and elasticity vary greatly. The variability of scalp elasticity has been found to be the most important factor relevant to the ease or difficulty in performing scalp flap procedures.

PATIENT SELECTION

The author believes that patient motivation is as important a consideration in the selection of candidates as physical characteristics. Physically, the ideal candidate should have a stable, somewhat limited balding pattern with good crown coverage and dense, thick donor hair. However, regardless of ideal physical characteristics, the patient whose dissatisfaction with baldness has resulted in a strong commitment to hair replacement has turned out to be the best candidate for flaps. These are men who, for personal or professional reasons, wear hairpieces but may prefer a permanent and reasonably aesthetic alternative solution to the prosthesis. They often have had some punch grafts but want greater density of hair than punch grafting alone can achieve.

Flaps of donor hair, like punch grafts, can be used on almost any balding scalp with predictable results. The ideal candidate for punch grafting is also the ideal candidate for flaps. The balding pattern should be evaluated to determine its greatest potential extent, especially when dealing with younger men. Usually by the age of 40, the balding pattern is well developed and relatively stable. Norwood[8] has provided a rather complete classification of balding patterns, and Juri[1] has described a simplified categorization. A slight modification of

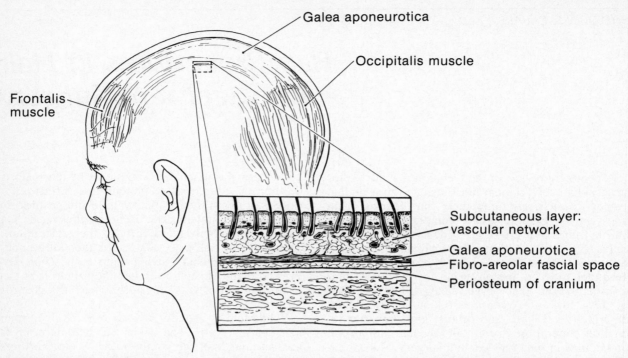

Figure 21–1. Anatomic highlights of the human scalp. Note that the vascular supply is superficial to the galea. The scalp is mobile over the fibro-areolar fascial space.

the Juri classification will be used in this chapter (Fig. 21–2).

The patient with frontotemporal recession and a stable balding pattern (Type I baldness) is a candidate for small flap procedures. These flaps are also useful in augmenting or revising punch-grafted hairlines. Most patients with a greater extent of baldness (Type II or IIIa) can be provided with dense frontal coverage using a large or small flap but cannot have

total coverage (see Fig. 21–5). Scalp reductions and punch grafting can aid with coverage in this situation. High-quality punch grafting along with scalp reduction might distribute limited donor hair better and result in a thin but natural-appearing hair cover, especially with Type IIIb baldness.

Flaps are usually the treatment of choice for black patients (unless the hair is racially atypical). Coiled hair follicles suffer a significant amount of transsec-

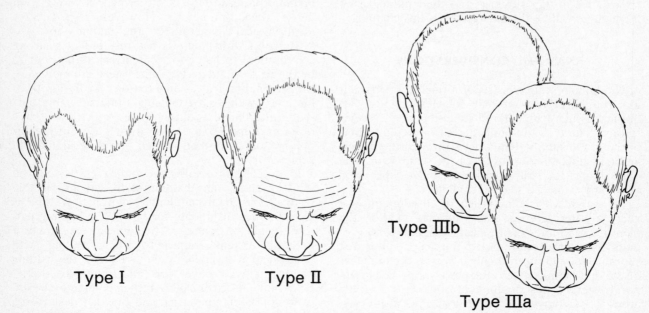

Figure 21–2. Male pattern baldness types. The more extreme Type IIIb with low fringe and recessed temporal points is an unfavorable candidate for flap operations.

tion in the punch-grafting process, and therefore, the yield is less satisfactory than with straight hair. The use of flaps eliminates this problem. The natural curly hair of blacks is also ideal for styling flap-grafted hair.

The relative tightness and flexibility of scalp tissue varies from one patient to another. Preoperative evaluation of this flexibility and therefore the ease of operation can be achieved by the experienced surgeon.

These comments on patient selection are not a complete inventory but represent the highlights of personal experience.

LARGE (JURI) DELAYED FLAPS

Hair-bearing scalp flaps have long been used for reconstructive purposes in burn or tumor patients to replace eyebrows, mustache hair, or hairlines. Juri described a lengthy series of cases wherein long, delayed pedicle flaps were used for the correction of male pattern baldness.[1] Previously, only isolated case reports on hair flap operations were described in the literature.[9]

The Juri flap procedure produces excellent cosmetic results. It is an exacting procedure with many fine details and subtleties that requires an efficient and imaginative operative technique. Utilizing the anatomic peculiarities of the human scalp, this operation (or series of operations) transfers the greatest amount of hair in the shortest period of time compared to other forms of surgical hair restoration. One Juri flap contains the hair equivalent of at least 450 4.0-mm punch grafts. The hair on the flap usually continues to grow and thereby bypasses the telogen phase of punch grafting. For instance, if the donor fringe hair were four inches long, it would still be that long after flap surgery. Punch-grafted hair would take 11 months to become four inches long, and that would apply only to the grafts from the first session.

Another aesthetic advantage is that the density of the hair is the same as the density of the fringe. The frontal hairline scar should not be easily detectable. An unsatisfactory frontline scar can usually be revised easily.

TECHNIQUE FOR LARGE (JURI) FLAP

The design of the flap is the most important phase of the operation. All other aspects of the operation coordinate this flap design into the final result.

Design

A hairline is first drawn on the scalp. This hairline should be placed in an aesthetically acceptable man-

ner with the peak midfrontal hairline no less a distance from the root of the nose than the measured distance between the base of the nose and the tip of the chin. It is wise to lace the hairline 2 to 3 cm above this point in the more severely bald individual, so there will be less bald scalp to be covered posteriorly, and the hairline will resemble a mature one. Some frontotemporal recession may be designed into the hairline, but if a large amount is desired and the hairline is located in a relatively posterior location, an inevitable dog-ear will result. The dog-ear, however, can be treated later. It is simply the price paid for a more aesthetic hairline. The rounded hairline lessens the technical difficulty of the operation.

After the hairline is designed, the posterior branch of the superficial temporal artery is located by palpation. It usually runs superiorly through the midportion of the sideburn and then curves in a posterior direction. Any doubt about its location can be alleviated by use of a Doppler flow detector. The artery need only be identified in the proximal 3 to 4 cm of the flap design (Fig. 21–3). The inferior edge of the flap should start at a point about 3 cm above the root of the helix (Point A), and the superior edge of the flap should start 4 cm from this first point—at an angle of 30 to 45 degrees to a line drawn from the horizontal (Point B). The posterior branch of the superficial temporal artery should be in the center of the origin of the flap.

Parallel lines 4 cm apart are then drawn on the scalp within the hair-brearing fringe. Calipers or a compass with two felt-tip marking pens attached can be used to make these lines.

The length of the flap design can be determined with the use of a template made of 3/8 inch foam rubber cut to simulate the length and curvature of the frontal hairline design. If one measures the frontal hairline and adds another 40% to 50%, one has the usual length of the flap.

The peak of the frontal hairline is usually at the junction of the posterior and middle thirds of the flap. The anterior third of the flap is relocated within the temporal hairline during the surgical transfer. Therefore, it is the posterior two thirds of the flap design that become the frontal hairline. The tail end of the flap design overlays the supramuscular flap, while the anterior portion of the flap design has the galea with it. It may be necessary to cross the midposterior scalp line to gain adequate length for the flap. These 4-cm-wide flaps have measured between 22 and 30 cm long.

Delays

Juri has described two delay procedures. The second delay is done one week after the first, and the transfer procedure is done one week after the

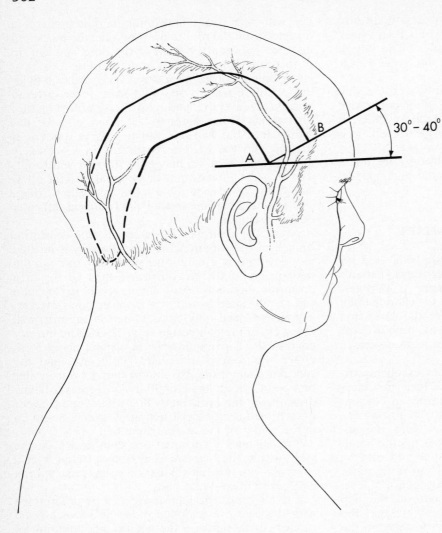

Figure 21–3. Design of the Juri flap: Classical delay procedures involve incisions along the solid lines on the first delay; dotted lines indicate undercut area of second delay.

second delay. The delay can be performed in the office.

The First Delay

The patient prepares for surgery by shampooing his hair with a hexachlorophene soap at home in the morning, and the hair is again washed with a povidone-iodine solution at the office. The hair is then bunched up in clumps using small rubber bands, and 1% lidocaine with ephinephrine (1:100,000) is infiltrated along the marked lines of the flap design. A special parallel knife is used to scratch in the incision lines. The cuts are then deepened through the galea by incising the proximal three quarters of the flap parallel to the hair follicles. The incisions are closed with a running 4-0 monofilament suture or staples. Undercutting is not performed now, nor is it necessary.

The first delay can be performed by cutting small segments and suturing them before proceeding. This segmental approach avoids blood loss. The effect of this first delay procedure is essentially the creation of a bipedicled flap whose posterior circulation is provided by the perforating branches of the occipital artery.

The Second Delay

This operation is performed one week after the first delay. The distal 6 to 8 cm of the flap are cut around and then undercut. The undercutting transects the occipital artery supply, which comes through the occipital musculature. There is no need to undercut the flap overlying the galea because little blood supply crosses that area. The second delay usually requires ligature hemostasis of the large perforating vessels before suturing the skin edges.

Postoperatively, a turban dressing is applied and worn for one day. The delay procedures can be compared to a session of punch grafting insofar as time, morbidity, and complications are concerned.

AUTHOR'S DELAY TECHNIQUE

Presently, the author still performs two delays with his modification of Juri's technique. A *bridge delay* has been performed on 24 patients without complication. Performing delays in the following manner allows the second delay procedure to be an insignificant undertaking. The first procedure involves cutting around the flap design, except for a 4 to 5 cm bridge on the midsuperior edge of the flap (Fig. 21–4). The distal end of the flap is undercut, accomplishing what is performed during the classical second delay described by Juri. One week later, the uncut bridge is transected and stapled shut (Fig. 21–5). A dressing is usually not needed. This second procedure takes five minutes and could even be done without local anesthesia; however, local anesthesia with epinephrine is used for the hemostatic effect. This bridge delay accomplished the same shift of blood supply as the classic delay: a bipedicled flap is created and converted one week later to a unipedicled flap while the peripheral circulation is being regained.

DISCUSSION OF DELAY PROCEDURES

The need for delay in these large flaps of a 7:1 length-to-width ratio has been challenged, and in-

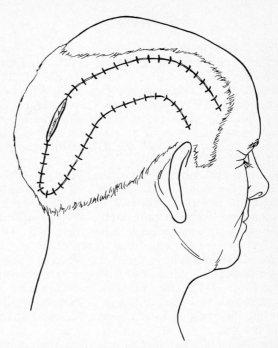

Figure 21–5. One week after the initial delay procedure with staples still in place. The bridge is cut through and then stapled closed.

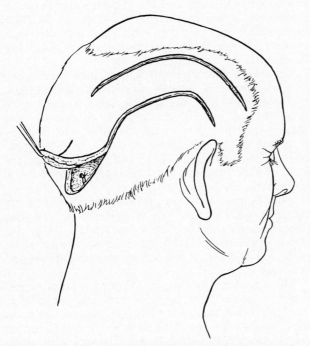

Figure 21–4. Bridge delay method preferred by the author. Distal end of the flap is undercut; edges are incised through the galea, leaving an uncut 5 cm bridge as shown. The occipital artery is often ligated.

deed, the operation has been performed without delay. Also, it has been done with one delay, so that all the steps in both delays of Juri's procedure were combined in one session—creating an unipedicled flap that is observed for one or two weeks before being transferred. This "testing" of the flap probably has some effect on increasing the viable length, especially if some bridges of the scalp are left untransected. Ohmori's reports on free flaps indicate that delays are not necessary.[10] The free flap only needs definite proximal arterial blood supply and is sewn into the recipient bed without tension or torsion.

The author believes that, in spite of occasional successful cases of large flaps done without delay, not all scalps have the favorable arterial directional anatomy for consistent results. Also, the fact that the pedicle of the flap is often sewn in place with some torsion on it, which causes some compromise in blood flow, adds to the argument for delaying the flap.

Experience with the smaller flaps, which are about as long as the anterior two thirds of a Juri flap, has shown that a *nondelayed* parieto-occipital scalp flap can almost always survive to create one half of a hairline. This much of a sclap flap is essentially an arterialized axial flap. The Juri flap is likely to have a randomized posterior portion that is less apt to survive completely in all cases. It is this posterior third of the Juri flap that benefits from delay.

FLAP TRANSFER

The major procedure of moving the flap into position is performed in a hospital of fully equipped office operating room under sterile technique. Endotracheal or intravenous anesthesia is used. Local anesthesia with a vasoconstrictor is infiltrated throughout the areas to be incised or undermined. Local anesthesia without a vasoconstrictor is used in areas near the base of the flap or into the flap itself.

The flap is elevated by sharp and blunt dissection deep to the galea (Fig. 21–6) and is carefully wrapped in saline-soaked sponges. The hairline incision is made with the knife handle tilted posteriorly at about a 45-degree angle with the scalp. This beveled incision is made to a depth equal to the length of the hair follicle and is deepened in a more perpendicular direction down to the subaponeurotic tissue (Fig. 21–7). The extension of this incision in the hair-bearing temporal scalp is beveled in the opposite direction in order to spare the hair follicles from trauma.

The parietal scalp is easily undermined in the subgaleal space (Fig. 21–8). Posteriorly, the scalp is undermined in the supramuscular plane, and once

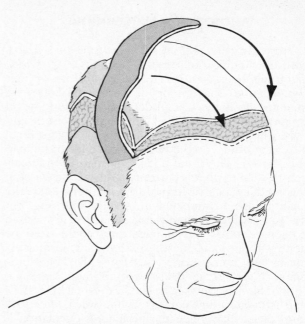

Figure 21–7. Juri flap is rotated toward the frontal hairline, which has a bevelled incision. Extensive undermining of subgaleal scalp is performed.

the hairline is reached, undermining in the neck is continued in the subcutaneous plane, similar to the dissection used in a facelift. The postauricular skin is undermined to the helical rim and into the lobule. The neck undermining should go at least halfway between the hairline and the clavicle—and in some cases even down to the clavicle (Fig. 21–9). The undermined areas are temporarily packed with large sponges. A suction cautery apparatus is used for hemostasis.

The donor site is partially closed with permanent or semipermanent sutures approximating the edges of the galea. Then, the leading edge of the flap is de-epithelized with sharp scissors. A strip of skin wide enough to uncover two or three hair follicles is removed. This maneuver allows hair to grow *through* the scar (Figs. 21–10 and 21–11). Irregularities of this trimming are desirable to produce a more natural hairline.

Undermining of the frontal and temporal scalp on the side toward the flap is performed, and the anterior edge of the flap is sutured in place by starting proximally and using an *advancing suture* to work out or lessen a dog-ear or to gain flap length, if necessary.

The advancing is done by suturing a point of the flap to a more distal point on the scalp edge (Fig. 21–12). A 5-0 monofilament interrupted suture is used by taking bites close to the skin edges and at the proper depth so the beveled frontal scalp edge overlays the de-epithelized flap edge.

The donor closure is completed with more buried, deep sutures in the galea. Even with extensive

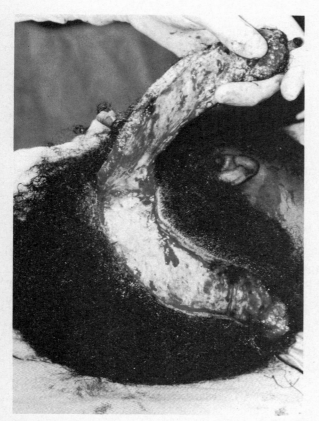

Figure 21–6. Juri flap (4 cm wide × 28 cm long) is raised from its bed. The galea is contained within the flap.

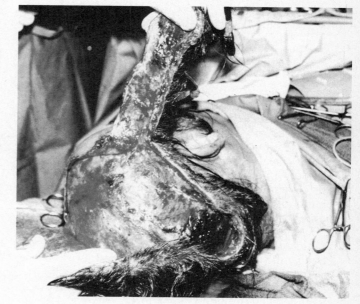

Figure 21–8. Juri flap with subgaleal undermining of the top of the scalp is demonstrated.

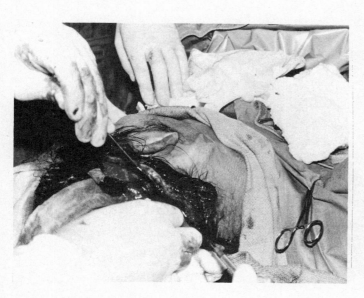

Figure 21–9. Neck undermining to facilitate donor closure is shown.

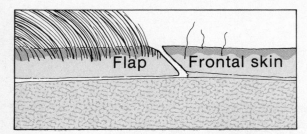

Figure 21–10. Frontal skin edge is bevelled, and the leading edge of the flap is bevelled and de-epithelized. Transected follicles grow through scar.

undermining, there can be tension on this part of the closure. The skin is closed with minimal tension using staples or 4–0 or 5–0 monofilament sutures (Fig. 21–13). One should emphasize that the tension is on the galeal closure, not on the skin closure.

On occasion, the most anterior portion of the donor closure will not come together. Often a full-thickness skin graft from the excised bald scalp, appropriately thinned, is sewn to the edges of the gap. Some months later, it can be removed if a cosmetic deficiency persists.

Finally, the excess bald skin is trimmed away in segments. The amount of scalp removed is usually less than the width of the flap because the scalp has been pulled laterally and posteriorly to cover the donor area. Enough scalp may be removed so that the closure line of the posterior edge of the flap has slight tension.

Closure of the posterior edge of the flap is attained with interrupted 4–0 monofilament sutures by taking bites through the full thickness of the bald scalp and

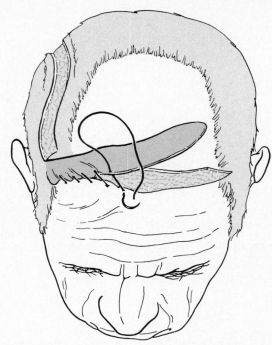

Figure 21–12. Advancing suture technique to gain maximum flap length and ease out dog-ear. An elevation or bulge often results at the proximal hairline.

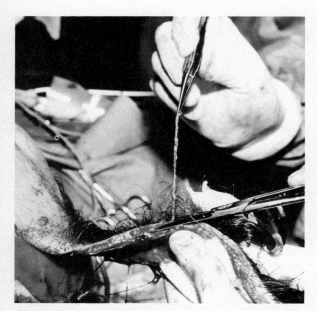

Figure 21–11. Scissors used to de-epithelize the leading edge of a Juri flap, an essential maneuver for the success of esthetic hair flap procedures.

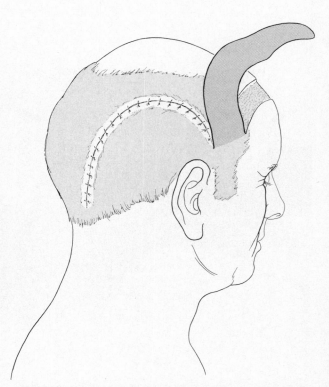

Figure 21–13. Donor site is closed in two layers; heavy buried sutures hold the galea under slight tension; skin is closed without tension.

through an *equivalent* amount of the posterior edge of the flap in order not to create a great step-off between tissues of different thicknesses, since the bald scalp is thinner than the flap. Staples may be used to complete the posterior flap closure line (Fig. 21–14).

A large suction drain is placed under the dissected neck skin. Two or three short Penrose drains are placed under the flap between the sutures of the posterior flap closure line, and a bulky but noncompressing head and neck dressing is applied. The drains are removed on the morning after surgery, and the dressing is reapplied and remains in place for three or four more days. Often the patient is surprised at how little pain there is, considering the extent of this operation. Pain not controlled with mild analgesics should be a warning of the possibility of expanding hematoma of the neck or impending necrosis of scalp tissues. Front-line sutures are removed five days after surgery, and the remaining sutures and staples are removed by 12 days after surgery. The hair may be carefully combed after one or two weeks.

Morbidity

As with extensive front-line punch grafting, forehead and eyelid edema with ecchymoses can occur on the third or fourth postoperative day. This presents no long-term problem and usually resolves in 10 days. This problem can be lessened by short-term steroid therapy, ice compresses, or a foam-rubber compression dressing on the forehead for the first three or four postoperative days.

Dog-ears or bulges of the elevated forehead skin

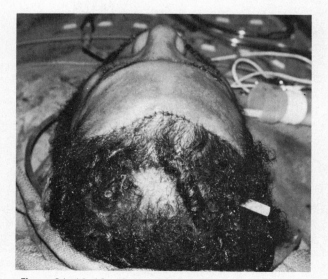

Figure 21–14. After the overlapped bald scalp is excised, the flap is sewn in place and the procedure is completed. Note the gradually peaked hairline; flap hairlines can be curved in esthetically acceptable configurations.

at the proximal side of the flap resolve greatly in five or six weeks. Then, half of the patients need an adjustment procedure done in the office as follows:

The proximal posterior suture line of the flap is opened, as is a limited area of the frontal proximal suture line. An anterior-posterior incision is made, and proximal and distal flaps are created. The surrounding tissues are undermined, and the flaps are pulled backward and relocated to flatten out any bulges. Bald skin resection and opening of the anterior donor closure site provide space where the flaps may be sutured. The dog-ear or bulge is an accepted part of this operation, and its adjustment is easy to perform (Fig. 21–15).

Operative bleeding problems lessen with experience. The tension of the galeal closure provides a great deal of the hemostasis in addition to ligation and cauterization. The operation should be performed before the vasoconstrictor wears off (1½ to 2 hours).

On occasions when it occurs, necrosis of distal flap ends and donor closure sites usually does not become apparent for about 10 days. By six weeks, the degree of full-thickness loss can be assessed. Treatment for this problem should be conservative in order to promote delayed healing. Broad-spectrum antibiotics, daily antiseptic applications, and sometimes dressings are utilized. Granulation tissue develops and epithelization is usually completed after 12 weeks. Donor closure defects (usually widened scars) may require late revisional surgery (six months or more postoperatively).

The Second Juri Flap

A second flarge flap procedure may be performed three to four months after the first one when the sclap has loosened somewhat. The design is similar to the front-line flap, but it may be taken higher or even at the edge of the fringe hair.

Delays are performed in the same manner as in the first flap operation.

The transfer procedure requires less meticulous suturing, and few dog-ear problems have been noted. The second flap is placed about 4 cm behind the frontal flap, except in cases of limited stable balding patterns where it may be placed immediately behind. Later, excision of intervening bald scalp and galeal removal beneath the flaps will allow stretching of the flap in the anterior and posterior dimension to gain greater scalp coverage (Figs. 21–16 and 21–17).

Donor closure problems with a second flap occur more often because circulation to the superior segment of the donor closure site must traverse old and new incision lines, and this is the area most distant from the blood supply. This same problem also occurs with the small flaps as described later. Bilat-

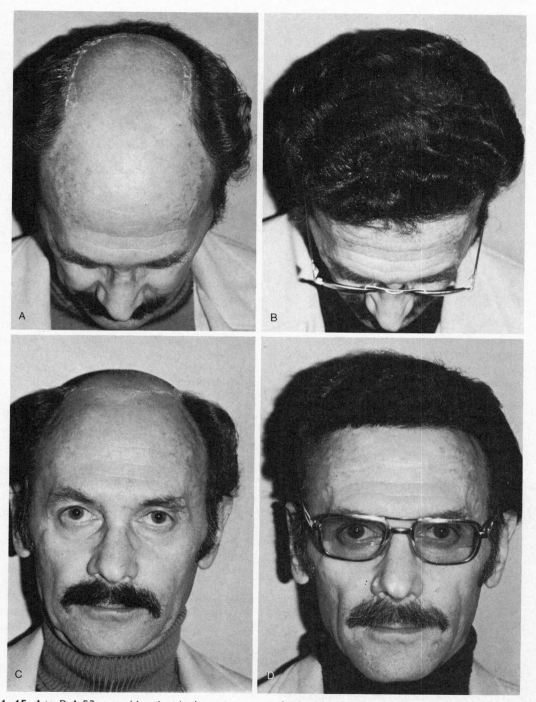

Figure 21–15. *A* to *D*, A 52-year-old patient is shown two years after one Juri flap procedure resulting in a dense frontal hairline with an imperceptible scar. Dog-ear was adjusted.

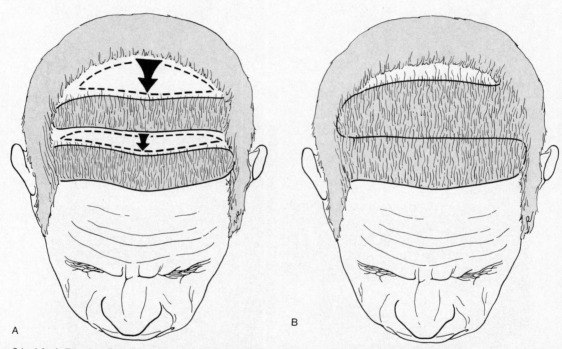

A   B

Figure 21–16. *A,* Two Juri flaps healed in place; arrows show excision and advancement possible with multiple scalp reductions. *B,* Schematic result of two Juri flaps after multiple bald scalp reductions. Because the flaps stretched 50%, two 4 cm flaps can cover 12 cm of the scalp.

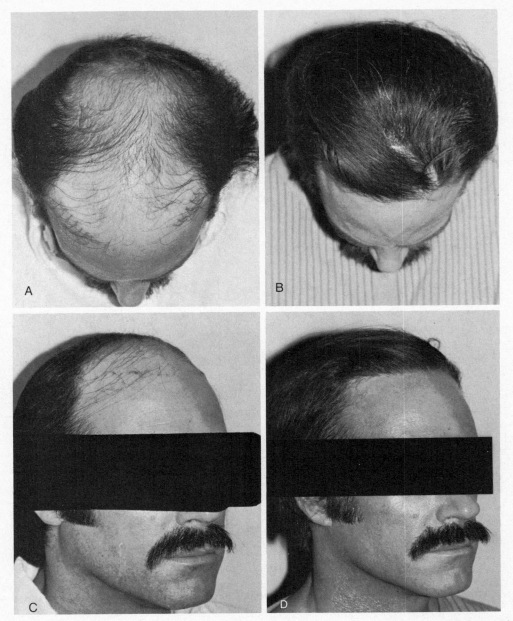

Figure 21–17. *A* to *D,* The 8-year postoperative result on a patient (now 43 years old) after two Juri flaps with three scalp reductions. Note the nonscarred hairline contoured along the old trial grafted hairline, which is styled with the hairline exposed.

eral scalp flaps essentially circumcribe the top of the scalp. Limited temporary hair loss may occur in the distal areas of the flap or in the donor closure area. If full-thickness skin loss has not occurred, the hair usually grows back in 12 weeks.

Third Juri Flap

Juri[1] has described using an occasional third flap for posterior coverage. The author prefers to do scalp reductions and punch grafting to cover the remaining cosmetic deficiency at the crown after two flap procedures (Fig. 21–18).

SMALL NONDELAYED (LATERAL) FLAPS

Publications by Elliott[2, 11] have stimulated interest and added refinement to nondelayed lateral scalp flaps used to form frontal hairlines. These procedures are less extensive than the large Juri flaps. The operations create the dense frontal hairline sought by many hair transplant patients. It takes two small flaps, one from each side, to make up a frontal hairline (Fig. 21–19). For purposes of brevity, the reader is referred back to the details on the design and surgery of the Juri flap. Most of those details apply to the small flap, so only the divergent points will be stressed in the following pages.

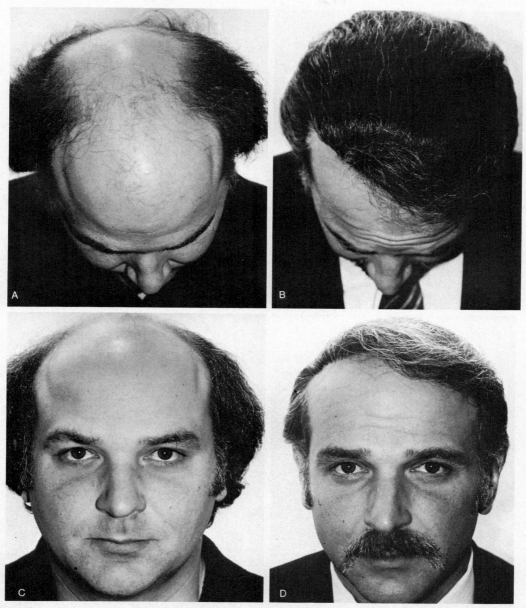

Figure 21–18. *A* to *H*, Multiple before and after views of a 40-year-old patient after two Juri flaps and three scalp reductions.

Illustration continued on following page

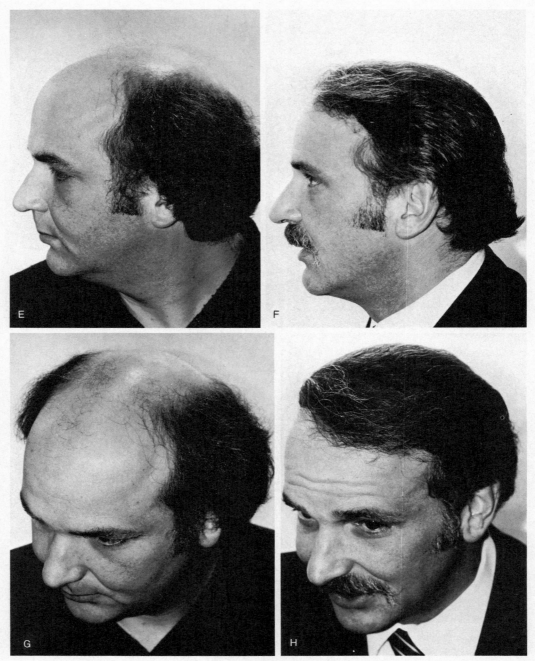

Figure 21–18 *Continued*

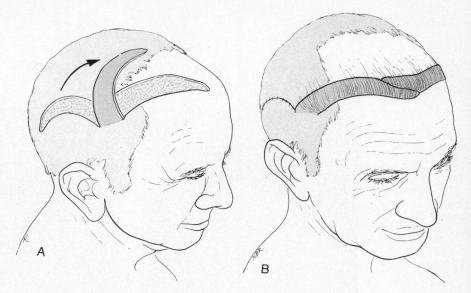

Figure 21–19. A, The first small nondelayed flap (lateral scalp flap, temporoparietal flap, or Elliott flap) is usually 2.5 cm wide. B, The second small flap is transferred about three months after the first procedure to complete the hairline. Junction of the flaps is in the midline.

As mentioned in the section on patient selection, small flaps are an excellent surgical treatment for limited Type I balding patterns. Ideally, a patient should be in his late thirties or forties, have a strong desire to fill in long-standing frontotemporal balding areas, and have a strong forelock of hair and a strong family history of this pattern (Fig. 21–20).

Another appropriate candidate is one who is primarily concerned with establishing a frontal hairline and who wants greater density than that achieved by punch grafting. These flaps may be ideal to revise unsatisfactory punch-grafted hairlines. Because the more posterior scalp has been harvested for grafts and is therefore scarred, these short flaps can contain nonviolated sections of the hair-bearing scalp, thereby allowing for a successful hairline reconstruction (Fig. 21–21).

The small flaps can be incorporated into a plan with punch grafting and possible scalp reduction. Scalp reductions may not be optimally useful under these conditions, since flap donor closures take up a good deal of the scalp elasticity. Scalp reductions should probably not be performed prior to flap surgery.

Small Flap Design

The hairline design is drawn on the scalp to satisfy the surgeon and the patient. A greater amount of frontotemporal recession can be achieved with the small flaps than with the Juri flaps because they are thinner and have greater flexibility. They do not have to be curved back again far past the midfrontal hairline, and nondelayed flaps have less stiffness. The flaps are 2.2 to 3.0 cm in width and taper slightly distally; the length is between 12 and 20 cm. The flaps are designed well within the assumed permanent fringe hair. A template can be useful. The origin of the flap is determined using the same geometrics as with the Juri flap, except for the smaller width. Although some state it is not necessary to have a named artery in the flap, the author insists on aligning the center of the base of the flap on the posterior branch of the superficial temporal artery.

Technique for Small Flaps

The hair is bunched up with rubber bands, and the scalp is prepped and draped. The areas around the flap and the forehad skin are infiltrated with 1% lidocaine with epinephrine (1:100,000). A special parallel knife is used to scratch in the incision lines of the flap. The incisions are deepened through the galea, and the flap is elevated and dissected to an anteriorly based pedicle. The frontal hairline is cut with a bevel. The leading edge of the flap is de-epithelized, and the flap is sutured in place using the advancing sutures as described for the Juri flap. Occasionally, closure of the donor defect can be accomplished without undermining, but one must be prepared to do fairly extensive undermining of the scalp cephalad and caudad to the donor defect, sometimes extending the dissection into the neck. Donor closure is best attained using strong, buried sutures, approximating the galea and using fine sutures or staples to close the skin. The most anterior portion of the donor defect can sometimes present a closure problem. This problem can also be handled using a small, full-thickness skin graft taken from the discarded bald scalp.

The bald scalp lying behind the flap is excised and discarded, and the posterior edge of the flap is sewn in place similar to the manner described for the Juri flap.

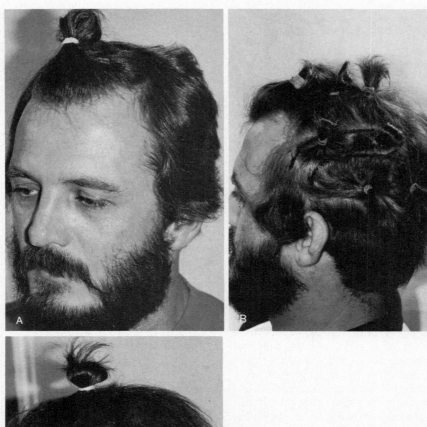

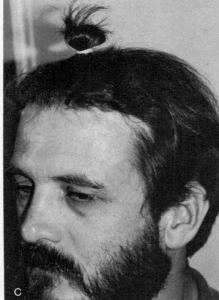

Figure 21–20. *A* to *C*, Small nondelayed left temporoparietal flap used to fill in the frontotemporal recess in a minimally bald, 35-year-old patient. A similar procedure was done on the other side.

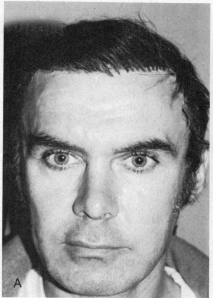
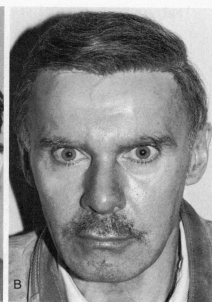

Figure 21–21. *A* and *B,* The eight-year result on a patient (now 53 years old) after two small flaps were used to revise an esthetically unpleasing punch-grafted hairline. Longer flaps containing extensively punch-grafted occipital scalp would not have been successful.

Often, drains are inserted underneath the flap and the closure line. A dressing is worn for 24 to 48 hours, and then the drains are removed and another light dressing is applied for another day or two. This operation has the same potential morbidity and complications as the Juri flap, but to a lesser degree.

Discussion of Small Flaps

A second small flap can be performed, preferably three or four months after the first flap has been completed, so that there is some return of laxity to the scalp to provide some ease for donor closure on the second side. Each flap should be designed long enough for some overlap in the midline in order to provide a greater amount of hair coverage in this region. The donor closure of the second flap, even if done after waiting, presents more of a problem than closure of the first flap.

Two small flaps can be performed at the same time but only under selective conditions. If there is a strong frontal forelock and if the flap does not have to go to the midfrontal scalp, the surgeon can transfer one of these nondelayed flaps and then, if the donor closure is easy, proceed to do the second side in the same sitting; however, the second donor site closure will be more difficult than the first. If these flaps are long enough so that they crisscross in the frontal midline, as described by Heimburger,[12] the incisions would nearly circumscribe the scalp and could lead the top of the scalp to slough. It is wisest to perform the two small flap operations with a significant time lapse between them.[13]

The small flap technique provides only a frontal hairline and largely eliminates the opportunity to have significant vascular supply to create further flap procedures, which can be performed in the second Juri flap. The main advantage and appeal of the small flap technique is that it may seem to be a lesser procedure than the Juri flap.

The problems and complications, such as necrosis of the flaps, donor closure problems, dog-ears or bulges, and temporary hair loss, are similar to the Juri flap procedure. Two flaps must be transposed and survive completely to create a hairline, but less hair is transferred than by one Juri flap operation. The author no longer performs the small flap procedure routinely.

The Extended Lateral (Small) Flap

The author proposes that the first flap can be designed as long as possible with the posterior branch of the superficial temporal artery in its origin. This nondelayed flap is designed so it becomes two thirds or even more of a hairline. One has little to lose even if there is some distal necrosis of the flap. Often, such a long nondelayed flap may survive in its entirety. If this flap does survive, the second flap can be relatively short and therefore sure to survive. There is the added advantage of having its junction to the side of the midfrontal hairline and allowing for a less obvious junctional scar. This shorter second flap also lessens the danger of compromising circulation to the top of the scalp. In the event that there is necrosis of the longer nondelayed flap, the second flap may be designed to compensate for it, and one might even consider delaying this second flap if necrosis makes a hairline short of the midfrontal region.

PREAURICULAR AND POSTAURICULAR FLAPS

These narrow flaps, based superiorly, have been described by Nataf[14] to augment grafted hairlines and to provide partial crown coverage. Since the flap is made so that the hair grows anteriorly, some theoretical cosmetic benefit is obtained, especially when combining this with punch grafts. Since these flaps are based opposite to the circulation of the scalp, delay procedures have been employed, but predictable survival of these flaps is not consistent. These flaps will rarely be long enough to produce half of a hairline. Marzola[15] advocates the use of the preauricular flap in conjunction with extensive scalp reductions and has presented some exemplary results.

FREE FLAPS

Ohmori[10] and Juri[16] report their experiences with free temporoparietal occipital flaps using microsurgical anastomotic techniques. Although most cases were for posttraumatic alopecia, free flaps were also successfully used in the treatment of male pattern baldness. These flaps are designed similarly to Juri's pedicle flap; then, anatomoses are made to the superficial temporal artery and vein on the contralateral side without delay procedures. When successful, the free flap has anterior hair growth most nearly approximating a natural hairline. Performed thus, the free flap would use up both superficial temporal artery systems, thereby precluding a second flap or a salvage flap in case of flap necrosis. However, Ohmori has described an operation that anastomoses the ipsilateral occipital vessels to the superficial temporal vessels and thereby allows for a potential second flap on the other side.

Needless to say, using free flaps involves exceptional training, skills, and preparation and will probably only find appropriate application in isolated situations.

SCALP REDUCTION PROCEDURES

This subject is covered extensively in this book by another author. Yet, these are flap procedures (advancement flaps), and their importance deserves mention in this chapter. Scalp reduction procedures are technically simple and relatively free of complications. They can be used between Juri flaps by excising the bald scalp in a horizontal direction (see Fig. 21–16).

When used with a plan of punch grafting, scalp reductions can lessen the number of punch grafts performed and provide coverage for the vertex of the scalp. Scalp reduction is performed under local anesthesia. An estimated excision is drawn on the scalp, and one side is incised. Extensive undermining of the subgaleal region is performed, and the flaps are advanced. The maximum amount of scalp is excised to allow for approximation with some tension. In case the scalp is not particularly flexible, a smaller-than-estimated amount of scalp is removed. A two-layer closure is advised with the deep layer being a permanent or semipermanent suture to hold the galea with tension. The skin should be sutured or stapled without tension. A width of 2 to 5 cm is usually removed in one session. Repeat reductions may be attempted at two- to three-month intervals.

Punch grafting can be performed in the same session with a scalp reduction. It is preferable that punch grafting be started prior to scalp reduction so that the donor grafts will not be taken from stretched scalp and thus have less density. The author often performs punch grafting in the same session with a scalp reduction, taking the donor grafts before performing the reduction.

EXPANDED SCALP FLAPS

The most exciting and significant adjunct to hair replacement surgery in the last seven years has been the application of tissue expansion to allow for scalp reduction procedures in those scalps that are inherently or postoperatively too tight to advance.[3, 4, 17, 18]

Tissue expanders are inflatable, strong silicone bags of various sizes that can be placed underneath tissue to be used for the flap reconstruction of an adjacent defect. One or more expanders can be used, depending on the situation. A rectangular, 200 or 250 cc expander of the Radovan design has been successfully used by this author on 19 patients.

One or two expanders are placed under the hair-bearing scalp adjacent to the non–hair-bearing defect (Fig. 21–22A). Saline is injected percutaneously into an injection port placed at a slight distance from the expander. Injections are made at three- to five-day intervals (Fig. 21–22B), and when the increase in distance across the expanded tissues equals the distance across the defect, the expanders can be removed (Fig. 21–22C). The flaps are then advanced, and the overlapped bald areas are removed (Fig. 21–22D).

Thus, in male pattern baldness, two lateral reduction procedures can be done with expanded flaps, and often complete closure of the crown and midscalp can be achieved. The major drawback of this procedure is the significant deformity that occurs in the process of expanding the tissues (Fig. 21–23). Therefore, scalp reduction using these expanded flaps for male pattern baldness would only be indicated for the highly motivated and demanding patient, who desires the ultimate in potential coverage

Figure 21–22. *A*, The location of the expanders with tubing and injection ports is shown. The injection port can be placed under areas other than those shown in the diagram. Incision sites are closed in two layers. *B*, View of inflated expanders. *C*, The expanders are removed, and lateral flaps are created and advanced toward each other. Potential scalp excision shown. *D*, Closure of advanced expanded flaps creating a double-Y configuration.

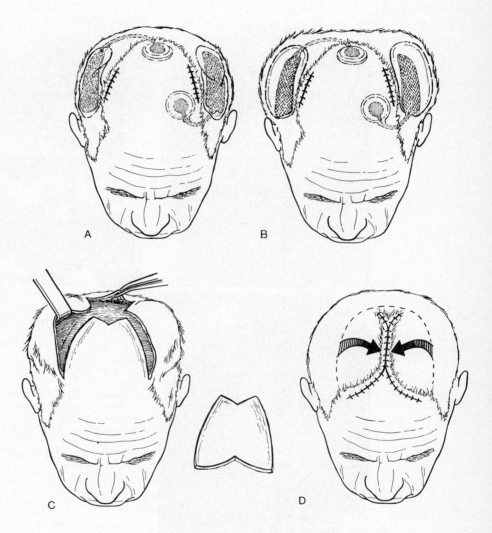

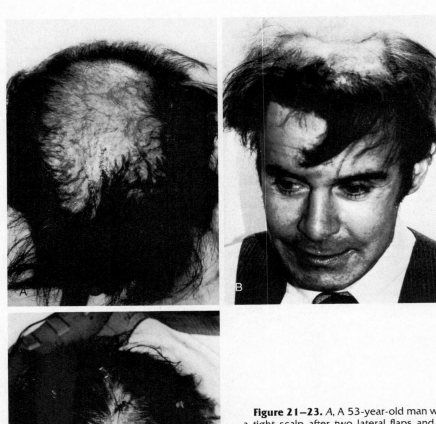

Figure 21–23. *A*, A 53-year-old man with a tight scalp after two lateral flaps and an attempted scalp reduction. *B*, Scalp expansion with two 250 cm rectangular expanders completely filled. *C*, Immediate postoperative view of the expanded flap closure.

and can stand both the temporary deformity and the discomfort. The patient should also be one who has had previous extensive scalp surgery because, as noted before, such patients' scalps expand with minimal discomfort, while virgin scalps expand with greater pain.

Preoperative tissue expansion in two cases of large pedicle flaps of the Juri design was employed on scalps that were inherently tight. Surgery was then performed with extreme ease of donor closure.

Patients who have tight cicatricial alopecia that is deemed inoperable have been successfully treated with tissue expansion techniques. It is the author's opinion that tissue expansion is the treatment of choice for such cases.

The use of the tissue expander in the scalp, as of this time, has not resulted in any significant complications.

HAIR STYLING

There have been comments that the pedicle flaps create visible scarred hairlines with the hair growing in the posterior direction. If the proper techniques are used and no complications occur, the scarring should be equivalent to or even less than that of punch grafting. The direction of the hair can be corrected by styling. The most useful styles are permanents or back-combing of the flap hair. The black patient, who generally has naturally curly hair, does very well with the flap techniques. The straight-haired patient can have a permanent in the flap hair which helps spread the hair over a greater area, blends it into the thinner remaining hair, and allows for the easiest of hair care: towel drying after a shower.

SUMMARY

Long or short, unipedicled transposition flaps for hairline re-creation and advancement flaps for scalp reduction are useful adjuncts or alternatives to the classic punch-grafting technique. These procedures require a thorough understanding of the dynamics of flap surgery, the anatomy of the scalp, and the variations in behavior caused by the degree of scalp elasticity of different patients. Except for scalp reduction, flap procedures cannot be done on an assembly-line basis, as can the punch graft technique. These hair-bearing flaps have to be highly individualized and require varied adjustment maneuvers. The positive aspect of transferring large amounts of continually growing hair must be weighed against the potential problems.

Flap operations for baldness have become accepted alternatives and adjuncts to the classic punch-grafting technique. It is because of increasing experience and understanding that consistently excellent results are achieved. Flap operations should be attempted only by those surgeons wo have had specific training in scalp flap surgery.

REFERENCES

1. Juri J: Use of parieto-occipital flaps in the surgical treatment of baldness. Plast Reconst Surg 55:456, 1975
2. Elliott RA: Lateral scalp flaps for instant results in pattern baldness. Plast Reconst Surg 60:699, 1977
3. Manders EK, et al: Skin expansion to eliminate large scalp defects. Ann Plast Surg 12:305, 1984
4. Kabaker S, et al: Tissue expansion in the treatment of alopecia. Arch Otolaryngol, July 1986
5. Kabaker S: Experiences with parieto-occipital flaps in hair transplantation. Laryngoscope, 88:73, 1978
6. Kabaker S: Juri flap procedure for the treatment of baldness. Arch Otolaryngol 105:509, 1979
7. Conley J: Regional Flaps of the Head and Neck. Stuttgart, George Thieme, 1976
8. Norwood OT, Shiell RC: Hair Transplant Surgery. Springfield, Ill, Charles C Thomas, Publisher, 1984
9. Lamont ES: A plastic surgical transformation. Report of a case. J West Surg Obstet Gynecol 65:164, 1957
10. Ohmori K: Application of microvascular free flaps to scalp effects. Clin Plastic Surg 9:263, 1982
11. Elliott RA: Treatment of male pattern baldness. In Curtis, EH (ed): Male Aesthetic Surgery. St. Louis, CV Mosby Co, 1982, pp 119–135
12. Heimburger RA: Single-stage rotation of arterialized scalp flaps for male pattern baldness: A case report. Plast Reconst Surg 60:789, 1977
13. Mayer TG, Fleming RW: Short flaps—their use and abuse in the treatment of male pattern baldness. Ann Plast Surg 8:296, 1982
14. Nataf J: Surgical treatment for frontal baldness: The long temporal vertical flap. Plast Reconstr Surg 74:628, 1984
15. Marzola M: An alternative hair replacement method. In Hair Transplant Surgery, ed 2. Springfield, Ill, Charles C Thomas Publisher, 1984, pp 315–323
16. Juri J, Juri C: The Juri flap. Facial Plast Surg 2:269, 1985
17. Radovan C: Tissue expansion in soft tissue reconstruction. Plast Reconstr Surg 74:482, 1984
18. Pierce HE: Possible use of the Radovan tissue expander in hair replacement surgery. J Dermatol Surg Oncol 11:413, 1985

22

CHARLES P. VALLIS, M.D.

The Strip Scalp Graft

The strip graft technique was first described by the author in an article published in 1964.[1] Several articles followed describing the combined use of the strip and punch grafts for hair replacement in male pattern baldness.[2-5] In carefully selected patients, transplantation of hair with free composite hair-bearing scalp grafts has been successful in replacing a significant amount of hair in prematurely bald areas of the scalp.

The strip graft operation, when executed properly, can produce an acceptable hairline of good density (Fig. 22–1). The strip graft can be used on many other areas of the scalp besides the frontal hairline. It may be placed in a step-wise fashion on the frontal scalp, parallel to the part line on the parietal scalp, or in other strategic areas on the crown.

On the scalp, the strip graft is used primarily for hair replacement in male pattern baldness. The strip graft requires an environment endowed with good circulation in order to survive. It does not fare well in scar tissue where circulation has been reduced severely. Strip grafts can be successfully employed in some cases of cicatricial alopecia. Coiffman suggests the use of thin strip grafts measuring 3 to 4 mm in width in some cases of cicatricial alopecia of the scalp.[6] An incision is made through the scar, which is slightly undermined, and the strip is placed into the scar on its side and sutured in position.

Strip grafts are used more often than any other method for replacing missing eyebrows and hair on the upper lip in the male. A successful take in these two areas depends on the existence of adequate circulation. The presence of atrophic scar tissue in the recipient site will require other methods of hair replacement.

The majority of patients with frontotemporal recession are treated first with a series of punch graft procedures. In most cases, patients are content with the result achieved by the punch grafts, and the use of any other method would be redundant. However, some individuals are anxious for a denser growth in the frontal hairline; others consider the tufted effect caused by the punch grafts unacceptable. In these patients, the strip graft increases greatly the amount of hair and enhances the natural appearance of the frontal hairline (Fig. 22–2).

Most of the problems that have been associated with hair transplant surgery are related to the reconstruction of a new frontal hairline. Regardless of which technique is used for the formation of this hairline, its position must be planned carefully and designed preoperatively. Improperly placed punch or strip grafts create an undesirable aesthetic effect. It is essential that the proposed new hairline does not run straight across the frontal region. There should be a widow's peak with some degree of posterior recession of the hairline on either side to give it a more natural appearance.

OPERATIVE TECHNIQUE

The strip graft operation is done as an office or outpatient procedure. A section of hair is shaved on the parieto-occipital scalp. The patient is placed in a prone position on the operating room table. The strip graft is marked on the scalp with an applicator dipped in gentian violet solution. Although the patient may have had several previous punch graft procedures, care is taken throughout the course of his treatment to preserve an intact area of hair growth on the parieto-occipital scalp suitable for taking a strip graft of adequate length and width.

The length of the strip graft is limited only by the existing donor site and the length of the frontal area to be spanned. However, the width of the graft is limited strictly. Since the width determines the continued viability of the graft, a very wide graft would fail to take. It was previously believed that the graft should be cut no wider than 5 mm. With experience, the author has increased the width of the graft to as much as 8 mm. Although the 8 mm graft takes very well in areas of the scalp untouched by previous surgery or trauma, it does not fare as well when placed close to previously implanted punch grafts. A graft 5 to 6 mm in width is used most frequently at present, since most patients have already had multiple punch grafts.

After the strip graft has been marked roughly, the local anesthetic (2% lidocaine solution without epinephrine) is injected. Pierce[7] has stressed the importance of not introducing a vasoconstrictor into the donor graft tissue. This probably insures quicker uptake of the circulation by the strip graft.

Strip grafts should be taken in a horizontal direction from the parieto-occipital areas of the scalp. The horizontal direction insures invisibility of the scar after healing. A simple instrument, called the

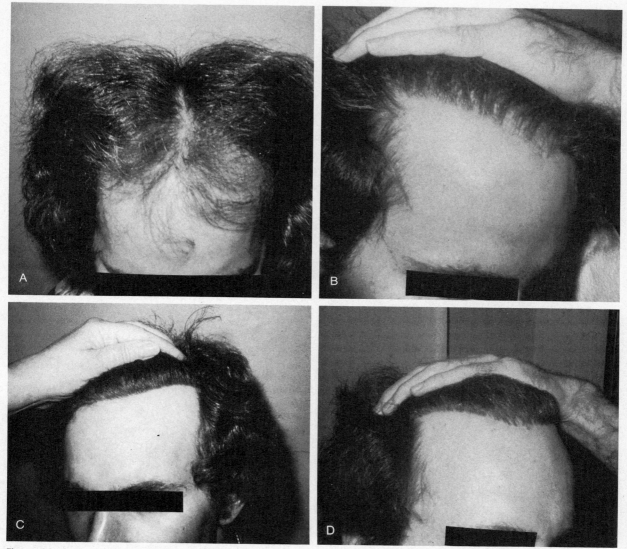

Figure 22–1. *A,* A 26-year-old man with frontotemporal recession. *B,* Result after 300 punch grafts. *C* and *D,* Result after strip grafts.

parallel double-bladed holder, was designed to allow the surgeon to take a strip graft of a predetermined and uniform width. This instrument, which takes two no. 15 scalpel blades and comes in varying widths from 5 to 10 mm, is used to make the initial incision in the donor site (Fig. 22–3A). This incision is carried through the epidermis no deeper than 1 mm. A single no. 15 scalpel blade is used to make the deeper incisions on either side of the graft (Fig. 22–3B).

When the deeper incision is made with the single blade, it is very important that it follows the slant and angulation of the hair follicles. Failure to do this results in the destruction of several rows of the underlying follicular bulbs and prevents a complete growth of hair in the graft. The incisions are carried down to the galea aponeurotica. The graft is lifted

off its bed with sharp-pointed curved scissors or with a scalpel (Fig. 22–3C). Care should be taken to stay below the level of the hair follicles when the graft is being elevated.

After the strip graft has been removed from its bed, no attempt is made at hemostasis, except for application of pressure on either side by the assistant. The wound is closed quickly with a continuous 3-0 nylon suture and a CE-10 needle (Fig. 22–3D). The graft that had been placed in a saline sponge is now carefully pared of excess fascia and fatty tissue (Fig. 22–4). The paring of the fat should not be excessive, and the hair follicles should not be exposed or damaged. The major circulation for the graft necessarily comes from the sides; consequently, an extra amount of fatty tissue under the follicles does not prevent the graft from taking.

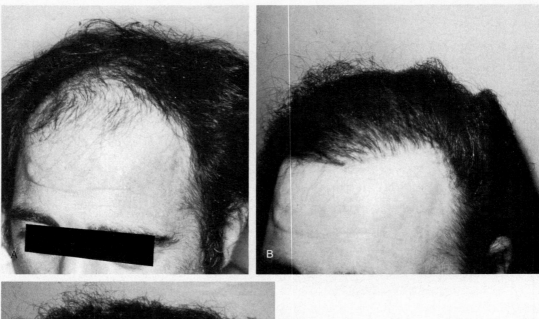

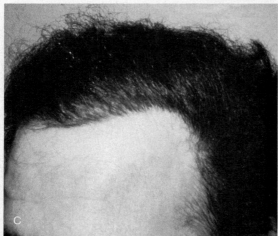

Figure 22–2. *A,* Preoperative appearance of a 40-year-old man. *B,* Result after 200 punch grafts. *C,* Result after a strip graft.

After the donor site has been repaired, the patient, who has been lying on his abdomen during this portion of the procedure, is asked to turn over and lie on his back. The head of the table is elevated to a 30-degree angle, and the recipient area on the forehead is then prepared.

The frontal hairline is reconstructed in two stages: One strip is used to span half the frontal scalp on one side, and about one month later, another strip is placed on the other side. It is wise to place the first strip on the side of the frontal scalp where the hair is parted. (In most males, it will be on the left side.) Some will be content with this single strip, since the other side can be easily camouflaged when the hair is combed over it (Fig. 22–5).

If strips are placed on both sides, it is essential that they form a complete hairline with no gaps. This is done by overlapping the grafts in the middle of the forehead. It is possible to span the entire forehead with one long strip, although this increases the operative time considerably.

When the entire forehead is spanned in one operation, the graft is cut into two segments and overlapped in the center of the forehead with a bridge of skin, measuring approximately 3 mm between the ends of the graft. This is done to prevent indentation of the graft in the center of the forehead, often resulting from contraction of a long uninterrupted graft across the entire width of the forehead.

The position of the graft has been previously designed and marked (Fig. 22–6A). (This is done with the patient in a sitting position before the operation is begun.) The line of incision is placed along the inferior edge of the front row of punch grafts. Shaving of the front row of grafts is done to facilitate placement and suturing of the strip graft. In some cases, the linear incision for the strip graft is placed through the front row of punch grafts. The incision actually transects the punch grafts, causing half of each graft to remain superior to the strip graft and the other half inferior to it. This maneuver creates enough irregularity in front of the strip graft

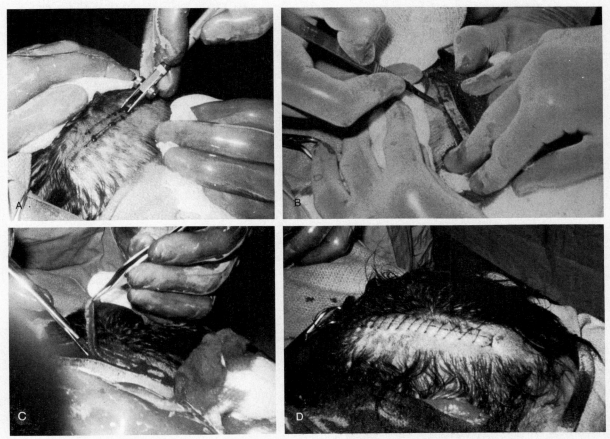

Figure 22–3. *A*, Superficial parallel incisions through the epidermis are made with a double-bladed instrument. *B*, The deeper incisions follow the angulation of the hair shaft. *C*, The graft is dissected off at the level of the galea with sharp curved scissors. *D*, Closure of the donor wound with a running suture.

Figure 22–4. Removal of fascia and excess fatty tissue from the graft.

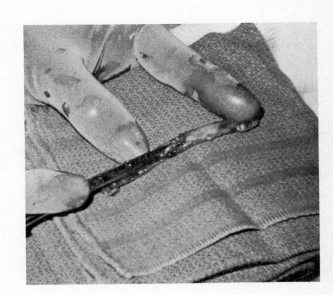

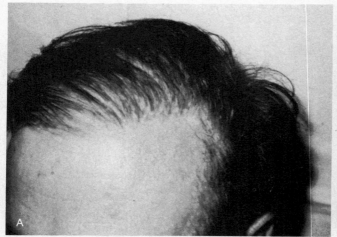

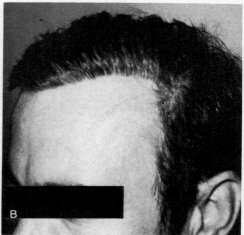

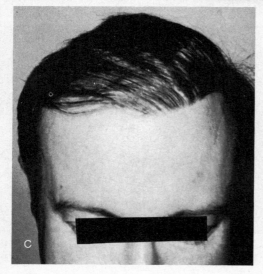

Figure 22–5. *A*, A 38-year-old man after 190 punch grafts for frontotemporal recession. *B* and *C*, Results following a strip graft on the left frontal side.

to eliminate any sharp linear effect that a solitary strip graft may produce.

A local anesthetic (a 2% lidocaine solution with 1:100,000 epinephrine) is injected subcutaneously along the line of incision. This effectively anesthetizes the ascending sensory fibers from the supraorbital nerves. The epinephrine helps greatly in reducing the amount of bleeding, but since the recipient area is not detached from the general circulation, any concentration of epinephrine will be eliminated in a few hours, thereby not hindering the reestablishment of circulation within the strip graft.

A simple linear incision is then made perpendicular to the skin, extending through the skin and subcutaneous tissue and the underlying fascia or galea aponeurotica (Fig. 22–6B). Inadequate splitting of the underlying galea in the recipient area does not allow the wound to open wide enough to receive the graft, and in the end, this causes constriction of the graft with resulting inadequate growth of hair.

Bleeding in the recipient wound varies with dif-

ferent patients. In some, the bleeding is profuse with multiple pumping blood vessels, whereas in others there may be only two or three actively bleeding blood vessels. Active bleeders are clamped with hemostats and ligated. The smaller bleeders can be electrocoagulated with the bipolar cautery (Fig. 22–6C). Excessive electrocoagulation should be avoided to prevent undue injury to the recipient area. Complete hemostasis is important and is further secured with weak epinephrine packs in the wound.

The carefully prepared strip graft is placed in the wound with the hair follicles pointed inferiorly. If the graft is placed thus, there will be a full growth of hair right to the edge of the inferior margin when the hair grows out. Also, when the patient combs his hair, the hairs will extend slightly downward before curving superiorly and thus camouflaging the linear edge of the graft. If the graft is not in this position, a pale white linear scar will result along the inferior margin of the graft.

The graft is sutured to the skin superiorly and

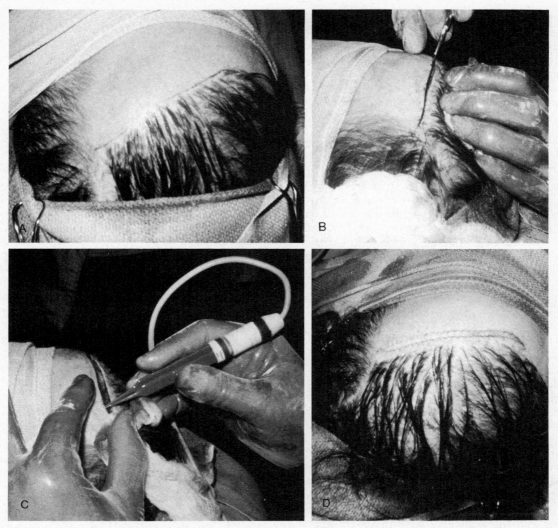

Figure 22–6. *A,* The strip graft incision site is marked with gentian violet solution. *B,* A single perpendicular incision is made through the skin, subcutaneous tissue, and galea. *C,* Control of small bleeders with bipolar cautery. *D,* Placement of the strip graft in the wound with hair shafts angulated inferiorly.

inferiorly with a continuous running 6-0 nylon stitch (Fig. 22–6D). Improper suturing of the graft in the recipient area frequently results in a poor take. A fine continuous suture, used in the superficial layers of the skin without strangulation but with close coaptation of the skin margins without overlapping, helps greatly in attaining a good take of the graft. When the suturing of the graft has been completed, a piece of gauze is gently but firmly rolled over the graft from one end to the other in order to eliminate any residual blood that may be present under the graft.

A circular head bandage is used for pressure over the graft, although a small stent tied over the graft can also be effective. It is important that the postoperative dressing not be placed too tightly, which may result in embarrassment of the circulation at the site of the graft. An excessively tight dressing

also causes marked periorbital edema and ecchymosis, which may last for several days after the operation. A rayon dressing is initially placed over the strip graft to prevent adherence to the dressing material. The pressure dressing is kept on for two days, then a small dressing is applied over only the graft.

The patient is allowed to go home immediately after the operation is completed. He is advised to refrain from overactivity for two weeks, to avoid excessive use of any alcoholic beverages, and to do nothing that would tend to raise his pulse or blood pressure. He is cautioned to avoid any physical contact, however minor, to his head. Early establishment of circulation to the strip graft is important for its complete survival. The patient is warned to keep his head elevated at all times and to use at least two pillows at night when sleeping.

The graft should be protected with a small gauze bandage for at least five days after the initial head bandage is removed. A thin layer of ointment, such as bacitracin, is placed over the graft with each dressing change. Dressings are usually not required after one week. All sutures are removed from both the donor and recipient sites in approximately nine days.

POSTOPERATIVE COURSE

The hair follicles in both the strip graft and the punch graft act alike. There is an initial false growth of hair for about three to four weeks. This hair is shed as the hair follicles go into a telogen phase, which lasts for two to three months after surgery. A new permanent growth then begins, and the new hair assumes the characteristics of the area from whence it came. Since hair growth proceeds at about 1 cm per month, six months or more are required before significant hair growth is noted.

COMPLICATIONS

If the patients are selected carefully and if the procedures are performed well technically, there should be few complications. Earlier in my practice, two strip grafts were lost completely because of infection. All patients are now placed on prophylactic antibiotics. Another graft was lost completely when the patient struck his forehead accidentally against a firm object a few days after the operation. In a small percentage of strip graft patients, there may not be a complete growth of hair in some areas even though the graft may have taken completely. As much as 50% of the total area of the graft may be involved. The smaller areas of alopecia can be corrected by the implantation of hair-bearing punch grafts. The larger areas can be corrected by excising the segment of alopecia and replacing it with a small hair-bearing strip graft.

Another complication is numbness of the scalp posterior to the grafts. This numbness is more marked following the strip graft operation. The transverse incision transects the sensory fibers of the supraorbital nerve, and the numbness lasts several months after surgery. Numbness can be very desirable at first, since subsequent punch grafts can be done with very little additional local anesthesia. Normal sensation usually returns after eight months to a year although residual numbness may persist for a longer period.

SUMMARY

Hair transplantation for male pattern baldness has been done on many patients by dermatologists and plastic surgeons during the past 25 years. In selected cases, hair transplantation has been successful for adequate replacement of hair in bald areas of the scalp. In most cases, the punch graft technique is used alone. However, in selected cases, especially in individuals desiring a dense growth in the frontal area, the strip graft in conjunction with punch grafts can be used. When the strip graft operation is properly executed, the results are gratifying. Strip grafts can be transplanted in any conceivable direction and to any area of the scalp. They may be twisted into any desired shape in order to conform to any recipient site. They can also be made short or long and may be cut into smaller strips or even into small square grafts. If careful attention is paid to the simple steps of the operation discussed in this article, a surgeon will usually be rewarded with a good take of the strip graft.

REFERENCES

1. Vallis CP: Surgical treatment of receding hairline: Report of a case. Plast Reconstr Surg 33:247,1964
2. Vallis CP: Surgical treatment of the receding hairline: Plast Reconstr Surg 44:271, 1969
3. Vallis CP: Strip graft. In Rees TD: Aesthetic Plastic Surgery. Philadelphia, W.B. Saunders Company, 1980
4. Vallis CP: The strip scalp graft. Clin Plast Surg 9:229–240, 1982
5. Vallis CP: The strip graft method in hair transplantation. In Vallis CP: Hair Transplantation for the Treatment of Male Pattern Baldness. Springfield, Ill, Charles C Thomas, 1982
6. Coiffman F: Square scalp grafts. Clin Plast Surg 9:221, 1982
7. Pierce HE: Problems encountered with the strip graft transplant procedure. J Natl Med Assoc 65:211, 1973

THOMAS H. ALT, M.D.

23

Therapeutic Facial Dermabrasion

Facial dermabrasion is an excellent procedure for the alleviation of facial scarring resulting from acne or traumatic incidents and for the correction of actinically damaged skin demonstrating solar elastosis, actinic keratoses, freckling, or senile lentigo. It is also therapeutically beneficial for the improvement or correction of chronic active acne, particularly in patients who have experienced therapeutic failure despite aggressive systemic therapy including potent antibiotics and isotretinoin (Accutane). Facial dermabrasion is a reliable procedure that has predictable results in all of the above conditions. To obtain excellent results, the surgeon must apply several principles of physics, which are simple to understand.

Physicians who criticize dermabrasion usually have little or no experience in applying these surgical principles. It is the author's belief that a surgeon cannot be a casual participant in performing facial dermabrasion. If the surgeon performs only one facial dermabrasion per month, an adequate experience level and the high degree of skill needed to produce predictable results will never be attained. It is a misconception that skill can be achieved from such limited experience. Also, the value of the technique should not be judged on results obtained by surgeons who have such limited experience.

Surgeons must devote a significant amount of their practice to perform this technically difficult procedure so that an adequate level of skill is obtained. The basic techniques applied in facial dermabrasion can be attained by attending the many national and international seminars conducted on this topic. One must also observe and participate in the pre- and postoperative care of patients under the tutelage of an established and skilled surgeon. To read a text or several articles on the topic is inadequate to provide the necessary knowledge and experience for even minimally adequate results with this procedure.

INDICATIONS FOR FACIAL DERMABRASION

The most common indication for facial dermabrasion is postacne scarring—a procedure described by Kurtin.[1] Burks[2] in his excellent monograph outlined its use for both postacne scarring and the therapeutic treatment of chronic facial acne. The procedure can provide excellent results for those patients who require continuing systemic antibiotic therapy for chronic acne and for those who have had treatment failures with potent systemic antibiotics or isotretinoin (Accutane). The treatment of actinically damaged skin has been reviewed recently by Field.[3] A partial list of indications for facial dermabrasion, including the correction of benign adnexal tumors, is presented in Table 23–1. Roenigk[4] obtained excellent results on many of these conditions, and every surgeon performing facial dermabrasion should be familiar with his article. Recently, Hanke[5] presented his results on therapy of multiple facial neurofibromas in patients with von Recklinghausen's disease. His results are truly remarkable, and every patient with significant facial disfigurement from this condition should be offered dermabrasion. Traumatic scars respond well to dermabrasion when performed four to eight weeks following the injury. Yarborough[6] demonstrated excellent results that, in many instances, eliminated the remaining scars after a dermabrasion. His results significantly alter the time-honored axiom, which plastic surgeons have espoused for years, to avoid any definitive reconstructive procedures for at least 12 months following the initial repair of an injury (Figs. 23–1 to 23–4).

CONTRAINDICATIONS

There are some patients on whom facial dermabrasion is contraindicated. These include neurotic or psychotic patients who have unrealistic goals. They are often highly manipulative and ignore much of the information presented by the surgeon. It is

TABLE 23–1. Indications for Dermabrasion

Postacne scarring	Chloasma
Traumatic scarring	Ephelides
Neurotic excoriations	Telangiectasia
Smallpox scars	Nevus flammeus
Chicken pox scars	Solar elastosis
Traumatic tattoo	Actinic keratoses
Decorative tattoo	Seborrheic keratoses
Scars from discoid lupus erythematosus (if disease is inactive)	Syringoma, multiple
	Trichoepithelioma, multiple
	Neurofibromatosis
Resistant or chronic acne	Adenoma sebaceum
Acne rosacea	Linear epithelial nevus
Rhinophyma	Basal cell nevus syndrome
Favre-Racouchot syndrome	Darier's disease
Pseudofolliculitis	Porokeratosis
Hidradenitis suppurativa	Lichen amyloidosus
Molluscum contagiosum	

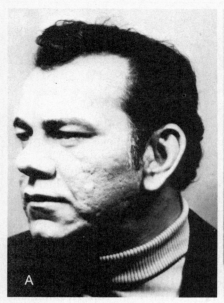
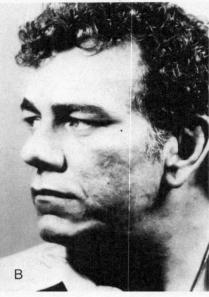

Figure 23–1. *A,* Patient, 35 years old, with atrophic and hypertrophic scarring of cheeks, chin, and mandibular areas. *B,* Significant improvement following two facial dermabrasions.

important to point out their denial of this information. An excellent paper by Wright[7] should be read by every surgeon performing facial dermabrasion. Patients who are perfectionists are not necessarily eliminated. These patients are often reasonable despite their desire to attain perfection. Limitations of the surgery must be carefully and thoroughly explained by the surgeon so that the perfectionist understands that some defects may persist, even after a dermabrasion performed by a skilled and experienced surgeon.

Patients presently on or having used isotretinoin (Accutane) during the preceding six months should be treated with extreme caution. It is the author's opinion that, at this time, these patients represent an absolute contraindication to facial dermabrasion. Since there is a significant alteration in the adnexal structures during and following the administration of Accutane, abnormal, inadequate, or delayed healing is possible following this procedure. The author has discussed this at length with Strauss,[8] a principal investigator studying Accutane, who recommends that facial dermabrasion be delayed for at least six months following the completion of its administration. He further recommends that a skin biopsy be performed to evaluate the status of the sebaceous glands and that a small spot dermabrasion be performed in an inconspicuous area if the number

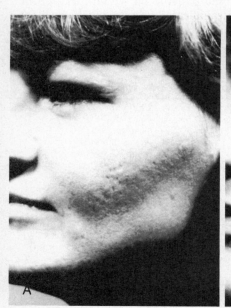
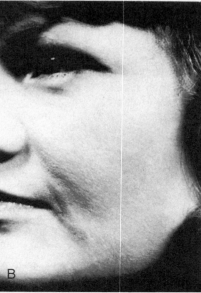

Figure 23–2. *A,* Patient, 34 years old, with moderate scarring of the cheeks. *B,* An almost perfect result following one dermabrasion.

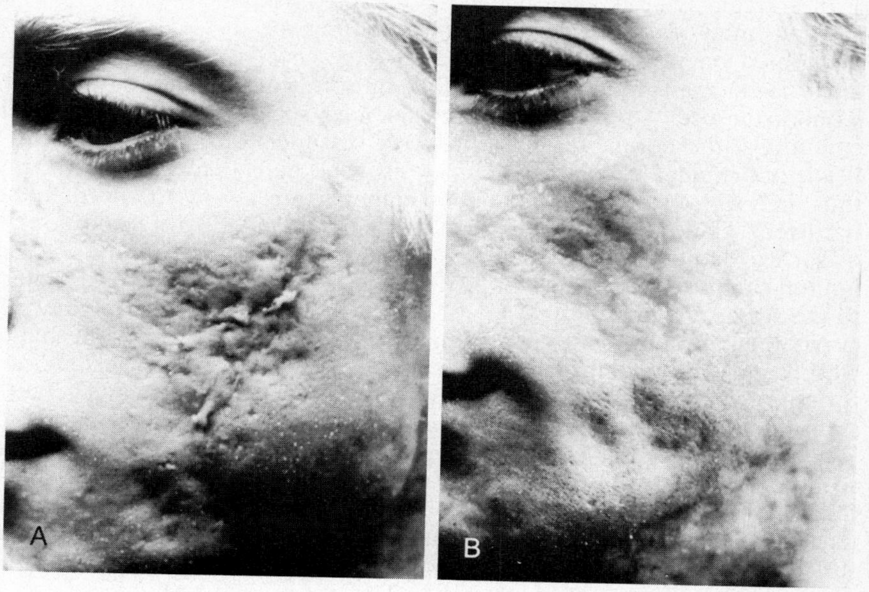

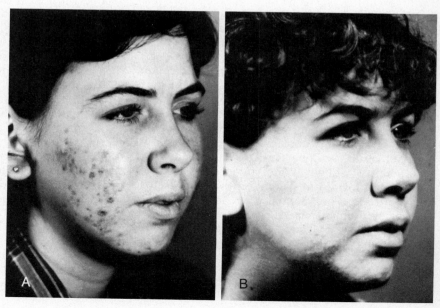

Figure 23–3. *A,* A 19-year-old man with severe atrophic and hypertrophic scarring and considerable bridging in the central cheek. *B,* Significant improvement nine months after first dermabrasion and immediately prior to second dermabrasion.

or size of the glands seems to be abnormal. The author has followed his recommendations and has had no untoward side effects or complications.

This caution was voiced by the author at the 1983 Dermabrasion–Chemical Peel Seminar of the American Society for Dermatologic Surgery held in Chicago. Roenigk countered with the statement that he and several others had performed facial dermabrasions without complications on patients who were either on or had recently concluded therapy with Accutane. A subsequent article by Roenigk and coworkers describes several such patients.[9] The author cautioned the editor of the journal that this article should not be published because the series

was too small and because Strauss had presented his observations. At the 1985 annual meeting of the American Society for Dermatologic Surgery, a paper was presented by Roenigk in which he reported on two patients who had sustained facial scarring from dermabrasion and who had undergone the surgery after using Accutane. Stegman commented from the floor that his group had also experienced two patients on Accutane who had developed similar scars. He noted that these scars were on the central cheek area which he thought was peculiar to Accutane, since the scars were not present in the danger zones. This author has previously cautioned others about this in the literature.

Figure 23–4. *A,* A 21-year-old patient with chronic cystic acne despite aggressive treatment with systemic and topical medications, including minocycline (systemically) and clindamycin (topically). *B,* Appearance six months after therapeutic dermabrasion showing excellent control of acne without the necessity of any topical or systemic medication.

In a recent issue of the Schoch newsletter, Lask also recommends that facial dermabrasion can be performed on patients undergoing Accutane therapy.[10] He suggests that this can be done on soft skin without the use of a refrigerant spray. Under such conditions, the dermabrasion is probably so superficial that minimal epidermal damage is done and thus, in his series of nine patients, no complications occurred. The author believes that the publication of such a small series as Roenigk's or Lask's is so limited that it can mislead and provide a disservice to the surgical community.

Another absolute contraindication is the patient who has severe uncontrollable acne that is actively forming hypertrophic or keloidal scars. Dermabrasion should be delayed until this phase is quiescent. When these scars are mature and no new similar scars are forming, the surgeon may cautiously perform a facial dermabrasion. Since the patient has this known history of abnormal scarring, both the surgeon and the patient must be aware of the risk of abnormal postoperative scarring. These areas almost always exhibit delayed healing because of significantly altered vascularity and epidermal structures. It is recommended that after reepithelialization these patients be seen regularly every two weeks so that topical, intralesional, or systemic corticosteroids may be instituted to prevent or correct the recurrence of abnormal scarring. Results in these patients have been gratifying, but the surgeon must remember to time the surgical procedure appropriately.

Chronic radiodermatitis, which demonstrates a diminution of hair follicles and an alteration in the epidermal structures, is another contraindication. Inadequate adnexal structures will lead to inadequate healing. This is not to suggest that patients who had earlier radiation therapy for acne be arbitrarily excluded. If facial hair is adequate or if significant facial acne persists, the surgeon knows that an adequate number of adnexal structures should be present to provide for normal re-epithelialization.

Cryoglobulinemia is an absolute contraindication. when topical refrigerants are employed. Vitiligo is a relative contraindication. Farber[11] and Sturm[12] recommend that patients with this condition undergo a spot dermabrasion to evaluate their response. Even this is not an absolute indication of the final result, so they must be cautioned about postoperative vitiligo in the surgical sites. A test area is also advised in patients with a past history of hypertrophic or keloidal scars following other surgical or traumatic injuries. The author has followed this advice and successfully dermabraded patients with both vitiligo and hypertrophic or keloidal scars without complications. Both surgeon and patient must realize there is a higher risk of scarring under these circumstances.

CONSULTATION

Consultation is critical in order to select appropriate patients for this procedure. Patients with all types of personalities present for evaluation. Adequate time must be allotted to satisfy both the surgeon and the patient. In the author's office, an experienced nurse displays photographic slides of before and after results from patients with varying degrees of postacne scarring and chronic uncontrollable facial acne. A photographic synopsis of the procedure and its postoperative phase is offered. The patient may ask the nurse any pertinent questions. This phase is generally completed in 20 to 30 minutes. The author then reviews the patient's history form and discusses his or her therapeutic goals. Some patients have unreasonable expectations based upon fantasy or sensational articles in the lay press. The surgeon must clearly articulate what the patient can and cannot expect, what the surgeon can and cannot do. Most patients who seek the author's advice because of disappointing results caused by another surgeon do so because they were never adequately assessed of the capabilities and limitations of facial dermabrasion. The patient's goals must be compatible with the predictable results of the procedure. The surgeon must require each patient to define and articulate a definitive goal that is reasonable considering the patient's personality and the degree of defect requiring improvement. This requires time and patience by the surgeon, but virtually eliminates postoperative dissatisfaction, since there are no surprises following surgery. A 15-minute consultation for this major surgical procedure is inadequate.

As demonstrated by the statistics presented later, patients undergoing dermabrasion in the author's office experience an average cosmetic improvement of between 65% and 85%. The author insists that a prospective candidate agree preoperatively to an improvement of 50% or less. In the author's experience, a patient has never stated that his or her improvement was less than 50%, so the author feels comfortable with this goal. However, each patient is cautioned that he or she may be the first to experience less than 50% improvement. Predictably, most patients initially state as their specific goal that any improvement at all would be worthwhile. Because the patient usually gains greater self-esteem and greater self-confidence, any cosmetic improvement will be beneficial.

Since the procedure is time-consuming, relatively expensive, and does require some risk, the author feels that a goal of "any improvement at all" is unrealistic, since it does not require a significant change to occur. However, these patients are highly motivated and will accept an improvement that may be less than what the surgeon or their friends and family hope for them. It is important to understand that the patient undergoes the surgery for his or her personal benefit and should not be influenced either positively or negatively by friends and family. Often, families discourage the patient from undergoing the procedure because they accept the individual as is. However, the family is not the person who must suffer the ridicule that often accompanies severe scarring. A spouse, family members, and friends should be supportive and allow the patient to arrive at a decision that is best for him or her personally.

The patient's stated goal is written on the chart along with any personal comments by the surgeon. Both are read back to the patient for approval. If the goal is unrealistic, the patient is told why it is unrealistic. This is not a matter of confrontation but rather patient education. Doctors have an obligation to teach every patient what can be expected and to provide sufficient information for patients to make an intelligent decision based upon their own personal needs.

After establishing specific goals, the patient's face is carefully examined, and the defects are recorded on the chart. This written description is read to patients so that they understand the severity and extent of their defects. The surgeon must educate them concerning the difficulty of correcting these defects. The author uses a checklist as a reminder to observe for evidence of vitiligo, chloasma, pseudofolliculitis, herpetic scarring, verruca plana, and evidence of cold allergy or cryoglobulinemia. The vaccinia scar is examined, and any other surgical or traumatic scars are studied for evidence of hypertrophic or keloidal response, hypopigmentation, or atrophic changes. The absence of each item is noted, and any abnormality is recorded on the chart.

Following the examination, a thorough discussion of the usual events during the preoperative, operative, and postoperative phases is conducted. The usual events such as erythema, edema, exudation, discomfort, crust formation, milia, acne exacerbation, and vasolability are discussed. Side effects, such as purpura, permanent hypopigmentation, and temporary postinflammatory hyperpigmentation, are reviewed. Complications such as infection and scar formation are reviewed in detail. A list of this discussion outlining each topic is present on the author's consultation sheet. As each subject is discussed, a check mark is made so there is evidence that the patient has received this information. Patients are then asked if they understand all of this information and if they have any further questions. An extensive typewritten list of the postoperative instructions is given to the patient to support, clarify, and in some instances amplify the information that was given concerning the procedure.

A proposal of the extent of the surgery and cost is then made by the author. Patients are asked if they are prepared to make a decision or if they would prefer additional time. Since most of these patients have considered this surgery for several years, a significant portion schedule the operation at the time of consultation. A tentative date for surgery is then set. The author generally requires a minimum of 30 minutes for his portion of the consultation, and this often extends to 45 minutes. The author sees too many unhappy patients who state that their surgeon spent only 10 to 15 minutes with them, that they did not understand what their needs were, and that the procedure was never fully explained to them. Fortunately, dermatologic surgeons are seldom guilty of this accusation.

PREOPERATIVE ORGANIZATION

Prior to surgery, laboratory evaluation, including a complete blood count and an evaluation of cryoglobulins and cryoprecipitins, is performed. The patient has a series of 20 standardized poses taken on slide film using photoflood illumination to adequately record the preoperative defect. This is done at least two weeks prior to the surgery so the film can be developed. The written postoperative instructions are reviewed in detail at the photographic session by a nurse experienced in dermabrasion.

Some patients with deep or large ice-pick scars or conspicuous linear scars can benefit from surgery performed four weeks prior to the dermabrasion. Ice-pick scars can be improved in three ways. The easiest is mere elevation of the depressed area using a sharp hair transplant punch. A cylinder of skin is incised at the site of the depressed scar to the level of the subcutaneous fat. This allows the scar enough mobility to be raised to a higher level where it is immobilized by normal clot formation. The surgeon must advance the punch deeply enough into the fatty layer to provide adequate mobility of the fibrotic band. Taping of these areas with Steri-strips or Clearon is optional. A second method is to replace these similarily cut cylinders of skin with small grafts harvested from the postauricular area. These grafts must be smaller than 3 mm in size. However, the texture and color of the skin usually do not match the recipient site, and the operation is much more time-consuming than just scar elevation. The third and least acceptable method is excision of the ice-pick scar using the punch biopsy technique followed by primary closure with a solitary suture. This often leads to a small hypopigmented scar that has two additional indentations created by the puncture wound from the needle during the insertion of the suture. Linear atrophic scars are improved by preoperative excision employing careful layered closure with a running subcutaneous suture. It is best to perform these procedures four weeks prior to the anticipated facial dermabrasion and to employ the principles outlined by Yarborough in his findings for treatment of traumatic scars.

On the day of surgery, patients arrive 1½ hours prior to the operation. They must be accompanied by an adult friend or relative since they will not be able to operate an automobile following the procedure. The postoperative instructions are reviewed again with the patient, and any individual who will be attending the patient during his or her postoperative period. The surgical release is reviewed with the patient and signed prior to the administration of any medication. If the patient requests a hypnotic for the night preceding surgery, the author requires that the surgical release be signed at an earlier date so that there will be no question of an inability to fully understand the surgical release. A 100 mg capsule of sodium pentobarbital (Nembutal) is given per os 60 minutes prior to the surgery. Men are asked to be cleanly shaven on the morning of surgery, and any significant facial hair on women is removed with an electric razor. The face is then surgically prepared with chlorhexidine gluconate (Hibiclens), and cotton is placed in the external auditory canals. Paper tape is used to cover the canal to prevent pooling of the liquid refrigerant on the tympanic membrane, which can cause cardiac arrest. Because of the bulky head dressing, the patient is instructed to wear a blouse or shirt which can be buttoned.

Thirty minutes prior to the surgery, an injection of 100 mg meperidine hydrochloride (Demerol) and 50 mg hydroxyzine hydrochloride (Vistaril) is given intramuscularly. This may be decreased to 75 mg of Demerol if the patient is light in weight. The patient must be adequately sedated and be at ease during the surgical procedure. Patients who are uncomfortable become uncooperative, and their level of concentration is readily lost causing the procedure to be difficult and lengthened in time.

The patient is then instructed to hold an ice-filled sterile glove on the right cheek (Fig. 23–5). The glove is placed directly on the skin of the cheek to provide maximum cooling, but a paper towel is placed over the glove for insulation where the hand will be held. This prechill is maintained for 30 minutes. The water in the glove has been frozen in the freezer section of a standard refrigerator. The author has never seen a patient have any detrimental effects from this prechill. One patient, age 69, did develop a frostbite on her cheek with a 30-minute prechill. The contralateral side was then prechilled for only 15 minutes, and following surgery, there was no difference in the healing time or final results between the two sides. The author cautions that elderly patients who have poor circulation should be prechilled for shorter periods.

The author's office has two surgical suites that are independently air-conditioned to control humidity and lower the temperature to 60°F. The temperature can be decreased from 72° to 60°F in approximately 20 minutes and maintained indefinitely, even during periods of high external temperature and high humidity and with five persons present in the room. Even in Minnesota, a cooler room during winter allows for more efficient freezing and improved results. This is logical since skin normally has a surface temperature of 92° F. Most rooms are maintained at 72°F. When the room temperature is decreased to 62°F there is a 30-degree difference between the skin temperature and the ambient room temperature, which creates a 50% improvement in the ambient air temperature. The patient's skin will freeze more rapidly, which is a distinct advantage for the surgeon. Conditions that alter this are an anxious patient in whom both the heart rate and systolic blood pressure increase, thus causing an increased peripheral vascular flow, which carries the cooling effect of the spray away more readily. Therefore, it is important to have a patient relaxed during the surgical procedure since it is difficult to freeze the skin on someone who is anxious. The humidity in the room is also a factor because it effects evaporation of the spray. Temperatures below 55°F are detrimental since they cause both the patient and the staff to shiver, which increases skin temperature.

After a prechill of 30 minutes, the ice pack is removed and the patient is placed in a sitting position. A solution of 1% gentian violet is applied on a sterile cotton applicator to outline the perimeter of the face, i.e., the inferior border of the mandibular ramus and angle (Fig. 23–6). It is strongly advised that any dermabrasion be extended to this area so that any subtle permanent color changes will be hidden in the shadow inferior to the mandible. Blending of skin color is usually excellent in the temporal regions and the periorbital areas. Frequently, there will be a permanent area of hypopigmentation if only the central cheek is dermabraded. This obvious color change leads to patient dissatisfaction. Even though scars may be absent in the

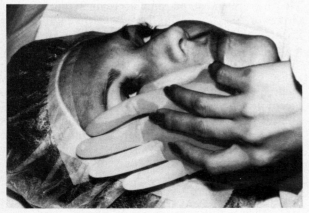

Figure 23–5. A sterile glove filled with water and frozen to 0°F. is held for 30 minutes against the cheek by the patient as a prechill.

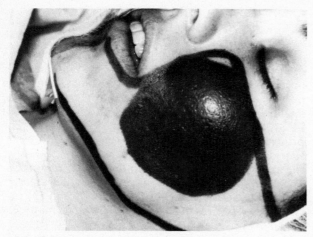

Figure 23–6. Preoperative marking of the perimeter of the area to be dermabraded using 1% aqueous gentian violet. The deeper area is painted in toto and dermabraded to the depth necessary to remove all scars. The remaining area is painted after the deeper dermabrasion is done and then dermabraded superficially to allow for excellent color blending.

lower cheek, the dermabrasion should be extended to the mandibular region. In many instances, the upper lip, nose, and forehead are free of postacne scarring. These latter regions are usually not dermabraded. Blending of color is excellent. In some instances, there is a small triangular area on the glabella that will demonstrate scarring. This is usually dermabraded and also blends very well.

In addition to outlining the boundaries of the area to be dermabraded, the gentian violet is used to delineate the regions that have significant scarring. The scarred areas are painted, but the regions with no significant scarring are initially left unpainted. After the borders of the dermabrasion are outlined and the areas for deep dermabrasion are chosen, the author completes a surgical scrub while the nursing staff applies Microfoam tape along the inferior border of the mandibular ramus and angle (Fig. 23–7). Microfoam tape, a product of 3M's Medical Products Division, is a foam tape that is thick but can be readily stretched.

The author prefers to dermabrade in a straight line along the mandibular ramus. The tape provides a template for this straight line. If no straight line is delineated, the beginning surgeon will frequently create a visually unattractive irregular or jagged line in this area. Although not readily perceptible, particularly in women, a straight line will appear similar to that line created by the application of cosmetics. Microfoam tape is superior to other types because it is a closed cell product and provides insulation to protect the skin adjacent to the area where the refrigerant is sprayed. This avoids frostbite and postinflammatory hyperpigmentation, which may occur. The thickness of the tape is also advantageous since it presents a raised border that acts like a

gutter preventing the liquid refrigerant from streaming down the patient's neck. If this is allowed, one will see areas of linear frostbite on the patient's neck, which leads to postinflammatory hyperpigmentation. At the mandibular angle, many cuts are made on one side of the tape so that it will follow the natural angle without buckling. A second piece of tape is then put over the exposed side of the first tape that has been cut.

At the completion of the taping, a new ice pack is placed on the left cheek where it is held by the patient, until the right cheek is completed. Since it takes approximately 30 minutes to complete one cheek, the author has arbitrarily chosen that length of time as a prechill. Thus, when the right cheek is completed and the author proceeds to the left cheek, the conditions are identical to those of the first cheek. While the second cheek is being completed, an Temp Aid* ice pack is taped to the forehead if that area is to be dermabraded. Thus, each segment of the face is prechilled identically, and the ice is removed immediately prior to the dermabrasion of that segment.

The author noticed in the past that, when the entire face was prechilled at the same time, there was a significant difference in postoperative results. The first cheek to be dermabraded always had the best cosmetic results. It was deduced that the prechill had a significant effect on the efficiency of the freezing. This was logical since, following the removal of the prechill, the skin warms and the vascular bed goes into a compensatory vasodilatation. Under these circumstances, it is difficult to freeze the skin with a refrigerant. In fact, a prechill that is applied and then removed for 30 to 40

---

*Temp Aid, Division of American Hospital Supply Corp., 134 Merchant Street, Suite 200, Cincinnati, Ohio 45246.

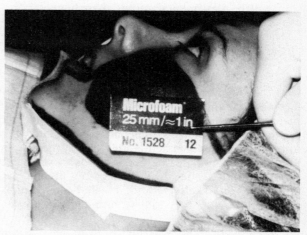

Figure 23–7. Microfoam tape delineates the inferior border of the mandibular ramus and angle to avoid a jagged appearance following dermabrasion.

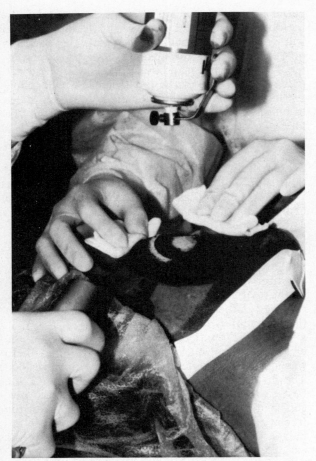

Figure 23–8. The most severely scarred area is frozen and dermabraded first. Only small segments are frozen and dermabraded to allow for "board hard" consistency. Note that the skin is not under tension during spraying. The gauze held by the nurse protects the nose and the eyes during spraying.

minutes prior to the commencement of dermabrasion will be detrimental rather than beneficial because of this compensatory vasodilatation.

The dermabrasion on the first cheek commences at the point where the scarring is most severe (Fig. 23–8). The author does not follow the outlines suggested by Burks[2] or Stegman and Tromovitch[13] who recommend that the face be dermabraded in a methodic manner with predetermined segments dermabraded sequentially. Often, these predetermined segments will not have significant scarring, and when following their recommendations, the surgeon may take 10 to 15 minutes before the most severe area is dermabraded. During this time, the prechill has lost some of its effect, and it will become more difficult to freeze the skin. Consequently, the dermabrasion will be less efficient. By commencing at the area where the scarring is most severe, the surgeon obtains the maximum advantage of the prechill.

PHYSICAL PRINCIPLES OF EFFECTIVE DERMABRASION

There are three principles that are important to effective dermabrasion. In seminars and previous articles on the topic, these principles have been poorly articulated or ignored altogether. If one analyzes the physics of mass and the vectors of force, certain principles become self-evident. The principles essential to the performance of an effective dermabrasion are: (1) the normal contour of the skin should be maintained during dermabrasion, (2) the skin should be changed to a solid state to provide effective abrasion (Fig. 23–9), and (3) one should be aware of danger areas that may scar readily (Fig. 23–10).

A cosmetic dermabrasion for postacne scarring is designed to improve the abnormal contour of the skin. Most scars are depressed leaving the adjacent normal skin higher. Dermabrasion does not elevate skin as does silicone or collagen, but instead it diminishes the level of the normal skin to the greatest amount safely possible, i.e., hopefully to the level of the depressed scars. The surgeon therefore selectively abrades the higher normal skin down to the level of the lower abnormal skin.

Most surgeons have been taught to stretch the skin prior to freezing. This is incorrect. Alteration of the abnormal skin by stretching it will flatten the

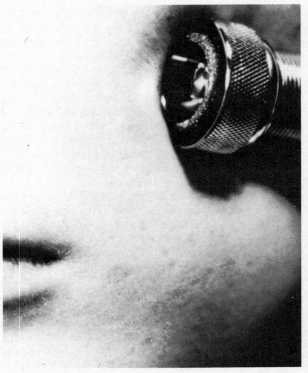

Figure 23–9. The firm substance of the abrading mechanism will definitely distort the skin if it is not altered to a solid state.

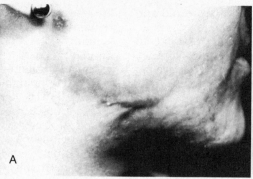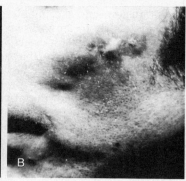

Figure 23–10. Danger areas that readily scar exist over bony prominences, such as the mandibular ramus (*A*) and the zygomatic arch (*B*).

contours, thus modifying and minimizing the difference in heights. When this pressure of stretching is released, the natural forces controlling the skin will spring back into effect, and the pre-existing contours will reappear. Thus, the dermabrasion must be accomplished without any tension to distort the abnormal contour. There are exceptions to this rule: One should stretch areas where marked natural contours occur to avoid excessive abrading on high areas while trying to abrade adjacent low areas. These regions include the philtrum, the cleft of the chin, the angles of the mouth, the nasolabial folds and the alae nasi. Other areas with marked contouring, such as excessive wrinkling, should be treated similarly.

Another procedure that may alter the contour of the skin is infiltration of a local anesthetic. If adequate time is not allowed for the anesthetic to disperse completely, the instilled liquid will distort the pre-existing contour. The author finds no need to use infiltration anesthesia or regional blocks, because the preanesthetic allays fear and the refrigerant spray when properly used provides total anesthesia in the area on which the dermabrasion is being performed.

The second principle in effective dermabrasion is the transformation of semisolid skin into a solid state—the most important factor in achieving superior results. The skin is soft and pliable and has a normal surface temperature of 92°F. It is a semisolid that is disturbed in contour when external pressure is applied to its surface by a firm object. Therefore, any solid object such as a fingertip, a pencil, or specifically a diamond fraise or wire brush will distort its contour. Since this distortion is detrimental to the objective, the skin must be transformed into a solid state in order to provide firm resistance to the abrading equipment. It is impossible to recontour a soft substance, such as a piece of gelatin, with a file and to obtain predictable results. However, when recontouring is done against a firm hard surface, such as a block of wood, the file will produce the desired results.

When using refrigerant anesthetics (Fluro Ethyl or Frigiderm), one can transform the skin into an insensitive solid state. The skin is frozen in small segments of approximately 1 square inch until it becomes absolutely firm. The refrigerant is sprayed in short blasts of 4 to 8 seconds. The initial point of freezing will probably require 3 or 4 blasts of spray before it is adequately frozen to allow effective dermabrasion. The author finds that this short series of spraying is better tolerated by the patient than a sustained spray of 20 to 30 seconds at the initiation of dermabrasion. When adequately frozen, the skin will maintain its usual contour and will not be distorted by the pressure of the abrading surface.

Inadequate freezing of the skin to a solid state is, in the author's opinion, the most common cause of inadequate results. Those using refrigerant anesthetics probably fail from timidity. This is unfortunate, because not only is adequate abrasion prevented but anesthesia is reduced, thus making the procedure uncomfortable. Some surgeons claim they can complete a full facial dermabrasion in 15 to 20 minutes. The author considers this to be impossible. Freezing small segments until they are absolutely solid and applying meticulous attention to every scar and its subsequent correction are time-consuming. At least one hour, and often more, is required for the author to complete a full facial dermabrasion. This attention to detail is rewarded by superior cosmetic and therapeutic results.

Two additional advantages accrue from transforming the skin into a solid state. The blood is frozen in the capillary loops and intense vasoconstriction of the arteriolar bed occurs, both providing a bloodless field during abrasion. The capillary loops and the papillary dermis are readily recognizable and provide a positive identification of the depth of abrasion. If dermabrasion goes deeper than the papillary dermis and into the reticular dermis, scarring may occur if all epidermal appendages are destroyed. It is easy to understand why surgeons performing dermabrasion using general anesthesia without freezing the skin with a refrigerant or those who inadequately freeze the skin produce inadequate results. Blood obscures the depth of the dermabrasion, and the pliable skin is distorted and responds poorly to an abrasive surface.

The third principle in effective dermabrasion is to be aware of danger areas that are overly susceptible to scarring. Skin, which has differing underlying structures, has varying but predictable freeze-thaw cycles. Skin overlying relatively avascular bone freezes rapidly and thaws slowly. Skin overlying abundant subcutaneous fat and muscle, both of which have a rich vascular bed, freezes slowly and thaws rapidly because the cooling effect is readily dissipated. Areas that freeze rapidly and thaw slowly are the mandible, particularly at the junction of its posterior and middle third, the bossing of both the chin and the forehead, and areas over the malar eminence and the zygomatic ridge. Caution must be taken in these areas because freezing occurs rapidly, which permits deep effective abrasion.

A major mistake made by the inexperienced surgeon is to freeze an excessively large area. The skin overlying highly vascularized subcutaneous tissue freezes slowly and thaws rapidly, both of which limit the depth of dermabrasion. In contrast, the skin overlying bone freezes rapidly and thaws slowly, which facilitates effective dermabrasion. Thus, when a large area is dermabraded, the abrasion will be carried deeper on the firmly frozen skin overlying the bone, but the depth is more superficial over the softer subcutaneous tissue. Repeated freezings and abrading of the entire area will finally carry the level of dermabrasion to an adequate depth in the skin overlying subcutaneous tissue, but a level too deep in the area overlying bone may be reached and result in scar formation. Therefore, these danger areas should be frozen in small segments and with caution by the surgeon.

These danger areas exist even for the surgeon who performs the operation on soft skin using general anesthesia. This is because the underlying bone provides greater resistance to the abrasive surface than the skin cushioned by the abundant subcutaneous tissue and underlying muscle.

As the freezing proceeds and the dermabrasion is completed in each segment, it is best for the surgeon to dermabrade to the desired depth without allowing the skin to thaw completely. The author uses both the 60,000 rpm Schumann High Speed Derma III Dermabrader and the 33,000 rpm Bell Hand Engine, both of which allow the operator to rapidly change the standard fraise to a pear-shaped fraise for special contouring of excessively deep ice-pick scars or high contour areas such as the nasolabial folds. Previously, the author did not do this special contouring with the pear-shaped fraise until the termination of the procedure; however, he found that refreezing of an area after complete thawing was impossible. Compensatory vasodilation, edema, and hyperemia prevented adequate refreezing.

In a specific segment, the painted scarred portions are dermabraded to an adequate depth, and the remaining unscarred skin is then painted with 1% gentian violet. These areas are then frozen and dermabraded to a more superficial level. This provides good blending of color and avoids a distinct area of hypopigmentation that occurs frequently when only the central portion of the cheek is dermabraded. To repeat, after the right cheek is completed, the ice pack is removed from the left cheek, the previously outlined scarred areas are painted with gentian violet, and an ice pack is taped to the forehead (if this area is to be dermabraded). The procedure proceeds in the exact manner as described above. Prior to beginning the abrasion on the left cheek, an additional injection of 25 mg Demerol is given. This maintains the patient at a high level of analgesia and permits the dermabrasion to progress without discomfort. If we presume that Demerol is completely metabolized over a 3- to 4-hour period, then 25% to 35% of the Demerol has been cleared and should be replaced with an additional injection. Upon completing the left cheek, a third injection of 25 mg of Demerol is administered before initiating any surgery on the forehead. If only a small triangle in the glabella remains to be abraded, this third injection is unnecessary. I have found that this regime is far more comfortable for the patient than when only one single injection of 100 mg of Demerol is given.

The forehead presents a particular challenge to the surgeon. Experience shows that this is the most painful area. There is a sensation of deep pain when the spray is applied over the frontal sinuses, which is very similar to that experienced when cold liquids or ice cream is eaten too rapidly. Some have suggested that this pain is due to supercooling of the supraorbital and supra-auricular nerves by the refrigerant. The author believes this explanation is correct because a regional block of these nerves using local anesthetic will eliminate this cold-induced pain.

The forehead may have many small hairs that should be removed with an electric shaver or clippers prior to the procedure. This is not to suggest any disfigurement of the normal hairline, but the fine hairs should be removed to decrease the buildup of debris on the wire brush or fraise. In individuals who have early balding, the dermabrasion should be carried to the hairline when possible to provide normal color blending. Since the forehead completely overlies bone, this area freezes rapidly and firmly, thus permitting a very efficient and rapid dermabrasion. The surgeon must be exceedingly careful not to carry the dermabrasion to a depth that may create a scar.

At the completion of the dermabrasion, the surgeon may choose to chemically peel the nondermabraded areas with trichloroacetic acid, using a 25% to 45% solution. The author has learned from others that 50% trichloroacetic acid can cause scarring, but 45% and lower does not. It has been the author's observation that this peel produces no specific improvement in color and provides only an additional irritant and a greater surface area that must heal during the postoperative phase. The erythema frequently subsides by the fifth postoperative day. These observations have been made on untaped applications.

Chemical peeling should be considered in the patient who has hyperpigmentation in the periorbital regions. This should be noted by the surgeon preoperatively, and a chemical peel employing Baker's phenol solution[14] should be applied without tape to these areas. This is necessary in less than 2% of the cases but avoids a possible color contrast in those patients affected. The chemical peel is treated in the same fashion as the dermabrasion, using postoperative wet packs and petrolatum until the area is re-epithelialized.

POSTOPERATIVE DRESSING

At the completion of the surgical procedure, the sterile gauze previously applied to the abraded areas to absorb the serosanguineous exudate is removed, and all clots are cleansed from the abraded surface using half-strength hydrogen peroxide diluted with tap water. Petrolatum-impregnated gauze is applied to the surgical sites and covered with approximately 10 layers of sterile gauze. A Kling bandage is applied to stabilize the underlying dressing. Patients are moved from the table and allowed to sit where they receive a soft drink for its caloric and caffeine effects. Their response is monitored and generally no narcotic antagonist is necessary, since it is desirable to have the patient slightly obtunded when returning to their residence. This allows them to sleep for several hours. If the preceding hypnotics and narcotics do not allow the patient to function adequately, 1 cc of naloxone hydrochloride (Narcan) is given to antagonize the Demerol.

POSTOPERATIVE CARE

Twenty-four hours after surgery, the patient removes the dressings and commences to apply wet packs using a terry cloth facial mask, which has been provided by the surgeon. A half-strength boric acid solution is made by combining equal parts of tap water and a saturated solution of boric acid. The patients use wet packs initially between 10 and 12 hours to reduce the erythema, edema, and crust formation. Late in the afternoon on the first postoperative day, patients are requested to call the office and report on their progress. The patients are seen in the office for the succeeding two weeks on

Monday, Wednesday, and Friday. All patients who have recently undergone dermabrasion or phenol chemical face peeling are scheduled at the same time so that a peer support group is formed. Patients further in their recuperative phase can advise and encourage the more recently treated patients.

The duration of wet pack use is progressively decreased so that, during the second postoperative week, it is four hours or less per day. When not using wet packs, the patient applies petrolatum covered with Saran Wrap to avoid drying of the treated sites. Most patients attain complete re-epithelialization some time between the eleventh and thirteenth day. Rarely, a patient who has undergone a very deep dermabrasion will require 16 to 18 days to heal selected areas, particularly regions of preexisting hypertrophic or keloidal scarring, which by their nature have diminished vascularity and poor recuperative powers. Using this technique, it can be predicted that areas which re-epithelialize in less than seven days will have no significant anatomic change, a fact that is commonly reported by patients who have undergone dermabrasion elsewhere and find that they have no anatomic improvement.

At the end of two weeks, following healing, the patient may return to work but should avoid sun exposure while any residual erythema persists in order to avoid irregular postinflammatory hyperpigmentation. At the beginning of the fourth postoperative week, small areas in each preauricular region are skin tested with sunscreens that have a sun protective value of 15. If no irritant or allergic response is noted after seven days of use, the patient is instructed to apply the sunscreen twice a day when sun exposure is anticipated. A 2½% hydrocortisone cream is applied two to four times per day to provide lubrication, decrease erythema, and diminish pruritus. Noncomedogenic water-based cosmetics, such as Almay or Allercreme, are used for the next three months by female patients. Heavy lifting and exercise is avoided during the first six weeks to diminish the Valsalva maneuver (this may not be necessary since patients employed in heavy physical labor seem to have no detrimental effects from lifting). Patients are seen on a biweekly or monthly basis until all the erythema subsides and the skin color has returned to normal. This is usually completed by the twelfth week.

USUAL COURSE, SIDE EFFECTS, AND COMPLICATIONS

The usual course has expected and predictable reactions. Every patient will experience erythema, edema, crust formation, and mild discomfort. The first three symptoms are controlled by wet packs, and the discomfort generally does not require any medication. The patient is given a prescription for

20 Demerol tablets (50 mg) and advised to use them on the first night of surgery and one half hour prior to dressing removal. The vast majority of patients do not use any analgesic.

Other anticipated responses include milia formation. Probably 100 percent of patients develop postoperative milia that are temporary and usually self-limiting. When stubborn milia persist despite the gentle use of a Buf-Puf, acne surgery can be performed. Approximately 50% of the patients with pre-existing acne will have a slight flare, which does not respond to systemic or topical antibiotics in most instances. This response is also self-limiting and generally begins by the sixth postoperative week and generally subsides by the fourth to sixth month. The author has never seen it extend beyond one year, and in all instances, patients have experienced therapeutic improvement of their pre-existing chronic acne (even severe cases).

Another anticipated response is a vascular flush that occurs in the previously frozen sites when a patient comes inside after exposure to cold during the winter. This flush signifies mild vascular instability. The author has never seen a patient become more susceptible to frostbite following dermabrasion although patients are warned to avoid excessive cold exposure during the first postoperative winter season.

Side effects are few and include purpura, hypopigmentation, and hyperpigmentation. Purpura is rarely seen and is almost universally experienced by women. This is the result of a torsional effect on the incompletely healed skin even though re-epithelialization is complete. In women, this is caused by whisker burn and is most frequently seen between the third and sixth postoperative week. Males are also cautioned of this effect, since it may occur from torsional forces involved in contact sports such as basketball, football, and wrestling.

Permanent postoperative hypopigmentation is not as prevalent as some believe. This is an anticipated side effect and not a complication as some authors claim. It is most commonly seen in dark-skinned Caucasion or Oriental patients. Although the author has no experience with black patients, Yarborough and Farber state that the darker the preoperative color, the less likelihood there is of any significant postoperative color change. Patients in whom permanent hypopigmentation can be anticipated usually resume their normal pigmentation within 12 months. Generally, only very subtle changes will occur, and these will be hidden under the mandibular ramus if the patient has been properly dermabraded. In the author's opinion, these subtle color changes have been greatly overemphasized by the critics of dermabrasion.

Patients are prone to postinflammatory hyperpigmentation if they are exposed to sunlight during the phase while erythema is persisting. This is a tem-

porary response, whereas hypopigmentation is usually permanent. Prevention consists of the regular application of sunscreens coupled with minimal sun exposure. Improvement is effected by the application of a bleaching cream consisting of equal parts of Eldoquin Forte and Retin A 0.1% Cream to the darkened areas, one to three times per day.

Complications consist of postoperative scar formation and infection from either bacterial or viral causes. These are complications rather than the aforementioned side effects, since they are not predictable or anticipated events. When the dermabrasion is properly performed, it is rare to produce postoperative scarring. Danger areas mentioned above should be dermabraded with caution. The patients on whom the author has seen scars develop either ineffectively used the postoperative wet packs and allowed thick crusts to form or rubbed the surgical site with wet sterile gauze so aggressively as to create an additional "dermabrasion" and the level of tissue damage was deeper than desired. One patient, who did not use wet packs for six days kept the surgical sites covered with petrolatum and cellophane. This allowed a thick crust to form, which subsequently caused scarring in the area of the mandibular ramus. Pre-existing scars of a severe nature were present in these areas.

Another patient was also ineffective in her use of postoperative wet packs, which caused a thick crust to form over her entire cheek. This crust was removed manually by curettage, and the patient was hospitalized for supervision of adequate use of wet packs. Upon examining the crust microscopically, it was noted that the deeper surfaces consisted of a fibrin clot containing many red cells and leukocytes. Covering this debris was a thin layer of newly formed epithelium. It is the author's suspicion that, had this crust been allowed to persist, the clot would have necessarily become organized and scar formation would have ensued. It is now the author's practice to remove any crusts manually using curettage when it is felt they are excessive. This occurs only occasionally, is usually not necessary before the fifth day, and is minimized by the use of wet packs and systemic antibiotics.

Bacterial infection is rare during the healing phase. However, infection with herpes simplex is not uncommon. Although Orentreich[15] claims that he has never seen scarring occur with a reactivation of herpes simplex when the involved area is kept moist with wet packs, the author has seen several patients who have developed very superficial scarring under these conditions. It is rare to observe any scarring when the herpes simplex infection is a reactivation of a patient's earlier herpes infection. However, when individuals are exposed to others having herpes simplex, the infection presents as a primary case rather than a reactivation. As such, there seems to be no pre-existing immune response, and these infections are quite severe and may result in significant postherpetic scarring. With acyclovir (Zovirax) capsules and topical ointment, this complication now causes less fear. Yarborough[16] has recommended that patients with frequent herpetic infections be dermabraded in two stages. The trigger areas of herpes simplex are not dermabraded until after all other areas are abraded and re-epithelialized. When there is a positive history of pre-existing facial herpes simplex, the author now uses 200 mg Zovirax capsules three times per day, beginning three days prior to surgery and continuing until 15 days after surgery. The trigger area is dermabraded with the uneffected areas. Although the series is very limited, no recurrence of herpes simplex has been encountered.

EQUIPMENT FOR DERMABRASION

There are several dermabrasion units that are available to the surgeon. The author has experience using three of these units (Fig. 23–11). All have advantages and disadvantages. The first effective unit was designed by Noel Robbins of Chatham, New Jersey, for Abner Kurtin, M.D., over 30 years ago. This is a modified cable-driven dental unit that has the capability of driving the dermabrasion fraises or wire brushes at a speed of 23,000 rpm. This unit is mounted on a movable stand and is controlled with a variable speed footpedal. A more compact wall-hung unit is available but provides only 18,000 rpm. This time-honored unit has been used for thousands of successful dermabrasions. Its major disadvantage is that the cable when bent during use becomes exceedingly hot and may rupture. This unit is ideal for the inexperienced surgeon, because it provides a moderate speed with adequate torque. The handpiece may be purchased with a modified safety sleeve designed for accurate and controlled dermabrasion to a predetermined depth by means of a rib that allows the handpiece to rest on the skin. This rib is adjacent to the fraise or wire brush and thus provides a very short fulcrum from this point to the abrasive surface (less than 2 cm). In addition, a fender covers the nonabrading surface of the fraise or wheel and markedly diminishes the spray that may result if the surgeon allows the skin to soften and bleed.

The most commonly used unit today is the compact Bell International hand engine. This consists of a very light, hand-held engine attached to a small console by a coiled electric cord allowing maximum flexibility without drag. Unfortunately, most surgeons using this device have purchased either Model 5-E (400 to 16,000 rpm) or Model 25-D (400 to 18,000 rpm), both of which provide a top speed considerably less than that of the larger Robbins unit. Also, there is no protective rib that may be

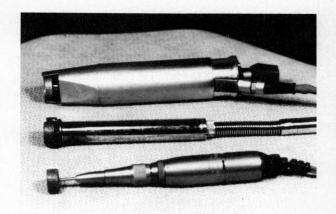

Figure 23–11. Handpieces have considerable differences in size and weight. The top unit (Schumann) weighs 19 oz.; the middle unit (Robbins) has a safety sleeve attached and weighs a total of 8½ oz.; and the bottom unit (Bell International Hand Engine) weighs 6½ oz. but, unlike the other two, has the distinct disadvantage of no safety sleeve or protective rib.

placed on the patient's skin to provide a guide for the inexperienced surgeon. Because there is no protective rib, the fulcrum that is created by the measurement of the abrading surface to the center of the surgeon's hand is considerably greater, i.e., up to 10 times that of the larger Robbins unit. Although Noel Robbins, the sole U.S. distributor of this unit, will supply a protective fender upon request, the accessory is not permanently attached to the hand engine and can vibrate loose during the surgical procedure. Also, the fender is so large in size there is considerable visual obstruction of the surgical site. These two disadvantages are significant.

A better handpiece, but often not recommended by the supplier, is from the earlier Model 8-AL, which provides 600 to 33,000 rpm, or from the latest Models 28-L and 2404, which provide 2000 to 35,000 rpm. These units can be used for hair transplantation and provide a much higher top speed, which is advantageous in dermabrasion. In addition, these higher-speed handpieces provide more torque than the 16,000 to 18,000 rpm units. The supplier cautions that these high-speed units must not be used at maximum rpm with a wire brush. Diamond-embedded fraises can be carefully balanced, but this is not possible with a wire brush. At speeds over 30,000 rpm, the shaft can fatigue and either bend or rupture.

Because the hand engine is an electrical apparatus, it must be sterilized by using a gas rather than an autoclave. Many surgeons employing this apparatus are probably not adequately sterilizing the handpiece between cases. An economical gas sterilizer is available from H. W. Anderson Products, Inc., Oyster Bay, NY 11771.

The latest high-speed dermabrasion equipment is the Derma III produced by A. Schumann of Düsseldorf, Federal Republic of Germany. This unit provides very high torque at a variable speed ranging from 15,000 to 60,000 rpm. This unit is an excellent addition to the science of facial dermabrasion, and it is presently the author's instrument of choice. The additional high speed allows the surgeon to decrease the operative time by approximately 25% to 35%. It is particularly beneficial on multiple deep scars or firm hypertrophic scars. The unit is provided with three protective sleeves, all of which enclose the abrading surface with a fender, thus decreasing the amount of debris which sprays from the operative site. The manufacturer provides high-speed diamond fraises of medium and coarse grit specifically designed to withstand the high rpm.

There are a few disadvantages of the Schumann device. First and foremost, the handpiece is exceedingly heavy, weighing almost 19 oz as compared to 6½ oz for the Bell hand engine and 8½ oz for the Robbins unit. The electric cord exits at an inferior position on the handpiece and thus can provide an obstruction and additional drag on the patient's body. The author has had both the handpieces modified so that the cord exits at a 90-degree angle from its usual position. Because the handpiece is so heavy and the abrasive quality so efficient, affected skin is dermabraded exceedingly quickly, which creates some ridging. Because of its weight, the fine work and final touches are now done by the author using the 35,000 rpm Bell hand engine. Together, these provide an excellent combination for rapid and efficient dermabrasion. The author does not use the Schumann machine for shallow scarring or the nose or generally in the danger zones, as previously mentioned. The Bell hand engine with its less efficient abrasive abilities and considerably lighter handpiece is the better choice in these regions. Since both of these units should be adequately sterilized, the surgeon must have gas sterilizing capability readily available for both the Schumann and Bell units.

Other disadvantages of the Schumann machine are the footpedal, which weighs over 14 pounds and is impossible to move without becoming contaminated unless assisted by a circulating nurse. The console itself is large and attached to a movable stand, which requires considerably larger storage space than the Bell hand engine but less than the Robbins unit. Probably the most disadvantageous aspect of the Schumann machine is its cost, presently retailing at about five times the cost of a Bell hand engine.

The abrasive surfaces used in dermabrasion consist of diamond fraises, stiff wire brushes, and serrated wheels. The author has no experience with the serrated wheel, very limited experience with the wire brush, and extensive experience with the diamond fraises. The fraise is easier for the inexperienced surgeon to use since it does not catch or "walk" on soft skin as readily as the wire brush. In addition, it is generally less abrasive and thus provides a greater margin of safety.

Robbins has recently introduced extra-coarse fraises that are superior to the previously available grits and are now the author's standard selection for the Bell hand engine. A major factor in the selection of the fraise over the wire brush is that it produces a flat surface during and at the conclusion of the abrasion, whereas the wire brush produces an irregular rugose surface that obliterates the capillary loops and sebaceous glands, both of which assist the surgeon in determining the depth of the dermabrasion. With a firm freeze and a diamond fraise, the surgeon can readily identify the papillary dermis by seeing the capillary loops and the deeper sebaceous glands, which reside in the upper reticular dermis. Dermabrasion carried to a deeper level than where the sebaceous glands reside generally invades the subcutaneous fatty layer and will produce a postoperative scar. These levels have been clearly identified by both Burks[2] and Stegman and Tromovitch.[13] The novice dermabrader should become familiar with this information. The author does not use the Schumann apparatus in the manner recommended by Robert Stolar of Washington, D.C.[17] He has advised that the Schumann instrument is best used on soft skin using general anesthesia. However, the skin is displaced by the abrasive wheel when unfrozen, bleeds readily, and requires considerable traction, which distorts the pre-existing scarred surface. Stolar further claims that, because of its high speed, the Schumann unit does not grab the skin as readily as a slower moving fraise or the wire brush. This may be true when the skin is under extreme traction; however, this cannot be expected when the skin is soft and under limited or no traction. The author has used the unit under the latter conditions and found it difficult to control, since it grabs the skin and rapidly traverses in the direction of the rotating fraise. The author finds this aspect to be dangerous rather than advantageous.

Many surgeons use a blower to more effectively evaporate the refrigerant spray. Because of the author's specially constructed surgical rooms, which provide a low humidity and a temperature of 60°F, the blower is unnecessary. To maximize the refrigerant spray, the skin is prechilled sequentially for a 30-minute period, as described earlier, using either a water-filled sterile glove frozen to 0°F or a special pack produced by the American Hospital Supply Company.

There are several refrigerant sprays that can be used for dermabrasion. The author's choice is Fluro Ethyl, which is a combination of 25% ethyl chloride and 75% Freon 114. This is dispensed from a pressurized metal container by a plastic nozzle to which a custom-designed handpiece is attached to aid in dispensing (Fig. 23–12). This product is very effective and evaporates so readily that a blower under usual conditions is not necessary. The spray should be held six to eight inches away to allow for adequate aerosol formation of the dispersed droplets. Under humid conditions, the dispenser must be held at a greater distance to promote proper aerosol formation. If this is not done, the material will condense on the skin. Another product used by many is Frigiderm, which is Freon 114. This product, like Fluro Ethyl, is noninflammable, nonexplosive, and less toxic than ethyl chloride. However, it is considered to be less effective by most surgeons when compared to Fluro Ethyl.

A new product introduced within the past five years is CryOesthesia −30C and −60C, which was touted by the supplier (Robbins) to be more effective than either Frigiderm or Fluro Ethyl. After trying the product for three months, the author discontinued its use because of the many disadvantages of CryOesthesia compared with Fluro Ethyl. The major disadvantages were that the patient experienced more pain during spraying, and the skin was frozen so rapidly and deeply that the author was concerned that it might cause irreversible tissue damage. In addition, there were disadvantages with the container, which was considerably larger and more difficult to grasp, the dispensing nozzle caused fatigue and could not be readily adapted to a custom-made handpiece, shipping time was great, and cost was considerably higher than that of Fluro Ethyl. Because of these factors and the concern that the cold injury to the tissue might be hazardous, its use was discontinued and Robbins was advised that problems might arise with other surgeons.

One year later at the international seminar on dermabrasion and chemical peeling held at the Northwestern University in 1983, three other surgeons voiced concern over this product. Each had observed that some patients experienced extreme pain during the spray, and all three had seen prolonged erythema of the surgical site lasting many months following a dermabrasion. The author interpreted this as minimal but definitive scarring in the involved areas. The three had also experienced overt scarring along the mandibular ramus. Because of this, the author joined the others in writing a cautionary letter to the editor of the *Journal of Dermatologic Surgery and Oncology*.[18] Hanke and colleagues have since conducted extensive studies on the contents of CryOesthesia −30C and −60C. They showed that both of these substances provided freezing that was considerably colder than that as stated by the manufacturer. Studies on laboratory animals showed that tissue damage was far greater using these substances than with the other refrigerant sprays. This information has been quite beneficial to the surgeon performing facial dermabrasion and has undoubtedly prevented a considerable number of detrimental results.

POSTOPERATIVE RESULTS

Postoperative evaluation may be divided into three categories: short-term, midterm, and long-term. Short-term evaluation is mentioned mainly as a caution to the patient, the surgeon, and the reader of surgical literature. This is the period from complete re-epithelialization (usually the tenth to the fourteenth days) to the twelfth postoperative week. During this period, there is varying erythema and edema. The latter gives a fullness to the remaining depressed scars, and the former masks the pre-existing hypopigmented areas. In most patients, the best cosmetic appearance is achieved within this interval. As edema and erythema subside, the true results of the surgery can be appreciated. Postopertive photographs taken during this period can be grossly deceptive, and no editor should allow these pictures to represent the final results.

During this short-term phase, some patients who have undergone a dermabrasion for chronic or uncontrollable acne experience a recrudescence of their active acne with pustule and cyst formation. This is not to be confused with milia formation,

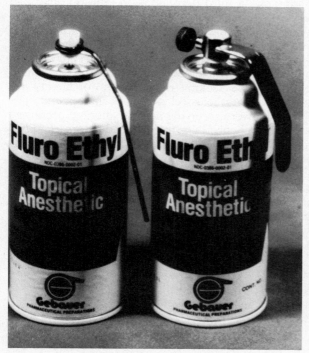

Figure 23–12. Fluro Ethyl, the refrigerant of choice, has a dispensing nozzle that may be modified with a custom-made handle to allow for less fatigue to the surgeon. Note that the dispenser on the left has the original wire handle, which is no longer available (probably because of legal implications).

which is an expected postoperative event. This flare subsides usually by the sixth postoperative month but will mask the cosmetic and therapeutic value of the surgery, at least temporarily.

Midterm results are those evaluated between the fourth and twelfth months. During the preceding short-term phase, all of the edema subsides, but some of the erythema may persist. A flare of active acne usually diminishes by six months, and a therapeutic benefit is almost universally achieved before the twelfth month. The compensatory seborrhea and milia formation have subsided by this time, and the patient has received maximal cosmetic and therapeutic benefit. The author usually, evaluates permanent improvement in the sixth month but has assessed this as late as one year following the procedure.

The long-term results are those evaluated more than one year following surgery. This may be too long an interval for objective evaluation to be possible. It is often difficult to get the patients to return, and they have difficulty in recalling their preoperative appearance. Without the aid of preoperative photographs, their evaluation is of little or no value, since it lacks objectivity. The passage of time dulls one's memory. Evaluation of results more than one year after the surgery, particularly with a written questionnaire and without the aid of preoperative pictures, cannot provide meaningful results.

Standardized methods of evaluation are elusive. Surprisingly, however, physicians and patient usually arrive at a similar percentage of improvement independently. Usually, neither the patient or the surgeon counts the individual scars that have been completely corrected or those remaining in estimating the relative percentage of improvement. If the patient looks at his face and likes what he sees, then it is better and he is improved. The old adage that "beauty is in the eye of the beholder" holds true. The author has never seen a patient who could thoroughly recall the degree and extent of his preoperative scarring. High-quality preoperative photographs that honestly portray the scarring are imperative. Shadowing is necessary to display scarring, but excessive shadowing distorts the natural appearance and exaggerates the defects.

To recall the preoperative appearance, both the patient and the author carefully review the standardized series of preoperative pictures. Then, with the aid of wall-mounted mirrors and overhead oblique light to accentuate remaining scarring, we independently arrive at a percentage of improvement. On occasion, several patients who are undergoing a final evaluation of improvement and postoperative pictures participate in the evaluation. When two evaluators are involved, it is rare that the appraisal varies more than 5%. When more participate, the variation is usually 10% or less. It should be remembered that these evaluations are made independently, so one assessment is not influenced by another.

Although the author has been performing facial dermabrasion since 1970, he has been keeping records of postoperative evaluation only for the past seven years. It is difficult for him to evaluate adequately patients who live a great distance from Minneapolis, particularly those who reside outside the continental United States. During the past seven years, none of his patients have evaluated their cosmetic or therapeutic improvement as less than 50%. Many have rated the improvement at 100%. Some of those undergoing cosmetic dermabrasion had obvious scars remaining. When asked why they rated their improvement at 100%, their answer was, "I achieved at least 100% of the improvement I had hoped for." This type of evaluation skews the statistics to the right but clearly demonstrates patient satisfaction with the results of the procedure.

To assess the cosmetic and therapeutic benefit of facial dermabrasion more closely, the author reviewed 100 consecutive cases that had been evaluated (Table 23–2). The ages of the patients ranged from 16 to 53 years with females outnumbering males 2 to 1. Fifty-six percent were between 20 and 29 years old; 53% of the patients were referred by their physicians. For 87% of the patients, the dermabrasion being evaluated was their first procedure. For 11% of the patients, the dermabrasion in question was their second procedure. One patient had undergone a third dermabrasion, and one had had a fourth procedure. Almost two thirds (65%) presented with some form of active acne, either under control but chronic in duration or uncontrollable with aggressive systemic and topical therapy. In addition to improvement of the acne, most of these patients were seeking cosmetic improvement; this group is nevertheless classified as therapeutic. The 35% who were receiving no acne therapy presented with no evidence of active acne; they are classified as solely cosmetic. Therapeutic improvement was judged no sooner than six months following surgery. Cosmetic improvement was judged no sooner than three months after the procedure and usually six months or later. Therapeutic improvement was based on four categories ranging from improvement with continued medication to complete control following cessation of all medication (Table 23–3).

As stated earlier, the range for cosmetic improvement was between 50% and 100%. The largest group of patients rated their cosmetic improvement

TABLE 23–2. Series of 100 Consecutive Cases of Facial Dermabrasion

Age Range	16 to 53 years
Female	64%
Male	36%
Physician Referred	53%

TABLE 23–3. Therapeutic Improvement From Dermabrasion

1. Previous uncontrollable acne now under good to excellent control on similar preoperative medication.

2. Good to excellent control of active acne on lower dose of medication.

3. Good to excellent control of active acne on less potent medication.

4. Previous acne requiring regular care now on no medication.

from 65% to 85% with the peak being between 75% to 80%. These statistics were not compiled during short-term recovery when edema, erythema, and the flush of initial enthusiasm can result in overly optimistic evaluation.

Therapeutic improvement of chronic or uncontrollable pustular or cystic acne was also judged by the patients to range from 50% to 100%. The average therapeutic benefit was less than the average cosmetic improvement, with the bulk of patients reporting from 55% to 80% improvement. No significant peak was identified. These statistics for therapeutic improvement are similar to those reported by many others who regularly perform dermabrasion. Unfortunately, little has been written about the therapeutic benefits of the procedure. The author suspects that those who see little or no therapeutic improvement are abrading too superficially.

These statistics also refute the recommendation that dermabrasion should not be performed until all of the acne is quiescent. Although it is advisable to obtain the best possible acne control prior to dermabrasion, it is detrimental to deny the therapeutic effects of facial dermabrasion to patients with active acne, particularly uncontrollable acne. To be sure, these patients may develop more scars after dermabrasion, but the subsequent scarring will be less severe, since the active acne is ameliorated or completely controlled by the procedure. The exception is patients with active acne keloidalis, in whom dermabrasion should be delayed until the process is totally quiescent.

Dermabrasion for facial scarring, particularly postacne scars, provides a definitive cosmetic improvement when performed by an experienced, skilled surgeon using the principles outlined. The results are gratifying for patient and surgeon alike. There is no alternative treatment to dermabrasion. Some other procedures correct acne scarring, e.g., collagen injection, scar excision, and punch grafting.

However, none of these techniques replaces dermabrasion; rather, they act as adjunctive procedures. Facial dermabrasion also provides therapeutic improvement for chronic or uncontrollable pustular or cystic acne and should not be denied during the active phase, despite the widely held belief that additional scars may form if dermabrasion is performed before the acne has subsided. In these patients, the improvement of active acne is hastened by facial dermabrasion. Dermabrasion has rightfully earned a proper place in the surgical armamentarium.

REFERENCES

1. Kurtin A: Corrective surgical planing of skin. Arch Derm Syph 68:389–397, 1953
2. Burks JW: Dermabrasion and Chemical Peeling in the Treatment of Certain Cosmetic Defects and Diseases of the Skin. Springfield, Ill, Charles C Thomas, 1979
3. Field LM: The value of dermabrasion in the management of actinic keratoses, in Epstein E (ed): Controversies in Dermatology. Philadelphia, W. B. Saunders Co, 1984, pp 96–102
4. Roenigk, HH Jr: Dermabrasion for miscellaneous cutaneous lesions: Exclusive of scarring for acne. J Dermatol Surg Oncol 3:322–328, 1977
5. Hanke CW: Dermabrasion of unusual lesions. Dermabrasion–Chemical Peel Seminar, Chicago, Ill, May 19, 1983
6. Yarborough JM: Patient selection. Dermabrasion–Chemical Peel Seminar, Chicago, Ill, May 19, 1983
7. Wright MA: How to recognize and control the problem patient. J Dermatol Surg Oncol 10:389–395, 1984
8. Strauss John S., Iowa City, Iowa. Personal communication, 1982.
9. Roenigk HH Jr, Pinski JB, Robinson JK, Hanke CW: Acne, retinoids, and dermabrasion. J Dermatol Surg Oncol 11:396–398, 1985
10. Lask G: No scarring from dermabrasion after Accutane? Schoch Letter 35:21, 1985
11. Farber, GA, New Orleans, La. Personal communication, 1980.
12. Sturm HM, Atlanta, Ga. Personal communication, 1980.
13. Stegman S, Tromovitch T: Cosmetic Dermatologic Surgery. Chicago, Year Book Medical Publishers, Inc, 1984, pp 47–76
14. Baker TJ: Chemical face peeling, an adjunct to surgical face lifting. South Med J 56:412, 1963
15. Orentreich N, New York, NY. Personal communication, 1978.
16. Yarborough JM: Complications of dermabrasion. Dermabrasion–Chemical Peel Seminar, Chicago, Ill, May 19, 1983
17. Stolar R: Abrasive planning with high-speed cutting tools (30,000 to 85,000 rpm). Dermatol Clin 2:285–291, 1984
18. Hanke CW, Pinski JB, Roenigk HH Jr, Alt TH: Caution—new skin refrigerants (letter). J Dermatol Surg Oncol 10:167, 1983
19. Hanke CW, O'Brien JJ, Salow EB: Laboratory evaluation of skin refrigerants in dermabrasion. J Dermatol Surg Oncol 11:45–49, 1985

24

Dermabrasion for Therapeutic Purposes

The cosmetic use of dermabrasion has been a controversial subject since its introduction in the mid-1950s. On the other hand, the procedure has been successfully used for the removal and control of actinic keratoses and other hyperkeratotic precancerous lesions. In addition to eliminating these conditions, it has been proven to have marked prophylactic effects against the development of new keratoses or other similar lesions. This type of surgery has been recommended for many other hyperkeratoses and/or precancerous lesions, but the main use is still for actinically damaged skin. The techniques vary in some instances from the cosmetic application of this modality, which is discussed below.

REGIONAL PLANNING

If most of the face is involved, the area can be planed using the cryoanesthetic techniques discussed in the previous chapter. It is possible to dermabrade practically every portion of the body, but the methodology must be altered according to the anatomic features of the region to be treated. Therefore, the use of dermabrasion for therapeutic purposes must be modified not only for the condition being treated but for the location to be planed. In this section, the latter factor will be discussed. These areas are the ones most often treated by planing for therapeutic reasons.

The Ears

The ears commonly suffer from solar damage resulting in atrophy of the skin, keratoses, and epitheliomas. These alterations occur most commonly on the rims of the ears. The entire cutaneous covering of the edges of the ears, especially the superior portion, can be removed easily under locally injected anesthesia such as procaine or lidocaine. This balloons the skin out a little, lifting it off the underlying cartilge. One must be careful not to plane too deeply, or the cartilage will be damaged. However, the subcutaneous injection of the local anesthetic adds to the protection against this hazard.

344

Lips

Planing of the lower lip may be indicated by the presence of keratoses and/or leukoplakia. Here, too, locally injected anesthetics are preferred to freezing. The cutaneous surface of the lip may be wiped off easily and rapidly by a whirling brush. This is a much simpler and quicker procedure than a lip shave. Healing is just as rapid as when this procedure is performed on other portions of the face. The bleeding stops spontaneously in a short time and then forms a crust. The cosmetic and therapeutic results of the surgery are excellent in this location. Healing is complete, and the crusts are shed spontaneously in about 10 days, as a rule.

Dorsa of Hands

Despite the thinness of the skin of this area in the geriatric patient plus the obvious superficial location of juicy blood vessels, nerves, and tendons, one can perform dermabrasion in this often-involved area safely with excellent results. Of course, the secret to success is found in the elevation of the skin from the important underlying structures by the subcutaneous injection of the local anesthetic. The therapeutic results, both curative and prophylactic, are successful and safe if performed expertly and carefully. Scarring with all these procedures is unusual since the operator does not carry the planing deep enough for this to occur. Lesions on the forearms can be eliminated by dermabrasion, but recurrences are frequent.

Planing can be performed with care in any portion of the body, even the genitalia. The actual techniqe varies somewhat depending on the cosmetic use. The anesthesia is more likely to be by subcutaneous injection rather than refrigerants. The area treated is smaller than a full-face planing, in most instances. Most surgeons use a smaller planer, such as the Dremel Tool, rather than the ordinary dermabrader used on a larger area, such as the entire face. This and other equipment is described in the next section.

In all of these locations, bloody oozing is succeeded by crusting, which is shed in 10 to 14 days leaving an erythematous surface that eventually returns to its normal color. As a rule, the skin is smoother than before the planing. Pigmentary changes, especially depigmentation, may result from this treatment (especially in the elderly).

EQUIPMENT

The only equipment needed to perform this procedure is a syringe and needle (25- or 30-gauge), a local anesthetic, and a planer. For most therapeutic uses, the Dremel Tool is adequate for this purpose but not if a full-face planing is contemplated. It is neither fast enough nor powerful enough for such an undertaking. A diamond fraise must be used with this equipment, since the lack of strength makes the application of a steel wire brush too slow to produce a satisfactory result. However, this set-up is excellent for spot planing or the removal of the skin from a limited area, such as the dorsum of a hand. It is lighter and allows for more accurate and more easily controlled limited dermabrasion. The Landau Instrument Company of North Hollywood, California, manufactures a more powerful, faster rotating instrument of this type, but it is much more expensive than the Dremel Tool.

The Dremel Tool was manufactured originally for use by hobbyists, but it can be converted easily to a planer. It can be purchased at nearly any hardware or hobby store. All of the equipment described herein can be purchased for a total outlay of about one hundred dollars.

A small adapter allows one to attach a diamond fraise to the tool. Since its use as a planer has gained acceptance, the manufacturers have modified the appearance to minimize the home-hobbyist look. It now sits on a base with the handle attached to the body of the equipment with a cable. It rotates about 25,000 rpm, an adequate speed for this purpose. A rectangular box contains the rheostat to control the speed of revolutions, and the tool can be plugged simply into this rheostat. A foot switch can also be used, and the speed can be altered by increasing or decreasing the pressure on this switch. The rheostat is preferable to the foot switch, since the speed can be accurately set before starting the procedure, thereby avoiding the vagaries of the torque produced by inconstant pedal pressure.

The actual surgical procedure does not vary greatly from that described for the full-sized planers. The difference resides basically in its application. As a rule, a local anesthetic is injected into and under the skin. The pathologic changes are wiped off by the diamond fraise. This allows for better control than the larger, more rapidly rotating brushes. If the skin of the entire area is eliminated, the prophylactic effect is enhanced, especially in the case of skin that has been damaged by external carcinogens, such as solar irradiation or x-radiation.

THERAPEUTIC APPLICATIONS

Actinic Skin

The most important and successful use of dermabrasion is in the treatment of actinically damaged skin including actinic keratoses and epitheliomas. Conversely, if one is interested in preventing recurrences of these changes, dermabrasion is the most successful treatment. Admittedly, the local application of 5-fluorouracil creams and lotions is an easier, less traumatic method of eliminating keratoses. On the other hand, it requires weeks of daily treatments, causes burns, and does not prevent the recurrences of further keratoses and epitheliomas.

By using dermabrasion, large areas of damaged skin can be removed quickly and comparatively painlessly, although healing does require 10 to 14 days to complete. Since the regeneration of new skin develops basically from the subsurface adnexa and since this new skin is of the same age and plagued by the same genetic weaknesses as the original cutaneous covering, these cells have not been damaged to the same degree by noxious radiation (solar or ionizing). Therefore, this skin does not exhibit as great a tendency to undergo premalignant or malignant degeneration. Therefore, if the patient uses common sense in avoiding these radiations by employing potent sunscreens (with a rating of 15 or more) and clothing (including caps with visors), recurrences are rare. Actually, the author has seen only one patient develop an epithelioma after such therapy. This was an ex-rodeo rider with an extensive malignant solar degeneration of the facial skin.

Furthermore, following full-face planing, the skin of geriatric patients shows mild erythema and edema and loss of the pigmentary changes of advanced age. The wrinkles are also minimized so the patient looks younger. Following this procedure, the skin looks younger in histopathologic sections also.

What can be accomplished in the aging skin by this procedure? The aims of this therapy must be considered both from the standpoint of cure and of prophylaxis. Planing will remove keratoses as simply and rapidly as any method at the surgeon's disposal. On the other hand, while it may be as effective as other approaches, it offers no significant advantage except that of speed in the treatment of multiple lesions. For instance, Zimmerman has stated that he removed 60 large seborrheic keratoses from the back of a patient by planing without anesthesia in three minutes! If one planes an epithelioma, the cancerous tissue is quickly reamed out by the planer. It requires much more pressure to plane normal skin than malignant alterations. The planing brush acts as an electric-driven curette. While dermabrasion does not spread cancer cells and even cures many epitheliomas, there are better methods for the treatment of skin cancers including electrosurgery, radiotherapy, Mohs' chemosurgery, cryosurgery, and scalpel excision.

From this, it can be readily seen that planing is not a great advancement in the treatment of premalignant and malignant alterations in the skin. Rather, its value resides in preventing the further development of keratoses and epitheliomas. It is well established that the patient who develops an actinic keratosis or an epithelioma is apt to manifest more of these lesions at a later date. This is due to the fact that the appearance of the first neoplasm indicates that the exposed areas of the skin have been damaged sufficiently by the passage of time and the relentless sun exposure to undergo malignant degeneration. Eradication of the new growths by surgical, chemical, or radiologic methods cures the lesion; it does not prevent the growth of other tumors in other portions of the exposed skin.

On the other hand, removal of the entire injured area of the skin, say, by excising the cutaneous covering of the back of the hand and replacing it by undamaged skin, such as a graft taken from the abdomen, would give the patient a new start. True, the graft would contain skin of the same age and hereditary faults that are inherent in the skin that was discarded. However—and this is crucial in understanding this procedure—the epidermis from the abdomen has *not* been damaged by 50 or 60 years of sun exposure. If the patient exposes the grafted skin to excessive sunshine, he could expect new keratoses and epitheliomas in the graft. Furthermore, because of the age of the skin, it would not take as much sunshine to cause a recurrence as it did originally. However, if the patient uses good judgment about solar exposure, recurrences would not be anticipated. Therefore, a potential dermatologic "cripple" would be given a second chance to lead a normal life without the constant threat of malignancy and the need for destructive therapy.

Unfortunately, such a procedure is a major one, necessitating hospitalization and loss of time from work. Furthermore, there is the possibility of such complications as infection and failure to obtain a take. Also, graft skin does not have the same appearance as normal epidermis. The cost of such an operation is not inconsiderable. Therefore, if the same effect could be obtained by a simple and safe office procedure, such as dermabrasion, certain advantages would be offered. In 1954, an attempt was made to study this possibility in three representative patients—one with a chronic radiodermatitis of the hand, one with multiple recurrent actinic keratoses and epitheliomas, and one with recurring cigarette-induced keratoses and epitheliomas of the lip. Two of these patients are still under observation seven years later; the other was followed for more than two years. All obtained marked benefit. The woman with the x-radiation damage has had several kera-

toses but considerably fewer occurrences than before the operation. The man with the actinic-damaged skin had no tumors in the planed areas during the more than two years that he was followed, but many such keratoses developed in the nonplaned areas. The man with the lip alterations suffered a leukoplakia three years after planing, but this responded rapidly and apparently permanently to x-ray therapy. Therefore, one could say that the procedure was successful in these patients.

Perhaps the term "successful" requires a little consideration in itself. If one expects 100% preventive results in every case, then successful is not the proper word to use. But then, this would mean that there were no successful procedures in medicine. All of these cases that the author has treated in this manner have obtained benefit—an absence or decrease in neoplastic changes in the planed skin despite the fact that one would have expected an acceleration in the degenerative process with advancing age. Furthermore, the unplaned skin acts as a control, since the changes continue in these areas while the abraded surfaces remain comparatively free of these complications.

Burks[1] went one step further. In an ingenious experiment, he planed only one side of the face in a series of patients with actinically damaged skin. He was able to demonstrate clearly and convincingly the cosmetic and therapeutic improvement on the treated side.

Chronic Radiodermatitis

This condition is more than a cosmetic defect. It should be treated as a threat to life and limb. Results in this condition should not be judged by the same standards applied to the treatment of an acne scar. The perfect restoration of normal-appearing skin is not the prime purpose of this therapy. The eradication of the tendency toward malignant degeneration is the aim of treatment. Radiation that produces a chronic burn, even so-called superficial therapy, penetrates sufficiently deep to injure the underlying adnexa, thereby delaying healing and increasing scarring. The depth of the process necessitates deeper planing, which increases the undesirable, but essential, features mentioned before. However, as a rule, the deeper epithelium is damaged less than the superficial layers. Regardless of whether the new epithelium regenerates from the remaining hair follicles, sweat glands or other structures or from the surrounding unirradiated epithelium, thereby producing scarring, the tendency of developing cancer and keratoses should be decreased. Such has been the author's experience.

The time required for healing is of no great importance. After all, the difference between 10 and 30 days is very little when one considers the improved prognosis. Surgical excision and skin grafting are the only other possible treatments in extensive cases of chronic radiodermatitis. The morbidity and cost are much greater with such procedures than with planing. Dermabrasion makes hospitalization unnecessary. It is wise to remember also that grafted skin does not resemble normal skin.

Leukoplakia

Leukoplakia on the lips can be planed successfully. Personal experience has confirmed this in many cases. Recurrences are uncommon if the procedure is carried to a sufficient depth. However, the postoperative use of a sunstick and the avoidance of smoking are recommended.

Xeroderma Pigmentosum

This disorder is basically due to a genetic weakness in the epithelium that is manifested by exposure to sunshine. When one considers that the surface epithelium and that of the deeper adnexa have a common embryologic origin, it is not surprising that the keratoses and epitheliomas recur quickly when planed skin is exposed to actinic radiation. Basically, the changes are due to intrinsic factors. Extrinsic factors are more important in such conditions as farmer's skin, or sailor's skin, although admittedly such contributing features as red hair, blue eyes, or fair skin play a role. One patient who had his face planed six years earlier developed some keratoses but no epitheliomas in the abraded areas.

Epitheliomas

Planing is a reasonably effective treatment for superficial basal cell epitheliomas. Apparently, it is more beneficial in squamous cell than in nodular cystic or ulcerated basal cell cancers. This is difficult to understand unless it is due to strands of basal cells being intermixed in the normal tissue and thereby protected from the brush. However, there is no question that a planing brush is more effective than a manual curette. When the whirling brush is applied to a cancerous mass, the brush seems to fall into the crater and cleanly reams out the neoplastic tissue. Although some claim that there is greater sensitivity of feel when the curette is used by hand, this is only true of gross masses only. The feel is not important in planing carcinomas since the removal is automatic.

The treatment of epitheliomas by planing is certainly not the treatment of choice. However, it should be stressed that it can be used safely in epitheliomas of the skin. Perhaps planing plus radiation will eventually give the best cosmetic results and the highest percentage of cures in superficial neoplasms. It will never replace x-radiation, mutilating surgery, or chemosurgery for far-advanced growths. Use of the planer might be an improvement over the curette in the modified Mohs' technique of chemotherapy suggested by Allington[2] and his co-workers. Possibly the most important finding is that planing does not spread skin cancers. Therefore, dermabrasion can be performed in the presence of epitheliomas.

REFERENCES

1. Burks JW, Marascalco J, Clark WH Jr: Half-face planing of precancerous skin after five years. Arch Dermat 88:572, 1963
2. Allington RR quoted in Mohs FE: Chemosurgery: Microcontrolled surgery for skin cancer, in Epstein E, Epstein E Jr (eds): Skin Surgery. Springfield, Ill, Charles C Thomas, 1982, p 628

25

LEON GOLDMAN, M.D.

Laser Skin Surgery

HISTORY

In 1985, the laser was 25 years old and laser skin surgery was 24 years old. There has been remarkable progress from the author's basement laser laboratory at the University of Cincinnati Hospital in 1961 to the elaborate laser operating rooms today. Laser dermatology has also gained in popularity and is now one of the four major segments of the laser market.

THE INSTRUMENTATION

Many more instruments are available for laser dermatologic surgery today, such as those for photoexcision, photocoagulation necrosis, and even complete photolysis of tissue. The laser reactions in tissue continue to be thermal coagulation necrosis and, for some of the new laser systems, photochemical reactions. The stalwart of laser surgical instruments in the past few years are the argon, the CO_2, and the neodymium-yttrium-aluminum-garnet (NdYAG) types. These lasers are becoming more flexible and smaller with more reliable outputs, but they are still expensive.[1, 2, 3] Argon flexibility is available in a low-output, air-cooled apparatus. The portable CO_2 battery-powered laser fits into a small suitcase, weighs about 12 kg, and has outputs (at times) of 8 watts. Waveguide RF CO_2 units are more popular and are moved easily from room to room. A superpulsed CO_2 laser permits more precise tissue destruction and is being introduced to dermatologic surgery. Surgical treatments using the NdYAG dermatologic laser began in the author's laboratory 13 years ago[1] and are now used mostly in other types of surgery. It was recently introduced into clinical dermatologic surgery especially by David,[2] and Landthaler,[3] and their colleagues.

Important new laser systems are being used in clinical investigative studies. These include 577 nm short-pulsed NdYAG lasers, the 1320 nm instead of the 1060 nm model. One half of the NdYAG laser, using so-called second harmonics (532 nm) is also used. Because of the present popularity of the NdYAG laser, current research has started with third harmonics (around 350 nm) and even fourth harmonics (with high enough outputs?) into the ultraviolet range (265 nm), a type of so-called "safe" excimer. In Europe, dermatologic surgeons use the Nath infrared coagulator as a control for CO_2 treatments (Fig. 25–1).

Other instruments are the currently investigational heavy metal vapor lasers, i.e., the copper vapor laser (CVL) especially for port-wine marks and vascular lesions, and the 628 nm goldhead vapor laser for the photodynamic therapy (PDT) program, which uses dihematoporphyrin ether (DHE) for cancer detection and treatment. These lasers are also being used for some controlled studies on the suppression of granulation tissue and for atherolysis.

Animal skin excisions have started with the excimer lasers, the so-called vacuum ultraviolet lasers, 193 nm, 248 nm, and chiefly 303 nm.[4] The 193 nm unit has been used for studies on epilation and the 248 nm unit for excisions. The safety aspects of the excimer lasers are of considerable importance; there are many concerns about possible leakage of hydrochloric acid and fluorine as well as mutagenesis with some of these ultraviolet lasers. They are the first laser systems with a carcinogenic potential in 24 years. None of the laser systems so far used are carcinogenic.

Incidentally, ultraviolet lasers are also of great interest because of the very superficial tissue reactions and the precise tissue excisions with the short pulses. The initial medical applications are in ophthalmology for radial keratotomy, corneal transplants, and astigmatism. Other current studies are in the ablation of atheromata in rabbits and pigs without perforation of the vessel walls. With the current work on animal skin, excimer lasers will have definite applications in clinical dermatology. Fortunately for dermatology, basic photobiologic studies with the excimer lasers are being done by Parrish.[4]

Fiberoptics are used to transmit lasers and to make laser surgery much more flexible so that many more applications can be developed. Such devices include hollow wave-guides now available for CO_2 lasers, and fiberoptics of varied compositions, including silver halide types, that can transmit beams from argon, NdYAG, and CO_2, lasers. Exposure to ultraviolet wavelengths causes deterioration. Considerable improvement is needed to develop significant transmission of CO_2 lasers. Nath has indicated that, with a special non-ionic liquid wave-guide, many current laser systems, including excimers, can be transmitted. Of course, there is less need of fiberoptics in laser dermatologic surgery. Both for

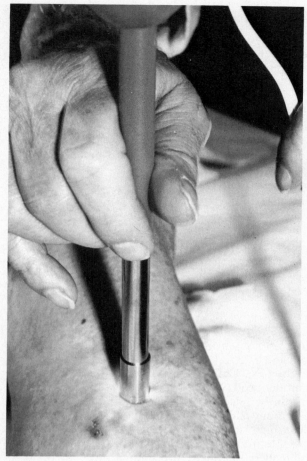

Figure 25–1. The Nath infrared lamp coagulator, used as a control for CO_2 laser treatments, has an air-cooled infrared lamp, a quartz rod, and a Teflon or sapphire tip.

actual need and easy availability, the skin will continue to be an excellent test area for the development of new laser systems.

Laser microsurgery will continue, not only for studies in photobiology, but also for clinical applications, such as the recognition and treatment of new tiny warts and residual bits of tattoo debris and the early recognition of skin malignancies.

Laser Safety

The skin is secondary to the eye in the laser safety program. The basic text about laser safety has been developed by the American National Standards Institute (ANSI). The Z136.3 Subcommitee on Safe Use of the Laser in Medical Institutions has a specific section in their guidelines on dermatology. With new powerful high-output laser systems, short-pulsed duration of laser impacts is possible in terms of nanoseconds 10^{-9}, picoseconds 10^{-12}, and now even femtoseconds 10^{-15}. Recent experiments in rabbit eyes have used 65 femtoseconds; the skin will

be the test area for the dynamics of these lasers in human tissues.

APPLICATIONS

Laser dermatologic surgery continues to be obligatory, preferred, or not to be used at all. The old sign still hanging in the author's laser laboratory reads, "If you don't need the laser, do not use it."

Obligatory laser surgery continues to be used for incurable port-wine marks, many tattoos, and many vascular lesions as well as the current photodynamic therapy (PDT) for inoperable tumors. The preferred list includes warts, especially extensive condylomata acuminata, adenoma sebaceum, actinic cheilitis, leukoplakia, and oral tumors. The laser is not needed and should not be used when there are current conventional techniques that are effective. This is confirmed by the data of the experiences of leading dermatologic surgeons, especially for nonvascular lesions. These dermatologic surgeons should have more experience with vascular lesions. A good laser dermatologic surgeon is, first, a good dermatologic surgeon and, second, someone who is trained and continues to learn about laser surgery. One of the current bits of laser philosophy is, "There are no good and bad laser systems, only good and bad laser surgeons."[5] Remember, laser surgery is precise, even into microsurgery (including microsurgery on chromosomes), and there is less bleeding with all laser systems.

Lasers will create new applications for dermatologic surgery. For good dermatologic surgery, there must be good controls. In addition to the usual physical modalities in dermatology as controls, one must consider the "hot scalpel," the microwave scalpel, and (for NdYAG laser control) the incoherent infrared coagulator. The new portable (battery-powered) CO_2 laser by Design Energy can be carried in a suitcase to nursing homes and private homes, but it must still be controlled with the high-frequency electrosurgical unit.

Port-Wine Marks

The port-wine mark is best treated with the short-pulsed 577 nm laser (Fig. 25–2). This is usually done with the flash-pumped dye laser. Next is the argon laser through the Dermascan[6] with its short pulse. This is the result of detailed and controlled studies of the Department of Dermatology at Harvard. Dark-colored port-wine marks of children can be similarly treated.

For a thick port-wine mark or a combined port-wine mark and persistent cavernous hemangioma, the CO_2 laser and the NdYAG laser may be used alone or in combination with the argon laser (Fig.

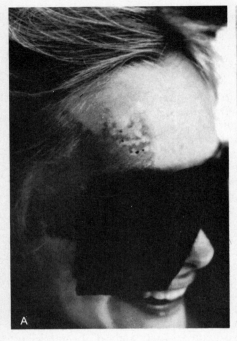
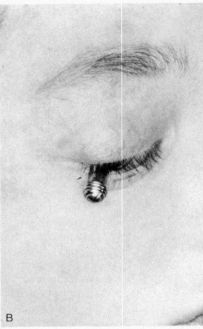

Figure 25–2. *A*, Patient with port wine mark. *B*, Appearance two years later before last treatment with the argon laser; polished steel shield in eye permits safe laser surgery directly to the eyelid.

25–3). Granuloma pyogenicum or, perhaps more properly, granuloma telangiectaticum that appears spontaneously or after any therapy (including argon laser therapy) is treated with the CO_2 or NdYAG laser with excellent results. Scarring, much less with the new laser systems, continues to develop about the nose, upper lip, and chin. Nevertheless, CO_2 lasers have successfully treated rhinophyma (Fig. 25–4).

In the author's experience, injections of corticosteroid suspension plus continued pressure (usually with a plastic prosthesis) is truly an important accessory for laser dermatologic surgery. Because of the short duration of the laser impact, chilling limits the thermal coagulation necrosis to precise areas. The author found the chemical chilling pack and an ice water plastic flowmeter, developed in his laboratory especially for argon laser therapy, superior to the ice pack or surface irrigation with ice water (Fig. 25–5).

Test areas, usually on the side of the face or forehead are done under local anesthesia. Plans for extensive treatments are made only after two to three months of observation. Extensive laser treatments of port-wine marks or of extensive vascular lesions are done by peripheral nerve blocks by those familiar with these techniques or by "come-and-go" anesthesia in the ambulatory surgical center.[7] These centers are an economic place for ambulatory laser surgery performed by multiple disciplinary experts.

Telangiectasia

The laser treatment of peripheral telangiectasia is another important application (Fig. 25–6). The ar-

gon laser is an important accessory and at 1 or 2 mm and 0.25 to 1.0 watt is effective for telangiectasia of the face. Chilling, if it does not redden the face, can be used without local anaesthesia. There is currently a lack of detailed data about the micropathology and vascular dynamics of the cosmetically disturbing superficial telangiectasia of the thigh and lower extremity, especially in women. Definitely controlled treatment procedures must be done to study this further. The test area should be a relatively large spot with multiple vessels of similar caliber (Fig. 25–7). For adjacent sclerotherapy, 20% saline is used. The second control, which the author has used for years, is intravascular galvanic current with a special 30-gauge needle 0.8 milliampere for one second (Fig. 25–8). The third adjacent, also used on the chilled skin, is a miniature intravascular argon probe 0.75 to 1.0 watt, at intervals along the vessel for 0.75 to 1.0 second. Protective glasses are required since there is bright transillumination through the skin. Perilesional, local anesthesia is used. An extravascular argon miniprobe treatment may also be used with thrombogenesis for a good cosmetic result without superficial epidermal damage. Postoperative chilling is done for 24 hours, and daily pressure bandages are continued for two and one-half to three weeks.

Warts

For laser treatment of periungual and subungual warts, nailplate removal is necessary. With digital block and a rubber-band tourniquet around the finger, the nail is removed with a nail elevator, a periosteal elevator, or even a mosquito hemostat

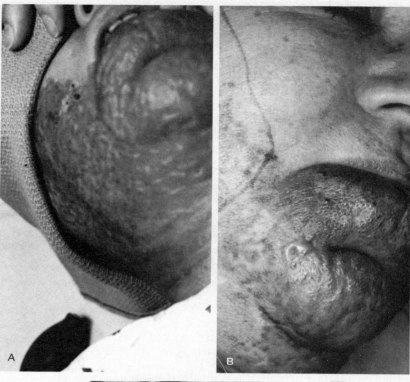

Figure 25–3. *A,* Large mixed port wine mark and cavernous hemangioma of the face and lip (test area is on right cheek). *B,* Same patient after repeated argon laser surgery with "come and go" general anesthesia. *C,* Appearance after bloodless CO_2 laser surgery and graft replacement to the lower lip. (Courtesy of Richard O. Gregory, M.D.)

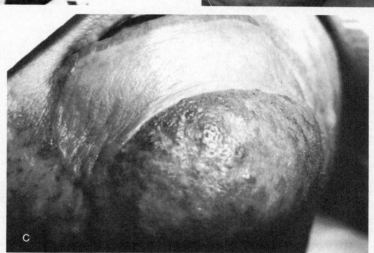

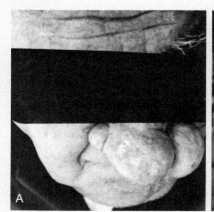

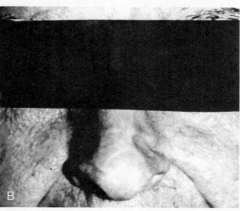

Figure 25–4. Patient with rhinophyma before CO_2 laser surgery (*A*) and postoperative appearance (*B*).

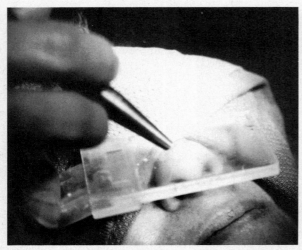

Figure 25–5. Argon laser treatment for a spider angioma on the tip of the nose given through a plastic chilling chamber with circulating ice water. Chilling localizes the treatment by reducing heat radiation and heat dispersion from the laser-treated spot.

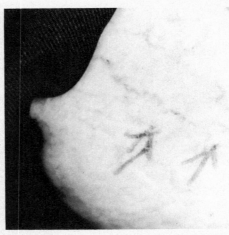

Figure 25–7. Mini-intravascular argon laser test area in the thigh of an elderly man (local anesthesia was used).

spread under the nail. Curettement is used beyond the edge of the wart area. Then, a 5-watt CO_2 laser at 1 or 2.0 mm is used to cover the entire area and 2 to 3 mm beyond with 2.5 watts. The tourniquet is removed. Telfa gauze with polymyxin B-bacitracin (Polysporin) is applied and a tubular gauze bandage applied after curettement. Minimal CO_2 and even less about the periphery all make for a good cosmetic result.

The early lesions of condylomata acuminata in both men and women are not only diagnosed under the skin microscope[8] or colposcope, but the condition is also followed by skin microscopy. Individual lesions may recur after adequate use of the CO_2 laser, but there is definitely less bleeding than with high-frequency electrosurgery. However, the real advantage is that new small infectious lesions can

be recognized early. The skin microscope also rules out folds, small hemorrhoids, polyps, milium cysts, and squamous acanthomas (seborrheic warts), which are often mistaken for condylomata acuminata. With the skin microscope, it is not necessary to use acetic acid to exaggerate the white swelling of small flat warts.

For extensive lesions, general anesthesia is preferred to caudal anesthesia. The patient is put in the lithotomy position. The area is cleansed but not shaved. The operating microscope is used. Large fungating lesions may be débrided, pressure hemostatic appliances (plastic, sterile paper clips attached to tongue blades) provide a dry base for the defocused CO_2 laser. Ebonized anoscopes help to check the anus for spread of lesions. If necessary, consultation with a proctologist and sigmoidoscopy may be necessary. In patients suspected of practicing oral

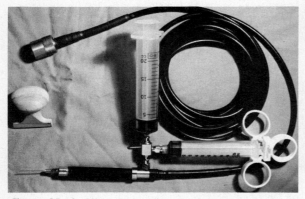

Figure 25–6. Mini-intravascular argon laser probe for the treatment of telangiectasia of the lower extremity. Coupler attaches to argon laser output on the console; saline purge clears fiber optics tube and needle of blood; external pressure knob limits thrombogenesis. (Patent No. 4,564,011)

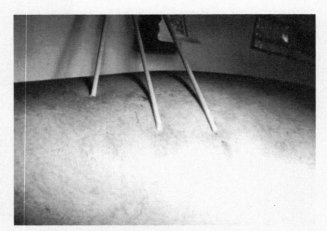

Figure 25–8. Results of simultaneous intravascular tests of superficial telangiectasia of the leg after one month. Upper pointer, sclerotherapy with 20% saline solution; middle pointer, galvanic electrosurgery with 0.8 ma for 1 second; lower pointer, argon miniprobe intravascular laser, 1 watt with a 5 W/cm^2 irradiance for 2 seconds.

sex, the oral cavity should be checked for condylomata acuminata. The condition may also spread to fingers and toes. Sexual contacts of the patient with condylomata acuminata must be checked with the skin microscope or the colposcope.[8] Postoperative therapy includes warm soapy soaks in the tub, topical nystatin (Mycostatin), and frequent observations using the skin microscope. Added immunobiologic interferon or interferon-inducers may help to prevent new lesions.

Adequate ventilation in the operating room is necessary for avoidance of air pollution. Iodine prep solutions are not used because of the irritant fumes. An effective plume evacuator is used close to the operating field. A loose gauze mesh over the vacuum aspirator prevents light objects such as gauze bandages from being sucked into the appliance. Operating room personnel should be assured that there is no hazard of developing oral condylomata acuminata, or even AIDS, from plume fragments.

For extensive warts about the fingers and toes,

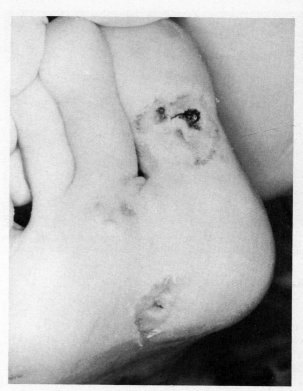

Figure 25–10. Extensive CO_2 laser surgery under Bier-Block anesthesia for warts of the ankle, toes, and plantar area; note the hemostasis after completion of the treatment.

Bier-Block anesthesia (Figs. 25–9 and 25–10) is used for lesions on the arms and legs and posterior tibial block for plantar lesions. Postoperatively, 20% to 40% aqueous solutions of urea are used. For broad extensive mosaic lesions, the first treatment is individual deep 10-watt CO_2 with débridement with 5 watt peripheral ring. A spotting technique is used rather than removing the entire plantar area. The patient is examined at two-week intervals to detect early recurrences.

For a huge recurrent cauliflower wart of the entire heel a plastic surgeon, Richard O. Gregory,[9] excised the entire area with a 10-watt CO_2 laser and applied a full-thickness graft. Complete healing followed.

Porokeratosis lesions, which are often mistaken for a miliary wart on the fingers, toes, and plantar areas may be treated effectively with the CO_2 laser and deep curettement down to the venous hamartomatous base.

Nails

Onychomycosis treated by a CO_2 laser does help if combined with griseofulvin (Fulvicin) therapy (Fig. 25–11). Using the CO_2 laser for matrixectomy should be avoided unless one desires a permanent matrixectomy.

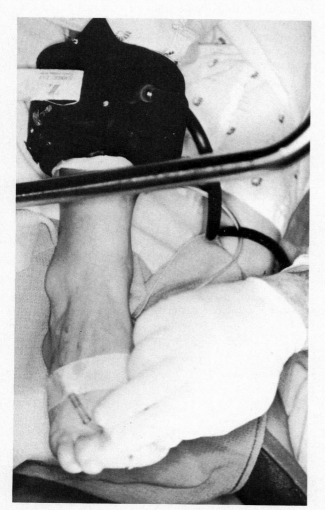

Figure 25–9. Bier-Block exsanguinating local anesthesia is especially helpful for laser surgery of an extremity.

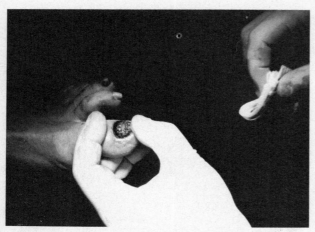

Figure 25–11. CO_2 laser treatment of onychomycosis of the big toe; when indicated, laser matrixectomy may also be done.

Tattoos

The laser treatment of tattoos is complicated by hypertrophic scarring, especially with the CO_2 laser on the forearm, sometimes as much as 10% (Fig. 25–12). The argon laser helps red marks; the NdYAG, black or blue; the ruby, red and blue; the CO_2, all colors. The author's studies with the Q switched ruby laser showed excellent small spots.[10] Current studies in Scotland[11] with the Q switched ruby laser also show good results on black and blue marks. The apparatus is still cumbersome, not flexible, and expensive.

Keloids

Except for keloidal nodules of the ear, laser treatment of keloids is still confusing.[12] Argon (excision and spotted), CO_2 excision, and NdYAG lasers have all been recommended. Detailed prolonged studies such as Bailin's[13] also help to solve the problem. Here, too, postoperative pressure prosthesis and intralesional injections of suspended corticosteroids are used.

EDUCATION

Learning laser dermatologic surgery cannot be done only with kodachromes or colorful video cassettes or tolerant pig's feet. The background in laser biophysics and photobiology must be acquired. Then, hands-on surgery, under instruction, must be done at a minimum with CO_2 and argon lasers on

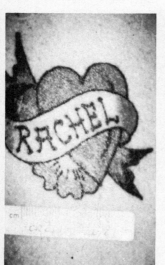

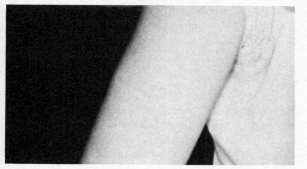

Figure 25–12. The cycle of effective argon laser surgery for an extensive tattoo of the arm. (Courtesy of Adriana Scheibner, M.D.)

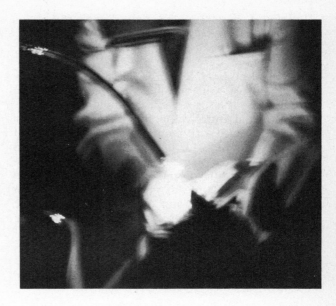

Figure 25–13. Laser-induced photodynamic therapy (PDT) for both cancer diagnosis and treatment. A hematoporphyrin derivative (DHE) is given intravenously and localizes in cancerous tissue. Three days later, 628 nm argon pumped dye laser or gold head vapor laser is used to expose the area with localized microvascular distribution and cellular cytotoxic reaction in the cancer. Picture shows laser beam transmission through a fiber optics tube to the cancer area. Often in dermatologic oncology, DHE may be either applied topically in mucous membrane lesions or in superficial lesions or injected locally into the tumor.

completely anaesthetized animals (pigs for incisions and flaps; rabbits for tattooing and veins). Certificates must be given for this introduction.

At present, the minimal requirements for preceptee training at the operating table, under supervision for treatment of patients should be four hours each with the CO_2, argon, and NdYAG lasers. As already indicated, the ambulatory surgical center has economic advantages for both patients and surgeons, with multiple disciplinary specialists using a variety of lasers and both nerve block and "come-and-go" anesthesia. Office practice can provide initial treatments for minor lesions.

THE FUTURE

The future for laser dermatologic surgery is great. The market will continue to be good. By 1987 or before, photodynamic therapy (PDT) with laser-induced fluorescence using dihematoporphyrin ether (DHE) and the goldhead vapor and the argon pumped dye lasers will be used for cancer diagnosis, including soft tissue metastatic lesions. All of these techniques will be used in clinical practice (Figs. 25–13 and 25–14). For dermatologic laser surgery, local implantation with DHE in Azone and other vehicles will be of value.[14, 15] For mucosal lesions, topical

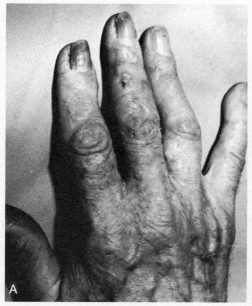
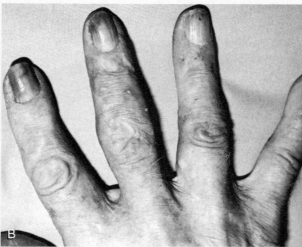

Figure 25–14. *A,* Physician's hand with x-ray dermatitis showing basal and squamous cell carcinomas and keratoses. *B,* Appearance two months later after laser-induced PDT.

applications of DHE with Azone and alcohol, as done by Berns, are possible. Research will continue, such as Oseroff's[16] on multiple exogenous chromophores.

Superpulsed laser systems, as established by adequate controls, will become available as dynamic experiments in laser surgery continue. The dermatologist of the future will use a comprehensive laser operating room with multiple laser systems and computer programs for information handling. With the continued development of nonsurgical applications of lasers, the dermatologist will have more detailed diagnostic means, more controlled data on laser wound healing, and more use of adjunctive treatments. In brief, the dermatologist should learn about, practice, and continue to perform well-controlled dermatologic surgery.

REFERENCES

1. Goldman L, Nath G, Schindler G, et al: High-power neodymium-YAG laser surgery. Acta Derm Venereol 53:45–49, 1973
2. David LM, Dwyer RM, Goldman RD: A Comparison of NdYAG and Argon lasers. Laser 85 Opto-Elektronik, July 3, 1985, Munich, Federal Republic of Germany
3. Lanthaler M, Haina D, Brunner R, Waidelich W: NdYAG Therapy of Telangiectasias. Laser 85 Opto-Elektronik, July 3, 1985, Munich, Federal Republic of Germany
4. John Parrish, personal communications
5. Peter Wolf Ascher, personal communications
6. Tang SV, Arndt KA, Gilchrest BA, Itzhasi I, et al.: Clinical Comparison of Millisecond Versus Conventional Argon Laser Treatment of In Vivo Vascular Lesions. Fifth Annual Meeting of the American Society for Laser Medicine and Surgery, May 29, 1985, Orlando, Florida
7. Goldman L: Dermatologic surgery in an ambulatory surgery center: ten years' experience. Cutis 34:65–68, 1984
8. Goldman L: Direct microscopy of the skin in vivo as a diagnostic and research tool. J Dermatol Surg Oncol 6:9, 1980
9. Richard O. Gregory, personal communications
10. Goldman L, Wilson R, Hornsby P: Radiation from a Q switched ruby laser: Effect of repeated impacts of power output of 10 megawatts on a tattoo of Man. J Invest Derm 44:69–71, 1965
11. Vance CA, McLeon PS, Reid WH, Evans JH, et al: Q Switched Ruby Laser Treatment of Tattoos, A Further Study. American Society for Laser Medicine and Surgery, May 29, 1985, Orlando Florida
12. Olbricht SM, Stern RS, Tang SV, Noe JM, et al: Complications of Cutaneous Laser Surgery: A Survey. American Society For Laser Medicine and Surgery, May 29, 1985, Orlando, Florida
13. Phillip Bailin, personal communications
14. Goldman L, Gregory RO, LaPlant M: Preliminary studies with PDT in dermatologic and plastic surgery. Lasers in Surgical Medicine 5:453–456, 1985
15. Goldman L, Gregory RO, LaPlant M, Taylor A, et al: Topical and Local Implantation of Dihemato-porphyrin Ether (DHE) for PDT. Presented at International Society for Laser Medicine and Surgery, Jerusalem, Oct 1985
16. Oseroff AR, personal communications

Zyderm Collagen

Since the last edition of this textbook, the indications and the technique for Zyderm collagen implants have been clarified and improved. Patients can be given an accurate prediction about what conditions respond to Zyderm collagen and about how many months the implant will probably last.

Unfortunately, a better explanation of why the implant retains correction for such a variable amount of time is not yet available. Factors as diverse as the patient's age, the anatomic location, the depth of the placement of the implant, and the mechanical stress across or around the implant all seem to affect the longevity of the correction. Conversely, the allergic granulomatous reaction of acquired immunity has been well studied, and the overall safety of the product, both short-term and long-term, are well established.

In November 1985, the FDA approved the release and distribution of Zyplast collagen, which is a glutaraldehyde cross-linked Zyderm collagen. The author participated in the studies that were submitted to the FDA for their approval. Although the length of experience is not nearly that as with Zyderm, the early indications are that this new product will last 12 to 18 months when placed in the immediate *subdermal* plane. Therefore, it will be used to treat more fibrotic types of lesions and for contour deformities. This material is so robust that it is quite successful in treating corns. A large study in the podiatry field has confirmed its ability to withstand the pressures of walking and has been successful in relieving the pain and clinical findings of hard corns. There are also studies using this application for gingival augmentation and osteogenesis stimulation. Other studies are looking into its use as a filling agent in patent and lax sphincters, such as the cardia of the stomach.

MATERIAL

It is the nonhelical portions of the mammalian collagen molecule that account for antigenicity, because these telopeptides are different among various species. The preparation of Zyderm collagen involves acid pepsin cleavage of these carboxyl and amino terminal ends, leaving the monotonously repetitious and tightly bound triple helix, which is a weak immunogen.[1, 2] Even though the central portion of the helix is not identical from species to species, the amino acid sequences are only slightly different, and probably because the stereochemistry of the molecule is so similar, not much allergic or foreign body reaction ensues. The chemically cross-linked product has even lower antigenicity, supposedly because fewer of these terminal radicals are exposed. The Zyplast is also much firmer and can resist pressures as well as collagenolysis.

Zyderm collagen is prepared from cowhides by purification, sterilization, and de-pyrogenation. The product is at least 95% Type I collagen, and the rest is Type III. This is very similar to the composition of human dermal collagen. Foreign-protein–induced immune reactions, which simulated rheumatoid arthritis in rats have been reported.[3] This study, however, was with the injection of Type II collagen and concluded, "Because of the lack of disease specificity, it is at present impossible to ascribe a definite pathogenic role to collagen autoimmunity in any human disease."

The product is delivered to the physician as a dispersion in buffered physiologic saline with lidocaine and with no preservatives. Some European countries do not have lidocaine in their preparation because its absence allows the implant to be classified as a medical device rather than a drug. Thus, approval through the regulatory agencies was less complex.

The dispersion remains fluid at a refrigerator temperature of 0 to 4°C, but it will congeal when warmed to body temperature. In the dermis, the implant loses the saline and lidocaine and becomes integrated into a dense collaginous mass. With present injection techniques (explained later), available human biopsies indicate that the collagen is usually found in several masses at different layers in the upper dermis.

The implant's identification with human tissue and staining abilities has been described by Ronald Barr and the author.[4] They were able to demonstrate that the implant can be identified in skin biopsies after routine paraffin fixation and hematoxylin and eosin staining. Although the Zyderm implant stains a pink very similar to natural collagen, it is much more amorphous and thus stands out in the section. The Zyderm implant stained with colloidal iron and counterstained with carbofuchsin is more magenta and thus discernible. With van Gieson's elastic stain, no fibrils or particles within the implant are visible, whereas normal dermis has multiple elastic staining fibers. Polarized light differentiates native collagen, which polarizes, from Zyderm collagen, which does not.

The longevity of the implant has been more difficult to study than previously expected. Animal skin and even human back skin are so different from the human facial skin, where collagen is used almost exclusively, that the earlier work was deemed unreliable. The author has recently completed a preliminary study in which Zyderm was injected monthly in the pre- and infra-auricular area of a human face for six months prior to the performance of rhytidectomy (face-lift). Sequential 30-, 60-, 90-, 120-, and 180-day biopsies of the implant in human facial skin were obtained. The implant was observed in skin with a spongy upper reticular and compacted deep reticular dermis as well as some areas which showed sun damage and some in the infra- and postauricular area and no sun damage. The preauricular test site is probably the most representative of the areas where Zyderm is used. Although this study is ongoing, the early (unpublished) results suggest that the implant is present at six months; there is no sign of allergic or foreign body reaction around the implant; there are very few fibroplasts growing through the implant but a few around the periphery; there seems to be little reduction in size of the implant between what is found at 30 days versus 180 days; and the implant placed in actinically versus nonactinically damaged skin shows no differences (Fig. 26–1). The specimens were also stained with colloidal iron in order to search for newly produced collagen products around the implant. Glucose amino glycans stain turquoise, which is easily recognizable on colloidal iron staining. At no time did any of the specimens show signs of excessive or new glucose amino glycans in or around the implant (Fig. 26–1B). This would suggest that Zyderm does not stimulate new native collagen production.

Burke and coworkers published electronphotomicrographs showing the collagen fibers 24 hours after implantation.[5] These fibers were randomly dispersed and formed an irregular matrix in contrast to the native collagen, which is a well-organized matrix and has a characteristic diameter and periodicity. Whether more fibrils are formed at longer times after the implantation or whether these fibrils function as native collagen bundles or as a matrix for the ingrowth of new fibroblasts that lay down new collagen is not now known.

The author's preliminary study differs from the findings of Burke and coworkers in that the implant is present and without signs of deterioration at six months after implantation. Also, if the colloidal iron stains are an accurate measure of the laying down of new collagen, there is no evidence that the implant is being replaced with glucose amino glycans or procollagen products.

Zyderm collagen is currently marketed in two

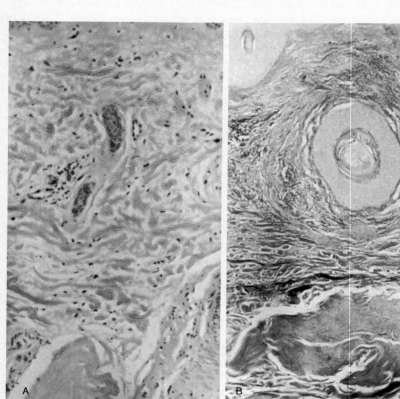

Figure 26–1. *A,* Human facial skin showing Zyderm implantations 180 days after injection. The implants are clearly distinguishable as more amorphous and lighter staining masses in the deep reticular dermis. There is no sign of allergic reaction. A few fibroblasts can be seen surrounding the implant, but they probably have not invaded the implant. *B,* The same specimen 180 days after implantation stained with colloidal iron to illustrate that there are not unusual amounts of new glucoseaminoglycans surrounding the implant. The outline of the implant is clearly distinguishable from that of native collagen.

concentrations. Zyderm I contains approximately 35 mg/ml collagen (by wet volume), and Zyderm II (introduced in 1983) contains approximately 65 mg/ml (by wet volume). Zyplast is like Zyderm II with 65 mg/ml wet volume. The Zyderm I is packaged in 0.5 ml and 1.0 ml syringes and the Zyderm II in 0.4 ml and 0.75 ml tuberculin syringes. The decision to market Zyderm II in a tuberculin syringe was made because all of the defects usually can be treated at one sitting with that volume and because the plunger in a tuberculin syringe becomes unstable when the syringe is filled beyond the 0.75 ml level. The hydraulic factors from the smaller plunger of the tuberculin syringe so greatly improved the facility of the injection techniques that many physicians feel Zyderm II is easier to inject from the tuberculin syringe than Zyderm I, which is about one half the concentration and is injected from a 1.0 ml syringe with a thicker barrel. Zyplast is packaged in a tuberculin syringe with 0.75 ml of material. Karagen is the product for treating corns and is packaged in a 0.5 ml tuberculin syringe.

INDICATIONS FOR CLINICAL USE

It is perplexing when other physicians say that Zyderm doesn't work, because for the author, it is working now better than ever. What makes Zyderm work is the proper selection of lesions, realistic expectations, and proper technique. Physicians must apply their knowledge of the characteristics of the material with their evaluation of the contours of the skin to select which lesions are most likely to benefit. Using Zyderm where one *hopes* it will work or where contour deformities need correction without a full understanding of lesion selection and proper injection techniques will guarantee failure and thus disappointment for both the physician and patient.

Most Zyderm is used to correct the early and specific changes of aging. Contour deformities secondary to disease and traumatic or surgical scarring

are the other two major areas for the use of this implant.[6-10]

GENERAL PRINCIPLES FOR INJECTION TECHNIQUE

For aging changes, the bevel of the needle can be either up or down and should be placed as closely as possible to the area to be injected. It is helpful to bevel the needle about 30 degrees at the hub. This helps to keep the injection very superficial. The needle should enter the skin at approximately a 30-degree angle and advance very slowly until the bevel is just in the high dermis. Sometimes the needle can be seen through the translucent epidermis. At this point, pressure is gradually placed on the plunger to test for where the collagen will flow. If it creates a puff blanch or a blanch of the dermis, placement is correct for most age-related changes. Klein and Rish have recommended a useful technique in which the guiding hand is placed on the skin to stabilize it and the syringe is placed on the thumb and forefinger of that hand.[11] It is then angled 30 degrees or less toward the skin and advanced just into the dermis. Klein then rocks the syringe up on his fingers so that the tip of the needle is lifted (Fig. 26–2A). He feels this assures him of injecting only into the high dermis. Sometimes, if the skin cannot be stabilized well enough with two- or three-point finger tension, the area to be injected can be pinched up between the thumb and index finger, and the needle enters at a very acute angle to the skin (Fig. 26–2B).

It is at this point that the plunger is depressed and the flow of Zyderm is carefully observed. If it should come out through the pilosebaceous opening, the needle is advanced just a little further into the dermis until the Zyderm is seen filling the dermis. If an area is being filled and the plunger suddenly depresses more easily, one should be aware that the Zyderm may be flowing into the subcutaneous

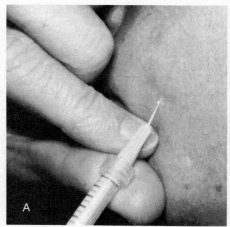
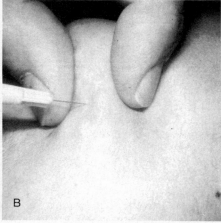

Figure 26–2. *A*, An injection technique showing the support of the syringe on the thumb and index finger, which is also stabilizing the skin. The needle can be rocked over the finger in order to keep the bevel and tip in the highest possible location in the skin. *B*, Another injection technique is to pinch up the skin, which not only stabilizes the injection site but also allows the needle to enter tangentially to the skin surface so that the material is placed only in the upper dermis. The thumb can act as a resting agent and a fulcrum for the syringe.

space. Sometimes several angles or different approaches will have to be used in order to place the Zyderm appropriately.

One does not have to inject very many patients before the fingers become sore from holding the syringe and the hands become tired from the pressure needed to inject the material. The company has helped to alleviate this problem by dispensing a circular disk which fits over the disposable syringe and provides a more comfortable platform for the second and third fingers. A better-designed disk is being readied for manufacturing that will be somewhat cushioned and provide even greater comfort. However, the real secret to prevent hand and finger fatigue is to push the plunger not with the pad of the thumb but rather with the thenar eminence—at the junction of the first metacarpal and proximal phalanx. The natural padding over the thenar eminence plus the increased leverage of the muscles of that area make depressing the plunger much easier and far less fatigue develops. This is an important adjustment in technique if one is ever to be comfortable treating very many patients.

Empirical findings have shown that a correction from Zyderm will last the longest if the implant is placed within the dermis.[6,7] Subcutaneous injections may correct depressed deformities temporarily, but seldom does the correction last longer than a few weeks or even a month. Anatomically, the dermis is a very small and rigid compartment. It is difficult to inject any solution in between the dermal collagen fibers, but this is exactly where it must go. Fluid-filled dermis becomes thickened and brawny and is described clinically as peau d'orange. The size of the compartment of the dermis is the natural limiting factor of how much collagen can be injected. If the dermis is fibrous or loose, it can be swollen above the surface of the skin—an overcorrection of the deformity, which more commonly happens in acne scarring than in aging changes. For depressed scars, overcorrection is encouraged in order to place as much of the implant as possible into the area and thus gain correction sooner. After the normal saline and lidocaine have been resorbed from the implant, as much residual collagen as possible will be left in place. This is the origin of the advice to overcorrect whenever possible. However, for most age-related changes, if Zyderm is placed properly within the dermis only, the injection end point will be when the skin develops the peau d'orange appearance. It is important to notice a white blanching of the skin first before much material is injected. If the skin elevates en masse, one is probably injecting below the dermis, in an area where there will be little implant longevity. The key to proper injection is seeing the skin blanch first then the gradual development of the peau d'orange.

The discovery that Zyderm is successful only if placed in the dermis has greatly increased the efficiency of the implant. In the early period, it was obvious that most physicians were injecting too much material in the subcutaneous plane.

Zyplast must be placed in the immediate subdermal plane. Should it be placed in the dermis, as is Zyderm, the implant will seem quite usual for several weeks but then often beads up and gives an irregular and obvious lump. This lump fades out after three or four more weeks, and the implant has the longevity in the dermis of 12 to 18 months. For this reason, it is felt that Zyplast should always be placed in the subdermal plane where it remains as a single bolus and serves to elevate depressions or contour deformities.

The implant is actually easier to place than Zyderm. It is not difficult to push the needle into the subdermal space. This can usually be detected by feeling less resistance on the needle as it is advanced through the skin. After the needle reaches the subdermal plane, one should use the fingers of the other hand to palpate the area where the implant is being positioned. It is as if the injecting hand is the brawn and the other hand is the brain because those fingers can be used to palpate or pinch or to direct the bolus where it will eventually lie. Once placed in the skin, the Zyplast bolus can be repositioned exactly where desired by pinching and massaging it within the first few minutes after being injected.

There is obviously much less bruising and pain with the placement of Zyplast; however, contrary to what one would expect, more material is required to achieve correction in most indications. It is obviously important to keep the tip of the needle just in the subdermal space so that larger vessels are not encountered.

TECHNIQUE FOR TREATING AGING CHANGES

Analysis of the skin to be injected will help the physician judge how much Zyderm can be placed at each spot. Sometimes wrinkled skin is thin, such as on the medial cheeks of older females and on the eyelids, whereas the nasolabial fold of men or on the glabella region the skin can be quite thick.

Most of the time, creases result from aging changes. The author's technique has changed over the past few years. Originally, he injected into the creases with a multiple puncture technique, advancing the needle up the long axis of the crease. Then he performed what is known as the double layer technique in which some Zyderm was placed at the dermal subcutaneous plane and more Zyderm was placed into the middle or high dermal plane. Seldom is the dermis thick enough to accommodate the two layers, and seldom is the physician able to discern exactly where the dermal subcutaneous plane is without injecting into the subcutaneous area.

Nowadays, it is more common for the author to hold the needle perpendicular to the long axis of the crease. Multiple pinpoint injections are made trying to disperse a little puff of Zyderm at the site of the crease. Most success is obtained when the immediate blanching of the skin is in a small circle around the point of injection. Often, however, the author achieves little globules of the Zyderm high in the dermis in a beaded fashion along the long axis. If entering the skin perpendicular to the long axis is unsuccessful, he reverts to injecting along the long axis with the needle pointed in the same direction. Only rarely does the author inject deeply into the dermis for age-related creases. The benefit of these technique modifications has resulted in corrections lasting 12 to 14 months.

Discrete creases and wrinkles associated with aging and senile elastosis can be divided into five areas that seem particularly well-suited for Zyderm: vertical glabellar lines, creases in the nasolabial and meilolabial areas, the radial creases or wrinkles of the perioral region, the secondary vertical creases of the nasolabial/meilolabial area, and the sleep creases found on the lateral forehead. Other areas respond with less predictability. These include the horizontal forehead creases, the chin, and crow's feet. The only controversy is about how long the correction persists after the dissolution of the lumpy appearance, which is not uncommon in fine skin or over bony prominences.

Most physicians who use Zyderm and those who use both Zyderm and silicone agree that the vertical glabellar lines are the most successful and responsive to Zyderm implants (Fig. 26–3). Surprisingly, little material is required to correct these lines, and frequently only one session is necessary to achieve full correction. The patient is placed in a supine position with the head only slightly elevated. For Zyplast, the same positioning is used, but usually only one treatment corrects the defect. The injection is made either with a multiple puncture technique

along the axis of the crease or with the needle entering perpendicular to the long axis of the crease. In sebaceous skin, the collagen may escape through the pores. Patience and perseverance are the keys when injecting into sebaceous skin. The creases can be outlined by pinching the glabella skin between the thumb and index finger or by asking the patient to knit the brow. At the conclusion of treatment, the folds will not appear when the patient knits the brow. As stated in the previous section, it is best to fill as much collagen as can be placed *within the dermis* of these creases. Usually, the skin is thick enough so that the Zyderm does not show through as a creamy, opaque, intracutaneous mass. However, there are some patients who have thin skin through which the material can be seen. For these patients, makeup may be necessary, or less concentrated Zyderm in smaller doses should be used in subsequent treatments.

Patients are advised that one or two treatment sessions may be necessary, but in the glabella, one session usually lasts six to nine months. In this area, it is important to differentiate between folds and creases. The latter are successfully treated whereas the former are only slightly modified. If the deep folds were in fact corrected, a protuberant mass would result. This is almost impossible to accomplish with Zyderm (another example of its goof-proof nature) and would not be desirable even if it could.

The nasolabila creases also respond well, but they require more material (Fig. 26–4). Usually two treatments are necessary with Zyderm II and sometimes three treatments with Zyderm I. It is important to differentiate between the nasolabial crease and a fold of the cheek overhanging the nasolabial area. The crease can be treated successfully. A mild nasolabial fold can be blunted so that it does not look as deep, but a true overhanging nasolabial fold could not (and should not) be treated with a dermal implant. The treatment for this overhanging fat is a face lift or a combination of a face-lift and liposuc-

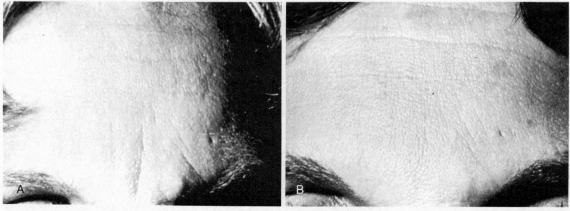

Figure 26–3. *A,* Patient prior to treatment; note the vertical glabellar creases. *B,* The result three months later after a second injection of Zyderm II.

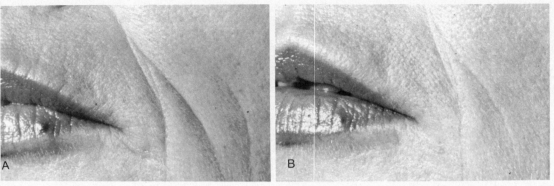

Figure 26–4. *A,* Patient prior to treatment. *B,* The result three months later after two treatments with Zyderm II. Notice the softening of the nasolabial and secondary nasolabial creases.

tion surgery. The deep grooves of the nasolabial area, particularly in the young person, can be significantly improved to soften the "hound-dog" or sad appearance. If a nasolabial area has deep grooves, they should be treated with Zyplast first. If there is a groove and a crease, both products can be used, first placing the Zyplast to obliterate the groove and then the Zyderm to obliterate the crease in the dermis. Some patients require only one or the other.

The grooves at the inferior borders of the oral commissure, commonly called the drool groove, are successfully treated with Zyplast. Zyderm is only partially successful here, but Zyplast will elevate that groove and completely eliminate it.

The fine wrinkles of the upper lip respond well, but the skin of the lip is such that it is difficult to place the collagen exactly into each of these fine wrinkles (Fig. 26–5). It may not be necessary to treat the specific wrinkles but rather treat the general area of the wrinkles, as described for the vertical glabella creases. Again, the needle can be directed along the long axis of the radial crease or perpendicular to it. In practice, usually both techniques

are necessary (Fig. 26–6). The very fine, short wrinkles originating at the vermilion border can be treated by placing collagen in the superficial skin along the border. Sometimes, the collagen will worm its way across this stromal space, and the puffiness at the margin will serve not only to stop the lipstick from running but also to give a more full definition to the lips. Both of these results are salutary.

The perioral region has a multitude of other creases and folds. Sometimes, the skin inferior to the oral commissure has multiple small creases. These respond to Zyderm, and the correction persists about six months. Chernosky has discussed that perlèche secondary to chronic maceration of this area is nicely corrected with Zyderm injections.[13] The radial creases on the lower lip respond, but less satisfactorily than those on the upper lip, and the deep folds on the chin are also treatable in some patients. But in others, there is no response or a short-lasting one. The author knows of no way to predict which wrinkles on the lower lip and the chin area will respond satisfactorily. The patient is usually told that one or two treatments will be tried and followed. If the correction was achieved and is

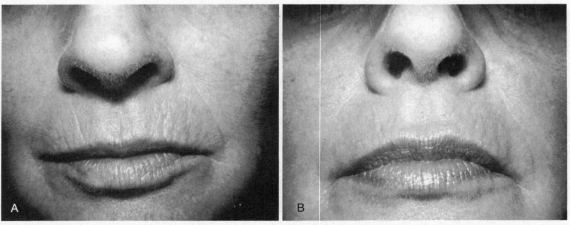

Figure 26–5. *A,* Patient prior to treatment. *B,* The result three months later after one treatment with Zyderm II. The vertical creases of the lip are obliterated.

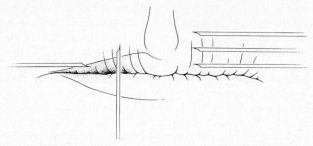

Figure 26–6. The injection of Zyderm into the upper lip area can be parallel or perpendicular to the creases or along the vermilion border.

persistent, then it is worth having maintenance therapy. If the correction was not achieved or lasted for a very short duration, then they should not have any further injections for those particular creases or wrinkles.

Secondary nasolabial lines are those found vertically on the midcheek (Fig. 26–7). They are parallel to the nasolabial lines and are usually more shallow. Whereas the nasolabial crease is a common finding in young people, the development of a secondary nasolabial line on the midcheek is one of the first distressing signs of aging. These creases can be completely cleared with one injection of Zyderm I or Zyderm II.

Other areas have a less predictable degree of success and, consequently, are more controversial as to whether they should be treated. Some physicians successfully treat crow's-feet and even the fine wrinkles on the lower eyelids with very tiny puffs of Zyderm I. The author has used Zyderm I on crow's-feet when they extend lateral to the lateral orbital rim, which is actually the temple region. The skin

is fairly thick, and by blunting the extensions of the crow's-feet, the patient's creases do not look nearly as bad. The author has been successful using tiny amounts of Zyderm I into the lower eyelid creases, but just as often, he has been unsuccessful in the sense that the patient had persistent lumpiness for several months. If the lumpiness does not bother the patient, several months of correction follow.

The same seems to be true of the horizontal forehead creases. The pull of the frontalis muscle is such that horizontal forehead creases are some of the first to appear with aging, sometimes even as early as the twenties. This is the most resistant to any therapy, even the coronal brow-lift, which requires extensive surgery and is successful more for drooping eyebrows than for horizontal forehead creases.

Either Zyderm I or Zyderm II can be used for the forehead. Small puffs are placed by the multiple-puncture technique along the long axis of the crease. The author's technique is usually to hold the needle parallel to the long axis. However, perpendicular is just as effective.

Zyplast is indicated when the vertical glabellar lines are actually grooves or furrows. Similar to the nasolabial area, the furrow can be filled with Zyplast, and if there is still a crease in the skin, Zyderm can be used in addition. The Zyplast bolus seems to interfere with the patient's ability to completely crease the glabellar area and thus is actually a treatment for the prevention of further wrinkling as well as a treatment for the creases and furrows formed.

Some patients, even at an early age, develop a crease across the malar prominence of the cheek. This is called the malar groove, and it usually runs

Figure 26–7. *A,* Patient prior to treatment. *B,* The result three months later after two treatments with Zyderm II.

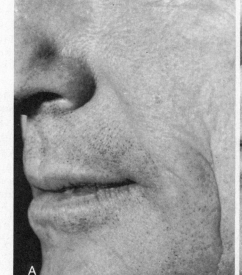
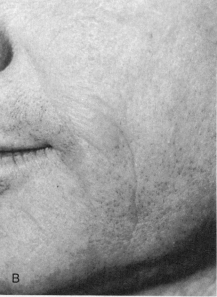

in an oblique fashion from the lower eyelid and cheek line over the malar prominence laterally. Sometimes, it runs directly vertically. This line makes the patient look sad or tired. Actually, clowns use makeup in this area to create a sad face. This is an unfortunate facial feature for some patients, and there has been no effective way to treat it. Zyderm I and II have been used and are only occasionally successful. Sometimes, this author has even plumped the skin as much as possible with Zyderm II only to find that the groove still persists.

All of this has been dramatically changed with the introduction of Zyplast. Different from any other material available, Zyplast safely and quickly fills this groove with a correction that lasts for almost a year. This is a tremendous improvement in the appearance for many unfortunate individuals. In addition to using Zyplast for some of the deeper and firmer acne scars, it has the unique ability to correct this groove.

Zyplast can also be used to contour other areas such as over the malar prominence, the orbital ridge, and in postrhinoplasty depressions.

TECHNIQUES FOR TREATING SCARRING

For acne scarring, the techniques may vary. Again, the goal is to place as much Zyderm as possible under the depressed area. But constant attention to the size of the dermal compartment is critical. Some depressed scars have normal or thickened dermis at the base that makes these particular scars the most amenable to treatment with Zyderm. Others may have atrophic bases. Not only will atrophic skin hold a small amount of the implant, but when that skin is elevated to the plane of the surrounding skin, it often has a whitish or scarred appearance. Thus, correcting atrophic scars is not much of an improvement cosmetically unless the patient wears makeup. Some depressed scars are fibrotic. The implant will not flow at all into fibrous tissue. It is possible to freeze fibrotic scars with liquid nitrogen and to inject collagen two days later while the area is edematous. It is also possible to force a little bit of collagen in, and at subsequent visits, the scar may be less fibrotic. Practically, however, because the material is prepackaged at 1.0 ml or 0.5 ml sizes and because repeat visits are troublesome for the patient, it is not a common approach. Most of the time, if there are many fibrous scars, dermabrasion is the technique of choice.

The needle is advanced into the base of the scar and placed just under the epidermis. The plunger is depressed to test where the flow of collagen is going. On a properly selected, soft depressed scar, the Zyderm will flow evenly into the base of the scar. As much Zyderm should be injected as the dermis will accommodate. If this will lead to overcorrection, all the better. It is difficult to overcorrect too much because of the subsequent, absorption of fluids and organization of the implant. Sometimes, if the depression is perfectly round, the needle can be placed at a 90-degree angle to the skin, pushed just into the dermis, and the plunger depressed. The collagen will flow in all directions and fill the implant evenly. More commonly, the needle is inserted from various points at the periphery of the depression.

Should the Zyderm flow to where it is not desired (and this is not an uncommon event), it can be squeezed or massaged back to the desired area. Also, some patients feel that massaging the collagen, once it is in place, leaves a smoother appearance in the first 48 hours. Some physicians believe that the collagen is better placed in this manner. The author considers all of the above to be true. Sometimes, he massages it back to where he wants it; sometimes, the edges are massaged so the lump is not quite as noticeable; and sometimes, in treating age-related lesions, it is massaged in order to make the whole area smoother.

On the other hand, it is usually appropriate to massage or shape Zyplast in the subcutaneous plane. It can be pinched or rubbed or squeezed into the exact proper position. It has the feeling of putty under the skin and can be maneuvered for a few minutes after injection, as desired.

It is important to realize that not all postacne scars are amenable to treatment with Zyderm. The older the scar, the less rigid and more pliable and thus the easier it is to distend. Generally, one should wait at least six months after an active lesion before trying to treat. Many patients are anxious for treatment as soon as they are over the active phase of acne. Indeed, all physicians try to reassure them during the active phase that, when it is over, they will be helped by the correction. However, if patients are under 22 years of age, it is wise to temporize as long as they will tolerate, so the scars will fully mature and the postinflammatory erythema and hyperpigmentation will resolve. Indeed, two to three years after active acne, many of the "scars" have resolved.

Before treating acne scarring, it is wise to analyze each of the scars. Some will be fibrotic and some soft and depressed. Some are not scars but only hyperpigmentation and persistent erythema. One must carefully analyze which lesions are amenable to implantation therapy. If there is a problem deciding whether a lesion will be pliable enough to expand, a test injection with normal saline is often helpful. If the lesion easily elevates, it would elevate with collagen. If, however, the normal saline cannot be pushed into the scar, it is unlikely that collagen will either.

Ice-pick scars have been studied histologically. Many times, there is a vertically oriented band of

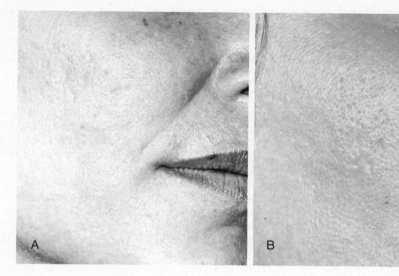

Figure 26—8. *A,* Patient with post-acne scarring prior to treatment. *B,* The result three months later after two treatments with Zyderm II.

fibrous tissue running from the papillary to the deep dermis. These fibers are perpendicular to the horizontal axis of the skin and, therefore, placing Zyderm in or around them does not elevate the dermis. These scars should be treated with other techniques, such as punch excision and grafting or dermabrasion or both.

The ideal scar for Zyderm is a broad-based, pliable scar with rolling edges that is fully matured and does not have significant inflammation (Fig. 26–8 and 26–9). Acne scars on the back can be treated with Zyderm, although many are fibrotic and so much material is required that it is usually not financially feasible.

DERMABRASION AND ZYDERM

Zyderm has been used successfully before and after dermabrasion, and the two are not mutually exclusive. The author tries to treat first with the modality that will give the patient the most benefit. If dermabrasion is anticipated, he will try to do that first and then treat those lesions that do not respond. However, sometimes it is important to establish rapport with the patient and to show them that, after the scarring is treated, they will indeed look and feel better. For patients who can afford it and want to try Zyderm first, there is no contraindication.

Dermabrasion causes an alteration in the organization and orientation of the collagen of the papillary dermis and of the mid-dermis.[14] Sometimes, scars that were too fibrotic for injection prior to dermabrasion are more amenable after. Dermabrasion lessens the sharp transition between the scar and normal skin, which makes a correction later with Zyderm more successful. With the removal of a certain number of scars by dermabrasion and the softening of the edges of other scars, those that still remain visible can be selected for Zyderm treatment. The author usually waits six months after dermabrasion before Zyderm because that time is necessary to see the final results of the dermabrasion.

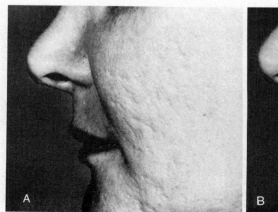
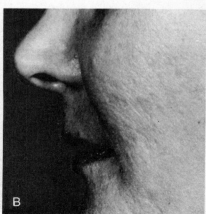

Figure 26—9. *A,* Patient prior to treatment. *B,* The result three months later after three treatments with Zyderm II.

POST-TRAUMATIC AND SURGICAL SCARS

If there is a contour deformity, Zyderm may be helpful. However, the physician must consider the anatomic location, whether the tissue is atrophic or missing altogether, the pliability of the tissue remaining, and the probable volume and maintenance schedules needed to produce correction (Fig. 26–10). If these factors are not considered, the patient and the physician may later be dissatisfied, whereas if they are considered, then both are happy with the contract and the results.

It is difficult to predict which surgical and traumatic scars will respond. The author's success rate at predicting good results with these types of scars is less than with acne scars or aging changes. Although not based on scientific evidence, his clinical impression is that probably one fourth of the postvaricella scars can be improved, one half of the matured, depressed postzoster scars will respond, and the response of postsurgical excision scars is completely unpredictable. Bailin and Bailin have written about the use of Zyderm after Mohs' surgery, and the author also finds this helpful.[15]

Occasionally, atrophy will develop after the injection of corticosteroids. It has been the author's experience that this atrophy is always self-limiting. However, some patients and physicians are quite distressed about it and want to treat it immediately. Zyplast collagen gives good results for this type of atrophy. By the time the Zyplast correction is lost, usually the atrophy has resolved spontaneously. If a patient who develops atrophy after the injection of corticosteroids is unhappy, a skin test can be placed, and during the one-month observation period, the physician and the patient have time to decide whether or not Zyplast treatment is desired.

There is only a slight difference in the injection technique between the two products. Some feel that Zyderm II is slightly more robust. The advantage of the more concentrated material is that, within a given compartment of dermis, the final result is that nearly twice as much collagen is deposited. Whether or not this has an effect on the longevity of the implant is questionable. The author's bias at the present time is that there is some greater persistence of correction after Zyderm II than Zyderm I. What is definitely true, however, is the deficiencies can be corrected with fewer office visits. What formerly took three or four visits for acne scarring or severe wrinkling now only takes one or two visits with Zyderm II. The vertical glabellar creases and some secondary nasolabial lines can be treated with one injection of Zyderm II, and that persists most of the time for approximately eight to 10 months.

Although the author has been using this product since 1978, it is only in the past four years that he feels the techniques have been properly worked out. But more importantly, in the past two years with proper selection of patients and by using Zyderm II, better techniques have been developed to consistently obtain a six- to eight-month correction for creases and wrinkles and slightly longer for acne scars.

The only problem with the more concentrated Zyderm II is that it remains palpable in thin skin, such as the eyelids. With Zyderm I, the recommendation for acne scarring was to overcorrect as much as possible. That is less true for Zyderm II. Also, in dealing with creases and wrinkles on thin skin, even though the implant is not raised above the surface of the skin, it may be visible if the skin is a slightly darker color than the collagen itself. This seldom happens in very fair skin.[16]

DIFFERENCES BETWEEN THE USE OF ZYDERM I AND ZYDERM II

Zyderm II has almost twice the amount of collagen per volume of injectable implant as Zyderm I.

EFFICACY AND PERSISTENCE

For postacne scars, the efficacy of this implant is measured in terms of the percent of correction and the duration of the correction. In age-related con-

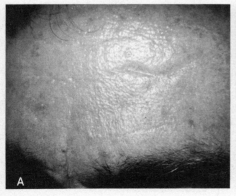
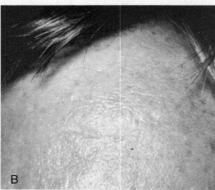

Figure 26–10. *A*, Patient prior to treatment. *B*, The result three months later after three treatments with Zyderm II.

ditions, the efficacy is measured in the cosmetic improvement of the patient and the persistence of correction. It is not necessary to remove all aging changes from the face or even desirable. It is not necessary to fully eradicate a crease or wrinkle but merely to soften or remove those creases and wrinkles that make the face look unhappy, tired, older than its years, and so on. For scarring, it is desirable to achieve 100% correction, and several visits two to four weeks apart during the beginning treatments are indicated. After correction is achieved, subsequent visits will depend on how well the implant holds. The author has seen patients who held post-acne scarring correction for a year to 18 months, while some have held it only for four months. Occasionally, patients require treatment at longer time intervals. Whether or not the scarring was maturing or whether new collagen was replacing the implant thus "eliminating" the scar cannot be determined. The need for less maintenance at longer intervals is something the author has observed in several patients.

The follow-up on aging changes seems more consistent. Further maintenance therapy is usually needed between six and 18 months.[17–19] Patients rightfully ask whether or not they will need collagen "forever." Some physicians who make value judgments for their patients (which may be appropriate for the physician to do) believe that maintenance therapy is needed once a year. This is an annuity for the physician and may be an unfair financial burden for the patient. The author's philosophy, however, has been to tell the patient that he will try to correct those aging changes that will respond to Zyderm and that the patient dislikes. Once they have been corrected, he and the patient will observe how long the correction remains. If it lasts long enough to be worth the money invested and if there is no sign of allergic reaction, then the patient can have the Zyderm whenever they want to budget that expense.

The author personally believes the patient should receive 12 to 18 months' benefit. However, when the cost and morbidity of the Zyderm injection are compared with some of the other ways patients spend money on their appearance, Zyderm competes well as a budget item. Patients seem to accept this, and they tend to budget repeat injections for special seasons, birthdays, and other special occasions. Also, neither patients nor the author envisions that the Zyderm will be given "forever." There are stages in life where certain aging changes are more noticeable. The first secondary nasolabial creases that appear on the cheek of a 40-year-old when there are few other signs of aging can be "erased" with Zyderm. The 30-year-old who has vertical glabellar creases making him or her appear angry is very happy to have these softened, and it is well worth the $200 a year to keep them softened for the next 5 to 10 years. The aging creases on some people are limited to certain areas, such as crow's-feet or the perioral area. If these can be corrected in a simple manner, no other major corrective surgeries are indicated.

Conversely, some people age in all areas of the face and have sun damage, sags, and accentuated folds secondary to movement. These individuals should not waste their time and money on Zyderm and be advised that such surgical procedures as face lifts, blepharoplasties, and chemical peels are better recourses. At the same time, the author has used Zyderm successfully to correct a specific crease or wrinkle that was bothersome to the patient. The author was comfortable with this decision because the patient was told that correction of this one area would not really change one's appearance or make one look younger. However, the patient was happy with this one bothersome crease or wrinkle being removed, and the author feels that it was a fair contract. Zyplast, even more than Zyderm, is able to radically change the appearance of some patients without the need for further major surgery.

Patient rapport can be developed easily while using Zyderm because it is such a simple, pleasant, and trouble-free experience. Many patients whom the author treated with Zyderm selected him to be their physician for further cosmetic work. In addition, many patients who are timid or embarrassed about seeking a physician for cosmetic surgery will start with a collagen consultation, because they are aware it is a nonsurgical office visit. Once they find a physician who is reasonable and professional, they accept the advice that more is needed than Zyderm. It is a good way to build a cosmetic surgical practice.

IMMUNOGENICITY AND SAFETY

Far more is known now about immunogenicity and safety than when this chapter was written for the previous edition. Zyderm has been used since 1978 and, at the time of this writing, 175,000 patients have been treated in the United States and Europe. With the exception of one case of sight loss, probably secondary to injecting too deeply in the glabellar region, there have been no major problems from the use of this implant. Concerns about developing a serious autoimmune condition have been a real and frequent question about the repeated injection of a foreign protein. Enough time has elapsed, and the number of patients treated with this product would seem to put those fears to rest. In addition, collagen products have been placed in the human body for many years in the form of heart valves. To the author's knowledge, there has never been any problem with autoimmune disease secondary to the placement of these valves. Granted, the skin is more likely to process a foreign protein, but the experience thus far does not show it to be of a serious nature.

As late as May 1984, there were publications decrying the use of this material.[20, 21] The arguments were the same as had been presented all along—surely some terrible autoimmunity would result from the injection of a foreign protein. So far, this has not happened, and hopefully, it never will. In these same past six years, meticulous studies have been done by Cooperman and Michaeli which indicate that those patients who exhibit local allergy to Zyderm develop antibodies only to Zyderm collagen.[22] These antibodies do not cross-react with human Type I and Type III collagen. They do not form precipitating antigen antibody complexes. They are only related clinically to patients who develop the acquired granulomatous allergic reactions at the treatment site and test sites.

Some of the fears about the use of implanted collagen are honest but fortunately misplaced because of the term "collagen." Charles Lapiere, M.D., of the University of Liège in Belgium has recently discussed the history of how "connective tissue" diseases were originally grouped.[23] In 1942, it was conceived that connective tissue was a system—an assembly of organ structures composed of similar elements combined from the same general function. The widespread involvement of connective tissue in rheumatic fever, polyarteritis nodosa, lupus erythematosus, and systemic sclerosis were all lumped into this connective tissue category. These were also called diffuse collagen diseases. Later, as the studies progressed, the changes of fibrinoid degeneration and inflammation around vessels led to the term collagen vascular disease. Further studies, however, have proven that the pathogenesis of these diseases is inflammatory and not related to any particular epithelial, endothelial, or parenchymal tissue. A collective term for all of these is no longer tenable. They should be called inflammatory diseases, and when autoantibodies exist, a more precise definition should be inflammatory autoimmune disease. If physicians can correct their thinking on the so-called collagen vascular diseases, then some of the ill-founded but understandable fears about the use of injectable collagen will be neutralized.

The development of allergy to the implant is the single most bothersome problem.[5, 24–26] From the early studies to more recent ones, about 3% of the population in the United States and northern Europe are allergic to the Zyderm implant. It is suggested that the consumption of beef has predisposed such a large percent of the population of this implant.[27] Nevertheless, the skin test is essential to discover the allergy in susceptible people. After the patient has been treated, the incidence of acquired allergy to the implant varies. In the author's practice, it has been around 0.5%, whereas others have reported it as high as 5%.[24]

The allergy manifests at the treatment site the same as it manifests at a positive skin test site.[29] There is swelling, induration, erythema, and pruritis. Some patients have all of the symptoms, some only one or two. The morbidity associated with the reaction is directly related to how intense it is and where it is. A swollen itchy spot on the arm is a lot easier to deal with than one on the midforehead. Sometimes, the reactions are so subtle that they are only palpable, and the patient is not inconvenienced. Other times, they are so noticeable on the face that they are difficult to cover even with makeup. These reactions last anywhere from three to 11 months on the average, although there have been some that lasted longer than a year. These reactions are associated with the presence of anti-Zyderm antibodies.

It has been the author's practice not to treat these reactions. The patient is assured that the reactions will resolve and the skin will be the same as prior to the reaction. If the physician carefully explains to patients before treatment that 0.5% to 1.0% are allergic to the implant, he or she is in the luxurious position of being able to remind them of this possibility. They can be assured that, in time, this reaction will go away. It would be much more difficult had the patient not been advised of the potential risks prior to the use of the material

The early in-house studies at the Collagen Corporation indicate that Zyplast is less allergenic than Zyderm. The total allergenicity to date seems to be around 1%, whereas for Zyderm it is between 3% and 4%. The theory is that the cross-linking of the implant before it is placed in the body hides the antigenic terminals from the immune surveillance system.

Another side effect is a transient swelling and erythema. This response is not related to the development of anti-Zyderm antibodies. It seems to be related to the ingestion of alcohol, exposure to sunlight, or becoming excessively warm such as in a sauna. These reactions are evanescent, and the patients can continue treatment. Such problems as infection at the treatment site and herpes reactivation are common.

Occasionally, a patient will develop bruising at the site of injection. This usually is noticed within the first 15 minutes of treatment. It is only a temporary nuisance. Some suggest that ice packs on the face prior to treatment prevent bruising. Patients do not develop it with each treatment, and it usually takes between five and seven days to resolve.

CONCLUSION

To the question, "Does Zyderm really work?" the author feels the answer is yes. For the amount and longevity of the correction that is presently being obtained in properly selected and treated patients, the author feels Zyderm is an appropriate medical device. There are many people who have received a great deal of benefit and many more who could benefit from it. The wish for a longer-lasting implant is a two-edged sword. Complications will last longer, the product will be less goof-proof, and materials placed where they are unwanted will be a nagging reminder for however long the longer-lasting implant persists. All faces change with time—even those young faces with acne scarring. A wrinkle or crease that may happily be eliminated with an intradermal implant for one decade might turn out to be an unhappy location for an implant in another decade of life. After practicing with injectable corrective materials for seven years now, the author finds that he is less desirous of having a permanent implant and more ready to accept an 18- to 24-month longevity of the material.

The development of the allergic reactions remains the only serious and difficult prlblem. There is some reason to hope that new forms of injectable collagen will be less allergenic. On the other hand, having a safe, approved material has been a boost to the author's practice, because it brings in people who are otherwise reluctant to talk to a cosmetic surgeon. A Zyderm consultation provides an opportunity to explain to patients what surgery might be appropriate and to minimize the misconceptions they may have about cosmetic surgery. It is a good way to develop a rapport with potential patients. On the whole, the author's experience with Zyderm has been a positive one, and there is no reason to believe that it will not become a permanent part of the armamentarium of the cosmetic dermatologic surgeon.

REFERENCES

1. Knapp TR, Luck E, Daniels JR: Behavior of solubilized collagen as a bioimplant. J Surg Res 23:96–105, 1977
2. Knapp TR, Kaplan EN, Daniels JR: Injectable collagen for soft tissue augmentation. Plast Reconstr Surg 60:398–405, 1977
3. Trentham DE, Townes AS, Kang AH, David JR: Humoral and cellular sensitivity to collagen in Type II collagen-induced arthritis in rats. J Clin Invest 61:89–96, 1978
4. Barr RJ, Stegman SJ: Delayed skin test reaction to injectable collagen implant (Zyderm). JAAD 10:652–658, 1984
5. Burke KE, Naughton G, Waldo E: Bovine collagen implant: Histologic chronology in pig dermis. J Dermatol Surg Oncol 9:889–895, 1983
6. Webster RC, Kattner MD, Smith RC: Injectable collagen for augmentation of facial areas. Arch Otolaryngol 110:652–656, 1984
7. Brehm G, Heite HJ, Jung EG, Zaun H: Xenogenic collagen for implants in treating pitted scars and cutaneous atrophies. Aktuelle Dermatologie 9:165–171, 1983
8. Zaren HA, Thomas DS: Injectable Collagen. Chicago, Ill, Year Book Medical Publishers, 1984, pp 241–252
9. Stegman SJ, Tromovitch TA: Implantation of collagen for depressed scars. J Dermatol Surg Oncol 6:450–453, 1980
10. Courtiss EH: Cosmetic defects and collagen injection. J Amer Acad Dermatol 247:3360, 1982
11. Klein AW, Rish DC: Injectable collagen update. J Dermatol Surg Oncol 10:519–522, 1984
12. Tromovitch TA, Stegman SJ, Glogau RG: Zyderm collagen: Implantation techniques. J Amer Acad Dermatol 10:273–278, 1984
13. Chernosky M: Presentation, Annual Meeting—American Society of Dermatologic Surgery, Maui, Hawaii, 1984
14. Stegman SJ: A comparative histologic study of the effects of three peeling agents and dermabrasion on normal and sun-damaged skin. Aesth Plast Surg 6:123–135, 1982
15. Bailin PL, Bailin MD: Correction of depressed scars following Mohs' surgery: The role of collagen implantation. J Dermatol Surg Oncol 8:845–849, 1982
16. Kaplan EN: Clinical variations in the utilization of Zyderm I and II. Plast Reconstr Surg 73:319, 1984
17. Robinson JK, Hanke WW: Injectable collagen implant: Histopathologic identification and longevity of correction. J Dermatol Surg Oncol 11:124–130, 1985
18. Rapaport MJ, Salit R, Rivkin L: Collagen injections for aging skin lines (wrinkles). J Amer Acad Dermatol 11:250–252, 1984
19. Nicolle FV: Use of Zyderm in the aging face. Aesth Plast Surg 6:193–195, 1982
20. Cohen IK, Peacock EE, Chvapil M: Zyderm (letter). Plast Reconstr Surg 73:857, 1984
21. Pharriss BB: Zyderm (letter). Plast Reconstr Surg 74:849, 1984
22. Cooperman L, Michaeli D: The immunogenicity of injectable collagen, Part I and Part II. J Amer Acad Dermatol 10:638–657, 1984
23. Lapiere C: "Connective tissue diseases" held misnomer. Dermatol Times, March 1985, p 3
24. Swanson NA, Stoner JG, Siegle RJ, Solomon AR: Treatment site reactions to Zyderm collagen implantation. J Dermatol Surg Oncol 9:377–380, 1983
25. Labow TA, Silvers DN: Late reactions at Zyderm skin test sites. Cutis 35:154–156, 1985
26. Rice D, Kamer FM, Chururkian MM: Complications of injectable collagen. West J Med, November 1984, p 676
27. Castrow FF, Krull EA: Injectable collagen implant—update. J Amer Acad Dermatol 9:889–893, 1983
28. Brook NA: Foreign body granuloma produced by an injectable collagen implant at a test site. J Dermatol Surg Oncol 8:111–114, 1982
29. Barr RJ, King FD, McDonald RM, Bartlow GA: Necrobiotic granulomas associated with bovine test site injections. J Amer Acad Dermatol 6:867–869, 1982

LAWRENCE M. FIELD, M.D., F.I.A.C.S. / RHODA S. NARINS, M.D.

Liposuction Surgery

HISTORY AND BASIC PRINCIPLES

Liposuction surgery (also called lipolysis, suction-assisted lipectomy, or blunt suction lipectomy) is historically of European origin.[32, 51, 53, 70] The suction concepts of the Fischers[32] were brilliantly evolved by Illouz[51] and modified by Fournier.[33, 34] The techniques and approaches of these originators of fat suction surgery continue to be refined by others. The major fact remains that the blunt cannula surgical techniques are remarkably safe for the removal of a variety of subcutaneous fat deposits.[8, 12, 23, 30, 33, 45, 46, 56, 80]

Compared to previous fat resection techniques, blunt fat aspiration has avoided most of the problems of seroma formation and bleeding associated with the more aggressive surgery utilizing sharp or curettage dissection of fat.[53, 82] It also avoids the unsightly scars of en bloc fat resection.[71] Suction lipectomy is applicable to varying fat deposits on the face and neck;[2, 26, 64, 79] proximal arms, axillae, and axillary extensions of the breasts; pseudogynecomastia in males;[66, 78] lateral thoracic fat accumulations; supra- and infraumbilical abdominal deposits; suprailiac crest areas; lateral and posterior buttocks; anterior, medial, and lateral thighs; and the posterior infrabuttock proximal leg, knees, and ankles. Other indications include lipomata, relapsing panniculitis, acquired and congenital lymphedema of the extremities,[84] and insulin-induced fat hypertrophy.[43] A variety of flaps have been defatted partially or completely using this technique.[74, 75] Liposuction reduction of a massively obese neck was performed to allow placement of an emergency tracheostomy tube.[73] A definite trend toward utilizing surgery on obese patients is apparently occurring, and continuing studies are underway.[6] These procedures are applicable to both outpatient and inpatient settings; however, the amount of fat that can be removed safely without significant hypovolemic problems or possible shock from blood loss has now been relatively established at 1500 to 2000 cc.[33, 45] We presently limit ourselves to this amount. Applications in the elderly are currently being defined. The senior author has performed abdominal suction lipoplasty in an 80-year-old female.[87]

EQUIPMENT AND PERSONNEL REQUIREMENTS

As dermatologic surgeons, the vast majority of our cases are performed on an outpatient basis,

although the first in-hospital liposuction procedure was performed by a dermatologist in December 1984.[66] The mainstays of the surgical team are the adequately trained surgeon and his or her assistant, who must be trained thoroughly in the maintenance of sterile techniques, although selected nonsterile nursing personnel may circulate. The surgery itself can require great physical strength and may result in extreme fatigue and even epicondylitis. A selective muscle training program may help prevent these problems.[31]

A variety of suction machines are now available. All are high-powered pumps that rapidly reach one atmosphere of pressure (30 pounds per square inch). Stainless steel cannulae are of varying manufacture, design, size, and configuration. Cannulae vary from 2 to 10 mm in diameter, have one or more blunt apertures, and may or may not curve distally. Modifications of cannula design continue to be made.[14, 22, 24] Instrumentation for sculpturing the face has undergone considerable change; a new flat-ended spatula has been developed to assist in the maintenance of higher negative pressures when working in open areas (i.e., under rhytidectomy flaps).[58]

A wide surgical table is preferable for many patients, allowing some margin of safety in shifting from back to side. A clean sheet placed under the sterile gowns and drapes is of significant assistance in lifting and changing positions of the patients. If general anesthesia is utilized, the accoutrements necessary for possible emergencies must be available, including a cardiac monitor, defibrillator, aspiration suction unit (separate from the liposuction machine), blood pressure apparatus, endotrachial tubes, Ambubag, the necessary pharmacologic agents for giving and counteracting anesthetics, a properly serviced anesthesia machine, and an intravenous stand to give both medications and fluid replacement as necessary. For the administration of general anesthesia in the dermatologic surgeon's office, both authors strongly prefer an anesthesiologist to a nurse anesthetist.[9, 47]

CONSULTATION

At the initial consultation, it is vital to determine if the patient's problem and expectations are realistic and amenable to the procedure. Explaining verbally the informed consent agreement and obtaining a written release are mandatory.[38, 49] Costs should be discussed beforehand, including charges for revision procedures. Preoperative photographs are necessary and may spare the surgeon considerable difficulty when reassuring a doubting patient. An evaluation of each individual's psychological makeup may be difficult, but an attempt to differentiate those likely to be unduly dissatisfied or troublesome is necessary.

With experience, we become better able to select the proper procedure or combination of procedures for a particular patient.[15, 21, 29, 38, 46, 50, 59, 80] The best aesthetic results are seen in the young, slim patient with localized deposits of fat.[1, 3, 5, 55] This presupposes taut skin overlying the contour deformity. However, good to excellent results can be obtained in older patients with less tight and less smooth skin who accept these limitations.[6, 29] Fat deposits that feel firm are better treated than those that are soft and malleable. Less-than-optimal candidates for this surgery should realize the primary benefits of the technique is to look and feel better in clothing. Although every effort is made for smooth contouring, some surface irregularity is possible, especially on the torso, abdomen, and thighs.[33, 71] Scars, varicosities, and the superficial irregularities of cellulite remain unchanged. Striae, though persistant, become less prominent as the underlying distension is lessened. If photographs of other patients are shared with the prospective patient, a variety of results should be included so perfection is not implied by the surgeon. Alternatives should be mentioned, as should the possibility of repeating the procedure if necessary. The latter is most common in procedures involving the abdomen, occurring secondary to dietary indiscretion and a poor exercise program.

Written preoperative instructions are presented to the patient. Aspirin-containing preparations and monoamine oxidase inhibitors should be discontinued at least two weeks prior to surgery.[9] Cyclic anovulatory drugs may cause venous thrombosis in the postoperative period, and might be discontinued in the preoperative cycle. If local anesthesia is employed, most systemic medication will have no impact. Prior to general anesthesia, it is important to have detailed information on all medications that the patient is taking to avoid any drug interactions, increased bleeding problems, or other unwanted side effects. It is the senior author's practice to rely absolutely on the anesthesiologist for this evaluation and for the subsequent selection of appropriate anesthetic drugs.[47] An antiseptic soap, such as Hibiclens skin cleanser should be used three days prior to and on the morning of surgery. If the surgical area is glabrous and the surgeon uses postoperative taping, hair in the surgical site should be shaved immediately before surgery, which lessens follicular inflammation and significantly decreases discomfort during tape removal. If a local anesthetic is used, a light breakfast is allowed provided heavy systemic medication is not given during surgery. If the latter course is contemplated or if the patient is to undergo general anesthesia, nothing should be allowed per os after midnight prior to surgery.

For all patients in whom blood loss may be significant, a preoperative hemoglobin or hematocrit is obtained. Patients undergoing general anesthesia must fulfill further requirements set down by the anesthesiologist. In the senior author's office, a baseline hemoglobin or hematocrit is obtained on all patients undergoing abdominal, large thigh, or large buttock procedures. Patients less than 50 years old and in good health require an electrocardiogram. Those older than this or with a history of significant medical problems require a physical examination by their own physician and clearance by the anesthesiologist for a general anesthetic.

All required laboratory tests, signed and witnessed consent forms, and preoperative photographs should be available.

Stool softeners taken for a day or two prior to abdominal surgery have been found to be helpful.[30]

PRELIMINARY PREPARATION—DAY OF SURGERY

The entire area is scrubbed and appropriate markings are made in the upright position with an indelible marking pen. Sitting is adequate for marking procedures above the waist, but the standing position should be adopted otherwise. Both vision and manipulation are used in the evaluation. The densest concentrations of fat should be demarcated, as should a peripheral zone in which partial lipectomy or blunt injury alone are used to smooth the transitional interfaces.

When the upper thighs are being reduced, it is preferable to extend the suction to both the lower buttock and infrabuttock prominences than to reduce only the lateral fat deposits. Areas to be specifically spared because they are devoid of fat should also be premarked.[42] Photographic documentation of all markings might be prudent in selected cases. The incision lines should be carefully delineated and pointed out to the patient. If additional incisions might be necessary during surgery, this fact should be made clear to the patient. It must be remembered that the marked areas will shift significantly with the patient supine. Therefore, the original markings should be followed in the contouring process rather than changing the surgical plan if the topography and markings have changed with positional shifts.

The patient is then rescrubbed and carefully positioned on the operating table. If a local anesthetic is to be used, it is administered within safety margins. Many observers believe injecting epinephrine reduces the amount of blood loss at surgery.[4, 41] Dolsky found that ice-packing an area for one hour or more lessened the requirements of local anesthetic.[20] Neither author utilizes drains now, although a suction pump drain left in place for two to three days may be required for pseudogynecomastia accompanied by resection of true glandular gynecomastia.

If general anesthesia is used, a cardiac monitor, an intravenous line, and an endotracheal tube must be in place. When the anesthesiologist is five minutes from the estimated incision time, the surgeon is called to the suite. Cap, mask, sterile gown, and gloves are donned. To handle both the cannula and tissue, a cotton heavy-mesh grasping glove may be used. Appropriate apertures are fashioned in the sterile drape. A last-minute check of all mechanical devices and positioning is done. The scalpel handle is grasped, the surgeon is in position, and awaits the anesthesiologist's permission to proceed.

SURGERY

The scalpel blade incises at the predetermined site, with individual anatomy and requirements determining each entrance. Any incision should be made just long enough to admit the size cannula being used. The cannula must reach the areas intended or additional and longer cannulae must be available. Some surgeons prefer to use a small blunt spreading instrument to assist the passage of the cannula through the skin and dermis.[48] Some use a nonaspirating rod to spread the subcutaneous fat before introduction of the suction cannula.[18] After the cannula has been introduced, the suction is turned on and a series of deep subcutaneous tunnels are made. The cannula is moved in a to-and-fro, piston-like movement—the number of strokes relating to the thickness and ease of removal of the fat. These vary from one or two passes in the more lateral nasolabial cheek fat pad to as many as 20 strokes in the periumbilical location where adipose tissue is very thick.

Tunnel depth should be just above the muscle and fascia. The hand without the cannula is used to palpate the precise location of the cannula tip, holding it at the proper depth. This tip should remain at least one cm below the surface of the skin, except in the face and neck where narrower margins may be permissible.[2, 3, 26, 61, 65] Elsewhere, enough adipose tissue is removed to leave 2.0 to 2.5 cm when opposing skin surfaces are pinched together. When forming the gluteal fold, less than one cm of fat might be left, and only in this maneuver might the aperture be turned upward against the dermal undersurface. Although sculpturing of the absent gluteal crease seems to be an established procedure, double infrabuttock creases have evolved in many people from buttock ptosis, so caution is urged in this location.[23]

According to Newman,[62, 64] the orifice may be turned toward the dermis in submental and neck work, for which he advocates the use of windshield-wiper–like, side-to-side movements in an attempt to completely remove the submental fat. Only in this area is this type of movement permitted.[26, 79] Depending on the site to be defatted, the cannula may enter the fat deposit from a distance to create tunnels in a radial fashion. Other deposits may permit a more central incision with a spoke-like tunnel configuration.[16, 40]

The surgeon must visually monitor the harvest from each tunnel as the fat passes through the transparent tubing, noting changes in the consistency and color of the aspirated material. More blood dictates moving to a different area. If tunneling is not carefully performed, the intervening fat islands may be too large and will leave an irregular contour. The larger the diameter of the cannula, the greater the chances for such irregularity.[21] To alleviate these isolated fat islands, they must be firmly grasped and secured for a smaller-sized cannula to enter and aspirate.[72] After the larger fat deposits have been removed, a smaller diameter cannula may be used to feather the area distally. Areas even more distal may be penetrated with a cannula without suction, the attendant traumatic fat atrophy allowing a smoother transitional topography. More than one incision may be made per area, with cannulae introduced from different directions to remove fat in a grid pattern. This crisscrossing lessens the likelihood of surface irregularities.[21] It must be emphasized that some septa to the skin and dermis should be preserved, and the area should not be completely undermined.

Suction lipectomy should be concluded when (1) the skin in the treated area is pinched between the index finger and the thumb with approximately 2 cm of tissue remaining between them ("pinch test"), or (2) the total amount of tissue removed approximates the safe, maximum allowable amount.

Experience is an excellent teacher in judging when the procedure is finished, but it is always best to err on the conservative side. While it is presently impossible to replace fat when too much has been aspirated, one can always remove more at a later date. When smaller volumes of fat are being aspirated, the level removed from one side may be marked with adhesive tape on the bottle before the second side is started. If large quantities are aspirated, different bottles may be used and compared.[29] Although some surgeons prefer the use of drains,[33] the authors' continuing experience and the quantity limitations involved in outpatient surgery have proven them to be largely unnecessary.

Incisions may be irrigated with saline solution, freshened by débridement, if necessary, and sutured. One may elect layered closure, interrupted sutures, or running sutures. It has been recently recommended that the wounds be irrigated with either saline or a combination of saline, adrenalin, bupivacaine, gentamicin, and chymotrypsine A. This combination supposedly lessens pain, hematoma formation, and the possibility of infection.[83]

Use of systemic antibiotics in the preoperative, intraoperative, and postoperative course is a matter of individual preference. The authors simply apply topical antibiotics to the incisions.

Choice of dressings is also an individual matter; the senior author prefers compression garments, and the junior author prefers redraping the skin with Flexiplast tape, but tape is far more difficult to apply and uncomfortable to remove. Both provide some hemostasis by pressure and redraping of the integument. Tape applied with tension should have the application started just short of the midline and never circumferentially without a break in its continuity.

A compression dressing similar to those used for face-lifts may be used for head and neck work, and a variety of special dressings have been developed for the nasolabial and malar fat pad areas. It is permissible to combine both tape and compression garments in selected cases. Depending on the area treated, sutures may be removed between five and 12 days.

Compression garments are left in place for a week. They may be removed at night after the first week and may be worn for several weeks after the sutures have been removed.

POSTOPERATIVE COURSE

Appropriate pain medications are prescribed; non-narcotic (i.e., non-triplicated) drugs are usually sufficient. Meals should be light the day following surgery; some surgeons restrict intake to fluids only. If the patient has had a general anesthetic, surveillance or assistance going to the washroom may be necessary. Relatively little physical activity is allowed for 24 to 48 hours. The ruby laser and ultrasound have been used to lessen the ecchymotic and fibrotic stage of hematoma formation.[39, 58]

Light exercise is generally possible after two weeks, and heavier exercise after four. Ecchymoses may not disappear for three weeks, while swelling slowly disappears over a two- to six-month period. Ankles may take a year or more for the swelling to decrease. Persistent abdominal tenderness, especially periumbilical, may persist for more than six months.

COMPLICATIONS

If the basic rules are followed, major complications are rare. At present, outpatient removal should probably be limited to 1500 to 2000 cc.[33, 42] Staged removals may be necessary if the rules of safety are not to be violated. Blood loss, critical drops in red cell mass, fluid shifts with hypovolemia, and electrolyte disturbances have not proven to be serious in the postoperative course.[19, 37, 57] If greater volumes are to be taken in an inpatient setting, probably a maximum of 2500 to 3000 cc should be removed in any single session. However, early unconfirmed reports (1985) of massive suctionings (to 10,000 cc) are coming from South American sources. Slight temperature elevations one to two days postoperatively have been noted, but these have been of no serious import. Swelling and bruising are universal, as are edema and discomfort. Infection, seroma, hematoma, dimpling, surface irregularities, residual prominences, hyperpigmentation, asymmetry, and sensory changes are all possible sequelae and should be mentioned in the preoperative consultation. Patients should be forewarned that swelling and tightness persist in the early weeks and may give rise to a period of disappointment. Patience is mandatory, as is dietary management. Failure to control caloric intake allows remaining fat cells to enlarge. If an area has been almost completely defatted, subsequent bulging will be minimal. In the more fibrous areas where adequate removal is difficult (supraumbilical, epigastric, and suprailiac waist regions), partial clinical recurrence may be seen. Repeat suctioning for residual irregularities in these areas will assist the contouring process, and serial removals may be necessary to accomplish contour relief for the compulsive eater. This recurrence problem is not applicable to the thin female with thigh deformities, to the individual with a congenital neck contour deformity, or to a variety of other problems routinely treated with a single surgical application.

Each anatomic area amenable to suction-assisted lipectomy requires focused concentration and study. These will be discussed in order from the head downward.

Face

The technique is applicable in submental, submandibular, preantral, preparotid, and malar fatty deposits. Cannulae varying between 3 and 6 mm are used with various incision points as described.

The most common submental incision is made in the midline within or just distal to the submental fold. Either separate fat compartments are individually treated,[25, 26] or the entire submental region may be swept in windshield-wiper–like fashion.[62] The submandibular and jowl areas can be reached from a central midline incision, or they may be reached by an infra-auricular or prelobular incision with the course of the cannula rigidly controlled by the placement of the surgeon's fingers above and below the mandibular prominence. Some prefer to lessen the vacuum pressure for facial work[3] while others see no advantage in this.[39]

The preantral area (nasolabial fold) may be approached through a lateral nasal vestibular incision or through the upper alar crease close to the nose.[2] The latter incision allows entrance to the fat compartment above the alar level. The number of strokes should be gradually lessened as one proceeds laterally from the more prominent medial aspect of the nasolabial fat.

Preparotid, submandibular, and jowl deposits are removed frequently in combination with rhytidectomy.[61, 67, 79, 85] Liposuction cannula dissections from submental, infralobular, pretragal, and mastoid incisions have revolutionized face-lift surgery, bringing a striking decrease in bleeding and nerve injuries.[59, 61] Dissections may be accomplished with a 3 or 4 mm cannula without suction, subsequently turning the suction on. Blunt dissection with the cannula forces one to stay safely above the level of the sternocleidomastoid region and thus above the level of the nerve. As the cannula proceeds along the mandible, one finger is locked under the mandible to hold the cannula tightly within the premarked tracks. Pressure from the cannula is inadequate to avulse the mandibular branch of the facial nerve in this location.[62] If a slightly dependent jowl is present, undermining should extend past this level.[5, 18, 85] Ancillary and appropriate undermining is then carried out at the level of blunt dissection in an essentially bloodless field.

Upper Extremities

This procedure is the treatment of choice for proximal upper arms of increased circumference due to fat deposits. Multiple incisions may be utilized with long 6 or 8 mm cannulae. Where there is significant collapse of skin and where there is dependent prominence of both skin and fat, the amount of improvement possible from suction alone may be inadequate.

Gynecomastia

For pseudogynecomastia, suction is the lipectomy procedure of choice (Fig. 27–1).[78] Entrance may be made via the anterior axillary line, periareolar area, inframammary area, and even from the lateral thorax. Suction with a 6 or 8 mm cannula is carried out, peripheral feathering being of significant import in this area. Residual masses of glandular tissue are frequently in evidence in the infra-areolar position, requiring sharp surgical dissection.[78] If resection of true gynecomastic glandular tissue is performed, the senior author utilizes a suction drain on occasion. Actual resection of skin is seldom necessary. In the large male breast, considerable difficulty will be noted in successfully aspirating the looser adipose tissue in the lateral breast area and below the axillary vault.[66, 83] The swelling and ecchymoses above the dressing, which may alarm the patient postoperatively, usually begin to fade by the fourth day.

Female Breasts

Although the female breast has been approached with this technique as an ancillary procedure, the authors have no personal experience with this and must refer the reader elsewhere. Appropriate use of this technique as an adjunctive procedure for the surgical treatment of mammary hypertrophy would seem to be established.

Abdomen

The abdomen is either the most popular or second most popular site (after thighs) for suction-assisted lipectomy. The rotund peri- and infraumbilical abdomen is most easily improved by this technique. The supraumbilical and infracostal fat roll is significantly more fibrous and much more difficult to remove. As the enlarged abdomen extends laterally

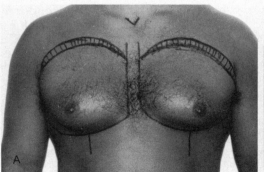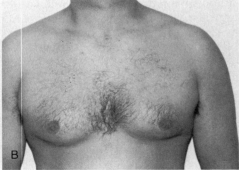

Figure 27–1. A male patient with adipose pseudogynecomastia: *A,* Preoperative appearance showing markings. *B,* Postoperative result with marked improvement.

to the suprailiac position, the adipose tissue becomes more fibrous and the difficulty of aspiration increases.

Because the abdominal skin is nourished by cutaneous perforating arteries, bleeding with abdominal liposuction may present some risk. Postoperative abdominal swelling demonstrates considerable resolution by five weeks, although fibrosis and retraction continue to occur in almost all patients for at least six months. Although some fibrotic retraction of the slightly pendulous abdomen is seen, significant skin overhang requires concomitant or delayed abdominoplasty procedures.[15]

The evolution of abdominal entrance incisions has led from a single umbilical or suprapubic incision to dual lateral abdominal incisions and now to multiple small abdominal incisions. Surgeons prefer cannulae of varying sizes, the present trend being toward smaller cannulae. "Love handles" may be present in either sex but are more frequently seen in males as isolated deposits; they are sex-related and probably controlled by a male hormone. The approach to these would be via the abdomen, if abdominal panniculus is to be removed, or via direct lateral flank or upper lateral groin incisions. The procedure in this area is physically difficult for the surgeon.

The belt line overhang may also be improved with this procedure. If suction is extended into the suprapubic area and beneath the mons veneris, one causes striking edema and ecchymoses that begin to resolve in five to seven days. In females, fatty collections above the iliac crests are amenable to this procedure as well. Combined with lateral thigh "saddle bags," this fat gives rise to the "violin deformity" that is encountered so frequently.[50]

Thighs

As with hormonal influences on the male flank, this area may be controlled by estrogen receptors on the fat cells, predisposing the area to fatty accumulation. Once removed surgically, this deformity should not recur in either obese or thin patients. A number of different entrances to the thigh fat have been proposed, including (1) through the bikini line and emanating radially, (2) from the infrabuttock line and extending anterolaterally, and (3) directly from the midpoint of the fat in spoke-like fashion.[16, 40, 44] With larger deposits, most authorities would simultaneously reduce some of the lower posterior buttock as well as the infrabuttock area of the upper posterior thigh.[18]

Large deposits of thigh fat situated anteriorly with convex bowing of the anterior thigh silhouette can be significantly reduced. A medial suprapatellar incision with suction toward the femoral crease serves well. This is then extended medially in a conservative fashion, combined with the more usual

lateral femoral or bikini line incision (i.e., the cannula crisscrossing slightly from lateral to medial and across the front of the thigh). A crisscrossing technique is also frequently used on the lateral thigh, combining the former with extensions to the iliac crest and flank deposits via more lateral buttock incisions.[23, 42]

It is important to stress to the patient who has superficial irregularities of the skin surface (e.g., cellulite or cascading) that these areas may not improve at all in texture or appearance. Stretch marks or dermal breaks in obese patients generally do show visual improvement as the protrusion lessens, but no promises should be made.

The infrabuttock creases are generally incomplete and fail to extend laterally because they are obliterated by the adipose accumulations in the thigh. They may appear upturned, square, or even turned downward. Asymmetry is frequent. Considerable skill is required to sculpture the fat in these areas to allow more normal infragluteal creases and to avoid creating double fold lines.[23]

The concept of circumferential sculpturing of the proximal distal lower extremities has appeared with up to 2000 cc being removed from the legs in single sittings through multiple incisions. This is difficult, requiring great experience and a close approximation of thigh symmetry.[23] Up to 3600 cc of fat have been removed in such legs using serial procedures.[23] The larger of asymmetric extremities may be reduced similarly.

Ankle and Calf

Women frequently complain of deposits in the more anterior and medial aspects of the knee. These may occur as an isolated phenomenon or as part of a diffuse enlargement of the lower extremity. These areas can now be approached for the first time by using small multiple incisions both anteriorly and posteriorly to sculpt this area with suction. Those experienced in the procedure can accentuate the contour of the gastrocnemius and remove fat around the Achilles tendon and from supramalleolar masses anteriorly and laterally. These are frequently combined with knee, lateral thigh, and iliac crest suctioning.[27] Cannulae of 4 to 6 mm are used. Extremity elevation and compression are required with swelling being present in some patients for more than one year.

LIPOMATA

Lipomata are the most difficult problem to aspirate, the fibrous stroma remaining after the procedure and requiring manual or instrument expression through the orifice.[29] In patients with multiple lipomatosis, the method allows blunt dissection. The larger the lipoma, the more appropriate liposuction aspiration seems to be, because a very large lipoma can be removed through a small incision. The senior author removed a lipoma 20 cm in diameter from the pretibial surface of a massively obese diabetic female through a 10 mm incision without comprising her systemically at all.

FLAPS AND MISCELLANEOUS

Blunt cannula aspiration represents a striking advance in the defatting of flaps.[57, 74, 75] The approach is simple and rapid and offers far better results than en bloc resections. The senior author had the opportunity to suction a myocutaneous flap that had been used to reconstruct the upper chest, neck, and chin of a woman burned some 60 years previously and whose flap had become selectively fat in later years. Residual adipose tissue in the lateral thoracic wall after radical mastectomy also responds to this approach. It is possible that suction aspiration of bulky myocutaneous flaps will become routine. The senior author has also described liposurgical debulking and cannula dissection for flap mobilization in reconstructive surgery following ablative procedures. Blunt suction lipectomy has also been used in insulin-induced fat hypertrophy[43] and in congenital lymphedema of the lower extremities.[84] At the time of this writing, no cases of adiposis dolorosa or Dercum's disease have been so treated and published. The presence of liposarcoma must be considered.[28]

TREATMENT OF OBESITY

Treatment of obesity by serial suction-assisted lipectomy is on the horizon.[6] One woman had 4000 cc removed during the first procedure and underwent two subsequent removals of 3000 cc each one week apart.[23] The senior author treated a patient whose buttock was so huge she could not sit in a chair, travel on public transportation, or stand up after she was in a sitting position without the assistance of others (Fig. 27–2). Three serial removals totaling 5500 cc allowed her to function normally.

SUMMARY

Liposuction (suction-assisted lipectomy, blunt suction lipoplasty, lipolysis) has proven to be a remarkably safe and efficacious method of removing fat in properly selected individuals.

In the patient who is educated about the procedure's limitations and who has realistic expectations based on age, skin tonicity, and size, satisfying results can be obtained. Remarkably, the single happiest group of patients for whom the authors have cared during their respective careers have been those in whom emotionally distressing areas of excess fat accumulation have been removed with relatively little pain and with relative simplicity.

Extensive reading, formal courses, and intraoperative experience are all considered mandatory prior to embarking on independent liposuction surgery careers.

REFERENCES

1. Alsofrom J: Lipectomy "magic bullet" for fat removal? Am Med News, May 27, 1983
2. Aronsohn R: Liposuction of the nasolabial fold: A preliminary report. Am J Cosmet Surg 2:51–56, 1984
3. Aronsohn R: Personal communication, June 1983
4. Askins S: Comparison of dry and wet liposuction techniques. Presented at The American Academy of Cosmetic Surgery Meeting, Los Angeles, Calif., January 1985
5. Berkowitz F: Personal communication, June 1983
6. Bestler J: Liposuction on obese patients—a preliminary report. Presented at The American Society of Lipo-Suction Surgery Meeting, Los Angeles, Calif., January 1985
7. Blue Shield, Medical Policy Guidelines Pamphlet. Suction-assisted lipectomy (lipolysis).
8. Body Sculpturing Through Lipo-Suction Surgery. The American Society of Cosmetic Surgery, Los Angeles, California
9. Braunstein M: Anesthesia, in Lipoplasty: The Theory and Practice of Blunt Suction Lipectomy. Boston, Little, Brown & Co, 1984, pp 105–114
10. Chajchir A, Benzaquen I, Wexler E: Suction curettage lipectomy. Aesth Plast Surg 7:195–203, 1984

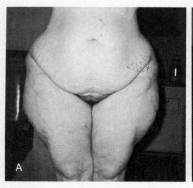
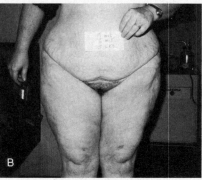

Figure 27–2. A 52-year-old woman with massive hip and buttock accumulations, which prevented her from sitting in a normal-width seat. A, Preoperative appearance. B, Appearance after three surgical sessions and serial reduction to a relatively normal contour and function.

11. Cosmetic Surgery. American Board of Cosmetic Surgery, Inc., Pacific Palisades, Calif.

12. Courtiss E: Suction lipectomy: A retrospective analysis of 100 patients. Plast Reconstr Surg 5:780–794, 1984

13. Courtiss E, LoVerme WE: Precision terminology for suction lipectomy. Plast Reconstr Surgery 75:132, 1985

14. D'Assumpcao EA: Cannula for liposuction. Plast Reconstr Surg 74:732, 1984

15. Dean J: Combined abdominoplasty and liposuction surgery. Presented at The American Society of Cosmetic Surgeons Meeting, Los Angeles, Calif., January 1984

16. Dolsky R: Spoke wheel liposuction technique. Am J Cosmet Surg 3:29–31, 1984

17. Dolsky RL: Body sculpturing by liposuction extraction. Aesth Plast Surg 8:75–83, 1984

18. Dolsky R: Personal communication, June 1983

19. Dolsky R: Fluid and blood dynamics of lipo-suction surgery. Presented at the Scientific Meeting of the American Society of Lipo-Suction Surgery, Los Angeles, Calif., January 1984

20. Dolsky R: Cryo-Lipo Suction. Presented at The American Society of Lipo-Suction Surgery Meeting, Los Angeles, Calif., January 1985

21. Drammis J: Fine Points and Pitfalls of Liposuction Surgery. Presented at The American Society of Cosmetic Surgeons Meeting, Los Angeles, Calif., January 1985

22. Drever J: The Helical Opening in Suction Cannula for Lipolysis, Plastic and Reconstructive Surgery 75(3):442–443, March 1985

23. Elam M: Personal communication, American Society of Liposuction Surgery Meeting, Los Angeles, Calif., January 1985

24. Elam M: Personal communication on the Cobra cannula, June 1983

25. Elam M: Personal communication, June 1983

26. Elam M, Berkowitz F: Submental and submandibular liposuction surgery. Am J Cosmet Surg 1:39–42, 1984

27. Elam M: Liposuction contouring of the knee and ankle. Am J Cosmet Surg 2:26–35, 1984

28. Enterline H, Culberson JD, Rochlin DB, Brady LW: Liposarcoma: Clinical and pathological study of 53 cases. Cancer 13:932–950, 1960

29. Field L: Dermatologic Plastic Surgery. Presented at the American Academy of Dermatology, Chicago, Ill., December 1983

30. Field L: Liposuction surgery: A review. J Dermatol Surg Oncol 7:530–538, 1984

31. Field L, Webb J: Kinesiology and Muscle Conditioning for the Liposuction Surgeon. Presented at The American Academy of Cosmetic Surgery Meeting, Los Angeles, Calif., January 1985

32. Fischer A, Fischer G: Revised techniques for cellulitis fat reduction in riding breeches deformity. Bull Int Acad of Cosmet Surg 2:40, 1977

33. Fournier P, Otteni R: Lipodissection in body sculpturing: The dry procedure. Plast Reconst Surg 72:598–609, 1983

34. Fournier P: Popularization of the Technique, in Lipoplasty: The Theory and Practice of Blunt Suction Lipectomy. Boston, Little, Brown & Co, 1984, pp 33–39

35. Fuerst M: Suction-assisted lipectomy attracting interest. JAMA 249(22):3005–3008, 1983

36. Grazer FM: Suction-assisted lipectomy, suction lipectomy, lipolysis and lipexeresis. The Western Journal of Medicine. 141:231, (Aug) 1984

37. Herhahn FT: Blood chemistry after lipolysis, in Lipoplasty: The Theory and Practice of Blunt Suction Lipectomy. Boston, Little, Brown & Co, 1984, pp 169–171

38. Herhahn F: Physical evaluation and informed consent, in Lipoplasty: The Theory and Practice of Blunt Suction Lipectomy. Boston, Little, Brown & Co, 1984, pp 95–104

39. Heschmati M: Personal communication, International Congress of Dermatologic Surgery, Jerusalem, Israel, October 1984

40. Heschmati M: Demonstration at the American Society of Lipo-Suction Surgery Meeting, June 1983

41. Heschmati M: Personal communication, June 1983

42. Hetter G: The effect of low-dose epinepherine on the hematocrit drop following lipolysis. Aesth Plast Surg 8(1):19, 1984

43. Hetter G: Surgical technique, in Lipoplasty: The Theory and Practice of Blunt Suction Lipectomy. Boston, Little, Brown & Co, 1984, pp 137–154

44. Hetter G: Treatment of insulin induced fat hypertrophy, in Lipoplasty: The Theory and Practice of Blunt Suction Lipectomy. Boston, Little Brown & Co, 1984, p 323

45. Hetter G: Lipoplasty: The Theory and Practice of Blunt Suction Lipectomy. Boston, Little, Brown & Co, 1984

46. Hetter GP, Herhahn F: Experience with "lipolysis": The Illouz technique of blunt suction lipectomy in North America. Aesth Plast Surg 7:69, 1983

47. Hindler H: General Anesthesia for the Liposuction Surgeon in an Office Setting. Presented at the Fourth International Congress of Dermatologic Surgery, Jerusalem, Israel, October 1984

48. Howes R: Personal communication, June 1983

49. Howes R: The "Howes and Whye" of liposuction surgery. Am J Cosmet Surg 1:49–51, 1984

50. Illouz Y: Body contouring by lipolysis: A 5-year experience with over 3,000 cases. Plast Reconstr Surg 72:620–623, 1983

51. Illouz Y: The origins of lipolysis, in Lipoplasty: The Theory and Practice of Blunt Suction Lipectomy. Boston, Little, Brown & Co, 1984, pp 25–32

52. Kesselring U: Regional fat aspiration for body contouring. Plast Reconstr Surg 72:610–619, 1983

53. Kesselring U, Meyer R: A suction curette for removal of excessive local deposits of subcutaneous fat. Plast Reconstr Surg 62:305, 1978

54. Lewis CM, Pruitt M: Massage and ultrasound, in Lipoplasty: The Theory and Practice of Blunt Suction Lipectomy. Boston, Little, Brown & Co, 1984, pp 175–178

55. Lipo-Suction Surgery Course. American Society for Lipo-Suction Surgery, Hollywood, California, June 1983

56. Martin N: Introduction of Lipolysis to the United States: A 3-year experience, in Lipoplasty: The Theory and Practice of Blunt Suction Lipectomy. Boston, Little, Brown & Co, 1984, pp 37–39

57. Nemetz J: Facial and Body Liposuction Surgery. Presented at the American Society of Cosmetic Surgeons Meeting, Los Angeles, Calif., January 1984

58. Newman J: New instruments, Concepts and Approaches in Facial Liposuction. Presented at the American Society of Lipo-Suction Surgery Meeting, Los Angeles, Calif., January 1985

59. Newman J, Dolsky R: Complications and pitfalls of facial lipo-suction surgery. Am J Cosmet Surg 2:8–12, 1985

60. Newman J: Liposuction surgery: Past-present-future. Am J Cosmet Surg 1:19–20, 1984

61. Newman J: Liposuction tunneling in conjunction with rhytidectomy. Am J Cosmet Surg 3:19–23, 1984

62. Newman J: Personal communication, June 1983

63. Newman J: Submental lipo-suction extraction with hard chin augmentation. Presented at the American Academy of Facial Plastic and Reconstructive Surgery meeting, Los Angeles, Calif., October 1983

64. Newman J: Facial profileplasty by lipo-suction extraction. Presented at the American Academy of Otolaryngology, Head and Neck Surgery, October 1983

65. Newman J: Combined lipo-suction and facial surgery with rhytidectomy. Presented at the Scientific Meeting of the American Society of Lipo-Suction Surgery, Los Angeles, Calif., January 1984

66. Pierce H: Personal communication, December 17, 1984

67. Plot S: Our new conceptions of the surgical treatment of cervical-facial lifting. Journal of Japanese Society of Aesthetic Surgery 22:211, (May) 1984

68. Reed R, O'Quinn S: Neoplasms of skin: Neoplasms of the dermis, adiposis dolorosa (Dercum's disease). In: Fitzpatrick, T. B., et al (eds.), Dermatology in General Medicine. New York, McGraw-Hill, 1971, pp 515–516

69. Schrudde J: Lipexeresis as a means of eliminating local adiposity. Aesth Plast Surg 4:215, 1980

70. Schrudde J: Lipexeresis in the correction of local adiposity. Presented at the First Congress of the International Society of Aesthetic Surgery, Rio de Janeiro, Brasil, 1972

71. Shaer WD: Gluteal and thigh reduction: Reclassification, critical review, and improved technique for primary correction. Aesth Plast Surg 8:165, 1984

72. Shippert R: The dynamics of fat breakdown and the role of progressive-diameter cannula technique and suction assisted lipectomy. Am J Cosmet Surg 1-15–18, 1984

73. Sonnenshine H: Emergency Cervical Liposuction to Facilitate Tracheostomy Placement. Presented at The American Society of Lipo-suction Surgery Meeting, Los Angeles, Calif., January 1985

74. Stallings J: Lipo-suction in reconstructive plastic surgery. Presented at the American Society of Lipo-Suction Surgery meeting, January 1984

75. Stallings J: The Defatting of Flaps by Lipolysis, in Lipoplasty: The Theory and Practice of Blunt Suction Lipectomy. Boston, Little, Brown & Co, 1984, pp 309–321

76. Stegman S, Tromovitch T: Liposuction in Cosmetic Dermatologic Surgery. Chicago, Yearbook Medical Publishers, 1983

77. Teimourian B, Adham MN, Gulin S, Shapiro C: Suction lipectomy—a review of 200 patients over a six-year period and a study of the technique in cadavers. Annals of Plast Surg 11:93–94, 1983

78. Teimourian B, Perlman R: Surgery for gynecomastia. Aesth Plast Surg 7:155–157, 1983

79. Teimourian B: Face and neck suction-assisted lipectomy associated with rhytidectomy. Plast Reconstr Surg 72:628–633, 1983

80. Teimourian B: A discussion of suction lipectomy: A retrospective analysis of 100 patients. Plast Reconstr Surg 5:795–796, 1984

81. Teimourian B, Kross S: Subcutaneous endoscopy in suction lipectomy. Plast Reconstr Surg 74:708, November 1984

82. Teimourian B, Fisher JD: Suction curettage to remove excess fat for body contouring. Plast Reconstr Surg, 68(1):50–58, 1981

83. Voukidis TE: Reply to suction lipectomy. Plast Reconstr Surg 75:137, January 1985

84. Winslow R: Treatment of congenital lymphedema of the lower extremities, in Lipoplasty: The Theory and Practice of Blunt Suction Lipectomy. Boston, Little, Brown & Co, 1984, pp 326–329

85. Chrisman B, Field L: Facelift surgery update: Suction-assisted rhytidectomy and other improvements. J Dermatol Surg Oncol 10:7, (July) 1984

86. Field L: Adjunctive liposurgical debulking and flap dissection in neck reconstruction. American Society for Dermatologic Surgery Meeting, Rancho Mirage, Calif., April 1986

87. Field L: Liposuction surgery in the geriatric age group—functional and cosmetic applications. International Society for Dermatologic Surgery Meeting, September 1986

Chemosurgery and Immunotherapy

28

FREDERIC E. MOHS, M.D.

Microcontrolled Surgery for Skin Cancer

Complete microscopic control of the excision of cutaneous cancers provides maximal assurance of the eradication of the neoplasms because the slender cancerous outgrowths can be located and selectively removed. The outgrowths may extend along various tissue planes for a considerable distance beyond the clinically apparent borders.[1] Moreover, the microscopic control permits maximal sparing of normal tissues since the excisions cease as soon as the terminations of the "silent" outgrowths are reached; hence, there is no need to remove the wide extra margin of apparently normal tissue that is customary with methods lacking complete microscopic control.

The complete microscopic control is achieved by the layer-by-layer excision of the tissues of the cancerous area with microscopic examination of the entire underside of each excised layer by the systematic use of frozen sections, as illustrated in Figure 28–1.[2] The tissues may either be subjected to chemical fixation in situ prior to excision of the layers (fixed-tissue technique), or a local anesthetic may be injected and the tissues excised in the fresh, unfixed state (fresh-tissue technique). The two techniques are described and their indications are delineated as follows.

THE FIXED-TISSUE TECHNIQUE

To produce in situ chemical fixation of the tissues, a zinc chloride fixative paste is applied and left in place under an occlusive dressing for one to 24 hours. The penetration of the fixative comes to a standstill in 18 hours. The depth of penetration is regulated by altering the depth and area of the applied fixative and the time it is permitted to act. The vehicle that carries the zinc chloride consists mainly of an inert, granular material (stibnite, 80-mesh sieve) that produces a matrix of granules held together by a binder (*Sanguinaria canadensis*) to produce a paste that releases the zinc chloride solution into the tissues in a controlled manner. A satisfactory preparation containing 45% zinc chloride by weight consists of: stibnite, 40 gm; sanguinaria, 10 gm; and a saturated solution of zinc chloride, 34.5 ml.[3]

Although the fixative may be applied directly to the surface of the neoplasm (as is usually done when treating melanomas), the usual procedure for carcinomas is to inject a local anesthetic and to excise and/or curette the main mass of the cancer. After this debulking procedure, hemostasis is achieved by rapid application of dichloroacetic acid, as originally described by Allington.[4] This keratolytic chemical is applied to a rim of skin at the edge to allow penetration of the zinc chloride, which does not readily penetrate the keratin layer.

Layers of tissue are excised without pain or bleeding because the incisions are through fixed tissue. Pain during penetration of the fixative usually is controlled with acetaminophen (300 mg with 30 mg of codeine phosphate), but stronger analgesics (up to 10 mg of morphine sulfate) may be prescribed as needed.

As each layer is excised, it is divided into specimens of a size that will fit on a microscope slide. The source of each specimen is marked on the lesion with 20% merbromin (Mercurochrome). The frozen sections, which are prepared by cutting through the flat underside of the specimens, are systematically scanned in the microscope, and the areas of cancer are marked in red pencil on a map of the lesion drawn on a pad of paper. Since subsequent applications of the fixative and excisions of the layers of tissue are limited to the areas of microscopically located cancer, the removal of the neoplasm is highly selective.

After completing removal of the cancer, a thin layer of fixed tissue remains for five to 10 days, after which it becomes demarcated so it can be removed exposing well-vascularized, granulation tissue. The wound may be left to heal by second intention or it may be closed with sutures or covered by a graft or flap. If an extensive defect requires a complicated repair, plastic surgeons often prefer to let the wound heal by granulation and to wait for six months or even a year if the neoplasm has recurred after treatment with other modalities that may have left outlying foci disconnected from the main tumor mass. If the neoplasm proves to be a melanoma, the wound almost always is permitted to heal by second intention to avoid the possibility that the repair might entail cutting through clinically invisible satellites and disseminating or covering small nests of melanoma cells.

verrucous carcinoma of the penis, which was previously called giant condyloma acuminatum or Buschke-Löwenstein tumor.[7]

Malignant Melanoma

In the author's opinion, melanoma is a prime indication for the fixed-tissue technique.[8–12] However, exceptions are melanomas that affect either the eyelid margins or the bulbar conjunctiva, for which the fresh-tissue technique with immediate cauterization of the excisional surface with dichloroacetic acid is indicated.[12] Since melanomas tend to invade the walls of blood vessels and lymphatics, and hence to metastasize rapidly, the technique varies from that used for carcinomas in two respects. First, the initial surgical excision of the main melanomatous mass is omitted because cutting through live melanoma tissue could conceivably disseminate malignant cells. Second, after a plane free of melanoma has been demonstrated microscopically, an extra margin of normal tissue is removed to encompass possible invisible satellites in the skin lymphatics. The width of the extra margin varies according to the type of melanoma, the depth of invasion (Clark's levels), the thickness (Breslow's thickness), the diameter and volume of the neoplasm, cellular anaplasia and pleomorphism, degree of adhesiveness of the melanoma cells, invasion of the walls of the blood vessels and lymphatics, extravasation of blood, number of mitoses, ulceration, rapidity of growth, anatomic location, and several other factors that affect the propensity of malignant melanoma to spread in a discontinuous manner.[11] The technique by which melanomas are excised includes application of dichloroacetic acid to the overlying skin to render the keratin layer permeable to the zinc chloride fixative (Fig. 28–4A). The latter is usually left on for 24 hours. Incisions always are

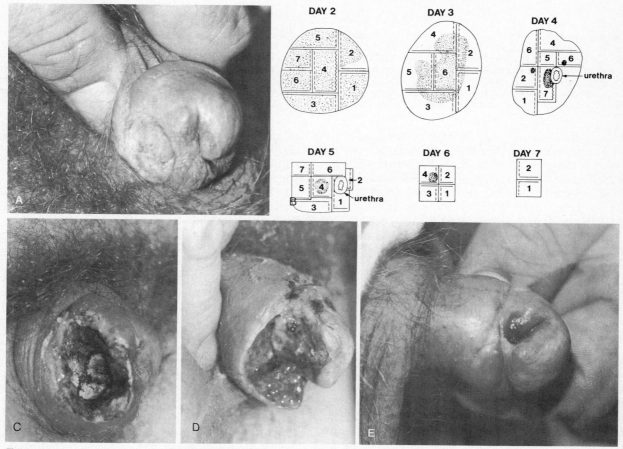

Figure 28–3. A, Squamous cell carcinoma of glans that recurred after four operations, three courses of x-ray therapy, one radium implant, and two treatments with electrodesiccation and curettage. B, Stippling in the diagram shows the location of the cancer on the maps of the lesion at successively deeper levels. C, The lesion after completing the excisions. D, Granulations two days later. E, The healed lesion. There has been no impairment of urinary or sexual functions and no recurrence in five years. (Reproduced with permission from Mohs FE et al: Microscopically controlled surgery in the treatment of carcinoma of the penis. Journal of Urology, 133:961–966, 1985.)

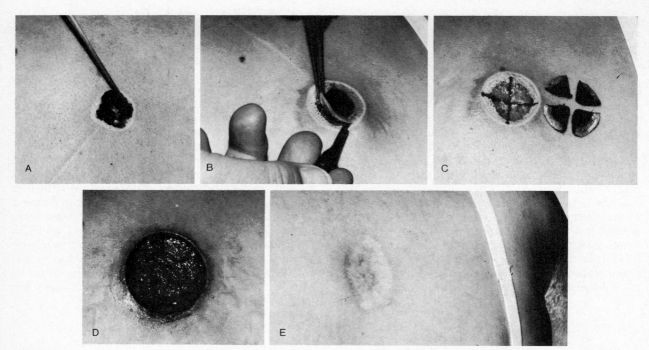

Figure 28–4. *A,* Superficial spreading melanoma, invasive to Clark's level III, on the interscapular back. The white border around the black melanoma is from the keratolytic action of the dichloroacetic acid that was applied prior to the application of the zinc chloride fixative. *B,* Excision of the second layer. *C,* Lesion after excision of the second layer; markings on the lesion indicated the sources of the four specimens. A cryostat was used to cut through the undersurfaces of the frozen sections. Although microscopic scanning of the sections revealed no melanoma at this level, an extra layer was removed and examined for possible satellites in the surrounding skin lymphatics. *D,* Granulation tissue after separation of the final layer of fixed tissues nine days later. *E,* Healed lesion after 18 months; no recurrence in 10 years.

through fixed tissue (Fig. 28–4B). After a plane of melanoma has been reached, an extra margin of tissue is removed, and the lesion is left to heal by second intention (Fig. 28–4E). The five-year cure rates reported in a consecutive series of 103 melanomas were: 100% for Clark's level II, 92% for level III, 64% for level IV, and 33% for level V.[3, 9] These results were achieved even though 69% of the neoplasms were nodular melanomas and 64% were invasive to Clark's level V.

INDICATIONS FOR THE FRESH-TISSUE TECHNIQUE

The fresh-tissue technique is used for most cutaneous cancers with the aforementioned exceptions of: (1) certain excessively extensive and complicated carcinomas, (2) penile carcinomas invading erectile tissue, and (3) malignant melanomas. Since the fresh-tissue technique varies somewhat in different situations, it is described and illustrated as used in the various anatomic areas.

Eyelid Cancers

Cancers of the eyelids were the first type to be treated with the fresh-tissue technique.[13] The reason

for adopting it was that the fixative used in the fixed-tissue technique had caused some problems with irritation of the eye, especially when the lid margins were involved.

In the treatment of cancers of the eyelid margins, a remarkable phenomenon is that a deep notch, produced by either the fixed- or fresh-tissue technique, is obliterated within a few weeks by the hammock-like, upward traction exerted by the contracting scar (Fig. 28–5).

In preparation for the excision of cancers of the lid margin, a local anesthetic is injected and 2% cocaine hydrochloride is instilled in the eye. A chalazion eyelid clamp is applied and held by an assistant to steady the eyelid and to provide hemostasis. Most of the grossly visible cancer is removed with the excision of the first layer. Vertical frozen sections of the first layer are made to establish the histologic diagnosis. Since the pearly appearance of neoplasm usually makes the diagnosis obvious, the second layer is often excised immediately. Hemostasis is achieved by the application of dichloroacetic acid to the excisional surface. However, before the clamp is removed, the dichloroacetic acid is thoroughly diluted with boric acid solution to prevent damage to the cornea. If cancer is observed as the frozen sections are scanned in the microscope, the process is repeated just in the involved areas until a plane free of cancer is reached (Fig. 28–5B). The thin layer of tissue that has been cauterized with dichloroacetic acid separates in a week or ten days, by which time the notch already is partly obliterated (Fig. 28–5C). After a month or two, the defect ordinarily has disappeared, and the previous site of the cancer can only be found by observing the lack of lashes in that area (Fig. 28–5D).

Extensive cancers that involve all of the lid margin respond remarkably well to this technique.[14] Care is needed to remove approximately equal amounts of conjunctiva and skin to prevent ectropion. If the cancer extends so close to the fornix that the eyelid clamp cannot be used, the eyelid is manually retracted and steadied by an assistant. After excision in this way, Oxycel cotton covered by Orabase and then by petrolatum serves to provide hemostasis.

Since cancers in the canthal areas are particularly prone to send out unpredictable ramifications, the microscopic guidance is important to ensure eradication of the cancer without causing excessive damage to the eyelids and eye (Fig. 28–6). With the fresh-tissue technique, extensions along the sclera can be followed without perforating the globe unless the cancer has invaded through to the choroid. Oxycel cotton used for hemostasis minimizes the danger of damage to the sclera.

Cancers on the lateral part of the lower eyelid and the adjacent cheek can cause downward traction and consequent ectropion if the wound is permitted to heal by second intention. However, this complication is readily avoided by a simple, diagonal closure that pulls the eyelid upward and laterally. This is possible because of considerable flexibility of the subcutaneous tissue in this area. The same procedure is effective for similar defects in the medial part of the lower eyelid.[15]

Defects of the upper eyelid margins do not rectify themselves quite as completely as those on the lower eyelid. Nevertheless, fairly extensive cancers can be removed without loss of adequate function. Cancers that originate in the conjunctiva can be excised by reversing the eyelid clamp so that the opening is on the conjunctival side. Dichloroacetic acid is used for hemostasis, and care is needed to dilute the acid and to apply an ophthalmic ointment before the lid is permitted to touch the cornea.

Extensive cancers that invade the eyeball or

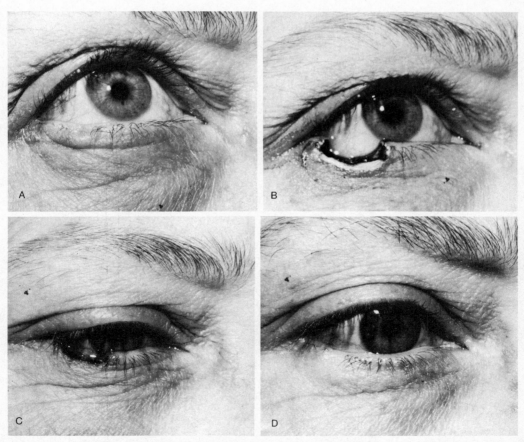

Figure 28–5. *A*, Basal cell carcinoma of the lower eyelid margin. *B*, Lesion after excision of the third layer when a plane free of cancer was demonstrated microscopically. *C*, Granulation tissue after eight days; the notch in the eyelid is already much more shallow. *D*, Healed lesion after 15 months; no recurrence in eight years. (Reproduced with permission from Mohs FE: Chemosurgery: Microscopically Controlled Surgery for Skin Cancer. Springfield, Ill, Charles C Thomas, 1978.)

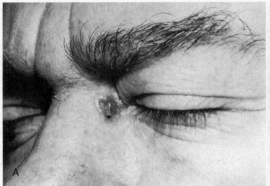

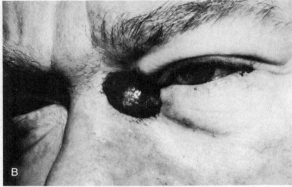

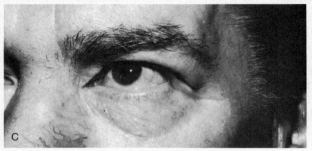

Figure 28–6. *A,* Basal cell carcinoma in the medial canthal area. *B,* Lesion after the excision was completed in three microscopically controlled stages. The medial ends of the eyelids as well as the canthus were invaded, but enough commissural tissue was left to obviate the need for a medial tarsorrhaphy. *C,* Healed lesion five months later showing how the scar contraction restored the canthus; no recurrence in five years.

around the optic nerve require removal of the eye. This is usually done by injecting lidocaine into the posterior orbit and removing the eye with the Bovie electrosurgical apparatus. If such extensive lesions involve bone, the use of the fixed-tissue technique may then be indicated.

Nasal Cancers

Many patients with cancers of the nose become candidates for microcontrolled surgery, not only because of the high incidence of carcinoma on this sun-exposed structure but also because most nasal neoplasms tend to grow inwardly and often send out silent extensions. These lead to a relatively high incidence of recurrence following treatment with methods lacking complete microscopic control of excision. In a series of 2711 cases of basal cell carcinomas of the nose, more than 25% of the patients had received previous treatment with some form of surgery or radiation.[3]

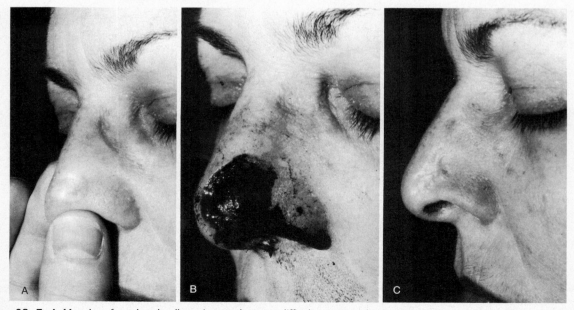

Figure 28–7. *A,* Morphea-form basal cell carcinoma that was difficult to see without manually blanching the area. *B,* Lesion after excision of the first layer. Three more excisions were required because of considerable peripheral extension of the cancer; only a small amount of cartilage had to be removed. *C,* Healed lesion after one year; no recurrence in five years.

A common site for basal cell carcinoma is the nasal ala; the ingrowing type is by far the most common variety. If the cancer does not invade through the full thickness of the ala, the lesions heal very well by second intention. This is exemplified by a morphea-form basal cell carcinoma that extended peripherally more than deeply (Fig. 28–7). However, if the cancer invades through or almost through the ala, a simple closure of the defect is cosmetically and functionally effective (Fig. 28–8). Cancers in the nasolabial fold area often extend deeply into the embryologic fusion plane. These lesions heal well by granulation, but if very deep and large, closure may be needed to prevent distortion of the upper lip.

Cancers of the tip and bridge of the nose may extend so deeply that a permanent depression may form if it is left to heal by second intention. This complication can be prevented by a simple transverse closure (Fig. 28–9). Lesions on the root of the nose heal so well by granulation that there is usually no need for closure (Fig. 28–10). However, if the cancer is so extensive that the nasal bone and septal cartilage are exposed, a simple vertical closure, or even a partial closure, can give very good results. The procedure not only covers the bone and cartilage to prevent desiccation necrosis but also brings the subcutaneous tissue up to the skin level and prevents deformity.[16]

Cancers of the Ear

Because the structure of the ear is so dependent upon the cartilaginous framework that supports the relatively thin overlying integument, it is important

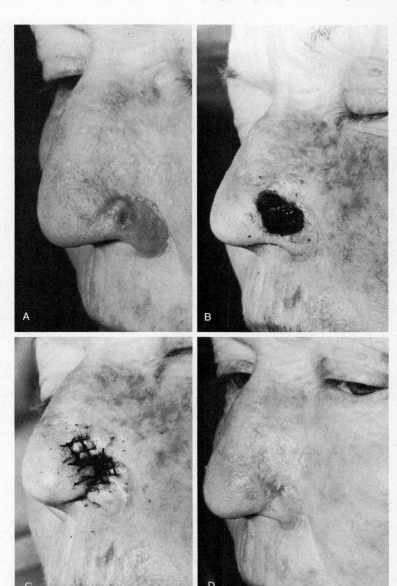

Figure 28–8. *A*, Basal cell carcinoma on the nasal ala. *B*, Lesion after excision in three stages; the cancer invaded so deeply that the tissue in the center was paper thin. *C*, Lesion after three-legged closure with the sutures placed to prevent upward traction of the rima. *D*, Healed lesion after five months; no recurrence in five years.

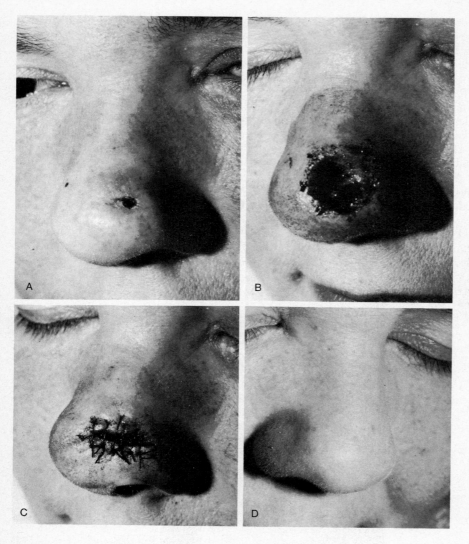

Figure 28–9. *A*, Basal cell carcinoma that arose in a chicken pox scar. *B*, Lesion after excision of the deeply invading neoplasm in three stages. *C*, Lesion after partial transverse closure that brought the subcutaneous tissue up to the skin level. *D*, Healed lesion after five years.

to save as much cartilage as possible without jeopardizing the assurance of eradication of cancers of these structures. Microscopically controlled surgery fulfills these requirements.

Cancers of the helix, unless very early, are likely to involve the perichondrium and require exposure of the cartilage. Often the cartilage can be kept intact by a simple anterior-posterior closure over the exposed cartilage (Fig. 28–11). Another way of coping with necessary loss of cartilage of the helix is by sacrificing some of the helix on both sides of the notch. Contouring of the ear in this way often produces a pleasing cosmetic result.[17]

Although cartilage provides a barrier through which cancer does not readily invade, extensive cancers, or two cancers on opposing sides of the ear, may require removal of a large segment of cartilage. In such cases, a satisfactory repair may be achieved by the removal of a wedge in such a way that a closure produces a well-shaped ear even though somewhat smaller than its opposite. Another

solution, when it has been necessary to produce a hole through the ear, is to fill the defect with a flap from the postauricular skin.[17]

Cancers of the antihelix and outer concha or on the opposing posterior surface of the ear usually are in areas where the cartilage impedes passage of the neoplasm to the other side. However, the perichondrium usually must be removed, exposing cartilage that would not support epithelialization. This requires removal of enough cartilage to produce a window through which granulation can develop from the opposite side.[14] However, care must be used to avoid removal of the perichondrium on the opposide side because the resultant vascular defect can cause a perforation through the full thickness of the ear.

In the inner conchal area the removal of any amount of cartilage is inconsequential because there is no chance of perforation. Cancers in the external auditory canal can be followed medially to the eardrum if necessary. A good headlight, slender instruments, and a loupe are essential. In some situations, an operating microscope is very helpful. If bleeding is too troublesome, despite suction, it may be expedient to change to the fixed-tissue technique to provide a bloodless field. Another possible advantage of the fixed-tissue technique is that the sharp demarcation that permits complete removal of the fixed bone and cartilage results in less formation of exuberant granulation tissue, which can be a cause of stenosis of the canal.

Cancers of the tragal and preauricular regions present no problems unless there is invasion of the temporomandibular joint, the external carotid artery, or the branches of the facial nerve. Entry into the temporomandibular joint is not a serious complication because ankylosis never develops, and if there is some destruction of joint structures, the adjacent fibrous and muscular tissue hold the structures in place and permit mastication. However, if appreciable amounts of the articular process must be removed, there may be some malocclusion. If the external carotid or superficial temporal artery is involved, the vessel is clamped with a hemostat as the layers are excised. Then, after a plane free of cancer has been reached, a suture-ligature is placed around the artery.

Invasion of cancer into the parotid gland requires care to remove only tissues that are invaded because of the proximity to branches of the facial nerve. Temporary salivary fistulas may result from the entrance into small parotid ducts. These usually can be caused to close by cauterization with dichloroacetic acid. This gives an advantage to the skin that then grows across since it is more suited to exposure to air than parotid duct epithelium.

Cancers of the Nonorificial Areas

Usually, there are relatively few difficulties in treating cancers in nonorificial sites. As in other areas, the assurance of eradication of the cancer and the lack of need to remove wide extra margins of tissues are important benefits of complete microscopic control.

Cancers of the scalp can be very troublesome because clinically inapparent outgrowths may extend for considerable distances in several strata including the dermis, lymphatic plexuses, fascial planes above and below the galea, and the pericranium. The microscopic control safely permits sparing of maxi-

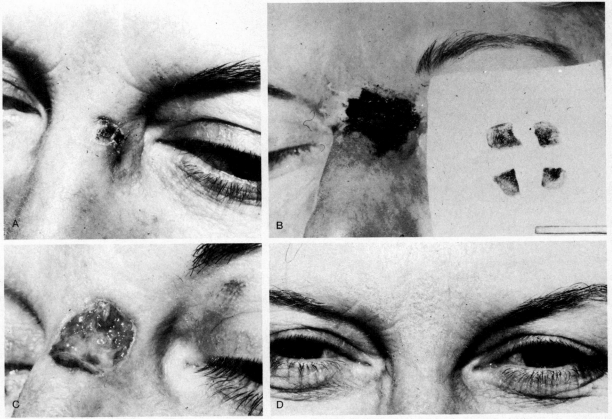

Figure 28–10. *A*, Basal cell carcinoma of the nasal root. *B*, Lesion with Oxycel cotton in place for hemostasis after the excision of the second layer; sections of the four specimens revealed two cancerous downgrowths, which required two more excisions. *C*, Granulation tissue after ten days. *D*, Healed lesion after two years; no recurrence in five years.

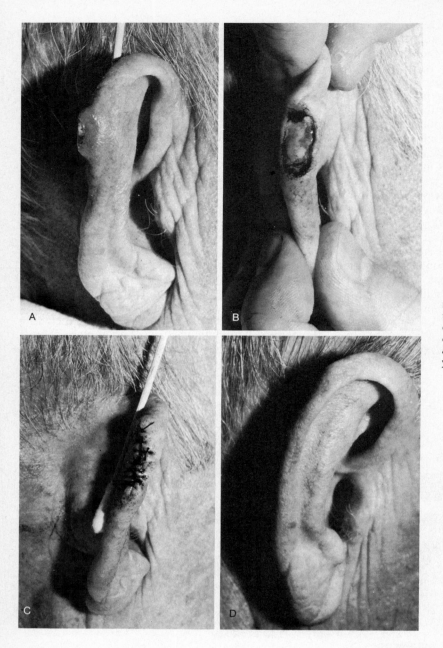

Figure 28–11. *A*, Squamous cell carcinoma on the helix. *B*, Exposure of cartilage that was necessary because the perichondrium was invaded. *C*, Anterior-posterior closure over the cartilage. *D*, Healed lesion after three months; no recurrence in four years.

mal amounts of normal tissues, and the scar contraction greatly reduces the hairless area. If cranial bone is involved, the affected bone can be removed with a chisel and, after decalcification, frozen sections can be prepared to povide microscopic control of the excision of the cancer in the bone. Even invasion through the inner table is not too serious, although sterile precautions are particularly important. Defects through the bone will become covered with granulations that support the ingrowth of epithelium or, if large, the take of a graft. The scar pulsates for several weeks, but as it becomes firm, the pulsation ceases. There is no need for insertion of metal or plastic plates. Entrance into large vascular structures such as the sagittal sinus are not overly serious because the hemorrhage can be controlled with a pledget of Oxycel cotton held in place with a pressure dressing. The resultant clot organizes to form a scar that closes these thin-walled vascular sinuses.

The outstanding reliability of microcontrolled surgery in the treatment of scalp neoplasms has been documented as follows: In a series of 576 patients with basal cell carcinomas, the five-year cure rate was 98.9% in the 444 patients in the determinate group, while in a series of 131 patients with squamous cell carcinomas, the five-year cure rate was 98.8% in the 83 patients in the determinate group.[18]

Large lesions on the temples and cheeks often heal by granulation with scars that are cosmetically acceptable. The sparing of tissue and the soft, smooth, well-vascularized scars are benefits, and the microscopic control is especially reassuring when the neoplasm is a treacherous, recurrent, morphea-form basal cell carcinoma (Fig. 28–12).

Large medial cheek lesions that may result in deformities such as upward traction of the upper lip or downward traction of the lower eyelid often can be repaired well with a simple vertical closure. If the patient had previous unsuccessful surgical and other treatments that may have resulted in clinically unrecognized outlying foci of cancer, such a simple closure can be safer than undermining to permit a more complicated repair or using grafts or flaps to cover the defect.[16]

Lesions on the forehead heal well by second intention, but since the whitish scars may be noticeable in this prominent part of the face, a transverse closure in a wrinkle line is often preferable. If the lesion is above the lateral brow, a rhomboid flap from the adjacent temporal area not only prevents a noticeable scar but also prevents upward traction on the lateral eyebrow.

Cancers of the skin of the upper lip commonly extend down to the vermilion border. Although these heal quite well by granulation with vertical linear scars, there is often better healing by vertical closure. Cancers of the skin of the lower lip and chin similarly often heal well by granulation, but in some situations, closures yield better cosmetic and functional results.

Cancers of the Extremities and Trunk

The complete microscopic control of excision is of particular value in assuring complete removal of cancers of the hands, where maximal sparing of

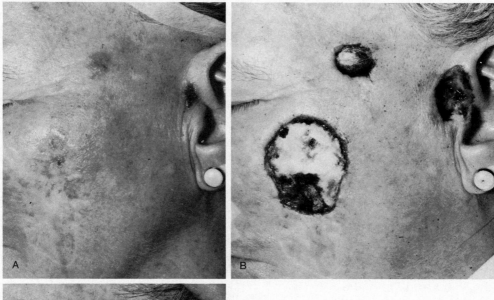

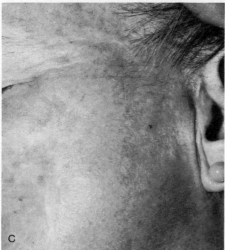

Figure 28–12. *A,* Morphea-form basal cell of mid-cheek of 15 years duration that had recurred after a course of x-ray therapy and four operations with grafting. There also were new basal cell carcinomas on the temple and the anterior helix. *B,* Lesions after the excision of the cheek lesion in three microscopically controlled stages and of the other lesions in two stages each. *C,* The lesions healed by granulation with a satisfactory appearance after one year. No recurrence in five years.

normal tissue is especially important. For example, physicians and dentists who develop squamous cell carcinoma of the hands and fingers from exposure to x-rays are in danger of losing their means of livelihood if these cancers cannot be controlled without extensive loss of structure and function. Cancers of the dorsum of the hand, even if they invade around the tendons, can be removed with no loss of the grasping function of the hand.

Cancers of the plantar surface of the feet can be removed and permitted to heal by second intention. Importantly, the patients can walk on the scars without discomfort. Verrucous carcinoma of the feet, formerly called epithelioma cuniculatum, can be removed with the fresh-tissue technique unless there is bone involvement, in which case the fixed-tissue technique may be preferable.[7]

Cancers of the Lip

Squamous cell carcinomas of the lower lip like cancers of the skin often send out clinically inapparent outgrowths for unpredictable distances from the main mass. Microcontrolled surgery provides a way to selectively follow these ramifications and to obviate the need for the removal of a relatively large portion of the lip. This sparing of normal tissue makes it possible to excise most cancers so conservatively that a simple anterior-posterior closure is often feasible (Fig. 28–13). However, if the cancer proves to be so extensive that a deep notch must be produced, a V-wedge closure is performed.[19] Of course, the regional nodes must be kept under observation, as is necessary with squamous cell carcinoma in other areas. Prophylactic node dissections are no longer practiced, but an effort is made to detect possible metastatic nodes before they reach a centimeter in diameter.

Cancers of the Vulva and Perineum

Squamous cell carcinomas of the vulva, perineum, and anal area as well as the uncommon basal cell carcinomas of these areas are amenable to treatment with fresh-tissue technique.[3] However, as with treatment of squamous cell carcinomas of the lips and other areas, precautions are taken to avoid implantation on the excisional surface. Usually, the surface is cauterized with dichloroacetic acid after the initial debulking excision, and as subsequent layers are removed, the wound is flushed with either boric acid solution or normal saline. The wounds heal so well by second intention that closure is only occasionally indicated. Every effort is made to have the patients return for follow-up examination so that if metastases should occur, they are detected very early, at which stage a successful regional node dissection is likely.

Verrucous carcinoma in the genito-gluteal area, although relatively less malignant than most squamous cell carcinomas, can still be troublesome because of the occurrence of silent outgrowths. Therefore, microcontrolled surgery provides the best chance of cure with the least loss of normal tissue.[7]

Extramammary Paget's disease in the vulvar and perineal regions is most effectively treated with the fresh-tissue technique, because the abnormal cells are often found a long distance from the clinically apparent disease. It is important to recognize the small, immature Paget's cells in the basal layer of the epidermis as well as the large, clear typical cells in order to be sure a plane free of neoplastic cells has been reached.[20]

COMMENTS

Advantages of Microcontrolled Surgery

Reliability. This is the most important attribute of microscopically controlled surgery. It is manifested by the high five-year rates of cure, some of which are presented in other sections in this chapter on melanoma and cancers of the penis, scalp, and lip. Crissey[21] has compared the five-year cure rates achieved with the fixed-tissue technique (99.3%) with the average of the best rates achieved by 12 other authors with other modalities including cold knife surgery (85.5%), curettage and electrodesiccation (92.6%), and radiation (94.7%). The same high rates of cure are being achieved with the fresh-tissue technique.

Recurrent basal cell carcinoma is a particularly good indication for microcontrolled study. In a series of 1387 determinate cases of patients treated with the fixed-tissue technique, the five-year cure rate was 96.8%.[3] In contrast, for recurrent basal cell carcinomas retreated with the original methods of curettage and electrodesiccation, surgery, or radiation, the cure rated was barely 50% in the series of 95 cases reported by Menn and colleagues.[22]

High rates of cure were also achieved with squamous cell carcinoma. In a series of 3299 cases of cutaneous squamous cell carcinoma removed with the fixed-tissue technique, the five-year cure rate was 94%.[3] As mentioned previously, the five-year cure rate of 94.2% was achieved in a series of 1448 cases of squamous cell carcinoma of the lower lip that were treated with the fixed- and fresh-tissue techniques.[19]

In general, the only circumstances that prevent successful results are invasion of vital structures or metastasis that cannot be controlled.

Sparing of Normal Tissue. This is an important benefit of the complete microscopic control because most skin cancers are on the face. Many facial lesions heal well by second intention, but if a repair is needed, the preservation of maximal amounts of

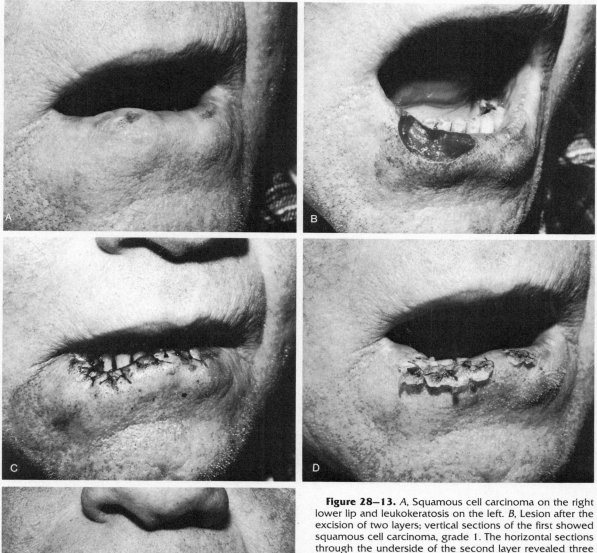

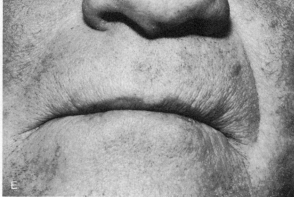

Figure 28–13. *A*, Squamous cell carcinoma on the right lower lip and leukokeratosis on the left. *B*, Lesion after the excision of two layers; vertical sections of the first showed squamous cell carcinoma, grade 1. The horizontal sections through the underside of the second layer revealed three downgrowths, the main one being posterior to the orbicularis oris muscle. Two more excisions were needed to reach a plane that was free of cancer. *C*, Lesion after anterior-posterior closure; collodion was applied and no other dressing was needed. *D*, Lesion one week later; the notch in the lip had already filled in considerably. *E*, Lesion after two years showed no defect and little visible scar; no recurrence in five years. (Reproduced with permission from Mohs FE, Snow SN: Microscopically controlled surgical treatment of squamous cell carcinoma of the lower lip. Surgery, Gynecology & Obstetrics, 160:37–41, 1985.)

normal tissue facilitates the reconstruction. The sparing of tissue is particularly important when the cancer approaches such important structures as an eye or the facial nerve. Only one or two millimeters beyond the furthest ramifications of the cancer must be removed.

Both the reliability and the sparing of normal tissues are consequences of the microscopic control that permits selective removal of the silent outgrowths that may extend for a considerable distance beyond the clinically observed borders of the neoplasm. These unpredictable outgrowths at times follow specific structures such as dermis, fascial planes, periosteum, perichondrium, lymphatic vessels, nerve sheaths, embryonic fusion planes, or the adventitia of blood vessels. However, some cancers have no special tissue affinity, but may spread unpredictably because of the countless mechanical and nutritive factors that affect the spread of cancer through the tissues.[1] Whatever the mode of spread, the microscopic control makes it possible to follow the ramifications in an accurate and controlled manner.

Low Operative Risk. This is partly a result of the lack of need for general anesthesia and partly because most patients remain ambulatory during treatment, with consequent decreased danger of pulmonary, circulatory, or embolic complications. Because many patients with cancers are elderly and in fragile general health, they tend to be more susceptible to these complications than the average patient. Other favorable factors are the lack of complications from the breakdown or infection of wounds, and the more conservative excision that is safely possible because the microscopic control obviates the need to remove a wide margin of apparently normal tissue.

In a series of 13,015 patients, many with extensive basal cell or squamous cell carcinomas, there were only 17 deaths during or shortly after treatment, a mortality rate of 0.13%.[3]

Excellent Healing. Following removal of cancers with either the fixed- or fresh-tissue techniques, the resulting scars are soft, smooth, and pliable. If a repair is needed, there is a maximum amount of well-vascularized tissue to favor good healing following the plastic repair. There is no danger of ulceration or malignant change in the scar.

Extension of Operability. Patients with cancers too extensive for hope of cure with other methods can be helped by the microscopic control and other technical advantages.

Disadvantages

Though excising cancer under complete microscopic control is simple in concept, its practice is somewhat more involved. Therefore, for optimum results, physicians who elect to enter this field should have a year's training in the operative technique and particularly in the interpretation of the microscopic sections. Also the preparation of the large, complete microscopic sections requires some special training and experience on the part of the tissue technician.

Pain from the penetration of the fixative with the fixed-tissue technique and pain from the multiple injections of the local anesthetic with the fresh-tissue technique are still present but to a decreasing extent as improvements evolve. For example, the debulking excision of the main cancerous mass under local anesthesia prior to the use of the fixed-tissue technique reduces the discomfort. In the treatment of melanoma where the fixed-tissue technique is used throughout, the injection of a local anesthetic a distance from the neoplasm reduces the pain of the initial application of the chemicals. The fresh-tissue technique with the use of a local anesthetic before the excision of each layer greatly reduces pain. The pain of injecting often can be minimized by making the first injection around the nerve supplying the area so that subsequent injections are relatively painless. Of course, analgesics ranging from acetaminophen to morphine may be used as needed with both the fixed- and fresh-tissue techniques.

CONCLUSIONS

The concept of excising cutaneous cancers under complete microscopic control is important because many of these neoplasms send out slender strands of cancer cells for considerable distances beyond the grossly visible and palpable borders. Whether the microscopic guidance is achieved with the fixed-tissue or the fresh-tissue technique, the procedure consists of the layer-by-layer excision of the tissues of the cancerous area with scanning of the undersurface of each layer in the microscope by the systematic use of frozen sections. The microscopic guidance makes it possible to remove the cancer with a high degree of selectivity, with a great assurance of the eradication of the cancer, and with the maximum sparing of adjacent normal tissues.

There are well over 100 physicians practicing microcontrolled surgery, but some larger centers of population still lack facilities and personnel for this much-needed procedure. Almost all dermatologists have some acquaintance with this method, and active interest is being shown by increasing numbers of otolaryngologists,[23, 24] facial plastic surgeons,[16, 25] surgeons,[26] head and neck surgeons,[27] oculoplastic surgeons,[13, 28-31] and plastic surgeons.[32, 33] With training centers, mostly university-based, in some 15 cities, it should not be long before physicians well-trained in microscopically controlled surgery will be available in all parts of the country.

Because of evolving changes in microscopically controlled surgery, there have been some attempts to devise a name that would be short and accurately descriptive. "Chemosurgery" has come to be synonymous with microscopically controlled surgery, but with the advent of the fresh-tissue technique, it became a misnomer. I have been using "microcontrolled surgery" because it could be an accurately descriptive term if it becomes generally recognized as meaning layer-by-layer, microscopically controlled excisions as described in this chapter. However, the possibility that uninformed individuals might say that conventional surgical excision and sending the specimen to the laboratory could also be called "microcontrolled" surgery recently led the members of the American College of Chemosurgery to vote to adopt the term "micrographic surgery," indicating that the specimens are examined in the microscope (micro) and maps are drawn to show where the flat, horizontal specimens originated (graphic). To be doubly sure, there would be no misunderstanding, they voted to adopt the name "Mohs micrographic surgery."[34] Some writers have shortened the name still further to "Mohs surgery."[35]

REFERENCES

1. Mohs FE, Lathrop TG: Modes of spread of cancer of skin. Arch Dermatol 66:427–439, 1952
2. Helm F, Milgrom H, Phelan JT, Klein E: Zur chemochirurgischen Behandlung der Hautkarzinome. Chemochirurgische Methode (nach Mohs) einer mikroskopisch kontrollierten Behandlung von Hautkrebsen. Derma Wschr, 150:451–458, 1964
3. Mohs FE: Chemosurgery: Microscopically Controlled Surgery for Skin Cancer. Springfield, Ill, Charles C Thomas, 1978
4. Lunsford CJ, Templeton HJ, Allington HV, Allington RR: Use of chemosurgery in dermatologic practice. Arch Dermatol Syph 69:148–156, 1953
5. Tromovitch TA, Stegman SJ: Microscopically controlled excision of skin tumors: Chemosurgery (Mohs): Fresh tissue technique. Arch Dermatol 110:231–232, 1974
6. Mohs FE, Snow SN, Messing EM, Kuglitsch ME: Microscopically controlled surgery in the treatment of carcinoma of the penis. J Urol 133:961–966, 1985
7. Mohs FE, Sahl WJ: Chemosurgery for verrucous carcinoma. J. Dermatol Surg Oncol 5:302–306, 1979
8. Mohs FE: Chemosurgical treatment of melanoma: A microsurgically controlled method of excision. Arch Dermatol Syph 62:269–279, 1950
9. Mohs FE: Chemosurgery for melanoma. Arch Dermatol 113:285–291, 1977
10. Mohs FE, Bloom RF, Sahl WJ: Chemosurgery for familial malignant melanoma. J Dermatol Surg Oncol 5:127–131, 1979
11. Mohs FE: The width and depth of spread of malignant melanomas as observed by a chemosurgeon. Am J Dermatopath 6:Suppl 1, Summer 1984, pp 123–126
12. Mohs FE: Microscopically controlled surgery for periorbital melanoma: Fixed-tissue and fresh-tissue techniques. J Dermatol Surg Oncol 11:284–291, 1985
13. Mohs FE: The chemosurgical method for the microscopically controlled excision of external cancer with reference to cancer of the eyelids. Trans Am Ophthalmol Otolaryngol, Course 483, Instruction Section 62:355–356, 1958
14. Mohs FE: Chemosurgery for skin cancer. Fixed tissue and fresh tissue techniques. Arch Dermatol 11:211–215, 1976
15. Mohs FE: Microscopically controlled excision of medial canthal carcinomas. Ann Plast Surg 7:308–311, 1981
16. Mohs FE: Chemosurgery. Clinics in Plast Surg 7:349–360, 1980
17. Mohs FE: Chemosurgery: Microscopically controlled surgery for skin cancer—past, present, and future. J Dermatol Surg Oncol 4:41–54, 1978
18. Mohs FE, Zitelli JA: Microscopically controlled surgery in the treatment of carcinoma of the scalp. Arch Dermatol 117:764–769, 1981
19. Mohs FE, Snow SN: Microscopically controlled surgical treatment of squamous cell carcinoma of the lower lip. Surg Gynecol Obstet 160:37–41, 1985
20. Mohs FE, Blanchard L: Microscopically controlled surgery for extramammary Paget's disease. Arch Dermatol 115:706–708, 1979
21. Crissey JT: Curettage and electrodesiccation as a method of treatment for epitheliomas of the skin. J Surg Oncol 3:287–290, 1971
22. Menn H, Robins P, Kopf A, Bart R: The recurrent basal cell epitheliomas. Arch Dermatol 103:628–631, 1971
23. Mohs FE: Chemosurgery for facial neoplasms. Arch Otolaryngol 95:62–67, 1972
24. Mohs FE: Chemosurgical techniques. Otolaryngol Clinics of North America 15:209–224, 1982
25. Mohs FE: New aspects of microscopically controlled surgery for facial carcinoma and melanoma, in Bernstein L: Plastic and Reconstructive Surgery of the Head and Neck. New York, Grune & Stratton, 1981, pp 46–59
26. Phelan JT: The usage of the Mohs' chemosurgery technique in the treatment of basal cell carcinoma. Ann Surg 168:1023–1029, 1968
27. Mohs FE: Chemosurgery for the microsurgically controlled excision of cutaneous cancer. Head and Neck Surg 1:150–164, Nov/Dec 1978
28. Mohs FE: Chemosurgical treatment of cancer of the eyelid. A microscopically controlled method of excision. Arch Ophthalmol 39:43–59, 1948
29. Cole JG: Histologically controlled excision of eyelid tumors. Am J Ophthalmol 70:240–244, 1970
30. Callahan A, Monheit GD, Callahan MA: Cancer excision from eyelids and ocular adnexa: The Mohs' fresh-tissue technique and reconstruction. CA—A Cancer J for Clinicians 32:323–329, 1982
31. Ceilley RJ, Anderson RL: Microscopically controlled excision of malignant neoplasms on and around eyelids followed by immediate surgical reconstruction. J Dermatol Surg Oncol 4:55–62, 1978
32. Shepard RA: Chemosurgery in the treatment of carcinoma of the skin. J Int Coll Surg 30:220–228, 1958
33. Becker FF: Reconstruction of facial defects resulting from Mohs' chemosurgical procedures. J Dermatol Surg Oncol 4:69–76, 1978
34. Mohs FE: Micrographic surgery for the microscopically controlled excision of eyelid cancers. Arch Ophthalmol. In press.
35. Swanson NA: Mohs surgery. Arch Dermatol 119:761–773, 1983

29

RICHARD B. ODOM, M.D.

Fluorouracil

In 1957, Heidelberger and his associates synthesized 5-fluorouracil (FU) as a member of a new class of tumor-inhibiting compounds. A few years later, FU became established as a useful chemotherapeutic agent in the palliative management of advanced carcinoma. In 1962, Falkson and Schulz reported inflammation and eventual clearing of multiple actinic keratoses in a patient treated with systemic FU for cancer. That same year, Klein and Dillaha and their coworkers described the selective cytotoxic effects of topical FU and introduced it into the therapeutic armamentarium of dermatologists.

Topical FU has become increasingly accepted because of its efficacy, economy, good cosmetic results, and relative absence of side effects in treating certain dermatoses, precancerous conditions, and various benign and malignant tumors. 5-Fluorouracil is a fluorinated pyrimidine belonging to the category of antimetabolites. Fluorouracil resembles the natural uracil molecule in structure, except that a hydrogen atom has been replaced by a fluorine atom in the 5 position. There is evidence that the metabolism of FU in the anabolic pathway blocks the methylation reaction of deoxyuradilic acid to thymidylic acid. In this fashion, FU interferes with the synthesis of deoxyribonucleic acid (DNA) and, to a lesser extent, inhibits the formation of ribonucleic acid (RNA). Since DNA and RNA are essential for cell division and growth, the effect of FU may be to create a thymine deficiency that provokes unbalanced growth and death of the cell. The effects of DNA and RNA deprivation are most marked on those cells that grow more rapidly and take up FU at a more rapid pace.

Results of several studies on percutaneous absorption of FU concluded that the amount systemically absorbed is too small to produce systemic side effects. Applying 2 gm of 5% FU cream daily would result in the systemic absorption of approximately 10 mg FU, which is well below the maximum daily dose of 12 mg/kg for cancer chemotherapy.

Fluorouracil is commercially available as 1% solution or cream, as a 2% to 5% solution, and as a 5% cream. A 20% ointment can be compounded by lyophilization of commercially available intravenous FU solution and incorporation of the resulting powder into hydrophilic petrolatum. For intralesional use, the intravenous solution of FU (50 mg/ml) is utilized.

Therapeutic response to FU depends on many factors, including the vehicle and concentration of FU, frequency of application, sites treated, patient's complexion, amount of sun exposure during treatment, and the extent and severity of the disease.

The patient is instructed to apply FU twice daily after the skin has been thoroughly washed. Early signs of inflammation appear on the face within three to five days and on the scalp, the neck, the back, and the chest within four to seven days following application; 10 to 14 days may elapse before a reaction is visible on the dorsa of the hands and forearms. For particularly hyperkeratotic lesions, pretreatment with a keratolytic preparation for one to two weeks is helpful. Occlusion under a polyethylene wrap enhances absorption and promotes more rapid clearing of the lesions. The guidelines for the choice of FU concentration and the duration of the therapy according to the site are as follows: face and lips, 1% to 2% FU for three weeks; scalp and neck, 5% FU for four weeks; back and chest, 5% FU for 4 to 6 weeks; arms and hands, 5% FU for six to eight weeks.

Evaluation of therapy at seven- to 10-day intervals by the physician will facilitate determining when a maximum reaction or peak response has occurred and when the lesions have been destroyed. The lesion disintegration phase is characterized by erosion and ulceration, intense inflammation, discomfort, pain, crusting, eschar formation, and evidence of re-epithelization that may occur during continued treatment. At this phase, a corticosteroid ointment is applied two to four times daily. Over the ensuing one to two weeks, healing takes place with residual erythema and occasional temporary hyperpigmentation.

Patients should be thoroughly indoctrinated regarding the possible undesirable cosmetic effects of FU — preferably through pictorial exhibits provided by pharmaceutical companies.

Special care should be taken when applying FU to areas near the lips, nose, and eyes because of the sensitivity of these areas. Light-complexioned persons undergoing this therapy should refrain from exposure to the sun, to avoid intensifying the skin reaction. When reactions are too vigorous, reduced frequency of application, a lowered concentration of FU, temporary interruption of treatment, and the use of lubricants or topical corticosteroids will

TABLE 29–1. Entities for Which FU Use Has Been Reported

A. Precancerous Conditions
   1. Actinic (senile, solar) keratoses
   2. Actinic cheilitis—leukoplakia
   3. Chronic radiodermatitis
   4. Xeroderma pigmentosum
   5. Bowen's disease
   6. Bowenoid papulosis
   7. Erythroplasia of Queyrat
   8. Paget's disease
   9. Lentigo maligna
B. Malignant Tumors
   1. Basal cell carcinoma
   2. Squamous cell carcinoma
   3. Metastatic carcinoma
C. Benign Tumors
   1. Keratoacanthoma
   2. Seborrheic keratoses
   3. Warts
D. Dermatoses
   1. Psoriasis
   2. Mycosis fungoides
   3. Porokeratoses
   4. Pityriasis rubra pilaris
   5. Darier's disease
   6. Vitiligo

ameliorate the irritant dermatitis within a few days. The dermatologic conditions for which FU has been used are listed in Table 29–1.

Precancerous Conditions

Actinic Keratoses. Topical FU is extremely effective in clearing multiple actinic keratoses. Besides clearing grossly visible multiple lesions as well as those that are only microscopically present, topical FU unmasks and outlines malignant lesions such as basal cell and squamous cell carcinomas.

Usually FU is applied sparingly twice daily and rubbed in well after the skin has been washed thoroughly. The duration of treatment is arbitrarily determined by the peak response of FU, since reliable criteria for the endpoint are not available. A change in color from bright to dusky red, evidence of re-epithelization, widespread crust formation, and increasing pruritus signal the endpoint. The patient who experiences the most pronounced reaction will have the best overall result and the least number of keratoses developing or recurring in subsequent months.

Concomitant use of a topical corticosteroid during FU treatment for noninflammatory elimination of actinic keratoses has been recommended. Extremely low concentrations of FU, such as 0.01%, applied once daily for several months, allegedly clears actinic keratoses without any visible dermatitis. Continuous use has been advocated for prophylaxis. Early studies question the efficacy of low concentrations of FU and cast doubt on the prophylactic

effect of such therapy. Most studies conducted to date report high recurrence rates after various concentrations of topical FU. Most patients will develop new lesions or recurrences within two to three years. Persistent, recurrent or new lesions can be managed by cryotherapy or electrosurgery.

Actinic Cheilitis and Leukoplakia

Several authors have reported success in treating actinic cheilitis and labial, intraoral, and vulvar leukoplakia.

Actinic cheilitis and leukoplakia of the lip treated with FU develop a prompt response, as manifested by erosion, inflammation, and moderate discomfort. Pretreatment biopsies for firm, indurated, ulcerated, or persisting lesions are recommended highly.

A 1% solution applied twice daily is adequate to elicit a vigorous response that is often complicated by moderate to severe discomfort and eschar formation. Soaking the lip 30 minutes before reapplying FU removes crusts, thereby permitting better penetration and efficacy of the preparation. Discomfort may be alleviated by liberal use of topical lidocaine gel.

Vulvar leukoplakia has been successfully treated with a 20% cream. Intraoral leukoplakia has partially or completely resolved following prolonged periods of treatment.

Leukoplakia of the genital tract and actinic cheilitis are excellent indications for treatment with topical FU and may preclude the necessity for surgery and its undesirable side effects.

Radiodermatitis. Topical FU in concentrations ranging from 1% to 5% are effective for the treatment of patients with keratoses and premalignant lesions developing in areas of radiodermatitis. Fluorouracil is useful in treating these components of extensive radiodermatitis.

Xeroderma Pigmentosum. Topical FU is useful in treating existing premalignant and malignant lesions in patients with xeroderma pigmentosum, especially when combined with sunscreens and restrictions of exposure to ultraviolet light. After such treatment, keratoses and tumors may continue to evolve, though more slowly and in reduced numbers. Cutaneous resistance to FU treatment may develop after prolonged treatment.

Bowen's Disease. Bowen's disease or carcinoma in situ has been treated successfully with topical FU in concentrations of 1% to 5%. The difficulty with this form of therapy in Bowen's disease is that there is residual disease in the depth of hair follicles that may lead to recurrences. Other causes for exacerbations include insufficient concentration of topical FU, inadequate length of treatment, and treating too small an area surrounding clinically apparent disease. Enhancement techniques including keratolytic agents, retinoic acid, and occlusion have been utilized to facilitate penetration of FU.

Fluorouracil therapy has been found to be as effective in treating Bowen's disease in genital areas (vulva, perineum, and penile shaft) as in nongenital locations. Usually, 5% FU cream is employed for two to 14 weeks. Some patients experience severe discomfort and pain that may necessitate temporary interruption of treatment. Topical lidocaine as a 2% gel or a 5% cream may alleviate pain and improve patient cooperation and compliance. Inadequate concentration of FU and too short a course may be responsible for poor results from FU treatment of in situ genital carcinoma. Post-treatment biopsies should be performed to verify a cure, and prolonged follow-up is mandatory.

Bowenoid Papulosis. This entity is felt to be caused by a human papilloma virus, and its status as a precancerous condition is controversial. Histologically, the changes are identical to those seen in Bowen's disease. Treatment with topical FU appears to be promising, but it occasionally fails to clear up the lesions, or the lesions may reappear. The 5% FU cream is recommended, and in men, condom occlusion has enhanced the therapeutic response.

Erythroplasia of Queyrat. Based on its natural history, erythroplasia of Queyrat is considered to be an entity separate from Bowen's disease. It lends itself ideally for FU treatment because of the absence of hair folliciles in the penile mucosa that serve as foci for recurrence of this disease. Patients should be treated with 1% to 5% FU for periods of four to 17 weeks. Higher concentrations of FU appear to shorten the course of treatment, and occlusive wrapping enhances the penetration and therapeutic response.

When combined with topical anesthetics, good patient rapport, encouragement, and emotional support, topical FU remains the treatment of choice for biopsy-proved erythroplasia of Queyrat despite its frequent unpleasant side effects. It is recommended that post-treatment biopsies be performed.

Extramammary Paget's Disease. Extramammary Paget's disease represents an intraepidermal adenocarcinoma that may extend contiguously into adnexal structures and, uncommonly, into the dermis. It may recur whether treated by surgical excision, vulvectomy, curettage and desiccation, or x-ray therapy. Despite apparently good responses to 1% to 5% FU for periods of up to 12 weeks, the disease may recur or be histologically proven to persist. In extramammary Paget's disease, FU at best has a palliative effect, and because of the high incidence of recurrences, FU is not recommended for treatment of this condition.

Lentigo Maligna. Lentigo maligna responds to 5% FU cream, but because of involvement of the adnexal epithelium in this condition, recurrences are common. Therefore, topical FU is not recommended for definitive treatment.

Malignant Tumors

Basal Cell Carcinoma. Several investigators have demonstrated that FU in concentrations ranging from 1% to 30% induce resolution of basal cell carcinoma in 56% to 86% of the lesions. Patients were treated for six to 10 weeks. However, the relatively high incidence of recurrence is alarming, and some authors have shown that, after apparently successful FU treatment, the tumor may continue to grow with extensions into the depth of the dermis. It is recommended that post-treatment biopsies be performed to confirm eradication of the disease after FU use.

In superficial multicentric lesions, concentrations of 5% to 20% result in tumor resolution in 95% of the cases without recurrence and with lessening of new lesions.

Experience with topical 5% FU and intralesional FU (50 mg/ml) for the treatment of recurrent basal cell epitheliomas has been disappointing because of the unacceptable recurrence rate.

In the basal cell nevus syndrome, FU is efficient in removing existing tumors, but new lesions continue to develop. Fluorouracil has possible prophylactic value in this syndrome, although this has not been established.

For patients who refuse surgery, FU in high concentration with long-term occlusive treatment offers some hope of palliation and tumor eradication.

Squamous Cell Carcinoma. Squamous cell carcinoma is not an ideal indication for FU use. However, when surgery is refused, a 20% concentration of FU applied under occlusion for six to 12 weeks may be used in an attempt to eradicate the disease. Post-treatment biopsies and careful follow-up are mandatory in such situations.

Metastatic Carcinoma. In most instances, cutaneous metastases from breast carcinoma, malignant melanoma, adenocarcinoma of the colon, leukemic infiltration, lymphoma of the skin, and hypernephroma have failed to respond to 5% FU or reacted slightly, only to recur following topical or intralesional FU administration. Topical FU therapy of metastatic disease appears fruitless.

Benign Tumors

Keratoacanthoma. Several studies attest to the efficacy of 5% to 20% FU with or without occlusion in the treatment of keratoacanthoma. Tumors usually involute in two to five weeks.

Intralesional injection of FU (50 mg/ml) has been shown to be highly effective in treating keratoacanthomas. The lesions are injected once weekly and usually result in significant regression after three to four injections.

Topical or intralesional FU is an excellent alternative for this condition because surgery is avoided and there are good cosmetic results, an excellent cure rate, and outstanding patient acceptance.

The potential drawback of confusing a keratoacanthoma with a squamous cell carcinoma can be avoided by adhering strictly to the following diagnostic criteria for keratoacanthomas: rapid evolution of the lesion (three to six weeks), characteristic tumor morphology, location (sun-exposed area), response to treatment with involution of 60% to 80% within three weeks, and clearing in five to six weeks. Failure to conform, particularly to the last criterion, should indicate the need for surgery.

Seborrheic Keratoses. Conflicting reports surround the results of 5% FU treatment for seborrheic keratoses. One report claims 100% success after 14 to 30 days of 5% FU under occlusion. Other authors report failures with topical FU.

Warts

Condyloma Acuminatum. Successful management of these neoplasms ranges from 10% to 72% with 5% FU. Marked irritation and discomfort, occasionally leading to painful erosions and ulcerations, may dictate interruption of treatment. Response rates from 57% to 95% for the urethral meatus have been reported. The treatment program may cause intense pain.

Verrucae Vulgaris. Success rates in the range of 50% to 60% have been reported in the management of verrucae vulgaris.

Plantar Warts. These warts have responded to topical and intralesional FU ranging from 50% to 90% of the lesions in various series.

Plane Warts. Flat warts of the face may be treated with 1% to 5% FU.

Miscellaneous Dermatoses

Psoriasis. Plaque-type psoriasis has been treated successfully with 5% FU under occlusion. Erosions tend to develop in treated lesions. Recently, intravenous FU has been reported to clear psoriasis effectively.

A 1% FU solution under an occlusive wrap for four to six months promotes some improvement in the nail dystrophy of psoriasis.

Mycosis Fungoides. A 5% cream causes improvement in lesions of mycosis fungoides but results in incomplete clearing. Topical FU appears to be of no value in treating this condition.

Porokeratoses

Mibelli-Type. 5% FU applied three times daily for two to six weeks has been efficacious in several reported cases of this entity.

Porokeratosis Palmaris et Plantaris Disseminata. It is unclear whether topical FU is of benefit in this entity.

Disseminated Superficial Actinic Porokeratosis. Topical FU appears to be of no value in the management of this condition.

Pityriasis Rubra Pilaris

Topical FU is apparently of no benefit in treating pityriasis rubra pilaris.

Darier's Disease

The value of topical FU in Darier's disease is uncertain.

Kyrle's Disease

Topical FU is ineffective in this disease.

Vitiligo

In one study, 5% FU cream was applied to vitiliginous lesions under occlusive dressings following an epidermal abrasion. The treated lesions became completely eroded after seven to nine days of treatment, and FU was stopped. Within 10 days, epithelization occurred, and repigmentation began one to two weeks later. Approximately 80% of treated patients showed complete or partial repigmentation. Patients with segmental vitiligo showed no repigmentation.

Side Effects of Topical FU Therapy

Irritation. After a few days of application, topical FU causes a mild, moderate, or severe dermatitis manifested by erythema, edema, burning, stinging, and discomfort and pain.

Hyperpigmentation and Hypopigmentation

Allergic Contact Dermatitis to FU. Up to 17% of patients previously treated with one or more courses of FU become hypersensitive to the medication.

Photosensitivity and Photoprotection of FU. FU is photoprotective; however, late in the course of FU treatment, the increased irritation upon sun exposure is attributed to FU-mediated damage of atypical cells and to heat.

Concealment of Residual Cancer. FU treatment may elicit a vigorous reaction in the skin, followed by re-epithelization with residual carcinoma growing in the depth of the dermis without surface changes.

Other Side Effects of FU

Uncommon side effects include reversible onycholysis with topical and systemic FU administration and prolonged telangiectasia after topical FU treatment. One case of hypertrophic scarring was reported on a patient's back after treatment of a superficial multicentric basal cell carcinoma. Another patient developed hair regrowth after treatment with 2% FU and 0.5% triamcinolone acetonide cream. One case of bullous pemphigoid was also reported following FU treatment.

Conclusion

Topical and intralesional FU is relatively simple, effective, and economical to use. With proper patient instruction and an explantation of expected results, it enjoys good patient acceptance. Usually, the cosmetic results are excellent. Occasionally, treatment with FU may avoid the need for surgery.

The advent of topical FU has introduced a new phase in treating precancerous conditions and certain malignant and benign tumors. The aforementioned advantages and the low incidence of side effects make it an almost ideal drug for treating certain dermatologic problems. The agent must be used with discretion, in combination with pre- and post-treatment biopsies when indicated, and with consistent follow-up examinations. Fluorouracil has become an indispensable therapeutic weapon in the dermatologic armamentarium.

SUGGESTED READINGS

Cohen JL, Stoughton RB: Pentration of 5-flourouracil in excised skin. J Invest Dermatol 62:507–509, 1974

Dillaha CJ, Jansen GT, Honeycut WM, et al: Selective cytotoxic effect of topical 5-fluorouracil. Arch Dermatol 88:247–256, 1963

Falkson G, Schulz EJ: Skin changes in patients treated with 5-fluorouracil. Br J Dermatol 74:229–236, 1962

Goette DK: Topical chemotherapy with 5-flourouracil. J Am Acad Dermatol 4:633-649, 1981.

Goette DK, Odom RB: Allergic contact dermatitis to topical fluorouracil. Arch Dermatol 113:1058–1071, 1977

Heidelberger C, Chaudhuri NK, Danneburg P, et al: Fluorinated pyrimidines: A new class of tumor-inhibiting compounds. Nature 179:663–666, 1957

Klein E, Milgrom H, Helm F, et al: Tumors of the skin. I. Effects of local use of cytostatic agents. Skin 1:81–87, 1962

Litwin JJ, Ryan RF, Reed EJ, et al: Topical chemotherapy of advanced cutaneous malignancy with 5-flourouracil creme. J Surg Oncol 3:351–365, 1971

Tsuji T, Hamada T: Topically administered fluorouracil in vitiligo. Arch Dermatol 119:722-727, 1983.

ERIC C. VONDERHEID, M.D. / EUGENE J. VAN SCOTT, M.D.

30

Topical Use of Nitrogen Mustard

Nitrogen mustard (mechlorethamine; N-methyl-2,2'-dichlorodiethylamine), an analog of the war gas sulfur mustard, was first used clinically in the early 1940s for intravenous therapy of lymphoproliferative neoplasms.[1] It was found shortly thereafter that mycosis fungoides lymphoma was also alleviated by intravenously administered nitrogen mustard.[2, 3] This drug was shown later to be efficacious when applied topically on the skin lesions of mycosis fungoides, as reported by Sipos and Jáksó[4] in 1956 and by Haserick and colleagues[5] in 1959. Subsequently it was demonstrated by Van Scott and coworkers[6–8] and by many others[9–13] that dilute solutions of nitrogen mustard, when applied to the entire body surface for extended periods, could provide complete and sustained remissions and possible cures for most patients with relatively early mycosis fungoides.

PHARMACOLOGIC BASIS OF TOPICAL THERAPY

Nitrogen mustard belongs to the group of drugs known as alkylating agents, which are characterized by their ability to form strong covalent bonds with various molecular groups. Important to the therapeutic effects of nitrogen mustard is its reaction with guanine and other bases in the DNA chain resulting in DNA-interstrand and DNA-protein cross-links.[14–16] Normal DNA replication and cell division are thus impaired or prevented. Although the action of nitrogen mustard on the cell cycle is not phase specific, its toxicity on cells is more often expressed during S-phase. The cycle is arrested at the G2-phase and mitosis is prevented. Rapidly dividing cells seem to be more sensitive to the toxic effects of nitrogen mustard, although this may be more apparent than real.

The high chemical reactivity of nitrogen mustard probably accounts for a virtual absence of systemic toxicity from daily whole body topical applications, even when cutaneous tolerance is exceeded. For example, in the authors' experience in treating hundreds of patients with mycosis fungoides, no evidence of bone marrow suppression has been encountered. The relatively high frequency of contact delayed hypersensitivity associated with topical nitrogen mustard indicates that the drug avidly reacts with epidermal proteins to form complete antigens. In contrast, carmustine, a chemically less reactive and more lipid-soluble alkylating drug, penetrates the epidermis more readily, has substantial potential for systemic toxicity, and is much less frequently associated with contact delayed hypersensitivity.[17, 18]

The pharmacologic mechanism by which topically applied nitrogen mustard causes lesions of mycosis fungoides to regress would seem to be the result of its direct toxicity on neoplastic T-lymphocytes in the cutaneous infiltrate. However, it seems odd that this pronounced effect is achieved usually without evidence of analogous toxicity to keratinocytes or melanocytes. An alternative possibility might be that nitrogen mustard interferes with other epidermal components or functions, e.g., Langerhans'-cell–T-lymphocyte interactions or keratinocyte-derived lymphocyte-activating factors,[19, 20] thereby inhibiting possible basic pathogenic mechanisms in mycosis fungoides.

THERAPEUTIC OBJECTIVES

Although occult extracutaneous involvement may occur in patients with extensive cutaneous lesions of mycosis fungoides,[21, 22] current evidence indicates that the disease begins in the skin and remains confined there for substantial periods before pathologic involvement of other organs. Therefore, aggressive therapy of mycosis fungoides during its early intracutaneous phase should be potentially curative. Indeed, experience to date with total-skin electron-beam radiation,[23, 24] methoxsalen photochemotherapy,[25] and topical nitrogen mustard chemotherapy[8] supports such a supposition. Since mycosis fungoides is almost always a progressive disease, intensive treatment at an early stage with the objective of cure seems justifiable.

TECHNIQUE OF TOPICAL TREATMENT

Because of the chemical instability of nitrogen mustard in aqueous solutions, the drug must be prepared immediately before use. The authors' preferred technique is accomplished by having the patient dissolve 10 mg of the drug in about 50 ml of tap water. The patient then immediately applies the solution to both normal and involved skin once daily after bathing. The palms are moistened with the solution, which is applied sparingly to other parts of the body. The patient is advised to moisten intertriginous areas ever so lightly in order to avoid primary irritation and not to apply the solution to the genital skin. Various ways may be devised for application to the back, e.g., via cotton gauze wrapped about the dipper end of a long-handled wooden spoon. Family members may assist the patient if necessary, and they are instructed to wear plastic gloves to prevent direct contact with the drug, which could cause sensitization. The patient must rinse the webs of the fingers at the end of each application to avoid irritation or wear gloves. Higher concentrations of the drug, e.g., 20 mg per 50 ml, or more frequent applications may be used if therapeutic response is slow. Thick plaques may be treated by application of extra amounts of solution.

An alternative formulation, but in the authors' experience less satisfactory, uses petrolatum as a vehicle. This must be made by a pharmacist who takes all proper precautions in handling the nitrogen mustard. An anhydrous formulation can be made by dissolving 10 mg of nitrogen mustard in absolute alcohol and blending it into 100 gm of anhydrous petrolatum to provide a 0.01% concentration. Such anhydrous formulations do have one advantage, that of chemical stability at room temperature over extended periods.[26]

Most patients with early mycosis fungoides will have objective regression of lesions from topical nitrogen mustard chemotherapy. Depending upon the intensity of treatment, the skin becomes free of visible lesions within periods varying from six weeks to six months.[7] The authors recommend continuing daily applications for six months beyond the time of complete clinical clearing to ensure complete histologic resolution. Thereafter, applications are made less frequently, decreasing gradually to once a week provided no new lesions emerge. Maintenance therapy is discontinued after a three-year disease-free interval.

ADVERSE REACTIONS

Irritant Dermatitis

There is substantial variability among patients in their propensity to have skin irritation from this administration, and this may be due entirely to the barrier properties of the skin. Body areas most prone to develop irritant dermatitis are the intertriginous areas and the scrotum. The problem of irritation can be minimized by a thorough explanation to the patient that such areas are to receive minimal amounts of the drug and that, if signs of irritation appear, applications of the nitrogen mustard solution to those areas are to be discontinued

temporarily. If general body areas of a patient become irritated, 10 mg of the drug may be dissolved in 100 ml of water, and half the volume is applied on one day. The remaining half is stored in the freezer and used the next day immediately after thawing.

Contact Allergic Dermatitis

Nearly half of all patients with early mycosis fungoides will develop delayed hypersensitivity to nitrogen mustard.[7] Rarely does sensitivity of immediate anaphylactic type (urticaria) develop.[27] A patient's advanced age, a later stage of disease, and simultaneous or prior use of immunosuppressant drugs or procedures[7] diminish the probability of sensitization. When contact sensitivity develops, the dermatitis usually appears two to four weeks after topical therapy is initiated. Differentiation from irritant dermatitis can be made by open patch testing with serial dilutions of the drug. Irritant or allergic dermatitis has not been encountered in persons in close contact with the patient, even spouses or sexual partners, with the use of nitrogen mustard solution.

Hyperpigmentation

To most patients, this consequence of topical nitrogen mustard chemotherapy is not considered to be an adverse event. The hyperpigmentation that follows topical therapy is not simply a postinflammatory event because, while sites of lesions may be later recognized by more intense pigmentation, uninvolved skin of all body areas develops a degree of hyperpigmentation in proportion to innate pigmentogenic potential. The authors also have witnessed substantial repigmentation of vitiliginous skin in patients who have both mycosis fungoides and vitiligo.

Epidermal Carcinogenesis

As with other therapeutic agents that alter DNA, the risk of carcinogenesis from nitrogen mustard is real. Carcinogenesis from the long-term use of topical nitrogen mustard chemotherapy has been observed only in the epidermis as an increased frequency of squamous cell carcinomas on sun-exposed areas and genital skin.[28, 29] Moreover, unpublished observations by the authors indicate that a markedly enhanced risk of epidermal cancer is associated with a combination of nitrogen mustard therapy and other carcinogenic agents in immunocompromised patients. For example, the authors observed the emergence of dozens of squamous cell carcinomas in several patients with advanced mycosis fungoides whose therapy had included prior exposure to ultraviolet radiation, topical nitrogen mustard, methoxsalen photochemotherapy, and total-skin electron-beam radiation. These carcinomas have arisen on both sun-exposed and nonexposed areas; growth of the tumors has been characteristically rapid; metastasis to regional lymph nodes has occurred in at least three patients. Although trial therapy with intralesional chemotherapeutic drugs (e.g., bleomycin and 5-fluorouracil) has caused variable regression of cutaneous carcinomas, surgical excision of the lesions is the treatment of choice.

TREATMENT OF OTHER CONDITIONS WITH TOPICAL NITROGEN MUSTARD

Beneficial responses of other reticulohistiocytic diseases to topical nitrogen mustard have been reported by several authors,[30-35] and use of the drug for such diseases seems appropriate. Its use on psoriatic lesions has been explored,[36-42] and while the risk of epidermal carcinogenesis conceivably might be acceptable for the treatment of some patients with psoriasis, the high risk of allergic sensitization to the drug disqualifies it for treatment, since psoriasis is worsened by delayed hypersensitivity reactions.

REFERENCES

1. Gilman A: The initial clinical trial of nitrogen mustard. Am J Surg 105:547, 1963
2. Henstell HH, Toberg JN: Treatment of mycosis fungoides with nitrogen mustard. J Invest Dermatol 8:183, 1947
3. Kierland RR, Watkins CH, Shullenberger CC: The use of nitrogen mustard in the treatment of mycosis fungoides. J Invest Dermatol 9:195, 1947
4. Sipos K, Jáksó, G.: A Mustárnitrogen Helyi Alkamázasa Néhány börgetegségben (Local administration of nitrogen mustard in some skin disorders). Borgyogy Vener Szemle 10:198, 1956
5. Haserick JR, Richardson JH, Grant DJ: Remission of lesions in mycosis fungoides following topical application of nitrogen mustard. Cleve Clin Q 26:144, 1959
6. Van Scott EJ, Kalmanson JD: Complete remission of mycosis fungoides lymphoma induced by topical nitrogen mustard (HN2). Cancer 32:18, 1973
7. Vonderheid EC, Van Scott EJ, Grekin DA: Topical chemotherapy and immunotherapy of mycosis fungoides: Intermediate-term results. Arch Dermatol 113:454, 1977
8. Vonderheid EC, Van Scott EJ, Wallner PE, et al: A tenyear experience with topical mechlorethamine for mycosis fungoides: Comparison with patients treated by total-skin electron beam radiation therapy. Cancer Treat Rep 63:681, 1979
9. Price NM, Constantine VS, Hoppe RT, et al: Topical mechlorethamine therapy for mycosis fungoides. Br J Dermatol 97:547, 1977
10. Grupper C, Durepaire R: Topical chemotherapy in mycosis fungoides. Bull Cancer 64:323, 1977
11. Molin L, Thomsen K, Volden G, et al: Mycosis fungoides plaque stage treated with nitrogen mustard with and without attempts at tolerance induction. Report from the Scandinavian mycosis fungoides study group. Acta Dermatol Venerol 59:64, 1979
12. Hemmings B, Noordijk EM, Van Vloten WA: Treatment of mycosis fungoides: Total skin electron beam irradiation versus topical mechlorethamine. Arch Dermatol 118:150, 1982
13. Ramsay DL, Parnes RE, Dubin N: Response of mycosis fungoides to topical chemotherapy with mechlorethamine. Arch Dermatol 120:1585, 1984
14. Lawley PD, Brookes P: Interstrand cross-linking of DNA by difunctional alkylating agents. J Mol Biol 25:143, 1967
15. Thomas CB, Kohn KW, Bonner WM: Characterization of DNA-protein cross-links formed by treatment of L 1210 cells and nuclei with bis (2-chloroethyl) methylamine (nitrogen mustard). Biochemistry 17:3954, 1978
16. Verushalmi A, Yagil G: The interaction of chromatin with alkylating agents. The monofunctional action of bis (2-chloroethyl) methylamine. Eur J Biochem 103:237, 1980
17. Zackheim HS, Epstein EH Jr: Treatment of mycosis fungoides with topical nitrosourea compounds: Further studies. Arch Dermatol 111:1564, 1975
18. Zackheim HS, Epstein EH Jr, McNutt NS, et al: Topical carmustine (BCNU) for mycosis fungoides and related disorders. A 10-year-experience. J Am Acad Dermatol 9:363, 1983
19. Patterson JAK, Edelson RL: Interaction of T cells with the epidermis. Br J Dermatol 107:117, 1982
20. Luger TA, Stadler BM, Katz SI, Oppenheim JJ: Epidermal cell (keratinocyte)-derived thymocyte-activating factor (ETAF). J Immunol 127:1493, 1981
21. Bunn PA Jr, Huberman MS, Whang-Peng J, et al: Prospective staging evaluation of patients with cutaneous T cell lymphomas: Demonstration of a high frequency of extracutaneous dissemination. Ann Intern Med 93:223, 1980
22. Scheffer E, Meijer CJLM, Van Vloten WA: Dermatopathic lymphadenopathy and lymph node involvement in mycosis fungoides. Cancer 45:137, 1980
23. Hoppe R, Fuks Z, Bagshaw M: The rationale for curative radiotherapy in mycosis fungoides. Int J Radiat Oncol Biol Phys 2:843, 1977
24. Hoppe RT, Cox RS, Fuk Z, et al: Electron-beam therapy for mycosis fungoides. The Stanford University experience. Cancer Treat Rep 63:691, 1979
25. Hönigsmann H, Brenner W, Rauschmeier W, et al: Photochemotherapy for cutaneous T-cell lymphoma. J Am Acad Dermatol 10:238, 1984
26. Taylor JR, Halprin KM, Levine V, Aoyagi T: Mechlorethamine hydrochloride solutions and ointment. Arch Dermatol 116:783, 1980
27. Daughters D, Zackheim H, Maibach H: Urticaria and anaphylactoid reactions after topical application of mechlorethamine. Arch Dermatol 107:429, 1973
28. du Vivier A, Vonderheid EC, Van Scott EJ, et al: Mycosis fungoides, nitrogen mustard and skin cancer. Br J Dermatol 99:61, 1978
29. Lee LA, Fritz KA, Golitz L, et al: Second cutaneous malignancies in patients with topical nitrogen mustard. J Am Acad Dermatol 7:590, 1982
30. Dolezal JF, Thomson ST: Hand-Schüller-Christian disease in a septuagenarian. Arch Dermatol 114:85, 1978
31. Zachariae H: Histiocytosis X in two infants: Treated with topical nitrogen mustard. Br J Dermatol 100:433, 1979
32. Berman B, Chang DL, Shupack JL: Histiocytosis X: Treatment with topical nitrogen mustard. J Am Acad Dermatol 3:23, 1980
33. Goodfellow A, Cream JJ, Seed WA: Histiocytosis X with unusual facial and axillary ulceration responding to topical nitrogen mustard. J R Soc Med 75:279, 1982
34. Brant F, Lipman M, Taylor JR, et al: Topical nitrogen mustard therapy in multicentric reticulohistiocytosis. J Am Acad Dermatol 6:260, 1982
35. Volden G, Falk ES, Wisløff-Nilssen J, et al: Successful

treatment of actinic reticuloid induced by whole-body topical application of mechlorethamine. Acta Dermatol Venerol 61:353, 1981

36. Van Scott EJ, Reinertson RP: Morphologic and physiologic effects of chemotherapeutic agents in psoriasis. J Invest Dermatol 33:357, 1979

37. Epstein E, Ugel AR: Effects of mechlorethamine on the skin lesions of psoriasis. Arch Dermatol 102:504, 1970

38. Zackheim HS, Arnold JE, Farber EM, et al: Topical therapy of psoriasis with mechlorethamine. Arch Dermatol 105:702, 1972.

39. Taylor JR, Halperin KM: Topical use of mechlorethamine in the treatment of psoriasis. Arch Dermatol 105:362,1972

40. Breza TS, Kechijian P, Taylor JR: Mechlorethamine in psoriasis: Further attempts to induce immunologic tolerance. Arch Dermatol 111:1438, 1975

41. Pariser DM, Childers RC, Kechijian P, et al: Intravenous desensitization to mechlorethamine in patients with psoriasis. Arch Dermatol 112:1113, 1976

42. Handler RM, Medansky RS: Treatment of psoriasis with topical nitrogen mustard. Int J Dermatol 18:758, 1979

31

CHARLES M. McBRIDE, M.D.

Regional Therapy for Cancers of the Limbs

Tumors on the limbs, which are relatively easy to detect by inspection and palpation and can often exist for long periods of time before becoming life-threatening, have been treated for centuries by various poultices, cauterizations, and amputations. In more recent times, the role of the lymphatic system in the spread and dissemination of malignant disease has been studied and control of disease in the regional lymphatics has been added to the surgical concept of treatment for cancers of the limbs (although the timing of this treatment has been questioned recently). Regional therapy for limb lesions has been advocated for many years, either in combined excision and lymph-node dissection or in major ablative procedures such as amputation. With the advent of chemotherapy, Creech and associates[1] suggested that regional chemotherapy would permit the entire limb to be treated in situ with minimal permanent sequelae. From this concept have grown the various forms of regional chemotherapy such as isolation-perfusion, intra-arterial infusion using the limb as an end arterial system, and endolymphatic therapy.

DIAGNOSTIC PROCEDURES

The diagnosis of cancers on the limbs is usually an office procedure, although formal treatment for most of these lesions may require a fully equipped operating room. An excisional biopsy is preferred for the diagnosis of smaller lesions. For the diagnosis of larger lesions, there is no proof that an incisional biopsy followed by adequate treatment within a reasonable period of time causes any adverse effects. There is, however, some suggestion that electrocoagulation of malignant melanomas may have an adverse effect,[2] and this is not recommended for most limb cancers.

For subcutaneous lesions, a needle biopsy usually establishes a diagnosis of malignant or nonmalignant neoplasm. This then permits the planning of definitive therapy without causing any major alteration in the lesion or the overlying skin that could make treatment difficult. For many of the lesions that commonly occur on the limbs (e.g., melanomas, sarcomas, and lymphomas, a frozen section diag-

nosis is not adequate. It is recommended that adequate tissue samples be obtained and submitted to the pathologist for permanent sections. Once a firm diagnosis is established, definitive therapy can be planned.

The staging of a disease is an integral part of treatment planning. For example, the staging system used for malignant melanoma at the University of Texas System Cancer Center, M. D. Anderson Hospital and Tumor Institute is given in Table 31–1. After initial inspection, palpation, and biopsy, a chest x-ray and liver function tests are recommended for most limb lesions. In cases of possible advanced disease, lymphangiography, arteriography, and CT-scanning should also be included as aids to accurate staging of the disease.

The gradations of malignant melanoma are open to various interpretations by different clinicians and pathologists who themselves may have difficulty in accurately classifying cutaneous as well as deeper lesions. Therefore, a thorough understanding of the classification used by any given investigator is necessary to evaluate treatment results and to compare them with the results of others.

Clark and colleagues[3] have done much to clarify this problem by microstaging malignant melanomas as to the level of invasion. Most institutions, however, do not consider a malignant melanoma involving Clark's level I as being other than a research classification. The author considers lesions to a depth of Clark's level III and less than 1 mm as superficially invasive malignant melanomas, and spread outside the local area from such a lesion should be minimal. Again, local treatment is all that is required. With invasion to level III and more than 1 mm thick, however, the probability exists that the melanoma has already invaded small lymphatics or blood vessels and has spread outside the local area. For this type of lesion, a regional form of therapy is required to treat the entire area of potential involvement by the melanoma.

As with any method of clinical staging, many lesions treated as Stage I will, in fact, have the clinical course of Stage III lesions, and it is obvious that these patients already had Stage III disease at the time they were first seen. Evidence of spread outside the local area, however, was not clinically apparent during workup, and any significant salvage

405

TABLE 31–1. University of Texas M. D. Anderson Hospital Staging of Patients with Malignant Melanoma

Stage 0	Superficial melanoma (Level II and level III lesions <1.0 mm thick)
Stage I	Primary melanoma only IA: Intact primary melanoma IB: Primary melanoma, locally excised IC: Multiple primary melanomata
Stage II	Local recurrence or metastases (All disease within 3 cm of primary site)
Stage III	Regional metastases IIIA: Tissues excluding nodes IIIB: Nodes IIIAB: Skin, etc., plus nodes
Stage IV	Distant metastases IVA: Cutaneous metastasis only IVB: Any visceral metastasis

of these patients can be obtained only by the use of a regional therapy.

TREATMENT INDICATIONS

Because the limbs represent readily identifiable body regions in which most malignant lesions will spread initially by direct extension or along lymphatic channels before dissemination occurs, prophylactic regional therapy in these cases provides the best opportunity for cure. Prior to the advent of regional chemotherapy, total ablation including the regional nodes was the only regional therapy available. This resulted in amputations being done, many on a prophylactic basis, to provide adequate therapy. Because of the morbidity associated with major ablations, attempts at regional surgical therapy were made using incontinuity dissections of the lesions and the intervening skin between the lesions and regional lymph nodes. This surgical treatment carries its own morbidity and is not truly a regional procedure.

Treatment of the entire limb by radiotherapy, other than through the endolymphatic route, requires larger fields than most radiotherapists believe are safe. Although not indicated as a regional treatment, radiotherapy using wide fields provides good control of local lesions, if there is in fact no spread of the disease out of immediately adjacent areas. Regional therapy of a limb via the vascular or lymphatic system permits treatment of the entire region. The efficacy of this therapy is limited only by the drugs and isotopes available, few of which at the present time are ideal for the tumors encountered. Prerequisites for regional therapy by isolation-perfusion are a normal blood supply to the entire limb and sufficiently good general health of

the patient to withstand a five-hour general anesthetic. Regional therapies by infusion and by endolymphatic therapy do not require this prolonged anesthesia; however, they do not carry as high a cure rate because of the lower drug concentrations obtained in the treatment area.

Although complete remissions of cancer of the limbs can be obtained by the use of isolation-perfusion alone (Fig. 31–1), local excision of the involved area (Fig. 31–2) should be combined whenever possible with regional chemotherapy. This will prevent recurrence of the lesion if a complete cell kill has not been obtained. Microscopic disease should be controlled as the entire anatomic region is exposed to the chemotherapeutic agent, and hence only a local excision of the tumor-bearing area is required.

REGIONAL TECHNIQUES

For regional therapy by isolation-perfusion, anatomic isolation of the limb must be obtained and circulation provided to the limb by a pump-oxygenator (Fig. 31–3) permitting perfusion of the entire limb with a high dose of the chemotherapeutic agent. A heat exchanger is used in the circuit, and hyperthermia may be added to the perfused limb as an adjunct to the chemotherapeutic agents. Care must be taken to avoid combining both thermal and drug damage to the limb. Excessive muscle breakdown from such damage may cause renal impairment after the limb is reconnected with the systemic circulation.

Because of the high incidence of malignant melanomas encountered on the lower extremities, the regional chemotherapeutic procedure most commonly done at the M. D. Anderson Hospital is an iliac dissection and perfusion.[4] A transverse incision is made at the level of the iliac crest, and the muscle is split to expose the peritoneum that is retracted medially to expose the vessels in the iliac fossa. The iliac and obturator lymph nodes are removed from the level of the femoral canal and obturator foramen to the bifurcation of the internal and external iliac artery and vein. Although these are not the regional lymph nodes for the lower limbs, they are checked by frozen sections for evidence of involvement, since metastases here would indicate dissemination outside the regional area and carry with it a correspondingly poor prognosis.

The branches and tributaries of the external iliac vessels just proximal to the femoral canal are divided to prevent bypass flow out of the limb. Bulldog clamps are placed across the obturator vessels, catheters are placed in the external iliac artery and vein and threaded down into the leg to a point near the take-off of the profunda femoris. A Steinmann pin is driven into the anterior superior iliac spine, and

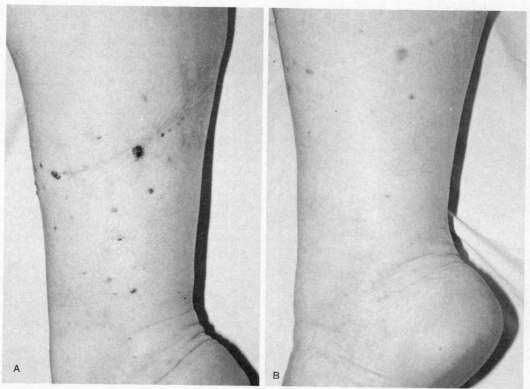

Figure 31–1. *A*, Intransit malignant melanoma on the calf of a patient following standard surgical treatment. *B*, Same patient five years after perfusion with a triple-drug regimen; the pigment is still in macrophages.

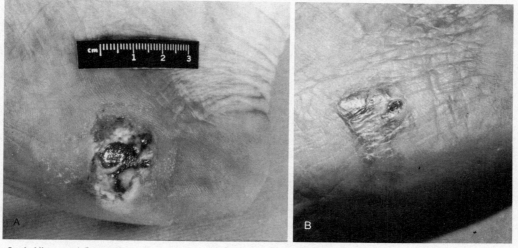

Figure 31–2. *A*, Ulcerated Stage IA melanoma on a foot. *B*, Six weeks after isolation-perfusion treatment, the lesion has healed and requires only a small local excision without a skin graft.

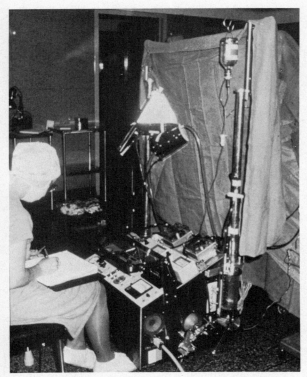

Figure 31—3. The double-headed roller pump with a small bubble oxygenator and heat exchanger used for perfusions.

an Esmarch bandage is wrapped tightly around the inguinal crease and held high on the hip by the Steinmann pin. The adequacy of the isolation is checked, using radioiodinated serum albumin in the pump circuit,[5] and is monitored by a collimator placed over the ventricular blood mass. In the majority of patients, the limbs will be isolated with less than a 5% leak over a perfusion period of one hour. The temperature in the limb is elevated to 102°F (38.9°C) during the period of drug perfusion by use of the heat exchanger. If the lesion is such that a local excision can be done following the perfusion, then a single drug such as l-PAM (l-phenylalanine mustard) or DTIC (dacarbazine)[6] is perfused for 45 minutes to one hour, following which the leg is washed out with dextran 70 and refilled with blood.

For treatment of Stage I melanoma, a prophylactic perfusion is performed, and the lesion or scar is excised immediately following the perfusion. Since this is a relatively small surgical procedure, no problem is encountered with subsequent healing. For patients with sarcomas and lymphomas in whom a combination of two drugs (PAM or DTIC and actinomycin D) are used, the potential for damage of the leg is greater and healing is slower as a result. In these patients, the tumor-bearing area is re-excised six weeks after the perfusion in order to

allow adequate time for stabilization of the tissues and to permit proper wound healing.

When a cure is expected, a local excision is always necessary, and only in a purely palliative case would the tumor be in situ. When treating patients with advanced disease in the limbs, such as Stage III melanoma, a combination of three drugs are used: l-PAM or DTIC with actinomycin D and nitrogen mustard. Combining the two alkylating agents permits a higher dose than is possible with either alone. Multiple drug perfusions may cause permanent tissue damage resulting in fibrosis and some weakness in the limb in the postperfusion period. No attempt is made to excise intransit metastasis when present, and many patients with advanced disease in the limbs have survived for more than ten years without a recurrence. With each succeeding year, it seems less likely that further disease will develop.

The technique, which is essentially the same for a femoral dissection and perfusion, is employed in patients who have multiple nodes present in the femoral triangle that are in danger of involving the overlying skin with subsequent ulceration. The inguino-femoral dissection prevents this ulceration, and the perfusion controls the disease in the remainder of the leg. When doing popliteal and axillary perfusions, it is not necessary to monitor the leak because of the excellent isolation obtained. With a popliteal perfusion, a pneumatic tourniquet is used proximally providing complete isolation. An Esmarch bandage high on the shoulder provides complete anatomic isolation for an axillary perfusion. Originally, the amount of leakage was checked during these operations, but it was never found to be significant.

On occasion, pelvic perfusions have been used to manage tumors in the skin of the genital and perineal regions. This is a much more extensive procedure (Fig. 31–4) that requires an abdominal operation, dissection of the aorta and vena cava, insertion of catheters down the common iliac vessels, placement of tourniquets around both limbs to prevent distal runoff, and an attempt to isolate the region by controlling the blood supplies via the aorta, vena cava, and mesentery. With careful dissection, it is usually possible to run the perfusion for an hour before a 100% drug leakage occurs, but it is necessary to reduce the drug dosage when this high leak is anticipated. Total-body tourniquets are available that can be used to improve isolation. These are not completely effective, however, and they add considerably to the time and stress involved in the operation.

When infusion therapy is used, the axillary or iliac vessels are exposed in the same manner as for limb perfusion. A small Teflon or Silastic catheter is placed in the vessel supplying the tumor-bearing area, tied securely to prevent displacement, and brought out percutaneously near a fixed bony struc-

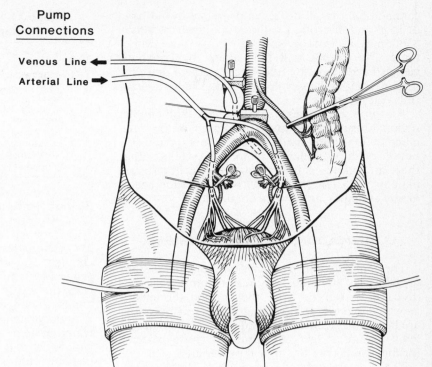

Pump Connections

Venous Line ←

Arterial Line →

Figure 31–4. Diagram representing the isolation technique necessary to insure an adequate pelvic perfusion.

ture, such as the anterior superiliac spine or attached to a subcutaneous access port (Fig. 31–5). Catheters placed percutaneously by a radiologist may also be used. A bedside pump with a varible flow rate that can exceed 500 cc a day is attached to the catheter initially; however, only the loading dose of the drug is delivered by this system. If DTIC is being infused for an advanced malignant melanoma, then five-day infusion courses are administered in this manner. At the end of the five days, the catheter is flushed with heparin and remains until it is time for the next course of therapy.

With care, it may be possible to keep these catheters functional for over two years. Percutaneously placed catheters are removed between courses of chemotherapy. Recently, cisplatin has been found to be an effective agent when used in intra-arterial infusions.[7] If Adriamycin is to be used, the heparin must first be removed from the circuit.

Endolymphatic therapy to a limb is provided by

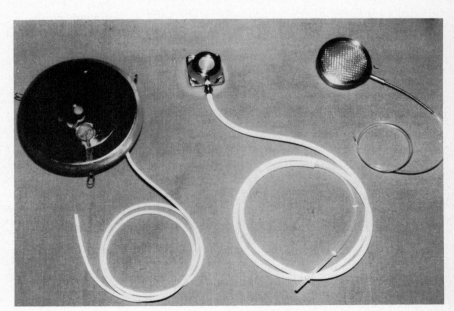

Figure 31–5. A selection of implantable devices for intra-arterial infusions.

cannulating a small distal lymph vessel in the hand or foot[8] and inserting a catheter to infuse a solution containing an isotope, such as ^{32}P over a period of time. The isotope will flow along the lymphatic vessels irradiating any tumor cells present and then be deposited in the lymph nodes and irradiate tumor cells trapped there.

All three techniques treat the entire limb and are regional forms of therapy. The efficacy of the treatment of the limbs varies with the anatomic distribution of the vascular or lymphatic systems. Since there are variations in the flow patterns in different patients, an even distribution of therapeutic agents in any system is not always obtained.

COMPLICATIONS OF REGIONAL THERAPY

The complications resulting from regional therapy for cancer of the limbs may result from the surgical procedure itself or from the specific therapeutic agents employed. In the first group of complications are hemorrhage, infection, and wound-healing problems that are, in fact, comparable to those expected for any similar major surgical procedure.

The problems related specifically to the therapeutic agents are tissue damage and skin slough, which can result from too high a dose or, more commonly, from an unequal distribution of drug flow. This results in the exposure of one area of the limb to a higher concentration of drug than other areas, with subsequent tissue destruction. Using high doses of drugs for perfusion results in some muscle fibrosis, which is similar in many ways to the fibrosis that occurs following radiation therapy. This fibrotic process usually stabilizes between three and six months and does not progress beyond that time. Most patients experience transient paresthesias from direct neural toxicity of the drugs; however, a permanently painful limb should not result from routine isolation-perfusions. Vascular complications such as thrombosis or intimal dissection are rare and usually recognized within 24 hours, at which time they can be corrected. In the event that an undetected leak of chemotherapeutic agents occurs into the systemic circulation, bone marrow depression may be a complication; this can be extremely severe with the use of high doses of alkylating agents, although leak monitoring should prevent this. The complications caused by isolation-perfusion observed over a 15-year period are given in Table 31–2.

When intra-arterial infusion of limbs is used as the regional form of therapy, the catheter can become dislodged or broken resulting in hemorrhage. Carefully securing the catheter at the time of insertion and leaving an expansion coil for movement adjacent to the vessel prevents this. A long-term catheter may plug, or it may erode through the wall of the vessel from the motion of the tip caused by

TABLE 31–2. Complications of Perfusion (January 1958 to September 1972)

Total Patients	728
Perfusions	897
Systemic Complications	
Death	6
Severe marrow depression	7
Homologous serum jaundice	11
Local Complications	
Tissue necrosis (amputation)	10
Thrombophlebitis	9
Necrotizing fasciitis	1
Peripheral neuritis	3

the turbulence in the vessel, however, this is usually such a slow process that hemorrhage does not result.

Thrombosis associated with catheter placement can occur and is usually associated with some intimal damage. The adverse responses in the limbs and the general systemic effects from infusion therapy vary with the drugs infused and are similar to those obtained with systemic chemotherapy.

Endolymphatic therapy, because of its use of the lymph system, may cause increasing fibrosis in the lymphatic and nodal areas with resultant lymphedema of the extremity, but this may be controlled if the disease itself is controlled. Transient pyrexia and occasional pulmonary problems may also be observed.

RESULTS OF REGIONAL THERAPY

The use of regional chemotherapy by isolation-perfusion in the treatment of malignant melanoma of the extremity may be expected to increase the ten-year survival rate of the Stage I patient from approximately 57% to more than 83%.[4] At the same time, it reduces the amputation rate and the number of skin grafts required to obtain control of the primary lesion. This same form of therapy may be expected to almost double the ten-year survival rate of patients with Stage III melanoma, as shown in Table 31–3.

With more advanced disease, as seen in patients with Stage III and Stage IV malignant melanomas, higher doses and a triple-drug combination are used. This produces some complications in approximately one third of the patients, but it would appear that this method may double the five-year survival rate, as shown in Table 31–4. The number of patients

TABLE 31–3. Raw Survival Rates for Patients Treated with Single Drug Perfusions

	Historical Controls			l-PAM Perfusion Only		
	2 yr	5 yr	10 yr	2 yr	5 yr	10 yr
Stage I	91%	73%	57%	94%	86%	83%
Stage II	56%	22%	22%	94%	55%	55%

TABLE 31—4. Raw Survival Rates for Patients Treated with Triple-Drug Perfusions

	Historical Controls		Triple-Drug Perfusions	
	2 yr	5 yr	2 yr	5 yr
Stage III	31%	16%	59%	40%
Stage IV	11%	7%	20%	0%

studied in these groups, however, is still small. Patients with disseminated disease can usually maintain a functional limb for the rest of their lives, and this contributes to their overall well-being and offers useful palliation. When used for sarcomas and lymphomas, regional chemotherapy by isolation-perfusion produces essentially the same five-year survival rate as the standard treatments of surgery or surgery combined with radiotherapy, but usually with less morbidity.

Treatment by intra-arterial chemotherapy for the patient who is a poor risk or who has not proven to be responsive to isolation-perfusion will often provide worthwhile palliation.[9] This often permits selected groups of patients to remain active for much longer periods of time than might otherwise be expected. Some excellent remissions and occasional cures have been obtained by the use of endolymphatic therapy in patients that have proven unresponsive to other forms of treatment.[8]

SUMMARY

The use of regional therapies for cancer of the limbs provides a method of treating the entire region involved, either as prophylaxis or for control of advanced disease and usually with less morbidity than is seen with standard surgical or combined procedures.

REFERENCES

1. Ryan RF, Winblad JN, Krementz ET, Creech O Jr: Treatment of malignant neoplasms with chemotherapeutic agents utilizing a pump-oxygenator. Bull Tulane Med Fac 17:133–143, 1958
2. Peterson NC, Bodenham DC, Lloyd OD: Malignant melanomas of the skin: A study of the origin, development, etiology, spread, treatment and prognosis. Br J Plast Surg 1:49–116, 1962
3. Clark WH, From L, Bernardino EV, Mihm MD: The histogenesis and biologic behavior of primary human malignant melanomas of the skin. Cancer Res 29:705–726, 1969
4. McBride CM, McMurtrey MJ, Copeland EM, Hickey RD: Regional chemotherapy by isolation-perfusion. Int Adv Surg Onc 1:1–9, 1978
5. Stehlin JS Jr, Clark RL, Dewey WC: Continuous monitoring of leakage during regional perfusion. Arch Surg 83:943–949, 1961
6. Pfefferkorn RO, Didolkar MS: Regional perfusion for melanoma of the extremities. J Ext Corp Tech 14:475–479, 1982
7. Pritchard JD, Mavligit GM, Wallace S, Benjamin RS, et al: Regression of regionally advanced melanoma after arterial infusion with cis-platinum and actinomycin-D. Clin Onc 5:179–182, 1979
8. Ariel IM: Malignant melanoma, its treatment by the endolymphatic administration of radioactive isotopes. Am J Roentgenol Radium Ther Nucl Med 111:310–322, 1971
9. Einhorn LH, McBride CM, Luce JK, Caoli E, et al: Intra-arterial infusion therapy with 5-(3,3-dimethyl-1-triazeno) imidazole-4-carboxamide (NSC 45388) for malignant melanoma. Cancer 32:101–107, 1973

32

JAMES J. STAGNONE, M.D.

Chemical Peeling and Chemabrasion

This chapter deals with light, intermediate, and deep chemical peeling with trichloroacetic acid; light peeling with an alternate resorcinol formulation; and a technique combining trichloroacetic acid peeling and dermabrasion referred to as chemabrasion. Light peeling is arbitrarily defined here as peeling done with 10% to 35% trichloroacetic acid and other mild acids; intermediate peeling is done with 35% to 50% trichloroacetic acid without taping; and deep chemical peeling is done with 50% to 75% trichloroacetic acid (with or without taping) or other strong acids, such as Baker's phenol formula.[1, 2]

LIGHT CHEMICAL PEELING

Light chemical peeling is the technique of periodically applying mild acids to the face for the treatment of acne, pigmentary changes, superficial scarring, fine wrinkling, and moderate actinic damage.

Indications

Acne

Light peeling is a safe and effective adjunct in the treatment of selected cases of acne vulgaris. The majority of acne patients are suitable candidates for light peeling. Chemical peeling affords good exfoliation compared to that obtained with liquid nitrogen, carbon dioxide, and ultraviolet irradiation. In actively scarring acne, light peeling produces a more rapid resolution and affords significant improvement in scarring in all cases and striking in many.

These patients derive a benefit that can be equaled to or surpassed only at the much greater cost, pain, and risk of deeper chemical peeling and dermabrasion. Depending on the severity, age, and sex of the acne patient, any part of the spectrum of acne therapeutics may be used in conjunction with light peeling. There are no absolute contraindications to light peeling, although the severity of the chapping induced by systemic and topical retinoic acids as well as other acne therapeutic modalities may exceed a patient's tolerance for the stinging, burning, and chapping caused by light peeling.

Pigmentary Changes

Chloasma, melasma, berloque dermatitis, and drug-induced and postinflammatory pigmentary changes usually respond rapidly and predictably to two or three light peels at weekly intervals and twice-daily use for two weeks of a bleaching cream recommended by Kligman and Willis.[3] As soon as it is tolerable following completion of this treatment, daily use of sunscreens and topical retinoic acid is recommended. For the two to three weeks of bleaching cream and light peeling therapy and for as long as a month thereafter, irregular peeling and migration of pigment often appear to be worsening. This is temporary, but often causes great concern to a patient who is not forewarned. Recurrences of pigmentation despite recommended sun avoidance and use of sunscreens may occur. The treatment may be repeated. Recurrences are less likely to occur and will be milder if retinoic acid is used each evening and sunscreens are applied each morning.

Fine Wrinkling and Moderate Actinic Damage

Many patients with fine wrinkling, moderate actinic damage, or simple weathering of the skin will benefit from light peeling. These patients benefit more from deeper chemical peeling or dermabrasion, but because of general health or the inability to handle the procedures emotionally or financially, they may elect the option of a light or intermediate chemical peeling.

Rejuvenation of the Skin Program. In the author's office practice,[4] a "rejuvenation" program has been used and modified over a number of years. The program, designed to alter sun-induced changes, is based on current knowledge of the normal physiology of the skin, the mechanism of so-called aging and sun-induced changes, and the knowledge of certain products that may alter these changes. This program influences mainly the uppermost layers of the skin that are the site of actinic keratoses and pigmentary changes of weathering and that are responsible for the surface appearance of the skin. Although the uppermost skin layers and some of the fine superficial wrinkles improve with the regimen, the deeper wrinkles are basically unaffected. Deeper wrinkling is treated best by rhytidectomy, phenol peeling, dermabrasion, and injections of medical filling fluids such as collagen and silicone.

The program results in a more youthful, healthy appearance and reverses some of the changes of prolonged sun damage that predispose to skin cancer. Treatment consists of several steps directed toward different aspects of these changes: (1) removal of weathered and dead cells, (2) stimulation of cell turnover, (3) rejuvenation of cells, (4) hydration of the skin, and (5) protection.

Because these steps may overlap or a step may be omitted to allow tailoring to the patient's needs, this brief discussion of the steps will not follow the sequence in which they are listed. With aging and actinic damage, there are irregular changes affecting epidermal cell turnover. An overall slowdown in cell turnover occurs with aging, but in areas of actinic keratoses, there is increased turnover resulting in dyskeratosis and hyperkeratosis. Not only keratinocytes but also melanocytes function irregularly resulting in blotchy pigmentation. These changes contribute to a weathered, tired, muddy, and dry appearance. Chemical peeling causes general exfoliation of epidermal cells in all areas of application stimulating cell turnover time.

In contrast, topical 5-fluorouracil affects specific areas of actinic damage rather than producing a general effect on all areas of application.[5] For this reason, the first step can be either a standard course of topical 5-fluorouracil or chemical peeling depending on the patient's needs and desires. The recommended first step is a course of 5-fluorouracil. After a variable recovery period, this is followed by chemical peeling of either the light or intermediate methods.

Throughout the program, vitamins or vitamin derivatives are used for possible rejuvenation and adjuvant anticancer properties. Vitamin A has the ability to cause developing cells to differentiate toward more plump, primitive, mucoid-like cells rather than to progress to keratinization.[6]

Vitamin A and its derivatives also have an ability to reverse metaplastic changes in epithelium and other cells.[7-10] In view of possible toxic or induced side effects of such vitamins, safe levels over limited time periods with periodic physical and laboratory examinations are recommended.

Another part of the rejuvenation program is hydration of the skin by using any of a number of excellent moisturizers nightly and sunscreens daily. A typical program for an average patient is illustrated in outline form in Table 32–1.

Intervals

Light peeling solutions are applied weekly or less often. Initially, the interval is once a week for one to two months. There is no set number of treatments, so patients may get twenty or more light peels in prolonged courses over a period of a year. There is no limit to the number of light peels a patient can receive unless complications occur. After the initial series of light peels and the usual excellent result, most patients decrease treatments for variable periods of time. Regardless of their problem—acne, pigmentary changes, or weathering—partial recurrences are likely, so patients have the option of returning for additional light peels at whatever interval they feel is necessary to keep their problem under optimum control. The average return rate for two or three weekly light peels is twice a year. Many patients sustain their improvement with home care, such as topical retinoic acid and sunscreens, and are seen annually until they are comfortable with self-treatment.

Preparation

The skin is prepared by cleansing it with alcohol and acetone to remove the cutaneous oils. Alcohol- and acetone-soaked sponges are squeezed out using gloved hands. The skin is scrubbed lightly first with alcohol until the dark film or accumulation on the sponge disappears or is significantly reduced. This dark film is a good indication of the amount of oil that needs to be removed. After two cleansings with alcohol, an additional single cleansing with acetone is performed. Removal of the surface oils standardizes the condition of the skin for an even absorption of the chemical solution.

TABLE 32–1. Rejuvenation of the Skin Program

Typical Patient:	45-year-old female with fair skin, fine wrinkles, scattered early actinic keratoses, and poikiloderma-like pigmentary changes.
Day 1:	A baseline complete blood count, sedimentation rate, and sequential multiple analysis are drawn. Topical 5-fluorouracil course of 30 days (three to six weeks) is started. Vitamins are taken with breakfast and supper (25,000 water-soluble international units of vitamin A or 10 mg of isotretinoin, B complex with 500 mg of vitamin C, 400 units of vitamin E, and a multiple-vitamin and -mineral tablet).
Day 32:	Intermediate peel (or six weekly light peels) is accomplished.
Day 40:	Evening applications of topical retinoic acid, as tolerated, and morning applications of an effective sunscreen are started.
Day 180:	Repeat lab tests. Discontinue vitamins A and E for a minimum of one full month. Peeling routine may be repeated. Daily applications of retinoic acid and sunscreen are continued indefinitely.

414 CHEMOSURGERY AND IMMUNOTHERAPY

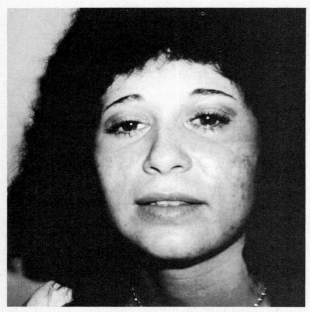

Figure 32–1. Typical appearance of reddening and whitening immediately after the application of a light peel; the color changes fade away, usually within a half-hour.

The therapist should be aware of the increased sensitivity of atopic, fair-skinned individuals as well as differences of sensitivity of the various segments of the face (e.g., the perioral area and eyelids are more sensitive than the forehead) and apply cleansers and solutions accordingly. It is not surprising that atopic individuals with darker skin have more complaints about excessively heavy peeling, because pigment is excreted with the exfoliate making the scales darker and more noticeable.

The usual precautions are utilized to avoid irritation of the eyes. Water-soaked sponges are readied to wash off any aberrant drops. The light peeling solution is tipped directly from the 16 oz stock bottle onto a gauze. If excessively saturated, the gauze is squeezed out by hand into a sink. For the face, 3 × 3 inch gauzes are used, and for the trunk, 4 × 4 inch gauzes. Small cotton swabs may be used for difficult-to-reach areas.

Application

For the first treatment, one coat of solution is applied evenly with smooth strokes using a wrung-out, damp gauze sponge. Because of the variations in skin sensitivity, the first application should be light. Reactivity as well as inherent characteristics, such as the atopic sensitive skin, varies slightly from week to week in the same individual. Some apparent factors are dryness, sun exposure, regular use of topical treatments, and perhaps premenstrual and other stress factors that cause hormone imbalance.

Since most patients begin topical treatments concurrently with their first light peel, a deeper take must be expected on the second treatment, so light application is again emphasized. The operator, who requests the patient to monitor the severity and duration of exfoliation, becomes familiar with the sensitivity of the patient's skin over a period of a few weeks and thereby decides whether or not to increase the concentration on subsequent applications. Stretching the skin, rubbing, overcoating, and using more moist gauze are methods used to increase the depth of the treatment.

Results

In most individuals, an almost immediate flushing or reddening of the skin will be followed by a dulling or whitening that usually lasts for less than an hour, but occasionally as long as a day (Figs. 32–1 and 32–2). Generally, the skin is slightly red until light exfoliation (which starts on the second day and lasts for three to five days) occurs. The peeling is equivalent to that seen after a mild sunburn. The patient is ready for a second treatment in one week.

Marked reactions causing prolonged redness and

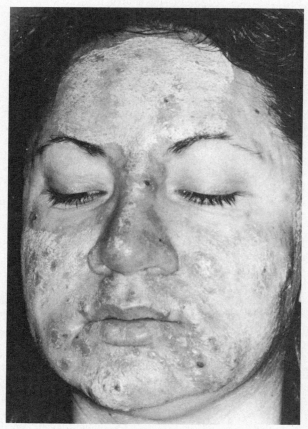

Figure 32–2. Extreme whitening immediately after a light peel that faded away within one hour.

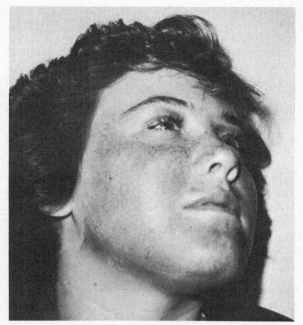

Figure 32–3. Unusual duration of reddening, which persisted until the completion of peeling on the sixth day.

crusting, which can be embarrassing for up to three weeks, have occurred in sensitive individuals who almost always were overzealously treated during one of the first three treatments (Figs. 32–3 and 32–4). Occasionally, in darker-skinned individuals, a large amount of pigment will be exfoliated during the first few peels (Fig. 32–5). This brownish flaking, which can be unsightly, can be somewhat disguised by using a light moisturizer.

Almost all acne patients are able to continue use of their regular acne topical medications without interruption. With the use of sunscreens and non-comedonogenic moisturizers, almost all patients are able to continue outdoor and indoor activities as usual.

In general, the more severe the reaction, the better the result. However, even where little or no visible reaction occurs, the author feels that microscopic benefits do occur. Although recovery from severe reactions and pigmentary changes in rare instances can be measured in weeks, no permanent damage has ever been seen as a result of light peeling.

Methods of Light Peeling

Trichloroacetic Acid Method of Light Peeling

In the office, trichloroacetic acid is used in strengths ranging from 15% to 35% for light peeling; however, 10% occasionally is used as a trial application or might be dispensed for self-administered

light peeling at home. The first treatment consists of an even application of 15% trichloroacetic acid for a timed period of one minute. Timing begins when the chemical is first applied to the treated area. An even redness or dulling or slight whitening is sought. If there is an uneven appearance after application, the areas showing no significant results are recoated. The treated areas are washed off with water in the same order as the acid was applied. After one minute, the area is sponged with a cool-water compress, or the patient may splash or sponge his or her face over a sink.

Treatments are given weekly or less often, and the time is increased by approximately 30 seconds each week depending on the results of the previous treatment. It appears that maximum benefit is obtained from about two minutes of undisturbed application. It follows that, beyond two minutes, the washing does not decrease the effectiveness of treatment. The washing affords the patient some relief from the discomfort of stinging.

The precisely defined and timed procedure reassures patients. When the time interval reaches two minutes at any concentration, and the patient appears to be ready for a stronger application, the concentration of the trichloroacetic acid is increased by 5%, and the time is set at one minute again. Most patients reach their tolerance and obtain maximum benefit at the 25% level.

Occasionally, the author sees patients who pro-

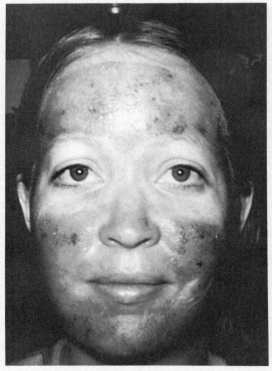

Figure 32–4. Appearance three days after an extremely deep "take" of a light peel; excellent end result one week later.

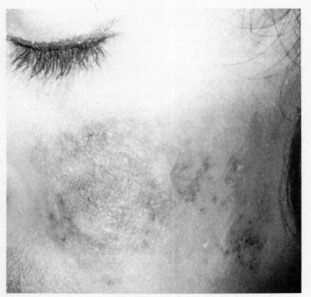

Figure 32—5. Brownish peeling five days after a light peel, occasionally seen in dark-complexioned patients.

gress all the way to 35% trichloroacetic acid for two minutes. The maximum concentration for any one patient may be repeated regularly, with some variation in saturation of the sponges and pressure of application. In general, with trichloroacetic acid, the depth of peeling is controlled by increasing the concentration of the acid and prolonging the exposure time.

Resorcinol Formula Method of Light Peeling

The Comb's formula is illustrated in Table 32–2. This formula and modifications of it have been used widely by lay peelers and in prestigious beauty salons on Fifth Avenue and in Beverly Hills. The author's modification of the method described by Horvath[11] follows.

As with trichloroacetic acid, the first treatment consists of an even light coat applied with a wrung-out gauze sponge. The same burning and color changes occur, but the method varies in that washing is not essential. Many patients fan themselves for a few minutes until the burning and stinging sensation subsides. Occasionally, sponging with water is necessary.

As with trichloroacetic acid, treatments are given weekly or less often. Assuming a slight-to-moderate reaction to the first treatment, two coats of solution are applied at the second treatment. Three coats are applied at the time of the third treatment. At subsequent treatments, depending on the previous take, three coats are applied with heavier pressure and wetter sponges. The depth of the take is gauged by the degree of flushing and whitening. In general,

with the resorcinol formula, the depth of peeling is controlled by the number of coats of solution applied. In addition, the operator stretches the skin while rubbing and overcoating areas to increase the depth.

Light peeling with resorcinol is limited to the face. The possibility of toxicity from resorcinol absorption has caused this limitation. When treatment is indicated on the trunk as well as the face, trichloroacetic acid is used on the trunk.

The advantages of this method over the trichloroacetic acid method are that there is no danger of using the wrong concentration of solutions, no need to neutralize the solution, and therefore, no need to time the duration of applications. The chances for mistakes are fewer, and the results appear to be comparable. A disadvantage is the limitation of its use only to the face.

Results and Summary

For the indications listed, the results of over 25,000 light peels over a 15-year period have been gratifying. The results are slow to occur and vary with the operator's experience and the patient's skin sensitivity. Since the technique does not allow double-blind evaluation and the diseases treated change with time and vary with light exposure, it is evident that peeling is not an exact science.

Light peeling is an inexpensive, safe technique that produces subjectively excellent results, has wide patient acceptance, is simple to perform, requires little or no postoperative care, and has virtually no complications.

INTERMEDIATE CHEMICAL PEELING

For our purposes, intermediate chemical peeling is the technique of applying intermediate-to-strong acids to the face as a single surgical procedure. Patients may electively repeat the procedure after a six-month rest. It is used mainly for the treatment of weathered, finely wrinkled skin, usually with moderate actinic damage, and occasionally for pigmentary changes or acne problems. In the author's office practice, intermediate peels are used most often in a skin rejuvenation program, as described earlier.

As an open procedure, i.e., without taping, 35% or 50% trichloroacetic acid is applied to the face.

TABLE 32—2. Comb's Formula

Resorcinol	14.0 gm
Salicylic acid	14.0 gm
Lactic acid (85%)	14.0 gm
Ethanol (95% q.s. ad.)	100.0 cc

In individuals with sensitive-appearing skin who usually have blue eyes and fair, freckled skin and who often suffer with atopy, 35% trichloroacetic acid is used over the periorbital and perioral skin, over bony prominences (such as along the mandible where tightness and movement might retard healing and increase the possibility of scarring), and on peripheral feathering areas. A 50% solution is used in all other areas. In individuals with normal-appearing skin, 50% trichloroacetic acid would be used over the entire face. It is wise not to exceed 35% trichloroacetic acid on all patient's necks.

Preparation

The skin is prepared in the same manner as that for light peeling. In most cases, no premedication is necessary, but this depends somewhat on the patient's apprehensiveness, which might dictate the same premedications used in deep peeling (e.g., meperidine hydrochloride, penetobarbital sodium, hydroxyzine pamoate, and diazepam). Stock bottles of 35% and 50% trichloroacetic acid are dated and, three months after preparation, discarded. About 10 ml are poured into a medicine glass that prevents any crystals at the mouth of the stock bottles from getting on the applicating swabs. Large swabs and small cotton swabs are thinned down by about 25%. The cotton applicator is immersed in the solution in the medicine glass, then elevated out of the liquid and pressed against the inside of the glass until the swab doesn't drip.

Application

The large swab is used over most of the face. The small cotton swabs are used to get within 1 mm of the eyelid margins and other curved or angled areas. It is convenient to start on the cheek with a large swab and to move quickly up from the mandible on one side to just below the eyelid margins, then to continue up the temple and across the forehead. The solution is applied with strokes in one direction and should be clearly seen wetting the skin evenly. Initially, there is no need to go over an area more than once. Approximately one third of the face can be painted evenly before the patient notices discomfort.

Over a period of a few minutes, the skin turns red and then white. After a minute or two, the patient senses stinging, burning, and pain that can be eased by applying dry gauzes with hand pressure. For the patient's comfort and to allow time to soak another swab as above, the author pauses for a minute or two. Then, the patient is ready to proceed with the next application to about one third of the face, and so on until nearly the entire face is treated

with the large swabs. Then the small cotton swabs are used. Soon, the patient's face should be uniformly bleached. In areas that are not white, another coat is applied. The patient's discomfort eases quickly. The application time, which varies inversely with the patient's pain tolerance, averages ten minutes.

Care and Results

Slight swelling is evidenced immediately after the procedure. There is no weeping or need for bandaging. Patients return home with pain and sleep medication, which is rarely utilized. Occasionally, blistering and edema are noted on the second day; in most cases, however, there is only slight swelling and a tenseness to the skin that patients note as a painless tightness. On the second day, they are instructed to compress the face with a solution of oil and water if there is vesiculation, and to use an antibiotic ointment. Ad lib showering is started on the second day, and copious flushing over the face relieves burning sensations. Desquamation commences on the second or third day and continues for about six days. Slight swelling, erythema, and flushing may persist for weeks. Patients are advised to avoid sunlight for three months. In nearly all cases where intermediate peeling is utilized, improvement is maintained by daily applications of retinoic acid starting about one week after surgery.

Summary

Intermediate chemical peeling is a conservative and safe technique used on hundreds of patients over the past 10 years without significant complications. It is simple to perform and postoperative care is minimal. There have been no permanent pigmentary changes as have been seen with 50% trichloroacetic acid under tape, phenol peeling, and dermabrasion. This method is recommended as the first conservative step beyond light peeling for those dermatologic surgeons who have limited experience with peeling and wish to expand their practice in this area.

DEEP CHEMICAL PEELING AND CHEMABRASION

Deep chemical peeling, dermabrasion, and chemabrasion are used when there is a need for dermal alterations deeper than that attainable with intermediate chemical peeling. At the initial consultation and examination, the patient and the surgeon must agree on the objectives of the surgery including the desired and safely obtainable depth, the probable

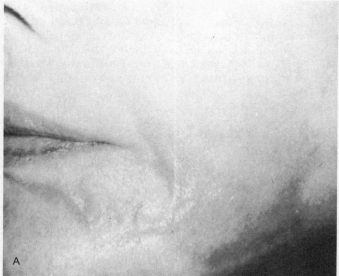

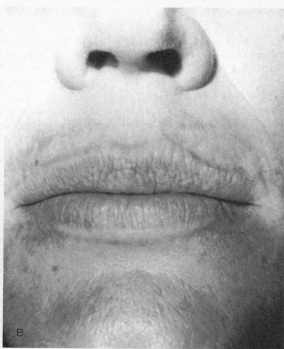

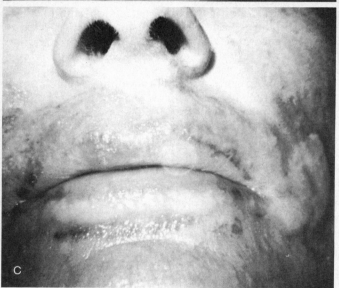

Figure 32–6. Complications: *A*, Hypertrophic scar six months after a chemical peel with 75% trichloroacetic acid. *B*, Hyper- and hypopigmentation four months after a chemical peel under tape with 50% trichloroacetic acid. *C*, Bacterial and viral infections after a dermabrasion.

results, the expected discomfort, the postoperative course, and the possible complications. The patient must accept that, in order to obtain sufficient depth of treatment to improve deep wrinkling, deep actinic changes, and various types of scarring, there will be a 100% incidence of what most patients consider adverse changes of pigmentation and texture. These changes should be amenable to the patients in exchange for improving their problems. Patients should understand that it is often necessary to repeat these procedures several times in order to obtain maximum benefit.

Deep Peeling

Deep chemical peeling is performed with Baker's phenol formula (see Chapter 33) and variations of it, 50% trichloroacetic acid under tape, and higher concentrations (up to 75%) of trichloroacetic acid with or without taping.

Except for segmental treatments, such as the perioral area which includes the lips and chin up to but not over the segmental line defined by the nasolabial folds, the author has discontinued phenol peeling because of the need for cardiac monitoring, which is not usually available in an office setting.

Experiences with persistent hypertrophic scarring, irregular thinning, and pigmentary changes after using 50% trichloroacetic acid under tape and after using higher concentrations with or without taping have convinced the author to discontinue deep chemical peeling with trichloroacetic acid and taping (Fig. 32–6). Some experienced cosmetic surgeons continue to utilize trichloroacetic acid for deep chemical peeling with good results.[12, 13]

Chemabrasion

When there is a need for a deeper peeling than intermediate chemical peeling, a technique that combines full-face intermediate peeling and dermabrasion has become the author's choice during the past ten years of practice (Figs. 32–7 to 32–10).[14] Occasionally, Baker's phenol is used in a segmental manner in the chemabrasion procedure allowing a more specific tailoring to patients' needs (Fig. 32–11).

Stegman's studies have demonstrated a scientific basis for individualization of the use of Baker's phenol, trichloroacetic acid, and dermabrasion.[15] However, even when used for segmental treatments, phenol causes such a high degree of pain for protracted periods that its use is discouraged, especially in view of the equally good results obtainable with chemabrasion using 50% trichloroacetic acid applications without significant complaints of pain. Experience with over 200 chemabrasions has demonstrated excellent results in nearly all cases where either deep chemical peeling or dermabrasion would have been indicated.

Technique

Chemabrasion is performed in the office approximately one hour after preoperative oral medication with pentobarbital sodium, meperidine hydrochloride, and diazepam. Skin preparation is the same as that described previously for light and intermediate chemical peeling. Immediately before starting the procedure, 2.5 mg of diazepam are slowly administered intravenously without drawing blood back into the syringe. Then, 50% trichloroacetic acid is applied over the face from just below the mandibular shadow line through the hairline, being careful to go slightly over the vermilion border and to within 1 mm of the eyelid margins. Application time is usually less than 10 minutes.

After a 10-minute delay, dermabrasion is accomplished in the usual manner (see Chapter 23). This delay allows time for coagulation of epidermal and dermal protein resulting in better visualization because of decreased bleeding. The coagulated tissue is more easily, quickly, and accurately abraded off. The entire procedure is easily accomplished in less than one hour.

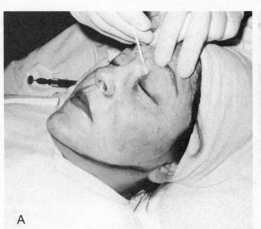
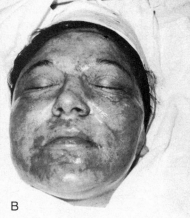
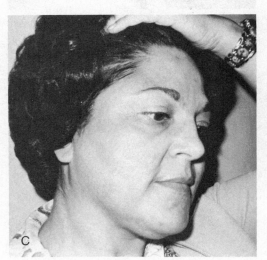

Figure 32–7. Chemabrasion: *A*, Application of 50% trichloroacetic acid over the face from the mandibular shadow line, through the hairline, and up to the eyelid margins; dermabrasion followed 10 minutes later. *B*, Appearance immediately after dermabrasion. *C*, Appearance nine months after the operation.

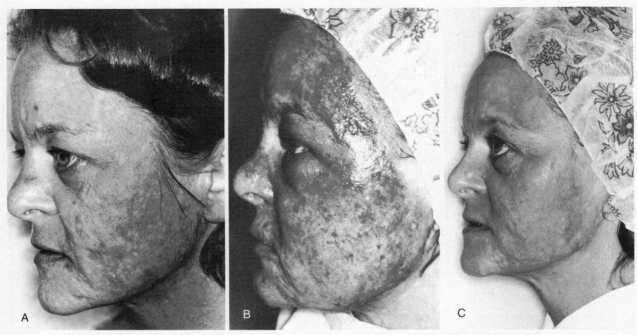

Figure 32–8. Chemabrasion: *A*, Preoperative patient with acne excoriée, fine wrinkling, weathering, and pigmentary changes. *B*, Appearance immediately after the chemabrasion. *C*, Appearance two weeks later with erythema caused by the surgery and the topical retinoic acid.

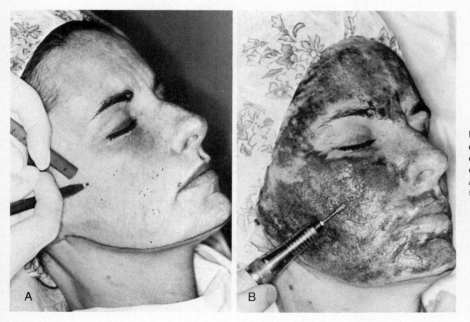

Figure 32–9. Chemabrasion: *A*, Use of gentian violet to mark the depths of acne scar pits before dermabrasion and after 50% trichloroacetic acid was applied. *B*, Appearance at the completion of the dermabrasion.

Figure 32–10. Chemabrasion: *A*, A 50% trichloroacetic acid solution was applied to the face from the shadow line, through the hairline, over the vermilion edge, and close to the eyelid margins; this was followed by gentian violet painting to mark the depths of the scars. *B*, Appearance immediately after sponging off with saline solution after the dermabrasion.

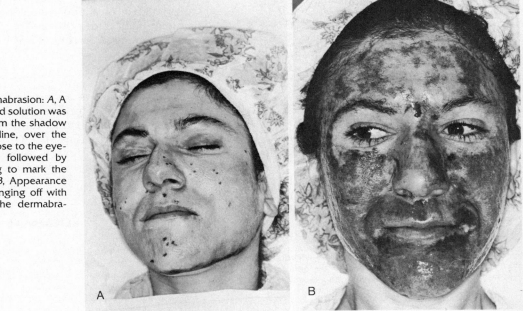

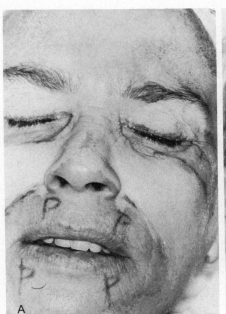
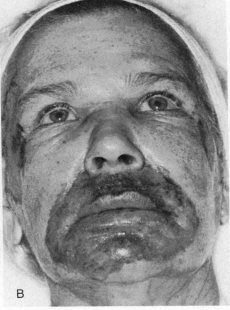

Figure 32–11. Chemabrasion: *A*, After 50% trichloroacetic acid was applied to most of the face, Baker's phenol solution was applied to the lower eyelids and perioral area for the deep lines; selective dermabrasion followed. *B*, Dermabrasion to perioral segment, which had pitted scars.

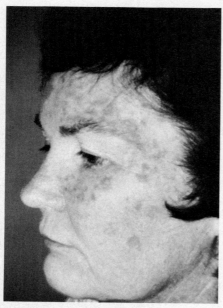

Figure 32–12. After 10 days of topical 5-fluorouracil therapy, no reactive actinic keratoses was seen in the perioral area, which had been chemabraded three years previously.

Complications

All the complications seen after dermabrasion including scarring, pigmentary changes, and infections can be seen after chemabrasion. There appears to be no additional risk because of the application of 50% trichloroacetic acid. The problems of blending treated and untreated areas as seen in dermabrasion are encountered less often after chemabrasion. Blotchy pigmentary changes seen between three weeks and three months after chemabrasion are nearly always self-correcting or are eliminated by the use of a bleaching cream.

Results

Often, for best results, the frequently coexisting problems of scarring, wrinkling, actinic damage, and pigmentary changes are treated by chemabrasion. Chemabrasion improves scarring to the degree expected with dermabrasion, but blending with normal skin is superior. Wrinkling improves, as one would expect with Baker's phenol, but with superior results

because of the ability of the operator to treat coexisting pitted and irregular lesions by varying the depth of the abrasion. Actinic damage, including keratoses, responds excellently (Fig. 32–12). Severe pigmentary problems unresponsive to bleaching preparations and light peeling frequently improve with chemabrasion (Fig. 32–7C).

Summary

Chemabrasion is a single procedure in which a full-face chemical peel is followed immediately by dermabrasion. Individualization of the chemical aspects of the procedure as well as the depth of the abrasion produces excellent results for the usual problems handled by deep chemical peeling and dermabrasion.

REFERENCES

1. Baker TJ: Chemical face peeling and rhytidectomy. Plast Reconstr Surg 29:199–207, 1962
2. Litton C: Chemical face peeling. Plast Reconstr Surg 29:371–380, 1962
3. Kligman A, Willis I: A new formula for depigmenting human skin. Arch Derm 111:40–48, 1975
4. J. R. Barkoff, J. J. Stagnone, and A. R. Ragaz (Albuquerque Dermatology Associates).
5. Dillaha CJ, Jansen GT, Honeycutt WM, Bradford AC: Selective cytotoxic effect of topical 5-flourouracil. Arch Derm 88:247–256, 1963
6. Montagna W: The Structure and Function of the Skin, Ed 2 New York, Academic Press, 1962
7. Mahrle G: Retinoids in skin cancer and hyperproliferative skin disease. J Derm Surg Oncol 9:631–632, 1983
8. Bollag W: Vitamin A and retinoids: From nutrition to pharmacotherapy in dermatology and oncology. Lancet 1(8329):860–863, 1983
9. Cristofolini M, Zumiani G, Scappini P, Piscioli F: Aromatic retinoid in the chemoprevention of the progression of nevoid basal cell carcinoma syndrome. J Derm Surg Oncol 10:10, 1984
10. Dicken CH: Retinoids: A review. JAAD 11:541–552, 1984
11. Horvath PN: The light peel. Bulletin Assoc Milit Derm 18 (2):5 Sept 1970
12. Resnik SS: Chemical peeling with trichloroacetic acid. J Derm Surg Oncol 7:549–550, 1984
13. Farber GA, Collins PS, Wilhelmus SM: Update on chemical peel. J Derm Surg Oncol 7:559–560, 1984
14. Stagnone J, Stagnone G: A second look at chemabrasion. J Derm Surg Oncol 8(8):701–705, 1982
15. Stegman SJ: A comparative histologic study of the effects of three peeling agents and dermabrasion on normal and sun-damaged skin. Aesthet Plast Surg 6:123–135, 1982

THOMAS J. BAKER, M.D. / HOWARD L. GORDON, M.D.

33

Chemical Peel with Phenol

Chemical skin peeling is a process in which chemicals are applied to the skin in order to produce alterations in the gross and microscopic anatomy of the dermis and epidermis. The procedure is primarily used for the removal of fine wrinkles in facial skin, pigmentation problems, and other minor skin blemishes. Synonyms for this process are chemosurgery, chemerasure, dermapeel, skin peeling, and chemexfoliation. Occasionally, it is referred to as chemical face-lifting;[1] however, this term is inaccurate since the face is not actually lifted as in a rhytidectomy.[16]

Trichloroacetic acid, salicylic acid, and phenol have been the most commonly used agents for the peeling process.[1-13] All of these agents are keratolytic and most are weak acids. The agent most frequently used is phenol, C_6H_5OH, commonly referred to as carbolic acid, although its formula does not contain the carboxyl (—COOH) group characteristic of an organic acid. The hydroxyl group indicates that it is nearer to being an organic base or an alcohol.

Since the fourth edition of this text was published in 1977, chemical peeling has become more widely accepted than previously. In the authors' opinion, it has withstood the test of time, and perhaps the reason for its sustained excellent results is due to careful patient selection. A buffered phenol solution remains the preferred agent in spite of some recent clinical evidence that cardiac irritability can be caused by phenol absorption from the skin.[21]

HISTORICAL BACKGROUND

Although there is, of course, no recorded evidence of beautification treatments among prehistoric people, they probably recognized and treated aging skin with abrasives, oil, and other simple drugs known at that time.

The Ebers papyrus (a well-known historical document, circa 1560 B.C.) contains a great deal of information on cosmetic treatments by early Egyptian physicians. This document discusses methods of removing wrinkles and moles, dying hair and eyebrows, correcting squints, and other procedures for beautifying the body. Some of the medications specifically mentioned are mixtures of alabaster, natron, salt, extracts of animal oils, and other similar items. Various agents to alter the gross appearance of the skin have been used since mankind had the ability to attempt such treatments. Early chemosurgery probably took the form of certain types of acid treatments. Exfoliation of the skin was effectuated by poultices from mineral and plant substances directly applied. Sulphur, mustard, and limestone were known to have been used. Indian women were known to have mixed urine with pumice and applied it to the skin to improve their appearance, although there is little evidence of significant value in this preparation. Turkish women used fire to singe the skin and lightly exfoliate it. However, despite frequent use of chemicals since the beginning of recorded history, little specific information is available on early methods of surgical and chemical treatments for aging skin. Yet, it is reasonably certain that similar oils, creams, and abrasives now employed for cosmetic purposes were probably prescribed by the medical men of those times.

During the early part of the twentieth century, chemical face peeling was principally used by lay operators and gained considerable publicity through newspapers and women's magazines in the late 1950s. The Fountain of Youth was proclaimed. The miraculous results were illustrated with spectacular before and after pictures and were exhibited in the advertising of these "lay clinics." By 1960, many patients began questioning their physicians about this process. Prospective patients were surprised to learn that medical doctors did not know the specifics of the procedure, since results appeared to be so spectacular in the eyes of the layman. Because of the clinical results observed from certain of these operations, there seemed to be an indication for adequate scientific investigation and evaluation of the process.

Personal conversation with operators of some of the lay clinics gave skeletal information regarding the use of their formulae. Initially, some basic animal studies were done, utilizing verious chemical solutions: specifically phenol, trichloroacetic acid, and salicylic acid. References in medical literature were sparse, but an article published by Bames[12] gave some background in clinical observations. The results of animal experiments could not be conclusive because it is necessary to substantiate the results by experimentation on human skin. Initial observations were made by treating small areas of human skin. The chemical formula was applied to areas of hyperkeratosis and brown aging spots. All of the basic experiments indicated that the procedure was effective and safe for use in clinical trials. Initially, the forehead was selected as the experimental site, since the skin is thicker in this area and it was felt that catastrophic results would be unlikely. Gradually, larger areas of facial skin were treated. Histologic studies have been carried out on a series of treated patients, and these individuals have been studied over a period of 13 years.[11]

Chemical face peeling offers physicians a partial answer to a problem that eventually confronts all of us, namely, the aging process. If medicine does not supply an answer to this problem in a controlled and scientific way, patients will turn to quacks and charlatans.

Nonmedical clinics still exist, particularly in some of the more densely populated metropolitan areas, and deaths have been reported as a direct result of chemical peeling by lay operators. It is unfortunate for unsuspecting patients that they are lured into these establishments through false and misleading advertising. Chemical peeling is a scientific process and should only be performed by physicians who are well versed in the characteristics of human skin as well as the overall physiologic response of the patient to various drugs utilized locally and systemically. A nonmedical individual should not be allowed to administer chemical peeling, and in many states, legislation has been enacted to prohibit lay operators from doing this procedure.

SELECTION OF PATIENTS

Patients with the following conditions were found to benefit the most from chemical peeling:
1. Those with fine wrinkling of the skin (Fig. 33–1).
2. Patients with abnormal pigmentation problems.
3. Those with skin damage due to radiation.
4. Patients with superficial acne scarring.
Selection of prospective patients is done only after a careful psychological and physiologic survey is completed. The ideal patient is best described as a fair-complexioned English woman who has spent most of her time indoors in a London climate with very little exposure to the sun. The opposite extreme would be a Sicilian fisherman whose complexion has been further darkened by constant exposure to the sun and the elements. Chemical peeling bleaches the skin and, therefore, the darker skin types present problems with the color contrast between treated and untreated areas, especially at the line of demarcation where the treatment terminates. The use of chemical agents on black patients is contraindicated.

The past 20 years of experience has substantiated that the selection of patients is of utmost importance. The bleaching effect of chemical peeling is absolute, and this must be stressed to prospective patients, especially if their complexion is either the freckle-faced and ruddy type or the dark type. The contrast between treated and untreated areas is significant, and it is up to the physician to use the procedure on the proper skin types and, furthermore, to properly advise the patient that the bleaching effect is permanent.

Chemical peeling of delicate, thin skin produces a smoother, more natural appearance with more uniform coloring than coarsely textured skin that is thick and oily. The latter tends to have less of a response to the chemical peeling and is more apt to undergo blotchy pigmentation with subsequent exposure to the sun, an undesirable sequela.

The usual complaints and requests of prospective patients for chemical peeling (Fig. 33–2) are:
1. Vertical lines on the upper lip.
2. Glabellar frown lines.
3. Multiple crow's feet in the periorbital area.
4. Fine mosaic lines in the face.
5. Irregular pigmentation of the facial skin.
Other patients may specifically request treatment for chloasma, ephelides, lentigo, weather-beaten skin, blotchy pigmentation, multiple hyperkeratosis of the face, and occasionally, superficial acne scarring. Although patients are often apprehensive about the process, chemical peeling is usually more acceptable to them than the surgical blade of the face-lift. A sufficient amount of time should be spent with patients before they undergo the chemical peeling process in order to adequately explain all facets of the procedure. This helps patients to tolerate the procedure, and they are apt to be more satisfied with the outcome.

The application of phenol is relatively simple and quick; however, it is followed by several days of restrictions, discomfort, and inconvenience. For example, the patient is not allowed to talk or eat for 48 hours, because these activities jeopardize the end results. These and other aspects of the treatment can create apprehension and lack of cooperation on the part of patients if they do not understand and anticipate their occurrence.

It must be carefully explained to patients just how much of an improvement may be expected, and they should be informed of the possible shortcomings of the procedure, including possible complications. Those facial features that will not be corrected by the chemical peel should be carefully stressed. For example, many patients erroneously believe that a chemical peel will substitute for a rhytidectomy. If the patient has sagging skin as well as fine mosaic lines on the face, the treatment will only produce smooth skin on a sagging face. Many prospective patients need a rhytidectomy as well as a chemical peel. The inevitable line of demarcation between the treated and untreated areas must be mentioned and stressed. Patients should be fully aware of the

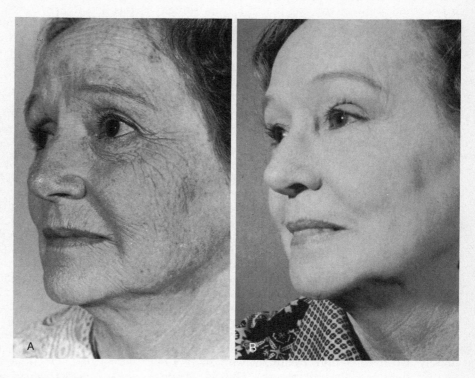

Figure 33–1. *A,* A 60-year-old prospective patient for face peeling. Note the fine lines radiating from the perioral area, the fine mosaic lines in the cheek, and the lines around the lower eyelids. This patient has a minimum of facial sagging for her age group and is an ideal candidate for a chemical face peel. *B,* Seven years postpeel. The chemically induced changes are long-lasting, as evidenced by the skin still being relatively smooth.

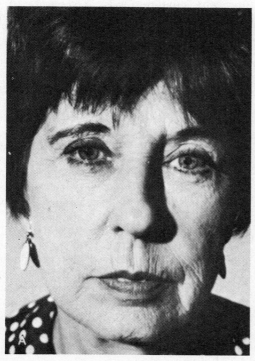

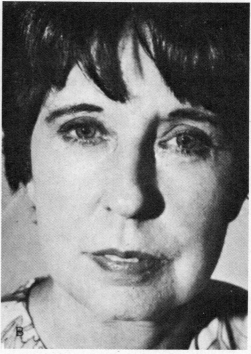

Figure 33–2. *A,* A 52-year-old prospective patient who complained about the "tired look" of her face. She specifically requested eradication of the superficial wrinkling in her face and was particularly interested in eliminating the lines on the upper lip and around the eyes. *B,* Ten months following chemical face peeling. Note the overall improvement in the facial configuration and that the expression appears refreshed.

time required for healing. In addition, they must be forewarned about protecting the skin from sun exposure for several months following the treatment. All of these factors should be discussed in order that patients may properly evaluate whether or not they are willing to make these personal sacrifices in order to achieve the anticipated end result.

TECHNIQUE

While there are many variations described in the literature with regard to the treatment of a patient undergoing a chemical face peel, the technique described herein has been found to produce satisfactory results and offers the fewest complications. The procedure should be carried out in a hospital or a clinic properly equipped to handle such patients. The initial four or five days of management are too complex to utilize this technique of total face peeling on an outpatient basis. It is unnecessary to use an operating room, since the treatment can be easily carried out in the patient's own bed in his room. The patient must be completely relaxed and tranquil prior to the application of the chemical solution, so the patient is premedicated approximately two hours before treatment with 200 mg of pentobarbital sodium by mouth. This is supplemented with 100 mg of meperidine hydrochloride given intramuscularly 45 minutes before treatment. If the patient is still apprehensive or excited, supplements may be necessary, and intravenous diazepam (Valium) in doses of 1 to 10 mg has proven to be adequate.

Since it has recently been reported that cardiac arrhythmias may be caused by the absorption of phenol,[21] a cardiac monitor should be used on all patients and their vital signs carefully observed. The authors' personal experience with over 2000 patients receiving partial or total chemical peel has shown no evidence of cardiac irregularities in the authors' patients. This is probably due to the extended time element involved in the application of phenol. Approximately 1 1/2 hours should be utilized to apply the solution. The procedure is frequently done in segments, for example, the forehead can be done initially and the tape applied. A period of 15 or 20 minutes is allowed to elapse and then one cheek is done. After an additional 20 to 30 minutes elapse, another segment of the face is done, which is followed by another time interval of 15 to 20 minutes before the total peeling is completed. Since the procedure takes about 1 1/2 hours, the concentration of systemic phenol absorption at any one time is reduced. By utilizing this technique, cardiac arhythmias have not been observed.

The skin is thoroughly washed with surgical soap followed by a cleansing with diethyl ether (the ether is applied on a 4 × 3 inch surgical sponge). Gentle cleansing of the skin removes all of the superficial oils and debris. Since ether is explosive, other patients in the room should be cautioned not to smoke. Adequate cleansing with diethyl ether is necessary, since the oils must be completely removed in order to prevent a separation of the adhesive mask that will be applied later. The oils, if left on the skin, are also a possible barrier to the effective contact of the phenol with the skin.

Formula

The mixture used is a saponified phenol suspension:
- 3 cc U.S.P. phenol (C_6H_5OH)
- 2 cc tap water
- 8 drops liquid soap (Septisol)
- 3 drops croton oil (from the seed of *Croton tiglium*)

The various ingredients are mixed fresh at the time of each treatment in order to be absolutely certain that the ingredients are correct and that the chemicals are fresh. All of the necessary ingredients for preparation of the formula are stored in dark individual bottles and kept in a small medicine bag, along with the other necessary materials, such as tape, scissors, gauze, and cotton-tipped applicators. Since the mixture tends to separate, it must be stirred vigorously with the tip of a cotton applicator immediately before each individual contact with the skin.

Application of the Formula

The peeling mixture is applied to the face with an ordinary cotton-tipped applicator. Care must be taken to apply the mixture evenly and uniformly over the entire area and into each wrinkle. The forehead is generally done first. On contact with the chemicals, the skin immediately becomes pearly white, and the patient experiences a mild burning sensation. This subsides within five to 10 seconds because of the local anesthetic quality of phenol. The application is carried well into the hairline to minimize the line of demarcation that could exist in that area. Chemical peeling does not affect the growth of hair folicles. The applicator is semimoist, rather than saturated, with the mixture in order to prevent the chemical from dripping on areas of the body where it would not be desirable. Lightly rolling the applicator onto a piece of gauze absorbs the excess liquid.

The applicator should be almost dry when treating the eyelids, since the conjunctiva and cornea could theoretically be damaged by contact with the mixture. To prevent this injury, the chemicals are applied with the applicator semimoist, and the eyelid skin is moistened to within 2 mm of the ciliary margin of the lower lid. The upper lid is held open until each of the lower lids has been treated, blotted, and allowed to air-dry. By using this meticulous method, no incidents of damage to the conjunctiva or cornea have occurred. It is unwise to use ointments on the conjunctival surface since the patient will squint and cause the ointment to spill over onto the skin, thereby making the phenol mixture ineffective and the adherence of the tape impossible.

It is a good precautionary measure to keep an irrigating syringe full of water close at hand in case some of the chemicals should inadvertently come into contact with the conjunctival surface. The upper eyelids are treated up to and including the tarsal plate, but not to the margin of the eyelid. This is done in order to prevent unnecessary edema of the upper eyelid. The mixture should be carried into the eyebrows, but no tape is applied over the brows since a temporary loss of hair would result when the tape is removed. The earlobes are usually wrinkled and are often treated if it is deemed desirable to remove the fine wrinkling from the lobes themselves.

The mixture is applied to the entire face down to a line 2 to 3 cm below the inferior margin of the mandible. If a natural skin crease is present in the upper area of the neck, this forms a logical line to terminate the peel. If there is no obvious crease in the upper portion of the neck, the mixture should extend only onto the neck far enough to camouflage the treated area as well as possible. Around the mouth, care should be taken to apply the chemicals at least to the vermilion border and preferably slightly onto it. Application there removes the vertical wrinkles of the upper lip, especially the smaller ones that radiate from the vermilion border. Such elimination is important because lipstick tends to run into these creases and gives an objectionable appearance.

Application of the Waterproof Mask

Once the skin has been completely covered with the chemical mixture, a mask of waterproof adhesive tape is applied directly to the skin. The eyes, eyebrows, nostrils, and mouth are left exposed. The first layer of tape is constructed of short pieces of half-inch tape. Careful application allows the mask to make good adhesive contact with the entire surface of the face. For the difficult areas, such as the lower eyelids, nostril rims, and upper lip, small lengths of quarter-inch strips are used for better adhesion. After the first layer has been applied, it is overlayed with one-inch tape to insure total coverage. Care should be taken not to apply the tape too tightly, since folds could be created beneath the

skin that would allow a small section to be left out of contact with the tape, thereby making the peel less deep in that area. After the entire face has been taped, the palms should be pressed lightly over the entire face in each individual area to insure adequate adherence of the tape to the treated skin.

Intensity of the burning sensation varies significantly from patient to patient and, in many instances, supplemental medication is needed. It is important that the patient be medicated sufficiently to maintain comfort during the ensuing three to four hours, which is the duration of the burning sensation. After three to four hours, the stinging of the skin stops and does not return during the treatment.

During the initial six to eight hours after the application of the mask, the face becomes edematous and the eyelids are frequently swollen shut. This should be explained to patients so they do not become apprehensive about their inability to see. The mask is left in position for 48 hours, during which time the patient is not permitted to talk and is instructed to keep the face as immobile as possible. Liquids are administered through a straw in sufficient quantity to maintain hydration and nutrition. The patient's head should be kept elevated at approximately 25 degrees. Bed rest is essential; however, bathroom privileges are allowed. The nursing service should be instructed that patients must be assisted to the bathroom, since there may be temporary difficulty with their vision from edema of the eyelids. Tranquilizers and other supportive drugs are given as indicated.

There is little change in the edema during the second 24 hours. The skin begins to weep, and patients experience sensations of fluid running beneath the mask. They should be instructed to expect this.

Removal of the Mask

The mask is left in place for 48 hours after its application. At the time of removal, additional medication is necessary; usually 5 to 10 mg of diazepam (Valium) is given intravenously just prior to removal of the mask. While this amount of medication is sufficient in most cases, clinical observation and judgment must identify patients whose low tolerance for pain requires more medication. It has been necessary on rare occasions to remove the mask under brief general anesthesia in the operating room. The edge of the mask is grasped with a forceps and underlying skin is gently pushed away with a sterile cotton-tipped applicator to tease the mask from the skin. Beneath the mask an edematous, weeping surface is seen that resembles a second-degree burn. The mask is carefully and slowly teased sway from the entire face and discarded.

Application of Thymol Iodide Powder

After the mask has been completely removed, the skin is covered with thymol iodide U.S.P. powder. A small amount of the powder is applied with a cotton-tipped applicator and carefully rolled onto the weeping surface. The powder adheres readily and forms a golden-brown crust. Reapplication of the powder is carried out three or four times during the next 24 hours until a heavy crust is formed. Thymol iodide acts as a bacteriostatic agent.

Separation of the Crust from the Face

At the end of 24 hours following the initial application of the thymol iodide powder (and 72 hours from the beginning of the treatment), a softening ointment is applied to the crust, hastening its spontaneous separation from the face. Use of the ointment should continue on a daily basis as necessary until the crust has separated. A and D ointment has proved to be quite satisfactory. Neosporin or Bacitracin ointment has also been utilized but seem to cause a high degree of skin sensitivity. Beginning on the sixth or seventh day following mask removal, the face is gently washed with cool tap water and a clean white washcloth. Most of the crust will have separated by this time and the face is seen to be red and edematous.

Peeling Without the Use of a Waterproof Mask

The expression "light chemical peel" is one which is often talked about and generally refers to the same process as described above but without the application of the waterproof adhesive mask. The function of the occlusive dressing (mask) is to cause a more profound effect. If the superficial mosaic lines are not deep and less of a peel is needed, the tape mask is not used. In younger patients with chloasma, the application of a complete facial mask does not seem to be necessary.

Early Post-Treatment Care

Approximately one week following removal of the mask, refrigerated hydrogenated vegetable oil will keep the skin greasy and comfortable. Crisco, for example, is a product that is well known to most patients and readily acceptable. Itching is often a problem during this phase of the treatment and is more prevalent during the night. This is apparently caused by the dependent positioning and venous congestion of the face. It is best treated with elevation of the head, ice packs directly in contact with the treated surface, antihistamines by mouth, and a topical steroid ointment. The use of adequate sleeping medication during the first few nights following treatment is helpful.

The length of confinement varies according to the intelligence, stability, and cooperation of patients as well as their individual progress and home situation. Most patients can leave the hospital or recovery facility on the fourth to the sixth post-treatment day.

From the seventh to the twenty-first day after initiation of the treatment, the skin has a somewhat granular appearance, and milia may form. No specific treatment is indicated except to keep the face well lubricated and clean. The reddish color persists from six to 12 weeks, and it gradually fades away to a pinkish hue that is usually not too objectionable. By the fourteenth day, most patients are able to wear cosmetics and are encouraged to do so for short periods of time. Lipstick may be used much earlier, since it is not appled to any treated area. At the end of three or four weeks, skillful application of cosmetics will comouflage the treatment almost completely. After the skin has regained its normal appearance and patients have returned to routine skin care, they are encouraged to use a moisturizing lotion or cream at night. Most patients will question the physician regarding recommendations on specific cosmetics. It is better psychologically to make specific recommendations rather than generalizations. Patients can thus be encouraged to maintain better skin care and give more attention to the proper use of cosmetics.

Late Post-Treatment Care

Since chemical face peeling removes a significant amount of the melanin cells in the basal layer of the epidermis,[7, 11] the process thereby lightens the skin color and reduces natural protection against the sun. Patients who have undergone chemical face peeling should be warned to avoid direct or even reflected sunlight for extended periods of time. The use of adequate sunscreens is recommended; here again, it is probably best to recommend specific products rather than to generalize. Opaque sunscreens appear to work better than the transparent ones. A sun protection factor (SPF) in the range of six to eight affords the patient sufficient protection against most exposure to sunlight, except direct sunlight which should be avoided.

Specific advice with reference to the sun should include the following:

1. Patients should stay out of direct sunlight for three to six months especially during the middle part of the day. If they must be in the sunlight, they should wear a wide-brimmed hat.

2. As a routine procedure, an effective sunscreen should be utilized daily for several months.

3. Patients should avoid reflected sunlight, which is particularly a problem when riding in an automobile for extended periods of time. Cases have been seen where patients developed irregular pigmentation on the side of the face exposed to the sun while driving.

No problems with blotchy facial pigmentation have developed in patients who have rigidly followed instructions on avoiding sunlight.

COMBINED CHEMICAL PEEL AND RHYTIDECTOMY

The older patient usually presents two basic problems: (1) generalized sagging of the tissue as a result of the body's losing battle with gravity (Fig. 33–3) and (2) fine wrinkling over the face along with deep lines in the forehead and around the mouth and eyes (Fig. 33–4). As previously stated, chemical face peeling puts smooth skin on a sagging face if the patient is in need of a rhytidectomy. Conversely, a rhytidectomy will only stretch the skin tighter on an otherwise finely wrinkled face and will not totally correct the problem. In patients having both problems, it is wise to advise ahead of time that neither procedure will totally correct the entire aging process. Therefore, they should be advised that it might

subsequently be necessary to undergo a rhytidectomy or, conversely, have the rhytidectomy before the chemical face peel. If both procedures are to be carried out, an interval of at least three or four months should separate them. Our personal preference is to do the rhytidectomy first and the face peeling second.[3, 5]

REGIONAL CHEMICAL PEELING

There are instances in which only an isolated area of the face needs to be treated,[6] most commonly the upper lip. Many patients requesting rhytidectomy are very concerned about the radiating lines on the upper lip and perioral area (Fig. 33–5). These are treated best by chemical peeling.[22] The skin of the mustache area is often of a different color from that of the rest of the face prior to treatment, and it will certainly be lighter following treatment. However, the "mustache area" is a rather circumscribed unit of the face, bordered by the nose, mouth, and nasolabial folds. The same formula and technique is utilized in regional peeling. Care should be taken to apply the mixture just onto the vermillion border and the entire upper lip and to include the nasolabial folds, extending the peel 2 to 3 mm beyond the nasolabial fold itself. If the peel stops at the naso-

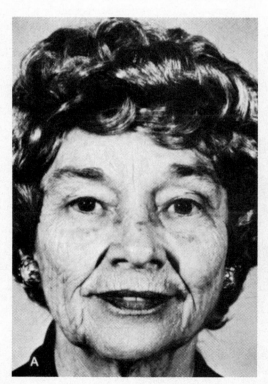
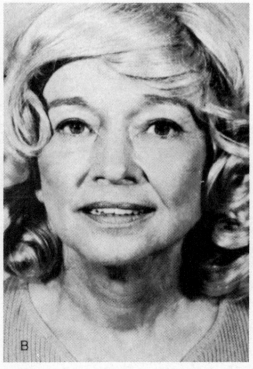

Figure 33–3. *A,* A 67-year-old prospective patient for combined rhytidectomy and chemical face peeling. Note the generalized sagging of the face as well as the aged look of the skin itself. *B,* Appearance 12 months following chemical face peeling and six months following rhytidectomy. The surgical lift corrected the sagging of the face and neck, while the chemical peel smoothed the fine wrinkling of the skin. This patient was also encouraged to wear a wig and to use more meticulous care with her makeup.

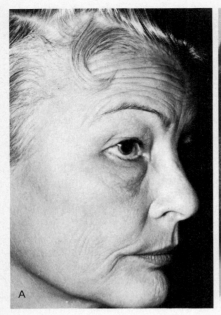

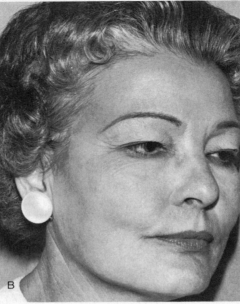

Figure 33—4. *A*, A 50-year-old patient with only fine wrinkling and very little sagging. *B*, Appearance six years postpeel. The fine lines have not returned, and the quality of the skin remains good.

labial fold, it will merely accentuate the line rather than partially eliminate it. The application of the tape to this area, the application of thymol iodide after removal of the tape, and follow-up treatment are the same as previously outlined for treatment of the entire face. Regional peeling can be done on an outpatient basis and is often done in the office as an isolated procedure.

On rare occasions, the glabellar area or periorbital area is treated as an isolated section of the face for peeling (Fig. 33–6), either with or without adhesive tape.[15]

PEELING IN ASSOCIATED SKIN CONDITIONS

Abnormal Pigmentation Problems

Chemical face peeling occasionally gives excellent results in correcting abnormal pigmentation problems (Fig. 33–7). It is effective in most cases, regardless of the cause of the condition. Chloasma, pigmentation due to drug reactions, brown aging spots, and freckles all respond to the treatment. The technique utilized for these procedures is exactly

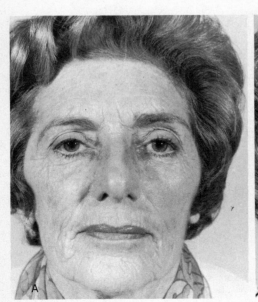

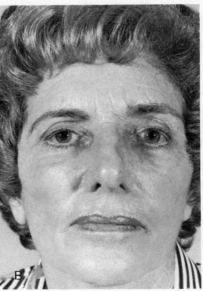

Figure 33—5. *A*, Note appearance of lip and perioral area. *B*, Postpeel appearance. Note the radiating perioral lines are markedly improved.

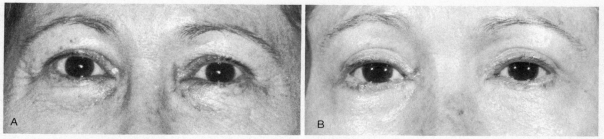

Figure 33–6. *A*, Note periorbital wrinkling. *B*, Four years following chemical peel of the upper and lower eyelids and periorbital area.

the same as described earlier in the text. Results appear to be permanent. Abnormal pigmentation often creates a greater social and psychological problem than the presence of wrinkles. Patients have been seen with such severe alterations in pigmentation that they would hardly venture from their homes and become socially withdrawn because of the problem. In most circumstances, the abnormal pigmentation is due to hyperpigmentation rather than a loss of pigmentation. The objective of securing a uniform color, whether dark or light, is preferable to a blotchy condition. The peeling results in bleaching the entire face, and the hyperpigmented areas will usually bleach to the same degree as the rest of the face thereby giving a homogenous appearance. In mild pigmentation problems, it is probably best to encourage patients to utilize cosmetics rather than subject themselves to an entire chemical face peel. This is particularly true in mild cases of chloasma.

Occasionally, patients will have extremely dark circles in the periorbital areas (Fig. 33–8). This discoloration can sometimes be removed by the topical application of the phenol solution. The patient must be warned about the lines of demarcation, especially since this is a limited, regional application around the periorbital area and is more apt to be noticed than the line of demarcation along the upper

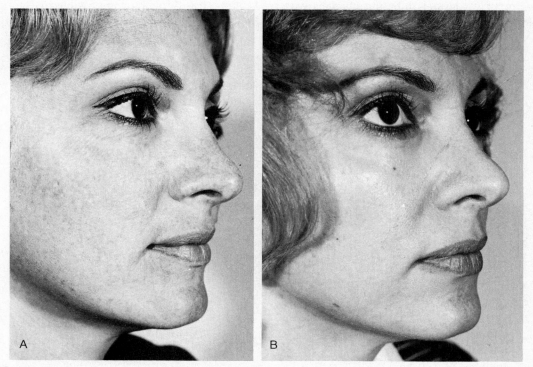

Figure 33–7. *A*, This 34-year-old patient had superficial acne scarring and mild hyperpigmentation problems associated with the acne combined with the use of oral medications. *B*, Appearance 18 months following chemical face peeling. There has been a significant improvement in the pigmentation problem as well as a tightening of the skin helping to improve the appearance of the superficial acne scarring.

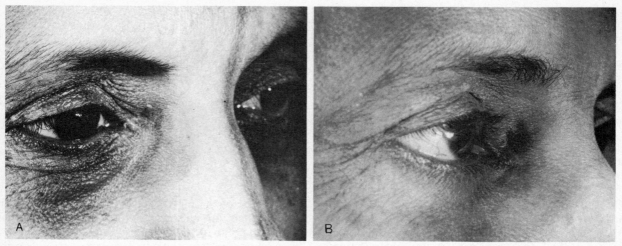

Figure 33—8. *A,* This patient has extremely dark periorbital circles. *B,* The chemical peel has served to bleach the periorbital skin and to improve her appearance.

portion of the neck following a total chemical face peel. In most instances, women find this line of demarcation more acceptable than the dark circles around the eyes.

Chronic Changes Due to X-Ray Radiation

The treatment of dermal radiation changes with dermabrasion has been disappointing. Response to chemical treatment appears to be much the same as with dermabrasion; however, the long-term effectiveness seems to be more permanent with chemical peeling. Physicians experienced in treating this type of condition with dermabrasion use the same criteria in the selection of patients as that for chemical peeling. Most patients have received x-ray radiation for the treatment of juvenile acne (Fig. 33–9). Usually, it is difficult or impossible to determine the amount of x-ray radiation patients have received,

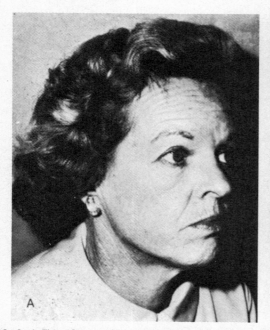
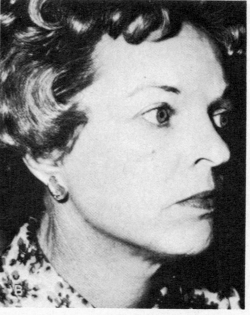

Figure 33—9. *A,* This 42-year-old patient had atrophy of the skin and other changes due to chronic radiation. In addition, she still had residual scarring following juvenile acne and was beginning to develop some of the superficial wrinkles in the skin characteristic of the aging process. *B,* Appearance one year following chemical face peeling. The acne scarring has improved, many of the lines of aging have been significantly eradicated, and a more homogeneous appearance to the facial skin has been created.

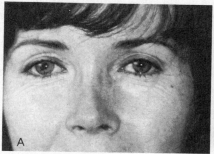
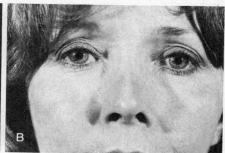

Figure 33–10. *A,* Appearance before chemical peel. Note freckles and periorbital lines. *B,* Appearance 11 years postpeel. Note that freckles have not returned and that the skin remains relatively smooth.

since many had the treatment several years previously and the clinical records are unavailable. However, the dosage does not appear to significantly influence the response to the chemical peel. Clinically, the response of the skin to chemical face peeling in this series has been the same as in patients who had not received radiation.

Freckles

Chemical face peeling does remove freckles permanently; however, it has not been used by the authors for the sole purpose of removing freckles. Coincidentally, many patients who were treated for other reasons had freckles removed at the same time, since peeling does effectively cause their disappearance (Fig. 33–10).

Telangiectasis

Litton stated that chemical face peeling was of considerable benefit in the treatment of telangiectasis.[1] This has not been true in this series of patients. An occasional patient shows some improvement in small telangiectatic spots of the face, but for the most part, these are not significantly altered, and peeling is not recommended for the alteration of telangiectatic areas. Some patients have demonstrated more telangiectasis following the peel.

Port-Wine Stains

A number of patients have presented themselves for treatment with this condition; however, a deep peel has no effect on the port-wine stain. Clinical tests have also been made with reference to hemangiomas. No significant benefit is seen, and therefore, it is not recommended.

Acne Scarring

Some patients with mild scarring from superficial acne have been treated with chemical peeling, and the results are encouraging (Fig. 33–11). However, peeling does not seem to offer as much to the patient as dermabrasion, and it has no significant benefit in the more advanced forms of acne.

Hypertrophied Scars and Burns

Chemical peeling of hypertrophied burn scars sometimes alters the pigmentation and makes the

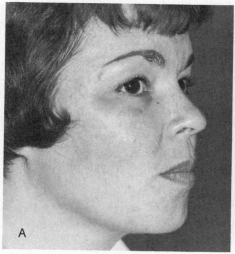
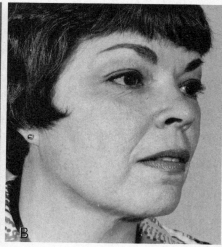

Figure 33–11. *A,* Mild acne scarring in a 30-year-old patient. *B,* Appearance 10 years following chemical peel.

area more homogenous with reference to the surrounding skin; however, it does not significantly alter the scars. Therefore, it is not recommended for this type of patient.

Hair

Chemical peeling does not alter the growth of facial or scalp hair. Routine face peeling involves applying the chemical solution into the hairline, along the eyebrows, and onto the fine hair of the face; however, in no case has there been any alteration in the hair pattern. Some patients have the mistaken notion that peeling removes hair; however, this is not true. The hair follicles are not damaged by the treatment, at least not to the extent that the growth of the hair is altered.

EFFECTIVENESS IN MEN

Chemical peeling has been done in a few male patients. Generally, men do not exhibit the necessity for peeling as do women. The fine radiating lines around the mouth and chin, for example, are a rare occurrence in men and therefore, requests for the procedure have not created a significant number of cases. The principal disadvantage in doing the peeling process in males seems to be the lack of response of the skin to the peel technique. Male skin is more oily and, therefore, theoretically cancels some of the effectiveness of the active ingredients. In addition, when a mask is applied on a man, the beard grows very rapidly and, in a matter of a few hours, pushes the occlusive dressing away from the underlying skin, thereby further reducing the effectiveness of the peel. For these reasons, the procedure is not recommended in male patients except in very unusual circumstances.

SYSTEMIC TOXICITY

The use of phenol raises the question as to whether or not systemic toxicity is produced through absorption. Numerous studies of this question indicate that such effects are unlikely.[17] Pure phenol is a colorless solution, having an aromatic odor and a burning taste. It can be obtained from coal tar or synthetically produced from monochlorobenzene. Pure phenol is a protoplasmic poison that affects the central nervous system. It is well known that it is absorbed through unbroken skin as well as through the mucous membranes.

An oral dose of phenol ranging from 5 to 15 gm can result in death within 24 hours. If there are systemic toxic manifestations from the application of phenol to the skin, they usually begin within a few minutes. The symptoms include faintness, muscular weakness, convulsions, weak and irregular pulse, depressed respiration, constricted pupils, coma, and even death. Deichmann studied detoxification and excretion of orally administered phenol and determined that it is removed from the body by three processes: excretion, oxidation, and conjugation.[17] Within 24 hours, the experimental animal will excrete 27% of a toxic (half-lethal) dose in the urine. Only traces are excreted in the feces at this time. At the end of 24 hours, 3% of the absorbed phenol may be found in the body.

Blood phenol studies were carried out by Litton in a series of 50 patients.[1, 18] Blood samples were drawn at one-, three-, and five-hour intervals and analyzed with a spectrophotometer. He demonstrated that with 3 cc of a 50% phenol solution applied to the entire face, the maximum blood phenol levels rose to 0.68 mg/100 ml within one hour after application. After two hours, the maximum level was 0.19 mg/100 ml, and after four hours, less than 0.1 mg/liter.

A case has been reported in the literature in which 23 mg/100 ml of blood phenol was found in a patient 15 minutes after oral ingestion of phenol.[1] The patient survived. Obviously, there is a large margin of safety between the 0.68 mg % in the series reported by Litton and the 23 mg % level demonstrated by this case.

Studies in this series concluded that no evidence of systemic toxicity existed either by routine laboratory analyses or clinical observations. The authors' series encompasses more than 2000 patients treated over a 20-year period. Their conclusion is that the formula utilized by the technique described herein does not lead to systemic toxicity. Both Ayres[23] and Brown[14] reported that liquid phenol can be used with relative safety when it is applied to a limited area of the skin in restricted quantities and at proper intervals. In applying phenol to the face in one sitting, MacKee and Karp[19] failed to find any systemic effects demonstrable by clinical or laboratory tests. Cardiac arrhythmias have not been observed in the authors' experience.

COMPLICATIONS

The untoward effects and complications that are encountered following chemical face peel include the following:

1. Reduction in the pigmentation of the skin (bleaching effect) (Fig. 33–12)
2. Increased sensitivity of the skin to sunlight
3. Milia
4. Hypertrophied scars
5. Scar contracture
6. Alteration of existing skin conditions

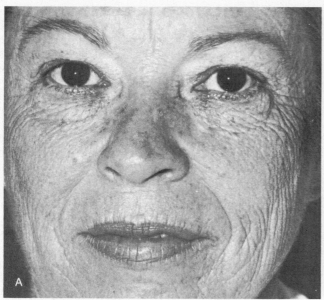 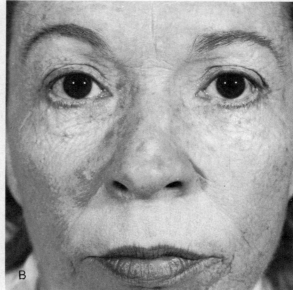

Figure 33–12. *A,* Note radiating lines on upper lip. *B,* Appearance five years postpeel. Note that lines have not returned and also that the bleaching effect of the peel is quite marked in this type of skin.

a. Darkening of existing nevi
b. Telangiectasia
c. Increase in size of the skin pores
7. Prolonged redness of the skin

While chemical face peeling has become an accepted form of therapy with a very low complication rate, complications do occur, and those planning to do the procedure should be aware of them.[9, 20]

Reduction in the Pigmentation of the Skin

Dark-complexioned patients show more bleaching effect than those with light complexions. Therefore, most of the problems associated with the line of demarcation can be avoided by proper patient selection. The ideal patient is one who has fair skin and a miminal amount of freckles or brown aging spots and who has not subjected the skin to excessive sun exposure. Many prospective patients are not good candidates for chemical peeling, and the consulting physician should not hesitate to refuse treatment. Since the bleaching effect following chemical peeling often causes a noticeable line of demarcation between the treated and untreated areas along the neck (Fig. 33–13), an attempt is made to minimize this at the time of treatment by extending the application of the mixture approximately one-half inch beyond the margin of the mask. Said in another way, after the solution has been applied, the mask is brought to within one-half inch of the treated margin. Tape on a treated area causes a deeper peel and, therefore, the technique of bringing the tape just short of the edge of the treated area tends to

make the line of demarcation less noticeable. The level at which the treatment stops is important, because there is frequently a natural line of differentiation in skin color just beneath the mandibular margin. This is an ideal place to limit the application of the chemicals. If the peel is brought down to the midportion of the neck, the treatment boundary will obviously be much more noticeable. Blotchy pigmentation of the face can occur following chemosurgery, but if sunlight is assiduously avoided, blotchiness is rare. If it does occur, the hyperpigmented areas will have to be repeeled. Normally, three or four months should elapse before a second peel is attempted. The original formula is applied directly to these blotchy areas and no tape is used.

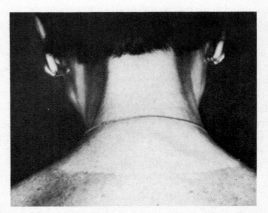

Figure 33–13. This 55-year-old patient exhibits the severe line of demarcation that can occur following treatment in certain types of skin. This particular patient had a chemical peel of the face and neck, but now has the problem of camouflaging the line across the shoulders when wearing a low-necked dress.

Increased Sensitivity of the Skin to Sunlight

Since there is a permanent reduction of the melanin-producing cells in the basal layer of the epidermis,[7, 11] the skin does not respond normally to sunlight, and tanning does not occur. None of the patients who undergo chemical face peeling are able to develop a suntan. Therefore, it should be stressed that they must avoid sunlight and use a sunscreen on the skin at all times. No cases of sunburn have been observed following chemical peeling.

Milia

Although milia have occurred following chemosurgery, the incidence is rare and certainly much less than after dermabrasion. Usually the milia will regress spontaneously, but if they do not after three or four months, the patients are advised to use a soft complexion brush on the skin several times daily. Those resistant milia that do not disappear may have to be opened individually in the office with a fine scalpel blade. In no instance have milia been permanent.

Hypertrophied Scars

Fortunately, hypertrophied scars are encountered rarely. Several cases have been seen in which severe scar contracture of the face and neck have occurred in patients being treated by "lay operators." The authors' personal experience is limited to four individuals who developed small, transverse hypertrophied scars in the midportion of the upper lip. This occurred between two and three months following treatment, and in each instance, the patient had undergone a segmental chemical peel of the upper lip at the time of rhytidectomy. No cases of hypertrophy of the scar of the upper lip have been seen when the upper lip was done as an isolated procedure, or when the lip was treated unassociated with any other surgical procedure. A conclusion has been reached that the scar hypertrophy was probably related to the excessive edema present from the rhytidectomy. A better technique is to treat the entire upper lip (if a rhytidectomy is being done at the same time) by applying the tape strip only along the skin just superior to the vermilion border, and not to tape the entire lip. Since this technique has been utilized, no instance of scar hypertrophy has been seen on the lip. While hypertrophied scarring has been reported following chemical peeling, it is very rare (less than 1%), but for medicolegal reasons, it is probably best to explain to the patient that it is a possibility. A consent form for chemical peeling should be utilized.

Alteration of Existing Skin Conditions

Darkening of Existing Nevi. Several patients have noted that moles have appeared on their faces following therapy. A review of the preoperative photograph shows that a pale nevus was present in the area prior to chemotherapy. Hyperpigmentation of nevi does occur following chemosurgery, and the patient should be forewarned.

Telangiectasia. Telangiectatic areas of the face are occasionally noticeable following the peel. In most cases, the telangiectatic spots were present prior to therapy, and since the skin appears somewhat thinner following treatment, they are almost always more noticeable. If the patient has telangiectasia prior to surgery, the possibility of the areas being more noticeable following treatment should be discussed.

Increase in Size of the Skin Pores. As in dermabrasion, pores appear larger following chemical peeling. There is no clinical problem associated with the enlargement, but it is important that the patient be aware of this possibility. Some patients will request chemical peeling for treatment of enlarged pores and have the mistaken idea that the chemical peeling will reduce the size of the pores. The reverse is true.

Prolonged Redness of the Skin

Under usual circumstances, the skin remains reddish or pink for six to eight weeks following treatment. However, an occasional patient has had redness for 12 to 18 weeks. In no case has the redness remained as a permanent condition. A clinical observation has been made that patients who maintain the redness for the longest period of time eventually have the best clinical result. If the redness persists more than six to eight weeks, topical steroids applied daily help diminish the erythema. Once again, the patient should be forewarned about the possibility of prolonged redness in order to avoid disappointment and misunderstanding.

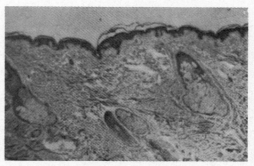

Figure 33–14. Hematoxylin-eosin stain of normal skin in a 60-year-old patient.

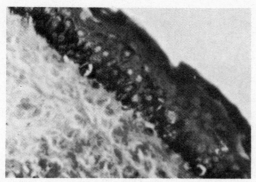

Figure 33–15. Fontana-Masson stain demonstrating the normal melanin-containing cells in the basal layer of the epidermis.

HISTOLOGIC CHANGES IN THE SKIN

Biopsies from patients have been secured ranging from three months to 13 years.[11] The biopsy material was secured from the neck encompassing an ellipse of skin that contained both treated and untreated skin at the junctional area. This allowed observation of the normal control skin contiguous with the treated skin. Three consistent findings have been observed, both in patients three months post-treatment and in others up to 13 years post-treatment:

1. Homogenization of the dermal collagen architecture (Figs. 33–14 and 33–15).

2. A marked diminution of the quantity of melanin granules present in the basal layer of the epidermis (Figs. 33–16 and 33–17).

3. An increase in the amount of elastic-staining tissue in the dermis as demonstrated by special elastic stains (Fig. 33–18).

The bleaching effect of the chemically treated skin can be adequately explained by the permanent reduction of the melanin-producing cells in the basal layer of the epidermis. The increase of the elastic-staining tissue in the dermis cannot adquately be explained; however, it probably represents a reaction to injury, since a similar histologic finding is

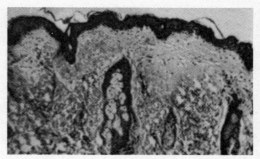

Figure 33–17. One year following chemical face peeling. Note the "smudging" of the dermal collagen layer.

noted in solar degeneration of exposed skin. It is speculated in a teleologic way that elastotic material in the superficial dermis is the body's response to injury, i.e, a means for protecting the underlying structures from further injury by ultraviolet or chemical penetration.

No deleterious effects, such as malignancy, were noted over the 15-year period of this study.

SUMMARY

Experience with chemical face peeling, utilizing the technique as outlined in this chapter, is relatively new in modern medicine. The authors' personal experience encompasses 22 years. It can definitely be concluded that chemical face peeling produces gross and microscopic changes in the skin that are permanent. This is grossly demonstrated by the elimination of wrinkles, the lighter color of the skin, and the change in its texture. At times, the pores may appear larger (a similar result occurs after dermabrasion). Microscopic alterations appear to be permanent and are predictable. The response of the skin to chemical face peeling varies rather widely according to skin type, color, and texture. However, proper patient selection, which has become increasingly precise in recent years, accounts for success more than any other factor. The thin-skinned, fair-complexioned woman who has only fine wrinkles and a minimum of gross sagging is the ideal candidate. A poor candidate is the patient with thick,

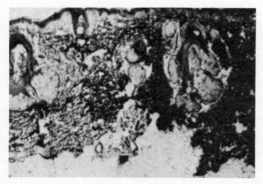

Figure 33–16. Verhoeff's elastic stain through junctional area. The treated area is on the right and nontreated area on the left. Note the increased elastic staining tissue in the treated section.

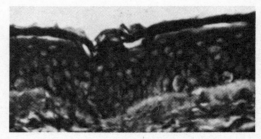

Figure 33–18. One year following chemical face peeling. Note the reduction of the melanin-producing cells in the basal layer of the epidermis. This is apparently a permanent alteration.

oily skin and an olive complexion and who has spent considerable time in the sun. Skin tanned and thickened from chronic exposure to the sun causes pronounced lines of demarcation between treated and untreated areas and a tendency towards lack of color homogeneity after peeling. The texture and color of the skin are of greater concern in the selection of patients than age. Chemical face peeling is a safe and accepted form of treatment with proper patient selection and careful attention to the utilization of the technique.

REFERENCES

1. Litton C: Chemical face lifting. Plast Reconstr Surg 29:371, 1962
2. Baker TJ, Gordon HL: The ablation of rhytides by chemical means, a preliminary report. J Fla Med Assoc 48:451, 1961
3. Baker TJ: Chemical face peeling and rhytidectomy. Plast Reconstr Surg 29:199, 1962
4. Baker TJ, Gordon HL: Chemosurgery of the face, some warnings and misconceptions. J Fla Med Assoc 49:218, 1962
5. Baker TJ, Gordon HL: Chemical face peeling, an adjunct to surgical face lifting. South Med J 56:412, 1963
6. Baker TJ, Gordon HL: Current approaches to facial rejuvenation. South Med J 58:1077, 1965
7. Baker TJ, Gordon HL, Seckinger DL: A second look at chemical face peeling. Plast Reconstr Surg 37:487, 1966
8. Baker TJ, Gordon HL: Chemical face peeling and dermabrasion. Surg Clin North Am 51:387–401, 1971
9. Baker TJ, Gordon HL: Chemical face peeling, in Goldwyn RM (ed): The Unfavorable Result in Plastic Surgery. Boston, Little, Brown & Co, 1972, pp 345–352
10. Baker TJ, Gordon HL: The chemical face peel: Indications, techniques, and complications, in Masters FW, Lewis JR Jr (eds): Symposium on Aesthetic Surgery of the Face, Eyelid, and Breast, vol 4. St. Louis, C V Mosby Co, 1972, pp 65–72
11. Baker TJ, Gordon HL, Mosienko P, Seckinger DL: Long-term histological study of skin after chemical face peeling. Plast Reconstr Surg 53:522, 1974
12. Bames HO: Truth and fallacies of face peeling and face lifting. Med J Rec 126:86, 1927
13. Batstone JHF, Millard DR Jr: An endorsement of facial chemo-surgery. Br J Plast Surg 21:193, 1968
14. Brown AM, Kaplan LM, Brown MA: Phenol-induced histological skin changes: Hazards, techniques, and uses. Br J Plast Surg, 13:158, 1960
15. Spira M, Dahl C, Freeman R, Gerow FJ, et al: Chemosurgery—a histological study. Plast Reconstr Surg 45:247, 1970
16. Hoopes JE, Wolfort FG, Dalton WE: Chemial rhytidectomy, in Masters FW, Lewis JR Jr (eds): Symposium on Aesthetic Surgery of the Face, Eyelid, and Breast, vol 4. St. Louis, C V Mosby Co, 1972, pp 73–75
17. Deichmann W, Witherup S: Phenol studies. VI. The acute and comparative toxicity of phenol and l-, m-, and p- cresols for experimental animals. J Pharmacol Exp Ther 80:233, 1944
18. Litton C: Observations after chemosurgery of the face. Plast Reconstr Surg 32:554, 1963
19. MacKee GM, Karp FL: Treatment of the post acne scars with phenol. Br J Dermatol 64:456, 1952
20. Spira M, Gerow FJ, Hardy SB: Complications of chemical face peeling. Plast Reconstr Surg 54:397, 1974
21. Truppman ES, Ellenby JD: Major electrocardiographic changes during chemical face peeling. Plast Reconstr Surg 63:44, 1979
22. Baker TJ, Gordon HL: Chemical peeling as a practical method for removing rhytides of the upper lip. Annals of Plast Surg 2(3):209–212, 1979
23. Ayres S III: Superficial chemosurgery in treating aging skin. Arch Dermatol 85:358, 1962.

BIJAN SAFAI, M.D. / PATRICIA L. MYSKOWSKI, M.D.

34

Immunotherapy of Cutaneous Tumors

With a better understanding of the development, evolution, structure, and function of the immune system, it is now possible for the first time to envision the use of the body's own immune mechanisms to fight infections and cancers. This has been made possible particularly by the modern advances over the past two decades, and we are now witnessing the initial steps toward development of practical and clinically applicable immunotherapy. Edward Jenner's observation that cowpox provided immunity against smallpox gave birth to immunobiology and resulted in the development of vaccination (a specific and effective form of immunotherapy), which has eradicated some life-threatening diseases and has controlled others.

The use of immunotherapy in the treatment of cancer is not a new approach. At the turn of the century, Dr. W. B. Coley, a surgeon at Memorial Hospital in New York, observed that five separate operations had failed to control the progression of the disease in a patient with cancer of the head and neck. However, an acute attack of erysipelas resulted in the regression of cancer in this patient. Dr. Coley's efforts to evaluate the effect of erysipelas in other cancer patients resulted in the development of Coley's toxin. This was used with some success in the treatment of certain malignant tumors by him and his colleagues.[1]

The introduction of radiation therapy and, later, chemotherapy brought to an end much of the initial enthusiasm for treatment of malignancies with immunotherapy. However, sporadic reports did appear, showing some continued interest in this field. A definite revival has come about during the past two decades, and a large amount of literature has emerged on the subject of immunotherapy.

The immune system has been shown to play an important role in both the predisposition to develop cancer and the way in which the host responds to malignancy once it is established. It is well documented that the immunodeficient patient is more likely to develop internal malignancy as well as skin neoplasms. Gatti and Good reported that patients with primary immunodeficiency states had nearly a ten thousandfold increase in their incidence of malignancy compared to that of the general age-matched population.[2] Individuals with secondary immunodeficiency states are also prone to develop cancers, as has been demonstrated by the high incidence of de novo squamous cell carcinoma of the skin in renal transplant recipients on immunosuppressive therapy.[3] Furthermore, patients with the lymphoproliferative malignancies have a sevenfold increase in skin cancers; basal cell carcinomas, squamous cell carcinoma, and malignant melanoma have the same relative amount of increase.[4] Thus, defects in immune surveillance may directly or indirectly contribute to the development of all types of malignancies, including skin cancers.

In the normal individual, there is also some suggestion that the immune system participates actively in fighting, or at least in modifying, the response to skin cancers. Bustamente and colleagues found an increased percentage of T-lymphocytes around basal cell carcinoma and squamous cell carcinoma.[5] A further humoral immune response to basal cell carcinoma was indicated by the presence of an increased number of immunoglobulin-producing cells around basal cell carcinoma. This would suggest an inverse relationship between lymphocytic infiltration of the skin cancer and biologic aggressiveness of the tumor. Similarly, in squamous cell carcinoma of the head and neck, an increased amount of lymphocytic tumor infiltration has been associated with a better prognosis.[6] This observation is consistent with a histologic response of skin cancers undergoing regression during immunotherapy.

Through the use of recent advances in the field of immunology, several different therapeutic approaches have already been developed, and their applications for skin cancer are being tested. However, it is widely recognized that any intervention in cancer utilizing the immunologic approach has to take account of the bulk of the tumor load, the presence of blocking factors for immune responses, and the immunologic competence of the host. The humoral or cellular immune response is only capable of handling a certain amount of antigenic load, indicating that cancer patients may be able to handle only a certain number of tumor cells.

Animal studies have shown that immunologically-induced prophylaxis is effective only against certain numbers of transplantable syngeneic tumor cells but not against larger numbers of the cells. Therefore, it is evident that immunotherapy is more effective if tumor reduction is achieved by other means, such as surgery, irradiation, or chemotherapy.

REPAIR AND REPLACEMENT OF AN INADEQUATE IMMUNE SYSTEM

This approach was initially tried in children with immunodeficiency diseases and was found to be quite successful and effective. It has been recently used in the treatment of certain types of leukemias and in patients with aplastic anemias. Fetal liver, thymic epithelium, and bone marrow transplantation have all been used for the correction of the immunodeficiency states. Bone marrow transplantation currently is the most promising modality for trial restitution of the immune system in these disorders, although the formidable challenge of graft-versus-host disease remains to be overcome.[7]

SPECIFIC IMMUNOTHERAPY (ANTIBODIES)

This approach involves the passive transfer of some of the products of the immune system, such as antibodies, with directed specificity for a given cancer. Prior to the development of antibiotics, serotherapy was practiced frequently for several different bacterial and viral infections. Recent investigations have indicated the possible role of humoral immunity in protecting the host against neoplasms. In vitro studies have shown that antibodies and complement may be cytotoxic for tumor cells.[8] Tumor cells may also be killed by antibodies in assays such as antibody-dependent cell-mediated cytotoxicity.[9] Protection against tumor growth has been observed in some in vitro experimental systems by administration of antisera. In addition, antibodies with direct specificity have been used in certain animal models (mouse leukemia).[10] Chemoimmunotherapy using drugs attached to tumor-specific antibodies has also been tried. Furthermore, antibodies as carriers of radionuclides have been used in some neoplastic processes.[11] Patients may have a functional defect that makes them unable to produce some of these antibodies or other products in sufficient amount, or they may have a defect in recognizing and rejecting the tumor cells as foreign. Thus far, however, serotherapy has been only effective if used prior to tumor inoculation, and successful therapy with antisera in already established tumors has been relatively rare.

ACTIVE SPECIFIC IMMUNOTHERAPY (TUMOR VACCINE)

The therapeutic advantages of active immunity, namely vaccination, over passive immunity in the area of infectious diseases provided a strong incentive for applying the same approach to cancer immunotherapy. Active immunotherapy with tumor vaccine has been attempted for over half a century. The presence of tumor-specific antigens and specific antitumor immunity was suggested by animal studies[12] showing that tumor growth could provoke host immune responses, which could actually prevent the growth of tumor cells. These observations have led to the development of tumor vaccines.

Tumor vaccines have been prepared for a number of tumors and used in a number of experimental trials. Tumor cells have been first inactivated by various means to make them incapable of proliferation. Mitomycin C treatment, freezing and thawing, irradiation, and heat treatment have all been used to inactivate the tumor cells.[13] However, these methods may also have the effect of inactivating the tumor-specific antigens. In an effort to increase the antigenicity of tumor vaccine, tumor cells have been coupled with highly antigenic carrier proteins such as rabbit gammaglobulin or treated with chemicals such as neuraminidase and concanavilin A.[14]

The clinical trials of tumor vaccines have mostly been in conjunction with conventional therapies as well as with other immunotherapeutic modalities. Thus far, the results of tumor vaccine therapy have not been impressive.

ADOPTIVE IMMUNOTHERAPY

This form of immunotherapy has involved: (1) nonspecific stimulation of lymphocytes with the use of agents such as phytohemagglutinin (PHA)[15]; (2) transfer of lymphocytes, which have already been sensitized by transplantation of tumors[16] (although some tumor responses have been reported, the problems of technique still have to be solved); and perhaps more promising, (3) the transfer of certain leukocyte products and molecular mediators, which are necessary for mounting specific immunologic responses in the recipient host (these include transfer factor, interferon, immune RNA, and a variety of thymic hormones).

Transfer factor, an extract of lysed leukocytes, was discovered by Dr. Sherwood Lawrence in 1955.[17] He took the peripheral blood from a subject who was skin-test–positive to purified protein derivative (PPD), separated and lysed the white blood cells, and then injected the extract into a recipient with a negative skin test to PPD. The recipient became skin-test–positive and remained so for several months. The factor obtained from the lysed leukocytes became known as "transfer factor" because it transferred positive skin tests. Little more was done until the demonstration that transfer factor would also transfer other parameters of cellular immunity such as migration-inhibitory factor[18] and increase the number of rosette-forming T cells.[19]

One problem with the use of transfer factor in malignancies has been the selection of suitable donors who can demonstrate a cellular immune response to the particular tumor in question. The suitability of possible donors can be determined by in vitro cell-mediated cytotoxicity assays. The dialyzable leukocyte extract of donors is tested in vitro against an established tumor cell line. If the cytotoxicity index is high, the donor is termed "immune" and transfer factor from his or her lymphocytes may be helpful to the cancer patient. Most donors are selected from the close household contacts of patients or from other patients who themselves manifest a high level of in vitro cytotoxicity to their tumor cells.[20]

Interferons are a series of inducible secretory glycoproteins produced by eukaryotic cells in response to viral infections or certain other stimuli, such as polyriboninosinic-polyribocytidylic acid (PolyI-PolyC).[21] All interferons are capable of inducing resistance to a broad spectrum of viruses in the cells.[22] Because of their effectiveness and the rapidity of action, interferons are an important line of defense against viral infections.[23] They may also protect the host against other intracellular parasites and even against neoplastic transformation and tumor growth.[24, 25] On an immunomodulating level, they may inhibit DNA synthesis in the lymphocyte proliferative responses to mitogens.[26] However, there is a marked increase in human cytotoxic natural killer cells and human antibody-dependent cell-mediated cytotoxic reactions in response to interferons.[27] On the basis of the actions of interferon on the behavior of killer cells and on the cytotoxic activity of T cells, its use has recently been approved for human cancers. Comparative in vitro studies and limited clinical trials indicate that lymphoid neoplasms may be particularly responsive to human leukocyte interferon, and nasopharyngeal carcinoma and osteogenic carcinoma to the fibroblast interferon.[28, 29] Leukocyte interferon has also been reported to cause regression of superficial breast cancer metastases when given intralesionally.[30] Human fibroblast interferon injected intralesionally has caused regression of skin metastases of malignant melanoma and breast and prostatic carcinomas.[28]

Immune RNA has recently joined the list of molecular products that may affect the host's response to tumor. Pilch and Ramming[31, 32] immunized guinea pigs with a specific tumor and extracted RNA from their lymphoid organs. This extracted RNA was incubated with spleen cells and then injected into inbred mice. They found that these mice were immune to tumor isografts, and that this was mediated by the extracted RNA ("immune RNA"). This material has found application in several malignant tumors of man and animals including malignant melanoma.[33] Immune RNA has certain advantages over other methods of adoptive immunotherapy. It does not contain histocompatibility antigens and thus could not result in sensitization. It carries no risk of inducing graft-versus-host disease in the immunosuppressed or immunodeficient patients, which could happen with lymphocytes. In addition, larger quantities of immune RNA could theoretically be obtained from animal, rather than human, donors. This method, however, is only recently being used in clinical trials in humans.

Thymic hormones have recently been investigated for their role in cancer. The high rate of malignancies in children with congenital immunodeficiency syndromes, as well as behavior of experimentally-induced tumors in congenitally athymic ("nude") mice, led to speculation that thymic hormones may exert a protective effect against tumors. Recently, thymosin, one of the several extracts of thymus tissue, has been shown to partially restore cell-mediated immune reactions in nude mice[34] and to promote prolonged survival in some animal tumor models.[35]

NONSPECIFIC IMMUNOSTIMULATION

Since the early 1960s, the approach of nonspecific immunotherapy has been widely studied and proven useful in animal and human cancers. This approach is based on the use of nonspecific immunostimulants such as viable microorganisms, nonviable bacterial products, and chemical compounds (Table 34–1).

Perhaps the most widely used agent is Bacillus Calmette-Guérin (BCG), a microbial material made of attenuated live mycobacteria. This has been used most frequently in the treatment of metastatic malignant melanoma It is important to note that there is heterogeneity in BCG preparations, since they are prepared through various techniques.[36] BCG has been used in the form of topical or intralesional preparations for the treatment of primary or metastatic skin tumors.[37] Different vehicles have been developed to allow the topical application of the antigen through the skin, and various concentrations have been tried. These topical preparations have been applied in an analogous manner to the rechallenge regimen of primary sensitizers and have been found to be effective. In patients with weak, or even absent, response to recall antigens, immunopotentiation may be achieved through the use of 20 to 40 mg of oral BCG vaccine. In most patients, conver-

TABLE 34–1. Nonspecific Immunostimulants

- *Mycobacterium* (BCG, PPD, MER)
- *Listeria monocytogenes*
- *Corynebacterium parvum*
- *Corynebacterium granulosum*
- *Bordetella pertussis*
- *Brucella abortus*
- DNCB
- Levamisole
- PolyI-PolyC

sion of negative skin tests to purified protein derivative (PPD) to positive ones, or augmentation of positive responses to PPD and other recall antigens, is achieved after a few doses of oral PPD and other antigens, even in patients with widely disseminated internal malignancies.[38] The effect of BCG, however, may be somewhat paradoxical since its excessive use may actually decrease the challenging response to other antigens. Therefore, patients receiving BCG immunopotentiation must be monitored by intermittent skin testing with several recall antigens. If the delayed hypersensitivity reaction begins to decline, BCG may be exerting an immunosuppressive effect and must be discontinued. The mechanism of this effect of BCG is not understood.

The use of BCG is not without risk, since the therapy does involve the injection of live organisms, and fever and draining subcutaneous abscesses have been reported.[39] In an effort to circumvent the problems that exist in using live organisms, efforts have been made to substitute an equally active, but nonviable, bacterial product. PPD has been used intralesionally in sensitized individuals, and recently a methanol-extractable residue (MER) of BCG has been developed that may prove to be an acceptable immunostimulant with fewer side effects.[40]

Other bacterial products have been used successfully in animal and some human studies include *Corynebacterium parvum,*[41] *Corynebacterium granulosum,*[42] *Listeria monocytogenes,*[43] and *Bordetella pertussis.*[44] Vaccinia virus has also been used intralesionally, again in metastatic malignant melanoma, as a local immunostimulant.[45]

Levamisole is a phenylimidazole thiazole derivative that has been used as an antihelminthic for many years. Levamisole was recently discovered to be immunotropic and helpful in restoring cellular immunity in some cancer patients. It has been successfully used both alone and in conjunction with chemotherapy in patients with metastatic disease to prolong disease-free intervals. Levamisole has proved to be less toxic and better tolerated than many other chemotherapeutic agents.[46, 47]

Another mode of therapy using nonspecific immunostimulation is a clinically practical and effective method of treating cancerous and precancerous cutaneous lesions that has been pioneered by Klein and coworkers.[48, 49] This involves the local use of skin-sensitizing chemicals such as 2-4-dinitrochlorobenzene (DNCB) to induce inflammatory responses (localized delayed hypersensitivity reactions) on and around some skin cancers. Although the antitumor effect is only local, this is the only truly curative immunotherapeutic approach to cutaneous malignancies available at this time.

The rationale for the induction of cell-mediated immune responses at the tumor site began with the work of Helm and Klein.[48] They first demonstrated that allergic contact dermatitis at the site of basal cell carcinoma resulted in tumor regression. Further studies of patients with multiple primary epidermal carcinoma showed that the delayed hypersensitivity reaction could be modulated to effectively eradicate malignant skin tumors.[49] Development of cutaneous delayed hypersensitivity reactions depends on two main steps: (1) the induction of sensitivity to primary antigens and (2) local challenge with the use of these antigens.

This approach represents an important example of application of immunologic memory to antitumor therapy.[50] It employs the host's previous experience (immune memory) in handling various antigens though rechallenge with the same agents. The antigens used thus far include DNCB and similar compounds as well as microbial antigens.

Prior to the beginning of the treatment, a patient's cellular immune status is usually assessed through skin testing with recall antigens to rule out possible anergy. The patient is also sensitized with a primary antigen, most commonly with chemicals such as DNCB. Two to three weeks later, the patient is challenged with the sensitizing agent. The vehicle containing the sensitizer is reapplied using an occlusive patch-test technique, beginning with very diluted concentrations, until the minimal concentration necessary to induce a delayed hypersensitivity reaction is determined. The range of minimal DNCB concentration necessary to elicit a challenge response in different individuals extends from 1 part in 1000 to 1 part in 10^{12} (1 trillion) parts of the vehicle. The concentration of DNCB is designated by different terms, i.e., T4 refers to 1 part DNCB in 10^4 parts vehicle, T5 refers to 1 part DNCB in 10^5 parts vehicle.

DNCB has been a model sensitizing agent, since natural exposure to it only rarely occurs, and initial application evokes a true primary sensitization. In addition, it has been shown that up to 94% of patients are capable of being sensitized to this agent. Potentiation of the local challenge response to DNCB has been achieved through the local use of chemotherapeutic agents such as 5-fluorouracil (5-FU). The enhanced inflammatory response through the combination of local chemotherapy and immunotherapy has been shown to be more effective in long-term follow-up of patients with multiple superficial skin cancers than either method alone.[49] Microbial antigens also have been used for induction of cell-mediated immunity at the tumor sites with successful results.[51] The recall agents include PPD, *Candida, Trichophyton,* pertussin, streptokinase-streptodornase (SK-SD), coccidiodin, mumps, and many other viral, bacterial and fungal antigens. These microbial agents have been especially important in the small percentage of patients in whom DNCB or other agents failed to establish primary sensitization. In a group of patient with multiple epidermal tumors who were unable to develop sensitization to DNCB, the immune response to recall antigens was nonetheless intact.[51] In addition, older patients (i.e., over 50) are frequently PPD-positive. Since the majority of patients with nonmelanoma skin cancer are older, PPD may readily be used therapeutically in this group.

IMMUNOTHERAPEUTIC APPROACHES TO SKIN TUMORS

While primary skin cancers are the most common cancers in man, an overall cure rate of 90% (excluding malignant melanoma) is usually achieved by the use of conventional therapeutic modalities such as surgical excision, electrodesiccation and curettage, cryotherapy, radiotherapy, and chemosurgery. These conventional approaches, however, are not practical in patients with multiple basal cell carcinoma, multiple Bowen's disease, basal cell nevus syndrome, and xeroderma pigmentosum. Thus, immunotherapy offers an exceptional approach in such cases and is being practiced as an effective adjuvant and/or alternate mode of therapy with increasing frequency. Immunotherapy has also been applied to metastatic cutaneous tumors.

Among the various forms of immunotherapy, nonspecific immunostimulation is the only one successfully applied to the treatment of skin cancers. Precancerous cutaneous tumors such as actinic keratoses are effectively controlled by the conventional modalities. Thus, there has been no real attempt to use immunotherapy for the treatment of this condition.

In the case of Bowen's disease (in situ epidermoid carcinoma), however, there has been a need for developing new approaches since the conventional ones have not always been curative.[52] Immunotherapy, namely the use of local sensitization with contact allergens, has effectively been used in the treatment of Bowen's disease. Furthermore, combined immunotherapy (topical DNCB) and chemotherapy (topical 5-FU) have been reported to result in complete clinical and histologic regression of multiple Bowen's tumors.[53]

Immunotherapy has also been used in the treatment of multiple basal cell carcinoma and in cases of basal cell nevus syndrome. Superficial spreading basal cell carcinomas are especially responsive to the use of local immunotherapy, while the nodular basal cell carcinomas are more resistant to this approach. The use of recall antigens, as previously mentioned, has also been applied to the treatment of multiple skin cancers.[54] Microbial products have been used intralesionally with good results. In addition, these antigens have been incorporated into a variety of vehicles (cream, ointment, or lotion) and utilized for induction of localized delayed hypersensitivity reactions at the sites of cutaneous tumors. The use of microbial antigens in topical form has made this approach more practical for both patient and physicians. For example, PPD preparations, in concentrations ranging from 500 to 100,000 units per gram of base, were found to be quite effective.[49, 55]

A modified, and more effective, method of treatment is the combination of local challenge regimens with topical chemotherapy, including 5-FU and other cytotoxic agents. Five-year follow-up studies have clearly demonstrated the superiority of combined topical chemotherapy and immunotherapy over either method alone in individuals with multiple epidermal cancer syndromes.[56] Studies of overall cure rates for groups of patients with multiple epitheliomas treated by this approach have shown that 60% to 90% of neoplasms were eradicated without recurrences. Follow-up periods were extended to five years. Residual tumors in these patients were treated with conventional modalities or in combination with immunotherapy.[49]

Local challenge regimens may add another advantage in the treatment of patients with multiple skin cancers through immunoprophylaxis. By producing an inflammatory reaction at involved sites, immunotherapy may reveal otherwise undetectable tumors, which then undergo resolution. It is likely that tumors too small to show clinically detectable inflammatory reactions still undergo regression. This is suggested by the findings of Klein and Holtermann that courses of immunotherapy are followed by a decreased incidence of new tumors.[56] Studies of patients with multiple skin cancer syndromes revealed that, following one or more courses of local immunostimulation, there was a marked reduction in the incidence of new lesions over a five-year follow-up period. This trend was contrasted with the known propensity of these individuals to develop new neoplasms as obtained from follow-up studies following standard therapeutic procedures. In addition, the incidence of tumors was reduced greatly by immunotherapy in seven of nine patients with xeroderma pigmentosum. These individuals had previously required several surgical procedures per year to control new cancers. However, during follow-up periods of five years or more, these patients required fewer surgical procedures.

To evaluate this hypothesis of immunoprophylaxis, studies of symmetrical sites were undertaken in which one was treated with challenge regimens and the other was treated with conventional modalities. When the control-treated and immunotherapy-treated sites were compared, significantly fewer lesions were observed on the site treated with local immunotherapy. In addition, progression of the new lesions to more extensive tumors was demonstrated to be reduced following immunotherapy. Similar findings were obtained in patients with late radiation dermatitis and the multiple basal cell carcinoma syndromes.[56]

Malignant melanoma represents 2% of all cancers in the United States, excluding nonmelanoma skin cancers, and is responsible for roughly 1% of all cancer deaths. In 1979, an estimated 13,600 new cases of malignant melanoma and overall deaths of 4000 were reported in the United States.[57] While the mainstay of successful therapy has been early detection followed by adequate surgical excision, there are nonetheless many cases with metastases to both the skin and internal organs. Historically, melanoma has been a relatively radioresistant tumor, so that radiotherapy has been used only in certain instances of palliation. Regional perfusion with chemotherapy (i.e., phenylalanine mustard) has also been tried but is still in the experimental phase.[58] Although several different systemic chemotherapeutic agents have been tried, only a few have been particularly effective against the tumor. Dimethyl triazenoimidazole-carboxamide (DTIC) has shown some promise, but it does not have good response rates in the majority of patients.[59] Therefore, other methods of therapy, especially in high-risk patients or those with established metastatic disease, have been tried.

The choice of adjuvant immunotherapy in malignant melanoma is a logical one. Primary melanoma will frequently exhibit variegation in color; white areas in the tumor correlate histologically with areas of tumor regression. In addition, the reports of spontaneous regression of both primary and secondary tumor deposits of malignant melanoma lend further support to the role of the host's cellular immune response in prevention of the tumor spread.[60]

The first use of intralesional immunotherapy with BCG in melanoma was reported by Morton's group.[60] They demonstrated that intralesional BCG could reproducibly yield tumor regression of skin metastases. Of the eight patients studied, five demonstrated regression of the injected lesions, and two of the five showed regression of adjacent but uninjected nodules. These clinical changes were accompanied by in vitro differences in antimelanoma antibodies. Similar observations were made following the use of intralesional vaccinia virus in skin metastases.[45] Eilber and colleagues[61] demonstrated the usefulness of adjuvant therapy with BCG in patients following excision of lymph node metastases. This retrospective report led to many further studies of this immunotherapeutic approach.

A significant increase in both the disease-free interval and survival time was shown by Gutterman and coworkers who used a combination of immunotherapy (BCG) and chemotherapy (DTIC).[62] Their patients had recurrent disease that was mainly confined to the skin and subcutaneous tissue.

Recently, Wood and colleagues[63] demonstrated the superiority of the combination of DTIC and BCG over either BCG or DTIC alone. Their findings in "high-risk" primary melanomas (lesions greater than 1.5 mm thick) were statistically significant. Clinical trials with other immunostimulants (i.e., levamisole, *Corynebacterium parvum*) as well as interferon (with and without chemotherapy) are currently in progress and will hopefully lead to better protocols of prevention and treatment of metastatic malignant melanoma. Attempts are also being made to develop a tumor vaccine for this neoplastic disease.

CONCLUSION

We can be confident that we are gaining new perceptions about the immunoregulatory mechanisms and some of the most perplexing facets of immunobiology. This knowledge has immense potential for clinical applications. One can readily foresee manipulations of the immune system to strengthen resistance to infections, to prevent and treat autoimmune disease, and to tilt the balance between the host's defense mechanisms and the neoplastic process in favor of the host. The status of immunotherapy in the 1980s is similar to that of penicillin in the 1940s—a powerful new weapon that is only beginning to be understood and utilized. As immunotherapeutic techniques are further expanded and refined, we can look forward to more advances in the treatment, and hopefully prevention, of skin cancer.

REFERENCES

1. Southam CM: History and prospects of immunotherapy in cancer: An introduction, in Southam CM, Friedman H (eds): International Conference on Immunotherapy of Cancer. NY Acad Sci 277:1–6, 1976
2. Gatti RA, Good RA: Occurrence of malignancy in immunodeficiency states. Cancer 28:84–98, 1971
3. Walder BK, Robertson MR, Jeremy D: Skin cancer and immunosuppression. Lancet 2:1282–1283, 1971
4. Berg JW: The incidence of multiple primary cancers. I. Development of further cancers in patients with lymphomas, leukemias and myeloma. J Natl Canc Inst 38:741–752, 1967
5. Bustamente R, Schmitt D, Pillet C, Thivolet J: Immunoglobulin-producing cells in the inflammatory infiltrates of cutaneous tumors. Immunocytological identification in situ. J Invest Dermatol 68:346–349, 1977
6. Bennett SH, Futrell JW, Roth JA, Hove RC, et al: Prognostic significance of histologic host response in cancer of the larynx or hypopharynx. Cancer 28:1255–1268, 1971
7. Fefer A, Thomas ED, Buckner CD, Cheever MA, et al.: Marrow transplantation in acute leukemia in man, in Southam CM, Freidman H (eds): International Conference on Immunotherapy in Cancer. NY Acad Sci 277:52–59, 1976
8. Wheelock EF, Toy ST, Weislow OS, Levy MH: Restored immune and non-immune function in Friend virus leukemia mice treated with Statalon. Prog Exp Tumor Res 19:369–389, 1974
9. Peter HH, Pavie-Fischer J, Friedman WH, Aubert C, et al: Cell-mediated cytotoxicity of human lymphocytes against a

tissue culture melanoma cell line (IGR3). J Immunol 115:539–548, 1975

10. Reif AE, Robinson CM, Smith PJ: Preparation and therapeutic potential of rabbit antisera with "directed" specificities for mouse leukemias, in Southam CM, Friedman H (eds): International Conference on Immunotherapy of Cancer. NY Acad Sci 277:647–669, 1975

11. Ghose T, Tai J, Guiclu A, Norvell ST, et al: Antibodies as carriers of radionuclides and cytotoxic drugs in the treatment and diagnosis of cancer, in Southam CM, Friedman H (eds): International Conference on Immunotherapy of Cancer. NY Acad Sci 277:671–689, 1976

12. McCoy JL, Fefer A, Glynn JP: Comparative studies on the induction of transplantation resistance in BALB/c and C57BL/6 mice in three murine leukemia systems. Cancer Res 27:1743–1748, 1976

13. Benjamini E, Theilen GH, Torten M, Fong S, et al: Tumor vaccine for immunotherapy of canine lymphosarcoma, in Southam CM, Friedman H (eds): International Conference on Immunotherapy of Cancer. NY Acad Sci 277:305–312, 1976

14. Takit H, Minowada J, Han T, Takada M, et al: Adjuvant immunotherapy in bronchogenic carcinoma, in Southam CM, Friedman H (eds): International Conference on Immunotherapy of Cancer. NY Acad Sci 277:345–354, 1976

15. Frenster JH, Rogoway WM: In vitro activation and re-infusion of autologous human lymphocytes. Lancet 2:979–989, 1968

16. Seigler HF, Shingleton WW, Metzgar RS, Buckley CE, et al: Immunotherapy in patients with melanoma. Ann Surg 178:352–359, 1973

17. Lawrence HS: The transfer in humans of delayed skin sensitivity to streptococcal M substance and to tuberculin with disrupted leukocytes. J Clin Invest 34:219–230, 1955

18. Levin AS, Spitler LE, Stites DP, Fudenberg HH: Wiskott-Aldrich syndrome; a genetically determined cellular immunologic deficiency: Clinical and laboratory responses to therapy with transfer factor. Proc Natl Acad Sci USA 67:821–828, 1970

19. Wybran J, Levin AS, Spitler LE, Fudenberg HH: Rosette-forming cells, immunologic deficiency diseases and transfer factor. N Engl J Med 288:710–713, 1970.

20. Byers VS, Levin AS, Hackett AJ, Fudenberg HH: Tumor-specific cell-mediated immunity in household contacts of cancer patients. J Clin Invest 55:500–503, 1975

21. Borden EC: Interferons: Rationale for clinical trials in neoplastic disease. Ann Int Med 91:472–479, 1979

22. Friedman RM: Antiviral activity of interferons. Bacteriol Rev 41:543–567, 1977

23. Rasmussen L, Farley LB: Inhibition of herpesvirus hominis replication by human interferon. Infec Immun 12:104–108, 1975

24. Priestman TJ: Interferon: An anti-cancer agent? Cancer Treat Rev 6:223–227, 1979

25. Krim M: Towards tumor therapy with interferons, Part II. Interferons: In vivo effects. Blood 55(6):875–884, 1980

26. Lindahl-Magnusson P, Leary P, Gresser I: Interferon inhibits DNA synthesis induced on mouse lymphocyte suspensions by phytohemagglutinin or by allogeneic cells. Nature 237:120–121, 1975

27. Zarling JM, Eskra L, Borden EC, Horoszewicz J, et al: Activation of human killer cells cytotoxic for human leukemia cells by purified interferon. J Immunol 123:63–67, 1979.

28. Horoszewicz JS, Leong SS, Ito M, Buffett RF, et al: Human fibroblast interferon in human neoplasia: Clinical and laboratory study. Cancer Treat Rep 62:1899–1906, 1978

29. Strander H, Adamson J, Aparisi T, Brostrom A, et al: Adjuvant interferon treatment of human osteosarcoma. Recent Results Cancer Res 68:40–44, 1978

30. Gutterman J, Yap Y, Buzdar A, Alexanian R, et al: Leukocyte interferon induced tumor regression in patients with breast cancer and B cell neoplasma. Proc Am Assoc Cancer Res 20:167, 1979

31. Ramming KP, Pilch YH: Transfer of tumor specific immunity with RNA inhibition of growth of murine tumor isografts. J Natl Cancer Inst 46:735–750, 1971

32. Pilch YH, Ramming KP: Transfer of tumor immunity with ribonucleic acid. Cancer 26:630–637, 1970

33. Pilch YH, Fritze D, deKernion JB, Ramming KP, et al: Immunotherapy of cancer with immune RNA in animal models and cancer patients, in Southam CM, Friedman H (eds): International Conference on Immunotherapy in Cancer. NY Acad Sci 277:592–608, 1976

34. Goldstein AL, Asanuma Y, Battisto JR, Hardy MA, et al: Influence of thymosin on cell-mediated and humoral immune responses in normal and in immunologically deficient mice. J Immunol 104:359–366, 1970

35. Khaw BA, Rule AH: Immunotherapy of the Dunning leukaemia with thymus extracts. Br J Cancer 28:288–292, 1973

36. Bast RC Jr, Bast BS: Critical review of previously reported animal studies of tumor immunotherapy with non-specific immunostimulants, in Southam CM, Friedman H (eds): International Conference on Immunotherapy of Cancer. NY Acad Sci 277:60–93 1976

37. Zbar B, Bernstein ID, Bartlett GL, Hanna MG Jr, et al: Immunotherapy of cancer: Regression of intradermal tumors and prevention of growth of lymph node metastases after intralesional injection of living Mycobacterium bovis. J Natl Cancer Inst 49:119–130, 1972

38. Eilber RR, Townsend CM, Morton DL: Results of BCG adjuvant immunotherapy or melanoma of the head and neck. Am J Surg 132:476–479, 1976

39. Sarks FC, Silverstein MJ, Hunt JS, Haskell, CM, et al: Complications of BCG immunotherapy in patients with cancer. N Engl J Med 289:827–830, 1973

40. Weiss DW, Bonhag RS, Leslie P: Studies on the heterologous immunogenicity of a methanol-insoluble fraction of attenuated tubercle bacilli (BCG). J Exp Med 24:1039–1065, 1966

41. Likhite VV: Rejection of tumors and metastases in Fischer 344 rats following intratumor administration of killed Corynebacterium parvum. Intl J Cancer 14:684–690, 1974

42. Milas L, Hunter N, Basic I, Mason K, et al: Non-specific immunotherapy of murine solid tumors with Corynebacterium granulosum. J Natl Cancer Inst 54:895–902, 1975

43. Bast RC Jr, Zbar B, Miller TE, Mackaness GB, et al: Antitumor activity of bacterial infection II. Effect of Listeria monocytogenes on growth of a guinea pig hepatoma. J Natl Cancer Inst 54:757–761, 1975

44. Likhite VV: Rejection of mammary adenocarcinoma cell tumors and the prevention of progressive growth of incipient metastases following intratumor permeation with killed Bordetella pertussis. Cancer Res 34:2790–2794, 1974

45. Roenigk HH Jr, Deodlar S, St. Jacques R, Burdick KH: Immunotherapy of malignant melanoma with vaccina virus. Arch Dermatol 109:668–673, 1974

46. Hoper DG, Pimm MV, Baldwin RW: Levamisole. Lancet 1:574–575, 1975

47. Perk K, Chirigos MA, Fuhrman P, Pettigrew H: Some aspects of host response to levamisole after chemotherapy in a murine leukemia. J Natl Cancer Inst 54:253–256, 1975

48. Helm F, Klein E: Effects of allergic contact dermatitis on basal cell epitheliomas. Arch Dermatol 91:142–144, 1965

49. Klein E, Holtermann OA, Helm F, Rosner D, et al.: Immunologic approaches to the management of primary and secondary tumors involving the skin and soft tissues. Reviews of a ten-year program. Transplant Proc 7:297–315, 1975

50. Stjernsward J, Levin A: Delayed hypersensitivity-induced regression of human neoplasms. Cancer 28:628–640, 1971

51. Holtermann OA, Papermaster BW, Walker MJ, Milgrom H, et al: Regression of cutaneous neoplasms following delayed type hypersensitivity challenge reactions to microbial antigens or lymphokines. J Med 6:157–168, 1975

52. Mohs FE: Prevention and therapy of skin cancer. Wis Med J 73:85–92, 1974

53. Raat JH, Krown SE, Pinsky CM, Cunningham-Rundles W, et al: Treatment of Bowen's disease with topical dinitro-

chlorobenzene and 5-fluorouracil. Cancer 37(4):1633–1642, 1976

54. Klein E, Holtermann OA, Case RW, Milgrom H, et al: Responses of neoplasms to local immunotherapy. Am J Clin Pathol 62:281–289, 1974

55. Klein E, Holtermann OA, Papermaster B, Milgrom H, et al.: Immunologic approaches to various types of cancer with the use of BCG and purified protein derivatives. Natl Cancer Inst Monogr 39:229–240, 1972

56. Klein E, Holtermann OA: Immunotherapeutic approaches to the management of neoplasms. Natl Cancer Inst Monogr 35:372, 1972

57. Sober AJ, Fitzpatrick TB, Mihm MC Jr: Primary melanoma of the skin: Recognition and management. J Am Acad Dermatol 2(3):179–197, 1980

58. Krementz ET, Ryan RF: Chemotherapy of melanoma of the extremities by perfusion: Fourteen years clinical experience. Ann Surg 175:900–917, 1972

59. Comis RL: DTIC (NSC-45388) in malignant melanoma: A perspective. Cancer Treat Rep 60:165–176, 1976

60. Morton DL, Eilber ER, Malmgren RA: Immunological factors which influence response to immunotherapy in malignant melanomas. Surgery 68:158–164, 1970

61. Eilber FR, Morton DL, Holmes EC, Sparks FC, et al: Adjuvant immunotherapy with BCG in treatment of regional lymph node metastases from malignant melanoma. N Engl J Med 294:237–240, 1976

62. Gutterman JU, Mayligit G, Gottlieb JA, Burgess MA, et al: Chemoimmunotherapy of disseminated malignant melanoma with dimethyl triazeno imidazole carboxamide and Bacillus Calmette-Guérin. N Engl J Med, 291:592–597, 1974

63. Wood WC, Cosimi AB, Carey RW, Kaufman SD: Randomized trial of adjuvant therapy for "high risk" primary melanoma. Surgery 83:677–681, 1978

Cryosurgery

35

RONALD R. LUBRITZ, M.D.

Superficial Cryosurgery

Freezing has been used to treat various skin conditions since before 1900. At that time, A. Campbell White was using liquid air.[1, 2] Pusey[3] popularized the use of carbon dioxide around 1905. Liquid oxygen began to be used from the late 1920s through the 1940s.[4] Liquid nitrogen was introduced as the cryogen of choice in the late 1950s and mid-l960s. Popularized by Allington[5] and others, it has remained the preferred cryogen to the present day. Cooper and Less[6] developed the cryoprobe technique for neurosurgery. Working independently, Torre[7] and Zacarian[8] modified and simplified these techniques for dermatologic use. Torre developed an efficient spray technique, while Zacarian developed copper-disc cryoprobe procedures. Not only was the groundwork laid by these two pioneers, but many of their developments and procedures have not been improved.

Basic principles of cryobiology and cryophysics have been established by various authors.[9–18]

The flow of temperature is always from a warmer to a colder object. Freezing of tissue occurs just below 0°C, and destructive effects are produced down to −50°C or lower.

Conductivity factors are important. Air is a poor conductor, water is a fair to moderate conductor, and most metals are good conductors. In addition, when ice forms, it is a better conductor than water. Thermal gradients or isotherms are set up within the ice ball itself.

The effect of freezing on human tissue depends upon several factors. The cooling rate is important. A slow freeze develops extracellular ice; a faster rate produces intracellular ice, which is more damaging to cells and tissue. The rate of rewarming, or thaw, is also important. A slow or normal thaw time produces "grain growth" or recrystallization, and as the tissue or cells thaw, ice crystals grow or expand in size. Also, a slow rewarming produces longer dehydration of cells. Both factors produce greater destruction. In addition, solute concentration occurs as ice forms, another factor that is damaging to cells. Repeating the freeze-thaw cycle increases the amount of destruction. It has been shown that the number of surviving cells decreases with each freeze-thaw cycle.

One of the most vital considerations is the minimum temperature reached in the target tissue by the freezing process. For maximum destruction, −50°C or lower should be obtained. There are several reasons for this. At these temperatures, no cells are likely to remain supercooled (without intracellular ice crystals). Most cells are killed during the initial freeze at these temperatures. Cell protective factors, such as damaged cell migration from the cryogen application and shielding of undamaged cells, are also less likely to exert major influence at these readings. Because of various low eutectic points of some tissue salts (the temperature at which there is no liquid phase left), these low temperatures should be reached for maximum destruction.

In summary, in order to maximize cryosurgical destruction, there should be a fast cooling rate (freeze), a slow rewarming rate (thaw), and a minimum temperature of −40 to −60°C.

For clinical applications, any cryosurgical method should: (1) provide rapid cooling of the target tissue, (2) allow for sufficient cooling of the entire target area, (3) permit normal thawing, and (4) allow for repeat freeze-thaw cycles if necessary.

It should be remembered that maximum destructive effects are *not* frequently needed for treating nonmalignant lesions, so procedures should be modified to accomplish this.

Consideration of tissue destruction levels can predict the amount of damage and subsequent cosmetic appearance following cryosurgical procedures. Nonmalignant lesions, in many cases, are epithelial in nature and, as such, do not require freezing past the PAS-positive membrane. This results in no scarring, which is also the case when treating the bulk of nonmalignancies, i.e., actinic keratoses and leukoplakia, seborrheic keratoses, warts, and lentigines.

Cryosurgery causes selective destruction of tissue. Cellular elements are more susceptible than stromal components. Rapidly growing cells are more sensitive, as are nerves and melanocytes. Stromal structures of blood vessels are usually preserved. Thus, even when treating nonmalignant lesions, care should be taken in areas where nerves lie superficially[19] or where excessive pigmentary changes would be undesirable.

Clinical effects of cryosurgery begin with erythema and edema. These start within a few minutes after application of the cryogen, as does urtication. With a superficial freeze, a vesicle or bulla will develop within a few hours. Vesiculation contains serous or hemorrhagic fluid. Cellular regeneration takes place starting at 48 hours or earlier, and crusting on the surface occurs after a few days and can last for two to three weeks.

Cryogen selection can be of prime consideration when treating nonmalignant lesions. Carbon dioxide remains in use by many dermatologists.[20] It can be obtained in blocks or produced as "snow" by CO_2 cylinders. Pencils can be made either from the solid chunks or snow. It is then applied directly to the target tissue or mixed with acetone and/or alcohol and applied with a type of mop or pompom. However, since CO_2 has minimum temperatures of only $-79°C$, it is limited in its applications to shallow, benign lesions.[21]

Nitrous oxide stores well. It reaches a minimum temperature of $-90°C$. Although it works well in a cryoprobe system, it is difficult to use in spray techniques. It also has a limited depth of penetration.

Freons produce a wide minimum temperature range, going as low as about $-90°C$.[22, 23] Freon 114 is used to cool skin for dermabrasion.[24] Freon 12 is another commercially available freon. Difficulties in delivery to and on the skin (Freon tends to pool) and potential cardiac toxicity limit its usefulness.[25, 26]

Of all cryogens available today, liquid nitrogen remains the freezing agent of choice.[27] It is inexpensive, generally available, and has a minimum temperature of $-196°C$. Its major drawback is the difficulty of storage. It must be stored in an insulated container or a Dewar flask and, even so, vaporizes whether or not in use. Dewar flasks from 10 to 35 liters are commercially available. Liquid is transferred to a smaller storage container or instrument for use during the day. Instruments varying from simple dippers to more sophisticated hand pumps, low pressure systems, rollers, or immersion heaters are available for this purpose. Because liquid nitrogen is the cryogen of choice, only techniques using it for treatment of specific conditions will be detailed in this chapter.

BASIC PROCEDURES

There are three popular techniques for using liquid nitrogen. The cotton swab technique employs these for application of the cryogen directly to the target tissue. Liquid nitrogen evaporates rapidly from the cotton, so it must be dipped into the reservoir at intervals for any treatment other than a brief application. The depth of freeze is limited.[28] This technique should be used for only superficial lesions (e.g., actinic keratoses, warts, and lentigines). Ready-made or handmade swabs can be employed. For small lesions, a small tight swab is selected. Larger and looser swabs are utilized for larger lesions. The swabs can be fashioned to a point or flattened on the ends, as desired. After selection, the swab is dipped into the reservoir of liquid nitrogen and applied directly to the lesion.

The second technique uses a cryoprobe and interposes a heat sink between the cryogen and the target.[29, 30] The cryogen in most instruments constantly circulates through the hollow probe and is vented out. The chilled probe is then applied to the target area. The capacity of a heat sink varies with its size, its composition, and the temperature difference created between it and the warmer target area.

Interface factors can be important when using cryoprobes. The interface is defined as the junction between the heat sink and the target. Because air is a poor conductor, a solid probe on an uneven, dry surface produces poor contact. It may be necessary to moisten the surface to improve the interface factors. In order to provide maximum beneficial interface factors and to increase heat transfer, cryoprobes are produced in various sizes and different contours and shapes.

The third procedure is spray freezing as refined by Torre.[31–33] Spray techniques are used in the majority of nonmalignant lesions. These methods allow the cryogen to be applied directly to the target area, thus eliminating or avoiding to a degree adverse interface factors. It is essential that freezing spread evenly throughout the target area for effective freezing. Various patterns of spraying have been developed to accomplish this.[34]

A spiral pattern of spraying produces a gradually enlarging circle of freeze. The spray is started at the center of the lesion and carried in an ever-widening spiral. This method is suitable for round lesions such as actinic keratoses.

The paint-brush pattern is started at the lateral point of the lesion and carried back and forth over the entire extent of the tumor. This may be applied in either a horizontal or vertical fashion. Rectangular or ovoid lesions are well suited to this pattern.

A third pattern occurs from concentration of the spray in a circle midway between the center and the periphery of the lesion. Superficial freezing proceeds centrifugally and centripetally. This pattern is suitable for large lesions.

It is generally accepted that instrumentation methods provide the most consistent results for many nonmalignant lesions and almost all malignant ones.[35–40] This allows more precise delineation of the temperature and depths needed. As previously mentioned, complete cryocongelation occurs around $-40°C$ to $-60°C$.[41–45] Frequently, these temperatures represent "overkill" of nonmalignant lesions. Instrumentation can make these factors easier to adjust and, in proper hands, help to minimize complications or aid cosmetic effect. Pigmentary problems,[46] nerve damage, and cartilage damage[47] can be minimized by proper technique. Hence, instrumentational liquid nitrogen procedures are given the vast bulk of attention in the following discussion.

The common measurement utilized to determine adequacy of freeze with these methods is the "thaw time." Freezing time is generally not used because freezing time is affected by too many variables. For instance, instruments from different manufacturers vary the freezing time, as does the size of the spray nozzle or probe.

There are two types of thaw times that provide the most consistent clinical measurement. The "halo" thaw time is used for malignant lesions;[48] the "total" thaw time is utilized for most nonmalignant ones.[49] The total thaw time is defined as the measured time from stopping application of the cryogen until all visual and palpable disappearance of the frozen area occurs.

SPECIFIC NONMALIGNANCIES

Angiomas

Selected angiomas respond well to cryosurgery. Osler-Weber-Rendu lesions usually disappear after a pointed cryoprobe is placed into the center of the lesion with solid freezing for several seconds. Venous lakes of the lips also respond well to a flat cryoprobe or spray. Lesions are frozen solid including the margins and adjacent skin. If a probe is used, a size slightly smaller than the lesion is selected.

Castro-Ron[50] has reported excellent results in the treatment of large hemangiomas that are symptomatic or deforming. Because of their vascularity, the lateral spread of freeze is not an accurate guide to the depth of freeze in these cases. Probes are used primarily to force the bulk of the blood out before and during the freeze.

Technique

Where possible, Castro-Ron uses a flat probe approximately the size of the lesion. For larger tumors, a flat or rounded probe can be moved from site to site in 1- to 2-cm areas until the entire lesion is frozen. For cavernous hemangiomas, he uses a flat probe with compression. The tumor is frozen 3 to 4 mm beyond the borders. Depending upon the instrument employed, several minutes of total freezing time may be necessary. Larger vessels require deeper and more solid freezing. For smaller sac-like tumors, one freeze-thaw cycle may be sufficient, but for larger tumors, a double freeze-thaw cycle similar to that employed in malignant lesions may be necessary.

Occasionally, spray freezing may be employed as an adjunct on rapidly growing lesions. Treatments may be repeated at eight- to 12-week intervals.

Comment

Castro-Ron has also reported excellent results on selected lymphangiomas.[50] Spraying the superficial portions, the probe is reserved for the bulky portions. This technique can help in controlling the growth. Most large hemangiomas treated in this fashion heal in three to six weeks. Edema can occur; large lesions of the head and neck produce marked edema persisting for as long as 10 to 14 days. Bullae usually resolve around the fifth day. Bleeding is rare. If this occurs, pressure usually suffices for control, although occasionally a suture is necessary. Pain can be severe but infection is uncommon. Occasionally, preoperative analgesics may be necessary. Daily washing with liquid soap for the first few days is indicated.

Dermatofibroma

Many dermatofibromas can be treated effectively by simple surgical excision. However, when they occur in certain locations, e.g., the lower extremities, a comparatively large amount of surgery may result in less-than-satisfactory cosmetic result. Cryosurgery offers a viable and simple alternative. Torre[51] first presented a series of 79 lesions treated by cryosurgical methods. At the end of the follow-up study, 61 were no longer palpable, and 55 had attained excellent cosmetic results. Spiller and Spiller[52] later commented favorably on these techniques.

Technique

Both spray and probe techniques can be used. A spray can be centered into the biopsy site. The lesion must be frozen relatively hard. Thaw times approach 1½ to two minutes in some larger lesions. A spray method is satisfactory for larger lesions but does not work well for smaller ones, unless constricting devices to limit the lateral spread of the freeze are employed.

For most lesions, a cryoprobe is utilized. A flat-headed type, usually one half to two thirds the diameter of the lesion, is selected. The lesion is frozen until a 1 to 2 mm border beyond the lesion is obtained. Although it takes longer to obtain a solid freeze, probes are frequently necessary to obtain the depth of freeze desired, since these tumors are often quite deep in relation to the horizontal width on the surface.

Insulating neoprene cones, similar to those used for malignant lesions, can also be used.[53] In these cases, a cone slightly smaller than the tumor is utilized. Liquid nitrogen is sprayed evenly onto the surface of the tumor until a white rim appears at the outer margin of the cone. Two freeze-thaw cycles may occasionally be necessary for deep dermatofibromas.

Comment

Repeat treatments at approximately two- to three-month intervals may be required. The patient should be forewarned of this possibility.

Complications are occasionally seen in treating dermatofibromas. The most frequent are pigmentary alterations. Both hyper- and hypopigmentations are observed. Often, there is a surrounding halo of hyperpigmentation. Although these are usually transitory, it may take as long as one year or more for them to disappear. Hyperpigmentation occurring directly over the dermatofibroma can be permanent. More treatments with less freezing at each session might reduce this complication. Occasionally, hypertrophic scars develop. As with pigmentary complications, these are usually transitory but take many months to resolve.

Granuloma Faciale

Graham was the first to report that cryosurgery could be helpful in cases of granuloma faciale.[54, 55] Recently, Zacarian[56] has confirmed this. With these reports from two reliable and respected workers in the field, it can now be stated that at least selected cases of granuloma faciale should be considered candidates for cryosurgical management.

Technique

Zacarian uses an open spray technique after the biopsy is performed. In at least one case, a single freeze-thaw cycle was instituted. The lesion was frozen solidly.

Comment

Granuloma faciale has been difficult to manage. Dapsone, ultraviolet radiation, topical application of psoralen, and intralesional injection of steroids have all been tried. It would appear that if cryosurgery is effective in at least some cases, prolonged therapy might be avoided.

Keloid

Selected keloids respond favorably to cryosurgery. As with other techniques, younger, smaller keloids respond best. Cryosurgery alone does not usually produce adequate results as compared to combined methods, except in small lesions.

Technique

Various techniques are used for keloids, but most physicians use combination methods. For medium and large keloids, the author's procedure is similar to that of Graham.[57] The lesion is injected with intralesional triamcinolone (10 mg/cc) diluted one to two with saline (or occasionally a local anesthetic). The keloid is spray-frozen solidly. Multiple lesions can be treated in this fashion. Some author-

ities, including Allington[58] and Ceilley,[59] inject the triamcinolone after freezing rather than before. The temporary softening of the keloid after thawing allows the triamcinolone solution to be injected more easily and to spread further in the tissue.

Torre[21] also employs a combined method for larger keloids. Approximately 90% of the lesion is excised first. The borders and depth are then spray-frozen solidly. The lesions appear to heal well with this method.

Zacarian[60] has reported on simple spray-freezing of small keloids. He found varied results.

Comment

Varied results are reported no matter what combination of techniques are used. This does not differ from other methods used in the treatment of keloids. At times, several treatments are necessary, usually about four to six weeks apart. For multiple lesions in particular, some combination of different methods should be considered.

Actinic Keratosis Including Leukoplakia

After the popularization of liquid nitrogen as a cryogen by Allington,[5] cryosurgery has been advocated as one of the treatments of choice for actinic keratoses. The procedures are performed rapidly with relative lack of complications. For lesions that are few in number, a cotton-tipped applicator or dipstick is adequate. In those cases where multiple lesions occur, the dip-stick presents certain disadvantages. There is sometimes a lack of control of the spread of freeze with the dipstick. Because it must be dipped into the liquid nitrogen reservoir repeatedly, a drip problem can also occur. This could be particularly hazardous when working around the eyes. Instrument methods help solve these potential problems.

Technique

Local anesthetic is unnecessary. Depending upon the unit, a spray technique employing 16- to 24-gauge needles is selected. The lesion is frozen with one of the spray applications described earlier. A small amount of tissue is frozen just outside the borders of the lesion. Thaw times of individual lesions range from 20 to 45 seconds. Freezing times are so rapid that erythema may not develop completely by the time the procedure is completed. Hence, it is advisable to mark the lesions to be treated and to use a systematic pattern in advancing from one lesion to the next.

Leukoplakia of the lip and buccal mucosa lend themselves well to cryosurgical therapy. When treating the lip, after a biopsy is taken, a spray technique should be utilized. Because these lesions are usually linear, it is best to start at one end and work toward the other. The lesion is spray-frozen solidly. Total thaw times are usually one to 1½ minutes. When an entire lip must be frozen, it is best to freeze only one half at a time to give the patient some degree of comfort and convenience when eating.

Both probe and spray techniques can be used for leukoplakia in the mouth. These lesions should be frozen just outside the active border. Occasionally, the plaques are so large or numerous they cannot all be treated during one session. Probes can be used that are available from various companies[61] or can be handmade to fit into the mouth. When probes are used, it is best to chill the probe before using it on mucosal surfaces. As the probe is applied, it should be moved around over the surface of the target area. This simple maneuver helps prevent sticking to the mucosa. Particularly when spray techniques are used, vapors cloud the area being treated. If small areas are being frozen, the patient can be told to breathe in through the nose and out through the mouth. For larger areas, it is preferable to have a small dental suction apparatus available that will remove the vapors. Care should be taken not to allow the spray to touch the suction for long, or the suction tip will act as a secondary cryoprobe.

Comment

Many actinic keratoses can be treated at a single visit. The patient should be reminded of the course of events that often occurs after treatment: erythema, exudation, and crusting. In many instances, bullae develop also, particularly over friction points and loose areas of skin such as on the arms or hands. These bullae, if not too large, should be allowed to resolve naturally. Occasionally, a few need to be evacuated. It is wise to forewarn the patient that this is not a cause for alarm.

Extremely hypertrophic keratoses, particularly those over the dorsum of the hand, may need repeated freezing. If this is necessary, an interval of eight to 12 weeks between treatments should be employed.

Spray techniques for actinic keratoses produce good results on the ears and nose. Used in hairy areas such as the eyebrows, lesions can be removed without permanent loss of hair. Delicate areas such as the eyelids and periorbital areas are also well suited to a spray technique employing small portable units with small nozzle openings.[27] Control for intermittent spraying is available on most current portable units and is a decided advantage when working in these areas.

Although it is widely acknowledged that cryosurgery is one of the treatments of choice for actinic keratoses, actual statistics, oddly enough, are lacking in this regard. Partly for this reason, Smolewski and the author have recently completed a statistical study on the cure rate of actinic keratoses by cry-osurgical methods.[62] Evaluation of 1002 lesions was made after single cryosurgical treatments. In order to qualify for inclusion in the study, lesions had to have relatively well-defined borders and no previous treatment. Lesion size ranged from ⅛ to one inch. A minimum follow-up of one year was required (the longest was eight years). Results showed 13 recurrences, or approximately a 98.5% cure rate. This study supports statistically the common clinically observed success of cryosurgical management of this precancerous lesion.

Leukoplakias of the buccal mucosa can prove to be difficult to manage, particularly when large or numerous plaques are present. Cryosurgery is an effective, safe, and relatively simple treatment for these lesions. However, when working around the tongue, care should be taken because scarring and nerve damage have been reported.[7]

Recently, 50 cases of leukoplakia of the lip, ranging in size from ¼ to one inch, were reviewed.[63] In 40 of the cases, which were observed for six months or longer, only one recurrence has been noted. This supports the contention that cryosurgery is an effective method for treating leukoplakias.

Seborrheic Keratosis

Many seborrheic keratoses are amenable to cryosurgical techniques. These techniques may be used alone or in combination,[64] but spray techniques are employed almost exclusively.

Technique

Morphology dictates the optimum technique. Flat lesions respond best and can be spray-frozen quickly. The technique is to employ, without anesthesia, a spray lightly over the entire lesion with a small halo. Thaw times of 30 to 45 seconds usually suffice.

Frequently, total eradication of raised seborrheic keratoses is not achieved by simple spray-freezing. A more successful alternative consists of first spraying the lesion superficially until it is slightly firm, then curetting it off. After being lightly frozen, the lesion peels off easily. A hemostatic material is applied, and then the wound is covered by an adhesive bandage.

Comment

Multiple keratoses can be frozen at the same session using these methods. However, there are disadvantages to this procedure. Some lesions recur and must be retreated. Also, the pigmentation is not always eliminated when treating flat lesions by spraying. These limitations must be weighed against the advantages of usual cosmetic elegance and speed of eradication. Care should be taken not to freeze the lesions too firmly when used in combination with curettage. A curette is difficult to use if the keratosis is frozen solid. If this happens, the lesion must partially thaw before continuing. Also, too much freezing can result in scarring or hypopigmentation.

Senile Lentigo

Treatment for removal of senile lentigines can be a frustrating problem. Poor results are the rule. Cryosurgery may be used with a moderate degree of success in many cases. Even when not eradicating the lesion, cryotherapy frequently lightens the color.

Technique

Either probes or sprays can be employed. With the spray technique, the lesion is frozen very superficially including a small halo. Total thaw times of around 20 seconds suffice. With most small portable instruments, three to six seconds of freezing for each lesion is sufficient.

Comment

Although multiple lesions can be treated at a single session, it is probably best not to treat too many at the first visit. It is wiser to use several lesions as a test area. The patient can return in four to eight weeks for re-evaluation. If both the operator and the patient are satisfied, more lesions can then be treated. In the past, probes were preferred, but with the advent of newer portable hand-held units, many physicians are now using simple spray-freezing techniques on these lesions.

Mucocele

Spiller and Spiller[52] reported the first successful use of cryoprobes for treatment of lip mucoceles. It is apparent that at least in selected cases, cryosurgery offers a rapid and effective means of resolving these cysts.

Technique

Although a spray alone may be used, the author now favors the use of open or closed cryoprobes for treatment. It has not been determined that evacuation of the cystic material aids in faster or more effective resolution. The author suspects that evacuation of all or part of the contents would enhance the effectiveness of the procedure. The probe is applied and the lesion frozen solidly until the ice ball is palpated beyond all margins of the cyst. Edema is to be expected the first days after the procedure. As with buccal lesions, the probes should first be chilled and then moved around over the target area for the first few seconds of freezing.

Comment

Frequently, more than one treatment is needed for eradication. If so, they should be performed from six to eight weeks apart. A larger number of cases are needed to determine not only the overall cure rate but other questions raised, namely, if there is a limiting size to effective treatment and if evacuation of the contents is advantageous.

Porokeratosis Plantaris Discreta

Recently, both Limmer[65] and Waller[66] have reported successful therapy of this unusual condition. In a series of 21 lesions, Limmer has shown an excellent response to cryosurgery in combination with surgical paring.

Technique

His method includes local anesthesia. Paring of the surface lesion is carried out prior to an initial spray-freeze. After this is done, débridement of each lesion is performed at 14-day intervals. Any residual portion is refrozen at these visits. This is repeated at two-week intervals until there is no visible pathologic condition. Several treatments may be necessary for the desired results.

Comment

These lesions are described as sweat duct abnormalities by Taub and Steinberg.[67] Surgical management had been previously advocated for them. It now appears that a combination of cryosurgery and surgical paring can be regarded as a treatment of choice for this condition.

Prurigo Nodularis

Recently, Waldinger and colleagues[68] treated a 55-year-old black woman with an eight-year history of prurigo nodularis. Because of poor response to previous therapy, freezing was employed. Freeze-thaw technique was used to produce blisters. This management resulted in smooth macule formation and afforded extended relief of the pruritus to these multiple lesions.

Sebaceous Hyperplasia

Lesions of sebaceous hyperplasia are treated primarily for cosmetic reasons. However, a double problem is posed: There is a need for both effective eradication and minimal scarring with any treatment process. Cryosurgery is well suited for this.

Technique

The technique is simple. A pointed cryoprobe is placed into or on the small punctum of each lesion. Depending upon the unit used, three to eight seconds of freeze time is all that is required. Once a very small margin of frozen normal tissue surrounds the lesion, the process is terminated. No thaw times are needed using this process.

Comment

Many lesions may be treated at a single session. However, it is best to treat all lesions in one area before skipping to the next. It is difficult to recognize which lesions have been frozen because freezing times are so short. There is a slight interval before erythema occurs. It should be explained to the patient that refreezing may be necessary. In the author's experience, two to three treatments at six- to eight-week intervals usually suffice for the desired cosmetic effect. Results compare favorably to platinum-needle desiccation. Caution should be taken when using the cryoprobe in this way. Certain units have systems whereby the liquid nitrogen being circulated through the probes is vented out in a fashion that could splatter or drip on the patient. Care should be taken to insure that venting occurs away from the patient.

Trichiasis

Cryosurgery for the adequate treatment of trichiasis was first advocated by Sullivan and coworkers.[69] Shortly thereafter, Fraunfelder expanded our knowledge of, and set the parameters for, treatment of these lesions.[70, 71]

Technique

Fraunfelder uses a spray technique after properly shielding the conjunctiva with a Jaeger plastic retractor or Styrofoam protector. A thermocouple is inserted near the base of the follicles and horizontal to the lid. The lid is frozen to a temperature of $-15°C$, at which point the procedure is terminated. More than one treatment may be necessary for effective eradication.

Comment

Both the upper and lower eyelid can be treated in this manner, although the upper lids do not respond as consistently. Previous management of this highly inconveniencing and sometimes compli-

cating disease has not been satisfactory. Because cryosurgery offers a relatively simple and effective treatment, it can be considered the therapy of choice for many cases of trichiasis.

Miscellaneous Comments

For completeness, this section of the chapter ends with a few comments on conditions that have not been previously mentioned or covered completely in other sections. Although the studies may be anecdotal, incomplete, or unpublished, each is nonetheless meaningful.

Infectious granulomas are known to respond to cryosurgical therapy. Not only have Atkinson and Daniels[72] reported their success in swimming pool granuloma, but at least one recorded case has been cured of chromoblastomycosis with this modality.[73] One other case has been reported as responding to cryosurgery, but it was not clear whether this was performed for cure or palliation.[74]

In the author's experience, chalazions do not respond well to cryosurgery. In a small series of patients, it was found that recurrence occurred whether the lesion was frozen alone or after incision, drainage, and evacuation of the contents.

Cotton-tipped applicators are used for cryosurgery of most verrucae. However, it is fair to say that digitate warts, including digitate condylomata, are best treated by a small portable instrument spray system.

Although the author's results in plantar and palmar warts have been somewhat dismal, others get better results.[75, 76] Prieto reported a high cure rate in a series of 160 warts, some followed as long as three years. His technique is to carefully pare the wart and to follow this with spray-freezing. Multiple freeze-thaw cycles are used.

AFTERCARE

Aftercare of cryosurgical wounds for nonmalignant lesions is simple. In most cases, the patient is allowed to continue normal bathing and is advised to clean wounds daily after a bath or shower with a cleansing solution such as hydrogen peroxide or alcohol. Particularly for patients treated for warts, molluscum contagiosum, or lesions in the perineal area, daily washing with povidone-iodine skin cleanser is recommended. Topical antibiotics are indicated for application only in lesions suspected of being infected at the time of treatment or if infection is likely to occur during the postoperative course. Systemic antibiotics are advised only in those cases of frank bacterial infection. This occurs rarely in the treatment of nonmalignant lesions, but seems to have an increased incidence in geographic regions where the humidity is high. Usually, lesions are left open, but loose dressings may be applied if desired. Makeup is permitted over the dry crusts. Sunscreen application for six weeks postoperatively is frequently advised to lessen the possibility of pigmentary problems in localities or at times of the year when heavy sun exposure is anticipated.

MORBIDITY

Severe pain during cryosurgery is rare, particularly in the treatment of nonmalignant lesions where freezing times are short. Transient stinging and burning sensations are usual during both freezing and thawing phases. Mucous membrane lesions are hypersensitive. Treatment to the forehead can produce a migraine-type headache, which may persist for hours and require analgesics. Edema following treatment is usual but rarely severe. Edema is more common in loose skin such as in the periorbital area. Cold compresses may be beneficial for this.

Vesiculobullous reactions to freezing are more common following cryosurgery for nonmalignant lesions than for malignant ones. The reason is that one usually freezes more superficially; hence, separation at the dermoepidermal junction would be more likely to produce a bulla. Freezing for malignant lesions goes much deeper, and while the bullous stage is passed through, a more exudative or gelatinous phase takes its place. Blister fluid may be serous or hemorrhagic, and occasionally, the reaction may extend well beyond the areas of cold application.

Pigmentary changes are usually transitory but, in susceptible individuals, may be permanent. Although the changes are more common in treating malignant lesions, one can encounter a typical hypopigmentation toward the center with a surrounding halo of hyperpigmentation in treated areas. Dermatofibromas especially produce pigmentary changes. All of the color in seborrheic keratoses may not be eradicated with treatment. The same is true for lentigines. This can often be blamed on inadequate treatment.

REFERENCES

1. White AC: Liquid air: Its application in medicine and surgery. Med Rec 56(4):109, 1899
2. Whitehouse HH: Liquid air in dermatology: Its indications and limitations. JAMA 49:371, 1907
3. Pusey WA: The use of carbon dioxide snow in the treatment of nevi and other lesions of the skin. JAMA 49:1354, 1907
4. Irvine HG, Turnacliff DD: Liquid oxygen in dermatology. Archives of Dermatology and Syphilogy 19:270, 1929
5. Allington HD: Liquid nitrogen in the treatment of skin diseases. Calif Med 72:153, 1950
6. Cooper IS, Less AS: Cryostatic congelation: A system for producing a limited, controlled region of cooling or freezing of biologic tissues. J Nerv Ment Dis 133:259, 1961
7. Torre D: New York: Cradle of cryosurgery. NY State J Med 67:465, 1967
8. Zacarian SA, Adham MI: Cryotherapy of cutaneous malignancy. Cryobiology 2:212, 1966
9. Johnson RB, Daniels F Jr: Enzyme studies in experimental cryosurgery of the skin. J Cryobiology 3:222–232, 1974.
10. Merryman HT: General principles of freezing and freezing injury in cellular materials. Ann New York Acad Sci 85:503, 1960
11. Mazur P: Causes of injury in frozen thawed cells. Fed Proc 24(Suppl 15):5175, 1965
12. Farrant J, Walter CA: The cryobiological basis for cryosurgery. J Dermatol Surg Oncol 3:403–407, Jul/Aug 1977
13. Gill W, DaCosta J, Fraser J: The control and predictability of the cryolesion. Cryobiology 6(4) 347–353, 1970.
14. Leibo SP, Mazur P: The role of cooling rates in low-temperature preservation. Cryobiology 8:447–452, 1971
15. Mazur P: Physical-chemical factors underlying cell injury in cryosurgical freezing, in Rand RW, et al: Cryosurgery. Springfield, Ill, Charles C Thomas, 1968
16. Mazur P: The freezing of biological systems. Cryobiology 1970
17. Smith JJ, Fraser J: An estimation of tissue damage and thermal history in the cryolesion. Cryobiology 11:139–147, 1974
18. Whittaker DK: Ice crystals formed in tissue during cryosurgery. I. Light microscopy. Cryobiology 11:192–201. II. Electron microscopy. Cryobiology 11:202–217, 1974.
19. Gage AA: Deep cryosurgery, in Epstein E (ed): Skin Surgery, Ed 3. Springfield, Ill, Charles C Thomas, 1970
20. Brothagen H: Local freezing of the skin by carbon dioxide: An experimental investigation of tissue temperature movements in depth. Acta Dermatol (Suppl 44) 41:1, 1961
21. Torre D, Lubritz RR: Cutaneous cryosurgery: Treatment of nonmalignant lesions. Committee on Home Study Programs, American Academy of Dermatology. Courses in Clinical Dermatology, 1977
22. Torre D: Freezing with freons. Cutis 16(3):437–445, Sept 1975
23. Torre D: Alternate cryogens for cryosurgery. J Dermatol Surg Oncol 1:56–58, June 1975
24. Wilson JW, Luikart R, Ayers S: Dichlorotetrafluoroethane for surgical skin planing. Arch Dermatol 71:523, 1955
25. Nicholas W: Are freon propellants inert? NY Journal of Medicine 74:1939, 1974
26. Harris JD: Toxic effects of aerosol propellants on the heart. Arch Int Med 131:162, 1973
27. Lubritz RR: Cryosurgery of benign and pre-malignant cutaneous lesions, in Zacarian SA (ed) Cryosurgical Advances in Dermatology and Tumors of the Head and Neck. Springfield, Ill, Charles C Thomas, 1977
28. Grimmett RH: Liquid nitrogen therapy, histological observation. Arch Dermatol 83:563–567, April 1961
29. Zacarian SA, Adham MI: Cryotherapy of cutaneous malignancy. Cryobiology 2:212–218, 1966
30. Zacarian SA: Cryosurgery of Skin Cancer. Springfield, Ill, Charles C Thomas, 1966
31. Torre D: Cutaneous cryosurgery. J Cryosurgery 1:202–209, Oct 1968
32. Torre D: New York: Cradle of cryosurgery. NY State J Med 67:465–467, 1967
33. Torre D: Cryosurgery in dermatology. Physicians' Panorama 6:4–8, 1968
34. Lubritz RR: Cryo corner: Cryosurgical spray patterns. J Dermatol Surg Oncol 4(2):138–139, 1978
35. Zacarian SA: Cryosurgery of Skin Cancer and Cryogenic Techniques in Dermatology. Springfield, Ill, Charles C Thomas, 1969
36. Zacarian SA (ed): Cryosurgical Advances in Dermatology and Tumors of the Head and Neck. Springfield, Ill, Charles C Thomas, 1977
37. Torre D: Cryosurgery, in Andrade R, Gumport SL, Popkin

GL, Reese TD, (eds): Cancer of the Skin. Philadelphia, WB Saunders, 1976

38. Lubritz RR: Cryosurgery for benign and malignant skin lesions: Treatment with a new instrument. South Med J 69:1401–1405, Nov 1976
39. Lubritz RR: Cryosurgical management of multiple skin carcinomas. J Dermatol Surg Oncol 3(4):414–416, July/Aug 1977
40. Lubritz RR: Cryosurgery of benign lesions. Cutis 16(3): 426–432, Sept 1975
41. LePivert PJ, Binder P, Ougier T: Measurement of intratissue bio-electrical low frequency impedance: A new method to predict pre-operatively the destructive effect of cryosurgery. Cryobiology, 14:245–250, 1977
42. LePivert PJ: The measurement of low frequency electrical impedance as a guide to effective cryosurgery. J Dermatol Surg Oncol 3:395–397, 1977
43. Savic M, Zacarian SA: A new impedance-based method for controlled cryosurgery of malignant tumors. J Dermatol Surg Oncol 3:592–593, 1977
44. Torre D, Smolewski S: Congelation Cryometry in Cryosurgery. Exhibit at the Conference of American Academy Dermatology, San Francisco, Calif, December 1978
45. Gage A: Correlation of electrical impedance and temperature in tissue during freezing. Cryobiology 16:56–62, 1979
46. Graham GF: Cryosurgery in the treatment of acne and specific cutaneous neoplasia, in Zacarian SA (ed): Cryosurgical Advances in Dermatology and Tumors of the Head and Neck. Springfield, Ill, Charles C Thomas, 1977
47. Torre D: Cryosurgery in dermatology, in Von Leden H, Cahan G (eds): Cryogenics in Surgery. Flushing, NY, Med Exam, 1971
48. Torre D, Lubritz RR, Graham G: Cryosurgical treatment of basal cell carcinomas. Progress in Dermatology 12:11–16, 1978
49. Torre D: Cryosurgery of premalignant and malignant skin lesions. Cutis 8:123, 1971
50. Castro-Ron G: Cryosurgery of angiomas and birth defects, in Zacarian SA (ed): Cryosurgery for Skin Cancer and Cutaneous Disorders. St. Louis, C.V. Mosby, 1985
51. Torre D: Dermatological cryosurgery: A progress report. Cutis, 11:782, 1973
52. Spiller WF, Spiller RF: Cryosurgery in dermatologic office practice: Special reference to dermatofibroma and mucous cyst of the lip. South Med J 68(2):157–160, 1975
53. Torre D: Cryosurgical treatment of epitheliomas using the cone-spray technique. J Dermatol Surg Oncol 3(4):432–436, July/Aug 1977
54. Graham GF: Treatment of acne and specific cutaneous neoplasia, in Zacarian SA (ed): Cryosurgical Advances in Dermatology and Tumors of the Head and Neck. Springfield, Ill, Charles C Thomas, 1977
55. Graham GF, Stewart R: Cryosurgery for unusual cutaneous neoplasma. J Dermatol Surg Oncol 3:437–442, 1977
56. Zacarian SA: Cryo corner: Cryosurgery effective for granuloma faciale. J Dermatol Surg Oncol 11:11, 1985
57. Graham GF: Cryosurgery for keloids, in Lubritz RR, Torre D (eds): Outline Manual of Dermatocryosurgery. Cryosurgery Course, American Academy Dermatology, Chicago, Ill, December 1979 (published courtsey of Owen Laboratories)
58. Allington H: Cryosurgery, in Epstein E (ed): Skin Surgery, Ed 4. Springfield, Ill, Charles C Thomas, 1976
59. Ceilley R, Babin RW: The combined use of cryosurgery and intralesional injections of suspensions of fluorinated adrenocorticosteroids for reducing keloids and hypertrophic scars. J Dermatol Surg Oncol 5(1):54–56, 1979
60. Zacarian SA: Benign and pre-cancerous tumors of the skin, in Zacarian SA (ed): Cryosurgery of Tumors of the Skin and Oral Cavity. Springfield, Ill, Charles C Thomas, 1973
61. Torre D, Torre S: Gadgets and gimmicks. Cutis 12:93, 1973
62. Lubritz RR, Smolewski S: Cryosurgery cure rate of actinic keratoses. J Am Acad Dermatol 7:631, 1982
63. Lubritz RR, Smolewski S: Cryosurgery cure rate of premalignant leukoplakia of the lower lip. J Dermatol Surg Oncol 9:235, 1983
64. Lubritz RR: Cryosurgical management of nonmalignancies. Dermatology 2:44–47, Aug 1979
65. Limmer BL: Cryosurgery of porokeratosis plantaris discreta. Arch Dermatol 115:582–583, May 1979
66. Waller J: Porokeratosis Plantaris Discreta (Conical Callus): Cone Spray Freeze Method. Presented at First Annual American College of Cryosurgery Meeting, New Orleans, La, March 13, 1978
67. Taub J, Steinberg M: Porokeratosis plantaris discreta: A previously unrecognized dermatologic entity. Int J Dermatol 9:83–90, 1970
68. Waldinger TP, Wong RC, Taylor WB, Voorhees JJ: Cryotherapy improves prurigo nodularis. Arch Dermatol 120:1598–1600, Dec 1984.
69. Sullivan J, Beard C, Bullock JD: Cryosurgery for treatment of trichiasis. Am J Ophthalmol 82(1):117–121, July 1976
70. Fraunfelder FT, Wallace RR, Farris HD, et al: The role of cryosurgery in external ocular and periocular disease. Transactions American Academy of Ophthalmology and Otolaryngology 83:713–724, July/Aug 1977
71. Fraunfelder FT, Petursson GJ: The use of liquid nitrogen cryospray for treatment of trichiasis. Ophthalmic Surg 10:42–46, Aug 1979
72. Atkinson SC, Daniels F Jr: Swimming pool granuloma: Treatment with cryosurgery. Cutis 11:818, 1973
73. Lubritz RR, Spence JE: Chromoblastomycosis: Cure by cryosurgery. Int J Dermatol 17:830–832, Dec 1978
74. Ramirez MM: Treatment of chromomycosis with liquid nitrogen. Int J Dermatol 12:250, 1973
75. Limmer BL, Bogy LT: Cryosurgery of plantar warts. J Am Podiatry Assoc 69:713–716, Dec 1979
76. Prieto A: Cryosurgery for Plantar and Palmar Verrucae. Presented at Third International Symposium on Plastic Surgery of the Head and Neck, New Orleans, La, May 1979

36

SETRAG A. ZACARIAN, M.D., F.A.C.P.

Cryosurgery of Malignant Tumors of the Skin

Liquid air was the refrigerant initially used for the treatment of many cutaneous disorders. Through the curiosity of two American dermatologists, A. Campbell White[1] and H. H. Whitehouse,[2, 3] cryotherapy had its beginnings at the turn of the century. These early pioneers were not content to freeze warts, angiomas, and actinic keratoses, but sprayed liquid air, through makeshift laboratory wash bottles, upon malignant tumors of the skin. Despite their initial clinical success and satisfactory destruction of larger neoplasms, they abandoned liquid air for the treatment of skin cancers. The reasons were probably many, such as (1) lack of sophisticated delivery system of the refrigerant, (2) poor control of the quantity of liquid air spray, more significantly, (3) the inability to monitor the evolving temperature gradients within the cryolesion at the tumor target, and (4) the inability to assess the final depth of the ice front during cryosurgery. For over 60 years, cryotherapy in dermatology was an important therapeutic modality but essentially confined to benign and precancerous disorders. The cotton swab technique became the standard delivery system of liquid air and, much later, liquid nitrogen.[4, 5]

Irving Cooper, the distinguished neurosurgeon, initiated in 1962 the modern cryosurgical technique employed today. He devised a sophisticated cryosurgical instrument with a 2.2 mm diameter cannula, which delivered circulating liquid nitrogen designed to freeze a segment of the basal ganglia in patients for the amelioration of their symptoms from Parkinson's disease.[6, 7] Utilizing the same technique, Cahan[8] and Gage[9] independently subjected internal and external malignant tumors to cryosurgery.

In 1964, this author and Adham applied copper discs of various diameters chilled by liquid nitrogen for the treatment of cutaneous carcinomas.[10] The following year, Torre[11] introduced the first liquid nitrogen spray unit, the CE-8, for the dermatologist. During the subsequent three years, this author was responsible for the design and development of the first two hand-held cryosurgical units for the delivery of liquid nitrogen by means of spray or closed probe technique.[12, 13]

THE PATHOGENESIS OF THE CRYOGENIC LESION

Freezing is a physical phenomenon that by its very nature sets into motion a complex biochemical and biophysical chain of reactions within the cell. The heat transfer that takes place when a refrigerant such as liquid nitrogen is applied to a given tissue or tumor is the withdrawal of heat and the alteration of the liquid cellular milieu to its solid phase, namely, ice. As freezing is allowed to continue, more of the underlying tissue is transformed into ice in a geometric pattern, not unlike the development of the isotherm curve from emission of electron energy by irradiation, resulting in the eventual crystallization of cell electrolytes.

One cannot freeze indefinitely. The microcirculation of the blood will keep in abeyance the final extension of the ice front. If one were to monitor temperatures within the cryolesion at various levels below the interphase, i.e., below the refrigerant source, at the periphery and margins, one would plot diverse temperatures. These are referred to as temperature gradients. In 1961, Brodthagen[14] studied temperature gradients of both porcine and human cadaver skin, subjected to cold temperatures produced by carbon dioxide. This writer with Adham[15] were the first to report on the in vivo gradient studies in human skin, comparing the cotton swabs and copper discs chilled in liquid nitrogen.

The effects of subzero temperatures upon biologic tissue are not understood entirely. Freezing of cells and tissue is complex and interdependent upon the boiling point of the cryogen, rate of cooling, and subsequent rate of thawing. Cryogenic temperatures produce a lethal effect on the cells and upon the microvessels. The cellular effect, particularly in rapid freezing, is one of dehydration (from both extracellular and intracellular ice crystal formation) resulting in the abnormal increase of electrolyte concentration within the cells.

Denaturation of lipid-protein molecules and thermal shock augment the eventual rupture of the cell membrane and produce biologic death.[16-18] Slow thawing has proven more deleterious than rapid freezing.[19]

The adverse effects of cryogenic temperatures upon small blood vessels have been reported by Kreyberg.[20, 21] An extensive study upon the micro-circulation of the Syrian hamster cheek pouch[22] clearly describes the rapid development of thrombosis, stasis, and ischemic necrosis following the induction of nominal subzero temperatures upon the tiny vasculature. These physiologic alterations upon the microcirculatory system fundamentally contribute to cryonecrosis of both normal and malignant tissue, which would otherwise be spared from the effects of cold at the cellular level.

METHODOLOGY AND INSTRUMENTATION

For effective cryonecrosis of skin cancer, the freeze front must extend at least 3 to 5 mm in depth below the cutaneous surface. The simple application of cotton swabs saturated in liquid nitrogen will produce an ice front not exceeding 1.5 mm in depth.[23] Copper discs cooled in liquid nitrogen served a useful purpose[10] for the treatment of malignant tumors and for experimental control studies in cryogenesis. The effectiveness of a delivery system that allows the free flow of liquid nitrogen vapor has proven to be ideal for the management of malignant tumors of the skin.[24] Cryosurgical units that employ carbon dioxide, Freon, or nitrous oxide are incapable of freezing in depth and are ineffectual in the treatment of skin cancer.[25]

There are at least 10 cryosurgical instruments available to the clinician. All of them are capable of delivering liquid nitrogen spray, and some will provide additional adaptable probes and plastic cones. In the past 12 years, the author has used the CS-76 cryosurgical instrument and, more recently, the CryoSurge, a hand-held unit, by Frigitronics. A single filling of this portable unit with liquid nitrogen will last the entire day. This delivery system allows interchangeable intradermic plastic needles varying in gauges from no. 14 to no. 26. The latter is ideal, for it provides a fine and delicate spray of the coolant to strategic sites, such as the eyelids and medial canthus. The volume of nitrogen can be controlled further by a built-in valve within this unit as well as by the flow pressure. The nitrogen vapor is delivered intermittently, a desirable feature not available in other hand-held cryosurgical units. This avoids the usual run-off of bubbles of liquid nitrogen during long freezing of a tumor. The unit is provided with plastic cones of various diameters as well as closed probes or discs, which are attachable to the unit with a Luer-Lock syringe and useful particularly for freezing intraoral disorders. A built-in pyrometer with two outlets for the insertion of the leads for the thermocouples are provided with the CS-76 unit.

With the hand-held unit, the CryoSurge, the purchase of a monitoring device, as with any hand-held unit, is a must.

Liquid nitrogen spray offers more rapid freezing of malignant tumors as compared with closed probes. The utilization of a plastic cone for the spray of liquid nitrogen provides the most rapid and intense freeze and also minimizes the rapid and often undesired peripheral spread of the ice front on the surface of the tumor target. Using the cone spray technique will shorten the freeze time to at least half of the interval required with an open spray technique. The subsequent thaw period following the cone spray delivery of the refrigerant is often three to four times as long than with the open spray technique.

For example, if a tumor is 1 cm in size, with an open spray technique it may take 60 seconds to adequately freeze in depth and a subsequent thaw time of 120 seconds. Freezing a similar tumor with a cone spray requires only 30 seconds to achieve the same adequacy of depth and a thaw time between three and four times as long, i.e., 90 to 120 seconds.

The formula for correlating the measurement of the lateral spread of freeze to the central depth of freeze from the surface will not accurately apply when using the cone spray technique in which the plastic cone is attached to the cryosurgical instrument. In this instance, the spray is directed from the center of the delivery device on to the center of the tumor target. The above formula as devised by Torre[26] may be applicable when using an open neoprene cone placed upon the tumor target and the liquid nitrogen is sprayed on to the tumor from right to left with a fanning S-shaped spray pattern. Even with this technique, the lateral spread of freeze from the margin beyond the cone is, at best, a rule of thumb for determining the achieved depth of freeze and certainly not an accurate guide to the exact temperature of the ice front at the specified depth.[27]

During freezing, there develops an interchange of heat transfer; the warm temperature from the underlying tissue is directed upward toward the cold heat sink (the nitrogen source, whether probe or spray). During this interphase, an ice front develops that gradually penetrates deeper and deeper upon the tumor target. The hemisphere of ice formation, or the evolving cryolesion, presents a heterogeneous temperature, or thermal gradient. It is essentially similar to the isotherm curve when one employs radiation to a tumor target, as mentioned earlier. The temperature of the ice front nearest to the refrigerant will be extremely cold, perhaps -100 to $-150°C$, while the most advanced depth of the cryolesion may be at 0 to $-10°C$. The temperatures at the outer margins of the hemisphere of ice are considerably warmer. Since effective cryonecrosis is temperature-related, the colder the temperature the

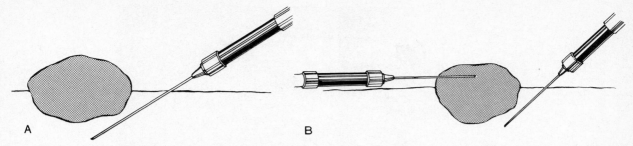

A   B

Figure 36–1. *A*, A single thermocouple inserted below the tumor. *B*, Placement of two microthermocouples for monitoring the cryolesion during freezing.

more lethal and destructive it is to the underlying malignant tumor. Destruction is dependent also upon the intensity of the freeze as well as the subsequent period of thaw, for it is during the thaw period that recrystallization of ice develops. This compounds the lethal effects of the freezing experience.

For the clinician who is a novice in the cryosurgical management of malignant tumors of the skin, the author strongly recommends that he or she monitor all tumors during freezing. Neoplasms overlying bone, such as on the forehead, temples, the regions of the zygoma, and the upper aspect of the nose, can be frozen to the depth of the periosteum. Once the overlying frozen skin and tumor bcome taut and immobile, freezing can be terminated. The clinician is now certain that the ice front has extended beyond the dermis and subcutaneous tissue and onto the periosteum, where carcinomas rarely extend. Immediately after thawing, a second freeze is applied. The second freeze will take less time than the first because the microvessels are still partially in vasoconstriction and will not offer the same resistance to the advancing ice front. To measure "halo-thaw time" is totally meaningless and provides nothing but confusion to precise and established cryosurgical techniques.

For larger malignant tumors of the head and neck, particularly those situated at critical anatomic sites, such as the ala nasi, nasolabial fold, medial canthus, and cheeks or those anterior to the tragus of the ear, one should monitor the advancing ice front. For more exacting and controlled cryosurgical procedures, the author advocates monitoring several sites within the cryolesion, particularly the margins beyond the visible tumor.

At present, there are two ways by which monitoring of the frozen tumor can be accomplished. The use of a single or a second thermocouple needle inserted at a predetermined depth centrally below the neoplasm and one at its margin is currently recommended (Fig. 36–1). The exact determination of depth at these focal points is aided by the use of an acrylic jig or template (Fig. 36–2). This is a plastic triangular device through which a thermocouple needle is passed. The template has calibrated

angles establishing the exact depth from the surface wherein the tip of the needle rests. Cryobiologists have theorized that a temperature of $-30°C$ is the lethal temperature to produce cryonecrosis.[28] Present opinion, however, considers a temperature of $-50°C$ to be more effective.[34]

The patient in Figure 36–3A was a 45-year-old man who presented with a biopsy-proven 22 mm nodular basal cell carcinoma of the left lower eyelid. The tumor nodule was anesthetized with 1% lidocaine solution, and a microthermocouple needle was inserted subcutaneously. After the patient's eye was anesthetized with 0.5% ophthalmic lidocaine solution, a plastic eyelid retractor was placed over the orbit of his eye to protect this site from possible liquid nitrogen vapor spray (Fig. 36–3B). After two minutes of open spray with liquid nitrogen, and when the underlying temperature of the tumor base was monitored at $-50°C$, the freezing was terminated. After a four-minute thaw period, a second freeze was executed. Bear in mind that with the second freeze, the interval to achieve the same adequate freeze time and/or temperature is a little less. As explained previously, the microvessels are still manifesting vasoconstriction and offer less re-

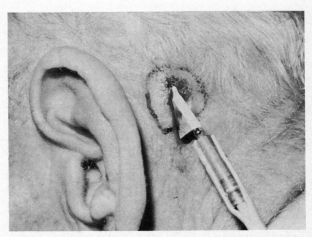

Figure 36–2. A template or acrylic jig in place through which a microthermocouple needle can be directed at a predetermined depth below the skin and tumor.

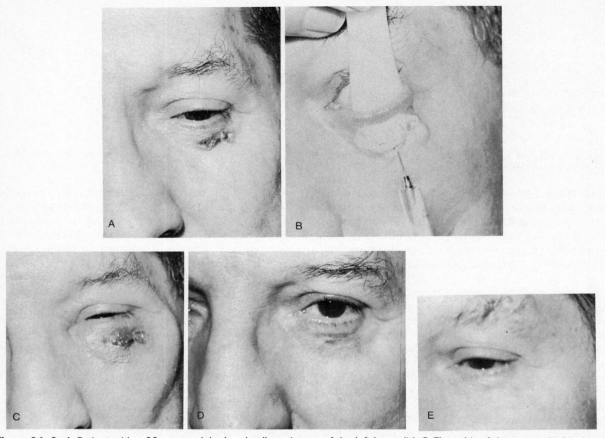

Figure 36–3. *A,* Patient with a 22 mm nodular basal cell carcinoma of the left lower lid. *B,* The orbit of the eye is shielded with a plastic lid retractor. A microthermocouple needle is inserted below the tumor to monitor the ice front during cryosurgery. After the initial freeze the temperature is monitored at −50°C, at which time the freezing is terminated. Immediately after thawing a second freeze is initiated. *C,* Forty-eight hours after cryosurgery the anticipated periorbital edema (which lasted six days) and the serosanguineous oozing from the tumor site appeared. *D,* Six weeks following cryosurgery the carcinoma is eradicated, but there is a residual hyperpigmentation at the site. *E,* Four years after cryosurgery there has been no recurrence of the carcinoma, and there is an excellent cosmetic end result.

sistance to the advancing ice front, as with the initial freeze.

About 48 hours after cryosurgery, the patient exhibited the typical periorbital edema with oozing and early crusting at the previously frozen site (Fig. 36–3C). Six weeks following cryosurgery, the patient showed no evidence of his basal cell carcinoma. A transient hyperpigmentation remained (Fig. 36–3D).

Four years after cryosurgery (Fig. 36–3E), there was no evidence of his skin cancer and little or no residual scarring, atrophy, or hyperpigmentation.

A more accurate and precise monitoring system was pioneered by LePivert.[29] He passed an alternating electric current through a series of parallel electrode needles inserted within the tumor target and measured the electrical impedance or resistance between the electrodes during freezing. This concept was based upon the existing tenet that, as one decreases the temperature within a cell or given tissue, there is a concomitant increase in impedance or resistance to the flow of electrical current within that cell or tissue. Once all the bound water within the cell is frozen and its electrolytes are crystallized, all electrical current through that cell ceases and impedance or total resistance is reached. This is referred to as the eutectic state and bespeaks of irreversible cell death.

LePivert's technique was modified by Savic and this author, who developed the Freeze Depth Indicator (Fig. 36–4). A modified direct current is generated by a 5 volt battery through multiple primary electrode needles inserted within the malignant tumor. During freezing, the electrical current flows through the primary electrode needles through the body of the patient to the secondary electrode cuff attached to the wrist. From there, the current flow passes and is registered upon the Freeze Depth Indicator. Through experimental and clinical studies, a close correlation was noted between temperature and electrical resistance.[30] There was a constant relationship between the achievement of −50 and −55°C and two million ohms (resistance), which was considered to be the eutectic state in which all bound water is frozen within cells and all electrolytes are crystallized, permitting no further flow of current and producing profound cryonecrosis. Further clinical studies have supported this concept of producing effective cryonecrosis of malignant tumors of the head and neck.[31] Other clinical investigators[32, 33] have corroborated the principles of electrical circuitry as a means of controlled monitoring of malignant tumors with cryosurgery.

The use of electrical circuitry to monitor malignant tumors of the head and neck is simple, effective, and more accurate; multiple tumor sites of the advancing ice front can be monitored simultaneously.

The patient in Figure 36–5A developed a slowly growing tumor of several years duration anterior to the tragus of her ear. The biopsy specimen was reported as being a basosquamous cell carcinoma. The tumor was nodular and measured 2.4 cm in size. A 3 mm margin of normal skin beyond the visible tumor was outlined. Two primary electrode needles were inserted within the tumor at a depth of 5 mm and subjected to vigorous freezing until two million ohms of resistance was achieved (Fig. 36–5B). The primary electrode needles are calibrated in millimeters, and the exact depth of penetration within and below the tumor can be determined accurately.

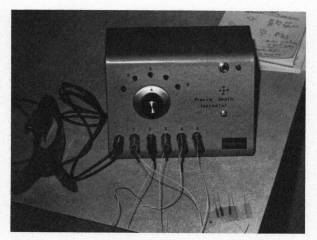

Figure 36—4. Current model of the Freeze Depth Indicator modified and engineered by Frigitronics Inc. of Shelton, CT, which is awaiting FDA approval. (Courtesy of S. A. Zacarian and from Journal of Dermatologic Surgery and Oncology, August 1980, 6(8):628–629. Copyright 1980, The Journal of Dermatologic Surgery and Oncology, Inc.)

In Figure 36–5C, the electric circuitry during cryosurgery is demonstrated. The primary electrode needles within the tumor monitor conductivity as electricity passes through the indifferent electrode on the left wrist and is registered on the Freeze Depth Indicator.

Six weeks following cryosurgery (Fig. 36–5D), the tumor was completely eradicated, and no recurrence has been observed after five years of follow-up.

As with all modalities for cancer therapy, certain criteria need to be established. There is no single best therapy for all cutaneous neoplasia, and one must individualize treatment choices for each patient, considering the patient's age, the histologic morphology of the neoplasm, and the tumor's anatomic site. Cryosurgery is effective for primary cancers of the skin—in particular, the nodular and nodular ulcerative types as well as superficial multicentric carcinomas. Tumors with ill-defined borders, such as morphea or sclerosing basal cell carcinoma and the adenoid type of basal cell carcinoma, do not respond as well to cryosurgery. In general, epidermoid carcinomas of the skin can be effectively eradicated with cryosurgery. Carcinomas of the scalp, ala nasi, and nasolabial fold demand vigorous freezing with a more generous margin than other sites, or the recurrence rate will be considerably higher. This applies also to tumors anterior to the tragus and medial canthus. The author would recommend monitoring neoplasms situated at these anatomic sites.

In the author's experience, carcinomas of the lower extremities subjected to cryosurgery take much too long to heal and can lead to secondary infection as well as atrophy of the frozen site. Therefore, freezing of tumors in these areas is not the first choice. The relative contraindications described herein may be waived, considering the age of the patient and the surgical risks the patient may face if cryosurgery is not employed. Lentigo maligna (or Hutchinson's melanotic freckle) is amenable to cryosurgery, but the recurrence rate is considerably higher than with basal cell or epidermoid carcinomas. A recent report by Dawber and Wilkinson[35] confirms this, but a longer follow-up would be desirable. In the author's series of 30 patients with lentigo maligna encountered during the past 12 years and subjected to cryosurgery, there have been only two recurrences (6.7%).[36]

Cancers of the eyelids, when properly selected, respond favorably to cryosurgery.[37] This is particularly true in tumors under 10 mm in diameter. In the author's series of 208 cases, the overall cure rate has been 92.5%.[38] One third of lower lid tumors are situated at the medial canthus, and the development of epiphora following cryosurgery is uncommon when compared to irradiation therapy or surgical ablation. Cancers situated upon the ears and the cartilaginous portion of the nose respond favorably

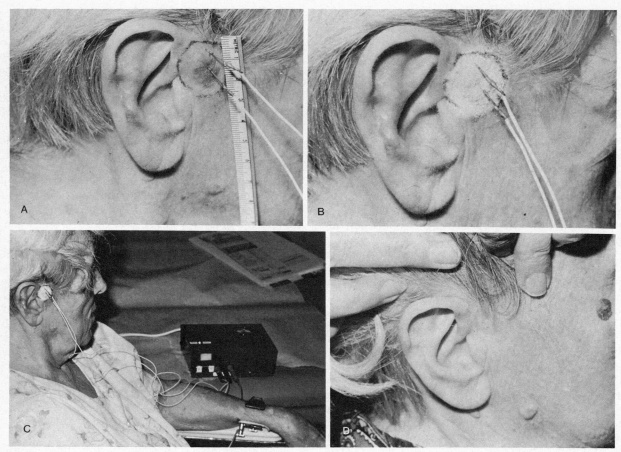

Figure 36–5. *A*, A 2.4 cm nodular basosquamous cell carcinoma with primary electrode needles inserted to a depth of 5 mm. *B*, Appearance at the end of freezing, during which two million ohms of resistance was registered on the Freeze Depth Indicator. *C*, The complete electrical circuitry between the primary electrode needles at the tumor site and the indifferent electrode upon the wrist cuff, which measures the decreasing electrical current flow until a resistance of two million ohms has been achieved. *D*, Six weeks following cryosurgery the carcinoma is completely eradicated with little to no scarring, except transitory hyperpigmentation.

to cryosurgery. Chondronecrosis subsequent to freezing of overlying tumor is rare. Several perforations of the ear have been verbally reported following cryosurgery. In these cases, the tumor had already invaded the cartilage.

A serious contraindication to cryosurgery is in patients who suffer from cold sensitivity, cryoglobulinemia, and cryofibrinogenemia and possibly in those with underlying autoimmune disease and pyoderma gangrenosa.

Complications from cryosurgery exist and have been reviewed exhaustively.[39] The most common and unavoidable permanent complication is hypopigmentation (unlike hyperpigmentation, which is transitory). Secondary infection and hemorrhage have been reported but are uncommon. Pseudoepitheliomatous hyperplasia and hypertrophic scars do occur, but the former is self-limiting, and the latter spontaneously involute and can be promptly eradicated with a single intralesional injection of triamcinolone. Keloid formation following cryosurgery has never been reported. Neuritis has been observed, but with time, nerve transmission returns, so this is not a permanent complication. It is important, however, to warn the patient of its possibility, if one anticipates intense freezing of a neoplasm overlying critical sites. Insufflation has been observed but is uncommon; a real possibility of this exists when a spray technique is used on an ulcerated or open lesion in which liquid nitrogen vapor burrows under the epidermis and expands it. This is observable, and immediately upon its occurrence, freezing can be terminated with no untoward reaction to the patient. The nitrogen is absorbed with no danger of an embolic phenomenon.

Freezing neoplasms close to the eyelid margin will increase the possibility of notching, a serious risk to consider. The same risk and complication is observed when freezing tumors too close to the vermilion border of the upper lip. Following freezing in that site, there is almost invariably a permanent tenting upward of the mucous membrane of the

TABLE 36–1. 3576 Patients with a Combined Total of 4845 Carcinomas of the Skin Subjected to Cryosurgery Between 1964 and 1984.[1]

Histology of Neoplasms[2]	Number	Percent
Basal cell carcinomas	4451	91.77
Epidermoid carcinomas	225	4.67
Basosquamous cell carcinomas	80	1.74
Bowen's disease (carcinoma in situ)	55	1.16
Lentigo maligna	34	0.66
	4845	100.0

[1]From Zacarian SA: Cryosurgery for Skin Cancer and Cutaneous Disorders. St. Louis, C. V. Mosby Co, 1985, Courtesy of the C. V. Mosby Company

[2]Of all carcinomas, 30% were under 1.0 cm, 60% were under 2.0 cm, and 10% were between 2.1 and 7.0 cm.

upper lip. This is not encountered when freezing tumors of the lower lip. If a tumor has not invaded the underlying cartilage of the ear or nostril (a rare occurrence), one need not fear permanently perforating the cartilage.

SUMMARY AND CONCLUSIONS

The author's cryosurgical experience of malignant tumors of the head and neck since 1964 is outlined in Table 36–1. Statistical data about recurrences have been summarized in Table 36–2.[40] In these cases, the highest rate of recurrences was observed in the treatment of recurrent carcinoma of the skin previously treated with either another modality or with previous cryosurgery. As pointed out earlier, higher recurrence rates have been observed in the author's experience with carcinomas of the scalp, ala nasi, nasolabial fold, postauricular tumors, and sclerosing basal cell carcinomas no matter where they were situated.

TABLE 36–2. Cure Rate of 4845 Carcinomas of the Skin in 3576 Patients Subjected to Cryosurgery Between 1964 and 1984.[1]

Of the total number of patients (3576):[2]	Cure rate
125 recurrences (3.8%)	96.2%
Of the total 4845 combined carcinomas:	
125 recurrences (2.7%)	97.3%
Of the 125 recurrences: 40 (32%) were recurrent carcinomas.	

When recurrences were noted:
43.3% appeared during the first year.
24.3% appeared during the second year.
<u>19.0%</u> appeared during the third year.

86.6% of all carcinomas demonstrating recurrences were observed within the first 3 years.

[1]From Zacarian SA: Cryosurgery for Skin Cancer and Cutaneous Disorders. St. Louis, C. V. Mosby Co, 1985. Courtesy of C. V. Mosby Company.

[2]165 patients have died or have been lost to follow up (error of correction: 0.03%).

The average dermatologist sees carcinomas quite early in their inception. For the most part, they are less than 2.0 cm in size and amenable to cryosurgery. For large tumors, one can combine curettage and electrodesiccation followed by cryosurgery for a higher yield of cure. Cryosurgery also offers a predictable safety in freezing recurrent tumors following radiotherapy without fear of delayed wound healing. In the hands of an experienced clinician who understands the principles of cryogenic surgery and its techniques and who will monitor the large tumors in critical sites, this modality offers the cancer therapist another tool to combat man's most common malignancy.

REFERENCES

1. White AC: Liquid air in medicine and surgery. Med Rec 56:109, 1899
2. Whitehouse HH: Liquid air in dermatology: Its indications and limitations. JAMA 49:371, 1907
3. White AC: Possibilities of liquid air to the physician. JAMA 36:426, 1901
4. Irvine HG, Turnacliff DD: Liquid air in dermatology. Arch Dermatol (Suppl) 19:47, 1929
5. Allington HV: Liquid nitrogen in the treatment of skin diseases. Calif Med 72:153, 1950
6. Cooper IS: Cryogenic surgery of basal ganglia. JAMA 181:600, 1962
7. Cooper IS: Cryogenic surgery for cancer. Fed Proc 24:S237, 1965
8. Cahan WG: Cryosurgery of malignant and benign tumors by freezing. Cryobiology 2:24, 1965
9. Gage AA, Emmings F: Treatment of human tumors by freezing. Cryobiology 2:24, 1965
10. Zacarian SA, Adham MI: Cryotherapy of cutaneous malignancy. Cryobiology 2:212, 1966
11. Torre D: New York, cradle of cryosurgery. NY State J Med 67:465, 1967.
12. Zacarian SA: Cryosurgery in dermatology. Int Surg 47(6):528, 1967
13. Zacarian SA: The cryogenic approach to treatment of lid tumors. Ann Ophthalmol 701–713, 1970
14. Brodthagen H: Local freezing of the skin by carbon dioxide snow. Acta Derma Venerol (Suppl) (Stockholm) 41(44):9, 1961
15. Zacarian SA, Adham MI: Cryogenic temperature studies of human skin. J Invest Derm 48:7, 1967
16. Meryman HT: Mechanics of freezing in living cells and tissue. Science 124:515, 1956
17. Meryman HT (ed): Cryobiology. New York, Academic Press, 1966
18. Lovelock JE: The denaturation of lipidprotein complexes as a cause of damage by freezing. Proc R Soc Med 147:427, 1957
19. Mazur F: Physical and chemical basis of injury in single celled micro-organisms subjected to freezing and thawing, in Meryman HT (ed): Cryobiology. New York, Academic Press, 1966
20. Kreyberg L: Local freezing. Proc R Soc Med 147:546, 1957
21. Kreyberg L: Stasis and necrosis. Scand J Clin Lab Invest 15(71):1, 1963
22. Zacarian SA, Stone D, Clater M: Effects of cryogenic temperature on microcirculation in the golden hamster cheek pouch. Cryobiology 7(1):27, 1970
23. Grimmett RH: Liquid nitrogen therapy: Histologic observations. Arch Dermatol 83:563, 1961

24. Zacarian SA: Cryosurgery of Skin Cancer (Chapter 9). Springfield, Ill, Charles C Thomas Publishers, 1969

25. Zacarian SA: Cryosurgery of Tumors of the Skin and Oral Cavity (Chapter 1). Springfield, Ill, Charles C Thomas Publishers, 1973

26. Torre D: Understanding the relationship between lateral spread of freeze and depth of freeze. J Dermatol Surg Oncol 5:51–54, 1979

27. Zacarian SA: Is lateral spread of freeze a valid guide to depth of freeze? J Dermatol Surg Oncol 4:561–563, 1978

28. Stone D, Zacarian SA, Peri DC: Comparative studies of mammalian normal and cancer cells subjected to cryogenic temperatures in vitro. Cryosurgery 2(1):43, 1969

29. LePivert PJ, Binder P, Ougiert T: Measurement of intratissular bio-electric low frequency impedance. A new method to predict preoperatively the destructive effect of cryosurgery. Cryobiology 14:245–250, 1977

30. Savic M, Zacarian SA: A new impedance-based method for controlled cryosurgery of malignant tumors. J Dermatol Surg Oncol 3:592–593, 1977

31. Zacarian SA: Cryosurgery for head and neck tumors. Comprehensive Therapy 5(2):48–54, Feb 1979

32. Gage AA: An experimental study of the correlation of electrical impedance and temperature of tissue. J Dermatol Surg Oncol 4:445–450, 1978

33. Torre D: Scientific exhibit, American Academy of Dermatology, San Francisco, 1978, and presentation of a paper on electric circuitry at the Second Annual Meeting of the American College of Cryosurgery, Grand Island, NY, June 1979

34. Gage AA: What temperature is lethal for cells? J Dermat Surg Oncol 5(6):459–460, 1979

35. Dawber RPR, Wilkinson DD: Melanotic freckle of Hutchinson: Treatment of macular and nodular phases with cryotherapy. Br J Dermatol 101:47–49, 1979

36. Zacarian SA: Cryosurgery for Skin Cancer and Cutaneous Disorders (Chapter 10). St. Louis, CV Mosby Co, 1985, pp 199–214

37. Fraunfelder FT: Cryosurgery of eyelid, conjunctiva, and intraocular tumors, in Zacarian SA (ed): Cryosurgery for Skin Cancer and Cutaneous Disorders. St. Louis, CV Mosby Co, 1985, pp 259–282

38. Zacarian SA: Cryosurgery for Skin Cancer and Cutaneous Disorders (Chapter 7). St. Louis, CV Mosby Co, 1985, pp 132–133

39. Zacarian SA: Cryosurgery for Skin Cancer and Cutaneous Disorders (Chapter 15). St. Louis, CV Mosby Co, 1985, pp 283–297

40. Zacarian SA: Cryosurgery for Skin Cancer and Cutaneous Disorders (Chapter 7). St. Louis, CV Mosby Co, 1985, pp 156–157

37

ANDREW A. GAGE, M.D.

Probe Cryosurgery

Cryosurgery is a method of producing tissue necrosis by freezing. For many years, its use was limited to the treatment of minor skin lesions by direct topical application of carbon dioxide snow or liquid nitrogen. As early as 1899, A. Campbell White[1] used liquid air as a spray or by swab dipped into the fluid to treat a variety of skin diseases, including lupus erythematosus, verrucae, and nevi. Additional experience with liquid air, including the treatment of skin cancer, was described by Whitehouse[2] in 1907. In the same year, Pusey[3] reported similar varied uses of solidified carbon dioxide, which was easier to handle and more easily obtained than liquified gases.

In 1950, liquid nitrogen was introduced into dermatologic practice by Allington[4] and thereafter slowly gained in clinical use as production for research and industrial purposes increased its availability. Still, cryosurgery remained a rather unimportant therapeutic modality because the freezing capability of cryogenic agents applied topically was limited. Depth of freezing was no more than 2 mm with liquid nitrogen, and solid carbon dioxide was even less effective.[5,6] This was scarcely the thickness of normal skin and explains why freezing in this manner was adequate for only superficial conditions. Wider applicability of cryosurgery was made possible by the development of apparatus that permitted continuous and rapid extraction of heat from tissues so that a large amount of tissue could be destroyed by freezing. As a result, the method acquired new importance and became established as an effective method of treatment for diverse conditions.

FREEZING WITH CRYOSURGICAL INSTRUMENTS

Renewed interest in the therapeutic potential of freezing followed the development of the cryosurgical apparatus by Cooper.[7] Originally designed to create a cryogenic lesion in the brain for the correction of Parkinsonism and other neuromuscular disorders, it was later modified for use as a means of achieving controlled destruction of tissue in other areas of the body. This stimulated the development of other types of cryosurgical apparatus using liquid nitrogen and other cryogenic agents as techniques of freezing were adapted to the problems of treating disease. Equipment now varies from simple and inexpensive hand-held devices to automated apparatus with probe heaters (Fig. 37–1). Choice between these should be made with some knowledge of the freezing capabilities of the instruments.

The cryogenic agents employed commonly in cryosurgical apparatus are liquid nitrogen, carbon dioxide, halogenated hydrocarbons (Freon), and nitrous oxide, all of which are nonexplosive gases in the normal state. The coldest agent is liquid nitrogen, which has a boiling point of about $-196°C$ at atmospheric pressure. It has the greatest freezing capability and is the best agent for destruction of large volumes of tissue, as is required in the treatment of cancer. The other cryogens are useful for less serious lesions, such as inflammatory or benign neoplastic disease, for which lesser degrees of freezing will suffice. The lowest attainable freezing temperatures with these agents follow: solidified carbon dioxide, $-78.5°C$; Freon 22, $-40°C$ (may produce temperatures as cold as $-70°C$); and liquid nitrous oxide, $-89°C$.[8] Although these cryogens lack the excellent freezing capability of liquid nitrogen, they are used in easily handled apparatus with rapid response time in comparison to some apparatus using liquid nitrogen. Additional information regarding the characteristics of cryogenic agents and the principles involved in the construction and operation of cryosurgical instruments may be found in general reference books on cryosurgery.

Choice of equipment depends upon the size and nature of the lesion being treated. Usually inflammatory lesions do not require deep freezing and hence may be treated with apparatus employing any type of cryogenic agent. The treatment of skin tumors, especially cancers, requires extensive freezing for a margin of safety and therefore liquid nitrogen apparatus should be used. Most of these, including the hand-held units, can be used to spray liquid nitrogen directly on the lesion or used as closed systems with cryoprobes so that liquid nitrogen is not released directly on the tissue.

Details of cryosurgical techniques vary with the type of lesion. Malignant tumors must be treated more aggressively than benign tumors or inflammatory lesions. In addition, techniques for using cryoprobes are somewhat different from those using a cryogen spray. No matter which technique is used, careful application is essential to be certain that the desired result, a localized area of tissue necrosis, will be produced by freezing in situ. Whether spray

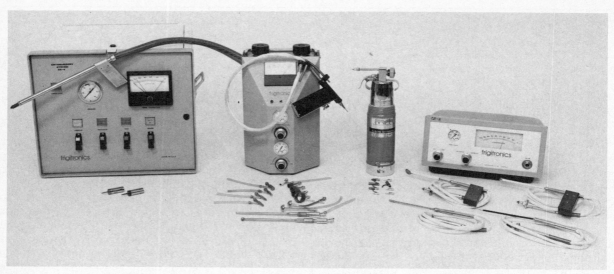

Figure 37–1. Different types of cryosurgical equipment: On the left is an apparatus cooled by liquid nitrogen with controls for preselection and automatic maintenance of freezing temperature. A flexible vacuum-insulated cable leads to the cryoprobe with a freezing surface at its tip. A thermocouple in the probe tip monitors its temperature, which is displayed on the console. The probe contains a heating element for quick removal after freezing. This apparatus is capable of extensive freezing of large skin cancers and has a wide range of uses, including freezing via endoscopy. The two pieces of equipment in the center are well suited to dermatologic practice. Both are cooled by liquid nitrogen and are satisfactory for the treatment of skin diseases in the office or clinic. Freezing may be done either with cryoprobes of various sizes or with an open spray of liquid nitrogen. A selection of assorted spray/probe devices are shown in front. On the right is shown an apparatus cooled by nitrous oxide, which is used in conjunction with probes of various sizes. It lacks the freezing capability needed for the treatment of invasive cancer but is satisfactory for other types of skin or mucosal diseases and for endoscopic use.

or probe is used, the basic features of technique are rapid freezing, slow thawing and, when thawing is complete, repetition of the freeze-thaw cycle. Holding the tissue in the frozen state for a few minutes will maximize the destructive effect.

CHOICE OF TECHNIQUE

The choice of technique is based in part on technical considerations in relation to the disease but also, in part, on personal preference because often either probe or spray, at least in skin cancer, will perform the task satisfactorily (Fig. 37–2). The advantage of a probe technique is that it produces a more predictable area of freezing and necrosis. The depth of freezing is related closely to the lateral spread of freezing from the probe. An additional advantage is the possibility of use of pressure on the probe, which increases the depth penetration of freezing because of compression of the tissue. Probe freezing is safer since the cryogen is not released on the tissues and therefore cannot run off into undesired areas and produce unwanted freezing. Probe freezing is necessary in endoscopic use.

The disadvantage of probe freezing is related to the fact that the probe becomes adherent to the tissue and careful attention must be given to avoid movement, because any fracture of the bond between tissue and probe will interfere with heat exchange and result in inadequate freezing. This bond is more difficult to achieve over dry or bony surfaces.

The advantage of the spray technique is that the cryogenic agent is used at its coldest possible temperature and that the spray can be moved freely about the lesion so freezing can be extensive and wide rather than deep. Therefore, the spray is superior to the probe in the treatment of extensive superficial inflammatory or benign lesions. The principal problem with the spray is that deep freezing is difficult to achieve. Prolonged use in one area results in troublesome run-off of liquid nitrogen from the tissue and undesired freezing of adjacent normal tissues may occur. The run-off develops after the surface tissues have been frozen so that vaporization of the liquid nitrogen no longer takes place quickly. This limits the ability of liquid nitrogen spray to achieve deep freezing quickly, especially since the spray does not compress tissue. Spray-limiting devices, such as open cones, are useful to control unwanted dispersion of the cryogen. The spray techniques may be used for large tumors, but ordinarily, the depth penetration of freezing by spray is too limited to use without first debulking the tumor by some surgical method.[9, 10]

FREEZING WITH CRYOPROBES

The manner of use is to apply the freezing surface of the cryoprobe to the lesion and allow liquid nitrogen to flow. The cold probe acts as a heat sink and produces tissue freezing by removing heat from the tissue faster than the blood supply restores it. A large thermal gradient is needed to freeze tissue to some distance, so the probe is used as cold as possible. As the temperature falls below zero, tissue quickly adheres to the probe and assumes a frosted appearance. Freezing is allowed to continue until the frosted appearance encompasses the entire lesion and, in the case of cancer, a margin of apparently normal tissue. Then the flow of liquid nitrogen is shut off and the probe is warmed for removal. The probe heater, if present, is used only to speed release from the tissue, which then is allowed to thaw without assistance.

No excision is performed except for a preliminary biopsy to establish the nature of the lesion. Treatments are performed with sterile equipment and technique. When no incision is made, there is little risk of infection, so sterility is not a critical matter. However, when there is an open wound, e.g., an ulcerating cancer, the usual precautions regarding sterile technique are necessary.

Cryoprobes may be either applied to the surface of a lesion or inserted into the tissues to be frozen. Surface freezing, with slight pressure on the probe to increase tissue-probe contact and increase depth of freezing, is used much more commonly. This technique, as compared with insertion of the probe into the tissue, has the advantages that no wound is caused, little or no bleeding occurs, the need for

anesthesia is lessened, and the danger of dissemination of tumor cells is minimized. On the other hand, some large bulky tumors are penetrated rather easily, and insertion of a pointed probe into the tissue increases efficiency of freezing because of greater contact with the freezing surface. The probe must be positioned carefully because when freezing starts, it can no longer be moved. Freezing is done as rapidly as possible. Tissue is frozen in increasing volume as heat is extracted, but the rate of extension of freezing slows as conditions at the periphery approach equilibrium between heat loss to the probe and heat supply by the circulation.

The amount of tissue frozen in a single application of the probe is related to the temperature of the probe, the area of contact between probe and tissue, the duration of freezing, and the blood supply to the tissue. It also depends on the quality of contact, because any fracture of the bond between probe and tissue interferes with heat exchange and insufficient freezing is almost certain (this is a major technical point in probe freezing). In freezing firm tissue or dry surfaces such as skin or tissue over bone, the probe contact is improved by the use of sterile lubricating jelly about the tip to serve as a conducting medium for heat transfer.

The shape of the frozen area depends on the area of contact between probe and tissue as well as the blood supply to the area and the pressure used in application. Small circular probes produce roughly hemispherical lesions. A larger probe, obtained by

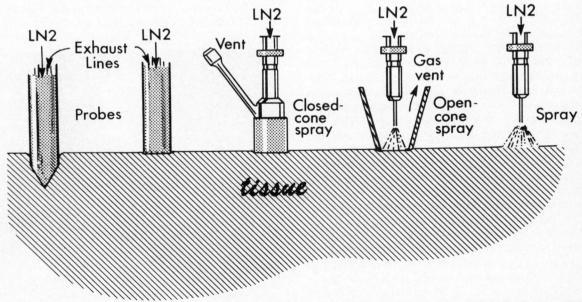

Figure 37–2. Diagram showing the differences and similarities in probe, closed-cone, open-cone, and spray devices. The two probes shown on the left are closed systems. During freezing the liquid nitrogen after change of phase is vented somewhere along the return line, perhaps even in the console. The pointed probe may be inserted in the tissue to achieve deeper freezing, but more commonly, surface freezing techniques are used. In both of the cone structures, the effect is to create an open probe (with some restriction of venting in the closed cone). The heat exchange surface is on the skin, instead of having metal interposed, and the venting is at the side or top of the device. When cooled, the walls of the cone act as a circular probe. The open spray has nothing to confine dispersion.

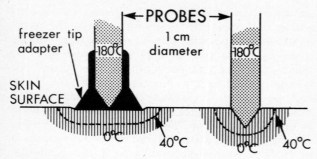

Figure 37–3. Diagram shows the effect of probe shape and area on the shape of the frozen tissue. In each instance the standard 1 cm probe, bluntly pointed, is shown. When used alone as on the right with some pressure on the probe to cause indentation of the skin or other tissues, the frozen area is roughly hemispheric. When the freeze tip adapter is added to provide a wider freezing surface, the resulting area is broadened and less deep at a similar stage in freezing.

adding an end adapter to the probe tip, will give a broader area with less penetration (Fig. 37–3). In general, the depth of freezing may be judged by the lateral spread of frost from the probe, and this is used as a guide in treatment.[11, 12]

Probe Techniques for Small Skin Cancers

Most skin cancers are small, less than 2 cm in diameter, and are well suited to a probe technique using a probe with a freezing surface as close as possible to the size of the cancer. The border of the cancer is outlined with skin-marking ink because the spread of the frosted appearance during treatment obscures easy determination of its extent. A second circle is marked 5 mm outside of the cancer border. A local anesthetic agent is injected beneath the tumor, which diminishes the blood supply to some extent and facilitates freezing. This fluid injection can be used to protect underlying structures such as cartilage or nerves from freezing by increasing the distance between the underlying structure and the carcinoma. Freezing is continued until the frost has spread to the outer circle. After thawing, the freezing is repeated. This is an effective conservative technique without thermocouples.

The use of thermocouples to monitor tissue temperature permits better control of treatment. Thermocouples may be used in several ways. For temperature beneath the tumor, the thermocouple is inserted through normal tissue a few millimeters outside of the cancer and passed through a subcutaneous position beneath its center. Freezing is accomplished until this thermocouple registers −40°C. Care is taken to freeze 5 mm beyond the border of the cancer at the skin surface. After thawing, treatment is repeated (Fig. 37–4).

An alternate technique of thermocouple usage is to place the thermocouple peripheral to the margin

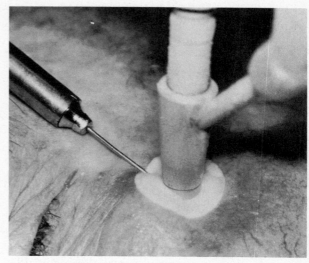

Figure 37–4. Basal cell carcinoma of the face below and lateral to the left eye being treated by freezing with liquid nitrogen. The probe (1 cm in diameter) is the same size as the surface of the cancer. The thermocouple is placed in a subcutaneous position beneath the cancer and freezing is continued until this thermocouple shows −40°C. The border of the frozen zone is 5 mm away from the edge of the probe. When both conditions (temperature and distance) are met, the tissue is allowed to thaw. Immediate repetition of the freeze-thaw cycle completes the treatment.

of the cancer. Since skin cancers tend to grow at their borders in the skin, the measurement of temperature at the border site is advantageous. In this technique, one or more thermocouples are inserted perpendicularly 2 to 3 mm deep into the skin, 5 mm from the margin of the cancer (Figs. 37–5 and 37–6).

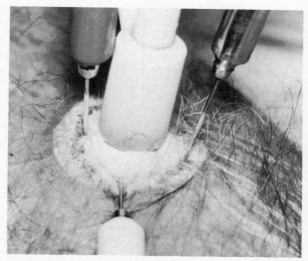

Figure 37–5. Basal cell epithelioma of the hand being frozen. Three thermocouples are used: One records surface temperature while the other two are inserted at the line drawn 5 mm lateral to the probe with the goal of achieving a temperature of −40°C at these sites. The frozen zone border is about another 5 mm lateral. This technique gives more extensive freezing than the alternate technique shown in Figure 37–4.

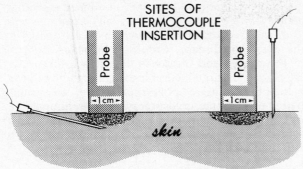

SITES OF
THERMOCOUPLE
INSERTION

Probe   Probe

|←1cm→| |←1cm→|

skin

Thermocouple is 5mm deep   Thermocouple is 3mm deep
and beneath the cancer   and 5mm from cancer

Figure 37–6. Typical sites and two useful methods of thermocouple insertion are shown. Either will yield satisfactory results when performed by an experienced practitioner. On the left is a thermocouple inserted at an angle from the side of the lesion through normal tissue. The thermocouple tip rests directly beneath the tumor at a depth of 5 mm. This thermocouple confirms the temperature at the depth of the tissue in the center of the lesion and is probably the most common method in skin cancer. On the right is an alternative method in which the thermocouple is inserted 5 mm from the border of the tumor, and 3 mm deep. The temperature registered at this thermocouple is interpreted as being the same temperature at the depth of the tissue beneath the tumor. This method assumes that the depth of freezing is approximately the same as the lateral spread of freezing from the probe. The advantage of this technique, the author believes, is that the thermocouple remains outside of the frozen area until the advancing ice front incorporates it so that it is relatively free of the error of conduction, which occurs with improper thermocouple usage. More than one thermocouple may be used, of course, and these two techniques may be used jointly.

When used in this way, assuming that the lateral spread of frost from the probe is about the same as the depth penetration of freezing, the temperature measured at the 5 mm border site should be the same as the 5 mm depth measurement. As the advancing edge of the frost comes to the thermocouple site, the temperature always measures zero. Freezing is continued until the border temperature

measures −40°C (Fig. 37–7). At that time, all cancer tissue is −50°C or colder. After thawing, freezing is repeated.

The difference among these techniques for small skin cancers is related to the extent of freezing. When the frost extends only to the 5 mm outer circle, the temperature at the circle is zero. This is conservative freezing, and the cosmetic result after healing will likely be favorable. However, when a thermocouple is used at the 5 mm outer circle to insure that a temperature of −40°C is reached, the frozen border is about 5 mm outside the outer circle. This is more extensive freezing and will destroy more tissue, increasing the chance for cure but at the cost of a favorable cosmetic effect.

A Probe Technique for Large Skin Cancers

Skin cancers 3 cm or larger in surface or diameter are ordinarily too large to be frozen in a single application of the probe. When multiple sites of application are necessary, freezing is continued at each site until the frozen border no longer advances, which is determined by observation and confirmed by the placement of thermocouples for temperature measurement about 2 cm from the edge of the probe. A near equilibrium of heat loss to heat gain usually occurs after five to seven minutes of freezing, and then the advance of the frozen border slows sufficiently so that it is best to discontinue freezing and move the probe to another site. Frozen zones are overlapped to insure that no area will be missed.

Bulky advanced cancers may be too large for treatment by cryosurgery alone, especially if the bulk of the tumor is more than 2 cm deep. If the cancer is soft, increased depth penetration can be achieved by inserting the probe into the tissue, but ordinarily, a better technique is to partially remove the cancer by excision with a scalpel or with curettage and electrocoagulation and then to treat the

Figure 37–7. Continuous temperature record of double freeze-thaw cycle produced during the cryosurgical treatment of a small basal cell epithelioma with the probe technique. The tissue temperature was recorded from a thermocouple placed 5 mm lateral to the border of the cancer, as shown in Figure 37–6. The freezing rate measured along the steepest part of the cooling curve was approximately 120°C per minute. Freezing was continued until the tissue temperature reached −40°C, then was held at this temperature for about a minute, then was allowed to warm above freezing. The second freeze-thaw cycle was similar.

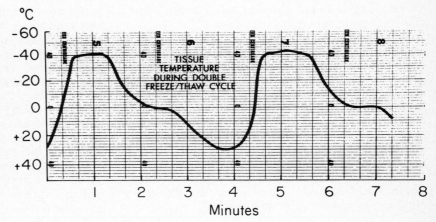

°C

TISSUE
TEMPERATURE
DURING DOUBLE
FREEZE/THAW CYCLE

Minutes

base of the tumor by freezing. This technique is especially useful when the tumor is based on underlying bone, because the effect of freezing extends into the bone and devitalizes any tumor that may be left. In such cancers, there often is some question about the adequacy of treatment, especially if cure of the cancer is the goal of treatment. The large open wound is observed carefully, and the need for repetition of treatment is judged by progress in healing. A biopsy is performed on any area slow to heal to detect persistent disease at the earliest possible moment. If persistent cancer is found, then cryosurgical treatment is repeated or an alternative treatment method is chosen.

FREEZING WITH LIQUID NITROGEN SPRAY

Spray techniques for diverse skin diseases are varied according to the type of disease. The technique required for the treatment of acne is different than that used for basal cell carcinoma. This section considers only the treatment of skin cancer.

Several techniques may be used for basal or squamous cell carcinomas.[13-16] One technique is simply an open spray of liquid nitrogen. After preliminary biopsy has established the nature of the disease, the margins of the tumor are marked with ink. A second marking is made 5 mm outside of the tumor margin, and a local anesthetic agent is injected. A thermocouple is placed beneath the tumor in the manner already described, and the liquid nitrogen spray is directed intermittently over the entire tumor until the temperature reaches −40°C. The spray pattern is planned to produce equal freezing in the entire area, including the 5 mm margin of normal tissue around the cancer. After thawing, the freeze-thaw cycle is repeated. During treatment, care must be taken to avoid nitrogen gas insufflation of subcutaneous tissues, which might occur if the spray is directed into an open wound, especially in the loose tissues about the eye. Ordinarily, insufflation will cause no problem, but fatal gas embolism has been described in dogs.[17] More likely is the possibility of infection, since liquid nitrogen may contain *Staphylococcus albus* and other organisms.

The cone-spray technique uses a plastic cone to limit the run-off of liquid nitrogen during use of the spray. The effect might be described as an open probe. In this technique, the margins of the tumor are marked with ink, and a local anesthetic is injected. Then, a cone with an inner opening as large as the lesion is selected. The contact edge is moistened and pressed firmly with the tumor in the opening. Liquid nitrogen is sprayed into the cone until a white rim of freezing spreads around its base and over an adequate margin of normal tissue. Thermocouples may be used to control this treatment in the manner already described.

Spray techniques may be combined advantageously with curettage. In basal cell carcinomas with ill-defined edges, the curettage aids in identifying the extent of disease. Curettage removes the bulk of the cancer and improves the chance of cure by cryosurgery. Large incurable cancers can be reduced in size by extensive spray-freezing, but it is usually better to combine cryosurgery with preliminary removal of the tumor using electrocoagulation. Cryosurgery is then used to treat residual disease and to maintain control.

USE OF THERMOCOUPLES AND OTHER MONITORING TECHNIQUES

Clinical judgment is the prime factor in controlling the volume of tissue freezing in cryosurgery and is paramount in determining the extent of disease and in deciding when sufficient tissue has been frozen. In non-neoplastic disease or in benign tumors, the margin of safety is great, and clinical judgment alone is adequate to control the treatment. Even in the treatment of cancer, those therapists with considerable experience in cryosurgery can achieve satisfactory results without the use of monitoring techniques. Observation and palpation of the frozen area are the determinants of judgment of the extent of freezing. Inferences about the depth of freezing are made by surface observations and supported by palpation. Fixation of frozen tissue to underlying bone or cartilage are important aids. Judgment about the depth of freezing is the major problem. To supply clinical judgment, methods of monitoring therapy have become important.[18]

The measurement of tissue temperature during the cryosurgical procedure is a method of controlling treatment, and its routine use should standardize methods of treatment and improve clinical results. The measurement is done by the use of needle-mounted thermocouples inserted into the tissue at the borders of the diseased tissue. The temperature is read on a pyrometer or other appropriate device. The measurement is used to supplement clinical judgment—an important consideration because the temperature of frozen tissue cannot be judged from its appearance and the use of thermocouples often leads to a longer treatment period. Especially in the treatment of cancer, it is of critical importance to know that temperatures lethal to cells are produced in the tissue. Under cryosurgical conditions, temperatures colder than −30°C must be achieved in order to be certain of cell death.[19] In the treatment of skin cancers, temperatures in the −20 to −30°C range at the borders of the lesions will produce severe tissue damage but are inadequate for safety. A better goal from the viewpoint of cure (though not in cosmetic effect) is a temperature of −40°C in normal tissue 5 mm lateral to the border of the skin cancer. This means that temperatures of −50°C or colder are achieved in the cancer.

Another method of quantification of cryogenic injury features the measurement of impedance to the passage of a small electric current in tissues during freezing.[20–24] The formation of ice crystals in tissue results in decreased electrical conductivity as water is removed from solution. Adequate freezing during cryosurgery is signalled by the rise in electrical impedance to high levels or the fall in current flow to negligible levels when all freezable water is crystallized. At this time, presumably all cells will be irreversibly damaged and would die. These alternative techniques of quantification can be used to predict tissue necrosis. Equipment to measure tissue resistance is still in evolution but has not been approved yet by the Federal Drug Administration for general use.

EFFECT OF FREEZING ON TISSUE

All types of cells are devitalized by freezing. The mechanism of injury is related to crystallization of water, solute concentration in the cells, and irreversible changes in cell membranes.[25] Cells containing ice crystals are considered damaged beyond the likelihood of survival. Damage from direct cellular injury is enhanced by the effect of freezing on the circulation. After freezing and thawing, the involved area becomes congested, effective circulation through small vessel ceases, hypoxic cells die, and necrosis follows. Many of these effects are well known from studies of frostbite in which the relative importance of direct cellular injury and vascular stasis have long been debated. In cryosurgery, microcirculatory failure is a major factor in cell dath. Although there are some differences in the sensitivity of different types of cells to freezing, the loss of blood supply deprives all cells in frozen tissues of any possibility of survival.

The mechanisms of tissue injury from freezing have considerable bearing on the technique of cryosurgery. Rapid freezing, promoted by good tissue contact with a cold probe, forms the more lethal intracellular ice. To maximize injury, the tissue should be kept in the frozen state for about three minutes. Slow tissue thawing is important to the lethal effect.[26] Tissues are allowed to thaw without assistance because prolonged phase transition (ice to water in thawing) increases cellular death. The time in phase transition is also increased by repetition of freezing immediately after thawing. When this is done, the critical temperature for cell death is altered, and necrosis almost always corresponds closely to the frozen area. A borderline of surviving cells remains just inside the edge of the frozen area.

The cryogenic lesion is characterized by sharply circumscribed necrosis. As thawing takes place, the previously frozen area becomes swollen and discolored because of congestion and slight perivascular hemorrhage. At the periphery of the dark red area, corresponding to the border of the previously frozen tissue, a narrow bright red zone due to hyperemia appears. Further evidence of injury develops slowly. The extent of damage depends upon the severity of freezing. If only the skin is frozen, as for benign superficial lesions, then the response will range from inflammatory reaction to superficial necrosis. The more extensive freezing required by large tumors is followed by greater destruction of tissue, and sharply demarcated necrosis becomes apparent in two ways. In the skin, an eschar forms, and two or more weeks may be required for separation. The time required for slough of the necrotic tissue depends in part upon its stroma. Cellular tissue sloughs quickly, but skin and other tissues with large quantities of fibrous stroma resists structural change, and the necrotic tissue requires many days for separation.

The effect of freezing on bone is pertinent. Experiments have shown that bone devitalized in situ by freezing is slowly resorbed and simultaneously replaced with new bone, a lengthy healing process similar to that which occurs with autogenous bone grafts.[27] During repair, the devitalized bone maintains form and continues function. Similar observations have been made on bone frozen in clinical cryosurgery, especially in the oral cavity.[28] Sequestration has been uncommon, even though healing required many months. Bone healing has been excellent with only slight loss of substance from resorption. This favorable response has permitted extensive freezing of bone in oral cancer in order to avoid excision. In skin cancer, it is of importance in the management of basal cell epitheliomas and other cancers growing next to bone and invading the foramina or eroding bone structure.[29, 30]

POSTOPERATIVE CARE AND COMPLICATIONS

Ordinarily, there is little pain after cryosurgical procedures. Some patients complain of burning sensations during thawing and even after. Freezing lesions about the forehead can sometimes be associated with a head pain, but severe pain is rare.

Care of the wound after freezing is similar to that provided for hot thermal injury. Edema forms soon after thawing and is especially severe on the face. Freezing of small skin cancers on the face is often associated with extensive edema, which usually lasts for a few days but may last for two weeks and cause considerable concern on the part of the patients. Before treatment patients should be informed of this occurrence. Reassurance is necessary during the postoperative period.

Weeping of serum from the cutaneous wound in the first week or two usually annoys patients and requires a small bandage, but then the wound dries and an eschar forms (Fig. 37–8). In the following days, the wound contracts and heals slowly but with an excellent cosmetic result.[31] Small wounds, such as those following treatment of basal cell epitheliomas 1–2 mm in diameter, may require a month for complete healing. During this time, when healing is advanced, the surface of the skin looks irregular and pseudoepitheliomatous but this response disappears without treatment. The wounds produced by extensive freezing for large cancers take longer to heal, but often, the final result is surprisingly good. With destruction of the full thickness of the skin, some scar formation must be expected. Hypertrophic scars are unusual. Secondary closure of extensive wounds should be delayed for several months to permit long-term observation for possible recurrences.

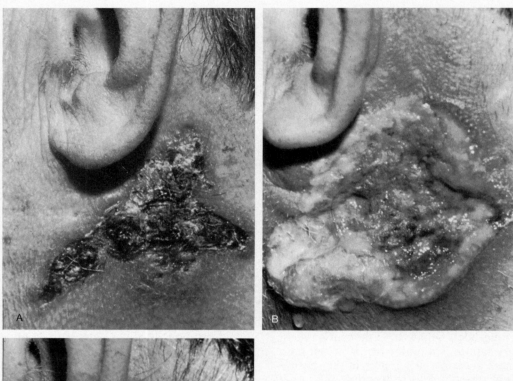

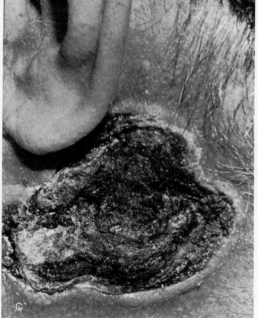

Figure 37–8. *A*, Basal cell carcinoma below and behind the left ear, which is of moderate size but still superficial and suitable for cryosurgery. Several successive applications of the probe were required to treat the entire area. *B*, Six days after freezing the previously frozen tissue has partially sloughed; serum is oozing from the wound. *C*, Three weeks after freezing an eschar has formed and the wound is contracting as part of the healing process. The eschar later separated, and the wound closed without need for operative intervention and healed with little scarring.

Most complications of cryosurgery are minor. Infection is unusual, but occasionally, the wound has an inflammatory response that extends beyond the area of cryogenic injury. Even less often, purulent fluid forms beneath the eschar, and surgical incision for drainage is required.[32] Hemorrhage during operation does not occur from cutaneous cryosurgery, and delayed bleeding, which may be associated with skin slough, is rare. Excessive scarring is infrequent but may follow excessive destruction of tissue or may be associated with uncommon conditions.[33]

Pigmentation of the skin may be altered by cryosurgery, and the patient should be informed in advance of treatment of this possibility. Melanocytes are very susceptible to freezing, and hypopigmentation of the skin may follow treatment. Repopulation with melanocytes occurs over several months and commonly restores natural skin tones. However, sometimes depigmentation is permanent; other times, excessive pigmentation may darken the skin.

An important potential complication is nerve damage. Neuropathy has been described after the treatment of digital warts.[34] Ulnar neuropathy followed freezing of a wart at the right elbow with cotton-swab application of liquid nitrogen.[35] Postauricular neuralgia has occurred after treatment of skin cancer close to the ear, and pain along the jaw has followed oral cryosurgery. Ordinarily, such symptoms subside in a few days. More disabling, but expected, was the facial nerve paralysis that followed extensive cryosurgery for cancer in the ear canal.[30] Long-term sensory losses have occurred from freezing lingual and inferior alveolar nerves during oral cryosurgery.[28] Nerves are as susceptible to freezing injury as any other tissue, but if continuity is not interrupted, a return of function is expected.

BENIGN LESIONS OF SKIN AND MUCOSA

Lesions that respond to topical application of liquid nitrogen via cotton swab are cured with greater certainty by the more efficient freezing possible via instrumentation. Verrucose and keratotic lesions, hemangiomas, and a variety of other benign lesions have been treated successfully.[15] Because of the simplicity of application and the infrequent need for anesthesia, freezing is the most convenient treatment for multiple seborrheic keratoses and for senile and other precancerous keratoses. Port-wine hemangiomas are resistant to treatment. Clinical use with benefit has been reported in the melanotic freckle and in junction nevi.[36–38] The effects of cryosurgery on keloids has been erratic, but reports of good results, which may include the intralesional injection of corticosteroids, merit continued trials.[15,]

[39, 40] Response of genital warts is sometimes good.[41] Tattoos are difficult to manage by cryosurgery if the foreign pigment is deep, but superficial tattoos may be treated successfully.[42, 43] Trichiasis has been treated effectively.[44] Rhinophyma and hyperhidrosis have responded to treatment.[45, 46] Pilonidal disease is treated simply by combined incision and freezing of the opened tract.[47] Pruritus ani has been managed successfully by this modality in some instances.[48]

Verrucae may be cured easily but sometimes persist after freezing, perhaps because the virus can survive extremely low temperatures. Failures are particularly likely to occur in plantar warts and periungual warts; nevertheless, these lesions may be treated with cryosurgery. For such small lesions, a pointed probe, somewhat smaller than the lesion, is applied to the center of the wart with sufficient pressure to indent the tissue and freezing is continued until the frosted appearance encompasses the wart and a small amount of normal tissue. After thawing, the wart is frozen again in the same way. No anesthesia is necessary if the patient is willing to tolerate the stinging sensation produced by freezing. Patient acceptance of this method is generally excellent, periungual wart therapy may be the exception because of pain. Spray and dip-stick techniques may also be used.[15]

Cryosurgery may be used to treat leukoplakia, papillary keratotic lesions, hemangiomas, mucoceles, and benign tumors of the oral cavity with excellent results. The only anesthesia needed is topical use of tetracaine (Pontocaine) or lidocaine infiltration. No excision is performed. The technique must be adjusted to fit the type of lesion. Treatment is usually given best with a cryoprobe of appropriate size that is cooled by liquid nitrogen. Excellent results are obtained in the treatment of hemangiomas of the buccal mucosa, tongue, or lip. Bleeding from these vascular lesions is avoided (Fig. 37–9). Benign tumors, even though large, respond well to freezing.[49] The element of risk is much less than in the treatment of cancer.

The most common lesion in this group is leukoplakia, a general clinical term that covers a variety of epithelial diseases, some of which are precancerous. The nature of the leukoplakia should be established by biopsy, since follow-up requirements are greater in dysplastic epithelial disease. Since the disease is superficial, cryosurgery for leukoplakia may be performed with nitrous oxide or liquid nitrogen. For small lesions, a cryoprobe is satisfactory. Commonly, leukoplakia occurs in wide patches over irregular surfaces, in which case using a spray of liquid nitrogen is better. In the oral cavity, the liquid nitrogen spray causes clouds of frozen water, which obscures vision. A high-volume vacuum is necessary to clear the field. In the posterior part of the oral cavity, the use of a probe is preferable. The results are generally good, but it must be remem-

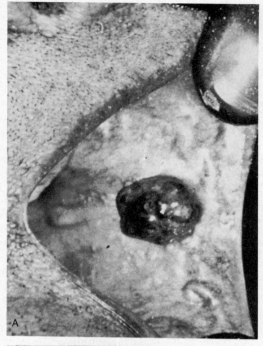

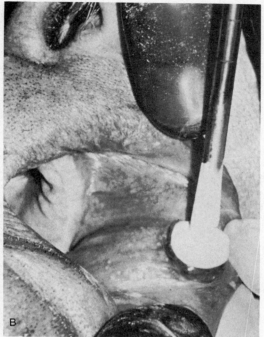

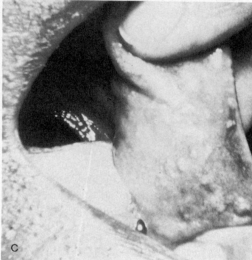

Figure 37–9. *A*, Hemangioma of the buccal mucosa; the diagnosis is obvious, so no biopsy is necessary or desirable. *B*, Hemangioma is frozen with 5 mm probe; no thermocouple is necessary in this type of lesion. *C*, Two months later the area is healed. (Reproduced with permission from F. Emmings, S. Koepf, and A. Gage: Cryotherapy for benign lesions of the oral cavity. Journal of Oral Surgery, 25: 320, 1967.)

bered that cryosurgery does not cure the underlying causes of leukoplakia, and unless these are corrected, new areas of disease may appear, especially with dysplastic disease.[49–52]

SKIN CANCER

The indications for the choice of cryosurgery in skin cancer are broad—almost all skin cancers are suitable for treatment with this technique. The histologic type of the cancer is not important to the choice of cryosurgery because there is no meaningful difference in the sensitivities of squamous cell and

basal cell carcinoma to freezing. From the treatment viewpoint, size, location, and extent of the tumor are more important than histologic type. Melanoma is also susceptible to freezing, but excision is preferable because the primary lesion is usually small. A preliminary biopsy is needed to establish the diagnosis, and in most melanomas, the biopsy is done by complete excision of the local growth.

Cryosurgery is widely used in the treatment of basal cell and squamous cell carcinomas. Some practitioners treat practically all basal cell cancers by cryosurgery. This is possible because most skin cancers are small (2 cm or less in surface diameter) and seldom extend beyond the skin surface more than 3 mm in depth. Since the cancer spreads at the margins rather than penetrates deeply, the disease is well within the destructive capabilities of cryosurgery. Freezing is capable of destroying small cancers easily with good cosmetic results and excellent cure rates.[16, 53, 54]

The special indications for cryosurgery are those skin cancers that present problems in treatment by excision. These include: (1) single small cancers of the head and neck, especially about the nose, eyes, and ears where surgical excision and closure is sometimes difficult, (2) multiple small superficial cancers, (3) cancers that arise in irradiated skin, (4) cancers that persist after radiotherapy or excision, (5) cancers that are located over bone, so that periosteal lymphatics may be infiltrated or the bone may be eroded by the growing cancer.

The use of cryosurgery for eyelid cancer has yielded excellent results in carefully chosen patients by practitioners experienced in the techniques.[55, 56] Eyelid cancer is difficult to treat by any method, and recognition of the problems in treatment is necessary. There is special reason for caution in the region of the medial canthus where deep infiltration of cancer may be unrecognized.[57]

Cancers arising in irradiated skin are often not large, but they are usually located in areas where tissue loss is costly, such as about the nose (Fig. 37–10). Freezing permits minimal tissue sacrifice in achieving a cure. Since new cancers may arise in the irradiated skin, conservative treatment acquires increased importance. The ability to repeat treatment, following the tumor growth wherever it becomes evident, is as useful in the treatment of small cancers in irradiated skin as it is in large rodent ulcers.

More difficult problems are infiltrating cancers that have resisted other methods of therapy and involve deep structures (especially bone) near the nose, eyes, and ears. Persistent cancer after radical excision or radiotherapy may still be treated with a chance for success by cryosurgery because the area is sharply localized and one can penetrate bony structures that cannot be easily excised. Some neglected extensive cancers originating on the external ear and invading the ear canal have responded very well (Fig. 37–11). In advanced cases, sometimes it is advisable to partially excise the tumor in order to facilitate freezing the deeper tissues. However, for patients with a high surgical risk, it may be preferable to perform no excision but to use freezing alone, repeating it every two or three weeks until all evidence of cancer is eliminated.

Relief of severe facial pain is an immediate benefit. Facial nerve paralysis occurs commonly after freezing lesions of the ear canal, but nerve function may return if nerve continuity is not interrupted. In general, the method of using cryosurgery for large cancers is to treat, observe, and re-treat if necessary, and to use biopsies to detect disease and to guide treatment. The wound is not closed, perhaps for months, to permit detection of persistent cancer at the earliest possible time.

Cryosurgery is useful for palliation of advanced cancer, such as bulky and ulcerating carcinoma or

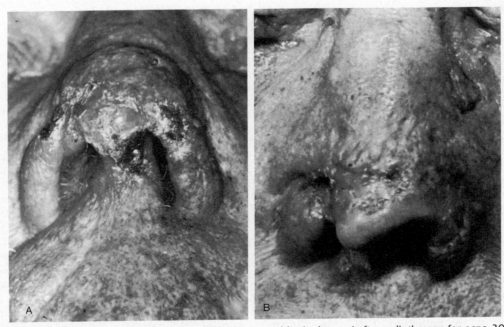

Figure 37–10. *A,* Squamous cell carcinoma in the nasal septum and both alae nasi after radiotherapy for acne 30 years ago. *B,* Three months after treatment the cancer-bearing area is healed with minimal tissue loss. There was no recurrence over years of observation.

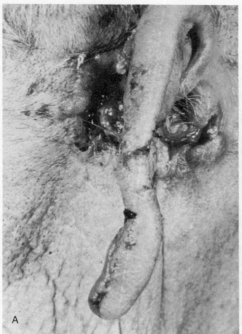
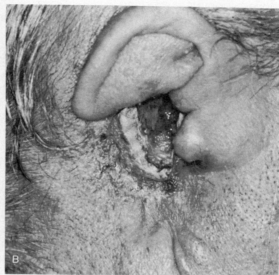

Figure 37–11. *A,* Basal cell carcinoma destroying the external ear and invading the face, neck, and ear canal. This was treated by partial excision (including mastoidectomy) and three cryosurgical treatments over a one month period. *B,* Six months later the wound is healing and no cancer is evident. (Reproduced with permission from A. Gage et al: Cancer cryotherapy. Military Medicine, 132:550, 1967.)

malignant melanomas eroding the face, neck, or other parts of the body. Tumor size is controlled, discomfort is relieved, and hemorrhage is prevented. However, except for pain relief, the palliation achieved is not impressive because invasion of the cancer continues, symptoms recur, and life is not prolonged. Treatment for ulcerating neck tumors must be given with care. Although it has been shown that normal large blood vessels are resistant to cryogenic injury and are not susceptible to rupture or thrombosis,[58] these findings do not apply when a devitalized artery is surrounded by a necrotic tumor. Under such conditions, hemorrhage is likely to result during the period of slough. Cancers treated for palliation grow again and require repetition of therapy every month or so. The author has not observed any clinical evidence of a cryoimmunologic response in such advanced cancers. In repeated treatments, only frozen tissue became necrotic, and any remote unfrozen tumor is not diminished.

ORAL CANCER

Cancer of the oral cavity is accessible to cryosurgery. This method of treatment may be considered in several situations. In some patients, cryosurgery may be used for the palliation of incurable cancer. In other patients, it may be used for the attempted salvage of patients who have residual localized ad-

vanced cancer after other methods of treatment have failed. Finally, it may be considered as a primary treatment for oral cancer when there is need for a safer or less disabling treatment than excision. The goal of treatment should be determined before treatment is begun.

Palliation of Advanced Oral Cancer

Cryosurgery provides palliation from advanced cancer by diminution in tumor bulk, desensitization of nerves, and reduction of malodorous secretions. Because radiotherapy offers substantial palliative benefits, patients should be chosen carefully for cryosurgery. The best indication for the use of cryosurgery is relief of pain. Some cancers, even though small, are painful, and extensive freezing desensitizes the nerve supply and provides comfort. In such patients, radiotherapy has commonly been administered in the past, but the exposed bone of the oral cavity becomes painful because of osteoradionecrosis. If the disease is still localized and still potentially curable, cryosurgical treatment provides a reasonable chance of benefit with low risk. Freezing with a cryoprobe is best. Surface contact freezing is used most often, but when the tumor is soft and bulky, the insertion of the cryoprobe into the tissue substantially increases the effectiveness of freezing. The technique is similar to that of freezing advanced skin cancer.

Problems in postoperative care are much greater than with the freezing of skin cancer because of interference with oral intake and respiration. Often, edema is sufficient to threaten the airway and to interfere with the swallowing of secretions. For these reasons, the freezing of large cancers in the posterior part of the oral cavity for palliative reasons is seldom advisable. In such cases, it is better to rely on radiotherapy. If cryosurgery is used, then a prophylactic tracheostomy should be established before freezing in order to protect the airway. Bulky tumors in the anterior part of the oral cavity do not require a tracheostomy, but still the edema may be troublesome for a few days.

Cancer Persistent After Excision or Radiotherapy

Sometimes, the amount of residual diseased tissue is small, still localized, and potentially curable. Commonly, both surgical excision and radiotherapy have been used so that further surgery is not possible and further radiotherapy is considered inadvisable. Such patients are reasonable candidates for cryosurgical treatment because the risk is small and the chance of benefit reasonably good, especially if pain is the predominant symptom. The cryoprobe technique is best suited to the treatment of such persistent cancers, and in well-chosen cases, the residual tumor can be destroyed and pain relieved. The occasional long-term survival of this type of patient is an indication of the usefulness of cryosurgery as a method of salvage when disease is persistent after other methods of treatment have been used.

Primary Treatment by Cryosurgery

Cryosurgery as a primary treatment for oral cancer should be considered in selected patients in whom conventional methods of treatment cannot be applied. The criteria for the selection of patients are: (1) The cancer is small to moderate in size, preferably without cervical lymphadenopathy, (2) the cancer is adjacent to bone so that excision would require removal of a portion of the mandible or the palate, and (3) the patient is a high surgical risk because of blood coagulopathy or severe cardiopulmonary disease.

The most attractive feature of cryosurgery for oral cancer is the possibility of avoiding a mutilating operation. Instead of resecting the mandible or palate, the neoplasm is frozen and excision is avoided (Fig. 37–12). The oral cancers ideal for cryosurgery are of small size and overlying bone such as the mandible, perhaps because the depth of cancer penetration is limited by the bone. For this reason, cryotherapy is the best choice for palatal tumors. The lethal effect of freezing penetrates the palatal bone destroying any tumor that is in the minute foramina, which traverse it. Small cancers of the anterior portion of the floor of the mouth or of the anterior two thirds of the tongue are also satisfactory because of easy accessibility to treatment. Those patients with large tumors on the floor of the mouth and the posterior part of the tongue, especially if they are already metastatic to cervical lymph nodes, should not be treated by cryosurgery unless necessitated by the general condition of the patient.

The technique for treatment is much the same as

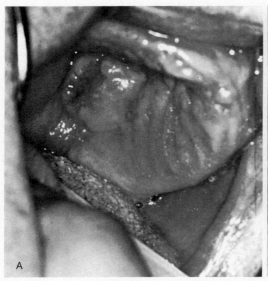 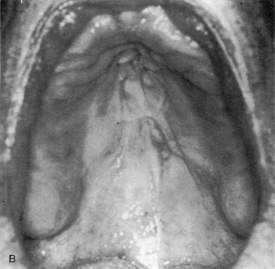

Figure 37–12. *A*, Adenocystic carcinoma of the palate. *B*, Three months after freezing healing is excellent and there is no evidence of the tumor. (Reproduced with permission from A. Gage et al: Cryotherapy for cancer of the lip and oral cavity. Cancer, 18:1646, 1965.)

already outlined, except that general anesthesia ordinarily is necessary for comfort and manipulation of the tumor. Special problems in postoperative care are related to the swelling that occurs in the oral cavity after freezing and to the mass of necrotic tissue that develops. Extensive freezing required by large oral cancers may cause problems in postoperative care related to deglutition and respiration. Careful attention to the airway is necessary, especially after freezing in the posterior part of the oral cavity. In the anterior part of the oral cavity, treatment is easy to give, but in the oropharyngeal region, vision is limited and treatment is more difficult. No excision is performed except for preliminary biopsy. After freezing, the tumor is allowed to slough, and the progress in healing is carefully observed. The need for repetition of treatment is determined as early as possible.

Five-year survival data for carefully selected patients are satisfactory, and the results are achieved with minimal risk and without sacrifice of bone.[28, 49]

COMPARISON WITH OTHER METHODS OF TREATMENT

Most benign and malignant skin lesions are managed easily by excision or electrosurgery. Most skin cancers can also be cured by surgical excision, which has the advantage that histologic examination of the excised tissue offers some evidence of the adequacy of treatment. For this reason, excision is the preferred treatment for single small lesions when excision and wound closure is simple, as is generally true for the trunk or extremities. Radiotherapy is equally suitable for most epitheliomas and has special application for those in areas difficult to treat by excision. Mohs' chemosurgery technique has yielded excellent results.

Cryosurgery must compete with these effective treatments and with other investigational techniques, such as lasers. Cryosurgery can cure small epitheliomas as surely as any other method of treatment. It is faster and easier to use than chemosurgery. It produces results faster than irradiation, and healing is much better because the blood supply peripheral to the lesion is preserved. Healing of soft tissue is more favorable after freezing than after electrocoagulation.[59] The advantages of cryosurgery include simplicity of use, little need for anesthesia, little bleeding, and few complications. Especially advantageous is the ability of freezing to penetrate bone, destroy any tumor that may be within it, and yet avoid the need for bone excision with its attendant deformity and disability. A specific immune response is stimulated by cryosurgery, and this has been shown to be of benefit in experimental tumor systems. Though clinical evidence of benefit is less clear, the potential use as a form of immunotherapy is an attractive feature that requires further investigation.[60, 61]

The principal disadvantages are that an entire specimen is not available for examination and that healing is slower than with excision and closure. The lack of a specimen is a circumstance shared by other methods of treatment, such as electrocoagulation and radiotherapy. In fact, only complete surgical excision produces a complete specimen for study. Slow healing is not entirely disadvantageous, since it provides time to study the open wound and is associated with favorable healing.

The chief limitation with cryosurgery, especially when dealing with cancer, is the difficulty of freezing sufficient tissue. The best presently available apparatus is hardly adequate for large cancers because such tissues are poor conductors of heat and are provided with a circulatory source of heat that limits the extension of freezing. The amount of tissue that can be frozen in a single application of a probe is small in comparison with the size of many cancers. Depth of freezing beyond 2 cm is difficult to achieve. Multiple applications of the probe, insertion of the probe into bulky tumors, and repetition of freezing at a later date are methods that compensate for the difficulties of freezing sufficient tissue, but these do not insure the capability of freezing large cancers. Inevitable advances in equipment design and improved techniques of freezing should eliminate some of these problems.

REFERENCES

1. White AC: Liquid air in medicine and surgery. Med Rec 56:109–112, 1899
2. Whitehouse HH: Liquid air in dermatology. JAMA, 49:371–377, 1907
3. Pusey WA: Use of carbon dioxide snow in the treatment of nevi and other skin lesions. JAMA 49:1354–1356, 1907
4. Allington HV: Liquid nitrogen in the treatment of skin diseases. Calif Med 72:153–155, 1950
5. Grimmet R: Liquid nitrogen therapy. Histologic observations. Arch Dermatol 83:563–567, 1961
6. Zacarian S, Adham M: Cryogenic temperature studies of human skin. Temperature recordings at two millimeter human skin depth following application with liquid nitrogen. Cryobiology 48:7–10, 1967
7. Cooper IS: A new method of destruction or extirpation of benign or malignant tumors. N Engl J Med 268:743–749, 1963
8. Torre D: Alternate cryogens for cryosurgery. J Dermatol Surg 1:56–58, 1975
9. Lubritz R: Advantages and disadvantages of cryosurgery and cryospray for malignancies, in Epstein E (ed): Controversies in Dermatology. Philadelphia, WB Saunders Co, 1984, pp 145–150
10. Gage A: Cryosurgery for skin disease: Variants in technique, in Epstein E (ed): Controversies in Dermatology. Philadelphia, WB Saunders Co, 1984, pp 151–161
11. Zacarian S: Is lateral spread of freeze a valid guide to depth of freeze? J Dermatol Surg Oncol 4:561–563, 1978
12. Torre D: Understanding the relationship between lateral spread of freeze and depth of freeze. J Dermatol Surg Oncol 5:51–53, 1979

13. Torre D, Lubritz R, Graham G: Cryosurgical treatment of basal cell carcinomas. Prog Dermatol 12:11–16, 1978

14. Spiller W, Spiller R: Treatment of basal cell carcinomas by a combination of curettage and cryosurgery. J Dermatol Surg Oncol 3:443–447, 1977

15. Kuflik E, Lubritz R, Torre D: Cryosurgery. Dermatologic Clinics 2:319–332, 1984

16. Zacarian S: Cryosurgery for skin cancer and cutaneous disorders. St. Louis, CV Mosby Co, 1985

17. Harvey HJ: Fatal air embolization associated with cryosurgery in two dogs. J Am Vet Med Assoc 173:175–176, 1978

18. Gage A, Caruana J, Garamy G: A comparison of instrument methods of monitoring freezing in cryosurgery. J Dermatol Surg Oncol 9:209–214, 1982

19. Gage A: What temperature is lethal for cells? J Dermatol Surg Oncol 5:459–460, 1979

20. Le Pivert P, Binder P, Ougier T: Measurement of intratissue bioelectrical low frequency impedance: A new method to detect preoperatively the destructive effect of cryosurgery. Cryobiology 14:245–250, 1977

21. Savic M, Zacarian S: A new impedance-based method for controlled cryosurgery of malignant tumors. J Dermatol Surg Oncol 3:592–593, 1977

22. Gage A: Correlation of electrical impedance and temperature in tissues during freezing. Cryobiology 16:55–62, 1979

23. Gage A, Caruana J: Current flow in skin frozen in experimental cryosurgery. Cryobiology 17:154–160, 1980

24. Gage A, Augustynowicz S, Montes M, Caruana J, Whalen D: Tissue impedance and temperature measurements in relation to necrosis in experimental cryosurgery. Cryobiology, 22:282–288, 1985

25. Farrant J, Walter C: The cryobiologic basis of cryosurgery. J Dermatol Surg Oncol 3:403–407, 1977

26. Gage A, Guest K, Montes M, Caruana J, Whalen D: Effect of varying freezing and thawing rates in experimental cryosurgery. Cryobiology, 22:175–182, 1985

27. Gage A, Greene GW, Neiders M, Emmings FG: Freezing bone without excision. An experimental study of bone-cell destruction and manner of regrowth in dogs. JAMA 196:770–774, 1966

28. Gage A: Five-year survival following cryosurgery for oral cancer. Arch Surg 111:990–994, 1976

29. Gage A: Cryosurgery for difficult problems in cutaneous cancer. Cutis 16:465–470, 1975

30. Gage A: Cryosurgery for cancer of the ear. J Dermatol Surg Oncol 3:417–421, 1977

31. Shepherd J, Dawber R: Wound healing and scarring after cryosurgery. Cryobiology 21:157–169, 1984

32. Greer K, Bishop G: Pyogenic granuloma as a complication of cryosurgery. Arch Dermatol 111:1536–1537, 1975

33. Stewart R, Graham G: A complication of cryosurgery in a patient with cryofibrinogenemia. J Dermatol Surg Oncol 4:743–744, 1978

34. Millns J, Fenske N, Pierce D: Neurologic Complications of Cryosurgery. J Dermatol Surg Oncol 6:207–209, 1980

35. Finelli PF: Ulnar neuropathy after liquid nitrogen cryotherapy. Arch Dermatol 111:1340–1342, 1975

36. Lorenc E, Woldridge W, Huewe D: The melanotic freckle of Hutchinson: Preliminary report. Cutis, 16:485–486, 1975

37. Graham G, Stewart R: Cryosurgery for unusual cutaneous neoplasms. J Dermatol Surg Oncol 3:437–442, 1977

38. Lindo S, Daniels F: Cryosurgery of the junction nevi. Cutis 16:492–496, 1975

39. Ceilley RI, Babin RW: The combined use of cryosurgery and intralesional injections of suspensions of fluorinated adrenocorticosteroids for reducing keloids and hypertrophic scars. J Dermatol Surg Oncol 5:54–56, 1979

40. Muti E, Ponzio E: Cryotherapy in the treatment of keloids. Ann Plast Surg 11:227–232, 1983

41. Ghosh AK: Cryosurgery of genital warts in cases in which podophyllin treatment failed or was contraindicated. Br J Vener Dis 53:49–53, 1977

42. Goldstein N, Penoff J, Price N, Ceilley R, et al: Techniques of removal of tattoos. J Dermatol Surg Oncol 5:901, 1979

43. Colver G, Dawber R: Tattoo removal using a liquid nitrogen cryospray. Clin Exp Dermatol 9:364–366, 1984

44. Fraunfelder FT, Petursson GJ: The use of liquid nitrogen cryospray for treatment of trichiasis. Ophthalmol Surg 20:42, 1979

45. Nolan JD: Cryosurgical treatment of rhinophyma. Case report. Plast Reconstr Surg 52:437–438, 1973

46. Ashby E: Cryosurgery for axillary hyperhidrosis. Br Med J 2:1173–1174, 1976

47. Gage A: Pilonidal disease—incision and cryocoagulation, in Ablin R (ed): Handbook of Cryosurgery. New York, Marcel Dekker, 1980, pp 257–365

48. Detrano S: Cryotherapy for chronic nonspecific pruritus ani. J Dermatol Surg Oncol 10:483–484, 1984

49. Gage A: Oral disease, in Ablin R (ed): Handbook of Cryosurgery. New York, Marcel Dekker, 1980, pp 233–256

50. Gongloff R, Gage A: Cryosurgical treatment of oral lesions: Report of cases. J Am Dent Assoc 106:47–51, 1983

51. Drouby H: Oral leukoplakia and cryotherapy. Br Dent J 155:124–125, 1983

52. Lubritz R, Smolewski S: Cryosurgery cure rate of premalignant leukoplakia of the lower lip. J Dermatol Surg Oncol 9:235–237, 1983

53. McIntosh G, Osborne D, Li A, Hobbs K: Basal cell carcinoma—a review of treatment results with special reference to cryosurgery. Postgrad Med J 59:698–701, 1983

54. Zacarian S: Cryosurgery for cutaneous carcinomas. An 18 year study of 3022 patients with 4228 carcinomas. J Am Acad Dermatol 9:947–956, 1983

55. Fraunfelder F, Zacarian S, Wingfield D, Limmer B: Results of cryotherapy for eyelid malignancies. Am J Ophthalmol 97:184–188, 1984

56. Liu D, Natiella J, Schaefer A, Gage A: Cryosurgical treatment of the eyelids and lacrimal drainage ducts of the Rhesus monkey. Course of injury and repair. Arch Ophthalmol 102:934–939, 1984

57. Anderson R: A warning on cryosurgery for eyelid malignancies. Arch Ophthalmol 96:1289–1290, 1978

58. Gage A, Fazekas G, Riley E: Freezing injury to large blood vessels in dogs. Surgery 61:748–754, 1967

59. Li AKC, Ehrlich HP, Trelstad RL, Koroly MJ, et al: Differences in healing of skin wounds by burn and freezing injury. Annals of Surgery 191:244–248, 1980

60. Neel HB: Cryosurgery for the treatment of cancer. Laryngoscope 90 (suppl 23): 1–48, 1980

61. Fazio M, Airoldi M, Negri L, Marchesa P, Gandolfo S: Specific immunological stimulation induced by cryosurgery in patients with squamous-cell carcinoma of the oral cavity. J Max-fac Surg 12:153–156, 1984

Special Location
of Diseases

PART

7

Eyelid Skin Surgery

The skin of the eyelids, one of the thinnest of the body, is separated from the underlying orbicular muscle by a layer of loose areolar tissue that is fat-free in all but very obese individuals. The orbital septum lies beneath the preseptal portion of the orbicular muscle. Under this lies the orbital fat, which is important in cosmetic blepharoplasty.

The skin of the lids is somewhat elastic, and its accordion-like conformation to the underlying structures allows for the movement necessary in opening and closing the eyelids. In older individuals, much of the elasticity is lost, and the lids become redundant, even to the point of overhanging the palpebral aperture and obstructing vision.

The eyelid skin contains many small hairs that are almost invisible to the naked eye. Near the lid margins, there are numerous coarse hairs, the lashes, which lie in three or four indefinite rows in any given cross section of the upper lid and are somewhat more sparse in the lower lid. The longer and coarser brow hairs overlie the superior orbital margin. The skin of the eyelid also contains both sweat and sebaceous glands that may become the sites of cysts or infections.

While the skin of the mobile eyelids is quite thin, that beyond the level of the orbital margins becomes thicker. Here, there is an abundance of subcutaneous fat.

There are horizontal creases in the skin of the lids that represent the level of the attachments of the upper and lower lid retractors to the underlying muscle septa.[1] The most constant of these is the upper lid crease, which usually lies at about the level of the upper tarsal border. The upper lid crease deepens on upgaze and disappears on downgaze or eyelid closure. In most individuals of Oriental extraction, the lid crease of the upper lid is either quite low or absent. The upper lid fold is formed by a double layer of skin overlying the principal crease.

Radiating from the lateral canthi, in all but young individuals, there are a varying number of "laugh lines" or "crow's feet" that deepen with age and are cosmetically troublesome to some.

SURGICAL CONSIDERATIONS

Placement of Incisions

When there is a choice, it is best to make incisions along wrinkle lines or creases. The resulting scars will be less noticeable. Incisions or closures made in other directions (necessary in some traumatic or tumor removal cases) form more evident scars; but these tend to fade with time, and "cross-wrinkle" closures are not necessarily bad.

Control of Bleeding

The blood supply of the eyelids is abundant. This is fortunate because it lessens the chance of post-operative infection (a rarity after eyelid surgery). However, the abundance of blood vessels in the area creates a surgical nuisance. Operative bleeding can usually be controlled by light cautery, pressure, and time. The local use of thrombin may be useful. Only very rarely are ties necessary.

Sutures

Unless there is undue tension, skin closure in the eyelid region can usually be done by skin suturing alone. If there is tension, subcutaneous traction sutures may be needed to lessen the width of the resulting scar. The skin can be closed with either fine silk or nylon. Silk is placed in either running or interrupted fashion. Nylon can be used in interrupted, simple running, or subcuticular serpentine-type placement. For small children, the author usually performs skin closures with 6-0 plain catgut in order to avoid the anesthesia or "strong-arming" necessary for the removal of nonabsorbable sutures. The author has not noted undue resultant scarring.

If there is but a small amount of tension on the skin edges, it is best to use closely-placed interrupted sutures with small bites and tight ties. These sutures will necrose the tissue within the loops and can often be wiped off with an applicator in four or five days. Minimal scarring results. If the sutures are tied loosely, there is a tendency for epithelial cysts to form in the suture tract, which requires "unroofing" and exteriorization for relief. Simple running or locked running sutures are good, but removal may create a problem in some instances.

Subcutaneous sutures for the lessening of tension on the skin closure are usually placed in interrupted fashion with the knots tied on the deep side. While plain or chromic catgut (4-0 to 6-0) has been used for many years with little or no trouble, there is a current trend toward the use of 4-0 or 5-0 Dexon and Vicryl, which are as good but not necessarily better.

Surface sutures should be removed fairly early (not longer than one week). Some wound separations are caused by unreasonably early suture removal. If sutures are to be removed in three or four days, **Steri-Strips** should be used to prevent the wound edges from separating.

Flaps

While upper eyelid skin defects can usually be closed by direct suturing and with little or no undermining, lower lid defects require some undermining in most instances. If additional skin is needed in lid repair, it can be furnished by advancement, transposition, rhomboid, rotation, or island flaps, by Z-plasty, X-plasty, YV-plasty, or VY-plasty, or perhaps by other plastic maneuvers.

Grafts

If there is a question about adequate skin being available for flaps, one should not hesitate to use free grafts. These are accepted well by the eyelids.

Split-thickness grafts take well but result in poor color and texture matches. They are used as a last resort or when infection cannot be controlled preoperatively. These grafts should be about 1½ or more times the size of the defect, because they tend to shrink and wrinkle as they heal.

Full-thickness grafts take almost as well as split-thickness grafts if there is a good vascular base and no infection. They shrink and wrinkle much less than split-thickness grafts and need to be only slightly larger than the defect. They can defy detection if properly chosen and placed.

Upper lid skin should be replaced by skin from the opposite upper lid, if available. If not, retro-auricular skin is the best substitute; however, it is thicker and less pliable than upper lid skin, and the cosmetic and functional result will not be as good. If an upper lid defect must be filled, and neither upper lid nor retroauricular skin is available, it is better to use split-thickness skin than to use supraclavicular or upper arm donor sites.

Lower lid skin is slightly thicker than upper lid skin and can best be replaced by a retroauricular graft. There are few instances when retroauricular skin is unavailable, but if this occurs, a graft taken from the upper lid immediately beneath the brow makes a good match. Supraclavicular and upper arm skin can be used in this area in a pinch, but the result is apt to leave much to be desired.

While the trend is away from the use of tarsorrhaphy following skin grafting to the lids, it does prevent graft shrinkage and leads to a better-appearing and better-functioning eyelid than a graft without tarsorrhaphy. There are instances when tarsorrhaphy will be inconvenient, and it is satisfactory to omit it. Early massage should be instituted if this is done.

Dressings

If simple closure without tension has been performed, dressings are not needed. If the surgery has been complex and it is desirable to reduce the mobility of the lid, an eye patch for two or three days will suffice. If flaps or grafts have been used, it is essential that the mobilized skin be held firmly against its new base, which requires some type of pressure dressing. This not only aids in nutrition of the flap or graft, but it helps to reduce postoperative bleeding and tissue swelling. The more complex the surgery, the more a pressure dressing is necessary.

Pressure can be applied over the closed eye by the application of two or three fluffed 4 by 4 inch gauze bandages held in place with two or three layers of firmly applied adhesive tape. Wraparound head dressings are usually not needed. If the surgeon feels that pressure is indicated, the first dressing should be left unchanged until the second or third postoperative day, then reapplied for three or four days longer.

A bolster of moistened cotton can be applied for pressure over a free graft. It is held firmly in place by tying some of the ends of the interrupted sutures used to secure the graft over it. This type of pressure is particularly useful when the eye must be left uncovered for the sake of vision or to enable one to instill medication, as in the case of glaucoma.

Massage

This simple and valuable postoperative maneuver has been badly neglected. Scars and grafts tend to contract as healing progresses. This can damage the final cosmetic and functional result of a well-performed surgical procedure. The fibrotic contraction of tissues can be prevented, or at least reduced, by massaging the area after surface healing has occurred. It is carried out for about five minutes several times daily. The skin can be protected with petrolatum or cocoa butter. When cutaneous and subcutaneous thickening can no longer be felt, the massage can be discontinued.

SURGICAL CONDITIONS AND THEIR TREATMENT

Congenital Defects

While congenital defects involving the deeper layers of the eyelids are common, those involving

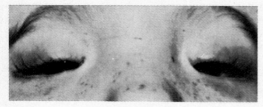

Figure 38–1. Epicanthal folds arising from lower lids in blepharophimosis syndrome. (Reproduced with permission from C. Beard: Ptosis. St. Louis, C. V. Mosby, 1969.)

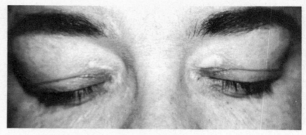

Figure 38–3. Xanthelasma of both upper lids extending to the medial canthi.

only the skin are rare. Those involving the deeper tissues will not be discussed in detail in this chapter.

Epicanthus. This fold of skin overlying the medial canthus may arise from the upper lid, the lower lid, or from both lids. It may be a normal part of an eyelid in Oriental people, in which case it arises from the upper lid. It may arise from the lower lid, in which case it is usually a part of the blepharophimosis syndrome, a dominant somatic hereditary condition characterized by ptosis, horizontal shortening of the palpebral fissure, telecanthus, lateral displacement of the lower puncta, ectropion of the lower lid, and epicanthus inversus (Fig. 38–1). It may arise from both lids, in which case it is a residual of the folds of fetal life (Fig. 38–2). In any of these types, it can be severe enough to cover the nasal sclera giving the patient the false appearance of having convergent strabismus.

Epicanthus arising from both lids is apt to become less marked as the bridge of the nose develops. If this improvement is insufficient, it can be relieved by double-Z-plasties[2] or by YV-plasties.[3]

If epicanthus arising from the upper lid is part of the normal eye in an Oriental, alteration is usually not requested. If it is, it can be flattened by Z-plasties, but the scar may take many months to fade.

Epicanthus inversus repair may be accomplished as part of the extensive surgery required for the blepharophimosis syndrome. It is usually combined with shortening of the medial canthal tendon for the purpose of lessening the telecanthus.

Congenital Ectropion. This is caused by a deficiency of lower lid skin and requires a skin graft, as previously discussed, for relief.

Metabolic Lesions

Xanthelasma. Soft yellowish deposits of xanthomatous material in the skin of the eyelids may be raised or flat, minute or large, even to the extent of involving a large part of both the upper and lower lids (Fig. 38–3). These deposits seem to result from an error of fat metabolism. The condition is frequently seen in diabetics or in people with high cholesterol or triglyceride levels. More often, no abnormalities are found.

Xanthelasma is a cosmetically deforming condition usually requiring treatment. While the lesions can be reduced in thickness by applications of trichloroacetic acid or by cryosurgery, surgical removal is the treatment of choice. Small lesions are easily removed by eliptical excision and primary closure. Larger lesions may present a problem in closure without creating malposition of the lid margins, lagophthalmos, and keratitis. Surgical judgment is needed in deciding what procedure to utilize in order to prevent these complications.

Xanthelasma lesions on the upper lid, even though extensive, can often be closed by undermining and direct closure. If there is more than a little trouble in eyelid closure when sutures have been placed, they should be removed and the defect covered with the skin obtained by flaps or grafts.

Xanthelasma removal on the lower lid is prone to result in ectropion if closed directly. If the surrounding skin is thin and redundant, it may be possible to undermine it and to advance the edges satisfactorily. Skin grafts from the retroauricular area are the best alternative.

If xanthelasma lesions are extensive, it may be wise to partially remove them and to wait for the skin to stretch and loosen for several months before removing the remaining portions. In any case, the patient with extensive involvement should be examined by an interested internist, because treatment for a metabolic condition may be indicated.

Degenerative Skin Changes

As a person ages, the skin undergoes degenerative changes resulting in a loss of elastic tissue, thinning,

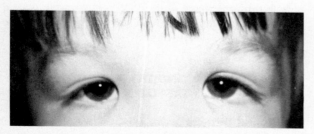

Figure 38–2. Congenital epicanthus arising from both lids in a patient originally seen because of "crossed eyes."

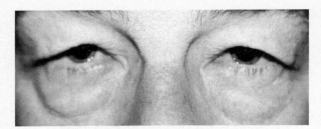

Figure 38–4. Dermatochalasis—the upper visual fields are restricted, and fat protrudes into the lower lids.

and stretching. The eyelid skin often undergoes these changes earlier and to a more significant degree than skin elsewhere on the body. Dermatochalasis may follow a familial pattern and, if pronounced, may be cosmetically distressing. If severe, it may result in a fold of skin overhanging the palpebral fissure obstructing vision and requiring blepharoplasty for functional purposes (Fig. 38–4). Coincidentally, the orbital septum may become thinned and stretched allowing the anterior orbital fat to protrude causing typical "bags" of the eyelids.

A large percentage of eyelid skin surgery consists of blepharoplasty. This is a large subject and is discussed fully in Chapter 39. Blepharoplasty is performed by several types of specialists: plastic surgeons, oculoplastic surgeons, head and neck surgeons, and dermatologic surgeons. All are capable of doing this operation, but they must be fully trained in the procedure and fully aware of the complications.

The actual removal of eyelid skin and plastic repair is rather simple. The judgment required in determining how much skin and fat (if any) to remove cannot be described and takes training and experience before the pitfalls can be avoided. The removal of too little skin is ineffective. Removing too much of the upper lid skin leads to lagophthalmos and keratitis. Inadequate blinking and impaired eye closure may also result from overexcision of upper lid skin. This is particularly distressing if there is a deficiency of tear formation, which is common in the age group requesting blepharoplasty. A Schirmer tear production test should be done preoperatively. If it indicates low tear formation, the amount of skin to be removed should be lessened or the operation cancelled. If lagophthalmos and keratitis occur, treatment with artificial tears should be tried. Often, skin grafting is needed. The availability of satisfactory donor skin may present a cosmetic problem.

The removal of too much skin of the lower lids leads to "scleral show" or ectropion, which may require skin grafting for relief if it is more than mild.

The removal of fat must be done very carefully to avoid operative and postoperative bleeding. Although a rare complication, deep postoperative bleeding can lead to an intraorbital pressure increase sufficient to impair the retinal circulation and lead to blindness. Much has been written about this complication.[4, 5] It must be understood by any surgeon who elects to perform blepharoplasties.

Trauma

The eyelids serve as delicately balanced curtains for the eyes. It is not unusual for them to be involved in trauma. Surgeons who attempt eyelid repair must be well oriented in eyelid anatomy. They must also be able to recognize injury to the eye and, preferably, evaluate and repair it. If uncertain about their skills in these regards, they should not hesitate to call upon an ophthalmic surgeon.

The eyelids contain the lacrimal puncta and canaliculi. Failure to repair traumatic defects of the lacrimal excretory system will lead to epiphora, which will eventually require the sevices of a surgeon accustomed to operating upon these structures.

Scars

The eyelids resist scarring better than most body tissues. However, after extensive loss of tissue, burns, or infections or after poor approximation of the skin edges, there may be deforming scars. These scars often result in malposition of the lid margins and cause tearing as well as cosmetic deformity. After a period of waiting and massaging and after the surgeon feels that all spontaneous improvement has occurred, surgery may be indicated. If the loss of tissue has not been too great, the scars may be excised and the fresh edges approximated in layers. Excellent functional and cosmetic results are usually obtainable. Extensive tissue loss and scarring may necessitate surgical procedures involving more than the skin. Skin grafting is usually a part of this type of repair.

Benign Tumors

Benign tumors of the eyelid include such conditions as nevi, papillomata, verrucae, various keratotic lesions, and cysts. These can be treated by cautery or by cryosurgery. If the diagnosis is not certain from the clinical appearance and if a pathological specimen is desired, the lesions can be excised with minimal margins and repaired by skin sutures. In lower lid lesions, some undermining of the edges may be needed to prevent ectropion formation. If the lesion is more than 5 to 6 mm in size, some revision of the defect to convert it to a crescent, or some more complicated skin plasties, as previously described, can be used on the eyelids.

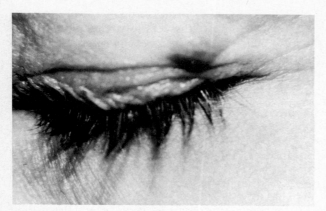

Figure 38–5. A small cavernous hemangioma in an adult that is confined to the superficial layers of the lid.

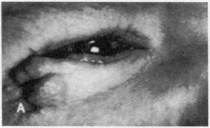
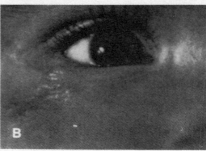

Figure 38–6. *A,* Small neurofibroma on the lower lid of a two-year-old child. *B,* Appearance following excision and advancement flap repair. (Reproduced by permission from C. Beard: Congenital Anomalies of the Eye. Presented at the New Orleans Academy of Ophthalmology's *Symposium on Surgical and Medical Management of Congenital Anomalies of the Eye,* 1968. St. Louis, 1968, The C. V. Mosby Co.)

Hemangiomas. Capillary hemangiomas (port-wine stains) that include the eyelids are usually extensive and involve the surrounding areas to a varying degree. They are extremely disfiguring and distressing and do not respond well to surgery unless quite small. They have been treated by tattooing, but the author has not seen striking results. They may do better with camouflage directed by a skilled cosmetologist. Contact argon laser treatment has been used recently on a limited number of patients. Early results are encouraging, but the follow-up periods are short.

Cavernous hemangiomas (Fig. 38–5) may be superficial and small, involving the eyelid alone, or may be extensive, involving deeper tissues and large periorbital areas as well as the lids. They are not ordinarily confined to the skin. In the infant, they may grow rapidly for a year or so, but the majority of them then regress slowly over the succeeding four or five years. Therefore, unless they are small and easily removable, it is considered best to observe them for a period of time, anticipating spontaneous regression, which will hopefully go on to complete resolution. If there is growth, these lesions are usually treated by steroid injections directly into the tumor, and many of them respond dramatically. The mode of action is in some doubt. Cavernous eyelid hemangiomas that interfere with eye movement or with the visual axis should be first injected with steroids. If they fail to regress rapidly, surgical excision is indicated to prevent amblyopia and to permit fusion.

Neurofibromas. Small neurofibromas confined to the eyelids are occasionally seen and are removable (Fig. 38–6). The usual neurofibroma tends to grow slowly until the patient reaches maturity, sometimes becoming gigantic (Fig. 38–7), and then to show no further growth. Some of them continue to grow during the first part of adult life. These tumors are usually accompanied by café au lait spots and by sessile and pedunculated neurofibromas on other areas of the body. They may extend into the orbit and cause defects in its bony walls resulting in pulsating enophthalmos or exophthalmos. They are usually subjected to repeated partial excisions, which may improve appearance. Unless the lesions are quite small, excisions are not complete or curative. On occasion, a neurofibroma will undergo malignant degeneration.

Keratoacanthoma. This rapidly growing benign skin tumor may occur on the eyelids (Fig. 38–8). It becomes a sharply defined, elevated lesion with a central verrucous crater. It may regress spontaneously or may grow to deforming proportions. A biopsy may be reported as squamous cell carcinoma. The clinical course is not consistent with this diagnosis. Keratoacanthoma can be treated by surgical excision (with small margins) and plastic repair (Fig. 38–9), by radiation, or by cryosurgery.

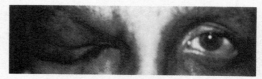

Figure 38–7. Neurofibroma of the right lids and orbit in an 18-year-old man. (Reproduced by permission from C. Beard: Congenital Anomalies of the Eye. Presented at the New Orleans Academy of Ophthalmology's *Symposium on Surgical and Medical Management of Congenital Anomalies of the Eye,* 1968. St. Louis, 1968, The C. V. Mosby Co.)

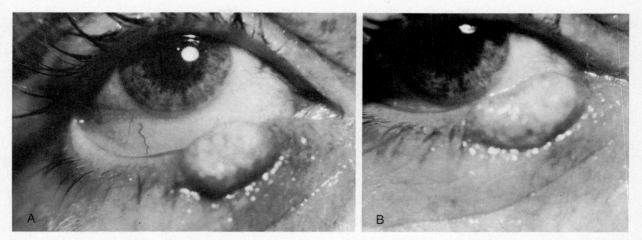

Figure 38–8. Keratoacanthoma on the right lower lid: *A*, Two weeks after first noted. *B*, Appearance one week later—note growth.

Malignant Tumors

The eyelids, particularly the lower eyelids, are favorite sites for the formation of malignant lesions. The great majority of these are basal cell carcinomas (Fig. 38–10). Squamous cell carcinoma (Fig. 38–11) is rare, and malignant melanoma (Fig. 38–12) is very rare. Sebaceous carcinoma arising from meibomian gland cells is not infrequent but involves the skin only secondarily.

Basal cell carcinoma is endemic in some areas that have a very sunny climate. Fair-skinned individuals are particularly prone to developing these tumors and should avoid excessive exposure to the direct rays of the sun, or at least, should use sunscreening lotions. Head protection by broad-brimmed hats is also helpful. The fad of tanning seems to be becoming less popular in some social sets, and this may help to reduce the frequency of these tumors. Since basal cell carcinoma is visible at the onset and is malignant by extension (only very rarely does it metastasize), it should have a very high rate of cure. Unfortunately, it is often neglected until its treatment becomes a major, rather than a minor, issue (Fig. 38–13). Lesions in the region of the medial canthus are particularly prone to deep extension and may become lethal.

Treatments. Basal cell carcinoma can be treated by surgical excision and plastic repair, by radiation, by curettage combined with cautery, by chemosurgery, or by cryosurgery.

Surgical Excision and Plastic Repair. This technique offers the greatest chance of cure but sometimes not the best cosmetic result. The tumor must be excised with wide margins that should be checked by frozen section. Then, and not until then, the repair can be planned. Extramarginal lesion excisions can be repaired by direct sutures, flaps, or

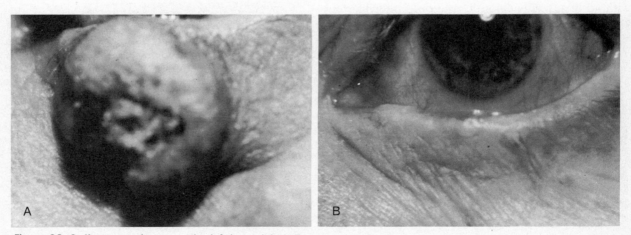

Figure 38–9. Keratoacanthoma on the left lower lid. *A*, Two months after first noted. *B*, Four years after excision with small margins and plastic repair.

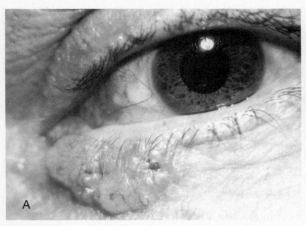
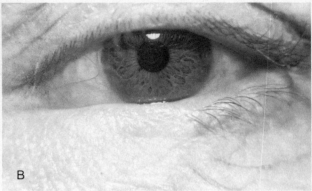

Figure 38—10. Basal cell carcinoma on the right lower lid. *A,* Preoperative appearance. *B,* Appearance six years after wide excision and plastic repair with a transposition flap from the upper lid.

grafts. Marginal lesions involve full-thickness lid excisions. There are many operations described for almost any type of full-thickness eyelid defect, and their descriptions, which would require a good-sized book, do not belong in this chapter.

It is of interest that incomplete excision is not always followed by recurrence. Indeed, one large series showed that only about 35% of incompletely excised lesions were followed by tumor recurrence.[6] Apparently, the immune system is sufficiently locally stimulated by the surgical trauma to eradicate the remaining malignant cells. This phenomenon cannot be relied upon, though, and its possibility does not justify incomplete excision.

The most certain way of avoiding the embarrassment of incomplete excision is by using graduated or layered tumor excision, using Mohs' fresh tissue chemosurgery technique followed by plastic repair.[7, 8] This is best done by specially trained dermatologic surgeons who do their own frozen section control without in situ zinc chloride fixation. Following the excision, if the defect is extensive, a plastic or an oculoplastic surgeon is usually called upon for the repair.

Radiation. Radiation has been successfully used for many years in the treatment of basal cell carcinoma. It is effective in most instances. A few tumors are radioresistant. Treatment must be fractionated over a period of time resulting in both a nuisance and an expense factor. The cosmetic effect may be poor because of skin changes and the loss of lashes; the lacrimal excretory system may be damaged. Despite these possible disadvantages, the treatment of basal cell carcinoma by radiation is good, and the prejudice against it by some physicians is unwarranted, providing that the treatment is given by skilled radiotherapists using modern methods.

Curettage and Cautery. Curettage and cautery is practiced by many and is undoubtedly effective,

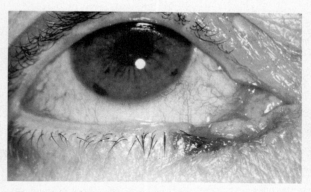

Figure 38—11. Squamous cell carcinoma on the right lower lid.

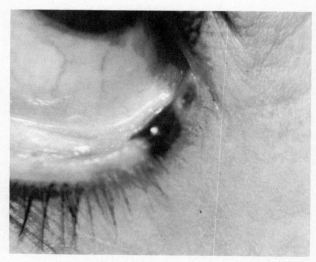

Figure 38—12. Malignant melanoma on the left lower lid.

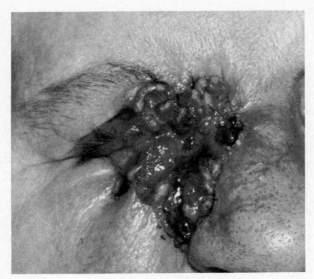

Figure 38–13. Neglected basal cell carcinoma on the right medial canthus with orbital invasion.

especially for extramarginal lesions. Since healing is by third intention, the effect following its use on the eyelids is not always good. The treatment of large lesions is apt to lead to ectropion. The author recommends that this type of treatment be used only for small extramarginal eyelid lesions.

Cryosurgery. This is a useful method of treatment for basal cell carcinoma. Adequate cold temperatures for treating malignancy are best obtained by liquid nitrogen applied by spray or by contact application through a closed metal tube. The tumor and a margin of normal tissue must be frozen, not just to whiteness but to a temperature of $-30°C$ as proved by a thermocouple placed beneath the tumor. The tissues are allowed to thaw and are then refrozen to the same temperature. A hemorrhagic blister is apt to result. When it resolves and the area has epithelialized, rebiopsy usually shows no sign of tumor. Cryosurgery has the disadvantages of depigmentation of the treated area and, if used near the lid margin, the loss of eyelashes. For some patients, these factors contraindicate its use. For older patients or those who are not otherwise good surgical candidates, it is often the best treatment. For those who care little about appearance and desire simplicity and rapidity of treatment, it may be the treatment of choice. It is unlikely that it will damage the lacrimal excretory system and is given in one session. For these reasons, it has an advantage over radiation therapy.

Regardless of the type of treatment, the patient has one golden opportunity for cure, and that is during the first procedure. The percentage rate of success drops significantly when recurrences must be treated.

COMPLICATIONS OF EYELID SKIN SURGERY

All surgery has potential complications. The surgeon who has none either does little surgery or fails to recognize them. While those that follow surgery of the eyelid skin are relatively rare, when a complication occurs, one should know what to do, or what not to do.

Inadequate Tumor Excision

In spite of precautions, inadequate excision may occur. Because some basal cell tumors fail to recur after apparent incomplete removal,[6] careful observation may be in order. Patients should be told of the problem and of the need for periodic examination. Otherwise, they may fail to report until a major recurrence is evident. If tumor becomes apparent, it should be treated the same as a primary lesion.

The alternatives to observation are early reoperation, radiation, cryosurgery, or chemosurgery. Early reoperation may be requested by the patient and should be insisted upon if squamous cell carcinoma or melanoma is involved. Each instance must be weighed and treated individually.

Undue Tissue Reaction

Any surgical procedure on the eyelid is apt to result in some postoperative swelling and ecchymosis. This is usually insignificant and requires no treatment. If the surgery has been extensive and excessive reaction is anticipated, it can be reduced by pressure dressings and/or cold compresses.

There is a feeling among many who do eyelid surgery that tissue reaction can be reduced, or its resolution hastened, by the use of oral trypsin (Ananase, Chymoral, Orenzyme). This has not been proved, to the author's knowledge, by double-blind studies. Fortunately, the answers to many of life's problems are often apparent and generally acceptable without rigorous scientific evidence. Those patients who receive this medication seem to fare better than those who do not. Sensitivity to trypsin is rare. It should not be used in patients with blood clotting abnormalities or with renal or hepatic disease.

Steroids are often used to reduce tissue reaction. However, the side effects can be more of a problem than the presence of the reaction.

Hemorrhage

If despite careful hemostasis at the operating table and the use of light or heavy pressure dressings there is still postoperative bleeding, it must be controlled. Less damage results if the bleeding occurs to the outside than if it infiltrates the operated tissues or "floats" a skin flap or graft from its base.

The wound must be inspected. Reapplication of pressure and perhaps the application of thrombin may be sufficient to stop the bleeding. If a point persists in spurting blood, it should be cauterized. Rarely is a tie indicated.

After the hemorrhage has been controlled and the area has healed, the damage must be assessed (there may be none). If there is tissue slough resulting in scarring and deformity, it may respond to time and massage, or it may require further surgery (but not until after all spontaneous improvement has occurred). Early reoperation, done upon unhealed tissues, usually leads to further deformity.

Infection

Infection is rare after eyelid surgery. The abundant blood supply helps to prevent it. The lids cannot be rendered bacteria-free by routine preps. One should not do elective surgery in the presence of active infection of the skin, lash margin, conjunctiva, or lacrimal apparatus. If postoperative infection should occur it is usually due to *Staphylococci* and will respond to appropriate antibiotic therapy. Ordinarily, the result of the surgery will not be compromised.

Necrosis of the Skin

Sometimes, the skin of the lids becomes necrotic after surgery. This may follow hemorrhage or infection, be caused by excess pressure, or occur without apparent cause. Missing skin will have to be replaced by flaps or grafts. The flap or graft used for replacement may undergo the same fate. Split-thickness skin grafts are less apt to do so, and they should be considered, at least as a temporary measure.

Deforming Scars

Following the most careful surgery, there are instances of undue scar formation. These may be due to idiosyncrasy. If anticipated, scarring can be reduced by the injection of steroids into the tissues at the time of surgery. If the scar becomes apparent later, it can be injected with steroids. Time and massage will help. On occasion, the scar will have to be carefully excised and the defect repaired in layers. Steroids should be injected at the time of this secondary surgery.

Ectropion

Excision of too much vertical skin of the lower lid may lead to ectropion. The amount of excision in this area does not have to be great to be excessive. If ectropion occurs, the area should be massaged for several weeks. If it persists after improvement has ceased, additional skin must be supplied by flap or graft.

Trichiasis and Entropion

Occasionally, the surgeon and patient will be surprised and annoyed by the presence of lashes touching the cornea. These can vary from one or two to all of the lashes of the lid. A few lashes can be removed by galvanic epilation. If there are from five to 10 offending lashes, surgical excision of the lashes and their follicles may be necessary. Stubborn aberrant lashes can be eradicated by surgically exposing the follicles and carefully cauterizing each bulb.

Cryosurgery has also been successfully used in treating trichiasis.[9] A measured temperature of −20°C will permanently remove the aberrant lashes (as well as some normal adjacent ones). Some depigmentation of the treated skin results and may be a cosmetic annoyance.

If all or most of the lashes are turned inward following an eyelid procedure, a careful examination to determine the cause must be made. Entropion following eyelid surgery limited to the skin is rare. Following full-thickness lid surgery, it is not uncommon. It is caused by malposition of the layers of the lid and requires surgical revision. This may include excision of some skin and suture fixation of both the skin and the underlying layers to the tarsus.

Loss of Lashes

Surgery of the eyelid skin near its margin may lead to the loss of lashes. If this should happen, it may be distressing, particularly to the female patient. Artificial lashes may satisfy some patients. Lash grafts leave much to be desired. There are no good donor sites. Brow hair is too long and must be constantly trimmed. It has a stubbly appearance in most instances. If the area of alopecia is not too wide, a full-thickness excision of the involved lid area with reapproximation of the edges containing normal lashes may be indicated.

The author has occasionally tattooed a line of pigment to simulate lashes. Initially, this looks good, but the pigment tends to disperse and fade with time and to need a touch up. This has led the author to be skeptical of the present fad of cosmetic eyeliner tattooing. The long-term results may not be as good as the early ones. And besides, who knows whether the fashions in eyeliner color and the desired extent of application will be the same five or 10 years from now?

REFERENCES

1. Collin JR, Beard C, Wood, I: Experimental and clinical data on the insertion of the levator palpebrae superioris muscle. Am J Ophthalmol 85:792–801, 1978
2. Mustardé JC: Repair and Reconstruction in the Orbital Region. Edinburgh, Churchill Livingstone, 1980, p 337
3. Hughes WL: Surgical treatment of congenital palpebral phimosis—the Y-V operation. Arch Ophthalmol 54:586–590, 1955
4. DeMere M, Wood T, Austin W: Eye complications with blepharoplasty or other eyelid surgery: A national survey. Plast Reconstr Surg 53:634–637, 1974
5. Waller RR: Is blindness a realistic complication in blepharoplasty procedures? Ophthalmol 85:730–735, 1978
6. Gooding CA, White G, Yatsuchashi M: Significance of marginal extension in excised basal-cell carcinoma. N Engl J Med 273:923–924, 1965
7. Tromovich TA, Stegman SJ: Microscopically controlled excision of skin tumors. Arch Dermatol 110:231–232, 1974
8. Anderson RL, Ceilley RI: A multispecialty approach to the excision and reconstruction of eyelid tumors. Ophthalmol 85:1150–1163, 1978
9. Sullivan JH, Beard C, Bullock JD: Cryosurgery for the treatment of trichiasis. Tr Amer Ophthmol Soc 74:189–202, 1976

39

Blepharoplasty

RONALD P. GRUBER, M.D.

There has been confusion in the literature as to the meaning of certain terms such as blepharochalasis and dermatochalasis. For this reason, it is best to define and use the terms that are properly employed by plastic surgeons to describe the phenomenon to be treated. Rhytids refer to wrinkles. Elastosis refers to the looseness of the skin that is clinically palpable. Protrusion of the orbital fat is often incorrectly referred to as herniation of the orbital fat; it is not a true herniation but simply an anterior bulging of the fat through a weakened orbital septum. Hypertrophy of the orbicular muscle, which is often seen as a thickening of the tissues along the infraciliary margin, is due to chronic muscle spasm and squinting and is accentuated when the patient smiles forcibly. Redundant skin with protrusion of orbital fat, the most common condition seen by the anesthetic plastic surgeon, is noted in both sexes and is of unknown etiology, although it is occasionally familial.

PREOPERATIVE EXAMINATION

A history and physical examination is performed and includes an evaluation of desires and expectations. If the surgeon is unable to fulfill these expectations, an unhappy reaction is sure to follow. Moreover, the nature of the procedure and potential complications must be discussed with the patient preoperatively. Some plastic surgeons are now discussing even the potential problem of blindness following blepharoplasty, although it occurs but rarely. Whether it is advisable to discuss this potential problem for fear of causing unnecessary apprehension with every candidate for blepharoplasty remains to be determined. It is important to ascertain whether or not the patient has medical problems, in particular hypertension, because of the known higher incidence of hematoma following this surgery in such patients. The hypertension must be under the best possible control preoperatively and followed carefully in the immediate postoperative period. In addition, patients are instructed to avoid aspirin-containing products 10 days prior to surgery for their known anticoagulating powers and for its potential of creating a hematoma postoperatively.

The patient also requires a check of visual acuity. Many plastic surgeons insist upon a complete eye examination by an ophthalmologic colleague, because the patient may later complain of a visual acuity loss that might have been present preoperatively. They also may note dry eye syndrome, which although minor prior to the blepharoplasty, may become exaggerated.

Other conditions to look for in a preoperative examination include exophthalmos, because overzealous removal of skin in this area exaggerates the exophthalmos and leads to a worsening of the aesthetic appearance, not to mention the problems of lagophthalmos and dry eye. Pre-existing ptosis of the upper eyelid should be noted because it too can be exaggerated following a blepharoplasty.

It is important to be certain that the cause of the patient's droopy upper eyelid is not due in large part to brow ptosis. The eyebrow is normally at a level at or above the supraorbital ridge. Very often in these patients, the eyebrow is found to be inferior to that level. This can be confirmed when the examiner elevates the eyebrow with his thumb and notes an improvement in the appearance of the eye. Such an elevation of the brow can improve not only appearance but also the superior peripheral vision, which is obstructed by redundant skin resting on the eyelashes in addition to a ptotic brow. When this is present, both a blepharoplasty and a browlift procedure (the technical details of which are not discussed here) should be considered. Occasionally, a browlift procedure will correct the aesthetic appearance without necessitating a blepharoplasty.

Another aspect of the examination includes searching for the level at which the supratarsal fold is located. In some patients, it is in the normal position (8 to 10 mm from the ciliary margin); in others, it is recessed in the very superior portions of the palpebral area (15 mm from the ciliary margin). In still others, it may be located at less than 8 mm or even absent (Fig. 39–1). If the fold is abnormally low, consideration must be given to a tarsal fixation procedure to be performed at the time of the blepharoplasty. Basically, this involves recreation of the supratarsal fold at a level appropriate for the patient (8 to 10 mm from the ciliary margin). Finally, asymmetry of the upper eyelids is a condition that must be diagnosed preoperatively so that it too can be corrected or improved.

Examination of the lower eyelid involves a search for pre-existing scleral show (Fig. 39–2). With ad-

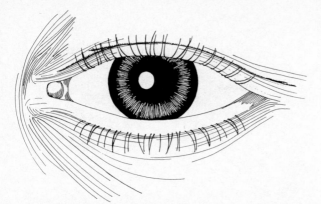

Figure 39—1. The eye should be examined for an abnormally low supratarsal fold, which is normally at 8 to 10 mm from the ciliary margin.

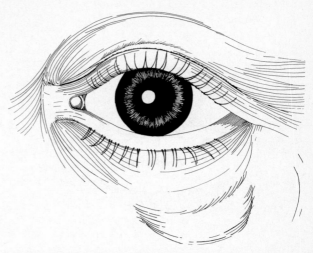

Figure 39—3. Secondary fat pads are a fullness on the cheek area, not necessarily due to fat pads, and are often not correctable by the standard blepharoplasty.

vancing age, this is more common and manifests itself as frank ectropion. This condition should forewarn the surgeon that lower blepharoplasty is fraught with a potential of converting the scleral show to ectropion if steps are not taken at the time of the surgery to prevent this problem. This is particularly important because the number one complication following lower blepharoplasty is ectropion. Another common condition to look for in the lower eyelids is referred to as secondary fatpads (Fig. 39–3). This is a prominence of what may be fat or simply edema located at the level of the malar eminence. Since it is not really part of the lower eyelid anatomy, it is not improved by the standard lower blepharoplasty alone. A separate treatment, which may be both medical and surgical, is required to correct this fullness in the cheek-eyelid region. It includes such approaches as the administration of diuretics, direct excision of the prominence, and lipolysis of the redundant fat.

Examination of both lids is next performed for such things as crow's-feet, which are simply a marked exaggeration and fanning of the rhytids at the lateral canthal area. Blepharoplasty usually fails to completely correct this deformity. Specific treatment for this condition includes chemical peel and

excision of portions of the orbicular muscle in this vicinity, the exact technical details of which are not discussed in this chapter. Finally, the patient may also have a hypertrophied orbicular muscle that manifests itself as a thickening or bunching up of the skin just beneath the ciliary margin when the patient forcibly smiles.

The patient may also exhibit myxedematous skin in the upper and lower eyelids, suggesting a thyroid condition. Therefore, a euthyroid condition would be required preoperatively. Those patients who are on long-standng steroid therapy may exhibit a considerable degree of periorbital edema, making blepharoplasty contraindicated if edema is the cause of the aesthetic problem.

Finally, it is advisable that preoperative photos be taken not only to aid the surgeon who might not remember all the preoperative details but also to remind patients of their appearance should they be unhappy with some of the secondary changes or minor degrees of asymmetry that occur.

METHOD

Preoperatively the patient is advised to wash his face and shampoo his hair with either pHisoHex or pHisoDerm on the day before surgery. The patient is also warned to avoid aspirin-containing products for ten days prior to the operation.

Before premedication, markings are drawn on the patient's upper eyelids. There is a wide variety of markings that have been used by various surgeons. The type described here is one of the more common ones that is utilized by the author. A slightly sigmoid-shaped ellipse of skin is outlined from the upper eyelid by placing the inferior markings in the area of the anticipated supratarsal fold. This inferior

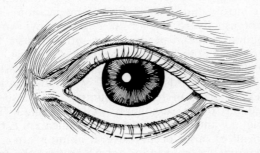

Figure 39—2. Examination should include a search for a pre-existing "scleral show," which predisposes a patient to postoperative ectropion.

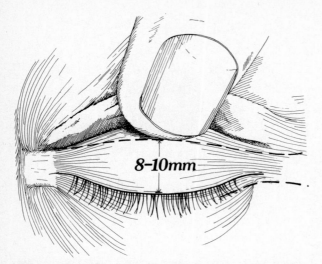

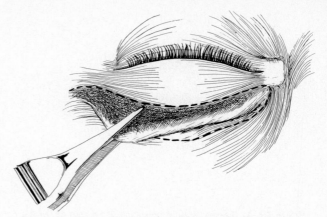

Figure 39–6. The exact amount of upper lid skin to be removed can be estimated by gently grasping the redundant skin with forceps.

Figure 39–4. The inferior marking of the upper lid corresponds to where the supratarsal fold should be (8–10 mm above the ciliary margin). It is marked while elevating the eyelid skin and brow with the examining finger.

marking is not necessarily in the existing supratarsal fold itself, but rather approximately 8 to 10 mm superior to the ciliary margin after elevating the brow skin with the examining finger (Fig. 39–4). The line should then sweep laterally and superiorly rather than follow Langer's lines, which might otherwise point inferiorly or straight laterally. The upper marking is made somewhat parallel to the lower one with a width of 5 to 12 mm, depending upon the amount of skin to be resected (Figs. 39–5 and 39–6). This can be ascertained by pinching the skin together very gently with forceps in the unanesthetized patient. After performing many blepharoplasties, this judgment can be established by elevating and depressing the eyebrow skin to ascertain the amount of elasticity in the upper eyelid. It is generally agreed that there is a tendency to remove too much skin from the upper eyelid, particularly from the central and medial portions of the eyelid.

The amount of skin that should be removed is often in the lateral third of the upper eyelid area where it cannot hide in the supratarsal fold and tends to become redundant. The other reason the skin markings should sweep laterally and superiorly is because this is the general flow of the aesthetically pleasant upper eyelid.

Care is taken to avoid drawing the line much beyond the lateral border of the orbital rim for fear of causing a scar in the thicker skin of the temporal area. One should also carefully avoid extending the markings into the concavity of the medial aspect of the upper eyelid because a scar band contracture could develop and result in an epicanthal fold.

A lower eyelid marking is made approximately 2 mm inferior to the level of the ciliary margin extending medially to the punctum and keeping it within one of the lateral crow's-feet. Some surgeons prefer to make a downward curve at the lateral canthal area so that, when a lateral pull is applied to the eventual skin flap of the lower eyelid, the redundant skin in this area can be resected avoiding a dog-ear.

The type of premedication varies widely depending on the surgeon's preference. This author has preferred slow push intravenous premedication on the morning of surgery because of the great flexibility, control, and reversibility of medication. The patient usually receives 1 to 2 cc fentanyl citrate (Sublimaze) administered slowly intravenously followed by 2.5 to 20 mg diazepam (Valium). As intravenous medication is given, the patient is asked to count backwards from 100. When the patient makes an error in reverse counting, he or she is considered to be reasonably well medicated. The distinct advantage of intravenous medication is that the peak of onset occurs several minutes after administering the medication, at which time the local anesthesia can be given. Should the need arise for reversal because of the patient's excessive drowsi-

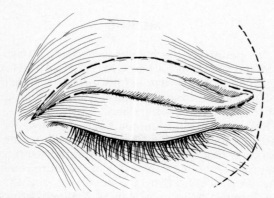

Figure 39–5. The superior marking on the upper lid runs somewhat parallel and 5 to 12 mm above it, which results in a sigmoid-shaped piece of skin to be removed.

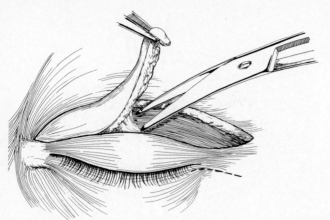

Figure 39–7. Skin is removed with tenotomy scissors; varying amounts of orbicularis muscle in the bed of the wound are also removed.

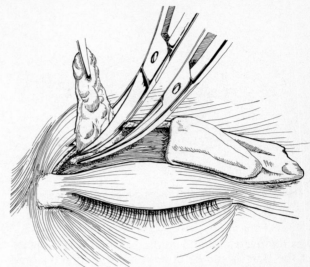

Figure 39–8. After incising the septum orbitale, the fat pads protrude and can be amputated at the level of the orbicularis muscle.

ness and inability to verbally respond to questions, the fentanyl citrate can be reversed with naloxone hydrochloride (Narcan). If necessary, one can also use physostigmine to reverse, or at least partially reverse, diazepam effect. During the procedure, 0.5 cc droperidol is given intravenously to prevent postoperative nausea. If hypertension develops during surgery, 1.25 mg chlorpromazine hydrochloride (Thorazine) is given intravenously every five to 10 minutes until a normal blood pressure is established. One should never inject more than a total of 5 mg intravenously.

Local anesthesia is established for the purpose of prolonging the duration of anesthesia. Thus, 1% lidocaine (Xylocaine) containing epinephrine is added to 0.25% bupivocaine containing 1:200,000 epinephrine. The anesthesia is administered with a 3 cc syringe and a no. 30 needle. Although it may not be the practice of many surgeons, the author prefers to do the entire blepharoplasty with the aid of magnifying lenses (approximately 2.5 power).

Upper blepharoplasty is performed by sharply excising the skin and usually most of the underlying orbicular muscle as well (Fig. 39–7). Different surgeons resect various amounts of muscle. It has become apparent that, without resection of the underlying muscle, one is simply concealing an unnecessary bulge of soft tissue beneath the wound and hindering the development of an aesthetically pleasing recessed supratarsal fold. Because there is often a redundancy medially, a small triangle of skin can be excised.

If it has been determined preoperatively that there are protuberant fat pads, an incision is made through the orbital septum at this time, over the point of maximum bulge (Fig. 39–8). This is determined by gentle digital pressure on the globe, which accentuates the bulging fat pad. Rather than making small stab wounds to allow the herniated fat to protrude,

a long incision is employed because better exposure is obtained for hemostasis. It cannot be overemphasized that the hemostasis must be complete in this area, and magnifiers or loopes have been found to be helpful for this purpose. Occasionally, the lacrimal gland will seem to be protruding into the area, but its color and lobulation is distinct from the fat of the upper eyelids, and it should not be inadvertently resected. If it should cause an unaesthetic bulge in the upper lateral eyelid, techniques are available (which are not described here) to return the lacrimal gland to its recess inferior to the lateral supraorbital ridge.

At this point, some modified form of supraorbital fixation has been advocated by a number of surgeons to accentuate the existing supratarsal fold, if not to create one if none is present. The details of this surgery can be found elsewhere. In essence, the inferior edge of the resultant wound margin following skin resection is fixed to the tarsal plate and becomes the edge of the supratarsal fold. The level of this fixation can be controlled to a great extent by the surgeon. Most important is the realization that the supratarsal fold often has to be recreated or shifted superiorly to achieve the aesthetic goal.

Closure of the wounds is straightforward without the necessity of closure of the orbicular muscle or the orbital septum through which the fat pads protrude. Therefore, closure of the overlying skin is performed with an interrupted or running 6–0 nylon suture or a subcuticular suture (Fig. 39–9).

At this point, patients should be asked to close their eyes, and it should be possible for them to barely do so. If not, consideration has to be given to the possibility that too much skin was resected. If there is any doubt, then some of the skin that

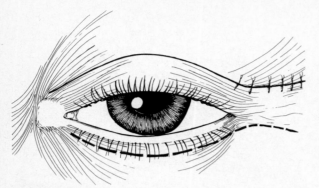

Figure 39–9. The upper lid wound is closed with interrupted or running 6-0 nylon sutures.

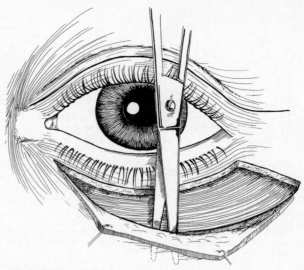

Figure 39–11. The skin-only flap can be elevated no further than the infraorbital rim. Alternatively, a skin-muscle flap (skin and orbicularis) has the distinct advantage of involving a relatively bloodless plane that can be elevated higher.

was removed should be either sutured back in place or the skin should be at least be banked and stored in the refrigerator in the event it is required in the near future to correct any lagophthalmos.

The lower blepharoplasty is performed by making an incision 2 mm inferior to the ciliary margin (Fig. 39–10) and extending it laterally into a rhytid in the crow's-feet area. There are two basic methods of approaching the removal of reduntant skin. One involves the elevation of a skin flap alone, drawing it superiorly and laterally and then resecting the redundant skin; the other involves the elevation of the skin muscle flap during the same maneuver. Each is discussed in detail.

For the skin-only technique, the skin is elevated from the underlying orbicular muscle of eye with the help of small tenotomy scissors or some other type of scissors that avoids inadvertent perforations of the skin flap (Fig. 39–11). Dissection is extended to the orbital rim. Bleeding is controlled best with a fine-tip needle electrocautery. Next, a search for the protruding fat is done by gently placing the examining finger on the globe noting the point of

maximum bulge. At this location, the muscle can be split with small scissors either from one side of the eyelid to the other or in two or three separate stab wound incisions (Fig. 39–12). The author finds it easier to split the muscle from one side to the other in order to facilitate hemostasis and quick removal of the fat pad. For the same reason that local anesthesia has to be given for the upper eyelid fat pad, it is injected here into the lower fat pads.

There are three distinct compartments; the medial one tends to have lighter colored fat. Not all of the fat compartments need to be removed, only those causing an unpleasing appearance. Commonly, the lateral fat pad is neglected and if the prominent fat

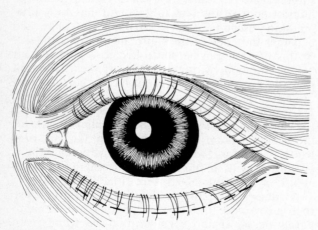

Figure 39–10. The lower eyelid marking is made 2 mm below the ciliary margin and extends laterally into the crow's-feet area.

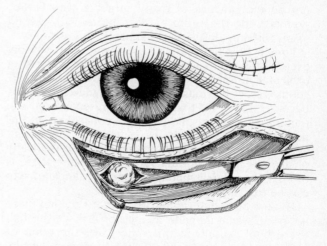

Figure 39–12. After the flap is elevated, the orbicularis or septum orbitale muscle or both are split (depending on the type of flap that was elevated) in order for the fat pads to protrude.

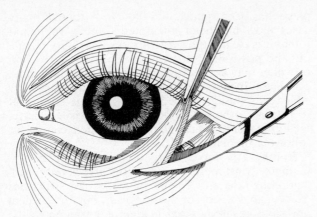

Figure 39–13. Redundant skin is removed from the lower lid flap by first asking the patient to open the mouth and to look upwards.

from this compartment is not adequately removed, it is conspicuous postoperatively. Resection of the fat is done in a similar fashion as that for the upper eyelid. The skin flap is then pulled superiorly and somewhat laterally while the patient is asked to open his or her mouth and to look upwards. This maneuver is done to maximize the size of the wound in order to avoid inadvertent removal of too much skin and cause an ectropion postoperatively (Fig. 39–13). After the patient performs this maneuver, the redundant skin can be removed, making certain that the skin flap abuts the ciliary margin wound as accurately as possible (Fig. 39–14). There has been a tendency for surgeons to remove too much skin at this time. Recalling that ectropion is the number one complication of lower blepharoplasty, conservation is in order.

Pulling the skin laterally helps provide support to the lower eyelid as well as smoothing out the rhytids that would otherwise develop. Unfortunately, it sometimes leaves a small dog-ear laterally, which

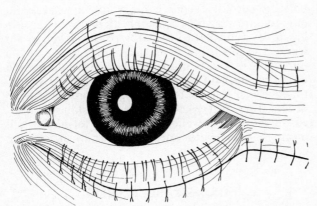

Figure 39–14. The lower lid wound margins must abut perfectly without tension prior to closure with interrupted or running 6-0 nylon sutures.

cannot be chased too far or the resultant scar will go well beyond the lateral orbital rim. Consequently, some surgeons remove a small vertical wedge of skin in the medial aspect of the lower eyelid incision to help provide more support for the lower eyelid and, at the same time, remove redundant skin.

Closure of the wound is similar to that for the upper eyelid because the orbital septum need not be repaired nor is it necessary to repair muscle that was split to gain entrance to the orbital fat pads.

If it was diagnosed preoperatively that the patient has a strong tendency toward an ectropion, it is at this time—prior to the wound closure—that corrective measures such as a vertical wedge removal of the tarsal plate from the lateral third of the lower eyelid (a modified Kuntz-Zymonowski procedure) is performed. Since removal of a vertical wedge from the lower lid often foreshortens the intercanthal width, many surgeons are now using a lateral canthopexy at the level of the bony orbital rim in order to support the lower lid without shortening it.

The skin muscle flap procedure employs the same infraciliary incision. Dissection is extended to the orbicular muscle into a plane that is virtually bloodless between the orbicular muscle and the orbital septum. Entry into this bloodless plane can be performed either laterally, which requires transection of a few of the orbicular muscle fibers, or in the central section of the infraciliary margin. In either event, once the plane is entered, a very rapid elevation of the skin muscle flap is possible with immediate and greatly facilitated visualization of the fat pads. Cotton applicators can be helpful peeling away the skin muscle flap from the underlying fat pads. As was the case previously, the fat pads should be injected with local anesthesia prior to electrocoagulation and excision. Again, one cannot overemphasize the need for hemostasis in this area, particularly in view of the fact that when retrobulbar hemorrhage has occurred postoperatively, it has usually occurred in those patients who had lower lid fat pad removal.

The excess skin is removed in a fashion similar to that suggested for the skin flap procedure. One can also resect a small extra portion of muscle from the edge of the flap if the patient was diagnosed preoperatively as having a hypertrophic orbicular muscle along the infraciliary area.

After completion of both the upper and lower blepharoplasty procedures and prior to final closure of the skin margins, it is helpful to have the patient sit upright at a 45-degree angle to judge the results. Examination of the upper eyelids often reveals that there is redundant orbicular muscle in the upper eyelid that could easily be resected to enhance the result with a slightly more defined supratarsal fold. Occasionally, it also becomes apparent that not enough eyelid skin has been removed in the lateral aspect of the upper eyelid. Also, the upright position tends to allow the fat to protrude because of gravity, and one might see a protrusion of the fat pads necessitating further resection. A patient sitting upright also facilitates the correct draping of the lower eyelid skin, because sometimes the flap has been pulled too far laterally or not laterally enough, resulting in the formation of rhytids simply from positioning of the skin flap or skin muscle flap. This can then be corrected prior to terminating the procedure.

POSTOPERATIVE PERIOD

In the immediate postoperative period, a removable dressing can be applied, but not a pressure dressing. This is changed every one or two hours. At that time, patients are allowed to remove the dressing and to use their eyes to determine if there are any unusual abnormalities such as swelling from hematoma or diminished visual acuity.

Ice bags are employed to minimize swelling in the first 24 hours only. The eye should not be in direct contact with the ice, which could be injurious to the soft tissue. It is suggested that the head of the bed be elevated to diminish venous pressure. It is important to follow the patient closely for any changes in the blood pressure, particularly if there is a history of hypertension.

The patient is seen the following day and examined for any small hematomas, or less common problems such as corneal irritation. If the patient has lagophthalmos in the immediate postoperative period, preventive measures should be taken to protect the cornea from exposure. The patient is again seen on the third to fifth postoperative day, at which time skin sutures are removed.

COMPLICATIONS

Immediate complications include hematoma (retrobulbar hemorrhage) as well as small hematomas that occur beneath the skin flaps. Retrobulbar hemorrhage is one of the most serious complications that may occur. It is encountered only rarely, but is generally associated with surgical removal of the fat pads, particularly from the lower eyelids. It is manifested by proptosis and firmness to palpation of the globe. Perhaps the single most important preventive measure for this complication is awareness of the problem and vigilance by both patient and doctor for unusual pain and swelling. Patients are reminded that discomfort is a part of the procedure, although this should respond to analgesics. However, continuous pain is abnormal and should not be tolerated by the patient. Rather, the physician should be notified immediately at any time of the day or night. The incidence of blindness following blepharo-

plasty has been reported at 0.04%. Although many cases have not been attributed directly to hematoma, it is clearly the surgeon's responsibility to rule out the possibility of such bleeding, the correction of which may prevent blindness. At the same time, ophthalmologic evaluation by one of the surgeon's colleagues should be performed. This is important to rule out other causes of decreased visual acuity, including acute angle glaucoma, which can occur following blepharoplasty.

Epiphora is encountered occasionally in the immediate postoperative period associated with lagophthalmos and edema of the eyelid structures causing an eversion of the punctum. Finally, corneal abrasions resulting from inadvertent trauma to the cornea are an occasional cause of discomfort to the patient in the immediate postoperative period and must be recognized immediately and distinguished from hematoma as the cause of pain.

In the early postoperative period, ectropion may be seen. If it persists into the intermediate and late postoperative period, it is due to resection of too much skin, particularly in a patient who is predisposed to ectropion, and one who exhibited scleral show in the preoperative examination. Small hematomas beneath the flap or in the subcutaneous tissue may manifest themselves in the first few days following blepharoplasty, if not on the first postoperative day. Sometimes, these can be drained through a small stab wound, but more often it is necessary to remove the sutures from the lower lid incision area and to evacuate the blood. If this is not done, the hematoma is replaced by scar tissue, and an unsightly irregularity and firmness of the eyelid develops. If this involves the lower lid, it can contribute to ectropion.

Infection is a rare complication but quickly diagnosed and usually treated easily. A nuisance complication is that of milia caused by sutures left in too long with resultant formation of epithelialized tracts in the subcutaneous area.

Late complications include ectropion, which has failed to subside despite conservative measures and may require surgical correction. In many cases, skin has to be returned to the area of the lower eyelid where too much has been taken. In other cases, a tightening or shortening of the horizontal dimension of the tarsal plate of the lower lid suffices. Lagophthalmos is a less common complication but usually occurs from overzealous resection of skin and muscle in the upper eyelids. Ptosis due to inadvertent injury of the levator mechanism is an uncommon complication.

UNDESIRABLE RESULTS

A common but much less serious undesirable result is that of residual fat pads, particularly in the lower eyelid and the upper medial eyelid areas.

Fortunately, these can be corrected by direct surgical intervention when the wounds have healed sufficiently. Occasionally, too much of the fat pads are removed, causing a depressed appearance with exaggeration of the orbital rim. This tends to occur in thin-skinned individuals, and the problem is difficult to correct, although some success has been obtained with fat grafts.

Redundant skin and rhytids may be seen in the lower eyelid and are a more serious problem if the patient anticipates complete removal of rhytids of the lower eyelid. This is especially true with crow's-feet, which are not readily corrected by standard blepharoplasty. Residual rhytids are more likely to be seen following the skin muscle flap procedure in an elderly patient where the skin does not stretch as much for the resection as in a skin-only flap. Fortunately, this condition is correctable.

The residual crow's-feet, which have traditionally not been completely amenable to blepharoplasty treatment, are treated with either chemical peel or resection of muscle in the lateral canthal area with improved results over the usual blepharoplasty technique. Details of this technique are not described here.

Finally, asymmetry between two sides is often noticed by the patient who tends to be a perfectionist. It is something that can be best avoided by paying close attention to details and informing the patient prior to surgery that there might be some residual minor asymmetries, which are common in people who have not had the operation.

SUMMARY

Blepharoplasty has proved to be one of the best procedures in plastic surgery to improve the aesthetic appearance of the face. Successful results, however, rely heavily on the surgeon's ability: (1) to diagnose the specific anatomic problems preoperatively, (2) to forecast which patients are most likely to develop problems postoperatively, and (3) to take specific measures preoperatively, intraoperatively, and postoperatively to avoid these potential complications. When these facets of the problem are appreciated, the surgical results are likely to be more satisfactory.

SUGGESTED READINGS

Baker TJ, Gordon JL, Mosienko P: Upper Lid Blepharoplasty. Presented at the 10th annual meeting of the American Society of Aesthetic Plastic Surgeons, March 22, 1977, Los Angeles

Graff WC, Smith JW (eds): Surgery of the Eyelids in Plastic Surgery. Boston, Little, Brown & Co, 1979, pp 404–409

Guy CL, Converse JM, Morello DC: Esthetic surgery for the aging face, in Converse JM (ed): Reconstructive Plastic Surgery. Philadelphia, WB Saunders Co, 1977, pp 1877–1898

Spira M: Blepharoplasty. Clin Plast Surg 5:121–137, 1978

40

DANIEL M. LASKIN, D.D.S., M.S.

Surgery of the Oral Cavity

Many of the lesions that occur on the oral mucous membranes are similar to those found on the skin, and essentially the same surgical techniques are involved in their treatment. There are sufficient variations in the types of conditions encountered and their management, however, for the subject of oral surgery to warrant separate consideration. The material in this chapter will attempt to show how some of the therapeutic procedures ordinarily used in dermatologic surgery must be modified because of anatomic and physiologic differences in the oral cavity. It will also deal with anesthesia for oral surgery, and special aspects of postoperative care. Finally, consideration will be given to the treatment of those pathologic processes that either occur only in the mouth or that present special management problems when they develop in that region.

ANATOMIC CONSIDERATIONS IN ORAL SURGERY

Surgical Danger Areas in the Oral Cavity

There are only a few major anatomic structures with which one has to be concerned when performing surgery in the mouth: the large blood vessels in the palate, tongue, and the region of the mental foramen; the lingual and mental nerves; and the parotid and submandibular ducts.

Blood Vessels. The oral tissues are highly vascular with excellent collateral circulation. Therefore, there is generally no need to worry about surgically interfering with the blood supply and producing tissue necrosis. Rather, the only concern is with excessive bleeding from inadvertently cutting a large artery or vein. Such vessels are found in the hard palate (anterior palatine artery), the tongue and floor of the mouth (lingual artery, ranine vein), and the region of the mental foramen (mental artery). When possible, incisions should be planned to avoid cutting these vessels. Otherwise, they should be isolated and ligated before being cut. Cauterization is usually inadequate for controlling such bleeding, and its use increases the chance for secondary hemorrhage.

Sensory Nerves. Whereas cutting minor sensory nerve branches during oral surgery causes no recognizable problem for the patient, injury to major sensory nerves results in a considerable area of

paresthesia or anesthesia. This can occur during surgical procedures in the region of the mental foramen and on the floor of the mouth. When it occurs in the former, the patient complains of numbness or altered sensation in half of the lower lip and chin; damage to the lingual nerve causes sensory changes on one side of the anterior two thirds of the tongue. Because of the frequent sensory stimulation of the lips and tongue, loss of sensitivity in these structures is extremely annoying to patients. When operating in these areas, the nerves should be isolated and retracted out of the way with umbilical tape. Since traction alone can produce transient sensory deficit, the patient should always be told of this as well as the possibility of more serious loss of sensation when surgery is contemplated in the region of the mental or lingual nerves.

Salivary Gland Ducts. The location of the parotid and submandibular salivary gland ducts must be taken into consideration when operating on the cheek or the floor of the mouth. If cut, the duct can be anastomosed over a small polyethylene tube kept in place for seven to 10 days. A more simple procedure, however, is to leave the wound loosely sutured and allow the proximal end of the duct to create a new opening at that point. When incisions are made in the region of the parotid or submandibular ducts, even if they are not involved in the surgical procedure, care must be taken to avoid encompassing these structures with the sutures used to close the wound since this will cause obstruction of the gland.

Influence of Muscle Pull on Intraoral Incisions

Making incisions parallel to the direction of muscle pull is only a consideration in the tongue and lips. In the cheek, where one would think muscle pull should be an important factor, decussation of the buccinator fibers distributes tension relatively equally in all directions so that incisions can be made in any desired location. The presence of the buccinator muscle, however, does provide a clearly delineated anatomic plane for governing depth when excising benign lesions of the cheek.

In the lip, when the lesion is large, cosmetic considerations may make it necessary to violate the principle of paralleling incisions to the direction of

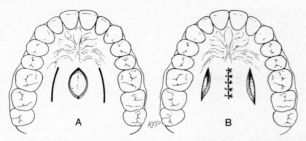

Figure 40–1. *A* and *B*, Closure of a palatal wound by the use of lateral relaxing incisions. The area of each secondary defect is less than that of the original wound, and therefore healing will be more rapid.

muscle pull. If vertical incisions extend across the mucocutaneous junction, suturing skin to skin and mucous membrane to mucous membrane is essential to produce an even lip line. A proper approximation is insured by placing the first superficial suture precisely at the mucocutaneous junction.

Influence of Relationship Between Soft Tissue and Bone

The close proximity of a large area of the oral mucosa to the underlying jaw bone is another factor modifying the management of oral lesions. In the excision of benign lesions arising from the overlying soft tissues, the periosteum and the bone provide distinct anatomic boundaries for determining the proper depth of the wound. On the palate and alveolar ridges, the proximity of the mucosa to the bone also influences the method of wound closure. The lack of elasticity of the thin submucosa in these regions results in a limited capacity for stretching, and incisions often cannot be closed even when undermining techniques are used. Such wounds generally are permitted to heal by secondary intention. If covering of the bone is desired or if hemostasis is a problem, Surgicel can be placed over the wound and held in position with a few transmucosal sutures.

When it is important to cover the area with mucosa, this can be accomplished by using a combination of undermining and relaxing incisions to permit a medial shift of the tissues (Fig. 40–1).

In other parts of the mouth, except the tongue, the submucosa is very elastic, and large defects can be closed simply by undermining the adjacent mucous membrane. Although this is not possible on the tongue, the underlying muscle will stretch sufficiently to permit most of these wounds to be closed primarily.

The close proximity of the jaws to the oral mucosa also influences the types of lesions seen in the oral cavity. In addition to those entities that arise from the mucous membrane, the submucosal tissues, and the minor salivary glands, there are soft tissue and osseous lesions arising within the underlying bone that may bulge into the oral cavity and resemble mucosal lesions. The former include various types of odontogenic and nonodontogenic cysts, ameloblastoma, central fibroma, central giant cell reparative granuloma, histiocytosis X, osteogenic sarcoma, and metastatic carcinoma (Fig. 40–2). Radiographs of the area are helpful in recognizing bone involvement and preventing inadequate surgical management.

Relationship of Teeth to Management of Oral Lesions

The presence of teeth plays an important role in determining how oral lesions will be treated. One must be aware of the fact that some lesions that appear to arise from the gingiva actually have their source in the periodontal ligament or adjacent alveolar bone. In such instances, removal of bone as well as soft tissue, and sometimes extraction of a tooth or teeth, is necessary to completely eradicate the lesion and prevent its recurrence. In this regard, the dermatologist also should be cognizant of the fact that infections arising from certain teeth can perforate extraorally and produce lesions on the

Figure 40–2. *A*, Central giant cell reparative granuloma appearing clinically as a gingival mass. *B*, Radiograph showing resorption of alveolar bone and displacement of teeth.

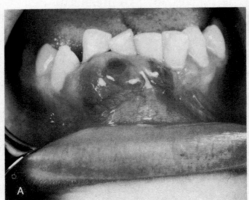
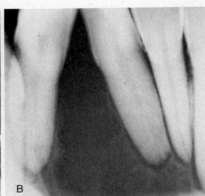

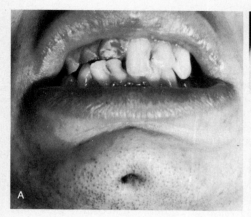

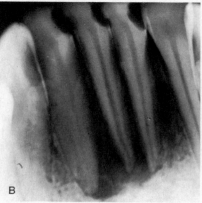

Figure 40-3. *A,* Chronic sinus tract in the skin caused by an infection from the lower teeth. *B,* Radiograph showing carious involvement of mandibular incisors and bone resorption caused by infection.

skin (Figs. 40–3 and 40–4). Such lesions cannot be managed successfully without either extracting the offending tooth or treating it endodontically.

PHYSIOLOGIC CONSIDERATIONS IN ORAL SURGERY

Blood Supply

The exceptional vascularity of the oral tissues provides a favorable environment for postsurgical repair. As previously mentioned, one seldom has to be concerned about compromising tissue healing as a result of interference with blood supply. The excellent blood supply also makes the tissues very resistant to infection. Although the mouth is a contaminated cavity, postoperative infections are rare unless there has been excessive trauma or if foreign organisms are inadvertently introduced by the surgeon. For this reason, prophylactic administration of antibiotics following oral surgery is seldom indicated.

Healing Rate of Oral Tissues

One of the favorable factors with intraoral surgery besides the excellent resistance of the tissues to infection is the rate of wound repair. Studies have

shown that the epithelial turnover in oral mucous membranes is much quicker than in skin.[1, 2] Clinically, this is reflected by a more rapid healing of surgical defects. This makes complete closure of oral wounds less important than skin wounds.

Another problem occurring on the skin, but not with mucous membrane, is the formation of heavy scars or keloids. Intraoral wounds generally heal with minimal scarring. When scars do develop, they usually become quite pliable within a few months. From a cosmetic standpoint, the presence of scars within the oral cavity obviously is not a problem.

Influence of Saliva

Although one might expect the presence of saliva to have an adverse effect on the healing of oral wounds, the reverse is actually true. The saliva not only has a cleansing action, but it also contains antibacterial substances that help prevent infection.[3, 4] Moreover, as demonstrated experimentally, moist wounds heal more rapidly than dry ones.[5]

The moist environment, however, does have an effect on treatment methods. Wounds produced by cauterization or electrocoagulation often have a tendency to become macerated. For this reason, excision of lesions with a scalpel or by electrosection is preferred.

The presence of saliva also influences the type of

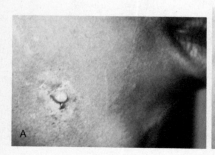

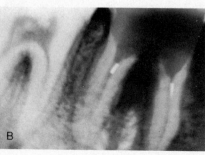

Figure 40-4. *A,* Pus draining from a sinus tract in the cheek. *B,* Radiograph showing the infected tooth causing the problem.

suture that should be used for final closure of intraoral wounds. Catgut sutures tend to become soft and untie very readily. Nonresorbable monofilament sutures, such as those made from nylon, also untie easily. Silk sutures are able to hold a knot well and are tolerated well by the tissues. However, they do have a tendency to accumulate debris. They also absorb fluid and therefore have a wicking effect that can result in bacteria being carried into the tissues. Polyglycolic acid sutures are tolerated best by the oral tissues. Although they are a polyfilament suture similar to silk, experiments have shown that they have less tendency to transmit organisms into the tissues.[6]

ANESTHESIA FOR ORAL SURGERY

Most soft tissue lesions in the oral cavity can be treated satisfactorily using local anesthesia. With extensive procedures or in uncooperative patients such as infants or children, however, a general anesthetic may be necessary. In these instances, nasotracheal intubation is preferred since it removes the endotracheal tube from the field and permits a gauze pack to be placed in the oropharynx to prevent aspiration of blood or foreign material. When cautery is to be used, a nonexplosive anesthetic agent must be selected.

An infiltration or field block technique can be used for local anesthesia. However, when injection in or near the lesion is to be avoided, or if it is undesirable to distort the tissues, a regional nerve block can be used. Description of the technique for such blocks can be found in any of the textbooks on dental anesthesia.[7]

A solution such as 1% lidocaine or mepivacaine with minimal concentrations of vasoconstrictor is generally employed. The vasoconstrictor is necessary not only for hemostasis but also to prevent the rapid absorption of the anesthetic agent. Because of the extreme vascularity of the oral tissues, absorption of anesthetic solutions can be very rapid, and toxic reactions may occur if excessive amounts are injected or if a vasoconstrictor is not used.

POSTOPERATIVE CONSIDERATIONS FOLLOWING ORAL SURGERY

Several considerations in the postoperative management of patients who have had intraoral procedures do not apply when surgery is performed in many other parts of the body. These relate mainly to the maintenance of diet and oral hygiene. The pain or discomfort that accompanies chewing and swallowing following oral surgery makes normal dietary intake very difficult. Such patients can become dehydrated very readily, and healing can be impaired. It is important, therefore, that adequate attention be given to maintaining proper nutrition and fluid balance. In the hospitalized patient, this can be accomplished with intravenous fluids to supplement oral intake. In the ambulatory patient, specific instructions should be given regarding the type and consistency of diet to be eaten. Soft, bland, nonchewy foods are tolerated best, and frequent small feedings are better than attempting to maintain a schedule of three meals daily. Immediately after surgery, a clear liquid diet may be preferable for a few days.

Maintaining cleanliness of the wound is another important consideration in promoting conditions for proper healing. The mouth should be rinsed at least four times daily, particularly after eating, with a solution containing a half-teaspoon of salt in a glass of warm water. Most proprietary mouthwashes contain alcohol and can be irritating to the surgical site. If hydrogen peroxide is used, it should be diluted to half-strength with water. In addition to rinsing, patients should be instructed, when possible, to brush their teeth as usual. The lips can be kept from drying by applying mineral oil, glycerine, or petroleum jelly.

The looseness of most of the oral tissues and their high degree of vascularity make them particularly

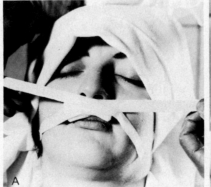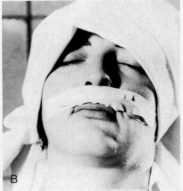

Figure 40–5. Application of an external pressure dressing to the upper lip using gauze and adhesive tape or Elastoplast. *A,* Crisscrossing of tape. *B,* Completed dressing. A similar technique can be used on the lower lip and chin. (From D. M. Laskin: The prevention of frequent complications in oral surgery. The Fortnightly Review of the Chicago Dental Society 35:5, 1958.)

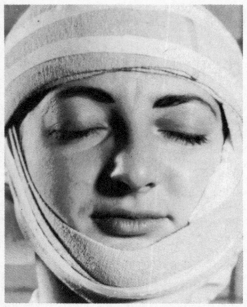

Figure 40–6. External pressure dressing to prevent swelling of the cheek.

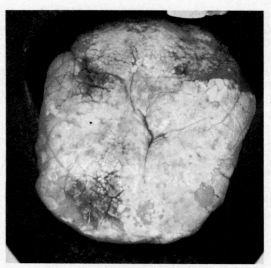

Figure 40–7. Severe leukoplakia of the tongue in a patient with tertiary syphilis.

susceptible to postoperative swelling. Such swelling not only adds to the difficulty in eating but also can cause dehiscence of the wound. Although pressure dressings cannot be applied directly to intraoral wounds, external pressure dressings can be used to limit swelling in the cheeks, lips, and gingival tissues (Figs. 40–5 and 40–6). Application of ice packs to the face, 30 minutes per hour during the first 24 to 48 hours after surgery, is also helpful in controlling swelling.

SPECIAL PROBLEMS IN ORAL SURGERY

As previously discussed, the treatment of most oral lesions requires only small modifications in the basic surgical techniques used on the skin. There are a number of lesions, however, that occur only in the oral cavity that require special attention in order to be treated successfully. Frequently, proper dental care plays an integral part in the management of these lesions.

Leukoplakia

Leukoplakia is a white lesion resulting from an altered maturation of the oral mucosa. Preferably, the term is used as a clinical diagnosis since histologically the changes may vary from a mild parakeratosis to a severe dyskeratosis.

Leukoplakic lesions can occur on any part of the oral mucosa as well as on the lips. They range from soft, milky areas to rough, leathery plaques that may become ulcerated. Although it has often been stated that the more roughened lesions are the most serious, there is no proven correlation between the character of the lesion and the incidence of premalignant change or malignant transformation. Some of the lesions that appear most innocuous clinically sometimes turn out to be the most serious. In fact, the small, slightly reddened lesions, referred to as erythroplasia, can be the most dangerous of all since the cellular changes in such lesions occur in the basilar layers rather than in the more superficial regions.

Chronic irritation from rough teeth or dental appliances, heavy smoking, and excessive alcohol intake are all factors that can predispose to leukoplakia. It is also seen occasionally in association with syphilitic glossitis (Fig. 40–7). In the latter instance, a positive diagnosis of syphilis does not eliminate the possibility that malignant transformation of a leukoplakia also may be present; the incidence of such transformation is actually greater in leukoplakia associated with tertiary syphilis than that caused by other factors.

Because leukoplakia is a precancerous lesion, definitive treatment should not be delayed for a long period of time. In early lesions, when the etiologic irritant is known and can be eliminated, the condition may reverse itself. If there has been no change after observation for 7 to 14 days, however, the lesion generally should be excised. Small lesions can be completely removed surgically. The specimen should include a border of normal mucosa and at least a portion of the submucosa. In most parts of the mouth, the adjacent mucous membrane then can be undermined and primary closure achieved. Diffuse leukoplakia can either be treated over a

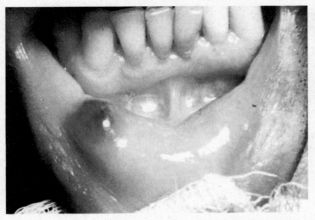

Figure 40–8. Mucocele of the lower lip caused by retention of mucus within the tissues.

period of time by multiple excisions or totally destroyed by electrocautery in a single operation. When the latter method is used, multiple biopsies should be taken to reduce the possibility of inadequately treating a carcinoma. In vivo staining with toluidine blue can be used in conjunction with clinical appearance as an aid in determining the proper biopsy sites.[8]

Mucocele (Mucous Retention Phenomenon)

A mucocele is neither a cyst nor a neoplasm. It results from the pouring of saliva from a ruptured minor salivary gland duct into the surrounding tissues where it becomes encapsulated and forms a bluish cyst-like lesion (Fig. 40–8). Mucoceles can occur almost anywhere in the oral cavity where mucous glands are found, but are seen most commonly in the lower lip, palate, and cheek.

Since a mucocele has a fibrous connective tissue capsule rather than an epithelial lining, removal of the lining is unnecessary. In fact, excision of the fluid-filled sac is not curative since it leaves behind the feeding gland. Proper treatment involves incision of the lesion and removal of the underlying mucous glands (Fig. 40–9). Visualization of the orbicularis oris in the lip and the buccinator muscle in the cheek serves as an indicator that the glands have been removed to the proper depth.

Ranula

A ranula is actually a mucocele arising from the sublingual gland in the floor of the mouth (Fig. 40–10). Treatment involves removal of the gland.[9] In performing the surgery, consideration must be given to preservation of the submandibular duct and avoiding injury to the lingual nerve.

Gingival Cyst

The etiology of this relatively rare lesion is not known. It has been suggested that they are actually implantation cysts.[10] Generally, they occur in the anterior part of the mouth, especially in the mandibular canine and premolar region. Clinically, they appear as a small bluish prominence in the papilla between the teeth. The radiograph usually shows a circumscribed radiolucency not associated with the

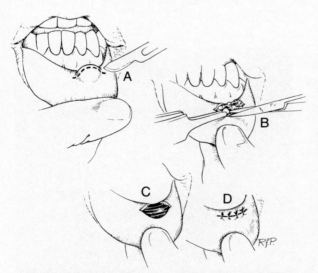

Figure 40–9. Technique for treatment of mucocele: *A*, Incision of the mucous membrane overlying the lesion. *B*, Removal of the underlying glands. *C*, Glands removed; the orbicularis oris muscle forms the base of the wound. *D*, Primary closure of the wound margins.

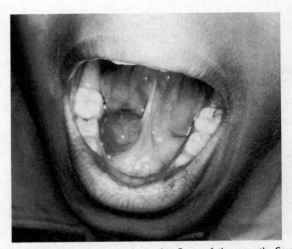

Figure 40–10. Large ranula in the floor of the mouth. Saucerization is not curative, since the lesion is a pseudocyst and will reform as the mucosa regenerates and the underlying gland continues to pour saliva into the tissues.

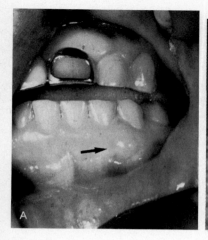

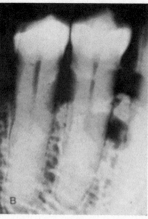

Figure 40–11. *A*, Gingival cyst (arrow) in mandibular canine region. *B*, Radiograph shows the resorption of bone caused by the pressure of the expanding lesion.

teeth (Fig. 40–11). When the cysts are small, they can be excised with the gingival papilla. Larger cysts are exposed by reflecting a mucosal flap and then are enucleated.

Eruption Cyst

Hemorrhage into the follicle of an erupting tooth gives rise to this bluish colored pseudocystic lesion that occurs on the crest of the alveolar ridge (Fig. 40–12). Usually, no treatment is indicated since they will rupture spontaneously as the tooth enters the oral cavity. However, if the child complains of pain or discomfort, the lesion can either be incised or marsupialized.

Fibrous Hyperplasia

This is one of the most common lesions found on the oral mucous membranes. It is not a neoplasm but merely a tissue reaction to chronic irritation. It may be sessile or pedunculated. Usually, it is relatively soft with a normal mucosal covering (Fig. 40–13). Occasionally, however, the surface may be white due to hyperkeratinization.

Treatment consists of simple surgical excision. The important thing to remember is that a sharp tooth or dental restoration, or an edentulous space into which the tissue is sucked, may be the causative agent, and the lesion will recur unless the condition is corrected.

Dilantin Hyperplasia

Epileptic patients on long-term Dilantin (phenytoin) therapy often develop gingival hyperplasia especially if they do not maintain proper oral hy-

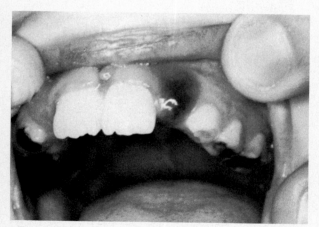

Figure 40–12. Eruption cyst over a maxillary incisor; the lesion usually feels fluctuant on palpation.

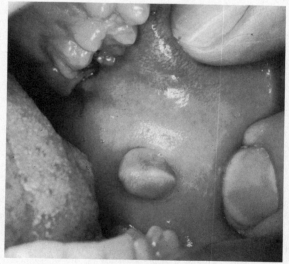

Figure 40–13. Fibrous hyperplasia of the buccal mucosa. The surface is slightly hyperkeratotic from rubbing against the teeth.

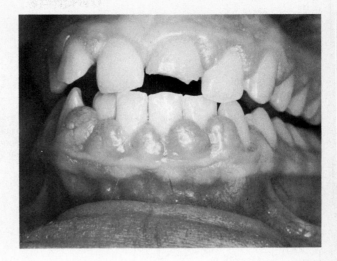

Figure 40–14. Dilantin hyperplasia of the gingiva. The condition tends to be worse in areas of poor oral hygiene. It often recurs gradually after surgical removal and must be retreated periodically.

giene (Fig. 40–14). Treatment requires special recontouring of the tissues after the excessive gingiva has been excised.[11] Preferably, this should be done by someone with dental training. Because poor oral hygiene is a predisposing factor, the lesion will recur rapidly unless proper periodontal care is maintained by the patient postoperatively.

Epulis Fissuratum (Denture Hyperplasia)

Irritation from ill-fitting dentures can lead to the formation of pendulous, lobulated, inflamed folds of tissue in the labial and buccal vestibule (Fig. 40–15). Since surgical excision and primary closure of the wound may significantly reduce vestibular depth and make wearing a denture difficult, the free mucosal edge is generally fastened at the height of the

vestibule with catgut mattress sutures, and the denuded periosteal surface is allowed to become re-epithelialized. To prevent recurrence of the lesion, either the old denture must be relined to produce an accurate fit or a new denture must be made.

Papillary Hyperplasia (Papillomatosis of the Palate)

Whereas freely movable mucosa usually forms relatively large hyperplastic masses when subjected to chronic irritation, the attached palatal mucosa forms multiple small nodules. Frequently, the tissue is very red and has a velvety feeling (Fig. 40–16). The condition is caused by accumulation of debris under a denture that is worn constantly without proper cleaning.

Since papillomatosis of the palate is a benign condition, complete removal of the mucosa down to the periosteum or bone, as sometimes recommended, is an inappropriate form of therapy. Much more rapid healing with less discomfort can be achieved by using mucoabrasion, a technique

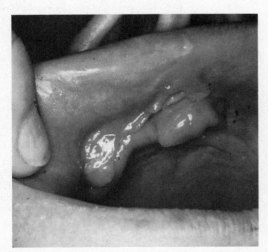

Figure 40–15. Large mass of hyperplastic tissue in the anterior maxillary vestibule resulting from a poorly fitting denture. The lesion may occasionally become ulcerated and painful.

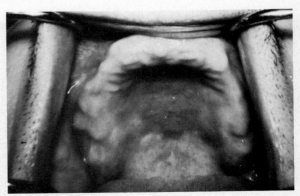

Figure 40–16. Papillary hyperplasia of the palate. The patient wore the denture constantly and failed to keep it clean.

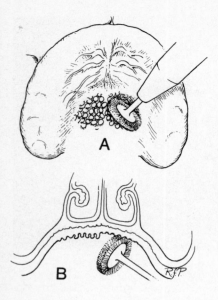

Figure 40–17. Treatment of papillary hyperplasia of the palate by mucoabrasion. *A*, Nodules are removed with a dermabrasion brush; care must be taken not to abrade the tissue too deeply and expose the underlying bone, since this prolongs the healing process. *B*, Coronal view showing the nodules removed and the remaining islands of mucosa.

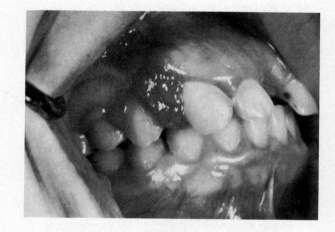

Figure 40–18. Pyogenic granuloma caused by food impaction between the teeth and improper oral hygiene. The patient's presenting complaint was recurrent gingival bleeding.

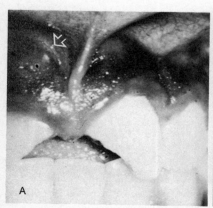
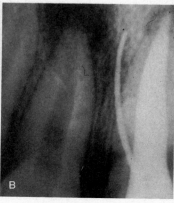

Figure 40–19. *A*, Sinus tract (arrow) over a fractured central incisor. *B*, Radiograph shows how chronic infection from the tooth produced bone resorption and led to the formation of a sinus tract.

similar to dermabrasion (Fig. 40–17). This procedure removes the hyperplastic tissue but retains the intervening normal mucosa so that palatal reepithelialization occurs within a week to 10 days. Postoperatively, the denture should be relined or remade, and proper oral hygiene should be encouraged.

Pyogenic Granuloma

When a gingival papilla between the teeth becomes irritated from calculus, an improperly contoured dental restoration, or food impaction, the tissue may ulcerate and become secondarily infected. Poor oral hygiene adds to the problem, and the chronic irritation leads to exuberant proliferation of highly vascular granulation tissue resembling a tumor. The lesions frequently occur in pregnant women where the associated hormonal changes predispose to gingival inflammation. In such cases, it is referred to as a pregnancy tumor.

The pyogenic granuloma has a purplish-red granular appearance. It is very friable and bleeds easily (Fig. 40–18). Proper treatment consists not only of surgical excision of the mass but also in the removal of calculus and institution of proper oral hygiene. In instances where the associated tooth or teeth have become extremely loose from alveolar bone resorption, extraction may be necessary.

Chronic Sinus Tract

This lesion clinically resembles a small pyogenic granuloma except that it occurs near the depth of the oral vestibule rather than at the gingival margin (Fig. 40–19). It is caused by chronic drainage of infection from the apex of an abscessed tooth. Excision of the exuberant granulation tissue will not effect a cure since it does not remove the causative factor. Instead, treatment should consist either of extraction of the offending tooth or endodontic therapy. Such procedures lead to spontaneous healing of the sinus tract.

REFERENCES

1. Meyer J, Medak H, Weinmann JP: Mitotic activity and rates in growth of regions of oral epithelium differing in width. Growth 24:29–46, 1960
2. Cutwright DE, Bauer H: Cell renewal in the oral mucosa and skin of the rat. Oral Surg 23:249–271, 1967
3. Jenkins GN: The Physiology and Biochemistry of the Mouth, Ed 4. Philadelphia, JB Lippincott Co, 1978, pp 340–343
4. Kraus FW, Sirisinha S: Gamma globulins in saliva. Arch Oral Biol 7:221, 1962
5. Winter GD: Movement of epidermal cells over the wound surface, in Montagna W, Bellingham RE: (eds): Advances in Biology of Skin, vol 5. New York, McMillan Co, 1964, pp 113–127
6. Lilly GE, Osbon DB, Hutchinson RA, Hefich RH: Clinical and bacteriologic aspects of polyglycolic acid sutures. J Oral Surg 31:103–105, 1973
7. Bennett CR: Local Anesthesia and Pain Control in Dentistry, Ed 7. St. Louis, CV Mosby, 1984
8. Niebel HH, Chomet B: In vivo staining test for delineation of oral intraepithelial neoplastic change: Preliminary report. JADA 68:801–806, 1964
9. Catone GA, Merrill RG, Henny FA: Sublingual gland mucous-escape phenomenon—treatment by excision of sublingual gland. J Oral Surg 27:774–786, 1969
10. Bhaskar SN, Laskin DM: Gingival cysts. Oral Surg 8:863–867, 1955
11. Goldman HM, Cohen DW: Periodontal Therapy, Ed 6. St. Louis, CV Mosby, 1980, pp 1056–1064

41

ROBERT W. KISTNER, M.D.

The Surgical Treatment of Lesions of the Vulva

The vulva, or external female genitalia, includes the following structures: labia majora, labia minora, clitoris, vestibule, hymen, vestibular bulbs, mons veneris, urethral meatus, vulvovaginal glands, and paraurethral ducts. The outer portion of the vulva is covered by somewhat altered skin that contains hair follicles and sweat and sebaceous glands. This is modified on the inner surface so that the inner portions of the labia minora are moist and do not contain hair follicles. The vulva serves as the entrance to the vagina and, in the normal state, covers and protects the urethral orifice. The labia have specific importance in the process of urination since it has been found that, following vulvectomy, uncontrolled "spraying" is a common complaint.

The anatomic location of the vulva predisposes its structures to unusual and occasionally rare disorders. At the same time, systemic diseases such as diabetes, amemia, Addison's disease, and gout may manifest themselves first by vulvar changes and complaints therefrom. The importance of veneral diseases as a major cause of symptomatology from these structures is obvious. Since a good portion of the vulvar area may be properly classified as skin, it is at once evident that any specific cutaneous disease may occur here; but because of certain variations, diagnosis may be difficult or even impossible. Difficulty in diagnosis is aggravated by the tendency of the patient to procrastinate and to utilize self-medication when the lesion involves the genitalia. Patient delay is of extreme importance when the disease is malignant since carcinoma involving these structures has a poor prognosis unless discovered early. Of equal importance is the physician's responsibility. Numerous studies have shown that "physician delay" may actually exceed "patient delay" by many months.

The diagnosis and treatment of lesions of the vulva is successful only if the physician completely investigates all possible etiologic factors and performs a meticulous examination. A thorough interview should determine the exact site and duration of specific complaints as well as generalized symptoms. Inquiry should be made about diarrhea or discharge; applications of lotions, medications, or soaps; systemic medications; contraceptives; sexual habits; clothing changes; and, of major importance, events that might be causative in producing mental stress, worry, or anxiety. The examiner should scrutinize closely the oral mucosa, fingernails, scalp, and pubic hair as part of the gynecologic examination. It is not sufficient to allay symptoms, since recurrence is commonplace. Therefore, the cause of the disorder must be found and specific therapy instituted.

THE KRAUROSIS-LEUKOPLAKIA COMPLEX

Medicine has been plagued for decades with confusing terminology due, in large part, to the perpetuation of error and the tenacity of clinicians to cling to terminology because of long association. Such is the case with certain so-called precancerous dermatoses of the vulva, occasionally labeled the "leukokraurosis complex." Confusion of terminology in this group of vulvar diseases dates from 1885 when the first cases of leukoplakic vulvitis were associated with marked sclerosis and narrowing of the vaginal outlet. The constriction was thought to be an essential feature of the disease, so that the term "kraurosis" (to shrivel up) was applied. This was unfortunate since kraurosis, like pruritus, is only a symptom, not a disease. Leukoplakia, by prolonged usage of the term, is a disease entity with specific histologic characteristics. Although the term really means "white plaque," its present connotation is much broader since white plaques may be present in several chronic dermatoses or even in kraurosis. As will be seen, microscopic leukoplakia bears a definite relationship to the development of vulvar carcinoma, and it may or may not be associated with a kraurotic vulva. Stated simply, many sclerosing vulvar diseases may be accompanied by kraurosis, but unless true leukoplakia supervenes, the malignant potential is small. With the hope of simplification, the following classification has been suggested: (1) simple kraurosis, (2) lichen sclerosus et atrophicus, (3) leukoplakia, and (4) carcinoma in situ.

Simple Kraurosis

Simple kraurosis of the vulva is a primary sclerosing atrophy limited to the labia minora, vestibule, urethra, and clitoris. It occurs most commonly in postmenopausal women. Usually, the labia majora, perineum, and perianal regions are not involved. In early stages, the skin may be red and glistening with isolated dark red or dull purple patches (kraurosis rouge). In later stages, the skin becomes pale yellow and has a smooth glistening surface, obliterated labial folds, atrophic mons veneris, and scanty broken-off pubic hairs. The vaginal orifice is narrowed and barely admits the index finger.

Histologically, there is hyperkeratosis (excess keratin above the epithelium) with flattening of the rete ridges, edema, and homogenization of the cutis collagen, separation of the elastic fibers, and mild arteriosclerotic changes in the deeper blood vessels. Simple kraurosis bears no known relationship to carcinoma of the vulva.

Leukoplakia

Leukoplakia may be defined as a chronic inflammatory condition, affecting either the entire vulva or a small part thereof, characterized by the formation of whitish plaques of thickened epidermis with sclerosis of the subjacent connective tissue and by the absence of elastic fibers, producing a parchment-like consistency of the skin (Fig. 41–1). Another requisite is various epithelial cellular changes including parakeratosis, dyskeratosis, and atypism. The plaques may be single or multiple, and sometimes bluish areas are found on the inner surfaces of the labia, around the clitoris, and on the perineum. Generally, leukoplakia does not involve the outer surfaces of the labia or anal area. The diagnosis can be made definitely only by microscopic

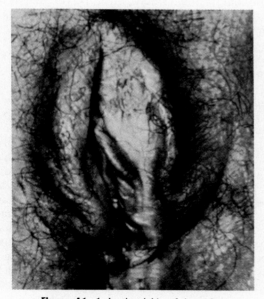

Figure 41–1. Leukoplakia of the vulva.

examination, and even then, the failure to appreciate certain histologic details has led to incorrect diagnoses. The most common errors have been in designating simple kraurosis or lichen sclerosus as a leukoplakic lesion. Because of the precancerous implication of this diagnosis, many unnecessary vulvectomies have probably been performed. In order to select biopsy sites, the vulva should be painted with toluidine blue and then washed with acetic acid. Areas retaining the blue stain should be sampled.

In about 90% of the cases of leukoplakic vulvitis, there is pronounced itching, whereas in the other 10%, only a feeling of burning, chafing, or discomfort is present. The exact relationship of vulvar carcinoma to leukoplakia is unknown, although Taussig wrote in 1926 a very pointed opinion: "I believe it [leukoplakia] will inevitably proceed to the development of cancer, but the rate at which this change takes place may be so slow that death supervenes before its accomplishment."[1] He therefore recommended surgical excision of the entire vulva including perineal and perianal skin for all cases of leukoplakia. That this will not completely prevent vulvar cancer is evident from the cases reported to have developed in recurrent areas of leukoplakia which, by definition, is a hypertrophic process. (Previous classifications of an atrophic type were usually lichen sclerosus.) It may develop in the previously mentioned sclerosing atrophy diathesis, in simple senile atrophy, or in normal vulvar skin. The process of its development has been described as similar to that of a senile keratosis on a mucous membrane—in other words, precancerous.

The important histologic changes are believed to be in the epithelium in the form of hyperkeratosis, acanthosis, dyskeratosis, cellular atypism, and absence of polarity. Some surface differentiation may be present. This is at variance with the opinion of Taussig, who believed the important changes to be the loss of elastic tissue in the dermis.[1] Changes of increasing degrees of anaplasia, ranging from dysplastic leukoplakia through Bowen-like dyskeratosis to carcinoma in situ and finally to microinvasive carcinoma, explain the pathogenesis of vulvar carcinoma from this entity.

The incidence of vulvar carcinoma in situ is increasing in younger patients. The etiologic importance of herpes simplex virus type II in cancer of the cervix is well established, and an association between vulvar and cervical malignancy has been suggested. Patients with in situ or invasive cervical cancer should be carefully screened for vulvar atypias.

From the literature, it has been apparent that the tendency for leukoplakia to develop into carcinoma is great, varying from 23.1%[2] to 50%.[1,3] The author's own experience at the Boston Hospital for Women can be cited. An adequate follow-up of three to 25 years was available on 35 patients with what was considered to be definite leukoplakia. Seventeen had some form of excision; in seven of these, either there was no improvement or a recurrence developed. Six of the seven patients were reoperated upon. In three of the original 35 patients (8.5%) squamous cell carcinoma developed. A safe conclusion seems to be that many (and perhaps most) squamous cell carcinomas of the vulva arise in true leukoplakia (not lichen sclerosus), but figures are not available to state in what percent of vulvar leukoplakias (treated or untreated) carcinoma will develop.

Treatment is variable depending on the extent of the disease and the symptomatology. Simple destruction by electrodesiccation or wide excision suffices if the lesion is small. If widespread, simple vulvectomy is indicated, but this should be extensive since the recurrence rate is high. The importance of proper diagnosis of a premalignant lesion of the vulva is evident, and follow-up examinations with repeated biopsies of suspicious areas are the only means of prophylaxis against cancer.

BENIGN NEOPLASMS

The most common benign neoplasms of the vulva are papillomas, lipomas, fibromas, and hidradenomas. Less common are neurofibromas, lymphangiomas, hemangiomas, and myxomas.

Papilloma

The dermal papilloma may occur on the vulva as a brown benign skin tumor of verrucous type. It may be single or multiple, and histologically, it shows striking hyperkeratosis with acanthosis and elongation of the rete ridges. Although the proper name for this lesion is nevus verrucosus, nevus cells are not present in the usual case. It is cured by simple excision.

A more common type of papilloma is condyloma acuminatum (venereal wart). These lesions should not be confused with condyloma latum, the lesion of secondary syphilis. They are frequently associated with chronic vaginal discharge, such as from trichomoniasis or moniliasis, and are benign epithelial growths of viral origin. Their size varies from 0.5 mm to 1 to 2 cm, and they tend to be grouped in clusters. If extensive, a cauliflower-like appearance is evident. During pregnancy, they enlarge rapidly and may occasionally completely fill the vagina and cover the labia, whereas during the puerperium, regression occurs. The histologic appearance is characteristic although, on occasion, a close similarity to a papillary squamous cell carcinoma is present. There is light thickening of the stratum corneum

epidermidis with extensive parakeratosis, marked acanthosis, and papillomatosis with thickening and elongation of the rete ridges. This gives an arborescent pattern on low power. Cells of the rete Malpighi demonstrate intracellular edema with a fairly large number of mitoses. However, the cellular pattern is orderly, polarity is retained, and the junction of the epidermis and corium is sharp—all of which differentiate this lesion from early carcinoma. The corium contains many dilated blood vessels and a dense infiltration of lymphocytes and plasma cells.

Diagnosis is usually evident on gross inspection, but biopsy should be done in atypical cases or if the lesion does not respond to treatment. If the lesions are small or scanty, the local application of 25% podophyllin in mineral oil or sandarac varnish may result in rapid disappearance. If the lesions are extensive, electrocoagulation is preferable to simple excision since the base may be lightly touched with the cautery as the lesion is removed. Although condylomata acuminata are generally believed to be benign, several recent reports have noted the development of vulvar carcinoma in such lesions.

Lipoma

This benign tumor arises from the fatty tissue of the labia majora or mons veneris and usually grows slowly and causes no symptoms except when its size is excessive. When this occurs, the mass acquires a pedicle and hangs from the groin or vulva. If the pedicle is wide, it may resemble a hernia. Some lipomas have attained gigantic size, but the usual one is not larger than 10 to 12 cm. The histologic appearance is that of normal fat cells with a connective tissue framework and capsule. The incidence of liposarcoma is extremely rare. Nevertheless, the lesion should be excised since difficulty in walking or in coitus eventually occurs.

Fibroma

This lesion usually develops as a firm nodule on the labia majora that then enlarges, develops a pedicle, and may hang down for several inches (or feet) so that ulceration and necrosis of the distal portion may occur. The histologic picture is that of any dermatofibroma, with a well-circumscribed lesion made up of intertwined collagen bundles and fibroblasts. In rare cases, the number of nuclei is excessive so that a suspicion of fibrosarcoma is raised. The circumscription of the lesion and absence of mitotic figures and giant cells are usually sufficient to indicate a benign condition. These lesions should be surgically removed both for cosmetic effect and for their malignant potential even though it may be small.

Hidradenoma

This is a benign, slow-growing, sweat gland tumor, whose histology simulates that of an adenocarcinoma. It is usually about 1 to 2 cm in diameter with a slightly raised, brown surface that may be umbilicated. This lesion may become quite large, and cystic change may occur. Histologically, this is an adenoma of the vulvar apocrine glands. It is not connected with the epidermis and is usually well encapsulated. The basic pattern is that of a cyst-like space in which numerous interlacing villous structures project. These structures as well as the wall of the cyst, are lined by a single layer of high cylindrical cells with eosinophilic cytoplasm and a large, oval, pale-staining nucleus. The cells are regular, and no anaplasia or atypism is evident. A characteristic finding is the layer of myoepithelial cells under the secretory cylindrical cells—a finding similar to that of apocrine tumors in the mammary gland. The lesion is almost always benign, but since few hidradenocarcinomas have been reported, all should be excised and submitted to pathologic examination.

MALIGNANT NEOPLASMS

This broad terminology includes a variety of lesions of separate structure, the most common and most important of which are the squamous cell carcinomas of the labia majora, labia minora, and vestibule. Other lesions, fortunately rare, are carcinoma of the clitoris, adenocarcinoma of the Bartholin glands, adenocarcinoma of the sweat glands, sarcomas, melanosarcomas, teratomas, and Paget's disease. The entire group is said to account for about 1% of all cancers in the female (1.4% of all primary malignant tumors at the Boston Hospital for Women) and for 5% to 10% of all cancers involving the female genitalia.

Carcinoma

Vulvar cancer (Fig. 41–2) usually occurs in postmenopausal women; about 70% of the author's patients are between 51 and 70 years old, with an average age of 61.6 years. Youth does not afford complete protection, however, since Way has reported 18 patients between 21 and 40 years of age.[4] Although postmenopausal bleeding will frequently bring the patient to the physician for examination, abnormalities of the vulva go unnoticed or, if discovered, are self-treated for long periods. A dangerous modesty seems to prevail, which accounts for serious patient delay. Added to this is the unexplained hesitancy of many physicians to biopsy vulvar lesions when they are first seen and when opportunity for cure is best. Many months are lost, during which time ointments, salves, lotions, and other medications are unsuccessfully tried.

It has become apparent that vulvar carcinoma is not only a disease of the aged but that, as age advances, the incidence of the disease rapidly increases. As the proportion of elderly individuals increases in our population, an ever-growing number of vulvar carcinomas will be seen. Thus, the importance of diminishing the patient delay is obvious if increased salvage is to be realized.

The correlation of leukoplakia, carcinoma in situ, and invasive carcinoma has been discussed. It should be reiterated that intelligent observation and treatment of leukoplakia should materially aid in lowering the incidence and mortality rate of vulvar cancer. In most series in which this correlation has been determined, leukoplakia preceded carcinoma in 12% to 40% of the cases. However, Hunt followed 95 patients with leukoplakia and found that carcinoma developed in only five; and in the author's series at the Boston Hospital for Women, follow-up of 35 patients with definite leukoplakia revealed that only three subsequently had invasive cancer. Other vulvar diseases such as granulomas and virus-induced condylomas have also been found to predispose a patient to the development of a malignancy. Factors such as family history, parity, marital history, and race do not predispose one to the development of malignancy. In a study of chronic dermatoses both with and without sclerosis, McAdams and Kistner were not able to indict any of these lesions as being precancerous. It is of interest, however, to note that 6% to 7% of all vulvar carcinomas occur in patients who have another primary carcinoma, usually in the breast, cervix, or urethra.

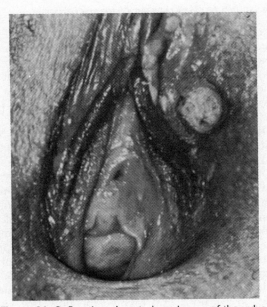

Figure 41–2. Everting ulcerated carcinoma of the vulva.

The symptoms complained of most commonly are a localized mass or lump, painful ulcer, discharge, vulvar irritation, dysuria, or bleeding. The duration of symptoms in some series has been as long as three or four years, but in the cases analyzed at the Boston Hospital for Women, it was 13.8 months. Physical examination reveals the lesion to be extremely variable in appearance since, in its early form, it may merely be an elevated papule or small ulcer. The lesion may be a typical everting, ulcerating mass, or it may be hypertrophic and resemble a papilloma. Another variety is the nonulcerating, superficial type that produces severe edema and a peau d'orange effect. About two thirds of the lesions are found on the labia majora and the remainder on the labia minora, clitoris, and posterior commissure. The majority of carcinomas are confined to the anterior half of the vulva, including the clitoris, and in most cases, the external skin surfaces are far more commonly involved than are the medial surfaces of the labia.

Diagnosis is usually obvious except in very early and nonulcerated lesions. Condylomata acuminata, papillomas, ulcerated chancroid, gummas, and tuberculous ulcers may be confusing, but biopsy, Gram's stain, and serologic tests will aid in the final diagnosis. The histology is usually that of a moderately well-differentiated, grade I or grade II squamous cell carcinoma. Way, however, found a rather large number of his cases to be of the anaplastic type and stated that these lesions were rapidly growing and rapidly metastasizing.[4] In early lesions, the microscopic pattern is that of irregular masses of epidermal cells invading the corium. These masses are composed of differentiated squamous and horn cells and dedifferentiated (atypical or anaplastic) squamous cells. Such anaplasia is expressed by variation in size and shape of the cells, hyperplasia and hyperchromasia of nuclei, loss of polarity, absence of prickles, keratinization of certain cells, presence of mitotic figures, and particularly atypical and bizarre mitoses. Differentiation is evident as an increased tendency toward keratinization with the formation of "pearls" composed of concentric layers of squamous cells with increased cornification toward the center. In the Boston Hospital for Women series, 21% were classified as grade I tumors, 68% as grade II, and 11% as grade III.

Clinical staging of carcinoma of the vulva is important, since it refers to the degree of extension of the disease as determined by physical or x-ray examination. It is obvious that survival should be directly correlated with this staging, and this is true not only of carcinoma of the vulva but also of the cervix, breast, and endometrium. A workable clinical staging has been proposed by McKelvey:

Stage I   Tumor is 10 cm² or less.
Stage II   Tumor is more than 10 cm².

Stage III   Tumor of any size that also involves surrounding structures, such as urethra, vagina, anus, or rectum.
Stage IV   Tumor of any size with clinically demonstrable intra-abdominal or other distant metastases.

In 1971, the General Assembly of the International Federation of Gynecology and Obstetrics (FIGO) approved the recommendations of the cancer committee for a new classification and staging system.

Clinical Stages of Carcinoma of the Vulva

Stage 0. Carcinoma in situ.
Stage I. Tumor confined to vulva—2 cm or less in diameter. Nodes are not palpable or are palpable in either groin, not enlarged, and mobile (but not clinically suspicious of neoplasm).
Stage II. Tumor confined to the vulva—more than 2 cm in diameter. Nodes are not palpable or are palpable in either groin, not enlarged, and mobile (but not clinically suspicious of neoplasm).
Stage III. Tumor of any size with: (1) adjacent spread to the urethra and any or all of the vagina, the perineum, and the anus and/or (2) nodes palpable in either or both groins (enlarged, firm and mobile, not fixed, but clinically suspicious of neoplasm).
Stage IV. Tumor of any size: (1) infiltrating the bladder mucosa or the rectal mucosa or both, including the upper part of the urethral mucosa, and/or (2) fixed to the bone or other distant metastases. There are also fixed or ulcerated nodes in either or both groins.

Tumor-Node-Metastasis Nomenclature

Primary Tumor (T). T1S, T1, T2, T3, and T4 (see corresponding FIGO stages).
Nodal (N) Involvement. NX, not possible to assess the regional nodes; N0, no involvement of regional nodes; N1, evidence of regional node involvement; N3, fixed or ulcerated nodes; N4, juxtaregional node involvement.
Distant Metastasis (M). MX, not assessed; M0, no (known) distant metastasis; M1, distant metastasis present.

Dissemination of vulvar carcinoma is usually by way of lymphatic metastases, probably by tumor emboli rather than by direct permeation. The most common route of spread is via the superficial inguinal nodes to the node of Cloquet (the most superior deep femoral node that lies in the upper portion of the femoral canal under the inguinal ligament) and from there to the external iliac nodes. Lesions of the clitoris drain directly into Cloquet's node, and lesions that involve the posterior vulva and lower vagina may also bypass the superficial and deep inguinal nodes and drain directly into the external iliac nodes. It is important to realize that contralateral and bilateral spread may occur with a unilateral lesion, so that a bilateral node dissection should be done if surgery is performed. Furthermore, negative findings in superficial nodes do not necessarily mean that the deep nodes are not involved. This situation is more common with lesions involving the posterior labia, posterior vestibule, and clitoris. A summation of many reported series shows that involved lymph nodes are found in 55% to 60% of all cases.

The natural history of vulvar cancer is, in general, that of a slowly growing lesion with spread to the groin and pelvic nodes and with localization in these areas for long periods. Remote metastases are not common until late in the disease when blood-borne spread may occur. If untreated, there is a subsequent fungating, ulcerative process that destroys the vulva, urethra, and anus, resulting in painful fistulas. Death may occur from ulceration of large blood vessels, from sepsis, or from widespread metastases.

Ideals of treatment must emphasize prophylaxis, early diagnosis, and early, complete therapy. Although isolated reports have suggested certain dyes, fibers, 3-methylcholanthrene, and smegma as carcinogens, no definite evidence exists to support this. Recently, a correlation between vulvar cancer and cigarette smoking has been noted. It was suggested that carcinogenic agents present on the fingers of habitual smokers may be transferred to the labia and act as a local irritant.

The role of scratching, or other trauma, is uncertain since carcinoma is not a sequela of the chronic dermatoses in which pruritus is present. The importance of leukoplakia has been emphasized, and it should be treated as a premalignant state. Chronic discharges, granulomas, syphilis, or condylomas should receive prompt and thorough attention. The important point is that any vulvar lesion should be biopsied, watched carefully, and rebiopsied whenever necessary. Recent reports have indicated that up to 35% of the patients with vulvar cancer also show dysplasia, carcinoma in situ, or invasive cancer of the cervix. Thus, careful screening is indicated in these patients.

Definitive therapy in most cases is surgical, and despite the age of the patients, a single-stage radical vulvectomy and bilateral groin resection is almost always possible. The operability rate varies from 50% to 90% and depends on the stage of the lesion and the courage of the surgeon. (It has been 83% at the Boston Hospital for Women.) The operation is extensive, although superficial, and to be complete, resection should include the mons veneris, groin, and inner thigh down to the muscle and fascia, together with the inguinal, femoral, and external iliac nodes and the upper 5 to 7 cm of the greater saphenous veins. No attempt is made to preserve the inguinal ligaments or the deep epigastric vessels in the adequate exposure of the deep nodes that are situated anterior and medial to the external iliac vein. The skin flaps may usually be pulled together under moderate tension, but Way insists that, if this is possible, an adequate amount of tissue has not been removed.[4] Necrosis over the symphysis almost always occurs and may require secondary grafting if the defect is extensive.

Five-year survival depends on the stage of the disease and, therefore, on the incidence of node involvement. In the series at the Boston Hospital for Women, only 7% of patients who had nodal metastases survived five years, whereas without metastases, the survival rate was 90%. McKelvey reported an 86% operability rate, an absolute five-year cure rate of 44.4%, with an 8% mortality rate.[5] Way has reported an 87% operability rate, with an operative mortality rate of 14.6%.[4] The five-year survival rate in patients surviving the operation was 90%. The average five-year survival of 286 patients who had radical vulvectomy and lymphadenectomy (reported by five authors) was 65.2%. In those patients in whom the lymph nodes were negative, the five-year survival was 83%. Extension of the disease to the vagina, urethra, or rectum indicates a grave prognosis, although ultraradical surgery to include partial or total exenteration may increase the survival rate in this group.

X-ray and radium are not used as primary therapy unless the disease is so extensive that surgery is not technically feasible. In such patients, judicious use of radium may be of great palliative value. Diathermy coagulation may be used as palliation in large, bulky tumors that distort the vulva and adjacent orifices.

OTHER VULVAR MALIGNANCIES

Carcinoma of Bartholin's glands is a rare finding, and its treatment is that suggested for other carcinomas. It may be mistaken for a benign tumor or a chronic bartholinitis because of its location. A high degree of malignancy exists because of the rich drainage of the gland lymphatics into the deep as well as the superficial lymphatics. Only 109 cases of this entity have been reported, with only nine patients living without disease at the end of five years. About one half of the tumors were adenocarcinoma, one third were squamous cell carcinoma, and the rest were mixed or undifferentiated.

Basal cell carcinoma of the vulva is also rare—just over 100 cases have been reported. It tends to recur locally rather than to spread by lymphatic and blood channels but, unlike basal cell carcinomas elsewhere on the skin, the prognosis is poor. There is some evidence that these tumors do not arise from the basal cells of the epidermis but from hair sheaths or distorted primordia of dermal adnexae. Lever believes them to be nevoid tumors derived from arrested, embryonal, primary epithelial germ cells. No relationship between leukoplakia and basal cell carcinoma has been demonstrated. Treatment should include a wide and deep local excision, best performed as a unilateral vulvectomy.

Only about 30 cases of sarcoma of the vulva have been reported. This tumor may arise from the connective tissue of the vulva or from a fibroma. Several cases of reticulum cell sarcoma and lymphosarcoma have recently been added to the literature. The prognosis is poor despite radical surgery. Melanomas are malignant tumors arising from a lentigo or pigmented nevus and characterized by a gradually enlarging, deeply pigmented nodule that is usually surrounded by an erythematous area (Fig. 41–3). Later on, the lesion ulcerates and satellites may appear. Since most melanomas involve the anterior vulvar structures, clitoral involvement is common, and lymphatics from this region drain directly to the deep pelvic nodes. Metastases occur first through lymphatics with involvement of adjacent nodes. Invasion of the bloodstream is a late event, but when it occurs, widespread metastases appear. Treatment should be radical vulvectomy and bilateral groin dissection unless distant metastases have been demonstrated.

Paget's disease of the vulva merits mention as a possible precancerous or early malignant lesion (Fig. 41–4). As a disorder of the mammary gland, it is a well-known entity, having been described by James

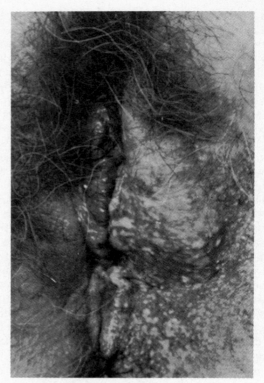

Figure 41–4. Paget's disease of the vulva.

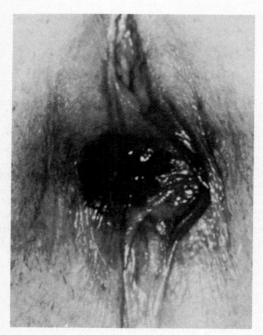

Figure 41–3. Melanoma of the vulva.

Paget in 1874. It is accepted that mammary Paget's disease is a primary duct cancer that has extended to the epidermis where it causes a cutaneous lesion. Woodruff, however, feels that Paget's disease of the vulva is an intraepithelial lesion and that Paget's cells arise de novo in the epithelium or in its appendages. It is possible that this lesion may progress to invasive carcinoma in much the same fashion as Bowen's disease if one accepts the histogenesis as being autochthonous, as suggested by Woodruff.[6, 7] Huber, in describing three new cases of vulvar Paget's disease, found a definite adenocarcinoma of the underlying apocrine sweat glands in one.[8] The fact remains that, even if a subjacent or adjacent apocrine carcinoma is not discovered, this by no means rules out the possibility that Paget's cells may have arisen therein. Another apocrine adenocarcinoma, carcinoma of the breast, has been reported in 14 patients with vulvar Paget's disease.[9] Therefore, mammography is indicated in all patients with vulvar Paget's disease.

In the vulva, the lesion occurs in women in the later decades of life whose presenting complaint is usually pruritis. Its macroscopic appearance is sharply demarcated, florid, red, and moist with occasional crusting. Little islands of whitened skin appear between the reddened areas (Fig. 41–4). The entire vulva may be involved, with spread to the perineum, mons, and thighs. The histologic appearance is characteristic. There is acanthosis with elongation and widening of the rete ridges. Paget's cells may be scattered or grouped in clusters, usually in the basalis. They are large cells, lacking prickles, and are surrounded by clear spaces. The cytoplasm is very light, and the nuclei are large, round, and pale. Paget's cells do not invade the corium, a fact that argues somewhat against their intraepithelial origin. Treatment should be a wide and deep excision with careful follow-up, despite the long interval that usually elapses before definitive treatment is employed. Bilateral pelvic lymphadenectomy is not usually employed as adjunctive therapy for Paget's disease of the vulva. Because local recurrences are common, repeated observations and biopsy of suspicious areas are suggested.

REFERENCES

1. Taussig FJ: Leukoplakia vulvitis and cancer of the vulva. Am J Obstet Gynecol 18:472, 1929
2. Miller NF, Riley GM, Stanley M: Leukoplakia of vulva: II. Am J Obstet Gynecol 64:768, 1952
3. Taussig FJ: Leukoplakia and cancer of vulva. Arch Dermatol Syph 21:431, 1930
4. Way SC: Carcinoma of the vulva. Am J Obstet Gynecol 76:692, 1960
5. McKelvey JL: Carcinoma of the vulva. Am J Obstet Gynecol 5:452, 1955
6. Woodruff JD, Hildebrandt EE: Carcinoma in situ of the vulva. Am J Obstet Gynecol 12:414, 1958
7. Woodruff JD, Novack ER: Premalignant lesions of the vulva: A pathological and clinical survey. Clin Obstet Gynecol 5:1102, 1962
8. Huber CP, Gardiner SH, Michael A: Paget's disease of the vulva. Am J Obst Gynecol 62:778, 1951
9. Friedrich EG, Wilkinson EJ, Steingraeber PH, Lewis JD: Paget's disease of the vulva and carcinoma of the breast. Obst Gynecol 46:130, 1975

SUGGESTED READINGS

Green TH, Ulfelder H, Meigs JV: Epidermoid carcinoma of the vulva. Am J Obstet Gynecol 75:834, 1958
Hertig AT, Gore H: Tumors of the Female Sex Organs: Part 2. Tumors of the Vulva, Vagina and Uterus. Washington D.C., Armed Forces Institute of Pathology, 1960
Jeffcoate TNA, Davie TB, Harrison CV: Intra-epidermal carcinoma (Bowen's disease) of vulva: Report on 2 cases. J Obstet Gynaecol Br Emp 51:377, 1944
Kindler T: Lichen sclerosus et atrophicus in young subjects. Br J Dermatol 65:269, 1953
Kottmeier HL: Carcinoma of the female genitalia. The Abraham Flexner Lecture Series, no. 11. Baltimore, Williams & Wilkins, 1953
Langley II, Hertig AT, Smith GV: Relation of leukoplakic vulvitis to squamous carcinoma of vulva. Am J Obstet Gynecol 62:167, 1951
Lever WF: Histopathology of the Skin. Ed 4. Philadelphia, Lippincott, 1967
McAdams AJ Jr, Kistner RW: The relationship of chronic vulvar disease, leukoplakia and carcinoma in situ to carcinoma of the vulva. Cancer 11:740, 1958
Newell JW, McKay DG: Clinical review of carcinoma of vulva. West J Surg 60:388, 1952
Pund ER, Cole WC: Carcinoma of Bartholin's gland. Am J Obstet Gynecol 43:887, 1942
Rubin AR: Granular-cell myoblastoma of the vulva. Am J Obstet Gynecol 77:292, 1959
Ulfelder H: Radical vulvectomy with bilateral inguinal, femoral, and iliac node dissection. Am J Obstet Gynecol 78:1074, 1959

42

GEORGE R. MIKHAIL, M.D. / RIAD N. FARAH, M.D.

Surgery of the Skin of the Male Genitalia

The phallus has symbolized since ancient times the generative power in nature. This is well depicted in an engraving in an ancient Egyptian temple that depicts Min, the god of fertility (Fig. 42–1).

The diseases that may involve the skin of the male genitalia and that may require surgical intervention are broadly classified into four categories: (1) benign lesions, (2) premalignant conditions and carcinomas in situ, (3) pseudomalignancies, and (4) malignant neoplasms.

BIOPSIES

In no other part of the body is histopathologic diagnosis of cutaneous lesions as important as when the genital area is involved. Because many of the diseases that affect the genitals closely mimic one another, the importance of tissue diagnosis cannot be overstressed so that premalignant and malignant lesions may be detected and treated at an early stage.

Biopsies can be easily performed in this area. When the tissue is to be obtained from the prepuce, the shaft of the penis, or the scrotum, excision through an elliptical incision is recommended. The edges of the wounds can be easily approximated with sutures because of the loose subcutaneous tissues in these areas. The direction of the long axis of the incision should be, whenever possible, across the shaft of the penis in order to minimize tension on the suture line in case of an erection. Since there is only a very thin fibrous tissue layer between the mucosa of the glans penis and the corpus cavernosum, suturing of the wound is usually not feasible. A superficial excision with the knife cutting in a slanted direction through the mucosa of the glans and the outermost part of the corpus cavernosum (shave biopsy) is usually adequate to obtain tissue from a nonexophytic lesion. Exophytic lesions may be excised for diagnostic and therapeutic reasons, and in such cases, thicker biopsy material may be obtained from the glans. The electrocoagulating current promptly controls bleeding, and wound healing by granulation is satisfactory.

BENIGN LESIONS

Benign lesions include inflammatory conditions, which may require only biopsy diagnosis, and growths that need definitive diagnosis or excision. Epidermal cysts, hemangiomas, angiokeratomas, verruca vulgaris, molluscum contagiosum, condyloma acuminatum, fibrolipoma, cutaneous horns, nevi, and hirsutoid papillomas are examples of benign tumors. The majority of these lesions may be merely a source of anxiety or, when large, may interfere with function. One should keep in mind that condyloma acuminatum and molluscum contagiosum of the genital area are usually acquired through venereal contact and that examination for other venereal disease in the patient and in the sexual partner should be instituted.

Cystic lesions of the penis may be congenital or acquired. Congenital cysts are seen in the area of the frenoscrotal junction and, histologically, may be epidermoid or, rarely, mucinous in type. Epidermal inclusion cysts are similar to those encountered on other parts of the body. They do not usually require treatment unless they become symptomatic or interfere with function. Simple excision is adequate. Sebaceous cysts of the scrotum are common and may be multiple (Fig. 42–2). Excision is simple to perform owing to the redundancy of the skin in this region, which permits easy closure of the wounds after removal of large portions of skin.

Penile hemangiomas may be superficial or deep. The superficial angiokeratomas appear as papular or macular reddish-blue lesions and are asymptomatic. These vascular spaces may be obliterated by the fulgurating current. Larger and deeper hemangiomas may require surgical excision, with or without grafting. When changes in size or consistency are observed, an excisional biopsy is recommended to rule out the development of a malignant hemangioendothelioma.

Nevi of the genital area may be pigmented or nonpigmented and, histologically, may be junctional, intradermal, or compound. Excisional biopsy is recommended when the development of a malignant melanoma is in question.

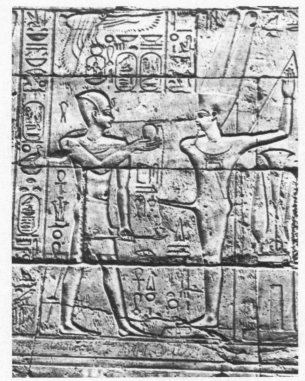

Figure 42–1. Pharaoh Ramses II (circa 1298 to 1231 B.C.) presents offerings to Min, the god of fertility.

Keloids may occur at the site of circumcision or trauma. Other rare lesions are fibromas, myomas, and lipomas.

Condylomata acuminata consist of fairly soft verrucous nodules that may coalesce into cauliflower-like masses (Fig. 42–3). Histologically, there is pro-

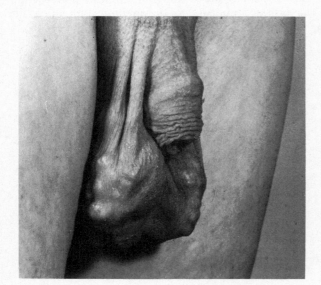

Figure 42–2. Multiple sebaceous cysts of the scrotum, which were removed by excision of a large portion of redundant scrotum.

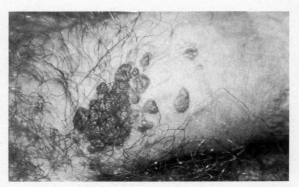

Figure 42–3. Condylomata acuminata of the penile shaft, which did not respond to topical podophyllin. Successfully treated by electrosurgery.

nounced papillomatosis and acanthosis, many of the keratinocytes are vacuolated and have round hyperchromatic nuclei, and an appreciable number of cells are in mitosis (Fig. 42–4). When these tumors occur on the glans penis and prepuce of noncircumcised patients, they may reach a considerable size and may become destructive. They are then known as giant condyloma or Buschke-Löwenstein tumors (discussed later). Ordinary condylomata acuminata respond well to topical podophyllin (15% to 20% in alcohol or in tincture of benzoin) when they occur on the moist mucosa of the prepuce and glans. Lesions on the shaft of the penis do not respond as well to this treatment and usually need to be surgically removed. Superficial shave excision followed by fulguration or local excision with primary closure are adequate. This serves to obtain biopsy material and, at the same time, removes the lesion. Superficial conditions that are clinically self-evident, such as molluscum contagiosum and verruca vulgaris, may be destroyed by fulguration, electrocautery, cryocautery, or chemical cauterization.

PREMALIGNANCIES AND CARCINOMAS IN SITU

Bowen's Disease

Bowen's disease is an epidermoid carcinoma in situ. Clinically, the lesion presents as a solitary, dull red plaque, often with areas of crusting and oozing. Th histopathologic picture is the key to the diagnosis. When it occurs in the skin of the shaft of the penis, the scrotum, or the inguinal areas, Bowen's disease may be treated in the same way as when it occurs in other hairy areas of the body. Because Bowen's disease tends to involve the adnexa and hair follicles (Fig. 42–5) and is prone to develop into invasive carcinoma in 51% of the cases, it is advisable to excise the entire lesion.[1] A surgical margin of 3 to 5 mm should be allowed in order to

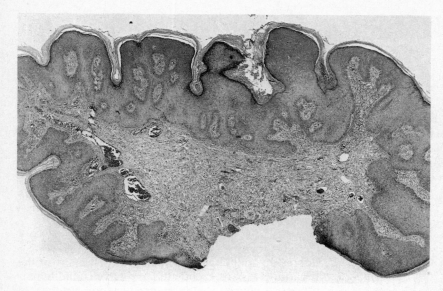

Figure 42–4. Histologic section of a condyloma acuminatum. There is pronounced acathosis with branching of the rete ridges. Some of the epidermal cells are vacuolated (hematoxylin-eosin × 42).

ascertain that any underlying carcinoma will also be removed. For the same reason, the use of topical chemotherapy with 5-fluorouracil is not recommended in this condition. Belisario, a pioneer in topical chemotherapy, has warned of the possibility of burying an active carcinoma below an apparently healed surface when such therapy is used for Bowen's disease.[2] The authors have used the Mohs fresh tissue chemosurgery technique with good results. This method assures complete removal of the lesion and any underlying carcinoma. Healing of the wounds by granulation tissue after this type of surgery is satisfactory (Fig. 42–6). It is important to keep in mind that Bowen's disease is occasionally associated with internal malignancies, especially when it occurs on covered areas of the body. The authors have encountered this association in three

patients with Bowen's disease of the genital region. One had carcinoma of the lung, and two had carcinoma of the colon.

Erythroplasia of Queyrat

Erythroplasia of Queyrat (EQ) is an epidermoid carcinoma in situ occurring on mucosal surfaces. Its location is on the inner surface of the prepuce and on the glans penis, almost exclusively in men who have not been circumcised during infancy. The lesion presents as a red, velvety plaque that occasionally may be elevated or papillary. It may become ulcerated and is then associated with discharge and pain. Irritation due to smegma retention underneath the prepuce appears to be an important etiologic

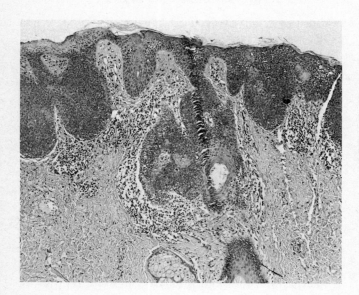

Figure 42–5. Bowen's disease: The epidermal cells are disorderly; many are dysplastic. Note the involvement of the hair follicle (hematoxylin-eosin × 105).

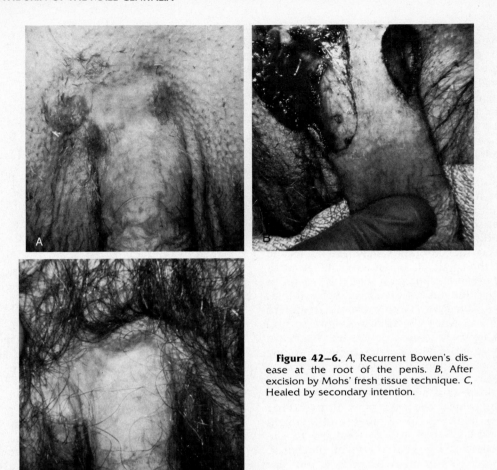

Figure 42–6. *A,* Recurrent Bowen's disease at the root of the penis. *B,* After excision by Mohs' fresh tissue technique. *C,* Healed by secondary intention.

factor. EQ has the same histologic features as Bowen's disease but occurs on a mucosa (Fig. 42–7) and is characterized by different biologic behavior. While Bowen's disease is associated with a high incidence of internal malignancy, this is infrequent with EQ. Also, metastases occur with greater frequency with the latter. These two attributes make EQ a distinct entity.[3] In the authors' experience, EQ has been the most common premalignant lesion of the glans penis. Squamous cell carcinoma had

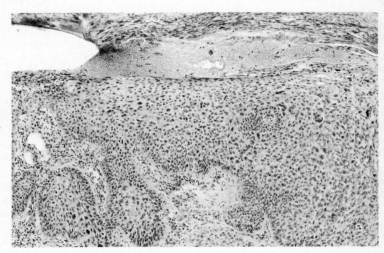

Figure 42–7. Erythroplasia of Queyrat of the glans penis. Note the similarity to Bowen's disease except for absence of adnexa (hematoxylin-eosin × 120).

developed in five of 15 cases (33%) at the time they were seen. An erythematous, velvety plaque of the glans penis or prepuce of nonfungal etiology that is unresponsive to topical anti-inflammatory therapy is a strong indication for biopsy.

The treatment modalities for EQ are mainly topical chemotherapy with 5-fluorouracil (5-FU) and surgical excision. In contrast to Bowen's disease, topical 5-FU is effective in EQ because of the absence of adnexal structures at the involved site. In early cases without nodules or ulceration, a 5% cream preparation of 5-FU is recommended. This is applied twice a day for three to four weeks.[4–6] A severe inflammatory reaction results, and it takes four weeks or so for the dermatitis to heal after the treatment is discontinued. Because of the location of the disease, the dermatitis may extend to the scrotum and the inguinal regions by spillage of 5-FU from the area of application. For this reason, it is advisable that the patient wear a rubber condom. Occlusion by this means also shortens the treatment period.[6] This modality is effective, but several courses, as many as four, may be needed to achieve a satisfactory result. The general agreement among dermatologists is to employ 5-FU in this disease.

However, in 14 patients with this disease, the authors obtained satisfactory results in only two cases by using topical chemotherapy. In two other cases, excision had to be done because of a violent reaction to 5-FU. When EQ is localized to the prepuce, circumcision is the treatment of choice. Small lesions on the glans may be excised, the base electrocoagulated, and the wound left to heal by granulation. Larger lesions on the glans may be excised, and the wounds grafted. If the patient has not been circumcised, circumcision may be undertaken at the same time, and the cutaneous portion of the dorsal prepuce may be retained and used as a pedicle graft to cover the defect in the glans (Fig. 42–8).[7] Those who practice Mohs' fresh tissue chemosurgery technique[8] can apply this method with gratifying results (Fig. 42–9).

During the last four years, the authors have treated four cases with this type of lesion with the fulgurating current. The rationale for this is that the mucosa in this area, unlike the skin of the shaft of the penis, does not contain adnexa along which the neoplastic cells may spread into the dermis as in Bowen's disease. The results have been gratifying. Even large areas of fulgurated, denuded mucosa healed well in a comparatively short time, and with minimal discomfort. One case has also been treated by the defocused beam of the carbon dioxide laser. The result appears promising, but the authors do not feel that this modality is superior to the ordinary fulgurating current.

Cancer is likely to develop in about 21% of the cases of EQ. The presence of ulceration or infiltration makes surgery mandatory. Excision has definite

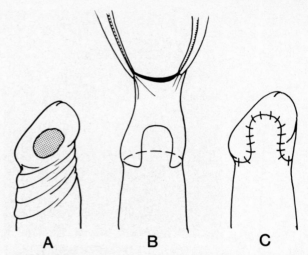

Figure 42–8. *A* to *C,* The Happle technique using preputial skin for grafting defects after excising the lesions on the glans.

advantages over topical chemotherapy. It helps to detect and remove a concomitant carcinoma if this has developed in the lesion. Graham and Helwig have found that 10% of cases will have evidence of squamous cell carcinoma and 2% will have lymph node metastases by the time the patient seeks medical advice.[3] Also, the morbidity time is brief after surgery. Circumcision is indicated in all cases, whether the prepuce is involved or not. This eliminates a major portion of the mucosal surface of the penis where EQ may later develop and also prevents further irritation by smegma. Penectomy is too mutilating, while fulguration and radiotherapy have a failure rate of 83%.[3] Morbidity in the form of edema, meatal stricture, and chronic radiodermatitis may follow radiation therapy.

Whatever the modality of treatment, patients that have had EQ should undergo periodic examination for the rest of their lives. As long as the penis has a mucosal surface left, the possibility of recurrence always exists. This has prompted Mato and Vilalta to devise a surgical technique they call decortication of the glans.[9] In this procedure, the entire mucosal covering of the glans and the prepuce is removed, and the skin of the prepuce is advanced to cover the glans to the urethral meatus. The steps of the technique are illustrated in Figure 42–10. The procedure is rather complicated but may be justifiable in unusually extensive EQ of the glans.

Extramammary Paget's Disease

Extramammary Paget's disease (EMPD) of the male genitalia is rare. The lesions present as erythematous, dermatitic patches, which may ulcerate (Fig. 42–11). The most common sites are the inguinal folds and the scrotum. The diagnosis can only

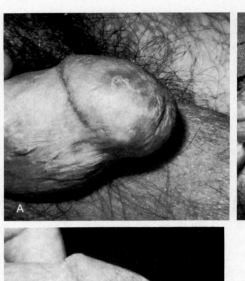
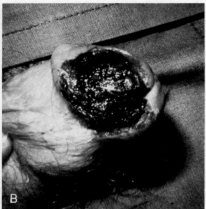
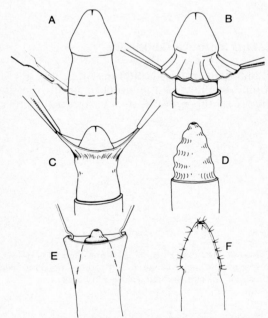

Figure 42–9. *A*, Erythroplasia of Queyrat of the glans. *B*, Result after excision by Mohs' fresh tissue technique. *C*, Wound healed by secondary intention.

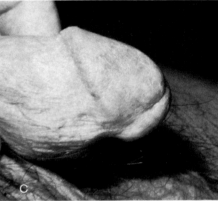

Figure 42–10. Diagram showing steps in the decortication of the glans technique. The entire mucosal surface of the prepuce and the glans is dissected away (*A* to *D*), then the cutaneous portion of the prepuce is used as a graft to cover the defect (*E* and *F*).

be established by histologic examination (Fig. 42–12). Unless localized to a small area, the results of treatment of EMPD are unsatisfactory because of the multicentric nature of this condition.[10] The preferred treatment is excision whenever this is feasible. It eliminates the disease and permits the exclusion of an underlying apocrine adenocarcinoma. The wound may be closed primarily or a graft may be applied. Extensive lesions that are not amenable to excision may be managed with topical 5-FU or bleomycin. Topical bleomycin has also been reported effective in the treatment of EMPD of the vulva.[11] In one of the authors' cases in which both inguinal regions, the shaft of the penis, and the scrotum were all involved, symptomatic and clinical improvement was achieved by using alternating courses of 5-FU and bleomycin. However, repeat biopsies demonstrated the persistence of foci of the disease, which also involved hair follicles (Fig. 42–12). This may account for the failure of treatment. Although the lesion is not radiosensitive, regional radiation of the skin lesion and the corresponding lymph nodes is recommended in inoperable cases. Concomitant carcinoma of the urinary bladder, rectum, or colon should be removed in every case if possible. Since mammary Paget's disease metasta-

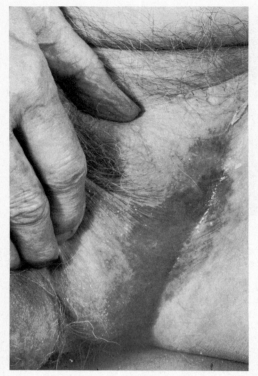

Figure 42–11. Extramammary Paget's disease—recalcitrant, erythematous, eczema-like plaques.

sizes to regional nodes in 50% of the cases,[10] comparable findings could also be expected with extramammary lesions.[12]

Leukoplakia

Leukoplakia of the glans penis is so rare that no mention of it is made in most dermatology textbooks. However, urologists recognize it as a distinct entity.[13] Clinically, the lesions consist of one or several whitish, opalescent patches that may not be raised and are ill-defined. If elevated, they appear sharply demarcated (Fig. 42–13). The condition is usually asymptomatic and appears to occur more frequently in diabetics. The clinical differential diagnosis includes chronic dermatitis, lichen sclerosis et atrophicus, candidiasis, and lichen planus. The lesions may become bullous as in lichen sclerosis et atrophicus. When ulceration takes place, the possibility of malignant degeneration should be seriously considered. Involvement of the urethral meatus is common and tends to cause strictures and even obstruction. Histopathologically, epithelial changes resemble those of the hypertrophic type of actinic keratosis of the skin. There is hyperkeratosis or parakeratosis, irregular acanthosis with disorderly arrangement of the keratinocytes, and cellular atypia (Fig. 42–14). However, some lesions may show atrophy of the malpighian layer.

Squamous cell carcinoma of the mucosa that has developed from a leukoplakia has a great tendency toward metastases. Therefore, leukoplakia should be considered and a biopsy obtained whenever a lichen-sclerosis-et-atrophicus–like lesion is seen on the glans, especially when other such lesions are not present on other parts of the body. A lesion on the glans of one of the authors' patients was labeled and treated as lichen sclerosis et atrophicus for eight years before squamous cell carcinoma developed. The treatment of leukoplakia is excision or destruction by electrocautery, cryocautery, or chemical agents.

Balanitis Xerotica Obliterans

Balanitis xerotica obliterans presents as white atrophic patches on the prepuce or on the glans. Stenosis of the urethral meatus frequently results.

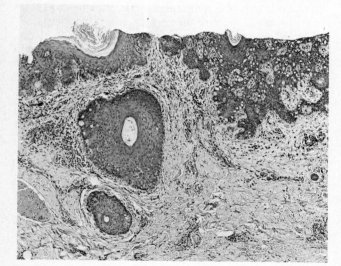

Figure 42–12. Paget's disease: The epidermis is permeated with large round cells, singly and in groups; note the involvement of hair follicles (hematoxylin-eosin × 66).

PSEUDOMALIGNANCIES

Bowenoid Papulosis of the Genitalia

Bowenoid papulosis of the genitalia (BPG) has been reported in recent years and was initially identified as Bowen's disease occurring on the genitalia of relatively young men and women. The condition appears as small, multiple papules, the nature of which is usually made after biopsy and not by clinical examination (Fig. 42–15).[14] The histologic features are identical with those of Bowen's disease but the lesions are distinctly small (Fig. 42–16). It has been shown that lesions of BPG may spontaneously regress.[15] Viral particles have been demonstrated in some cases.[16] Therefore, the condition may be regarded as benign, but until there is definite proof of this, conservative surgical ablation or local destruction by cryocautery or electrocautery is recommended.

Giant Condyloma Acuminatum

Giant condyloma acuminatum (Buschke-Löwenstein tumor, verrucous carcinoma) occurs mostly on the penis and is thought to be a variant of ordinary condyloma acuminatum, which is induced by the papovavirus. However, there is no evidence as yet for the viral etiology of the Buschke-Löwenstein tumor.[17] Because of this, it has been postulated that the lesion represents from its inception a low-grade malignancy, a so-called verrucous carcinoma, a term used to designate carcinomas with slow, locally aggressive growth but without a tendency toward metastasis.[18] The tumor occurs in noncircumcised patients and presents as an exophytic, fungating, wart-like mass that may attain a considerable size. The growth characteristically penetrates into the

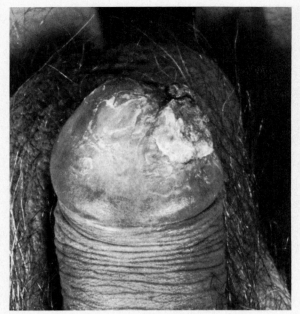

Figure 42–13. Leukoplakia of the glans penis—extensive scaly plaque, which encroaches on the urethral meatus.

Erosions and fissures of the glans may also occur. Patients may complain of pain, discharge, pruritus, painful erections, and urinary obstruction. The lesion occurs in circumcised and uncircumcised middle-aged males. Most cases represent lichen sclerosis et atrophicus. However, chronic irritation in the uncircumcised and other lesions, such as benign mucosal pemphigus, may result in a similar clinical picture. Carcinoma has developed in some cases. Treatment is directed at the relief of meatal stenosis by meatotomy, circumcision when the prepuce is involved, or excision of lesions on the glans.

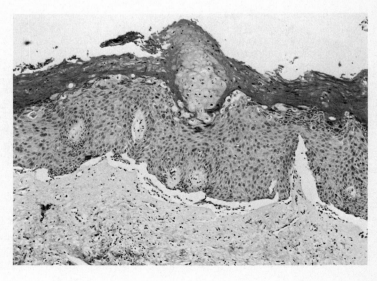

Figure 42–14. Leukoplakia of the penis—disorderly arrangement and atypia of the keratinocytes, individual cell keratinization, and abnormal mitoses (hematoxylin-eosin × 90).

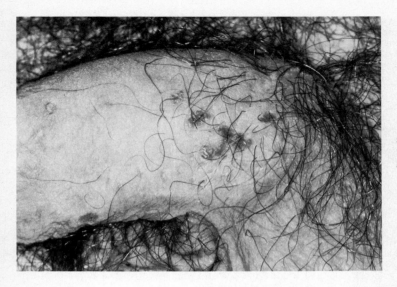

Figure 42–15. Bowenoid papulosis of the penis—small, hyperpigmented, verrucous papules in a twenty-six-year old patient (cf. Fig. 42–3). (Photograph courtesy of Dr. A. W. Kopf.)

Figure 42–16. Bowenoid papulosis of the penis—histologic section shows the epidermal changes of Bowen's disease, but the lesion is a small papule (hematoxylin-eosin × 90). (Slide courtesy of Dr. A. Mehregan.)

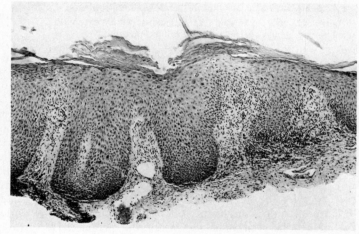

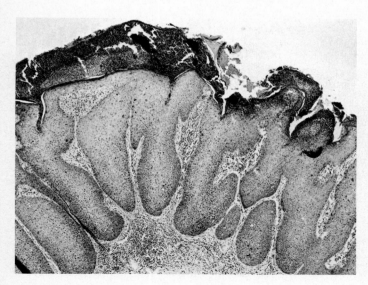

Figure 42–17. Giant condyloma acuminatum (Buschke-Löewenstein tumor). Histology is similar to that of ordinary condyloma acuminatum. In this case, numerous mitoses are prominent.

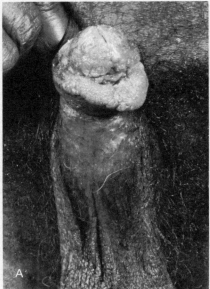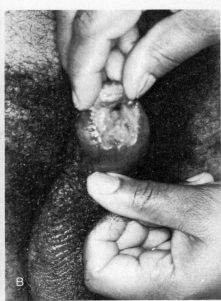

Figure 42–18. Giant condyloma acuminatum (Buschke-Löwenstein tumor) in a man who had painful and difficult marital relations for eight years. *A,* Tumor involves glans, urethra, and coronal sulcus. *B,* Appearance after excision by Mohs' microscopically controlled chemosurgical technique. Note the urethral opening in the center of the defect. Wife became pregnant for the first time three months after surgery.

deeper tissues causing extensive tissue destruction and clinically behaves like a malignant tumor. Because rare examples of malignant transformation of condylomata acuminata have been reported,[19] caution should be exercised so that the true pathologic diagnosis is established. Although the histology is similar to that of ordinary condyloma acuminatum, multiple biopsies may be necessary to arrive at a definitive decision (Fig. 42–17). Review of the literature indicates that the only satisfactory treatment is thorough but conservative surgical ablation. The Mohs microscopically controlled chemosurgery technique satisfies both of these requirements and is well suited for the treatment of this lesion.[8] One of three cases successfully treated by this method is shown in Figure 42–18. When the tumor is extensive and involves the shaft, partial or complete penectomy may be necessary. The tumor does not respond to podophyllin, caustic agents, or radiotherapy.

MALIGNANT TUMORS

Squamous Cell Carcinoma

Squamous cell carcinoma of the penis is relatively rare but is still the most common type of penile cancer. The tumor occurs most frequently on the glans and in the coronal sulcus and, less commonly, on the prepuce and the shaft. Like erythroplasia of Queyrat, the incidence is highest among those who are not circumcised at birth. It is most commonly diagnosed during the sixth and seventh decades of life but has been seen in patients under 40 years of age and even in children.[13] The neoplasm may appear as an indurated, erythematous plaque, a warty growth, an ulcer, or an exophytic lesion. Phimosis may obscure the lesion. Thus, prolonged neglect may result. Because the dermatologist is more apt to be consulted about penile lesions that may be precancerous or early malignancies, one cannot overemphasize the importance of obtaining a histologic diagnosis of lesions that are recalcitrant or suspected of being malignant so that early treatment may be instituted. The differential diagnosis includes syphilitic chancre and gumma, chancroid, condyloma acuminatum, herpes progenitalis, lyphogranuloma venereum, granuloma inguinale, erythroplasia of Queyrat, Bowen's disease, leukoplakia, and traumatic ulceration.

The treatment of cancer, especially when the penis is involved, should not be undertaken by the inexperienced physician. The staging system of squamous cell carcinoma of the penis by Jackson has been universally adopted (Table 42–1).[20] This system is recommended as the guide to deciding what surgical procedure is required, and for evaluating

TABLE 42–1. Staging of Carcinoma of the Penis*

Stage I	Neoplasm limited to prepuce or glans penis or both without evidence of lymph node involvement.
Stage II	Invasion of shaft or corpus cavernosum by the malignancy, but without nodal or distant metastases.
Stage III	Biopsy-proven regional node metastasis.
Stage IV	Inoperable regional node involvement or distant metastases.

*Adapted from Jackson SM: The treatment of carcinoma of penis. Br J Surg 53:33–35, 1966.

the prognosis. Because the dermatologist's domain may include cases in Stage I, only the treatment applicable to this stage will be discussed. When the tumor is limited to the prepuce, circumcision is adequate. When the neoplasm involves the glans or the coronal sulcus, the standard treatment advocated by urologists is amputation at a minimum of 2 cm beyond the visible or palpable tumor.

The probability of development of inguinal node metastasis, which may be unilateral or bilateral, in patients with Stage I carcinoma is less than 20%, and if metastases develop, they usually do so within three years of the appearance of the tumor. Because the determination of the presence or absence of lymph node metastasis by physical examination of lymphangiography is not reliable, the question arises whether prophylactic inguinal node dissection should be performed at the time of excision of the carcinoma. The consensus among urologists favors clinical examination of the patient every two months for at least three years. However, in obese patients in whom it is difficult to palpate lymph nodes, prophylactic node dissection is advisable.[13] The authors have experienced the value of this plan in a patient where one out of 20 nodes showed metastatic carcinoma, although none could be palpated preoperatively by several examiners. In this case, the involved node was in a contralateral position. This indicates the necessity of bilateral lymphadenectomy when this procedure is indicated.

There are few malignant lesions, if any, that evoke emotional repercussions equal to those of cancer of the penis. Since the majority of squamous cell carcinomas occur on the glans, amputation at 2 or more cm proximal to the clinical tumor can cause severe mental anguish. A practical and, at the same time, effective treatment for Stage I carcinoma is Mohs' chemosurgery technique.[8] This method is ideal because it assures complete removal of the cancer and yet provides maximal preservation of normal tissues and function. The authors have practiced this technique in six cases with gratifying results. Four patients were treated by the fixed tissue method and two were treated by the fresh tissue method. Figure 42–19 illustrates one such case. The patients treated have retained good sexual function. The patient illustrated here was alive and without metastasis after an eight-year follow-up period. It is

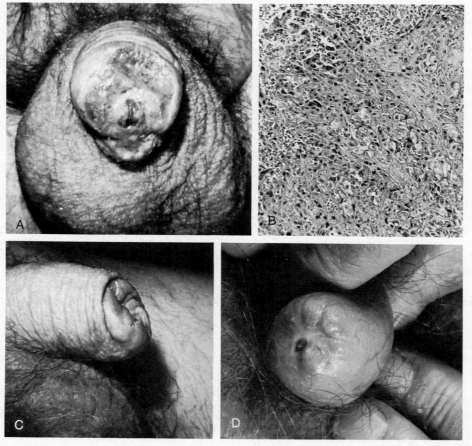

Figure 42–19. Squamous cell carcinoma of the glans penis. *A,* Preoperative appearance. *B,* Poorly differentiated squamous cell carcinoma (hematoxylin-eosin × 175). *C,* Appearance after Mohs' chemosurgical excision. *D,* Patient's urethral opening after healing by granulation. Note that stricture of the urethra did not result. Patient was alive and well seven years after surgery.

worthy of note that in none of the cases where the urethra was involved did stricture of the urethra develop. The rules concerning lymph nodes also apply when chemosurgery is undertaken. In only one of the cases mentioned did metastases develop, and this had obviously taken place by the time the patient presented for treatment.

Basal Cell Carcinoma

Basal cell carcinoma of the penis is extremely rare. The treatment modalities applicable to similar tumors on other parts of the body also apply here.

Malignant Melanoma

Malignant melanoma of the penis is rare. Less than 1% of all primary penile cancers treated at the M. D. Anderson Hospital were malignant melanomas.[21] Early metastases occur by lymphatic permeation to the ilioinguinal nodes and through the vascular corpora cavernosa. The recommended treatment of Stage I melanoma (localized lesion without metastasis) and Stage II melanoma (metastasis confined to one regional area) is excision of the primary tumor by partial or total penectomy together with en bloc bilateral inguinal node dissection. Immunotherapy and chemotherapy are used as adjunctive treatment. The prognosis of this neoplasm is poor owing to the frequency of early metastases.[13]

Other malignant tumors of the penis include sarcomas, fibrosarcoma, myosarcoma, hemangioendothelioma, leiomyosarcoma and Kaposi's sarcoma. The treatment in all such cases is aggressive surgical excision, radiation therapy, and chemotherapy.

Metastatic Lesions

Metastatic lesions to the penis are infrequent despite its rich vascular composition and its proximity to the prostate, the bladder, and the rectum, which are common sites of primary carcinomas. Renal, osseous, and pulmonary tumors have metastasized to the penis. The corpora cavernosa are usually involved; consequently, priapism may be the presenting complaint. Nodular and chancriform lesions have been observed, and urinary obstruction and hematuria may occur.

The most common malignancy of the scrotum is squamous cell carcinoma. Historically, it was common in chimney sweeps but is still occasionally seen (Fig. 42–20). Wide excision is the treatment of choice and was successful in this case. Inquinal lymphadenectomy is indicated when the nodes are palpable.

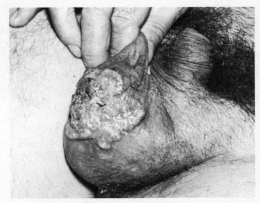

Figure 42–20. Squamous cell carcinoma of the scrotum that was successfully treated by a wide excision.

ANESTHESIA OF THE MALE GENITALIA

The methods of induction of local anesthesia for operations on the male genitalia are different from those used in other parts of the body by virtue of the anatomic innervation, which is specific to this area.

In the case of a localized lesion of the shaft of the penis or the scrotum, local anesthesia (local block) will suffice for the purpose of biopsy or complete excision. For circumcision and other operations on the foreskin or on the glans penis, anesthesia can be achieved by partial block. The anesthetic is injected subcutaneously around the circumference of the penis, immediately proximal to the corona. When the lesion involves a large portion of the glans and when a malignancy of the glans penis is under consideration for biopsy or excision, complete regional block of the penis is recommended.

Anatomically, the penis is innervated by the right and left dorsal nerves of the penis, which are divisions of the pudendal nerves (S 2-4) in the perineum. The two main nerves run along the dorsal surface of the penis and give off smaller branches that extend to the ventral surface. The frenulum receives its nerve supply through branches that lie between the deep fascia (Buck's fascia) and the corpora cavernosa. To undertake the block, the spines of the pubic bone are palpated and two intradermal wheals of anesthetic are raised on each side. These two points are then connected by intradermal and subcutaneous infiltrations from the skin to the bone. This requires about 5 ml of solution. Intradermal and subcutaneous infiltration is then carried out between each of the previous points and a third point on the median raphe of the scrotum at the base of the penis (Fig. 42–21A); 10 ml of solution are required for this. The penis is then held in a vertical position and the anesthetic is injected fanlike from each of the three points at the base of the

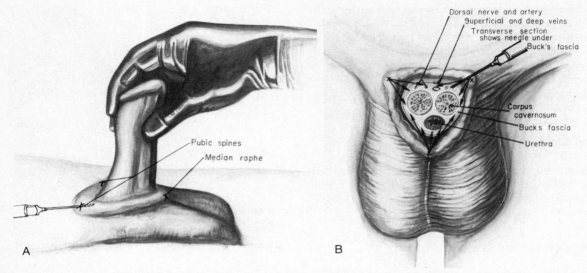

Figure 42–21. Regional block anesthesia of the penis: *A*, First stage—the base is infiltrated with anesthetic in a ring-like fashion. *B*, Second stage—the anesthetic is injected below Buck's fascia.

penis. The solution should reach the level between Buck's fascia and the corpora cavernosa (Fig. 42–21B). This last step requires another 10 ml to anesthetize the frenulum. It may be omitted if the frenulum is not included in the operative site. The anesthetic the authors use is lidocaine. The total amount needed is about 15 to 25 ml of 0.5% to 1% solution. Operating analgesia is established in five to 15 minutes and lasts one to three hours. Infiltration of the prepuce is to be avoided since sloughing results from such practice.[22]

CIRCUMCISION

Circumcision can be traced to antiquity. It is mentioned in the Old Testament and has always been practiced by Jews and by some primitive peoples of the Orient, Africa, and Polynesia. In ancient Rome, both pagan and early Christian priests were required to be circumcised, and it is mandatory for all Moslem male children.

Although the advantages of a foreskin seem minimal, while the medical benefits that might be derived from its removal appear significant, the propriety of routine circumcision has been questioned in recent years.[23]

The main indications of circumcision are (1) phimosis, (2) paraphimosis, (3) benign lesions (such as condyloma), (4) premalignant lesions, (5) superficial malignant lesions of the foreskin, and (6) inflammatory disorders of the glans (balanitis). Furthermore, neonatal circumcision does assure the newborn of relative freedom from the hazards of penile cancer in later years, and prevents most of the above conditions. The technique depends on the age of the patient.[24]

In the neonate, the use of a mechanical device such as the Gomco clamp is convenient and very popular in most nurseries (Fig. 42–22). A dorsal slit is first made to allow the foreskin to be retracted, and adhesions between the foreskin and the underlying glans are then freed. The bell is placed over the glans, and the foreskin is drawn forward over the bell and clamped in position. The degree of advancing the foreskin over the bell is important. If too little, the circumcision is inadequate, and if too much, the shaft of the penis may be denuded. The skin distal to the clamp is cut away with a scalpel. No suturing is needed.

There are three techniques that are applicable in children and adults. They are the guillotine, the dorsal slit, and the sleeve resection techniques.

The guillotine technique is the oldest and is still in use (Fig. 42–23). The foreskin is clamped at the frenulum and at an opposite point on the dorsum. A straight hemostat is then applied obliquely across the drawn foreskin, and the excess skin is excised with a scalpel. Excess mucosa is trimmed, and the bleeding points are controlled with 4-0 catgut ligatures. The skin and the mucosa are approximated with interrupted sutures of 4-0 chromic catgut. A strip of petrolatum gauze is placed around the base of the glans. This is to be removed within 24 hours. The sutures do not have to be removed because they slough off within a two-week period. Sitz baths are recommended 48 hours postoperatively.

In the dorsal slit technique (Fig. 42–24), the foreskin is first completely freed of any adhesions that may hold it to the glans. With two hemostat forceps placed on its freed end, one at 3 o'clock and the other at 9 o'clock, the foreskin is drawn over the glans. An incision is made in the midline of the dorsal aspect of the foreskin up to but immediately

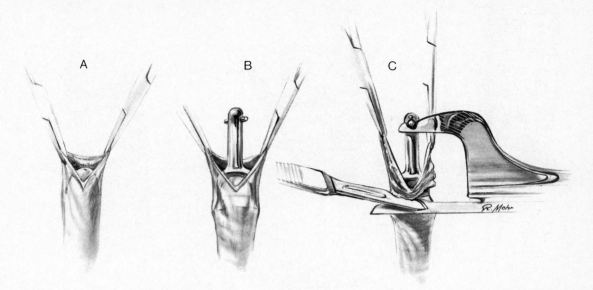

Figure 42–22. Circumcision by the Gomco clamp technique: *A*, The foreskin is drawn distally. *B*, The bell is placed on the glans penis all the way down to the coronal sulcus. *C*, The clamp is applied, and the foreskin is resected.

distal to the base of the glans. An oblique incision is made between this point of the dorsal slit and the frenulum on each side, thus removing two flaps of skin. The bleeding points are ligated. A mattress suture placed on the frenulum helps to control the bleeding. Excess mucosa is excised. The skin and the mucosa are then approximated with interrupted sutures of 4-0 chromic gut.

The sleeve resection technique is illustrated in Figure 42–25. A circumferential incision is made in the penile skin opposite the coronal sulcus. The foreskin is then retracted and a similar incision is

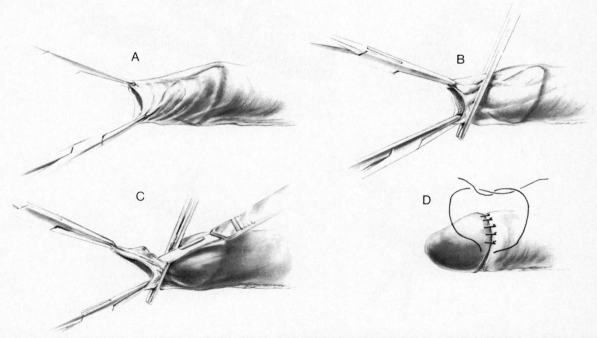

Figure 42–23. Circumcision by the guillotine technique: *A*, The foreskin is drawn distally. *B*, A straight hemostat is applied obliquely just distal to the tip of the glans. *C*, The foreskin distal to the clamp is excised. *D*, The edges are approximated.

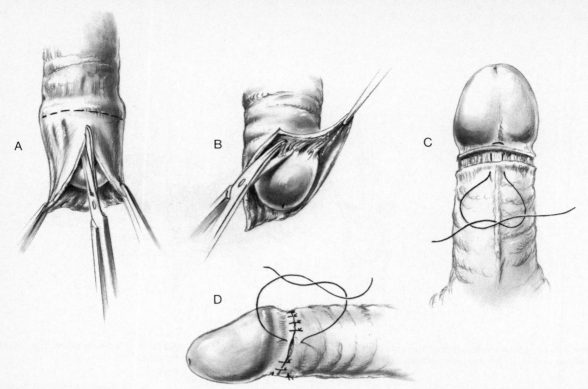

Figure 42–24. Circumcision by the dorsal slit technique: *A,* A dorsal slit is made. *B,* The lateral flaps are resected. *C,* A mattress suture is placed at the frenulum. *D,* The skin edges are approximated.

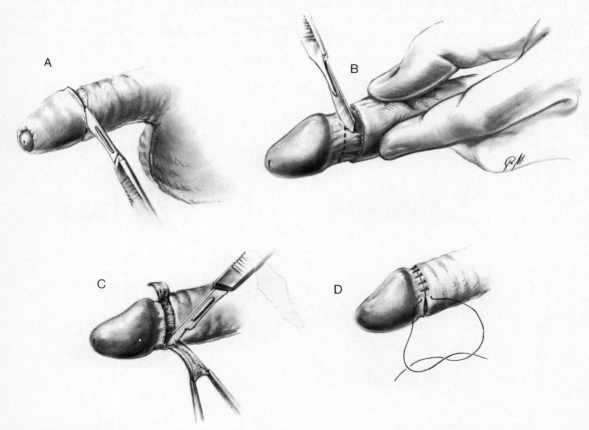

Figure 42–25. Circumcision by the sleeve resection technique. *A,* A circumferential skin incision is made opposite the coronal sulcus. *B,* A similar incision is made over the mucosal skin. *C,* The sleeve of skin between the two incisions is excised. *D,* The skin edges are approximated.

made in the mucosal skin a few millimeters behind the coronal sulcus. The sleeve of skin between the two incisions is then excised and the skin edges are approximated with interrupted sutures of 4-0 chromic catgut.

As Shulman and coworkers emphasize, the operation does have its complications, and at one time or another, severe complications have been reported. The most common complication is perimeatal ulceration and subsequent meatal stenosis.[25]

REFERENCES

1. Graham JH, Helwig EB: Premalignant cutaneous and mucocutaneous diseases, in Graham JH, Johnson WC, Helwig EB (eds): Dermal Pathology. Hagerstown, Md, Harper & Row, 1972, pp 581–597
2. Belisario JC: Topical use of 5-fluorouracil. Med J Austral 2:91, 1973
3. Graham JH, Helwig EB: Erythroplasia of Queyrat. A clinicopathological and histochemical study. Cancer 32:1396–1414, 1973
4. Honeycut WM, Jansen GT, Dillaha CJ: Topical antimetabolities and cytostatic agents. Cutis 6:63–72, 1970
5. Klaus GD, Elgart M, DeVillez RL: Erythroplasia of Queyrat. Treatment with topically applied fluorouracil. JAMA 232:934–937, 1975
6. Goette DK, Carson TE: Erythroplasia of Queyrat. Cancer 38:1498–1502, 1976
7. Happle R: Surgical treatment of erythroplasia of Queyrat. Plast Reconstr Surg 59:642–645, 1977
8. Mohs FE: Chemosurgery: Microscopically Controlled Surgery for Skin Cancer, Ed 2. Springfield, Ill, Charles C Thomas, 1978
9. Mato J, Vilalta A: Decortication of the glans. Presented at the I International Congress of Dermatologic Surgery, Lisbon, Portugal, October 7–10, 1979
10. Klingmuller G, Ishibashi Y: Extramammary Paget's disease, in Andrade R, Gumport SL, Popkin GL, Rees TD (eds): Cancer of the Skin. Philadelphia, W B Saunders Co, 1976, pp 662–678
11. Watring WG, Roberts JA, Lagasse LD, Berman ML, et al: Treatment of recurrent Paget's disease of the vulva with topical bleomycin. Cancer 41:10–11, 1978
12. Duperrat B, Mascaro JM: Maladie de Paget extra-mammaire. Presse Med 73:1019–1024, 1965
13. Schellhammer PF, Grabstald H: Tumors of the penis and urethra, in Harrison JH (ed): Campbell's Urology, Ed 4. Philadelphia, W B Saunders Co, 1979, pp 1175–1188
14. Wade TR, Kopf AW, Ackerman AB: Bowenoid papulosis of the penis. Arch Dermatol 115:306–308, 1979
15. Berger BW, Hori Y: Multicentric Bowen's disease of the genitalia. Spontaneous regression of lesions. Arch Dermatol 114:1698–1699, 1978
16. Lupulescu A, Mehregan A: Bowen's disease of genital areas. J Cutan Pathol 4:266–274, 1977
17. Friedman-Kien AE: Giant condyloma of Buschke-Loewenstein, in Andrade R, Gumport SL, Popkin GL, Rees TD (eds): Cancer of the Skin. Philadelphia, W B Saunders Co, 1976, pp 814–820
18. Kraus FT, Perez-Mesa C: Verrucous carcinoma. Cancer 19:26–38, 1966
19. Dawson DF, Duckworth JK, Bernhardt H, Young JM: Giant condyloma and verrucous carcinoma of the genital area. Arch Pathol 79:225–231, 1965
20. Jackson SM: The treatment of carcinoma of the penis. Br J Surg 53:33–35, 1966
21. Johnson DE, Ayala AG: Primary melanoma of penis. Urology 2:174–177, 1973
22. Adriani J: Labat's Regional Anesthesia, Ed 3. Philadelphia, W B Saunders Co, 1967
23. Preston EN: Whither the foreskin? A consideration for routine neonatal circumcision. JAMA 213:1853–1858, 1970
24. Devine CJ Jr: Circumcision, in Harrison JH et al (eds): Campbell's Urology, Ed 4. Philadelphia, W B Saunders Co, 1979, pp 2401–2406
25. Shulman J, Ben-Hur N, Neuman Z: Surgical complications of circumcision. Am J Dis Child 107:149–154, 1964

43

ROBERT BARAN, M.D. / ECKART HANEKE, M.D.

Surgery of the Nail

Most of the following techniques fall within the province of the dermatologist. Although some would normally be carried out by a hand surgeon or podiatrist, they are useful in the armamentarium of the dermatologic surgeon. The objectives of nail surgery are to facilitate diagnosis when a biopsy is indicated, to alleviate pain, to treat infection, to correct deformities, to remove local tumors, and to ensure the best cosmetic result.

ANATOMY

The nail plate is the product of constantly differentiating ectodermal tissue (Fig. 43–1). Its normal appearance and growth depend on the integrity of: (1) the four epidermal structures: matrix, nail bed, hyponychium, and proximal nail fold and (2) the bony phalanx that forms part of the nail apparatus. The nail is set into proximal and lateral nail grooves formed by invaginations in the corresponding nail folds. The periungual tissue and, above all, the distal bony phalanx determine its gross form.

The nail plate emerges from beneath the proximal nail fold, which adheres closely to the nail for a short distance and forms a gradually desquamating tissue, the cuticle, which seals the cul-de-sac. The matrix from which the nail is derived extends approximately 6 mm under the proximal nail fold, but its most distal part is visible as the white semicircular lunula. For most of its length, the nail plate, which has a loose attachment to the matrix, lies distally on a firmly adherent nail bed of highly vascular connective tissue containing glomus organs. It is colorless but translucent, transmitting the pink color of the underlying nail bed. The nail bed epithelium presents with parallel longitudinal rete ridges. The subepithelial capillaries run longitudinally at different levels, one upon the other. Distally adjacent to the nail bed, the hyponychium, which is an extension of the epidermis under the nail plate, ends at the distal groove. The hyponychium marks the point at which the nail plate separates from the underlying tissue. There is very little space between the nail and the bone of the distal phalanx, and this space is occupied only by the nonkeratinizing nail epidermis and dermis.

The dermis under the matrix and nail bed is composed of loosely arranged connective tissue fibers. There is no subcutaneous tissue.

The circulation of the nail unit is supplied by two digital arteries that course along the digits and give off branches to the distal and proximal arches. The proximal matrix is also supplied by a branch of the digital artery coming off at the midportion of the middle phalanx and proceeding directly to the matrix, providing a collateral circulation.

Fingernails grow at a rate of 0.1 mm a day; toenails grow much more slowly. The thickness of fingernails varies from 0.5 to 0.75 mm, while toenails are normally 1 mm or more. Individuals doing heavy manual labor usually have thicker nail plates.

The sensory nerves to the dorsum of the distal phalanges of the second, third, and fourth fingers are derived from fine, oblique dorsal branches of the volar collateral nerves. Longitudinal, dorsal branches of the volar collateral nerves supply the fifth digit and the thumb.

The functions of the nail are multiple: (1) to protect the normal nail bed, (2) to act both as a weapon and as a tool for scraping or gripping small objects, (3) to provide counterpressure for the pulp that is essential to the tactile sensation involving the fingers, (4) to enhance the appearance of the fingers, (5) to provide a protective covering for the wounded nail bed, (6) to maintain a smooth, even nail bed for the regenerating nail plate, (7) to enable accurate repositioning of damaged subungual tissue, and (8) to act as a splint for fractures of the phalangeal tuft.

EXAMINATION OF THE PATIENT

History

The history may reveal systemic disease. Dermatologic conditions, vascular disease, diabetes, blood dyscrasias, collagen diseases such as scleroderma, allergy, chronic pulmonary disease, and the compromised host may all be significant. Surgery of the nail is not recommended in high-risk patients, but the importance of systemic disease in nail abnormalities is often overemphasized.

A history of concomitant administration of drugs may be relevant. They may affect anesthesia (such as monoamine oxidase inhibitors or phenothiazines), prolong bleeding (such as aspirin or anticoagulants), delay healing (such as steroids), or have toxic effects on the nail (such as demethylchlortetracycline).

534

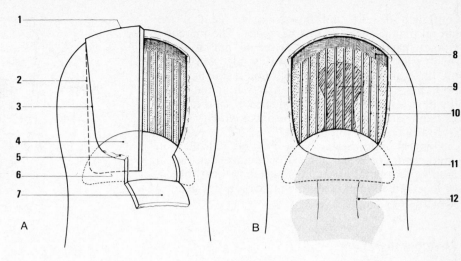

Figure 43–1. Anatomy of the nail. *A*: 1 = Distal free edge of the nail plate; 2 = lateral edge of the nail plate running along the lateral nail groove; 3 = lateral nail fold; 4 = lunula; 5 = cuticle; 6 = proximal edge of the nail plate; 7 = proximal nail fold. *B*: 8 = hyponychium; 9 = distal bony phalanx underneath the nail bed; 10 = nail bed; 11 = nail matrix with lateral horns; 12 = extensor tendon.

There may be a history of allergy to lidocaine or mepivacaine (Carbocaine) or Parabens (which is contained in both as a preservative). A knowledge of previous antitetanus immunization is important since tetanus toxoid may be advisable in association with surgery in the toenail area or in traumatic lesions that come into contact with soil.

Examination of the Diseased Nail

A magnifying lens may be useful to observe the color, surface structure, and periungual tissue and, when practicable, to compare the unaffected contralateral digit. It may be necessary to probe in order to localize pain or to x-ray for suspected bone involvement.

NAIL OPERATIONS

The basic requirements for nail surgery include a detailed knowledge of the anatomy and physiology of the nail apparatus, full aseptic conditions, regional block anesthesia, and local hemostasis.

The hand is prepared for surgery to the fingernail using a surgical scrub with povidone-iodine or alternative disinfectant soap.

The foot should first be soaked in appropriate antiseptic solutions before any surgery is performed on the toenail.

A sterile surgical glove with the tip of the appropriate finger removed provides an aseptic covering of the patient's hand. The foot is draped with sterile towels which are secured with towel clamps.

Instruments

The instruments used in nail surgery are the same as those used in cutaneous surgery with the addition of nail elevators (dental spatula or Freer septum elevator), skin hooks (flexible retractors), double-action nail splitter (bone rongeur), nail-splitting scissors, pointed scissors (Gradle scissors), curved iris scissors, small-nosed mosquito hemostats, disposable biopsy punches (2, 3, 3.5, and 4 mm), Penrose drains, Luer-Lok syringe, and 27-gauge needles.

Anesthesia

Type of Anesthesia. Lidocaine is widely used because the incidence of allergy to this agent is very low. It should be given without epinephrine because the resulting ischemia could cause gangrene. It has been claimed that using tepid lidocaine will minimize the burning sensation associated with its administration. Unlike lidocaine, mepivacaine is not a vasodilator and may be preferable. Although emergencies related to minor surgery occur rarely, the ready availability of resuscitative equipment and knowledge of proper procedures are essential.

A tourniquet is unnecessary prior to a punch biopsy. If a bloodless field is required, a Penrose drain may be placed around the base of the digit and used as a tourniquet. It should not be left on for more than 15 minutes.

Anesthesia is usually performed as a digital block. This is achieved by inserting the needle into the dorsolateral aspect of both sides of the digit at the web. About 0.3 ml of the anesthetic is placed near the dorsal digital nerve and 0.7 ml near the palmar or plantar nerve. Two ml of 1% mepivacaine is sufficient; more than 5 ml of anesthetic may interfere with the circulation. Anesthesia may take five to 10 minutes to become established. Local distal digital anesthesia, which is an alternative, should never be used if the distal phalanx is infected. Using a 30-gauge needle, the injection is started near the junction of the proximal and lateral nail fold. It is continued distally and downward to deaden the lateral digital nerve and its branches. The injection is then carried across the proximal nail fold, to involve the transverse nerve at this side, and finally to the other side of the digit. For distal nail bed operations, a supplementary injection at the tip of the digit is necessary. Regional anesthesia is favored by hand surgeons using metacarpal or axillary block, or brachial plexus anesthesia.

General Anesthesia. This may be indicated in children or for psychological or medical reasons in adults. Peripheral arterial insufficiency, heart block, or local infection may also be indications for general anesthesia.

Postoperative Care

At the end of the operation, the digit is either cleansed with a sterile 10% hydrogen peroxide solution and sprayed with a colorless disinfectant, or an antiseptic with hemolytic action may be used. The nail area is then covered with an antiseptic or antibiotic ointment on gauze or pads. A bulky dressing gives a cushion against local trauma. Tubegauz is put over the bandage.

Postoperative pain may be severe and is alleviated by elevating the extremity as much as possible for two days. Pulsating pain beginning after 36 to 48 hours may indicate an infection that should be treated according to the results of culture of the organism. Any bulky dressing, blood-stained after 24 hours, should be changed, but usually the dressing may remain for a week. Stitches are removed after seven to 12 days.

DIAGNOSTIC PROCEDURES

Biopsy of the Nail Area

The type of biopsy selected will depend on the information required. In onychomycosis, it is helpful to use sturdy scissors to take specimens that include a portion of the distal nail plate and the underlying hyponychium. A 3 mm punch biopsy limited to the nail plate can be performed when a suspected mycotic lesion is not confined distally. Routine periodic acid–Schiff stain is mandatory to identify fungal organisms and to rule out psoriasis. Note, though, that dual pathologies do exist.

Punch biopsies are also useful for small lesions or for diagnostic purposes. A 3 to 4 mm disposable punch, cutting through the nail plate, must reach the bone before it is withdrawn. The tissue cylinder is then released from the bone with fine, curved scissors (or Gradle scissors). Histologic orientation is greatly facilitated if the nail plate is left in place, although distortion often occurs during the prepa-

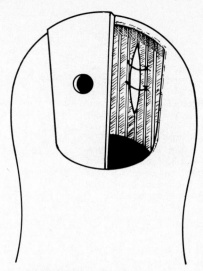

Figure 43–2. Nail bed biopsy.

ration for histology. When the nail is thickened, it should be thinned before biopsy.

Longitudinal Nail Bed Biopsy (Fig. 43–2). It may be advisable to avulse the nail plate fully or partially for the diagnosis of a tumor or an unusual lesion. A longitudinal elliptical wedge of tissue down to the bone is removed. Then, the edges of the ellipse are undermined to facilitate primary closure with 6-0 Dexon. Relaxing incisions at the lateral margins of the nail bed may be necessary if primary closure is not possible.

Transverse Biopsy of the Matrix (Fig. 43–3). The proximal third of the nail plate is removed after reflection of the proximal nail fold. An elliptical or a crescent-shaped biopsy is then performed. If the

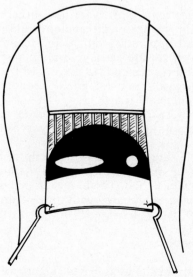

Figure 43–3. Nail matrix biopsy.

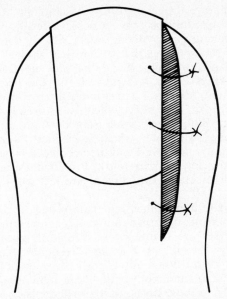

Figure 43—4. Lateral-longitudinal nail biopsy.

wedges of the incisions are undermined, the wound can be sutured, without tension, using 6-0 Dexon. It is cosmetically important to maintan the curvilinear configuration of the distal margin of the lunula because it plays an important role in shaping the free edge of the nail plate. If the proximal matrix portion has been left intact, no nail fissure results, and the plate is merely thinned.

Lateral-Longitudinal Biopsy (Fig. 43–4). This elliptical biopsy could be done on either side of the nail plate and proximal nail fold. For the most part, the incisions parallel the lateral edge of the nail plate. Beginning in the lateral nail groove, the incisions should include a 3 to 4 mm nail segment reaching to the bone. This ensures that a full-thickness fragment of the matrix with its lateral horn is obtained. Slightly curved iris scissors are useful for releasing the tissue from the bone. Starting at the tip of the digit, one proceeds proximally while maintaining contact with the bony phalanx. Under-

mining the nail bed aids in primary wound closure. Polypropylene sutures (6-0) are used.

Nail Fold Biopsy. Biopsy of the proximal nail fold may be useful for the diagnosis of connective tissue disease. This may be performed as a 2 to 3 mm wide crescent-shaped biopsy of the edge of the proximal nail fold. A 2 mm punch biopsy and a shave biopsy are alternative procedures for the location of uncommon conditions. Punches should not involve the free edge because these might lead to distortion of the proximal nail fold. Healing is rapid by secondary intention.

NAIL AVULSIONS

This is the most common nail operation and is usually unnecessary and is frequently contraindicated because of the possible resultant damage to the nail organ. The nail plate is the physiologic cover of the matrix and nail bed. Nail avulsion always tears off the superficial cell layers of the matrix. The nail bed epithelium becomes epidermoid with a granular and a horny layer. The whole nail bed may shrink, thus increasing the transverse curvature of the nail. This is particularly important in the great toe. The pulp of the hallux is pushed dorsally owing to its rolling motion during walking, and this results in the formation of a distal nail fold overriding the toe.

In the distal nail avulsion technique (Fig. 43–5), a septum elevator is inserted under the proximal nail fold, which is separated from the proximal portion of the nail plate. Then, the elevator is slid under the distal edge of the nail plate, freeing it from the hyponychium and nail bed. Back and forth motions of the instrument facilitate the separation of the nail, but special care is necessary at the proximal corners. Finally, the nail plate is grasped with a sturdy hemostat and peeled off with a twisting motion.

Cordero's proximal nail avulsion method (Fig. 43–6) starts by freeing the nail from the proximal nail fold. The nail elevator is then cautiously moved

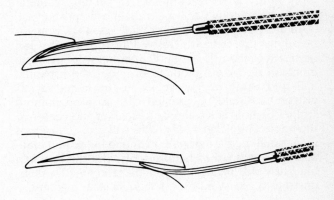

Figure 43—5. Classic nail avulsion starting distally and proceeding proximally.

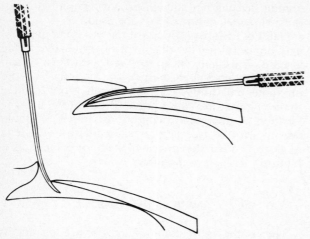

Figure 43–6. Cordero's technique starting proximally and proceeding distally.

around and under the proximal nail edge. The corners of the nail plate are firmly attached to the lateral nail sulcus under the proximal nail fold and must be freed before the base of the nail plate is placed on the proximal nail fold. Then, the nail elevator can be pushed easily between nail plate and nail bed up to the hyponychium.

Since nail avulsion is commonly performed for onychomycosis, it is mandatory to remove subungual keratoses and debris from the nail bed and sulci with a smooth curette. In the management of high-risk patients, nonsurgical removal of the nail should be considered when necessary. This can be effected by the use of urea paste (40%) applied directly to the nail after the surrounding skin has been protected by adhesive tape. The paste is left in place for three to eight days, and the dressing is then removed. Sometimes much of the affected nail comes away, and the remainder, which has lost its nail bed attachment, can be removed with scissors.

SUBUNGUAL HEMATOMA

Subungual hematoma is a frequent phenomenon. Only rarely is its resemblance to subungual melanoma close enough to pose a diagnostic problem.

Acute trauma with severe pain is always remembered by the patient. Depending on the site and intensity of the injury, the hematoma will be visible immediately or grow out from under the proximal nail fold within a few weeks. If the hematoma is visible, it should be drained with a sharp pointed scalpel or hot paper-clip cautery over the center of the hematoma (Fig. 43–7). This will give relief from pain. Small hematomas are included in the nail plate and not degraded to hemosiderin, and the Prussian blue test will be negative in these cases. To demonstrate the true nature of this blackish pigment, a benzidine test (Hemostix) with scrapings boiled in a small test tube will give a positive result.

A hematoma involving over 25% of the visible nail is the warning sign of nail bed injury. X-rays are mandatory since the bone may be fractured. The nail is carefully removed and the hematoma evacuated. Hemostasis facilitates the reconstruction of the torn nail bed, which is sutured with 6-0 Dexon. Blood and tissue remnants are removed from the nail plate, which is cleaned, shortened, and slightly narrowed and then replaced by suturing it to the lateral nail folds. Provided there is no wound infection, the stitches are left for 10 to 12 days.

Chronic hematomas are mainly due to repeated trauma from ill-fitting footwear or sporting activities. They are painless and frequently escape the notice of the patient. The repeated hemorrhage may grow out in a longitudinal fashion, thus mimicking longitudinal melanonychia. Some hematomas persist, and in these cases, partial nail avulsion may be necessary.

PARONYCHIA

Acute subungual paronychia that does not respond to penicllinase-fast antibiotics within 48 hours should be treated surgically by removing the proximal third of the nail plate. It is cut transversely with nail-splitting scissors (Fig. 43–8).

In distal subungual infection, probing will determine the most painful area and provide an indication for the site of fenestration of the nail plate. Soaking the finger in antiseptic solutions, such as chlorhexidine, twice daily and dressing with wet compresses usually result in rapid healing.

Sometimes the evacuation of a bullous pyoderma brings to light a narrow sinus that may communicate with a deeper, necrotic inoculation zone. This must be laid open and excised. Bacterial cultures and sensitivity studies are of paramount importance.

Chronic paronychia manifests as a red and painful swelling with retraction of the perionychial tissue

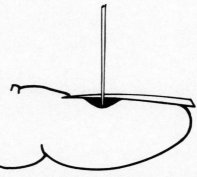

Figure 43–7. Drainage in acute partial subungual hematoma.

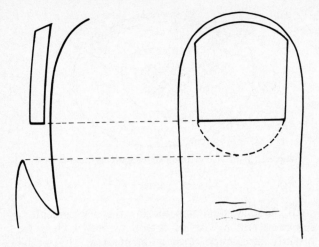

Figure 43–8. Acute paronychia—removal of the base of the nail plate.

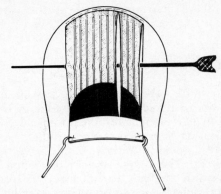

Figure 43–10. Post-traumatic split nail deformity—the scar is excised, and relaxing incisions are made at the lateral margins of the nail bed.

accompanied by loss of the cuticle and separation of the nail plate from the undersurface of the proximal nail fold. It may be due to *Candida albicans* infection or foreign bodies such as hair, bristle, or wood splinters. Conditions not responding to medical therapy are treated by the excision of a crescent-shaped full-thickness piece of the proximal nail fold that is 5 to 6 mm at its greatest width and extends from one lateral nail fold to the other and includes the entire swollen portion of the proximal nail fold (Fig. 43–9). Complete healing by secondary intention takes about two months.

POST-TRAUMATIC SPLIT NAIL DEFORMITY

Wounds running longitudinally through the matrix (and nail bed) may cause a split in the nail. To correct this unsightly deformity, oblique incisions are made at the lateral corners of the proximal nail

fold and are brought proximally toward the extensor crease of the distal joint (Fig. 43–10). The nail fold is then elevated and the matrix exposed. After the nail has been avulsed, the scar is excised from its most proximal portion in the matrix to the distal margin of the nail bed. The incision is made to include a full thickness extending down to the bone. The entire elliptical defect is undermined in order to facilitate closure. If the wound is under tension, relaxing incisions are made at the most lateral margins of the nail bed. This allows the central margins to be approximated more easily with interrupted sutures of 6-0 Dexon. The proximal nail fold is replaced into its normal position, and the two angular incisions are closed with 5-0 nylon sutures and then removed after seven days. Nonadherent gauze is packed under the proximal nail fold to separate it from the matrix. The exposed surface of the nail bed is covered with the nail plate, which has been trimmed and sutured in position. The new nail, which will regenerate, will be slightly narrower than the normal contralateral nail. If the split is close to the lateral margins of the nail plate, the most reliable method is to use the technique recommended for the lateral-longitudinal nail biopsy without reflecting the proximal nail fold.

INGROWING NAILS

Ingrowing nails mainly occur in the great toe and rarely affect the second toe. Fingers are only involved in exceptional cases, and a search for underlying pathology, such as a tumor, foreign body granuloma, exostosis, or osteoarthritis is indicated.

There are nearly as many different hypotheses concerning the etiology of ingrowing toenails as physicians treating this disorder. Irrespective of the initial cause, the condition finally presents with a nail bed that is too narrow for its nail plate. Fre-

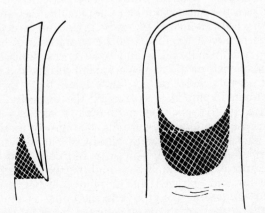

Figure 43–9. Chronic paronychia—excision of the proximal nail fold.

quently, there is overcurvature of the overlying plate.

Infantile Ingrown Toenails

The infantile type of ingrown toenail usually shows a rim of tissue at the distal edge of the nail plate and hypertrophic lateral nail folds. A crescent wedge excision is carried out all around the distal phalanx to a distance of about 2 mm from the nail (Fig. 43–11). The wedge should be 4 mm at its greatest width and has to be dissected from the bone. The defect is closed with 5-0 monofilament sutures, which should be removed after 10 to 14 days. In addition, this is the only technique suitable for treating distally embedded toenails after avulsion.

Juvenile Ingrown Toenails

The juvenile type is the most common one. It is often found in tall, thin adolescents with hyperhidrosis and acrocyanosis. The nail is usually embedded medially, although both sides of the nail may be affected. In an effort to relieve the pain, the patient often tries to cut off the offending lateral corner of the free edge under the inflamed, swollen soft tissue. The most lateral part, however, usually remains, giving rise to a nail spicule piercing through the epithelium of the lateral nail sulcus. Granulation tissue and secondary infection follow.

Treatment of the early stages is conservative. The foot is soaked in warm water with povidone-iodine

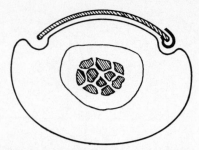

Figure 43–12. Guter treatment for an ingrown toenail.

soap. Under local anesthesia, the nail spicule is removed and a wisp of cotton wool, which is frequently moistened with a disinfectant, is put between the lateral nail edge and sulcus. If possible, inserting a plastic gutter (such as the one provided in the toenail treatment kit available from Portex Ltd., Hythe, Kent, Great Britain) is a good alternative (Fig. 43–12). This relieves the pressure and avoids infection. The center of the nail may also be ground to render it more pliable. After removal of the spicule, the granulation tissue may resolve spontaneously. Another kit containing a rubber wedge is aimed at pushing the nail fold laterally. Conservative management usually relieves pain and inflammation but demands a high degree of compliance. Recurrences are very frequent, and a definite surgical cure is necessary in about two thirds of the cases. Nail avulsion is not advisable.

For definitive cure, at least two different types of operations are performed: wedge excisions of the whole nail apparatus and selective matrix excisions leaving the rest of the nail organ intact. The most common wedge excision includes the lateral portion of the nail, the corresponding hyponychium, nail bed, matrix, and the proximal and lateral nail fold. The incisions have to be carried down to the bone, and in order to remove all of the lateral nail portion, the wedge has to be very wide in its proximal part. This renders primary suture very difficult. If the wedge is too narrow and does not include the lateral matrix horn, which is the most important structure to be removed, remnants of the lateral matrix horn give rise to nail spikes and recurrences. Since the pathogenesis of the ingrown toenail results in a nail that is too wide for its underlying bed, logical treatment is aimed at correcting the disparity. Selective matrix excision permanently narrows the nail, resulting in a safe cure for the ingrown toenail.

The nail plate is cut longitudinally at its lateral fifth, after the lateral nail strip is freed from the proximal nail fold, nail bed, and matrix with a nail elevator and extracted. A no. 1 needle is inserted along the lateral nail groove to the bone, as a guide to the corner of the lateral matrix horn, then an incision is made in the proximal nail fold to expose

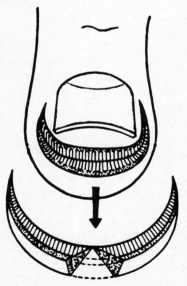

Figure 43–11. Howard-Dubois soft tissue resection for the infantile type of ingrown toenail.

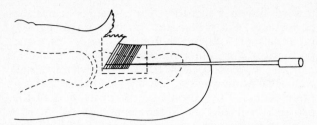

Figure 43–13. A no. 1 needle is inserted along the lateral nail groove to the bone, as a guide to the lateral horn of the matrix (after Austin).

the lateral matrix area, and the matrix is dissected out around the needle that marks the most proximolateral matrix area that has to be excised (Fig. 43–13). The resulting wound cavity is filled with small tapered antibiotic tablets, and the proximal nail fold is closed with a Steri-Strip. Usually, granulation tissue disappears within three to five days after removal of the piercing nail spicule. No nail avulsion is necessary prior to this small but definitive operation.

As an alternative to a surgical approach, the lateral matrix portion may be cauterized with liquefied phenol (88% solution). After removal of the lateral strip of the nail, hemostasis is accomplished with a tourniquet, and the blood is carefully cleaned from the space under the proximal nail fold using sterile gauze.

Curettage of the lateral matrix before phenol cautery usually guarantees the result. Antibiotic tapers are put into the wound cavity as described above. An antimicrobial ointment is applied with a dressing that is changed after two days. It is essential to have a completely bloodless field since blood inactivates phenol. The cautery has to be applied for three minutes in order to achieve a complete eradication of the matrix epithelium.

Postoperative pain after phenol cautery is minimal since phenol has a considerable local anesthetic action. It is also antiseptic. The matrix epithelium is sloughed off and usually exhibits slight oozing for two to three weeks. Daily foot baths with povidone-iodine soap will accelerate healing.

Some authors advocate a total ablation of the matrix and nail bed, resulting in permanent eradication of the nail organ. This radical operation takes several weeks to heal, and there is a surprisingly high rate of recurrence. First, the nail is avulsed. The proximal nail fold is reflected after lateral incisions expose the matrix epithelium. A no. 1 needle is inserted along each lateral nail groove to the bone, then the matrix (Fig. 43–13) is excised as a rectangular block of tissue, down to the periosteum, with special attention to the insertion of the extensor tendon beneath the matrix. The block extends distally to just beyond the edge of the lunular area, proximally almost as far as the joint line, and laterally until the fatty tissue of the pulp is reached. The proximal nail fold is replaced and the wound closed with a Steri-Strip. Dressings are changed every other day. The patient should keep the foot elevated as much as possible.

The Terminal Syme operation is still more radical. It is the removal of the matrix and nail bed with the amputation of the distal half of the terminal bone. The ridged skin of the pulp is then pulled dorsally and sutured over the defect of the former matrix. Recurrences are said to be less frequent and healing to be more rapid in the Terminal Syme amputation than with Zadik's procedure. However, personal experience of more than 15 years with the selective lateral matrix excision has shown that recurrences with this method are very rare, and both the functional and cosmetic results are excellent.

Hypertrophy of the Lateral Nail Fold

Some people have thick hypertrophic lateral nail folds (Fig. 43–14). They are usually the result of long-standing ingrown nails. Inflammation may range from the subclinical to the severe. About one fifth of the nail digging into the lateral nail fold is cut and avulsed; then, depending on the degree of hypertrophy and inflammation, different methods may be used. If hypertrophy is moderate (Fig. 43–15), one incises an elliptical wedge of tissue taken from the lateral wall of the toe to the bone, pulling the lateral nail fold away from the offending lateral nail edge. The lateral nail fold then gradually shrinks with decreasing inflammation.

If hypertrophy is marked (Fig. 43–16), an incision is made through the nail bed along the nail groove, including the granulation tissue, and the blade is carried up through the lateral part of the proximal

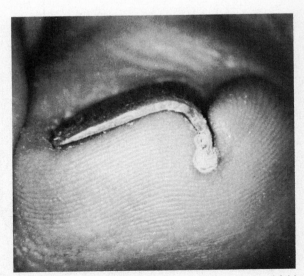

Figure 43–14. Unilateral hypertrophy of the lateral nail fold.

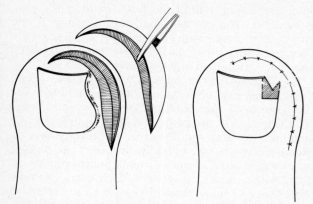

Figure 43–15. Treatment of moderate hypertrophy of the lateral nail fold.

nail fold to about 1 cm proximal to the cuticle. Distally, the incision reaches 2 to 3 mm inferior to the free nail margin. A parallel incision is then made through the nail wall, turning distally and proximally

toward the first incision. The incisions reach the periosteum except for the portion involving the proximal nail fold and the pulp. A wedge of tissue is removed, including the nail groove, the lateral nail fold with granulation tissue, and a sliver of nail wall. The wound edges are approximated, but sutured with 5-0 nylon only in the distal part of the proximal nail fold and in the distal nail bed.

When the lateral hypertrophic nail fold is associated with a nail distally embedded, the more radical soft tissue excision around the whole nail is indicated (see the section on infantile ingrown toenails) (Fig. 43–11). If infection is evident, nail avulsion is performed about one month prior to the operation.

Pincer Nails

Pincer nails (overcurvature or unguis constringens) are relatively common and may affect the big toe alone or all of the digits (Fig. 43–17). However,

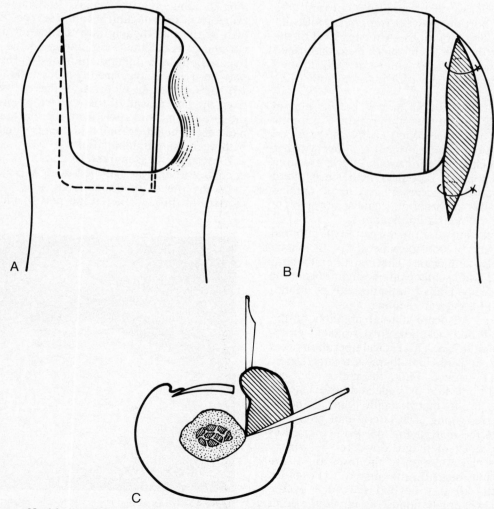

Figure 43–16. *A* to *C*, Surgical treatment for marked hypertrophy of the lateral nail fold in an ingrown toenail.

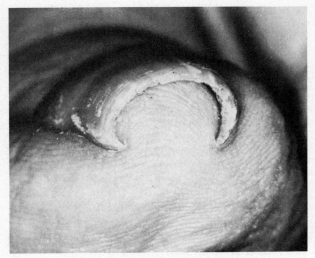

Figure 43–17. Painful pincer nail.

pain is usually produced only in the hallux. Pincer nails in young people are due to an inborn anomaly of the distal phalanx, which may be demonstrated radiologically. They are symmetrical and often involve several toes. Elderly people with overcurvature of the nail suffer from foot deformities or osteoarthritis of the distal interphalangeal joint of the fingers. Radiographs show irregular osteophytes at the base of the terminal phalanx. The widening of the bone under the matrix area probably causes the distally increasing overcurvature by pushing the lateral matrix horn laterodistally. This might be the cause of the distal dorsal tuft, since the overcurvature results in continuous traction of the distal nail bed portion. Traction is known to produce exostoses. There are different treatment approaches.

The nail brace technique (Fig. 43–18) is aimed at correcting the inward distortion of the nail by maintaining continuous tension on the nail plate. After cleaning the sulci, a firm but elastic nail brace made from stainless steel wire is fitted to the nail plate. A series of adjustments adapted to the gradual de-

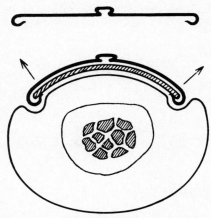

Figure 43–18. Nail brace technique—a conservative management in pincer nail.

crease of curvature is made over a period of six months and results in a painless correction of the pincer nail. However, since the underlying bone pathology remains untreated, the condition usually relapses.

Clipping of the lateral nail plate, as far proximally as possible, offers an alternative conservative approach. Since the pincer nail is very thick, the use of an emollient (3% salicylic acid in petrolatum) for two days is recommended as well as occlusive treatment dressing with a shaving soap. In early cases, grooving the nail plate throughout its entire length may temporarily relieve the pressure on the lateral sulci.

Surgical methods are usually necessary for a definitive cure. There are several alternatives:

1. A wedge excision including the lateral portion of the nail plate, nail bed, and matrix has been recommended. With permanent nail narrowing, the lateral nail strip cannot dig into the lateral groove.

2. Matrix resection prevents the nail from regrowing.

3. Howard-Dubois soft tissue resection (Fig. 43–11) consists of a preliminary nail avulsion and is complemented by removal of the distal tuft of bone. It is successful in most cases but should be supplemented by the nail brace technique as the nail regrows.

4. An attempt may be made to flatten the narrowed, swollen distal nail bed. After nail avulsion, a median longitudinal incision of the nail bed is made down to the bone. The nail bed is dissected from the bone and spread to both sides. It is held in position by reversed tie-over sutures put in the folds and tied over a pad on the plantar aspect of the digit. The lozenge-shaped defect in the nail bed is covered with split-thickness skin. A compression bandage is applied for one week. The tie-over sutures are removed after three weeks.

5. Bearing in mind the probable pathogenesis, the following synthesis of steps from different procedures is recommended (Fig. 43–19). The nail is narrowed by a bilateral excision or cautery of the lateral matrix horns. The distal half of the nail plate is carefully removed, and a longitudinal median incision of the nail bed is carried down to the bone. The nail bed is then dissected from the bone and mobilized. The dorsal tuft is removed with a rongeur. The nail bed is sutured with 6-0 Vicryl, and reversed tie-over sutures are put in the folds and tied over the plantar aspect of the toe. This procedure spreads the heaped-up distal nail bed and prevents regrowth of the nail from the lateral matrix horns.

CONGENITAL MALALIGNMENT OF THE HALLUX NAIL

Deviation of the longitudinal axis of the big toenail is not rare in infants. It may cause chronic

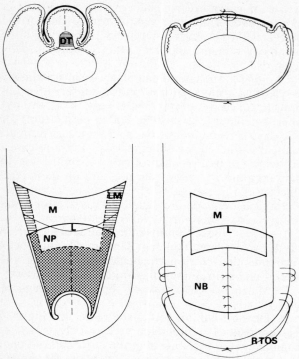

Figure 43–19. Haneke's operation for the correction of pincer nail. DT = dorsal tuft of terminal phalanx; L = lunula; LM = lateral matrix horn; M = matrix; NB = nail bed; NP = nail plate; RTOS = reserved tie-over sutures; ⫶⫶⫶ = nail plate portion to be removed; ≡ = lateral matrix horn to be excised or cauterized.

paronychia or ingrowing nails within the first years of life, but later onychodystrophy or onychogryphosis may develop. Management will depend on an accurate assessment of the degree and significance of the nail deviation and associated changes:

1. If the deviation is mild, the nail may overcome the initial, slight distal embedding as it hardens, and sufficient normal nail may grow to the tip of the digit to prevent further secondary traumatic changes. No surgical treatment is needed for these cases.

2. If the lateral deviation of the nail plate is marked, then many potentially disabling changes

may occur in childhood and in adult life. Surgical correction (Fig. 43–20) is essential in order to prevent permanent nail dystrophy.

A crescent wedge-shaped excision is carried out below the nail bed and matrix all around the tip of the toe. The crescent has to be larger on the medial aspect. A small Burow's triangle is removed at the start of the lateral incision. The nail bed and matrix are dissected free from the bone and the whole nail apparatus is swung to realign the nail's longitudinal axis. Then, 5-0 polypropylene sutures are used and the stitches removed after 12 to 15 days.

ONYCHOGRYPHOSIS

The nail in this condition is very much thickened and distorted; it often resembles a ram's horn (Fig. 43–21). It consists of irregular, obliquely arranged lamellae of nail material and remnants of serum. The matrix surface is papillomatous. The nail does not adhere to the shrunken nail bed, and the nail bed epithelium is keratinized like epidermis. Conservative treatment is indicated in high-risk patients (peripheral arterial disease, severe diabetes mellitus). The nail is softened with an emollient and clipped or trimmed with rotating grinders. This procedure is often unsatisfactory, and a surgical approach may be indicated.

In surgical treatment, the nail is avulsed and complete hemostasis is ensured. The matrix is cauterized with liquefied phenol—two to three minutes for the matrix, 30 seconds to the undersurface of the proximal nail fold and the nail bed. The matrix in onychogryphosis often extends more distally, and this has to be kept in mind during matricectomy. Phenol cautery is superior to cold steel surgery for matricectomy: it is simpler, demands less skill, takes less time to perform, and has a higher success rate. In addition, infection is far less frequent, postoperative pain is minimal, and postoperative morbidity is shorter. Onychauxis (nail thickening) and pachyonychia congenita may also best be treated with phenol cautery or electrofulguration of the subungual tissue.

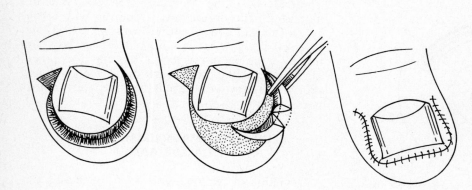

Figure 43–20. Nail malalignment treatment.

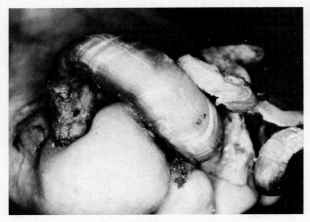

Figure 43–21. Onychogryphosis.

NAIL TUMORS

There are a considerable number of different nail tumors. Nearly all of them share certain difficulties in diagnosis that are peculiar to the nail region:

1. The unique anatomy of the nail apparatus modifies the tumor appearance, growth, and symptoms.

2. Either blood or melanin may produce atypical pigmentation.

3. Nail tumors often mimic infections or are themselves secondarily infected.

4. Nail changes due to the tumor are often noticed only after an incidental trauma and may therefore not be diagnosed.

5. Non-neoplastic swelling may occur.

An x-ray should always be performed when there is persistent inflammation, swelling, or a suspected tumor.

PERIUNGUAL WARTS

Periungual warts are unsightly, benign virus tumors with a rough keratotic surface. Fissuring may cause pain and infection. Subungual warts are rare and painful and may even erode the bone. Treatment of periungual warts is often frustrating. In children, they may respond to therapeutic suggestion. Saturated monochloroacetic acid applied sparingly, allowed to dry and covered with 40% salicylic acid plaster for two to three days allows blunt removal after three to four days. The procedure may be repeated until all the warts are cleared. No more than three fingers should be treated at the same time because pain, which is not caused at the time of therapy, is generally delayed.

Cryotherapy is another popular modality but is unsuitable for children. Treatment of the proximal nail fold has to be performed very carefully in order to avoid damage to the matrix. Curettage and electrodesiccation produces unsightly scarring. Cold steel should be avoided. Infrared coagulation and carbon dioxide laser surgery have been used with some success. The argon laser may be used for selective coagulation of the blood-filled capillaries in the papillae after the verrucous keratosis has been largely removed with keratolytic agents. Subungual warts are treated in the same manner after removal of the portion of the nail protecting the wart.

DORSAL MYXOID CYST

The nature of this lesion is still unclear. It usually develops in the proximal nail fold just beside the median axis and is much more frequent in fingers than in toes. Osteoarthritis of the distal interphalangeal joint is often present. Repeated incisions or punctures and drainage; simple excision; electrocautery; chemical cautery; injection of proteases, steroids, and sclerosing agents; x-rays; and other methods have all been used with varying effect.

A careful extirpation of the cyst-like lesion is recommended. A drop of sterile methylene blue solution is mixed with fresh hydrogen peroxide, and 0.1 to 0.2 ml is injected into the distal interphalangeal joint via the volar joint crease. This will clearly identify the stalk connecting the joint with the cyst and the cyst itself, which may show tentacle-like extrusions. The skin over the cyst is incised, and the lesion is meticulously dissected. The pedicle is traced to the joint capsule and resected; osteophytic spurs of the terminal phalanx are removed with a fine chisel or bone rongeur. A small rotation flap may be used to cover the skin defect. A split-thickness graft is an alternative as well as healing by secondary intention.

For small myxoid cysts in a distal location, nail fold excision, which involves a technique similar to that employed in chronic paronychia, may be used. Cryosurgery was reported to give an 86% cure rate.

SUBUNGUAL EXOSTOSIS

Subungual exostoses are painful osseous growths mostly occurring in the big toe of young people. The differentiation from osteochondroma is somewhat academic. Trauma is the major etiologic factor; x-rays are mandatory for diagnosis.

Treatment consists of removal of the exostosis under full aseptic conditions. An L-shaped laterodistal incision parallel to the nail is made. The exostosis is dissected free and removed with a bone chisel. The nail bed covering the exostosis is usually heavily altered and exhibits thinning, hyperkeratosis, and loss of elasticity. Therefore, treatment that involves incisions of the nail bed should be avoided if possible.

SUBUNGUAL GLOMUS TUMOR

This tumor is rare but well known because of its characteristic radiating pain that may be spontaneous or evoked by minor trauma. It is seen through the nail plate as an indistinct bluish lesion. The nail plate is often thinned over it and may become ridged. Probing may aid in the exact localization. X-rays will reveal secondary bone involvement. Surgical extirpation is the only treatment.

Small tumors in the center under the nail may be enucleated after punching a 6 mm hole into the nail plate and incising the nail bed. Those in lateral positions are excised by an L-shaped incision. The nail bed dermis is dissected from the bone until the glomus tumor is reached. The recurrence rate is 10% to 20%, representing incompletely excised, multiple, or newly developed tumors.

BOWEN'S DISEASE AND SQUAMOUS CELL CARCINOMA

Bowen's disease is not as rare as might appear from the medical literature. It is an intraepidermal carcinoma and may progress to an invasive squamous cell carcinoma, hence the term "epidermoid carcinoma." Squamous cell carcinoma is of low-grade malignancy, and its development is slow. Pain, swelling, inflammation, elevation of the nail, ulceration, tumor mass resembling pyogenic granuloma or ingrown nail, and bleeding are typical features. A biopsy is necessary in order to confirm the diagnosis. Mohs' chemosurgery is the treatment of choice, ensuring radical excision and sparing the healthy, surrounding skin. Plastic surgery is an alternative.

LONGITUDINAL MELANONYCHIA

Longitudinal linear pigmentation of the nail by melanin may be due to benign melanocytic hyperplasia, lentigo simplex, nevocellular nevus, atypical melanocytic hyperplasia, or malignant melanoma. Pigmented nail strips are common in dark-skinned races but rare in Caucasians. In persons with fair complexion, they are more likely to be malignant than benign. Therefore, complete excisional biopsy is recommended for both diagnosis and therapy. Histology may be difficult, and sometimes only serial sections may reveal the true nature of the lesion.

The treatment depends on the size and site of the lesions (Fig. 43–22). For strips not exceeding a width of 3 mm, a punch excision is performed. The proximal nail fold is reflected, and a 3 or 3.5 mm punch can be cut through the soft nail plate into the matrix down to the bone at the beginning of the pigmented band. The tissue cylinder is then released from the bone with pointed iris scissors.

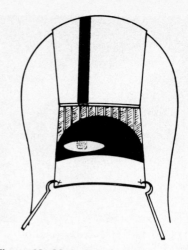

Figure 43–22. Longitudinal melanonychia.

Pigmented bands wider than 3 mm require a fusiform matrix biopsy with its greatest width over the center of the band. After reflection of the proximal nail fold, the proximal third of the nail plate is removed and the lesion excised. This may be difficult to see after avulsion of the proximal portion of the nail plate, and a marking on the proximal nail fold is a useful guide. Careful undermining will allow primary closure of the matrix. Lesions located at the margins of the nail are excised as a lateral-longitudinal nail biopsy.

Subungual melanomas remain asymptomatic for a long period. Incidental trauma, secondary infection, nail dystrophy, ulceration, and bleeding may cause the patient to seek medical advice. About a quarter of subungual melanomas are amelanotic. Pigmented tumors may present as a brown spot in the matrix, nail bed, or plate, a longitudinal pigmented band, or brownish-black discoloration spreading from under the nail or nail fold to the surrounding skin. The latter is called Hutchinson's sign and is an almost certain indication of melanoma.

Longitudinal melanonychia with periungual pigmentation, nail dystrophy, ulceration, or a mass that bleeds readily should be treated a priori as a malignant melanoma. Complete removal of the whole nail organ is sufficient for early melanomas (level II = pT 1), but tumors reaching or penetrating the dermis usually demand amputation. Defects after ablation of the nail apparatus may be closed with a distant flap or graft.

MINOR PLASTIC SURGERY OF THE NAIL

Correction of Racket Thumb

This condition is due to an abnormally short and broad terminal bony phalanx (Fig. 43–23). The nail

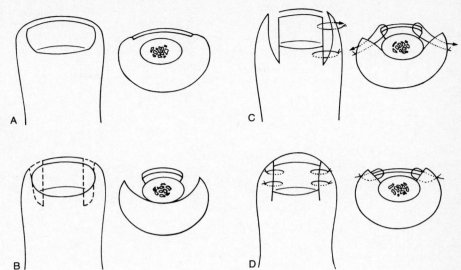

Figure 43–23. *A* to *D,* Surgical treatment for racket thumb. *C* and *D,* Reconstruction of the lateral nail fold.

is very short and wide; the lateral nail folds are usually lacking. Treatment is aimed at narrowing the terminal phalanx to about the normal length-to-breadth ratio using the technique described for lateral-longitudinal nail biopsies. The lateral aspects of the thumb are mobilized and sutured as described for the reconstruction of the lateral nail fold.

Reconstruction of the Proximal Nail Fold

Minor lacerations may be adequately treated by excision of a crescent-shaped full-thickness piece of the proximal nail fold and by secondary healing (Fig. 43–9).

Reconstruction of the Lateral Nail Fold

Loss of the lateral nail fold results in an uneven, unsightly appearance (Figs. 43–23 *C* and *D*). It is caused by wedge excisions and also by lateral-longitudinal nail biopsies. This can be prevented by a slight modification of the suture. The lateral nail wall is freed from the bone. The needle is first inserted into the midst of this wall in between the dorsal and volar aspects of the terminal phalanx and pulled through the nail bed and nail plate, then turned back to the lateral nail fold and inserted again at the level of the nail groove. The wound margins are approximated, and this results in an elevation and restoration of the lateral nail fold.

SUGGESTED READINGS

Baran R: Removal of the proximal nail fold, Why, When, How? J Dermatol Surg Oncol (in press)

Baran R, Bureau H: Congenital malalignment of the big toenail as a cause of ingrowing toenail in infancy. Clin Exp Dermatol 8:613–623, 1983

Baran R, Haneke E: Diagnostik und Therapie der streifenförmigen Nagelpigmentierung. Hautarzt 35:359–365, 1984

Bureau H, Baran R, Haneke E: Nail surgery and traumatic abnormalities, in Baran R, Dawber RPR (eds): Diseases of the Nails and their management. Oxford, Blackwell Scientific Publications, 1984, pp 347–402

Douglass MC, Krull EA: Diseases of the nails, in Conn HF (ed): Current Therapy. Philadelphia, W B Saunders Co, 1981

Fosnaugh RF: Surgery of the nail, in Epstein E, Epstein E Jr (eds): Skin Surgery, Ed 5. Springfield, Ill, Charles C Thomas, 1982

Haneke E: Behandlung einiger Nagelfehlbildungen, in Wolff HH, Schmeller W (eds): Fehlbildungen—Naevi—Melanoma. Fortschritte der operativen Dermatologie, vol 2. Berlin, Springer-Verlag, 1985, pp 71–77

Haneke E: Pathogenesis of pincer nail. Paper read at the 5th Congress of the International Society for Dermatologic Surgery, Jerusalem, 1984 (in press)

Haneke E, Baran R, Bureau H: Tumours of the nail apparatus and adjacent tissues, in Baran R, Dawber RPR (eds): Diseases of the nails and their management. Oxford, Blackwell Scientific Publications, 1984, pp 403–452

Morkane AJ, Robertson RW, Inglis GS: Segmented phenolization of ingrowing toenails: A randomized controlled study. Br J Surg 71:526–527, 1984

Scher RK: Nail surgery, in Epstein E, Epstein E Jr (eds): Techniques in Skin Surgery. Philadelphia, Lea & Febiger, 1979, pp 164–170

Special Diseases

PART

PART

8

44

ERVIN EPSTEIN, M.D.

Thoughts on Melanoma

Melanoma is both an interesting and puzzling neoplasm. In addition to its reputation as a ruthless killer, its incidence has increased at an alarming rate. Concurrently, with this basically unexplained explosion in its frequency, a great deal of academic and clinical research has enriched our knowledge of this tumor. To this might be added the results of deductive reasoning and serendipity to bring us to our present level of knowledge and ignorance.

INCIDENCE AND ETIOLOGY

We can all agree that the incidence of melanoma has been increasing. However, no one really knows how to explain this phenomenon. There is no dearth of theories to explain it. On the other hand, it is possible that most of these explanations are based on statistical freaks. By this I mean that a fortuitous grouping of cases has led to conclusions that have not withstood the test of scrutiny or confirmation by other investigators. For instance, what seemed to be a logical explanation resulted from a report on fertility drugs. The reporting physician claimed that he used these medications in nine women, and eight of them developed melanomas. This certainly was an exciting theory and one that even had some theoretic backing to lend credence. However, although the use of these agents has increased, this report lacks confirmation. The great American philosopher Mark Twain perhaps said it best when he remarked, "Science is a wonderful field. For a very small input of fact, you get such an overwhelming return of theory."

What about ionizing radiation as a cause? The Livermore Laboratory, which is concerned with the development and utilization of nuclear energy, had an "epidemic" of melanomas. This problem was studied very carefully by the scientists at the laboratory, and the U.S. government even dispatched a blue-ribbon committee to investigate this problem. The committee's report was never completed because the Department of Energy was disbanded as an economy move inspired by Reagonomics, but their unofficial explanation was that this was a statistical aberration of no significance. Most of the sufferers had no contact with the ionizing radiation generated at this facility. There was no increase in the incidence of skin cancers, which are thought to be caused by solar or ionizing radiation. They had no unusual exposure to solar irradiation.[29] The so-called epidemic vanished rather than accelerated. There was no epidemic of melanoma in Livermore's sister laboratory in Los Alamos.[1]

A search of the available books and the literature was disappointing as far as shedding light on the possibility of ionizing radiation being a cause of this malignancy. Only Traenkle mentioned four cases of melanoma occurring in patches of chronic radio-dermatitis, i.e., patients who had physical evidence of an overdose of ionizing radiation. However, he admitted that this might not be of significance.[29] In an unimpressive presentation, Conley claimed that he saw five patients who developed melanoma from x-radiation therapy.[8] Although all received such treatment, it was obvious from the photographs that two originally had lentigo maligna, two cases occurred after other injuries (one being a thermal burn), and the fifth developed in an area that had received a large dose of such therapy for a squamous cell carcinoma of the lip. When you consider that the preceding conditions may have had more to do with the development of the melanoma than the therapeutically applied radiation, one must be skeptical of Conley's interpretation of the etiology of these melanomas. A note placed in the *Schoch Letter* asking its 6000 subscribers for case reports of melanomas caused by ionizing radiation resulted in only three letters suggesting one case each, none of them convincing.

If the linear hypothesis suggesting that low-level radiation may cause cancer were true, then such radiation might cause melanoma or anything else since we are all exposed to low levels of radiation from normal background irradiation in the atmosphere, including televisions, microwave ovens, medical diagnoses and therapy, industrial exposure, and atomic bombs.[11] Basically, this theory claims that all x-rays are carcinogenic and that the incidence occurs in a straight line. In other words, if 100 rads caused 100 cancers, one rad would cause one cancer.

I consider the linear hypothesis to be absurd. If one accepts the proposed logic for this concept, then one must believe that if a 100 mile an hour wind will blow the roof off a barn, a 10 mile an hour wind will blow 10% of the roof off.

This brings us to another possible cause, sunshine. There is no question that this energy plays some part in the production of melanomas. There is no dearth of studies proving this, which consider such parameters as incidence in sunny versus cloudy areas of the globe, relation to sunspots, times of the year, and increased occurrence on the lower legs of women compared with men's. There is no question that melanoma is more apt to occur in sun-exposed portions of the body when accompanied by other malignancies commonly blamed on overexposure to this energy, such as sailor's skin, farmer's skin, and xeroderma pigmentosum. Cases of melanoma apparently caused by PUVA therapy have been reported. Brodthagen reported on a melanoma apparently caused by exposure to a UV-A suntan bed.[5] However, considering the overall problem, evidence such as this must be considered to be circumstantial.

After all, the devotees of the concept of sunshine being the cause of melanoma have been unable to solve the 64-thousand-dollar question: Why is melanoma encountered more commonly on the covered parts of the body than on exposed areas? Despite the work of Kripke showing that exposure to ultraviolet light increased the possibility of transplanting melanomas to unexposed areas in mice, it hardly solves the problem of the occurrence of this neoplasm on non–sun-exposed locations in human beings.[20] While it is true that the incidence of melanoma is increasing in sunny climates, it is also increasing in other climates.

Beral and coworkers, who studied office workers, claimed that fluorescent lighting is a potent cause of melanomas.[3] However, even Beral admits that most of her cases occurred on the covered parts of the body. She ignored the fact that fluorescent lights give off a minimal amount of ultraviolet radiation. It was suggested that the reason that exposed areas were not affected more often is because the sunlight causes some thickening of the epidermis that protects the exposed areas from the irradiation from the fluorescent lights. These authors noted that fluorescent lights burning at home did not increase the incidence of melanoma. They admit that the incidence of melanoma is less in Australia and Great Britain in people working outdoors. They found that melanoma occurred less frequently in those exposed to sunlight the most. All of this work suggests that neither sunlight nor fluorescent lights hold the key to the increased incidence of melanoma.

Under other statistical freaks, we might consider the reports of "epidemics" in New York policemen using Mace or other reports incriminating diet as the explanation for this increase.

It has been suggested that improved diagnostic methods might constitute the sought-for explanation. The clinical diagnosis of this tumor will be discussed later. At this time, it should suffice to say that our clinical acuity has not improved much. The histologic diagnosis of superficial spreading melanoma (Level I) is being made more frequently than in the past. Also, we can hope that an increased

level of awareness in both physicians and laypersons has led to the uncovering of more cases. Unfortunately, we still see patients with this malignancy wandering from doctor to doctor, receiving only reassurance until someone finally recognizes the need for a biopsy, and a histologic confirmation establishes the diagnosis of melanoma.

Traditionally, trauma has been considered to be a causative, precipitating, or aggravating factor in all cancers. This is true in melanomas also. Both acute and chronic injuries were considered to be important in these neoplasms. However, this concept has become much less fashionable today after prolonged study and experimentation. On the other hand, I doubt if one can deny the possible influence of injury, especially chronic irritation, in maximizing the appearance of the growth and in some instances, the dissemination of melanomas.

Inheritance also plays a part in the development of melanomas. These tumors are found in certain inherited conditions such as xeroderma pigmentosum and B-K mole syndrome. There does seem to be a cancer diathesis. Patients with multiple cutaneous malignancies, such as basal cell and squamous cell cancers and sarcomas, may also manifest melanomas. Multiple cutaneous malignancies are noted not infrequently, and they may all be of the same type or any mixture of the lesions mentioned above. Also, congenital nevi may be a forerunner of melanoma.

There is a great deal of evidence that some cancers may be caused by viruses. This is also true of melanomas; however, this has not been established at this time to be the cause of this tumor.

The separation of the Allen-Spitz juvenile melanoma from the melanoma group should actually have decreased the number of melanomas presented.

PREMELANOMATOUS LESIONS

Traditionally, the junction nevus has been considered to be the basic premelanomatous lesion. But this concept leaves something to be desired. For instance, the neonate presents basically junction nevi, but in the elderly junction nevi are rare. What happened to all these junction nevi in the meantime? They have disappeared—not the moles, the junctional elements. Certainly, they have not all become melanomas. Perhaps the signficance of these nevi depends on the age of the patient and exposure to other factors that may be active in the production of these tumors. Furthermore, melanomas arise de novo in at least 50% of the cases.

At the present time, interest has evolved concerning the malignant potential of congenital melanocytic nevi. Solomon feels that all these lesions are premalignant and should be removed as early in life as possible.[28] On the other hand, Kopf points out the impossibility of applying such a campaign in a universal manner since there are not enough surgeons or dermatologic surgeons to carry out this project.[18] In addition to the psychic trauma, this policy would inevitably lead to a race of iatrogenically scarred adults. Furthermore, not all melanocytic nevi become melanomas. However, Kopf does admit that such lesions may eventuate in melanomas and recommends removal of those over 2 cm in diameter. While it is true that the larger the tumor, the greater the risk, it should be realized that there is nothing magical or sacred about the 2 cm measurement. Individual judgment is still the important deciding factor in the course to be followed in the management of these benign growths.

The B-K mole is a familial type of premelanomatous lesion. The lesions appear somewhat later in life and show a dyskeratotic type of nevus histologically. The sufferers from this condition have a high incidence of melanomas, although the tumors are of reduced malignancy.

PROGNOSIS OF MELANOMAS

From the standpoint of prognosis, melanomas may be divided into two categories: those with or without metastases. The outlook in the former is dismal, while in those confined to a single lesion, it is hopeful to very good. However, it is very difficult to determine if metastases have occurred in a patient clinically free of such unfortuante dissemination. For instance, Knutson and coworkers reported that in their series of 127 patients, lymph node dissection established that the clinical examiner was incorrect in 37.5% of those thought to have clinical lymph node metastases and in 22.2% of those in whom the clinician felt that these nodes were not affected.[16] Even after the most thorough examinations on the patients and laboratory testing, the absence of lymph node involvement cannot be determined without serial sectioning of the nodes (an unrealistic procedure in clinical practice). Microscopic involvement may be present but undetected by any available test other than prolonged study of serial sections. Yet, the differentiation between involvement of the nodes and freedom of the nodes is crucial in establishing the prognosis.

But, of course, we have other measures of prognosis. Studies of Clark's[7] or Breslow's[4] levels, whether classified as I, II, III, or IV or actual measurement of maximum penetration, are of great value in revealing the outlook for recovery or tragedy. Still, statistics do not apply to individuals. The incidence of cure or death in a patient is 100% in that individual. Not only is the cure rate in Levels I and II patients not quite 100%, but not all the patients with Level IV penetration perish. It should

be remembered that these measurements of penetration do not establish the basic malignancy of the tumor. They merely indicate whether the neoplasm has penetrated deeply enough to lodge in areas of increased vascularity, increasing the possibility of metastatic spread. This, of course, is of great value in suggesting therapeutic approaches and the chances of curability or palliation to be gained by the indicated therapy. The same can be said of volumetric measurements or the visible size of the tumors.

Day and coworkers state that histologic classification of melanomas is a more accurate measurement of prognosis than Breslow's levels.[10] Braun-Falco and colleagues find that the mitotic index (a comparison of the number of mitotic figures per cell group) is the most accurate indicator of prognosis in patients with these neoplasms.[25]

On the other hand, certain other factors are of importance in predicting the outcome from the moment they appear. For instance, amelanotic melanomas and pedunculated melanomas have a more ominous future than that borne by the patient with a banal melanoma.[26] The sex of the patient makes a difference; the prognosis is more favorable in women. Age is a crucial factor; probably most so-called melanomas in small children actually are examples of benign juvenile melanomas. In the aged, many melanomas are of the lentigo maligna type with a better prognosis than most. Furthermore, in my experience, melanomas in those past the age of 70 behave in a much less aggressive manner than in younger patients.

An 88-year old man had the largest melanoma that I have ever seen. It was of 18 years duration and had never been treated. If Clark had established a level classified as one million, I presume that this patient could qualify for such a rating. There were histologically proven metastases to the skin of the back. This patient died of pneumonia about two weeks later. At autopsy, not a single internal metastasis was found.

Another patient, 94 years old, consulted me because of a large black tumor on the cheek. Histopathologic examination revealed that this lesion was a metastasis from an undisclosed melanoma. The lesion was excised comparatively conservatively and did not recur. In addition, he had a large number of lesions that clinically resembled comedones. Examination under the microscope showed that these blackhead-like lesions were also metastatic melanoma. These lesions were destroyed by electrodesiccation and curettage under local anesthesia. The patient survived at least three years after the operations, and a primary melanoma was never discovered. He did give a history of a preceding eye operation but a report from the operating ophthalmologist revealed that this procedure was performed for a retinal detachment only.

The location of the primary tumor makes a difference also. For instance, tumors on the lower legs or in areas where more than one lymph node chain may be active in draining the site of the melanoma, such as near the midline of the trunk or on the genitalia, have a more serious prognosis. Melanoma of the eye tends to be comparatively benign.

Chronic melanoma occurs also. In these individuals, metastases occur but are relieved by simple excision of the primary tumor and the metastatic nodules. More metastases succeed the eradicated ones, and this may continue for many years, even for more than 20 years, before the patient finally succumbs. I have no explanation for this prolonged course except the vague statement "immunology," but it does indicate that the treatment of the metastases, if possible, may be a worthwhile procedure. One should not withhold therapy merely because evidence of metastatic spread is available.

I have been following a group of patients with melanoma without apparent metastases for more than 25 years. To the best of my knowledge, there are no other studies in the literature extending for more than 10 years. This group has furnished some very important information about the outlook for the patient without obvious metastases. For instance, 40% of these patients were alive after 25 years regardless of the eventual cause of death. Of the patients who died because of melanoma, 92% did so within the first decade after the diagnosis and treatment of their malignancy. None of the patients died of melanoma after 15 years, so it can be said that 15 years can be used as proof of cure in patients with *primary* melanoma. Only 20% of those perishing succumbed to their melanoma. This certainly offers a hopeful outlook and indicates that primary melanoma is not the ruthless killer it becomes after it has spread past its original manifestation. The 20% of deaths could be explained by the presence of occult metastases at the time of treatment. The findings in this series will be discussed further in other sections of this chapter.

DIFFICULTY OF DIAGNOSIS

It must be emphasized that a black color is not synonymous with malignancy. I have heard nondermatologists state at tumor boards over and over again, "The lesion is black. It may be a melanoma. We'd better remove it, widely and deeply." This is a lot of nonsense. In 559 patients with black lesions on the skin, only 2% of the lesions proved to be melanomas.[13] Furthermore, 85% were benign. Are we justified in subjecting all or many patients to morbidity-causing procedures that result in mutilation because such surgery is indicated in 2% of such patients? I doubt it.

Despite the writings of Mihm and others that a melanoma can be diagnosed clinically by the irregular shape of the plaque, the mixture of colors including reds, blues, blacks, and browns and by the rough surface, I submit that most melanomas do not show this characteristic appearance and that benign tumors may mimic these same features.[21] The diagnosis may become obvious by the finding of a rapidly growing, black, bleeding tumor with metastases, but by that time, it is too late to promise the patient a good prognosis. Therefore, early diagnosis is a must.

Clinical diagnosis is very unreliable. Most published series indicate that the clinical diagnosis is made correctly in only 40% to 50% of the cases.[17, 19] After reviewing all of the cases in which I entered melanoma as a possible diagnosis or those in which I did not suggest this possibility on the chart and histologic examination established that the lesion was a melanoma, I discovered that my batting average was only 400 (40%)—great for an outfielder but gruesome for a clinician.

While on the subject of the difficulty of diagnosing a malignant melanoma, I would like to allude to two rare tumors that may cause considerable confusion. First, is the capillary aneurysm, a small flat black lesion that grows rapidly and probably disappears spontaneously after a period of months. It does not attain a great size. The lesion is dark black and does not present the bluish or purplish coloration of a vascular lesion. On biopsy, a single enlarged subepidermal capillary is noted. A thrombus may be present in the vessel. There are no tortuous vessels such as one sees in the banal cutaneous varix. Serial sectioning reveals a fusiform swelling of the involved capillary.

Another rare tumor is the cellular blue nevus. This grows slowly and may reach a surprising size. The tissue is dark black and at surgery is nearly always diagnosed as a melanoma because of the hue and the depth of spread. Histologically, it does not resemble a melanoma. As a rule, the tumors are found in the midline of the lower back and buttocks but may occur in other locations as well. As an example, I would like to mention an 18-year-old black woman who consulted me for a flat black lesion on her lower back. The clinical diagnosis was a nevus, either junctional or the ordinary blue nevus type. However, when I cut into the presumably superficial lesion, I found that it extended deeper and deeper. The clinical diagnosis was changed to melanoma but, fortunately, the histologic diagnosis was of a benign cellular or giant blue nevus.

There are many other cutaneous conditions that can produce black lesions and so are confused with melanoma including pigmented basal cell epitheliomas, junction nevi, ordinary blue nevi, seborrheic keratoses, glomus tumors, and a host of other conditions. In most instances, the clinical differentiation is reasonably clear. In some cases, it is very difficult to distinguish clinically a pigmented basal cell epithelioma from a melanoma.

Therefore, we must realize that the clinical diagnosis of melanoma is definitely one that must be confirmed by the histopathologist. But, is it safe to biopsy a melanoma? I think so.

To illustrate that clinical diagnosis of melanoma may be fraught with difficulties, I would like to recount this true story. On D-day in World War II as the invasion of the European mainland was progressing, General Dwight D. Eisenhower had his shirt off. A surgeon on his headquarters staff noticed a black lesion on the general's back and told him that it was a melanoma and should be removed immediately if not sooner. Eisenhower refused pointing out that he was busy that day, but the surgeon was insistent. Somebody suggested that the dermatologic consultant should be consulted before surgery was performed, but he was not immediately available. Because of the surgeon's insistence and persuasion, the surgery was performed that very day while the gods of war bellowed along the French coast. The lesion was excised widely and deeply, and the specimen was put in a bottle of formalin for histopathologic study. Finally, the dermatologic consultant, the late Dr. Donald Pillsbury of the University of Pennsylvania, arrived and was shown the specimen.

He took one look at the lesion in the bottle and exclaimed, "Why that's nothing but a seborrheic keratosis, a very benign growth."

The surgeon was understandably annoyed and turning to Pillsbury asked, "And how would you have treated this?"

"I probably would have removed the growth with my fingernail," and plucking the specimen from the bottle, Pillsbury did just that.

Several years later, as president of the United States, Eisenhower dedicated a new hospital. His speech took the form of praise for the surgeon who, as the patient told one and all, "Saved my life."

EFFECT OF BIOPSY ON PRIMARY MELANOMAS

Biopsies may be incisional (e.g., using a punch, curettage, or a scalpel) or excisional. Certainly, the latter is to be preferred if feasible. Theoretically, cutting into a melanoma increases the probability of spreading the tumor—or at least this is what I was taught in medical school nearly a half century ago.

About 30 years ago, I developed a rapidly growing, small flat black lesion below my left eye. About 10 or 12 physicians, including dermatologists, surgeons, radiologists, and oncologists, saw the growth and told me that it was probably a melanoma and should be removed stat. The surgeon wanted to remove half my face as was the custom in those

days. Anticipating the morbidity and mutilation that would follow such a procedure, I talked the physician into performing a conservative removal. This was difficult indeed. Histolpathologic examination of the specimen revealed a benign capillary aneurysm so I do not face you today resplendent in my scars. However, I did wonder what would have happened if the neoplasm had been a melanoma. Would I have blown my chances of a cure?

This inspired me to study a group of patients with presumably localized melanomas through the cooperation of the California Tumor Registry, as mentioned earlier. The 193 patients who were followed for 10 years had no significant difference in survival time whether they had radical surgery at the outset or histopathologic examinations followed by definitive therapy at a later date, even one week later.[13] On this basis, it was claimed that a biopsy could be performed prior to the definitive treatment. This would prevent the mutilating surgery performed so commonly in those days on lesions suspected of being melanomas. This was done because of the commonly held belief that anything less than a wide and deep removal would allow the melanoma to enter the bloodstream and be peppered all over the body. The follow-up study after 25 years confirmed the conclusion of the 10-year study.

Other investigators have confirmed the safety of biopsy in melanoma. Paslin studied the problem in hamsters and found that incisional biopsies did not exert a deleterious effect on survival of these animals. Jones and colleagues established the same in 111 patients whose melanomas were subjected to incisional biopsies, as judged by five-year survival rates. Knutson and coworkers compared patients who had incisional biopsies with another group who suffered excisional biopsies. They, too, were unable to demonstrate any untoward effects from doing an incisional biopsy prior to the institution of definitive therapy.

Therefore, if it is safe to perform a biopsy, morbidity and mutilation can be avoided in suspected cases until a definitive histologic diagnosis of melanoma can be established.

VALUE OF PROPHYLACTIC LYMPH NODE DISSECTION

The literature is replete with conflicting evidence regarding the value of prophylactic lymph node dissection in primary melanoma. Some claim that the lymph nodes are a wall stopping the melanoma cells and preventing their spread, at least temporarily, to other more vital structures and therefore should be spared. Others claim that this procedure is indicated since the spread of a melanoma is basically through the lymphatics, and removing them rids the body of the lymph nodes with subclinical metastases. Das Gupta claims 98% success in five-year cures when this procedure was added to the surgical extirpation of the primary cutaneous lesion.[9] These are the best statistics that I have seen, and perhaps this view is the justifiable one.

In my 25-year study, 46.4% of the patients who had such a dissection were still alive at the conclusion of the study as compared with 34% of those denied this procedure.

Impressive as this comparision may be (approximately a 30% improvement in the prognosis), there is still a weakness in its interpretation. The quoted study is on nonmetastatic tumors. In those having a lymph node dissection, patients manifesting even microscopic metastases were no longer considered to be primary and were eliminated from the series. However, some of those in whom this possibility existed but was not established or disproven by surgical and histopathologic means might have already developed metastases. Since this possibility was not investigated except by clinical examination, the tumors were classified as primary and retained in the series. The differentiation between patients with localized neoplasms and those who had seeded metastases and who were spared the procedure was based on the presence or absence of grossly enlarged, hard lymph nodes, an unscientific and inexact method. As stated earlier, Knutson showed that this method was incorrect in approximately 30% of the cases.

We must consider the possibility that such therapy is of greater prognostic than therapeutic import. In other words, where there was no clinical evidence of such dissemination and lymph node extirpation was avoided, there might still have been microscopic extension so that the tumor was no longer confined to the primary site. In fact, it may have spread far and wide prior to the excision of the seemingly localized melanoma. This factor could explain the differences in survival between the two series, those subjected to lymph node dissection and those denied this operation.

LABORATORY DIAGNOSIS

The clinical pathologist is of assistance in establishing the diagnosis and prognosis of melanomas. This assistance is crucial in interpreting the microscopic features of the tumors. He or she is the one who should make the definitive diagnosis. By establishing the level or depth of its penetration, the surgeon can be furnished with important clues as to the choice and the extent of the projected therapy. However, the pathologic diagnosis of melanoma is not always a simple task or one devoid of hazards. Incorrect interpretations are possible even under the microscope. Furthermore, the biopsy may include a reasonable amount of normal tissue. Therefore, the slide may not show the definitive pathology unless several sections are made at different levels and studied. I have seen only only one section in nearly 25 that presented the typical characteristics of a melanoma. One should not rule out the possibility that a lesion may be a melanoma on the bais of only a few sections.

Melanuria may indicate advanced involvement and is a sign of a poor prognosis.

Experiments with skin tests have been interesting but not pathognomonic of the diagnosis of melanoma.[6] An extract from a melanoma is injected intradermally on the forearm. An indurated reaction is considered to be a positive result. In most instances, a positive test indicates the presence or history of a melanoma; a negative one, the absence of this tumor. However, false positives and negatives occur, which make this test unreliable.

Since we have inspection and histologic methods for determining the diagnosis, one may wonder why these tests are necessary or desirable. It would be great if we could establish the presence or absence of metastases by chemical or immunologic means. Some melanomas are not subject to biopsy, for example, tumors occurring within the eyeball. In order to biopsy such a lesion, it would be necessary to enucleate that organ. In the case of a negative biopsy, this would be a terrible loss, unless the eye were not functioning, because a physician erred in the diagnosis. Fortunately, melanoma is a low-grade malignancy in retina. The ophthalmologists I consulted do not treat such melanoma unless they are very sure of the diagnosis and the tumor seems to be growing actively. However, it is difficult to advise this course of inaction considering that melanomas can kill.

Another interesting approach is liquid crystal thermography.[25] These crystals change color indicating differences of temperature in various tissues. Rapidly growing lesions such as malignancies are warmer than the surrounding skin. This is reflected in the colors of the crystals. Of course, this is a nonspecific reaction since it does not differentiate between melanomas and other active lesions. It does not tell one how deep the tumor extends. Of greater interest, subcutaneous metastases may be demonstrated by this method. If there is a "hot" subcutaneous mass occurring in the region of a melanoma, one can presume that the clinically apparent or inapparent lesion is probably a metastatic melanomatous one. This may also be true in apparent lymph node metastases. Radiologic examination by magnetic resonance imaging, computed tomography, or ultrasound, may reveal involvement of the lungs, the gastrointestinal tract, liver, bones, and other organs. But these examinations demonstrate nothing but alterations in the shadows that are interpreted as metastatic lesions, the nature being assumed by the features of the primary lesions.

However, it must not be forgotten that melanomas may coexist with other metastases that have different prognoses or different responses to therapy.

MEDICOLEGAL IMPLICATIONS

Malpractice litigation is assuming gargantuan proportions nationwide. We find that the cases are filed by one of two types of lawyers. We have a plethora of nonspecialized attorneys who are scraping for crumbs and who will take any case in hope of finding the pot of gold at the end of the rainbow. However, their knowledge of medicine and personal injury law is usually limited and their activities result in disappointment for the plaintiff in most instances. On the other hand, we also have an abundance of personal injury lawyers who specialize in such cases. They study the pros and cons of the suit for long periods of time. They review appropriate medical books and articles and obtain consultations with physicians. They are skilled in cross-examination and other courtroom niceties. They have a staff of investigators who gather evidence for them, some of whom are very clever in their work. Many of them offer referrers a "finder's fee," a split of the action and have more work than they can handle. Furthermore, they accept cases on a contingency basis. If they win, they get 30% to 50% of the judgment and the plaintiff pays all of the expenses out of his or her share. On the other hand, if the lawyer loses, he or she receives nothing and must shoulder all the costs.

Under this system, attorneys must carefully consider the case before accepting it. If they do not win, they may even face a malpractice suit from their client or a countersuit from the accused. Therefore, most specialists turn down more suits than they accept. And how do they decide which one to take? I have been told that they want cases that qualify in two particulars: a reasonably obvious mistake on the part of the doctor and enough damage so they can try for a large amount of money—which, after all, is the name of the game.

There is no condition in dermatology that qualifies in these two respects as well as a melanoma. The damages are the greatest (death), and it often occurs in a young individual who may be the mother of small children or the sole support of a family. Futhermore, the diagnosis of melanoma is not easy. Clinically, it is fraught with inexactitudes. Histologically, there can well be a difference of opinion before the metastases appear. Furthermore, doctors cannot diagnose a condition unless they consider the possibility. It might be surprising to learn how many practitioners of medicine have little or no knowledge of melanoma and its implications. Many generalists tell me that they have never seen a melanoma. One must suspect the tumor before

being inspired to take a biopsy. One must also know that therapy does not consist of a simple conservative excision. As a rule, all suspicious-appearing lesions should be subjected to histopathologic examination by a qualified histopathologist, and treatment should be handled by someone experienced, trained, and skilled in the management of such cases.

Be alert to this possibility of melanoma for the good of the patient. But if one is concerned about medicolegal entanglements, be alert for one's own sake too.

THERAPY

The name of the game for the patient and the doctor is producing a cure or at least comfort and palliation for the patient with a melanoma. The question is, how do we treat a patient after we establish by histopathologic means that the patient does indeed have a melanoma?

While there are many approaches available, the primary lesion should be excised. This can be done with conventional cold steel surgery. The removal should be wide and deep. The exact margins of normal skin and depth differ according to various authorities. The present feeling is that the older methods of removing 5 cm of normal-appearing tissue is excessive and more than what is required. The depth of the excision seldom needs to be extended down to the fascia. Treatment of lesions where extensive areas of skin are not available for eradication, such as the eyelid, has shown that one need not be as radical as once thought. Furthermore, in my frequently quoted series of 193 patients followed for 25 years, all of the patients were treated by surgery alone. The removals were accomplished by many physicians, some specialists, some generalists, who sacrificed different amounts of tissue to varying depths, and yet the results (as judged by the survival figures) indicate that basically all methods were successful. The skill of the surgeons ranged from excellent to passable. Certainly, lymph node dissection should be employed if there is evidence of involvement of the regional glands. Prophylactic removal of these structures must still be a matter of individual choice.

The lesions may also be removed by electroexcision performed by the hot cautery, as exemplified by the Post and Percy cauteries, or by cold endothermy excision. The latter has the advantage of speed and the possibility of closing the wound. The cautery is slower, but there is less bleeding during this procedure. The defect produced by a cautery cannot be closed by suturing. The wound resulting from either method of electrosurgery is slow to heal and is accomplished by secondary intention if suturing is not employed. As a rule, the degree of scarring is acceptable except on the chest, the paranasal area, or the feet. Skin grafting is seldom, if ever, necessary in such cases. Furthermore, there is a theoretic advantage to this approach because it seals the blood vessels and decreases the opportunity for dissemination of the tumor. However, this is probably of more theoretic than actual value.

Radiotherapy is the treatment of choice in many European countries. The dosage is great—a cauterizing dose of a total of 10,000 rads or so. This results in a slow-healing reaction that is replaced by scar tissue and a chronic radiodermatitis. It must be stressed that such small areas of radiodermatitis seldom, if ever, undergo malignant degeneration. Recently, I became aware that work is being done in Canada indicating that melanomas are radiosensitive in doses comparable to those employed for epitheliomas.[15]

Mohs believes that his method of microscopic control is the treatment of choice in melanoma, and his statistics are suggestive.[23] On the other hand, it must be remembered that melanomas do not spread by extension in the manner of a basal cell epithelioma, so that eradication of the primary lesion and its microscopic extensions does not always save the patient. The fresh tissue technique with the cryostat may also be used for this purpose. Incidentally, Bailin has shown that superior sections can be produced by using a cutting laser to obtain the necessary specimens.[2]

Chemotherapy, immunotherapy and laser treatments are still in the experimental stage. They have been used most frequently in advanced cases. Rightfully, they have not been recommended as a substitute for surgical excision. However, palliative chemotherapy and/or immunotherapy are indicated in those individuals manifesting metastases. There is no evidence that either should be substituted for lymph node dissection, whether of the therapeutic or prophylactic type. The results of surgery plus one of these two methods have not been established as an advance in the saving or prolonging of life over surgery alone at this time. However, once dissemination has occurred, there is no reason for not trying every available approach.

Laser surgery offers hope that primary lesions can be eliminated by this modality.[14] Some of the lasers have an affinity for dark-colored tissues. Melanomas can be destroyed by this energy. However, lasers are not used universally, and this technique is still in the investigative stage. To the best of my knowledge, it has been used only experimentally on metastatic lesions.

It seems clear that excision by either of the methods described above, cold steel or electrosurgery, is the preferred approach in controlling this condition. The other methods can be used as adjuncts. On the other hand, we do not have a completely satisfactory method for treating melanomas. Further research and studies are not only indicated but essential.

NEED FOR EDUCATION

Melanoma is being diagnosed earlier than ever before. Our therapeutic methods are giving us better and better results. Yet, the number of people dying each year from this neoplasm is increasing. This seeming paradox can be explained by the increase in frequency of melanoma. Therefore, one might say that we are diagnosing cases earlier and obtaining superior therapeutic results but are still losing the war.

We must educate more people regarding this condition so that they will consult us earlier, while methods of treatment can save their lives. Diagnosis prior to metastatic spread is essential to attain the optimum results. I believe that more can be accomplished by bringing our message to physicians than by bombarding the public with information about this malignancy. However, neither direction of attack should be neglected. Certainly, it should be emphasized and re-emphasized to patients that a black lesion on the skin may be very dangerous, expecially if it is growing. But the late signs of melanoma should not be overlooked either, such as bleeding or elevated tumors. In addition, one should not forget the signs of early superficial spreading melanoma—a jagged edge, a mixture of colors, and a rough surface—since these lesions may progress to advanced levels of involvement if neglected.

If the patient consults the physician early in the course of the malignancy, the physician should display an index of suspicion, biopsy the neoplasm, and consult a dermatopathologist or a competent general pathologist about the specimen. Then, if the lesion is adequately removed, the percentage and numbers of fatal results should decrease despite the increase in incidence.

I have been told that the incidence of melanoma in Australia is very high but that their mortality rate is less than ours. They credit education of the population for this favorable balance, saying that everyone in Australia knows about the dangers, signs, and symptoms of melanoma. It is certainly true that we no longer see the formerly common gigantic epitheliomas. It is possible that this resulted from the publicity given these tumors by our cancer societies. Perhaps we do need to expand this educational campaign to include melanoma.

FURTHER CONTROVERSIES

I would like to briefly mention or emphasize a few other controversies regarding melanoma: Is it necessary to remove a large amount of grossly normal tissue when excising a primary melanoma? Why do we need a margin of 5 cm of such skin, subcutaneous tissue, and possibly even fascia? Does this make more sense than the hemipelvectomy and other mutilating surgery of earlier days? My aforementioned study suggests that primary melanoma can be cured with very conservative excision. The reported series of 193 patients followed for 25 years contained subjects in which practically only the tumor was excised, and yet the patient lived for more than 25 years after the surgery. For example, one patient presented with a gigantic melanoma of two years duration, and excision was confined to the lesion without any sacrifice of normal tissue. There was still no recurrence six years later.

Is local infiltration anesthesia apt to cause dissemination of the tumor? Not likely when you review such neoplasms removed under local injection anesthesia.

Is removal of the draining lymph nodes by dissection in continuity from the primary lesion to the nodes necessary? Theoretically, this approach seems reasonable, but most evidence supports the concept that it is safe to biopsy a melanoma, even by an incisional biopsy. Although this practice is not accepted in Europe, the studies of Rampen in the Netherlands support the latter viewpoint.[24] But then, we can find a dissenting study to everything that we believe in medicine.

What about old age and melanoma? In my experience, melanoma runs a more benign course in geriatric patients. Yet, most of the books state unequivocally that this malignancy is more aggressive in the elderly. If one looks carefully at the quoted statistics in these publications, one finds that this disagreement is based on semantics. In those claiming that this neoplasm is more malignant in the group under discussion, their dividing line indicates that old age begins at 50 years. However, if 70 years old is considered as the dividing line, then one must admit that melanomas (and, in fact, most tumors) are less aggressive in the elderly.

There are many immunologic tests that can be performed to strengthen the concept of an immunologic factor in melanoma. Mastrangelo, Bellet, and Beard discuss these in the book *Human Malignant Melanoma* by Clark, Goldman, and Mastrangelo.[31] They list the following tests as being of some value in this regard: delayed cutaneous hypersensitivity, lymphocyte-mediated cytotoxicity in vitro, lymphocyte transformation response to melanoma antigens, production of lymphokines in response to melanoma antigens, immunofluorescence, immune adherence assay, cytotoxic antibody, dinitrochlorobenzene reactivity, response to recall antigens, and others. Some of these tests may be of value in establishing the diagnosis of melanoma or hinting at the prognosis in a given case. Unfortunately, none of these tests are pathognomonic or completely reliable.

Melanoma is still a mystery. I have pointed out some areas of disagreement and aired the views of the contributors and of this iconoclast. Until the riddle of melanoma is solved, one should keep an open mind about its many facets.

REFERENCES

1. Acquavella Tietjen GL, Wilkinson GL, et al: Malignant melanoma incidence at the Los Alamos National Laboratory. Lancet 1(8277):883, 1982
2. Bailin PL, Ratz JL, Lutz-Nagey L: CO_2 Laser Modification of Mohs' Surgery. J Dermat Surg Oncol 7:621, 1981
3. Beral V, Evans S, Shaw H, Milton G: Malignant melanoma and exposure to fluorescent lighting at work. Lancet 2(8293):290, 1982
4. Breslow A: Tumor thickness level of invasion and node dissection in stage I cutaneous melanoma. Ann Surg 182:572, 1975
5. Brodthagen H: Malignant melanoma caused by UV-A suntan bed? Acta Derm Venereol (Stockholm) 62:356, 1982
6. Char DH, Hollingshead A, Cogan DG, et al: Cutaneous delayed hypersensitivity reactions to soluble melanoma antigen in patients with occular malignant melanoma. N Eng J Med 291:274, 1974
7. Clear WH Jr, From L, Bernardino EA, et al: The histogenesis and biologic behavior of primary human malignant melanomas of the skin. Cancer Res 29:705, 1969
8. Conley, J.: Irradiation as an Etiologic Factor in the Development of Melanoma, Arch. Otolaryng. 92:627, 1970
9. Das Gupta TK: Results of Treatment of 269 Patients with Primary Cutaneous Melanoma, Ann Surg 186:201, 1977
10. Day CL Jr, Harrist TJ, Gorstein F, Sober AJ, et al: Malignant melanoma. Prognostic significance of microscopic satellites' in the reticular dermis and subcutaneous fat. Ann Surg 194:108, 1981
11. Effects in Populations of Exposure to Low Levels of Ionizing Radiation. Nat Acad Sci, Nat Res Council, 1972
12. Epstein E, Bragg K: Curability of melanoma: A 25-year retrospective study. Cancer 46:818, 1980
13. Epstein E, Bragg K, Linden G: Biopsy and prognosis of malignant melanoma. JAMA 208:1369, 1969
14. Goldman L: Laser surgery, in Epstein E, Epstein E Jr: Skin surgery, Ed 5. Springfield, Ill, Charles C Thomas, 1982
15. Johanson CR, Harwood AR, Cummings B, et al: Radiotherapy in nodular melanoma. Cancer 51:226, 1983
16. Knutson CO, Hori JM, Spratt J: Melanoma. Cur Prob Surg, 3–55 Dec 1971
17. Kopf AW, Bart RS, Rodriguez-Sains RS, et al: Malignant Melanoma. New York, Masson Publishing USA, 1979
18. Kopf AW, Bart RS, Hennessey P: Congenital nevocytic nevi and malignant melanomas. J Amer Acad Dermat 1:123, 1979
19. Kopf AW, Bart RS, Rodriguez-Sains RS: Malignant melanoma: A review. J Dermat Surg Oncol 3:341, 1977
20. Kripke ML: The role of UVR-induced immunosuppression in experimental photocarcinogenesis. Prog Dermat 16:1, 1982
21. Clark WH Jr, Goldman LI, Mastrangelo MJ: Human Malignant Melanoma. New York, Grune & Stratton, 1979
22. Mihm MC Jr, Clark WH Jr, Reed RJ: The clinical diagnosis of malignant melanoma. Semin Oncol 2:105, 1975
23. Mohs FE: Chemosurgery: Microscopically Controlled Surgery for Skin Cancer. Springfield, Ill, Charles C Thomas, 1978

24. Rampen FHJ, Van Houten WA, Hopp WCJ: Incisional procedures and prognosis in malignant melanoma. Clin Exp Dermat 5:313, 1980.

25. Ratz JL, Bailin PL: Liquid crystal thermography, in Epstein E, Epstein E Jr: Skin Surgery, Ed 5. Springfield, Ill, Charles C Thomas, 1982

26. Schmoeckel C, Braun-Falco O: The prognostic index in malignant melanoma. Arch Dermat 114:871, 1978

27. Shapiro L, Bodian EL: Malignant melanoma in the form of pedunculated papules. Arch Dermat 99:49, 1969

28. Solomon LM: The Management of congenital melanocytic nevi. Arch Dermat 116:1017, 1980

29. Traenkle HL: X-ray induced skin cancer in man, in Urbach F (ed): First Internat Conf Biol Cutaneous Cancer. NCI monograph no. 10, 1963

30. Voelz GL, Hempelmann JN, Lawrence JNP, et al: A 32-year medical followup of manhattan project plutonium workers. Health Physics 37:445, 1979

31. Clark WH Jr, Goldman LI, Mastrangelo MJ: Human Malignant Melanoma. New York, Grune & Stratton, 1979.

45

Acne Surgery

Under the generic term of acne surgery, a heterogeneous group of surgical procedures employed in the treatment of acne vulgaris are included. These include the removal of blackheads and whiteheads, emptying pustules, the eradication of cysts, and the improving of scars. As far as the last named is concerned, dermabrasion and superficial chemosurgery are the treatments of choice. However, since these modalities are also of value in certain conditions other than acne scarring, they are considered to be worthy of separate chapters.

The inclusion of this chapter in this book does not constitute a blanket recommendation for the employment of this type of surgery. Under each manifestation of this disease, the advisability of the approach is considered separately. On the other hand, it is recognized that many dermatologists employ these procedures in the treatment of this dermatosis. Therefore, it must be realized that the recommendations made in this section are those of the author. Many dermatologists can be found who will agree with him; many can be discovered who will disagree. With the full realization of this controversy, the following descriptions and advice are offered.

COMEDONES

Each pustule of acne originates in a comedo (or blackhead). Therefore, it would appear to be a wise maneuver to remove blackheads as they appear. However, the extrusion of the follicular plug is of temporary benefit only—prompt recurrences are the rule. Permanent eradication of the enlarged pore requires excision. Even electrosurgical approaches do not remove the dilated duct since it is tortuous, and the desiccating needle cannot be inserted throughout its entire course. Excision, by a scalpel or a biopsy punch, even if followed by expert suturing, leaves a scar. The purposes of acne therapy are threefold: cure of the presenting lesions, preventing of new pimples, and the avoidance of scarring due to the disease or its treatment. One should never sacrifice *eventual* cosmetic results for temporary benefit. Furthermore, with the passage of time, the comedones tend to disappear. Therefore, it is felt that there is no necessity of producing scars merely to eradicate comedones.

The black plug can be removed by a comedo extractor. There are several types available. The most commonly used, and best, is a small metal bar with a hole in the end. This aperture is placed over the lesion, which is then expressed by the application of pressure. The crucial aspect of the maneuver is to be certain that the dark area is positioned near the edge of the opening. Pressure, then, results in the extrusion of the plug including its black surface by the application of a small amount of force and causes minimum or no damage to the adjacent skin. On the other hand, if the black mass is placed in the center of the hole, much more pressure will be required to remove the sebaceous material, causing greater trauma to the skin. Damage to the skin irritates the epidermis and often leads to the formation of pimples.

It requires a certain amount of practice to remove the plugs with the minimum of trauma. However, patients, or their parents, can be trained to do this satisfactorily by a demonstration followed by some practice doing it. The physician can perform this maneuver, but it is a time-consuming task. One can have the office nurse do it, but again, it is felt that the removal of comedones should be performed daily. The busy dermatologic office will encourage patients and their families to take over this task.

As previously stated, expression of the blackheads is of temporary benefit only. The patent duct tends to refill, and the contents must be expressed again and again. On the other hand, the proper removal of comedones is considered to be comparatively effective in preventing pustules and is indicated in the treatment of this often disfiguring disease that produces so much psychic trauma in the impressionable teenager. Vitamin A acid creams and gels may be beneficial in removing comedones and in preventing their recurrences.

MILIA

Milia (or whiteheads) are blackheads covered by a layer of skin. The black color, which comes from dirt caught on the exposed sebaceous plug, is therefore absent in milia. Basically, the technique and problems discussed in the comedones section also apply to milia. The only difference is the necessity for puncturing the overlying skin, which can be accomplished by a hypodermic needle, and then the contents can be expressed with a comedo extractor.

Actually, there are fewer recurrences than after the removal of a blackhead plug. This condition is a common postoperative complication of planing. Some cases of acne consist mainly of milia. This approach does not cause scarring or pustulation unless too much trauma is exerted in removing the plug or if secondary infection supervenes—a very rare occurrence.

At times, it will be found that the so-called whiteheads are not milia but actually tiny sebaceous cysts. In these instances, it is necessary to make an opening sufficiently large to express the entire cyst wall, which is preferably kept intact.

PUSTULES

Many dermatologists feel that the opening and expression of pustules is of benefit in the treatment of acne vulgaris. There is no question that the individual lesion heals more quickly if the contents are removed. However, the author definitely feels that this procedure *increases scarring*. Furthermore, the scarring that results from the incision of these pustules tends to be of the "ice-pick" variety and is resistant to such cosmetic procedures as planing or chemosurgery. It is felt that the medical treatment of acne will ultimately do more with less damage in pustular cases. X-radiation, antibiotics, Accutane, and antiacne local therapy are recommended over the scalpel attack on pustules of this dermatosis.

However, since apparently many skin specialists disagree with this concept, the surgical therapy of pustular acne is included. The lesions can be opened without resort to either local or systemic anesthesia. A no. 11 scalpel blade is inserted into the lesions, and the contents are evacuated by gentle pressure with the opposite end of the blade. Drainage can be increased in many instances by inserting a small mosquito hemostat and opening it widely in the cavity. Rubbing alcohol may be applied with pressure after the lesion has been emptied. Washing the entire are area with alcohol will decrease the probability of new lesions developing from autoinoculation. The postoperative use of a lotion containing rubbing alcohol (oz. viii) and mercury bichloride (gr. i) is recommended in these cases.

Many practitioners feel that a combined scalpel and comedo extractor would be of value for the performance of acne surgery. The author has used a combined instrument for many years; however, the scalpel end is used only for the treatment of cysts (see next section). Savitt recommended a gadget in which an ordinary comedo extractor was welded onto a Bard-Parker scalpel handle with a no. 11 blade. However, a much simpler way of securing the same result is to drill a small hole in the scalpel handle. This takes about two seconds to accomplish and is quite satisfactory for the dual purposes for which this "monster" is intended. Perhaps the oral use of retinoids will make this type of surgery extinct.

CYSTS

Cysts may be of several types in acne. Tiny sebaceous cysts resembling milia may be present. They may be treated in the same manner as whiteheads, except that it is necessary to incise the skin more widely than the aperture produced by a hypodermic needle. However, the opening is very superficial and should not result in scarring. At times, it is wise to insert a little trichloroacetic acid and lavage it out with alcohol, as mentioned later.

The cysts may reach a respectable size. The methods of removing such cysts are almost numberless. The author's approach is to excise them completely with an elliptical incision that is then closed with sutures. This is preferable if they are in an area in which scarring is not too objectionable, such as a covered portion of the body as exemplified by the back. On the other hand, if such a scar would be conspicuous, the cyst is opened, and the contents are expressed by pressure applied by the scalpel handle. At times, the cyst wall pops out after the cheesy material has been evacuated. This is true especially if the cyst has never been opened before—surgically or spontaneously. If the wall does not come out in a cooperative manner, the remaining portion is attacked by pressure, pulling with a hemostat, curetting, or whatever approach seems advisable. Then, a saturated solution of trichloroacetic acid is introduced into the wound. This is diluted within a few seconds by alcohol. A palpable mass will remain caused by the acid and the bleeding. In most instances, though, this will diminish and disappear over a period of one to two months. It is necessary to encourage drainage during the early postoperative period. This can be accomplished by the patient or the physician by keeping the crust removed and separating the edges of the wound manually, inserting a rubber or gauze drain, and using wet dressings (such as Alibour water).

Lesions clinically resembling cysts may prove to be acne pustules containing purulent matter rather than the cheesy contents of a sebaceous cyst or a combination of the two. In such instances, there is no cyst wall to facilitate surgical separation of the lesion from the surrounding tissues. While these masses are more superficial than true cysts of the same size, they lead to scarring regardless of the therapeutic approach. In fact, scarring can be reduced in such cases by judicious employment of incision and drainage. The opening should be of the minimum size consistent with easy evacuation of the pus. On the other hand, many of these pustules will heal without drainage following nonsurgical measures such as the systemic administration of antibiotics (250 mg of tetracycline four times a day, for example). A word of warning is necessary at this point. Chloramphenicol (Chloromycetin) should not be used orally in acne. It is doubtful if this preparation should even be applied topically because of the possibility of absorption through the skin. This disease requires long-term therapy, and the effect of long administration of this drug on the blood cells may be disastrous. Therapeutic perspective is essential in treating acne—a benign dermatosis that heals spontaneously in most instances. It is unwise to use a drug with the potentiality of causing aplastic anemia for the control of such a condition, especially when there are many equally efficacious agents available.

At times, one may wish to remove the entire top of the cyst or large pustule. This can be done by shaving off the dome with a scalpel or scissors or by dermabrasion. Marsupialization, which leaves a cyst wide open, has also been recommended. The cyst may be opened with a biopsy punch, leaving a gaping hole for drainage. All of these methods are acceptable but unnecessary. Furthermore, they leave more of a cicatrix than conservative incision. One should remember that acne is only a cosmetic problem, and surgical approaches tend to leave permanent scars. Therefore, conservatism is recommended in acne surgery.

Some physicians prefer to use electrodesiccation instead of the scalpel to promote drainage, but this is apt to produce more hypertrophic scarring. Also, according to patients, it is more painful than the emptying of the purulent material by a comedo extractor, a needle, or an incision. Intralesional injections of antibiotics and/or corticosteroids are often beneficial.

SCARRING

Scarring commonly follows acne, especially in severe cases or those in which injudicious surgical intervention has been practiced. The scarring may be of the pitting or depressed type or may be hypertrophic in appearance. Commonly, the three forms coexist. Some of the therapeutic agents, especially for the raised lesions, are not included in this book, since they are not surgical approaches. Examples of such modalities include x-radiation and the intralesional injection of hydrocortisone or triamcinolone salts.

In addition to dermabrasion and cosmetic chemosurgery, certain approaches are of value. Excision with or without grafting is one of the more successful means of minimizing unsightly scars. Shaving hypertrophic scars to the level of the skin results usually in prompt recurrence, although in some instances, postoperative radiation or the local administration of corticosteroids may prevent the reappearance of the keloidal neoplasm.

Cryosurgery is a valuable approach. The author's personal preference is for a carbon dioxide "slush" that is prepared by crushing dry ice to a fine powder. This can be accomplished with a hammer or an automatic ice crusher that contains no glass (the extreme cold will break the glass) and has an escape valve (otherwise, the vapor pressure will increase and might cause the crusher to explode). Carbon dioxide powder can be gathered from a cylinder and used in the same manner, although dry ice blocks are less expensive and more convenient to use. A small amount of acetone is added to the powder so that a mass is formed with the approximate consistency of sherbert.

This mixture is painted on the scarred skin repeatedly until the area turns white. As a rule, this is followed by erythema and desquamation. Small areas can be maintained in a deeply frozen state so that blistering will follow. The entire face may be treated during a single session. In fact, this approach is of value on the chest and back also. The degree of freezing necessary and the time it should be maintained can be judged accurately after a little experience. These factors can be increased or decreased on subsequent treatments depending on the degree of reaction and benefit obtained. Repeated applications are necessary, usually after an interval of one week. As the scarring improves, the treatments may be spaced further and further apart. This approach is of value in active acne also; dermabrasion is not. Obviously, scarring may coexist with active lesions. Liquid nitrogen may be substituted for the slush. Liquid nitrogen may be applied with a spray or a roller and is simpler to use since it requires no preparation.

There are certain precautions to follow in the adoption of this approach. The slush falls off the face and trunk without clinging so that severe burns do not result. However, if some of the dry ice is trapped on a portion of the body, a deep burn may develop. This is true for the nose, where it is necessary to wipe the ice off quickly after applying it. Nasty burns will occur on the neck or chest if the material falls under the dress or shirt of the patient. On the hands, burns can result in the same manner. Therefore, patients should stand up with their hands behind their back when the front of the body is being treated, and in front when the back is being frozen. The standing position is also advisable in order to prevent the slush from falling on the patient's lap. The acetone may cause stains or discoloration in clothing, to the patient's dismay.

At times, the results obtained by cryosurgery for acne scarring are excellent. The author has seen improvement equaling anything obtained by planing or chemosurgery. The disadvantage of this approach is the need for repeated applications of the therapeutic agent.

EVALUATION OF ACNE SURGERY

Dermatology allows for conflicting experiences and opinions. This is true especially in the management of acne, where there are many therapeutic conflicts: x-ray versus no x-ray, contraceptive pills versus no pills, diet versus no diet, and acne surgery versus no drainage.

Drainage *is* valuable in the management of the individual lesion, which heals more rapidly after evacuation. However, it does nothing to decrease the future development of new comedones, papules, or pustules. It is possible that drainage increases scarring, and the author believes that it does in most instances. Most patients with acne, including a high percentage of those with severe eruptions treated with Accutane, antibiotics, and other conservative measures, heal without cicatricial complications. It is well known that excoriating the lesions causes scarring. Pustules *may* cause scars; surgical intervention *will*. The hands-off policy seems to be a good gamble in most cases.

Acne surgery must be considered as an adjunct only in the management of this distressing dermatosis of the young. The use of nonscarring modalities, such as ultraviolet light, cryotherapy, drying local applications, and dietary control, should not be neglected in these individuals. In most instances, expert medical management will eliminate the need for the approaches described in this section. However, it is conceded that, in selected cases, these procedures may be of value in the optimal attack on scarring papules and pustules.

At this time, it seems likely that the oral use of Accutane and other members of the retinoid family will eliminate the need for a surgical approach in the control of acne.

46

Surgical Treatment of Nevi

Nevi (nevocellular nevi) are the most common tumors of the skin. The lesions consist of localized collections of nevus cells that are derived from melanocytes. Nevi are common in individuals of all races and ages, with the average Caucasian adult having over fifteen such lesions. Thus, it is not practical to surgically remove all such growths. Excision is usually performed for diagnosis or cosmesis, or if the lesion is irritated or subject to recurrent injury. Fortunately, there is a very low potential for malignant transformations in most nevi.

Nevi may be classified clinically and pathologically as junctional, intradermal, compound, and blue. They differ principally in the predominant location of the majority of the nevus cells. There is general acceptance that these cells arise from the neural crest of the embryo and migrate to the skin surface, thereby producing hamartomatous collections of melanocytic-type cells. Many nevi begin in the junctional stage, evolve through the compound stage, and eventually become predominantly intradermal. In some instances, the nevus cells may then seem to completely disappear from the dermis leaving behind only a fibrous or fatty stroma. The proper treatment of nevi depends upon their type, size, location, the age of the patient, and the likelihood of malignancy. A total surgical excision should be performed if malignant transformation is suspected. Worrisome signs include a recent change in size or pigmentation, inflammation, itching, pain, bleeding, or ulceration. If a suspicious lesion is too large for conservative total excision or is in a cosmetic area, an incisional biopsy is indicated, especially if extensive or possibly disfiguring surgery (as for malignant melanoma) is anticipated. Congenital and dysplastic nevi are considered precursors of malignant melanoma and should be completely excised.

Junctional Nevi

Clinical Description. Junctional nevi are flat, pigmented macular lesions that are light brown to black in color. Moles that occur in childhood are usually junctional in type. There is an increased incidence of these lesions during adolescence. Those nevi on the palms, soles, genitalia, and mucous membranes are almost always junctional nevi. There is general agreement that junctional nevi have some malignant potential. Perhaps the superficial location of the

melanocytic cells exposes them to more trauma, actinic damage, and other carcinogenic factors, thus making them more prone to develop into malignant melanoma.

Pathology. The nevus cells are predominantly located singly and in nests in the lower epidermis. Nests of cells may also lie below the epidermis in the upper dermis. With proliferation of the nevus cells in this location or by "dropping off," the lesion may become compound or eventually dermal.

Treatment. Usually surgical excision is performed with a fusiform excision placed in the preferred skin lines (wrinkle lines). Shave excision (tangential excision) followed by light electrodesiccation and curettage may result in a slight surface depression, but this may be preferable to linear scars resulting from elliptical excision for the treatment of multiple lesions. Specimens should always be examined histologically. Therefore, treatment with electrodesiccation and curettage, cryosurgery, or dermabrasion without histologic examination should be avoided.

Compound Nevi

Clinical Description. Usually, these lesions are raised and pigmented with a variety of surface configurations: macular, papular, nodular, verrucous, pedunculated, or with or without hairs. The color may vary from a flesh-tone to brown or black. Congenital nevi are usually of this type.

Pathology. Both junctional and dermal collections of nevus cells are seen. It is believed that compound nevi arise from junctional nevi by the "dropping off" of nevus cells from the epidermis. Congenital compound nevi often have considerable numbers of nevus cells deep in the dermis and along hair follicles.

Treatment. Suspicious-appearing lesions and those with large amounts of hair should be excised with full-thickness removal. Failure to completely excise a hairy nevus results in regrowth of the nevus from nevus cells located along hair follicles. If only a few hairs are present, shave excision followed or preceded by epilation may be done. If pigment persists or returns a few weeks later, this can be removed by a light liquid nitrogen freeze (about 15 seconds) or chemical peeling with 30% trichloroacetic acid. Recurrence may necessitate full-thickness excision. Shave excision is suited for the removal of multiple lesions on the face. Small pedunculated lesions may be removed with iris scissors.

Intradermal Nevi

Clinical Description. These lesions are often pale and dome-shaped. Hair may not be present. Older lesions are often pedunculated.

Pathology. Kopf and Adrade have demonstrated that most intradermal nevi are really compound nevi.[1] Careful serial sectioning shows the presence of some junctional component in nearly all such lesions.

Treatment. Treatment is the same as for compound nevi. Complete excision is indicated for suspicious lesions. Shave excision followed by light electrodesiccation or 20% aluminum chloride for hemostasis frequently produces a good cosmetic result. Hair must be removed with electrolysis if this technique is utilized.*

Blue Nevi

Clinical Description. These lesions are light gray, blue, or bluish-black with a macular, papular, or nodular configuration. The blue color is due to the depth of the melanin, which produces a Tyndall light-scattering effect. They are usually solitary lesions present from birth and clinically remain unchanged. Variants include the mongolian spot, nevus of Ota, and nevus of Ito.

Pathology. The *common type* of blue nevus contains fusiform or elongated nevus cells in the middle to lower dermis. Melanin is present in melanocytes and in surrounding melanophages. The *cellular type* of blue nevus contains closely packed collections of relatively large spindle-shaped cells containing little pigment. Numerous melanophages are seen interspersed in these collections of cells. The nevus cells on cross section appear rounded and have abundant pale cytoplasm.

Treatment. Malignant change is rare in the common blue nevus; however, malignant transformation may occur in the cellular blue nevus.[2] Silverberg and coworkers reported intracranial invasion by a cellular blue nevus of the scalp.[3] They stated that 5% of blue nevi metastasize locally without undergoing malignant histologic changes. When excised for cosmetic reasons, removal of the full thickness of skin with a margin of subcutaneous tissue is needed to assure complete removal. Shave excision with electrodesiccation and curettage will generally pro-

duce a poorer cosmetic result than conventional excision.

Congenital Nevi

Clinical Description. Most are compound nevi, usually presenting as raised hyperpigmented lesions that are often hairy and occupy large areas (e.g., giant hairy nevus or bathing trunk nevi). They are present at birth and become thicker with age. A significant percentage (2% to 30%) of these develop malignant melanoma, which more commonly arises in the dermal component than with ordinary nevi.[4–6]

Pathology. Junctional and intradermal nevi cells are seen. Usually, there is some papillomatosis. Some may lack a junctional component and have areas resembling blue nevi.

Treatment. Because of their malignant potential, the author feels that congenital nevi should be completely excised. Shave excision is not suitable treatment for congenital nevi because of their deep dermal involvement and malignant potential. Excision with a margin of a few millimeters of normal skin is advised. Giant lesions should be removed when the patient can tolerate the surgery and when conditions for reconstruction of the defect are optimal. Permanent removal of giant hairy nevi by dermabrasion early in life has recently been reported,[7] but further studies are needed to determine the efficacy of this method.

The selection of proper therapy for nevi in children is frequently complex. Often superimposed on this problem is significant anxiety in the parents concerning the possibility of malignancy and cosmetic deformity. In general, indications for biopsy or removal of a pigmented nevus include possible malignancy, significant parent or patient anxiety, and/or the presence of a cosmetic deformity. The proper timing of the procedure varies widely. However, the suspicion of malignancy requires immediate biopsy or excision. Significant anxiety in the parents and/or patient may be an indication to remove the lesion, but not necessarily immediate removal. Other factors affecting the timing of the procedure include the location and size of the lesion, the necessity of local or general anesthesia, and the availability of tissue to reconstruct the created defect.

SURGICAL TECHNIQUE

At present, there are three basic methods of surgical removal of pigmented lesions. These include complete excision, shave excision, and serial excision. In addition, dermabrasion and cryosurgery may be utilized. Again, the method utilized depends on the location and size of the lesion, the depth of

---

*It is important that the pathologist be informed if a lesion is recurrent since these lesions often have a pseudomalignant appearance histologically.

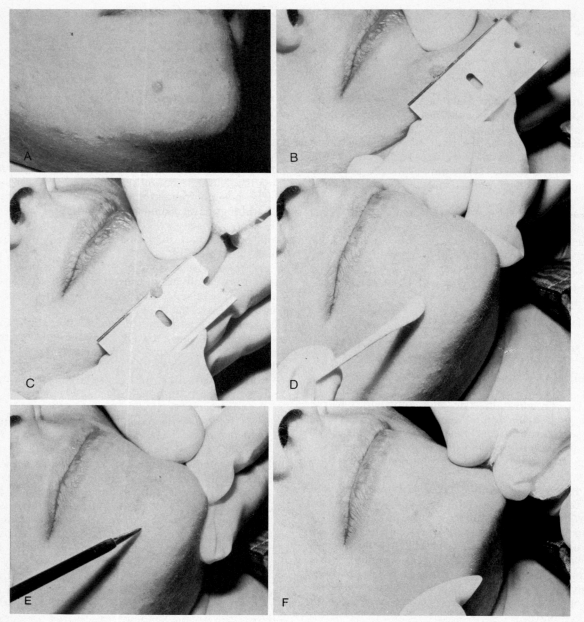

Figure 46–1. *A*, Preoperative appearance of a compound nevus on the chin of a young woman. *B*, After marking the margins and infiltrating the base with local anesthesia, the excision is performed with a razor blade. *C*, A sweeping motion is used to remove the lesion. *D*, Hemostasis is obtained by applying 20% aluminum chloride solution. *E*, Light electrodesiccation is used to complete the hemostasis or to level out any irregular edges. *F*, Immediate postoperative appearance.

the lesion, and the method of reconstruction of the created defect.

Shave Excision

This method is especially useful for small nevi or multiple facial nevi. It works especially well for elevated dermal nevi. After excision, the created defect is allowed to heal by secondary intention. Advantages include a minimal surgical procedure

and rarely the need for surgical reconstruction. Disadvantages include limited effectiveness for deeper lesions, the possibility of a poorer cosmetic result, and slower healing by secondary intention.

Technique

The skin is prepared with alcohol, Hibiclens, or other acceptable agent (Fig. 46–1). Excision margins are marked with 2% aqueous gentian violet using a scribe made from a broken wood applicator (a

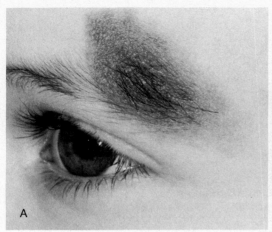
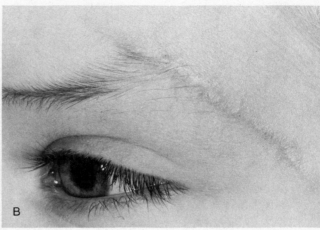

Figure 46–2. *A,* Supraorbital hairy nevus in a five-year-old child. *B,* Six-week postoperative result following an elliptical excision of the nevus. The defect was closed by wide undermining of the skin of the superior margin of the defect. This prevented excessive elevation of the eyebrow, which would have occurred if the skin of the lower margin of the defect was also undermined and advanced to close the defect. A long-lasting absorbable suture (Vicryl or Dexon) may be placed between the subcutaneous tissue beneath the eyebrow and the underlying periosteum to help maintain the correct position of the eyebrow and to prevent the tension of the skin closure from elevating the eyebrow.

twisting motion when breaking the applicator helps to produce a sharp point). Anesthesia is obtained by local infiltration of the anesthetic agent. A local anesthetic with a vasoconstricting agent, such as 1% lidocaine (Xylocaine) with 1:100,00 epinephrine, is preferred since it will prolong anesthesia and improve hemostasis.

The tissue is removed with a lateral sweeping motion using a no. 15 scalpel or a razor blade. One should start with the heel of the blade and remove the lesion with a smooth slicing motion. A sawing motion should be avoided since this may give an irregular, serrated wound base. The halved Gillette Super Blue Blade works well, has a very thin cutting edge (1 millionth of an inch thick), and is extremely sharp and flexible. The blade can be bent to allow

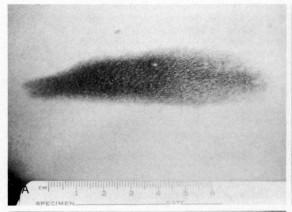
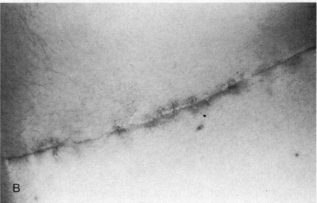
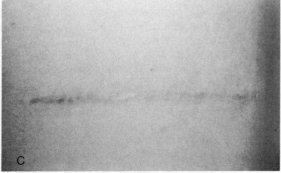

Figure 46–3. *A,* Preoperative appearance of a congenital nevus on the trunk of an eight-year-old girl. *B,* Appearance of the postoperative scar after the sutures were removed. *C,* Appearance of the same scar three months later.

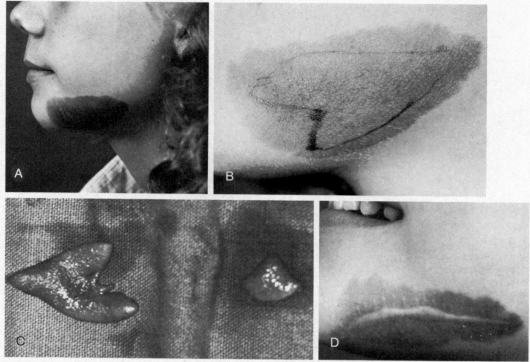

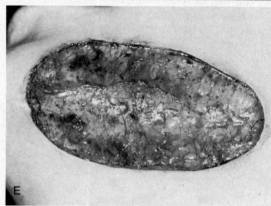

Figure 46–4. A, Large hairy nevus of the lower face and chin in a girl who desired removal for cosmetic reasons. Total excision would require a skin graft or flap for reconstruction to avoid severe distortion of the oral commissure, which would occur if primary closure was attempted. B, Gentian violet marking for the proposed margin of the initial excision of the nevus, which was removed by serial excision. Extensive undermining of the lower portion of the nevus and the skin of the neck may be advanced superiorly to close the defect. An additional part of the nevus may then be excised from the inferior margin of the partial excision, being careful that the closure of the defect will not distort the oral commissure. C, Specimen of the initial partial excision of the nevus. D, Result obtained two months after the initial partial excision. E, Defect following the complete excision of the remaining nevus, which was performed six months after the initial partial excision. Massaging the scar and skin of the neck on a daily basis for two months prior to the procedure helped to relax the scarring of the initial procedure and made the final closure easier.

Illustration continued on opposite page

excision in the exact arc needed to conform to the shape of the lesion removed. To avoid leaving a depression when removing a raised lesion (e.g., intradermal nevus), allow the subcutaneous swelling from the local anesthetic to subside. A saucerizing removal may be necessary for junctional lesions, though this results in a small depression. Hemostasis may be obtained by applying 20% aluminum chloride solution, Monsel's solution, pressure (pinching or stretching), or light electrodesiccation with a fine needle tip. Elevated or irregular edges that persist may be contoured with iris scissors or with a combination of light electrodesiccation and curettage.

Full-Thickness Excision

Complete excision involves the resection of the nevus and some underlying subcutaneous tissue, thereby creating a defect that usually requires surgical reconstruction. This method should *always* be used for lesions in which malignancy is suspected and for premalignant lesions including dysplastic nevi and congenital nevi. It also works well for large lesions that contain a significant amount of hair for junctional nevi. Primary advantages of this method are the availability of the entire lesion for histologic examination and the complete excision of the lesion.

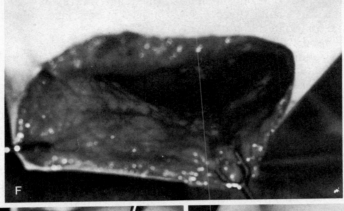

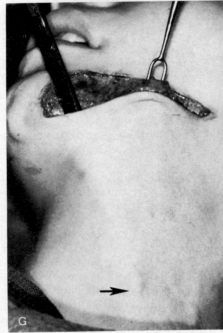

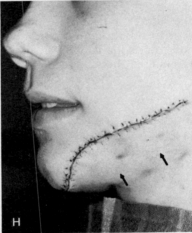

Figure 46–4 *Continued. F,* Extensive undermining of the skin of the lower margin of the defect and the neck created a flap that could be advanced superiorly to close the defect. Advancement of the skin of the upper margin of the defect would distort the oral commissure and must be avoided. *G,* Arrow marks the tip of the instrument demonstrating the inferior extent of undermining the skin of the neck. *H,* Completed closure of the created defect that utilized superior advancement of the skin of the neck; note the lack of distortion of the oral commissure. The placement of long-lasting absorbable sutures between the subcutaneous tissue of the inferior skin flap and the periosteum of the mandible minimizes the inferior displacement of the commissure. Care must be taken to place the suture in the deep skin (as shown by the arrows). The patient must be informed preoperatively that scar revision may be necessary in six to eight months.

When this technique is used, some method of reconstruction is usually necessary.

Technique

Small lesions may be excised in a simple ellipse placed in the preferred lines of closure, viz., wrinkle lines or lines of facial expression (Fig. 46–2). This allows the scar to be hidden in natural skin lines and also minimizes postoperative widening of the scar. Larger lesions may necessitate closure utilizing Z-plasty, W-plasty, skin grafts, or flaps. Primary closure should be utilized whenever possible because it often provides an excellent cosmetic result and is the simplest approach (Fig. 46–3). It is often necessary to undermine adjacent skin so that this tissue may be advanced without undue tension to close the wound. This results in a scar of minimal length and diminishes tension, which decreases postoperative widening of the scar. Care should be taken to avoid distortion of adjacent tissue (e.g., the eyelid or lip), excessive tension, and a long linear scar. After undermining, hemostasis is obtained and the wound closed in layers. Absorbable sutures (catgut,

Vicryl, or Dexon) should be placed in the subcutaneous tissue to approximate the wound edges without excessive tension and to obliterate the dead space. The skin is then closed with fine monofilament sutures utilizing an atraumatic technique with interrupted or subcuticular sutures.

Proper postoperative care is vital in obtaining optimum results. Excessive crusting, which may disrupt the skin margins when the sutures are removed or lead to stitch abscesses, must be prevented. The author instructs patients to clean the suture line twice daily with 2% hydrogen peroxide and then to apply an antibiotic ointment. Skin sutures should be removed in five to seven days, unless subcuticular sutures are used, in which case they may be left in place for two or three weeks. After removal of the sutures, tape closures may be applied (Steri-Strip or Clearon) and used for a two- or three-week period to provide additional support and to minimize widening of the scar.

Serial Excision

Serial excision involves the repeated partial excision of a large nevus that cannot be excised and closed primarily in a single procedure.[8]

Technique

This method requires wide undermining of skin margins and primary closure of the defect each time the procedure is performed (Fig. 46–4). The usual interval between excisions is six to eight months. Stretching of the skin and subsequent closure is facilitated by having the patient massage the area containing the scar for five minutes twice a day for the three-month period prior to the repeat excision. This technique may allow the excision of a large lesion without the necessity of a skin graft or local flap to reconstruct the defect. It also minimizes the amount of visible scarring. Care must be taken to prevent deformity of adjacent structures such as the nasal alae, lips, eyebrows, or eyelids. Frequently, a revision of the scar is necessary after complete removal of the nevus.

TISSUE EXPANSION

Serial excision and advancement flaps in the management of large congenital nevi may be replaced by more modern techniques utilizing tissue expansion (see Chapter 54.) Argenta and others have described the technique of expanding cutaneous tissue by implanting a prosthesis with an inflatable reservoir.[9–11] Following repeated injections of saline into the reservoir, the overlying tissue expands to the point that even very large lesions can be removed in one stage without the use grafts and flaps.

CRYOSURGERY

Removal of nevi by cryosurgery has been reported. Most nevi respond poorly or unpredictably to freezing.[12] Torre reports junctional nevi may disappear after cryosurgery.[13] Because a surgical specimen is not available for histologic interpretation, the author feels that this technique should be reserved for the removal of recurrent pigment after the histologic diagnosis has been established by a surgical excision.

CONCLUSION

Shave excision, full-thickness excision, and serial excision are the most common methods of surgically removing nevi. Other methods of reconstruction include primary skin grafting; delayed skin grafting; and local, regional, or distant flaps. In general, these methods of reconstruction are performed best by physicians with advanced training and experience in reconstructive surgery.

The increasing incidence of melanoma-associated mortality is alarming. Hopefully, early recognition and surgical removal of the precursors of melanoma will help reverse this trend. The two most important precursors are: (1) dysplastic nevi found in the general population and in certain melanoma-prone families and (2) certain congenital nevi.[14] A thorough examination, prophylactic excision of atypical dysplastic nevi, and careful follow-up are necessary in the familial form of dysplastic nevi. Solitary lesions should be completely excised (not shave-excised). Although the actual incidence of malignant melanoma appears to vary with the size of the lesion and other factors, it is probably prudent to remove all congenital nevi.[14–17] Complete full-thickness skin excision including a margin of normal tissue should be performed.

REFERENCES

1. Kopf AW, Adrade R: A histologic study of the dermo-epidermal junction in clinically "intradermal" nevi, employing serial sections. Annual New York Academy of Science 100:200, 1963
2. Hernandez FJ: Malignant blue nevus, a light and electron microscopic study. Archives of Dermatology 107:741–744, 1973
3. Silverberg GD, Hadin M, Dorfman RF, et al: Invasion of the brain by a cellular blue nevus of the scalp. Cancer 27:349–356, 1971
4. Reep WB, Becker SW Sr, Becker SW Jr, Nickel WR: Giant pigmented nevi, melanoma and leptomeningeal melanocytosis. Archives of Dermatology 91:100–119, 1965

5. Greeley PW, Middleton AG, Curtin JW: Incidence of malignancy in giant pigmented nevi. Plast Reconstr Surg 36:25, 1965
6. Sober AJ, Fitzpatrick TB, Mihm MC: Primary melanoma of the skin: Recognition and management. Am J Dermatology 2:179–197, 1980
7. Johnson HA: Permanent removal of pigmentation from giant hairy nevi by dermabrasion in early life. Br J Plast Surg 30:321–323, 1977
8. Webster RC: Cosmetic concepts in scar camouflaging-serial excision and broken line techniques. Trans Am Acad Ophthalmol Otolaryngol 73:256–265, 1969
9. Argenta LC, Watanabe MJ, Grabb WC: The use of tissue expansion in head and neck reconstruction. Ann Plast Surg 11(1):31–37, 1983
10. Radovan E: Tissue expansion in soft tissue reconstruction. Plast Reconstr Surg 74(4):482–492, 1984
11. Graham WP: Soft tissue expansion: Concepts and complications. Plast Reconstr Surg 74(4):493–507, 1984
12. Lubritz RR: Benign and premalignant cutaneous lesions, in Zacarian SA (ed): Cryosurgical Advances in Dermatology and Tumors of the Head and Neck. Springfield, Ill, Charles C Thomas, 1977
13. Torre D: Dermatological cryosurgery: A progress report. Cutis 11:782, 1973
14. Precursors to malignant melanoma. National Institutes of Health Consensus Development Conference Statement, Oct 24–26, 1983. J Am Acad Dermatol 18(4):1683–1688, 1984
15. Rhodes AR: The malignant potential of small congenital nevocellular nevi. J Am Acad Dermatol 6(2):230–241, 1982
16. Solomon LM: The management of congenital melanocytic nevi. Arch Dermatol 116:1017, 1980
17. Rhodes AR: Small congenital nevocellular nevi and the risk of cutaneous melanoma. J Pediatr 100(2):219–224, 1982

47

ROGER I. CEILLEY, M.D.

Surgical Treatment of Warts

Warts are one of the most common skin tumors seen in man. They are caused by a papilloma virus and affect about 10% of the population. The proper management of warts depends upon their location, depth, number, and previous treatment as well as the pain and discomfort they produce. The surgeon should be able to distinguish most warts from other skin tumors such as verrucous carcinoma and from deep fungal infections. Also, the surgeon should be able to choose from several different modalities since the therapy should be tailored to the individual patient, the type of wart, and its location.

Surgical treatment often is selected after other methods fail. *Of utmost importance is the fact that warts are an epidermal disease; thus, treatment should not produce dermal injury that might result in scarring and disfigurement.* Since most warts eventually resolve spontaneously, one might logically ask why treat at all. The principal reasons are that warts may produce considerable disability, cosmetic deformity, and dysfunction and may persist for long periods of time. Also, treatment may decrease the spread and transmission of these troublesome lesions.

The various reported methods of treatment are legion, and this attests to the fact that no one method is ideal in every instance. The following sections deal with the surgical approach to the treatment of warts. The most common surgical techniques include cryosurgery, laser surgery, electrosurgery (fulguration, electrodesiccation, and cautery), and excisional surgery (blunt dissection, sharp dissection, and curettage).

CRYOSURGERY

Cryosurgery is a simple, rapid, yet effective method of treating most warts in the office setting. The low temperature of liquid nitrogen ($-196°C$) does not destroy the wart but rather produces a separation at the dermoepidermal junction. A blister forms, and the wart with its infected cells sloughs off. The basement membrane persists, and re-epithelialization occurs in a matter of days. Usually, there is little or no scarring, but hyperpigmentation or, more commonly, hypopigmentation (usually transitory) may develop. Retreatment in one to three weeks is often needed; recurrence is common with warts on the palms, soles, and periungual areas.

Technique

The dip-stick cotton applicator or small cryosurgical unit may be used. The author prefers to use a larger, fluffy swab similar to those used for sigmoidoscopy. These larger swabs hold a greater amount of liquid nitrogen. The cotton tip is shaped into a point smaller than the wart (Fig. 47–1A). The swab is dipped in liquid nitrogen and applied to the wart for five to 60 seconds without pressure. Thick warts should be debrided first with a no. 15 blade or a razor blade. Freezing is continued until a zone of freezing, or "ice ball," extends 1 to 3 mm beyond the margins of the wart (Fig. 47–1B). One must be careful when freezing over the nail matrix because permanent nail dystrophy may develop. Freezing over nerves, such as the ulnar and digital nerves, may cause temporary or permanent neuritis. Also tendons, bursae, and cartilage on the fingers can be frozen and possibly damaged. When using a cryosurgical spray unit, the diameter of the tip should be small. An effective yet simple shielding device (to limit the lateral spread of freeze) can be made by drilling various sized and shaped holes in a collection of tongue blades (Fig. 47–2).

Digitate Warts. The stalk, base, and small rim of normal tissue is frozen solid for 15 to 20 seconds.

Periungual Warts. Trim away the overlying nail prior to freezing. One may need to use local anesthesia to allow adequate freezing, but excessive freezing may result in edema with severe pain in this area.

Warts on the Glabrous Skin. The best results with cryosurgery are achieved in this location. Freezing with liquid nitrogen and a cotton applicator is usually preferred.

Flat Warts. Only a brief freeze (five to 15 seconds) is required. Freeze individually or in a small group. Carbon dioxide and acetone slush may also be effective.

Warts on Palms and Soles. A high recurrence rate is seen with cryosurgery. The severe pain attendant with this treatment often discourages the patient from subsequent procedures.

Postoperative Care

No dressings are required. Printed postoperative instructions should be given to the patient outlining

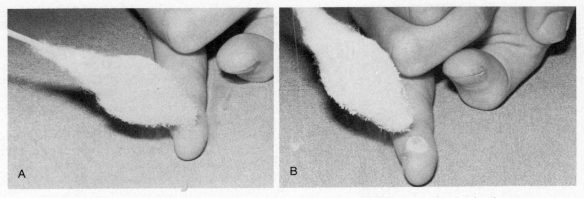

Figure 47-1. A, Cotton-tipped applicator used for freezing warts. B, Wart immediately after freezing.

what to expect and what measures to take. No dressings or ointments are needed. If a tense, painful, or awkward blister develops (Fig. 47-3), it may be decompressed with a sterile lancet or needle leaving the roof intact. Some dermatologists feel that removal of the vesicle roof is important in preventing recurrence and routinely do so three to five days after freezing. When the patient returns in two to three weeks, any remaining lesions should be debrided and retreated.

Condylomata Acuminata

Usually, podophyllin is the treatment of choice. Podophyllin-resistant warts, such as those on dry skin (buttocks, thighs, and the shaft of the penis), often respond well to cryosurgery. Also, cryosurgery and podophyllin may be used in combination.

ELECTROSURGERY

Warts may be treated effectively with electrosurgery. This method is useful especially for single warts that have been present for a long period of time and/or are refractory to other methods. Care must be taken to avoid excessive destruction of normal tissue because this leads to unnecessary scarring and pigmentary changes. One must restrain the impulse to stop bleeding with a strong coagulating current. The hemorrhage may be controlled by a biopsy ring or with pressure by pinching or spreading the skin with the thumb and forefinger.

Technique

The skin is cleansed with an antibacterial solution and the area injected with 1% lidocaine; one should be careful not to enter the wart and spread the virus along the injection tract.

Electrodesiccation and Curettage

The sharp electrode tip (a fine-pointed tip should be used so the destruction can be controlled with the least amount of current) is pushed into the wart, and a low-to-medium coagulating current is passed

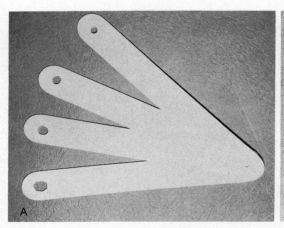

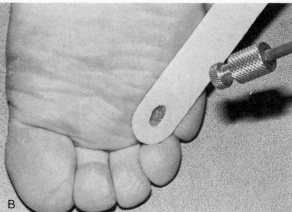

Figure 47-2. A, Cryosurgical shields made from wooden tongue blades. B, Using the shield for freezing a plantar wart with a liquid nitrogen spray.

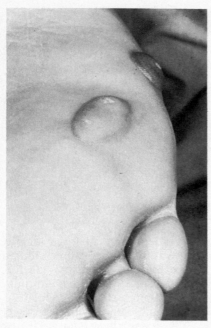

Figure 47–3. Tense painful blisters after cryosurgical treatment of plantar warts.

Filiform Warts. A fine electrode with short bursts of low current should be used and the charred tissue removed with iris scissors or a curette.

Periungual Warts. Extreme care must be exercised to avoid damaging the nail matrix or producing scarring of the nail bed. The author prefers curettage in this area. Extremely persistent or atypical lesions should be biopsied to rule out squamous cell carcinoma of the nail bed or periungual tissues.

Flat Warts. Very light electrodesiccation and/or curettage is used. The author prefers cryosurgery, curettage, or simple topical treatment. Scars or pigmentary changes are common on the face following treatment. If this method is used, a small test area in an inconspicuous area should be done first.

Palmar and Plantar Warts. If surgery is needed, the author prefers blunt dissection (see the next section) or cryosurgery. Again, extreme care must be exercised to prevent scarring, which in this location may be extremely painful and a greater problem than the wart itself.

Anogenital Warts. Electrosurgery may be necessary when podophyllin or other methods fail. Occasionally, hospitalization and general anesthesia may be required. Suspicious-appearing lesions should be biopsied. Large warts may be removed with the cutting loop and the base coagulated. Light charring without curettage is often effective for the tiny warts on dry surfaces, such as the shaft of the penis.

through the wart tissue until it becomes greyish and a small bubble forms on the surface. The soft wart tissue is then removed with a curette and the base touched with Monsel's solution, aluminum chloride solution, or light electrodesiccation. An alternative approach is to lightly electrodesiccate the surface with a low-to-medium current to soften the hyperkeratotic surface of the wart. The junction between the wart and the normal skin is then incised with small iris scissors, and a curette is used to remove the softened wart tissue. The base is then lightly desiccated and the process repeated if necessary.

Postoperative Care

Usually, no dressings are required. The wounds may be cleansed with hydrogen peroxide and an antibiotic ointment applied until healing is complete, usually five to 14 days. Again, careful follow-up is necessary with early retreatment if a recurrence is noted.

Electrocautery

The hot cautery tip is applied to the surface, producing a charred, gelatinous layer. This tissue is then curetted and the remaining tissue removed by repeated gentle curettage and light cautery (Fig. 47–4).

EXCISION

Standard excision with suturing is not advised since this entails damage to the dermis, results in

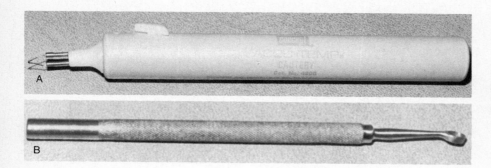

Figure 47–4. A, Disposable battery-powered cautery unit (Concept). B, Dermal curet used for removal of warts (Millibilt).

scarring, and often leads to recurrence of the warts in the excision line. The use of small curved scissors, curette, and blunt dissection may be useful in some instances.

Technique

Filiform Warts. These may be removed with the scissors or curette (usually without anesthesia); aluminum chloride or Monsel's solution is applied to the base for hemostasis.

Flat Warts. These may be effectively removed with the flick of a sharp curette; pressure or aluminum chloride or Monsel's solution provides hemostasis.

Periungual Warts. Under local anesthesia, the margin between the wart and normal tissue is incised with iris scissors or a dull scalpel. Overlying nail tissue is trimmed, and the wart is then removed with a large-handle curette (see Fig. 47–6). A pressure dressing is then applied, or aluminum chloride or Monsel's solution used. Mushy wart tissue at the base is curetted until the gritty feel of normal dermis is reached. The hyperkeratotic rim is then trimmed with small curved scissors.

Palmar and Plantar Warts. Pringle[3] and others[4, 5] have described a technique of blunt dissection that is very effective in treating these often recalcitrant lesions. Blunt dissection, if carefully carried out, separates the wart from underlying dermis relatively atraumatically and does not lead to scarring. This technique has been most effective in the author's hands for solitary or isolated warts of long duration (those present over six months).

Technique

The area is prepped with an antibacterial solution. If the wart is very large or thick (Fig. 47–5A), it is helpful to pare it down with a single-edge razor blade until a sharp margin between the wart and surrounding skin is visualized. The area is then infiltrated with 1% lidocaine using a 25- or 30-gauge, half-inch needle (Fig. 47–5B). One infiltrates until an edematous, blanched appearance is present. Lidocaine with epinephrine is used on the palms and soles but not on the digits. One must avoid passing the needle directly into the wart in order to avoid spreading it along the injection tract. Injecting from the side instead of directly perpendicular into the palm or sole is less painful. The needle should be advanced very slowly and gently, pushing the anesthetic ahead of the needle. The hyperkeratotic skin around the wart is then scored (not into the dermis) with curved scissors (Fig. 47–5C) or a no. 15 blade. The wart, if small, may be avulsed with a sturdy curette or separated (Fig. 47–5D to F) with

a nasal septum Freer elevator (Fig. 47–5G). Once the base of the growth is reached, the wart is carefully separated from the dermal layer. One can see the rete ridges that make the digit prints. A small curette is then used to remove any sections of verruca that remain (Fig. 47–5H). A slightly dull curette works well for this and ensures that one does not damage the dermis. The calloused margins of the wound are then trimmed with the iris scissors (Fig. 47–5I), and aluminum chloride or Monsel's solution is used for hemostasis (Figs. 47–5J and 47–6). A pressure dressing is then applied.

Postoperative Care

The pressure dressing is removed in 24 to 48 hours and the wound treated with the open technique of warm soaks and antibiotic ointment without dressings two times a day. The patient returns in seven days for trimming of the calloused edge and in 21 days for follow-up. Early recurrences are readily treated by removal with a small curette or freezing with liquid nitrogen. The management of hyperhidrosis following the surgery is helpful in preventing recurrences.

LASER SURGERY

The CO_2 laser is an effective modality for treating hypertrophic warts and warts that have been refractory to other modalities. Bailin feels that the CO_2 laser is the treatment of choice for plantar warts and condylomata acuminata.[6] With the advent of smaller portable laser units, such as the Ambulase unit by Xanar (Fig. 47–7), laser surgery for all types of warts in the office setting may become commonplace.

Technique

The skin is cleansed with povidone-iodine (Betadine) or Hibiclens and local or general anesthetic utilized.

Palmar and Plantar Warts. Long-standing and multiply recurring warts are biopsied utilizing iris scissors or the focused beam to cut off a representative specimen. Histologic analysis is obtained to rule out malignancy such as verrucous carcinoma. The remaining wart tissue is then vaporized using the defocused beam at low-to-medium power settings with the pulse mode at 0.1 seconds. A binocular loupe, 2.5 power, is used to help detect small satellite warts and to see precisely when the wart has been vaporized (Fig. 47–8). An anodized dermal curette is used to remove the surface char and to locate residual pockets of wart tissue (Fig. 47–9).

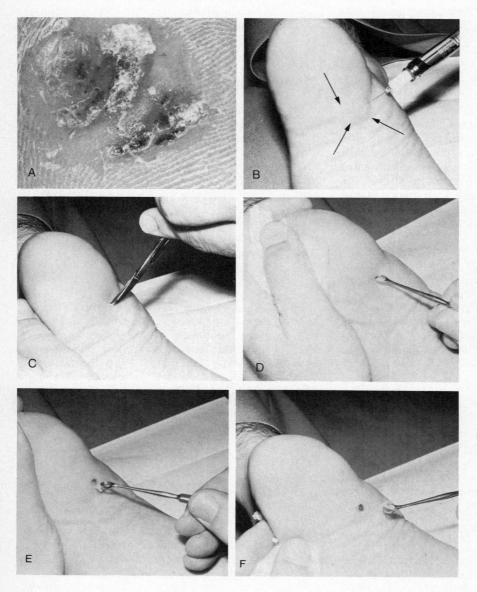

Figure 47–5. *A*, Large plantar wart. *B*, Technique for infiltrating local anesthetic. *C*, Trimming hyperkeratotic skin around the wart with curved iris scissors. *D* to *F*, Avulsing the wart with a curet.

Illustration continued on opposite page

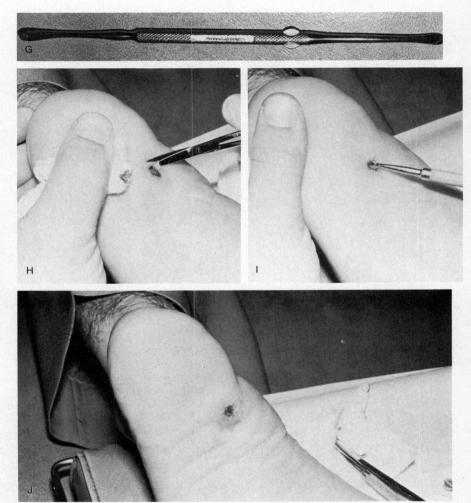

Figure 47–5 *Continued. G,* Freer-elevator used to enucleate plantar warts. *H,* A small curet is used to remove any remaining wart tissue around the perimeter. *I,* Trimming the calloused margins with iris scissors. *J,* Wound after the application of 20% aluminum chloride for hemostasis.

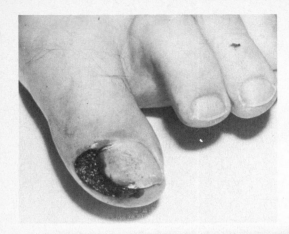

Figure 47–6. Wound after the removal of a periungual wart and the application of Monsel's solution for hemostasis.

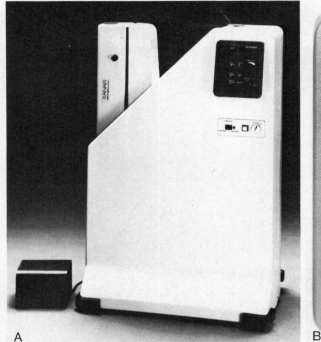

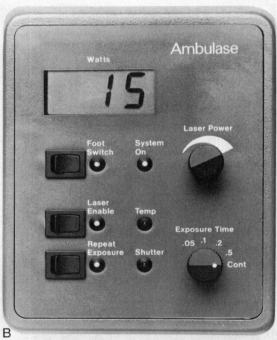

Figure 47–7. *A*, The Ambulase portable laser unit by Xanar. *B*, Close-up of the control panel.

Figure 47–8. Binocular loupe used in laser surgery.

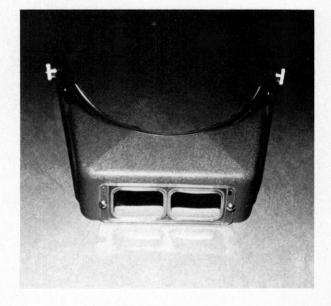

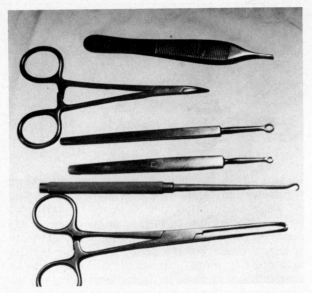

Figure 47—9. Anodized surgical instruments for laser surgery.

Hydrogen-peroxide–soaked 4 × 4 gauze is also helpful to wipe off surface char as the tissue is removed. After all the visible wart tissue is removed, the margins and base of the wound are lightly vaporized at a low-power density to sterilize the surface and to obtain complete hemostasis.

Anogenital Warts. Large pedunculated condylomata may be excised with the focused beam. The excised specimen is then sent for pathologic interpretation. The base and other small or flatter warts are vaporized as noted previously. For multiple perianal or intra-anal warts, general anesthetic may be required. Placing the patient in the dorsal lithotomy position is most convenient for the operator. A disposable plastic speculum can be used to assist destroying warts located deep in the anal canal. The removal of these lesions is essential in preventing recurrences. The CO_2 laser can also be used to remove intraurethral warts.

Periungual Warts. These are treated the same as plantar warts. The CO_2 laser can be used to vaporize the nail overlying subungual warts as well.

Flat Warts. Very light vaporization using a very low-power setting is sufficient. A test area should be done first in areas of cosmetic significance.

Postoperative Care

The wounds are allowed to heal by granulation and epithelialization. The wound is covered with an antibiotic ointment and a nonadherent gauze, such as Adaptic. A light pressure dressing is applied (a sanitary pad and belt or scrotal support may be used for anogenital wounds). After 24 to 48 hours, the wounds are treated with the open technique whenever possible.

CONCLUSION

Warts are often difficult to eradicate. A thorough knowledge of the pathogenesis and natural course of these tumors is essential in their intelligent management. Treatment should be tempered with a knowledge that these are epidermal tumors that eventually resolve spontaneously in a high percentage of patients. Thus, ideally, treatment should not result in scarring or cosmetic disfigurement. One should tailor the treatment to the patient, their lesion(s), and the operator's skill. One should choose the least destructive method that provides effective treatment. The most aggressive approaches should be reserved for the more refractory lesions.

REFERENCES

1. Lubritz RA: Cryosurgery of benign and premalignant cutaneous disorders, in Zacarian SW (ed): Cryosurgical Advances in Dermatology and Tumors of the Head and Neck. Springfield, Ill, Charles C Thomas, 1977
2. Burdick KH: Electrosurgical Apparatus and Their Application in Dermatology. Springfield, Ill, Charles C Thomas, 1966
3. Pringle WM: Treatment of plantar warts by blunt dissection. Arch Dermatol 108:79–82, 1973
4. Ulbrich AD: Warts: Treatment by total enucleation. Cutis 14:582–586, 1974
5. McGlamary DA: Verruca Surgery, A Nonscarring Technique. Presented at the annual meeting of American Society Dermatologic Surgery, April 1977
6. Bailin PR: Use of the CO_2 laser for non-PWS cutaneous lesions, in Arndt KA, Noe J (eds): Cutaneous Laser Therapy: Principles and Methods. New York: John Wiley & Sons, 1983, pp 187–201

48

ROGER I. CEILLEY, M.D.

The Treatment of Hypertrophic Scars and Keloids

Many factors influencing the quality of wound healing appear to be independent of surgical technique and routine pre- and postoperative management. The dermatologic surgeon operating in functionally or cosmetically significant areas of the body is concerned with the development of hypertrophic scars and keloids. Heredity, race, pigmentation, site, nature of the injury, wound tension, and a history of past healing may all be partial predictors of the likelihood of hypertrophic scar or keloid formation. The fact is, however, that these lesions may be the unfortunate result of surgical procedures on any patient.

Several medical and surgical techniques have proved to be successful when based on two premises: (1) Different modalities are appropriate in different stages of lesion maturation, and (2) one treatment modality may favorably influence a subsequent different treatment. Compulsive long-term follow-up as well as prophylactic and early treatment of other lesions is essential in the proper management of patients with these lesions.

Hypertrophic scars and keloids are unsightly bulky lesions that inhibit motion, cause pain, and itch. They have been shown to result from an increase in collagen synthesis as compared to normal wound healing.[1] An element of decreased collagen degradation may also be present.[2] Many authors have pointed out physiologic and clinical differences between these two lesions.[2, 3] Clinically, hypertrophic scars stay within the bounds of the wound, and keloids are, in a limited sense, locally invasive and grow beyond the boundaries of the original wound. Keloids appear metabolically more active and histologically more disheveled than hypertrophic scars. Hypertrophic scars are more likely to regress spontaneously and respond more consistently to treatment. Despite these differences, both lesions respond to the same therapeutic efforts, so for the sake of this discussion, the two are considered variants of the same pathologic process.

TREATMENTS

The varied and numerous treatment modalities reported in the literature for the management of these lesions suggests there is as yet no one entirely satisfactory method. In a large retrospective study of 340 lesions treated over 26 years, it was demonstrated that simple excision alone resulted in a recurrence in over 50% of the patients.[4] Also, the recurrent lesion was frequently worse than the original one. It should be noted, however, that no correlation was made between recurrence and age, the lesion location, or the mode of injury.

Pressure Therapy

Physical therapy through the use of pressure garments and stretching techniques has become an integral part of the management of postburn keloids and hypertrophic scars.[5, 6] These techniques help minimize scarring and help maintain function while maximizing cosmetic results. Johnson's recent monograph on this subject provides practical guidelines for the effective use of multiple pressure devices and stretching techniques.[5] Long-term (six to 12 months) application of pressure following keloid excision has been described as an effective means of reducing recurrences by forcing collagen deposition in a linear pattern.[7] Frequent massage of hypertrophic scars by the patient has proved to be a simple and effective adjunctive modality in many of the author's patients. Using an emollient cream or ointment, the patient massages the scar for five minutes, four to five times each day. A topical corticosteroid cream may be utilized in some instances as well.

Internal pressure, through the use of tissue expanders (see Chapter 54), has recently been shown to soften and flatten hypertrophic scars.[8] Reconstruction of burn scars utilizing tissue expansion techniques may revolutionize the surgical management of these patients.[9, 10] Even huge contracture scars can be removed and the defect covered by the adjacent flap of expanded tissue. Donor tissue is created utilizing a temporary, implantable silicone bag that is gradually expanded by injecting normal saline through a gel-filled valve system, which is also implanted. Internal pressure over a six- to 12-week period exerts its force on the overlying flap, and expansion occurs producing additional tissue for reconstruction. Interestingly, the expanded flap maintains full thickness with normal epithelial thickness, but the thinner dermis is supported by an additional fibrous capsule layer.

Cryotherapy

Cryotherapy was described at least as early as 1931 in the French medical literature.[11, 12] The technique at the time was limited solely to the application of carbon dioxide slush. Both temperature and treatment areas were difficult to control, and the method never gained wide acceptance. With the development of modern liquid nitrogen spray and probe units, cryotherapy has become a practical technique for removal of a variety of lesions. The physiology of freezing is described elsewhere in this text. Suffice it to say that cryotherapy has profound effects on both collagen and cellular elements. It is notable that a cryosurgeon with great experience states that he has never seen a keloid as a result of cryoexcision.[13]

Radiation Therapy

Superficial radiation therapy was first reported at the beginning of this century and has received steady attention up to the present. Since x-rays are most effective on rapidly multiplying cells, most techniques have evolved into early dosage following surgical excision.[14] It is at this time that the rapidly growing capillary buds and fibroplast proliferation of the healing process may be suppressed most easily, decreasing subsequent collagen deposition.[15] Most series suggest treating within one to two days postoperatively with a total dose of around 1500 to 2000 rads. Approximately a 20% to 30% recurrence rate may be expected.[16] Higher dosage decreases this rate but results in atrophy and telangiectasia in the treated area.[17] Recently, the interstitial implantation of an iridium 192 wire at the time of closure of keloid excision has been described. This can deliver 2000 rads while reducing dosage to adjacent tissues.[18]

Systemic Medical Treatment

A large variety of systemic medications used postoperatively have been tried in an effort to prevent keloid formation. Corticosteroids, methotrexate, penicillamine, colchicine, β-aminoproprionitril have all been used with mixed success in the past. Because these drugs all may have serious toxic side effects, they are not recommended for general use at this time. Safer drugs, such as antihistamines, have not proved to be reliably effective yet. Hopefully, fur-

ther research will provide a safe and effective drug to prevent and treat hypertrophic scars and keloids.

Immunotherapy

Another point of view is reflected by a recent report suggesting that keloids might form as a result of autoimmune reaction to sebum.[19] Twenty-nine patients were pretreated with a sebum antigen desensitization program before excision. The recurrence rate was one third of a control surgical group.

Intralesional Corticosteroids

Systemic and intralesional ACTH was suggested in a 1951 paper[20] that sparked great interest in intralesional steroid injection.[21-22] Currently, intralesional injection of triamcinolone acetonide seems to enjoy wide popularity for the treatment of hypertrophic scars and keloids. Corticosteroids are well known for their ability to inhibit protein synthesis and fibroblast migration. While some evidence exists that these agents enhance collagen degradation, the exact mechanism of hypertrophic scar and keloid reduction is unknown.[2] The pharmacologic effect of corticosteroids used at commercially available concentrations is not limited to keloids. They may have a profound effect on normal skin causing atrophy or depigmentation.[23-24] Side effects result primarily from spillage of the steroid out of the lesion, usually as a result of the great amount of pressure necessary to infiltrate the keloid matrix. Other side effects related to concentration or the total dosage include occasional sloughing of tissue or mild cushingoid symptoms. Clearly, when using intralesional steroids, the lowest *effective* concentration should be selected. Because of these problems, the author has been utilizing a technique of early treatment with cryotherapy and diluted triamcinolone injection, followed in a year or so by surgical excision if necessary.[25-27] Other investigators have also reported favorable results utilizing this combined approach.[28]

Technique

The keloid is prepared with any appropriate skin cleanser, such as 70% alcohol. Local or general anesthetic may be essential depending on the patient and the site of the lesion. If local anesthesia is necessary, a 1% lidocaine regional block is adequate. First, the keloid is treated in 1 to 2 cm segments with a cryotherapy unit until a distinct ice ball forms (Fig. 48–1). As the lesion thaws, it will rapidly become pink and edematous. This is not only therapeutic in itself, but greatly facilitates the subsequent steroid injection by loosening the tight keloid matrix. After the frozen lesion thaws, it is

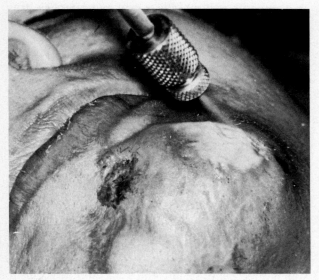

Figure 48–1. Freezing a keloid with a liquid nitrogen spray.

injected with corticosteroid suspension using a 3 cc, three-ring Luer-Lok control syringe and a 5/8 inch 25-, 27- or 30-gauge needle (Fig. 48–2A). Smaller lesions may be injected with a l cc Luer-Lok disposable syringe with an assist ring to provide additional injection force (Fig. 48–2B). Intralesional injections are usually triamcinolone acetonide at a concentration of either 10 mg/cc or diluted to 5 mg/cc. The spread of triamcinolone is monitored by observing the superficial blanching of the edematous keloid (Fig. 48–2A). Definite resistance must be felt during the injection, and the blanching should not be allowed to proceed into normal adjacent tissue. Injection should be administered as superficially as possible. The suspension within the syringe must be shaken frequently during the injection process to insure a uniform concentration of corticosteroid. Failure to do this may result in deposition of pockets of steroid crystals in the scar. The area is then lightly dressed, and the patient is given a petrolatum-based antibiotic ointment to use in case the freezing results in superficial blistering.

Usually, maximum softening and flattening occurs in four to eight weeks, although telangiectasia may

remain three to six months thereafter. Multiple injections are the rule, averaging a total of four or five per lesion. Subsequent injections may not require the freezing because of softening produced by the previous treatment. Concentration of triamcinolone acetonide may be reduced to 5 or even 2.5 mg/cc and injected with a 30-gauge needle. The patients set their own timing for subsequent injections. The best results are obtained when the keloid is first starting to enlarge. Expected results are shown in Figures 48–3 and 48–4. Should such a treatment regime not result in complete eradication of the lesion, surgical excision with postoperative steroid injection is utilized. The following case emphasizes the use of multiple modalities in the treatment of these lesions.

Illustrative Case

B. G. was a 55-year-old woman who sustained thermal burns of her upper and lower lips, right cheek, right hand, and both legs in a gasoline fire. She first consulted the author nine months after the injury with keloids and hypertrophic scars on her face and in the other previously mentioned areas (Fig. 48–5A). Over the course of one year, she received a series of three freeze-injection treatments as described above. This resulted in a decrease in size and a marked softening of lesions as well as a diminishing of their pain and pruritis (Fig. 48–5B).

Because of concern over the appearance of her upper lip, she was seen in consultation by Dr. Richard Babin in the Department of Otolaryngology and Head and Neck Surgery, University of Iowa School of Medicine.* Six months following her last injection (30 months after her original injury), a surgical revision of the remaining keloid on her upper lip was undertaken by Dr. Babin.

Bilateral, laterally based advancement flaps of her upper lip were fashioned, taking advantage of the nasal sills and alar facial creases superiorly. The vermilion border and nasolabial fold helped cam-

---

*Dr. Babin is now Professor and Chairman of the Department of Otolaryngology and Maxillofacial Surgery at the University of Tennessee Center for Health Sciences, Memphis, Tenn.

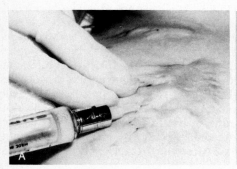

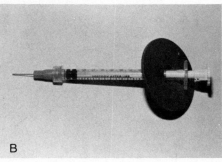

Figure 48–2. *A,* Injection of a keloid after the lesion thaws from freezing. *B,* Disposable 1 cc Luer-lok syringe with an assist ring.

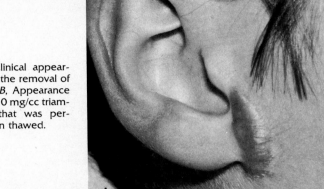
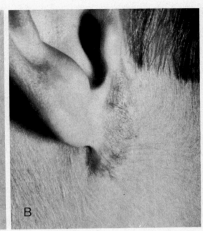

Figure 48–3. A, Clinical appearance of a keloid from the removal of an epidermoid cyst. B, Appearance after one injection of 10 mg/cc triamcinolone acetonide that was performed after the lesion thawed.

ouflage the incisions inferiorly (Fig. 48–5C). Burow's triangles, lateral to the nasal ala and within the nasolabial fold, facilitated advancement. It became apparent that complete excision of the scar tissue would result in a tight closure and a single vertical incision below the nasal columella. For these reasons, a superiorly based flap of remaining scar tissue was fashioned, carefully debulked, and oriented in a vertical position below the columella. This reconstituted both philtra and a cupid's bow at the vermilion border. The incision sites were injected with 3 cc of triamcinolone acetonide, 2.5 mg/cc. The results at six months were satisfactory enough that the patient was able to hide the residual scarring with makeup, and chose to defer any dermabrasion (Fig. 48–5D). Follow-up examination two years later showed no signs of recurrence.

Laser Surgery

Excision of keloids with the CO_2 laser appears to be an effective method of treating these lesions. The keloid margins are infiltrated with local anesthesia, and the lesion is excised with the continuous focused mode at a medium to high power setting. A saucer-like shave excision, as described by Bailin,[29] is utilized. After hemostasis is complete, the base margins are injected with 20 to 40 mg/cc of triamcinolone acetonide. Wounds are then allowed to heal by secondary intention. Early observations indicate some hypertrophic scarring, but not true keloid formation. The apparent advantage of the laser over conventional electrosurgery is the absence of damage to the adjacent dermis and attendant fibroblast stimulation. The nerve endings and blood and lymphatic vessels are sealed with minimal damage. This likely accounts for the reduced postoperative pain seen with the CO_2 laser surgery. Long-term studies are needed to determine the usefulness of this modality in the treatment of keloids.

Excision Techniques

In general, the results of *excision* and *primary closure* of keloids has been unsatisfactory. Pollock

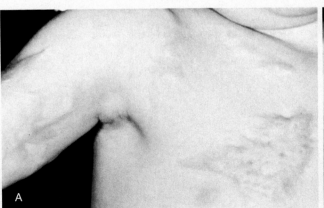
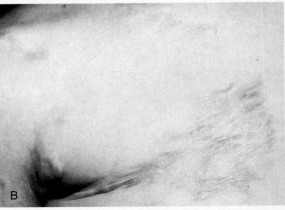

Figure 48–4. A, Clinical appearance of keloids on the chest and arm from a thermal burn. B, Appearance after two injections of 10 mg/cc triamcinolone acetonide after the thaw from freezing.

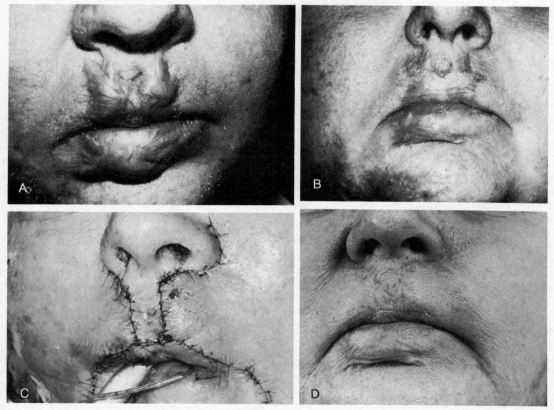

Figure 48–5. *A*, Clinical appearance of keloids on the lips and chin of a patient with thermal burns. *B*, Appearance after three freeze-injection treatments. *C*, Appearance immediately after surgical revision of the lip scars shown in B. *D*, Appearance six months after surgery.

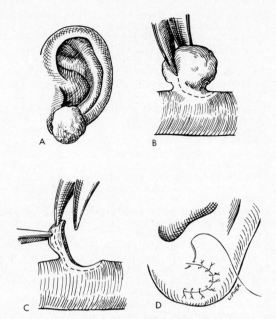

Figure 48–6. Keloid excision technique followed by flap reconstruction: *A*, Preoperative appearance. *B*, Excision of the bulk of the keloid with an outline of a small portion of skin for a flap to cover the defect. *C*, Dissection with iris scissors of residual keloidal tissue from the skin to be used as a flap. *D*, Suture of the flap in place without tension on the suture line. (Reprinted with permission from V. W. Weimar and R. I. Ceilley: Treatment of keloids on earlobes. Journal of Dermatologic Surgery and Oncology, 5(7):522–523, 1979.)

and Goslen report good results when treating keloids that are linear or characterized by a narrow attachment of the underlying skin and that can be closed without excessive tension.[30] A minimum of surrounding skin is removed, and the wound is closed parallel to relaxed skin tension lines. Adjunctive intralesional corticosteroid therapy is performed at the time of surgery and regularly afterwards.

Excision of Keloids with Skin Grafting. This procedure has been recently reported by Pollock and Goslen[30] and Apfelberg and coworkers.[31] The technique seems best suited for smaller lesions (less than 10 to 12 cm). An incision is made at the base of the keloid and the overlying epithelium is dissected off. The bulk of the keloid is then excised to a plane a few millimeters below the surrounding normal skin. The graft is trimmed and sutured in place utilizing a 5-0 or 6-0 monofilament suture. Postoperative care is the same as with routine skin grafting. Adjunctive intralesional corticosteroid injection is also utilized.

Excision with Flap Closure. This is another procedure that can be used for keloids. Multiple techniques have been reported, but the author prefers the method described in two articles.[30, 32] The technique (Fig. 48–6) is similar to the grafting technique described above except a semicircular incision is made on one side and then the overlying epithelium is dissected off, creating a very thin flap. The bulk of the keloid is then excised and the flap sutured in place. This technique has been especially useful for earlobe keloids but can be used in any location (Fig. 48–7). Adjunctive intralesional corticosteroid therapy is also utilized.

The major advantage of these techniques is that no separate donor site is needed, which might result in an additional keloid. Meticulous surgical technique with minimal use of pinpoint cautery (or none at all) and precise wound closure without significant dead space or wound tension is necessary for good results. Close follow-up with adjunctive pressure and intralesional corticosteroid injection help to reduce the likelihood of recurrence postoperatively.

DISCUSSION

The surgical management of keloids and hypertrophic scars remains a difficult problem for the cutaneous surgeon. Combined modalities in the treatment of these lesions have been popularized at

Figure 48–7. *A*, Earlobe keloid after preoperative intralesional triamcinolone acetonide injection. *B*, Postoperative appearance.

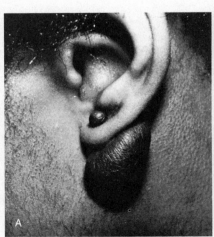
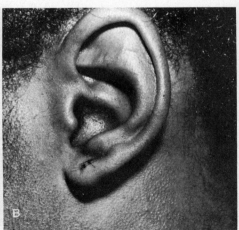

one time or another. Surgery in combination with steroid injection or radiation has its advocates. Cryosurgery and intralesional steroid injection have been shown to enhance results and minimize complications. Recently, CO_2 laser excision in combination with intralesional steroid injection has been found to be an effective method of treating keloids. Pressure therapy in various forms has been shown to be an effective, noninvasive method of treating keloids and hypertrophic scars. Unfortunately, immunotherapy and systemic medical treatment of these lesions has been disappointing to date.

The patient with a keloid or hypertrophic scar has a long-term management problem. Therapy inappropriate at the onset of the lesion may be successful later on. If lesions are treated early with pressure, stretching, cryotherapy, and intralesional steroid injections, softening and debulking may enhance or even eliminate the need for surgical reconstruction later on. With compulsive long-term follow-up, appropriate physical therapy, and intralesional injections, the long-term results are likely to be improved. Proper coordination of these procedures and interspecialty cooperation is needed to best serve these patients. The Duke University Keloid Clinic is a good example of the multispecialty effort encompassing both clinical and investigative studies.[30] With the proper effort and cooperation, a similar approach can be utilized in most medical communities.

REFERENCES

1. Cohen IK, Keiser HR, Sjooerdsma A: Collagen synthesis in human keloid and hypertrophic scar. Surg Forum 22:488–494, 1971
2. Cohen IK, Diegelmann RF: The biology of keloid and hypertrophic scars and the influence of corticosteroids. Clin Plast Surg 4:297–310, 1977
3. Hunter JAA, Finley JB: Scanning electron microscopy of normal human scar tissue and keloids. Br J Surg 62:741–744, 1975
4. Cosman B, Crikelair GF, Gaulin JC, et al: The surgical treatment of keloids. Plas Reconstr Surg 27:355–358, 1961
5. Johnson CL: Physical therapists as scar modifiers. Physical Therapy 64(9):1381–1387, 1984
6. Larson D, Abston S, Evans E, et al: Techniques for decreasing scar formation and contractures in the burned patient. J Trauma 11:807–823, 1971
7. Kischer CW, Shetlar MR, Shetlar CL: Alteration of hypertrophic scars induced by mechanical pressure. Arch Derm 111:60–64, 1975
8. Argenta CE: Tissue expansion in reconstructive surgery. Presented at the annual meeting of the Amer Soc for Derm Surg, Orlando, Fla, April 3, 1985
9. Tissue Expansion: "Future of Plastic Surgery for Next 20 Years." MEDICAL NEWS. JAMA 22(247):3039–3040, 1982
10. Radovan C: Tissue expansion in soft tissue reconstruction. Plast Reconstr Surg 74(4):482–490, 1984
11. Spillman L, Watrin J: Le Traitement des chéloïdes par la radiothérapie associée à la cryothérapie. Bull Soc Franç Dermat Syph 38:976–979, 1931
12. Lortat-Jacob F, Lortat-Jacob J: Traitement des chéloïdes par la cryothérapie. Bull Soc Franç Dermat Syph 38:983–990, 1931
13. Zacarian SA: Cryosurgery of Skin Cancer and Cryogenic Techniques in Dermatology. Springfield, Ill, Charles C Thomas, 1969
14. Ollstein RN, Seiger HW, Gilloley JF, et al: Treatment of keloids by combined surgical excision and immediate postoperative x-ray therapy. Ann Plast Surg 7:281–285, 1981
15. Levy DS, Salter MM, Roth RE: Postoperative irradiation in the prevention of keloids. Am J Roetgenol 127:509–510, 1976
16. Craig RDP, Phearson D: Early postoperative irradiation in the treatment of keloid scars. Br J Plas Surg 18:369–376, 1965
17. Van Den Brenk HAS, Minty CJ: Radiation in the treatment of keloids and hypertrophic scars. Brit J Surg 47:395, 1960
18. Malaker K, Ellis F, Paine CH: Keloid scars: A new method of treatment combining surgery with interstitial radiotherapy. Clin Radiol 27:179–183, 1976
19. Yagi KI, Dafalla AA, Osman AA: Does an immune reaction to sebum in wounds cause keloid scars: Beneficial effect of desensitization. Br J Plast Surg 32:223–335, 1979
20. Conway H, Stark RB: ACTH in plastic surgery. Plast Reconstr Surg 8:354–377, 1951
21. Maguire HC: Treatment of keloids with triamcinolone injected intralesionally. JAMA 192:125–126, 1965
22. Murray RD: Kenalog and the treatment of hypertrophical scars and keloids in negroes and whites. Plast Reconstr Surg 31:275–280, 1963
23. Kelchum LD, Smith J, Robinson DW, et al: The treatment of hypertrophic scar, keloid, and scar contracture by triamcinolone acetonide. Plast Reconstr Surg 38:209–218, 1966
24. Fishman EW, Finbert AR, Feinberg SM: Local subcutaneous atrophy. JAMA 179:971–972, 1962
25. Ceilley RI, Babin RW: The combined use of cryosurgery and intralesional injections of suspensions of fluorinated adrenocorticosteroids for reducing keloids and hypertrophic scars. J Dermatol Surg Oncol 5:54–56, 1979
26. Babin RW, Ceilley RI: Combined modalities in the management of hypertrophic scars and keloids. J Otolaryngol 8:457–460, 1979
27. Babin RW, Ceilley RI: The freeze-injection method of hypertrophic scar and keloid reduction. Otolaryngol Head and Neck Surg 87:911–914, 1979
28. Hirschowitz B, Lerner D, Moscona AR: Treatment of keloid scars by combined cryosurgery and intralesional corticosteroids. Aest Plast Surg 6:153–158, 1982
29. Bailin PR: Use of the CO_2 laser for non-PWS cutaneous lesions, in Arndt KA, Noe JM (eds): Cutaneous Laser Therapy: Principles and Methods. New York: John Wiley & Sons, 1983, pp 187–201
30. Pollock SV, Goslen BJ: The surgical treatment of keloids. J Dermatol Surg Oncol 8(12):1045–1048, 1982
31. Apfelberg DB, Maser MR, Lash H: The use of epidermis over a keloid as an autograph after excision of the keloid. J Dermatol Surg Oncol 2:409–411, 1976
32. Weimar VW, Ceilley RI: Treatment of keloids on earlobes. J Dermatol Surg Oncol 5(7):522–523, 1979

Pinch Grafting for Leg Ulcers

Leg ulcers are caused by a variety of local and systemic factors. A classification of ulcers based on the symptomatology and appearance of the ulcer and the surrounding skin is presented in Table 49–1.[1] The majority of leg ulcers seen in the office practice of dermatology, however, can readily be attributed to venous hypertension, chronic arterial disease, trauma, or a combination of these factors.

Successful management of a leg ulcer requires that the underlying cause be determined and treated and that the ulcer receive appropriate care. The great majority of ulcers can be healed by attention to these precepts. In most instances, however, this requires long periods of bed rest either at home or in the hospital, the use of pressure gradient dressings, and repeated visits to the physician's office or hospital. Although the necessity for frequent application of medication, compresses, and dressings has been reduced somewhat by the use of plastic occlusive dressings, chronic ulcer care occasionally presents a major problem. Some patients or their families are unwilling or unable to cope with an ulcer because of ignorance or apathy. Simply stated, the ulcer is too messy or offensive. Furthermore, in some instances, despite good conservative local therapy, the ulcer will fail to heal. For these patients, a surgical approach for covering the ulcer is indicated.

USES

A variety of skin-grafting techniques has been employed for re-epithelializing leg ulcers. Among those most commonly used are split-thickness grafts,[2] split-thickness mesh,[3] postage-stamp strips,[4] suction-blister transplants,[5] and pinch grafts.[6] All but pinch grafts require special equipment that is usually not available in the dermatologist's office.

Pinch grafting has other salubrious features as well. It is an office procedure, a simple, inexpensive form of therapy for which no special training is necessary. Pinch grafts will "take" on granulating ulcers, infected ulcers, and often those with a poor blood supply. Patients unfit for major surgery or vascular surgery because of underlying heart and pulmonary disease or obesity are candidates for this approach. There is relief of pain, minimal blood loss, and in most instances, healing within three weeks. The grafted site results in a durable scar in which ulcers are less likely to recur even when the underlying venous or arterial disease cannot be corrected.

Like most procedures, pinch grafting also has disadvantages. A poor cosmetic appearance often results in the donor and recipient site. In elderly patients, however, where the technique is applicable, this is often a secondary consideration. Furthermore, the cosmetic result in the recipient site can be improved by attention to the size and thickness of the pinch grafts. Bed rest or relative inactivity for two to four weeks after grafting might be detrimental to some patients subject to thrombophlebitis. This complication can often be prevented by foot and leg exercises for a few minutes every hour while awake. In some instances, low-dose heparin therapy may be indicated. Pinch grafting is indicated for ulcers that fail to heal after a period of appropriate therapy. The ulcer should be stable, preferably one that is beginning to heal and to show re-epithelization at the edges. An ulcer that is deteriorating should not be grafted. Patient cooperation is mandatory. He or she must be willing to keep the leg elevated for two to four weeks postoperatively, be able to maintain the dressing over the graft, and return for follow-up visits.

TABLE 49–1. Diagnostic Categories of Ulcers*

I. Punched-out, painful, ischemic
   A. Chronic arterial disease
   B. No preceding vascular disease
     1. Increased blood viscosity
     2. Embolization
     3. Vessel wall defects
       a. Functional
       b. Organic—either noninflammatory or
         inflammatory
II. Punched-out, anesthetic ulcers, ischemic
III. Associated with dermatologic disease
IV. Undermined edge
V. Ulcerated nodules
VI. Geometric shapes
VII. Purulent base—either with or without marked adenopathy

*(Modified from Lazarus GS, Goldsmith LA: Diagnosis of Skin Disease. Philadelphia, FA Davis Co, 1980, p 314.)

ETIOLOGY OF ULCERS

Before grafting, the cause of the ulcer should be determined and treated. For example, the venous stasis ulcer requires a reduction of venous hypertension. This can be accomplished by bed rest with elevation of the leg, pressure gradient dressings, elastic bandages, stockings with or without local compression over the ulcer, Unna's paste boot, compression sclerotherapy of incompetent perforators, and ligation or stripping. For the ischemic ulcer, improved perfusion of the extremity is necessary. In addition to bed rest with slight dependency of the legs, pentoxifylline (400 mg three times a day by mouth) is valuable.

Large vessel disease may be amenable to vascular surgery, while sympathectomy is beneficial in selected cases of small vessel disease. Other considerations include the presence or absence of malignant deterioration. For example, a biopsy is indicated to confirm squamous cell cancer, if suspected. Ulcers resulting from deep fungal infection, tuberculosis, or syphilis obviously should be treated appropriately. Grafting a factitious ulcer will usually be unsuccessful, and so self-induction should be suspected in any ulcer with a geometric shape.

PREPARATION FOR GRAFTING

The optimal local requirements for grafting are listed in Table 49–2. Edema can usually be alleviated by a period of bed rest, systemic diuretics, and pressure gradient bandages or the Jobst pump. Cool compresses followed by topical fluorinated steroids will often clear concomitant dermatitis. If the dermatitis is caused by discharge from the ulcer, protecting the skin with Lassar's (zinc) paste can be helpful. Although the ulcer bed need not be absolutely sterile for pinch grafting, cultures and sensitivity studies should be obtained.

Heavy colonization by such gram-negative organisms as *Pseudomonas aeruginosa* often causes graft rejection. Pinch grafting should, of course, be avoided when frank infection is present. If infection is diagnosed, appropriate local and systemic therapy should be instituted. Daily applications of porcine xenograft will often clear secondary infection. When the xenograft adheres to the bed it is allowed to remain in place for several days. Upon removal, the ulcer is ready for grafting.[7] Ideally, the ulcer bed should consist of cherry red granulation tissue. Necrotic material, crusts, and adherent membranes interfere with graft and should be removed to expose the capillaries of the ulcer bed. Large eschars are best removed surgically under local anesthesia.

TABLE 49–2. Requirements for Grafting

- Absence of leg edema
- Dermatitis free surrounding skin
- Absence of infection
- Absence of eschar and necrotic debris
- Cherry red granulation tissue

The use of plastic occlusive dressings for several weeks will clean most ulcers except those with tightly adherent eschars. An added benefit of these dressings is that they stimulate the production of granulation tissue. Smaller amounts of necrotic debris can be removed mechanically by application of wet to dry dressings or whirlpool baths.

HARVESTING SKIN GRAFTS

The anterolateral thigh is most often used as the donor site. In some instances, the lower abdomen is more appropriate. The area is shaved, if necessary, and then cleaned thoroughly with either chlorhexidine gluconate or povidone-iodine. After marking the site with a skin marking pencil, it is anesthetized with 1% lidocaine without epinephrine.

Several techniques may be used to obtain the grafts. When a small number are required, the skin can be pinched between the thumb and forefinger of the left hand while the specimens are shaved off with half of a Gillette Super Blue Blade held with the thumb and index finger of the right hand. A large number of grafts are more easily removed by elevating the skin with a skin hook or a 25-gauge needle mounted on a syringe and removing the graft with a No. 21 scalpel blade held parallel to the skin surface. Intradermal injections of sterile physiologic saline can also be used to raise the skin specimens before cutting.

Generally, grafts should be about 1 cm in diameter and 1 to 2 mm thick. This thickness is achieved when the edge of the blade used to cut the graft is just not visible through the graft. Subcutaneous fat should not be included with the graft because it interferes with the graft "take" and causes greater scarring of the donor site. The harvested grafts are placed on a saline-moistened 4 × 4 inch sponge. After all the grafts have been obtained, a temporary pressure dressing is applied to the donor site to effect hemostasis.

The leg and the ulcer are cleaned with chlorhexidine gluconate or povidone-iodine and rinsed with saline, after which a gauze wet with saline is applied. The grafts are placed on the ulcer bed with a straight needle and thumb forceps. They should be positioned next to, but not touching, until the ulcer is covered. A margin of 1 to 2 mm at the ulcer edge is left uncovered because epidermis growing in from the edge may prevent border grafts from taking. The ulcer is then covered with a polyurethane dressing. To maintain contact of the grafts with the ulcer bed, several layers of gauze-covered dressing sponges cut to fit the grafted site are placed over the adhesive semipermeable dressing.[8] The foot, ankle, and leg are then wrapped with elastic bandages to apply slight pressure to the ulcer. After hemostasis is achieved, the donor site is covered with a polyurethane dressing and several gauze dressing sponges can be held in place with adhesive tape.

POSTOPERATIVE CARE

The patient can return home where the leg should be kept elevated. When seen again at 48 to 72 hours, the elastic bandage and gauze are removed, and the grafts inspected through the plastic membrane. If the discharge is purulent, the dressing is trimmed to the edge of the ulcer to allow better drainage. This does not necessarily indicate frank infection. The pressure and elastic bandage is reapplied, and the patient is seen again at five days and at 14 days.

The membrane on the ulcer and donor site is allowed to lift off by itself or can be soaked off after 14 days. Upon removal, gentle cleaning with a mild soap and application of emollient cream and an elastic bandage are recommended. For venous ulcers, this is continued until definitive treatment can be undertaken. Elastic stockings are prescribed for those unsuitable for surgery. Ischemic ulcers often remain healed, despite lack of corrective surgery for the underlying problem.

CONCLUSIONS

Although pinch grafting or any type of grafting procedure will not recreate an unscarred area of skin, it does afford a good reparative possibility. When the indications for pinch grafting are followed, the success rate for treatment of such ulcerations is high, making pinch grafting a recommendable procedure.

REFERENCES

1. Lazarus GS, Goldsmith LA: Diagnosis of Skin Disease. Philadelphia, FA Davis Co, 1980, p 314
2. Michaolides P, Caniga C: The treatment of ulcers on legs with split thickness grafts. J Dermatol Surg Oncol 5:961–965, 1979
3. Chilvers AS, Freeman GK: Outpatient skin grafting of venous ulcers. Lancet 2:1087–1088, 1969
4. Vesterager L: Split-skin grafting for ulcers on legs. J Dermatol Surg Oncol 6:739–741, 1980
5. Hentzer B, Kobayasi T: Suction blister transplantation for leg ulcers. Acta Dermatovener (Stockholm) 55:207–209, 1975
6. Ceilley RI, Rinck MA, Zuchlke RL: Pinch grafting for chronic ulcers on lower extremities. J Dermatol Surg Oncol 3:303–309, 1977
7. Robson MC, Krizek TJ: Predicting skin graft survival. J Trauma 13:213–217, 1973
8. Gilmore WA, Wheeland RG: Treatment of ulcers on legs by pinch grafts and a supportive dressing of polyurethane. J Dermatol Surg Oncol 8:177–183, 1982.

50

JEROLD Z. KAPLAN M.D., F.A.C.S.

Cutaneous Burn Injury

Burn injuries are among mankind's oldest known afflictions. It is certain that shortly after man learned to tame fire that accidents involving this useful "gift of the gods" occurred. Treatment of burn wounds was mentioned in Ebers Papyrus, one of the earliest medical manuscripts. However, it is within the last century that modern burn care has truly developed and evolved.

TYPES OF BURNS

Burns may be due to flame, scalds, electrical or chemical injuries, contact with hot objects, and radiation. Flame burns may vary from extremely small, such as a match flaring on one's finger, to extremely massive, such as a victim trapped in a house fire. The depth of the injury may vary from relatively superficial to extremely deep. Smoke inhalation injury is a frequent concomitant complication of flame injuries. Scald burns may be due to high-temperature or low-temperature liquids. High-temperature scald burns due to molten metal, tar, hot grease or oil, or boiling water are generally uniform in depth and may have sharp outlines at the level of immersion. Low-temperature scald burns due to tap water of 135 to 160°F are usually caused by accidents in the shower and bathtub but may also be due to abuse. These injuries frequently are more severe than initially estimated because of the progressive nature of long exposure to a moderate temperature agent.

Electrical injuries may be due to either high- or low-voltage. High-voltage electrical injuries frequently result in massive, deep tissue destruction as the path of the current follows those structures with the least electrical resistance, i.e., blood vessels and nerves, but the most thermal damage is done along the path of greatest electrical resistance, i.e., the bones. High-voltage electrical injuries frequently have a small wound of entry and a relatively small but explosive wound of exit, yet may destroy two or more extremities in their path through the body. Low-voltage electrical injuries generally caused by house current are more dangerous in their potential for electrocution rather than a true burn, but small burns may occur at the point of contact. In addition to the electrical injury, flame burns may occur from ignition of clothing.

Chemical burns may be due to acids, alkalies, or other corrosive chemicals. Acid burns generally tend to be relatively self-limiting, and the extent of damage is generally apparent at initial examination. Alkali burns, such as those caused by potassium or sodium hydroxide, tend to be progressive, and the exact amount of injury may not be apparent immediately upon early examination. Toxicity of chemical agents may also be a complicating factor in the treatment of patients with chemical burns.

Contact with a hot object such as an iron at home or heated metal in an industrial situation frequently causes a very deep burn of limited extent that is treated best by early surgical excision. Radiation, either in the form of sunlight or ionizing radiation (e.g., that used in oncologic therapy) may also cause burns. Sunlight-induced burns are generally superficial, but they may be extremely extensive. Burns that result from radiotherapy are generally sharply demarcated but may involve damage to deeper tissue as well as the skin.

EXTENT OF THE BURN WOUND

The extent of the burn wound may be rapidly estimated or precisely calculated. Rapid estimation of the total body surface area (TBSA) is provided by the "rule of nines." This technique divides the body surface into areas of approximately 9% each. Each upper extremity comprises 9%, the head and neck 9%, the anterior and posterior torso each twice times 9 or 18%, and each lower extremity 18%. Totaling these areas yields 99%; the additional 1% is assigned to the genitalia. It must be emphasized that the rule of nines applies only to adults and becomes inaccurate as the victim's age decreases below 15 years old. With the use of the rule of nines, however, a rapid estimation of the extent of the burn wound may be made. In those patients with a massive burn injury, the use of the rule of nines on unburned areas and then subtracting from 100% may be more useful.

For more precise calculation of the total body surface area of the burn wound, the Lund and Browder[1] chart is utilized. This chart divides the body into multiple areas of varying small percentages. After the patient has been initially cleaned and débrided, the wounds are very carefully sketched and then an estimate made of the percentage of each small area. Dividing the body into multiple small areas permits a more precise estimation of the body surface involved and also allows correction for patients of any age.

In the child, the exact surface area in square meters should also be calculated. Fluid replacement in the child is based on surface area rather than weight because a child's surface-area-to-weight ratio is significantly different than an adult's.

DEPTH OF THE BURN WOUND

Burn wounds have generally been classified as first, second, or third degree with occasional use of the term "fourth-degree injury," but today they are characterized as partial- or full-thickness injuries. A partial-thickness injury implies that dermal elements have been spared, whereas a full-thickness injury implies complete destruction of the epidermis and dermis.

First-degree burns are the least severe burn injury. The skin is reddened and tender, but generally no medical therapy is required unless the burn is extremely extensive. First-degree burns heal in three to five days without residual scarring. Occasionally, erythema may persist for several days, but this too will resolve.

Second-degree burns have a wide range of depth and therefore vary in diagnosis and treatment. Superficial second-degree burns involve the epidermis and may involve the upper portion of dermal papillae. The wound is generally blistered, and when the blisters break or the area is débrided, the underlying tissue is moist or weeping, pink or red in color, and extremely sensitive. Treatment of this depth of burn wound is aimed at protection of the wound so that normal healing processes may occur. Healing time is generally between five to 15 days and residual pigment changes may occur but physical scarring is unusual.

Deep partial-thickness wounds (deep second-degree burns) result in complete destruction of the epidermis and varying levels of destruction of the dermis and dermal elements. These wounds are generally mottled pink and white, and they may still be soft to the touch. They are insensitive to light touch or pinprick, although there may be pain present in the burn wound. These wounds will heal in three to four weeks if protected from infection, dessication, and other deleterious effects, but significant scarring always results. Preferred treatment of the deep partial-thickness wound frequently involves surgical excision and grafting.

The full-thickness or third-degree burn injury results in complete destruction of the epidermis and dermis. The wound may be leathery or parchment-like and generally is white or tan in color. The skin is firm and inelastic. While extremely small full-thickness injuries may granulate and epithelialize, in general, the third-degree injury requires surgical excision and grafting.

Differentiation between deep partial- and full-thickness injuries is frequently difficult. The partial-thickness wound, however, is generally soft and moist as opposed to the hard, dry, full-thickness injury. The partial-thickness injury may be swollen from edema, whereas the full-thickness wound may be sunken because of contraction of the heat-tanned skin.

Many methods have been proposed in order to ascertain the depth of the burn wound, including injection of dyes and thermography; however, clinical assessment remains the method of choice.

ON-THE-SCENE EMERGENCY CARE

The first and foremost emergency procedure is to stop the burning process. If this is not done rapidly, the delay will allow for continuing damage to the skin with resultant deeper injuries. In the flame injury, this is simply done by extinguishing the flame. If the person whose clothes are on fire has the presence of mind and previous training to stop, drop, and roll, almost all flames will be extinguished. As is more often the case, the person panics and runs and must be tackled or tripped in order to drop and then roll on the ground. Smothering with a blanket, such as an asbestos blanket or other heavy blanket may be helpful, but blankets are often not available at the scene. Likewise, spraying with water or any fire extinguisher is acceptable. Again, the main point is to stop the flaming process.

In a patient who has sustained or who is sustaining an electrical injury, it is most important to realize that two processes may be going on at the same time. Sparks may have ignited clothing and a burn may be occurring in addition to a deeper electrical injury caused by the electrical source. The electrical source must be disconnected immediately, which may sometimes be accomplished by shutting off the power. However, in other instances, it is necessary to safely remove the wires from the victim or vice versa. Great care must be used in performing the rescue, or additional persons may be injured. Once the electrical source has been shut off, the flame should be extinguished.

In a chemical burn, it is most imperative to remove exposure to the chemical immediately. This is best accomplished by immediate removal of all clothing and flooding with water. A safety shower is an excellent method for performing this, but if not available, a garden hose or fire hose may also be used. It is important that large quantities of water be used both to remove the chemical and to dilute any chemical reactions that may occur from exposure to the water. In general, neutralization of the chemicals should not be attempted; however, if neutralization is performed it should be done with a weak base, such as ordinary soap for acid burns, and a weak acid, such as diluted vinegar, for alkali burns. In certain instances, a solvent may be used to remove the offending chemicals. The most common of these is the use of alcohol or alcoholic solutions for phenol burns or dilute copper sulfate solution for phosphorus burns. However, the most important factor is to remove all of the offending chemical.

Immediate cooling of the burn wound is the only on-the-scene care of the burn wound that should be performed. It must be emphasized that this should be immediate cooling of the burn wound and not of the burn victim. Any cold solution is satisfactory; ice water from the refrigerator being the optimal. If this is not available, any cold liquid, or, in fact, any liquid at or below body temperature may be utilized. Cooling of the burn wound has been alternately suggested and condemned over the 4000-year-old history of burn care, but it now has a firm medical basis. Immediate cooling tends to stabilize the lysosome membrane and therefore may protect from autolysis those cells that may not have been damaged irreversibly.

Cooling should be performed only as long as necessary to drop the burn-injured cell to or slightly below body temperature and should not be so extensive as to drop the temperature of the entire burn victim. Packing the patient in ice has no benefit and is, in fact, dangerous. Patients may develop frostbite on top of the burn wounds or drop their core temperature to such an extent that they may not have sufficient energy reserve to regain normal body temperature.

The next task that must be performed at the scene and in which significant errors may occur is assessment of associated injuries. The burn wound itself is never an acute emergency. Even a patient with 100% total body surface burns would survive a few hours without any care unless an associated injury results in death. Associated injuries, depending on the etiology of burn, include fractures of any of the bones, head trauma, chest or abdominal internal injuries, and massive lacerations. All these should be treated as appropriate for that injury, ignoring the burn wound. Fractures should be splinted and bleeding stopped by direct pressure. Head and internal injuries cannot generally be treated on an emergency basis, and their treatment must be deferred until definitive medical care is available.

EMERGENCY MEDICAL CARE AND RESUSCITATION

Emergency medical care of burn victims after they arrive at a medical facility is directed toward evaluation of the injury and appropriate treatment or referral. Of prime importance is to assess the burn victim for associated injuries. Even massive burns are never rapidly fatal, but a missed ruptured aorta, lacerated liver, or cardiac contusion may result in the rapid demise of a patient who would otherwise be salvageable. Treatment of these associated injuries takes precedence over the burn. Initial evaluation of burn size using the rule of nines and an estimate of the depth indicate the seriousness of the burn injury.

If the burn injury is minor, gentle cleansing of the wound and application of a protective dressing with appropriate follow-up at 48 hours is the only therapy required. If the patient is stable, has no associated injuries or significant associated illnesses, and can be transported to definitive care within one half hour, no specific therapy is necessary. A clean, dry sheet should be used to cover the patient, who should then be transported to the burn center.

If the patient will be admitted to the receiving hospital or if transportation will be longer than one half hour, minimal initial care should be performed in the emergency room. A peripheral intravenous line should be started with a moderate-sized (16- to 18-gauge) angiocath or similar device. Resuscitation fluids may be estimated by the Parkland formula of 3 to 4 cc of Ringer's lactate solution per percent of body surface burned per kilogram of body weight; one half is administered in the first eight hours after the burn injury. As a rough approximation in the adult, 15 cc of Ringer's lactate solution per percent per hour is an appropriate rate. Hypertonic lactated saline resuscitation is advantageous in the major burn victim for minimizing the burn wound and pulmonary edema, but this technique requires close monitoring and should be performed only in the burn center.

A Foley catheter should be inserted under aseptic conditions to monitor urine output. Baseline arterial blood gases including a carboxyhemoglobin level should be drawn and the patient then begun on nasal or mask oxygen therapy. Pain medication, only if necessary, should always be given intravenously and in small, repeated doses. The burn patient may have impaired peripheral tissue perfusion, and intramuscular injection may result in absorption of a large and unexpected dose of narcotic when peripheral perfusion is restored.

CHEMICAL, ELECTRICAL, AND SCALD INJURIES

Chemical, electrical, and scald injuries are different than the standard flame or contact burn for determining the depth of injury. A chemical injury may involve more than the pure physical destruction of surface tissue. Some chemicals, such as nitric acid, will form colored compounds upon reaction with the protein and other components of skin, and therefore color may not be an indicator of depth of burn. Other chemicals, such as hydrofluoric acid, may have a progressive and toxic effect due to highly reactive ions, such as the fluoride ion, and the wound that is pink or red from a hydrofluoric acid burn may actually represent an extremely severe injury.

Electrical injuries are significant in that a surface wound may represent only the tip of the iceberg as far as the extent of tissue damage is concerned. A relatively small surface injury visible in both palms may represent an electrical injury that will eventually necessitate bilateral shoulder disarticulation. With the electrical injury, it is extremely important to look for "kissing" wounds in the cubital or popliteal fossae and in the axillae. It is also vitally important to carefully examine what appears to be unburned or uninjured extremities for erythema, edema, and swelling as well as vascular and neurologic integrity. When in doubt, extensive, operative exploration with fasciotomy as necessary may be vital to maximize the chances for a limb's survival.

Scald injuries, particularly if caused by hot tap water, do not physically destroy even nonviable tissue. Hemoglobin or myoglobin may be released and fixed in nonviable tissue, imparting a pink or red color. Therefore, color is *not* a useful characteristic in determining the depth of a scald injury.

CLEANSING OF THE BURN WOUND

Cleansing of the burn wound and the burn patient should be done on admission and thereafter as determined by the need for dressing changes and type of dressings. Cleansing of the burn wound is initially performed in order to remove foreign material such as soot, dirt, or grass as well as loose, nonviable epithelium. Subsequent cleansing is necessary to remove the topical agent as well as exudate and/or additional nonviable tissue. Historically, patients were placed in a Hubbard tank filled with water for cleansing; however, it has been shown that immersion in a tank of water is conducive to an increased infection rate from migration of resident bacteria from the perineal and perianal areas to the burn wound. Although some people have advocated adding antibacterials such as iodophors or sodium hypochlorite to the water, the concentration cannot be antibacterial without also being toxic to nascent epithelial cells. A preferred method of cleansing, therefore, is to suspend the patient over an empty tub and cleanse the wound under a flow of water that allows continuous washing of nonviable or foreign material down the drain rather than onto the patient.

Bed baths of patients should be utilized to the minimal extent possible because they are an inadequate substitute for tubbings. Bed baths should be confined to those patients who cannot, under any circumstances, be moved because of medical or surgical reasons.

Removal of tar or similar materials from the burn wound presents special problems. The usual solvents or cleansers are too harsh to apply to burn-damaged skin. Specific solvents are available to remove tar or other non–water-soluble grime. It is important to use a solvent that is nontoxic and painless to the burn patient. Mineral oil is slow but effective. Commercial solvents based on citrus oil work very well.

ASSESSMENT OF THE BURN WOUND

Assessment of the burn wound is the key to successful care of the burn patient. Although the burn wound is immediately visible and accessible for inspection, infrequent and untimely assessment of it all too often yields less-than-optimal results with the burn patient. While laboratory determinations may be helpful, clinical judgment reigns supreme. Proper assessment involves the senses of sight, touch, smell, and hearing.

The burn wound should be visually examined at every dressing change, or daily if dressing changes are done more than once a day, by a physician qualified to assess the burn wound. The same degree of concern should be exercised as that for auscultation of the chest or palpation of the surgical abdomen. General appearance of the dressings and the burn wound should be noted. Purulent drainage on the dressings should be distinguished from the slimy, yellowish-green appearance of normal wound exudate combined with silver sulfadiazine. The green color of *Pseudomonas* and the black of *Aspergillus* are quite distinctive. The appearance of unburned tissue surrounding the burn wound should be noted and characterized. Erythema with or without edema may indicate an early streptococcal or staphylococcal cellulitis. Ecthyma gangrenosum, the hallmark of disseminated *Pseudomonas* sepsis, or similar lesions in unburned skin indicate massive and uncontrolled sepsis. Many topical agents stain the burn wound and it is important to recognize the normal grayish color induced by cerium silver sulfadiazine or the black staining of silver nitrate. Healthy granulation tissue should be firm and bright red. Epithelial buds may present as bright red dots poking through the base of a burn wound.

In addition to visual inspection, it is important to inspect the burn wound with the gloved hand. Loose eschar or subeschar pockets of purulence are frequently found by palpation rather than visual inspection. Palpation is often a better indicator of edema than visual inspection, and edema may be evaluated and rated the same as pretibial or pedal edema. Palpation of extremities may indicate the possible need for escharotomy, and the manually palpated pulse is far superior to one that must be identified with the Doppler. Checking the patient's sensation is also important following the progress of moderate to deep second-degree wounds. A sterile hypodermic needle is an ideal tool for testing sensation.

As in any field of medicine, listening to the patient is of prime importance. The patient who tells you about a significant change in the feeling of an area of the burn wound is requesting an extraordinarily careful examination of that area. Listening to the changes in the patient's comments also provides a valuable method of following progression of the burn wound.

While burn wards no longer have the stench associated with them as little as 20 years ago, the odor of a burn wound or burn dressing may provide 24- to 48-hour headstart over the bacteriology lab. The sickening sweet odor of *Pseudomonas,* the moldy bread odor of *Aspergillus*, and overpowering stench of nonsporulating anaerobes, and to the experienced observer, multiple other characteristic odors identify many microorganisms as surely as a culture. Decisions about whether a dressing change is necessary may frequently be made on the basis of the physical appearance of the dressing as well as its odor. Current high-tech machines identify microorganisms by gas chromatography of metabolic byproducts; this same technique is applicable at a much lower cost using a talented nose.

Laboratory assessment of the burn wound includes microscopic sectioning and pathologic examination and various techniques of culturing the burn wound. In their classic book, *The Burn Wound*, Order and Moncrief described the perivascular cuffing by *Pseudomonas* in burn wound sepsis.[2] Invasion of essentially normal tissue by bacteria is pathognomonic of burn wound sepsis. Modified Gram's and Giemsa's stains and routine hematoxylin and eosin as well as numerous special stains allow visualization of bacteria in the tissue. Unfortunately, significant invasion of bacteria and particularly of fungi is frequently not seen on microscopic sections until autopsy.

Bacteriologic assessment of the burn wound has been performed in many ways over the years, yet its clinical significance is still debated. Most burn wounds have surface growth of bacteria. MacMillan in the 1950s demonstrated that the burn wound is not sterile and that, even with the topical antimicrobial therapy of the 1980s, most burn wounds have bacterial colonization.[3] Surface colonization, however, does not invariably lead to burn wound sepsis and, in fact, rarely does so. Nonetheless, because of its ease and noninvasiveness as well as being an indicator of potential future invasive organisms, surface culturing is widely used. Semiquantitative techniques of surface culture including laying a saturated gauze sponge over the burn wounds, swabbing a measured area, or surface contact plate culturing, have not been shown to have a significant advantage over simple surface culturing with a swab.

Quantitative wound biopsies are used to determine numbers of bacteria *in* rather than *on* the burn wound, and burn wound sepsis has been defined as greater than 10^5 viable microorganisms per gram of tissue. Quantitative biopsies require removal of all surface organisms, so that the laboratory must be capable of sterilely weighing a tissue sample and then homogenizing it for a quantitative culture. The drawbacks to quantitative culturing are the slight increased cost compared to routine cultures, the necessity of a minimally (but nonetheless) invasive surgical procedure, and the fact that the burn wound is not an absolutely uniform lesion in which any given area is certain to be representative (thus necessitating the need for multiple biopsies). The 24- to 48-hour lag time is also a deterrent to its clinical rather than research use.

The time delay inherent in all culturing techniques has led to the development of several rapid, semiquantitative techniques for assessing the burn wound. Robson has recommended imprinting a fresh biopsy specimen onto a glass slide. The print is then fixed and stained. Greater than 1 bacterium per high-power field is felt to be indicative of a tissue count greater than 10^5 per gram of tissue.

In summary, assessment of the burn wound is a clinical evaluation supplemented by laboratory studies. Serial assessments with appropriate action based on those assessments will minimize morbidity and maximize survival of the burn victim.

TOPICAL CHEMOTHERAPY

The history of topical chemotherapy of burn wounds is essentially as old as the recorded history of medical care. In his writings, Hippocrates recommended a mixture of "swine seam and bitumen" (lard and pitch) on dressings applied to the wound. Ancient Arabic physicians used a poultice of burned pigeon dung as a topical wound-healing agent. As early as the 1800s, silver nitrate in a 10% solution was used on the burn wound. Wet dressings containing various solutions have likewise been used for over 100 years. Modern burn topical therapy dates to the 1920s when Davidson used tannic acid as an escharotic to tan the burn wound. The hard, dry eschar did indeed decrease the incidence of burn wound infection, but the hepatotoxicity of tannic acid soon brought this method into disfavor. The antibacterial effect of dyes was noted in the 1930s and such dyes as gentian violet, malachite green, scarlet red, acriflavine orange, and others were used, again to promote a dry and somewhat antibacterial eschar. The discovery and purification of penicillin by Fleming, Flory, and Chain in the 1920s and 1930s and Prontosil, the first sulfa drug, by Domagck in 1935 ushered in the age of specific antimicrobial therapy. Sulfa powders were used topically during World War II, but their relative inefficacy and systemic reactions limited their development as burn wound agents. The rapid developments in antibiotics in the late 1940s and early 1950s led to multiple antibiotics being applied to the burn wound without significant success. In the early 1960s, mafenide (Sulfamylon) in a hydrochloride form was first applied to animal and then human burn wounds at the Surgical Research Unit at Brooke Army Medical Center.[4] The striking reduction in morbidity and mortality in the small to medium burn wound initiated today's modern topical chemotherapy. Monafo and Moyer, in 1965, repopularized the use of silver nitrate dressing utilizing a 0.5% rather than 10% solution.[5] Charles L. Fox of Columbia University combined the oligodynamic antimicrobial effect of the silver ion with sulfadiazine to develop silver sulfadiazine (Silvadene or SSD).[6] The convenience of silver sulfadiazine combined with the relatively low incidence of significant side effects has led to its emergence as the number one topical antimicrobial agent in use today.

General Considerations for Topical Antimicrobial Therapy

Antimicrobial therapy is an adjunct to, and not a substitute for, good surgical wound care. Topical agents will neither cure nor prevent fatal wound infection if basic attention to wound care is not given. The dressings on a burn wound should be changed as necessary; not necessarily on a fixed schedule. As a general rule, daily dressing changes are adequate for most burn patients. If the dressing is intended to débride a wound, such as a wet to dry dressing, more frequent dressings may be necessary. If a wound is clean and free of infection and in the final stages of epithelialization or following a skin graft, changing the dressings more frequently than every two or three days may be contraindicated. It is imperative that good clinical judgment of a physician knowledgeable and skilled in burn care determine the frequency of dressing changes. It is likewise imperative that the burn wound be examined daily, or at every dressing change if dressings are done less than daily, by a physician trained in burn care.

Specific Topical Agents

Silver Sulfadiazine

Silver sulfadiazine (Silvadene, SSD) was developed by C. L. Fox and combines the oligodynamic

action of the silver ion with the antibacterial action of the sulfa moiety. Silver sulfadiazine is generally supplied as a 1% suspension in a cold-cream–like base.

Advantages. Silver sulfadiazine is convenient, stable, easy to apply, comfortable for the patient, and relatively nonstaining.

Disadvantages and Precautions. Silver sulfadiazine may cause an idiopathic leukopenia of uncertain clinical significance. The silver ion may leach out chloride and, with it, sodium. Therefore, patients with large burns being treated with silver sulfadiazine frequently require salt supplementation. Allergy to the sulfa component has been reported but is usually mild and only rarely requires discontinuance of the drug.

Mafenide

Mafenide (Sulfamylon) was first developed by the Germans in the late 1930s, and its use in burn patients developed at Brooke Army Medical Center by Moncrief, Lindberg, and others in the early 1960s. It is supplied as an 11.2% concentration in a thick, water-soluble base. Originally supplied as a hydrochloride form, it is now supplied as an acetate.

Advantages. Mafenide is a highly defusable, effective antibacterial agent. It is the agent of choice for electrical injuries, burns combined with crush injury, and for patients with old or infected burns at the time they are first seen.

Disadvantages. Mafenide is quite hygroscopic and may cause intense pain upon application; it is also a potent carbonic anhydrase inhibitor and may result in a severe metabolic acidosis. For this reason, mafenide should not be used to cover more than 15% to 20% of the body surface at any one time. A clinical picture resembling adult respiratory distress syndrome (ARDS) has been seen in patients who have had a significant portion of their body covered with mafenide. Sulfa allergy is not infrequent with the use of mafenide and may require its discontinuation.

Silver Nitrate

Silver nitrate in a 10% solution was used as early as the 1840s. Because of its damage to normal tissue, it was abandoned. Moyer, Monafo, and Bretano popularized its use in a 0.5% solution, which is the concentration currently used.

Advantages. Silver nitrate is antimicrobial against a wide range of organisms, and resistance does not develop. It is readily available, can be made on site, and does not cause allergic reactions. Silver nitrate may be used over grafts as well as acute burns.

Disadvantages. Silver nitrate is messy and stains linen, clothing, floors, and walls. The silver ion leaches out chloride and, with it, sodium necessitating frequent monitoring of electrolytes and replacement therapy. Methemoglobinemia may also occur in patients being treated over very large body surface areas.

Technique. Silver nitrate dressings should be made of at least 16 layers of gauze, kept continuously moistened, and changed at relatively frequent intervals.

Nitrofurazone

Nitrofurazone (Furacin, Actin-N) is supplied as a 0.2% preparation in a soluble cream base.

Advantages. Nitrofurazone is a broad-spectrum antibacterial with relatively minimal side effects. It is easily converted into a solution form by diluting with equal volumes of normal saline and is extremely useful for soaks to protect granulation tissue or new grafts. It is pain-free upon application, easily removed with water, and nonstaining. The polyethylene glycol base does not evaporate as rapidly as aqueous solutions; therefore, dressings rarely dry out.

Disadvantages. Rare instances of allergic reactions have been reported but usually do not require discontinuance of the drug. A report has been made of renal toxicity caused by the glycol base.

Topical Aminoglycoside Ointments and Creams

Topical aminoglycoside ointments and creams include gentamycin- and neomycin-containing preparations. Topical gentamycin was originally popularized by Stone in the 1960s, but it is rarely used on major burns today.

Advantages. These preparations are convenient, comfortable, and easy to apply.

Disadvantages. Resistance, particularly in *Pseudomonas,* is rapid to develop and has significantly minimized their use.

EARLY SURGICAL AND MEDICAL INTERVENTION

For many years, physicians treated the burn wound with topical agents and awaited the natural separation of the eschar that occurs two to four weeks after the injury. Because the nonviable eschar serves as a pabulum for bacterial growth and permits bacterial growth underneath it, the equivalent of an abscess results. Recently, aggressive removal of the eschar has been advocated.

Topical enzyme application allows rapid, nonsurgical dissolution of the eschar. Travase is the most widely used of these preparations.[7] A thin layer of the ointment is applied directly to the eschar and covered with a moist saline dressing or an antibac-

terial dressing that does not interfere with the action of the enzymes. Iodine will inactivate Travase and therefore must be thoroughly removed if used. These dressings are changed every six to eight hours. Deep second- or third-degree wounds are débrided in less than 24 hours by this technique. Early grafting is then performed, particularly on the hands.

Other enzyme preparations have been used on burns, but their specificity to collagen or nucleic acids has been a limiting factor.

Early surgical excision of the burn wound is optimal in certain specific indications.[8] Early excision to fascia with immediate grafting is the procedure of choice for small (less than 10% total body surface), deep, localized third-degree burns. The immediate or rapid removal of the burn-injured tissue lessens the metabolic stress to the burn victim, minimizes hospital stay, minimizes pain, and results in an excellent cosmetic result for a burn of this depth. Excision may be carried out using the cold scalpel, electrocautery unit, electrically heated scalpel, or laser. All of these techniques have their own advocates but clear-cut superiority of any specific excision technique has not been demonstrated. Utilization of early excision requires the availability of an operating room and team seven days a week and suitable donor sites to allow immediate coverage of the burn wound. Application of allograft, xenograft, or synthetic dressings have been advocated, but these diminish the advantages of early excision.

Tangential excision of the burn wound as originally described by Jackson and coworkers[9] and by Janzekovic[10] is a technique whereby multiple thin shavings of the burn wound are performed using a hand-held or power-driven dermatome. The wound is sequentially excised of nonviable tissue until a healthy, bleeding, viable base is obtained. Hemostasis is then obtained with a topical thrombin and epinephrine solution or with hot saline compresses, and split-thickness skin grafts are applied to the excised area. This technique is most applicable to areas of deep second- or mixed second- and third-degree injury.

Early excision of massive burn injuries combined with coverage of the excised wound with an allograft or a xenograft, or more recently with cultured skin has been reported in a very limited number of cases. These techniques are still experimental and limited to those centers that have the support and research facilities to carry them out.

TEMPORARY AND NONAUTOLOGOUS SKIN REPLACEMENT

Removal of nonviable skin is technically relatively easy and could rapidly be performed on any burn patient. Replacement of excised skin on both a temporary and particularly a permanent basis has occupied the attention of surgeons and researchers for over 1000 years. Temporary coverage of second-degree burns or excised burn wounds includes allografting, xenografting, semisynthetic, and synthetic dressings.

Allograft or human donor skin is generally obtained from cadavers but may, in some instances, be obtained from living donors. These grafts may be obtained fresh or may be procured from skin banks throughout the country. Unmatched allografts may be used to provide a temporary protective cover to superficial or moderate second-degree burns during their re-epithelialization or to provide a temporary biologic dressing to excised burn wounds prior to coverage with an autograft. Tissue typed and matched allografts have also been experimentally used as a permanent graft in patients with massive burns, but this is not yet in widespread clinical use.

Xenografts or cross-species grafts are used only on a temporary basis. Porcine xenografts are commercially available in fresh, frozen, irradiated, and lyophilized forms. Xenografts from other species have been used in the past, but are rarely used today. Silver-impregnated xenografts are available and have been reported to aid in preventing burn wound infection.

The technique for xenografts and allografts is the same. Frozen grafts need to be thawed or lyophilized grafts rehydrated. The grafts are then applied, dermal side down to the second-degree or excised burn wound and held in place with Steri-Strips or dressings. Topical antimicrobial therapy may be applied over these grafts. Xenografts or nonmatched allografts must not be allowed to "take" and are changed every three days.

Synthetic temporary skin coverings have the advantage of room temperature shelf storage, prolonged shelf life, uniformity of composition, and potentially unlimited availability. These dressings include both experimental and commercially available products. Polyurethane film dressings decrease pain and increase the rate of healing of second-degree burns and skin-graft donor sites. A semisynthetic dressing incorporating collagen and a synthetic backing has been reported on favorably by Frank and others.

BURN WOUND SEPSIS

Burn wound sepsis is a surgical, infectious emergency that may result in serious morbidity or mortality if not treated early and aggressively. Burn wound sepsis is a systemic disease of local origin. Massive local infection of the burn wounds may result in disseminated sepsis with resultant hypotension, hypo- or hyperpyrexia (depending upon the offending organism), hyperglycemia, thrombocytopenia, leukocytosis or severe leukopenia, and metastatic abscess formation. Burn wound sepsis is usually heralded by degeneration of the burn wound, and it is for this reason that daily evaluation of the burn wound is vital in the optimal care of the burn victim. A malodorous wound with a moth-eaten appearance and with surrounding erythema and edema either has or will develop burn wound sepsis. While "classic burn wound sepsis" was first described with *Pseudomonas aeruginosa*, essentially any microorganism may cause this complication. This includes gram-positive organisms such as a *Staphylococcus* or *Streptococcus*; gram-negative *Enterobacteriaceae* and *Pseudomonas*; fungi including *Aspergillus, Mucor,* and *Candida*; and viruses including the herpes and varicella-zoster group.

The treatment of burn wound sepsis requires a multifaceted therapeutic program. Systemic support of the burn victim may include intravenous fluid and antibiotics as well as massive doses of steroids and/or cardiotonic or vasoactive drugs. Simultaneous local care of the burn wound is a sine qua non. The microvascular circulation of the burn wound is absent or significantly impaired and cannot be depended upon to deliver therapeutic antibiotics to the burn wound. Topical antimicrobial therapy should generally be switched to mafenide (Sulfamylon) since this is the most effective, penetrating agent. Subeschar infusion of antibiotics consisting of an aminoglycoside combined with a semisynthetic penicillin also delivers antibiotic directly to the infection site. The dosage for these antibiotics should be equal to that recommended for a single dose of antibiotic therapy dissolved in 250 to 500 ml of saline or Ringer's solution. The antibiotic solution is then infused beneath the eschar for a clysis. Surgical excision of the burn wound or, in severe cases, amputation of the limb may be necessary.

REFERENCES

1. Lund CC, Browder NC: The estimation of the areas of burns. Surg Gynec Obst 79:352, 1944
2. Order SE, Moncrief JA: The Burn Wound. Springfield, Ill, Charles C Thomas, 1965
3. MacMillan BG: Local care and infection in burns. J Trauma 5:292, 1965
4. Moncrief JA, Lindberg RB, Switzer WE, Pruitt BA Jr: Use of topical antibacterial therapy in the treatment of the burn wound. Arch Surg 92:558, 1966
5. Monafo WW, Moyer CA: Effectiveness of dilute aqueous silver nitrate in the treatment of major burns. Arch Surg 91:200, 1965
6. Fox CL Jr: Silver sulfadiazine—a new topical therapy for *pseudomonas* in burns. Arch Surg 96:184, 1968
7. Dimick AR: Experience with the use of proteolytic enzyme (Travase) in burn patients. J Trauma 17:948, 1977
8. Burke JF: Primary burn excision and immediate grafting: A method for shortening illness. J Trauma 14:389, 1974
9. Jackson D, Topley E, Cason JS, et al: Primary excision and grafting of large burns. Ann Surg 152:167, 1960
10. Janzekovic Z: A new concept in the early excision and immediate grafting of large burns. J Trauma 10:1103, 1970

51

Local Surgical Treatment of Axillary Hyperhidrosis

It was over 20 years ago that the local surgical treatment of axillary hyperhidrosis was introduced independently by Skoog and Thyresson[1] and by Hurley and Shelley.[2, 3] Since that time, the local surgical approach has been used all over the world, and its efficacy is clearly established. Indeed it has replaced thoracic sympathectomy as the preferred surgical management of this disorder.

The purposes of this report are to consider the essential features of axillary hyperhidrosis (clinical and pathogenetic) and to describe the technique and results of the Hurley-Shelley operation for the amelioration of excessive axillary sweating. A preliminary section also deals with the history of axillary hyperhidrosis surgery and the variety of operative techniques that have been developed for this problem over the past two decades.

There has been an apparent reduction in the demand for surgical treatment of axillary hyperhidrosis[4, 5] because of the availability of effective topical treatment employing aluminum chloride hexahydrate in anhydrous ethanol (Drysol) applied at bedtime under occlusion.[6] A preliminary trial with this topical treatment should be prescribed for all patients with axillary hyperhidrosis before surgery is recommended. Moreover, as described later, this topical treatment can be used to augment the reduction in sweating achieved by local axillary surgery. Other forms of medical or dermatologic therapy are relatively ineffective or impractical in treating axillary hyperhidrosis. Oral anticholinergic drugs are generally inadequate and may produce unpleasant side effects. Calcium channel blockers, such as diltiazem, may reduce emotional eccrine sweating to a limited degree, but the sustained use of such medication is undesirable.[7] Topical scopolamine esters, which inhibit axillary sweating dramatically in normhidrotic individuals,[8] have not been studied in patients with axillary hyperhidrosis and may not be similarly suppressive. A more recent approach using topical local anesthetics under occlusion[9] appears to be less effective than the aluminum chloride hexahydrate in ethanol method. Finally, tap water iontophoresis[10] and biofeedback or behavioral therapy[11] should be considered as treatment alternatives, although they are less likely to control the problem satisfactorily.

HISTORICAL SURVEY

It is surprising that the local surgical treatment of axillary hyperhidrosis had not been developed earlier. General surgeons had long observed that a dry axilla often followed a radical mastectomy in which extensive axillary dissection was performed to remove lymph nodes or breast tissue within the "axillary tail of Spence." It was not until 1962, however, that Skoog and Thyresson introduced a local operative treatment using carefully placed incisions and reflection of skin flaps followed by dissection of the sweat gland layer over the entire axilla.[1] The authors claimed marked reduction in axillary sweating after this procedure, and stressed that any small islands of residual sweating could be easily ablated by additional localized surgery, which was apparently necessary in several of their patients.

Months later, in 1963, Hurley and Shelley described a simple surgical technique for the management of axillary hyperhidrosis in which a large elliptical excision was made through the heart of the major axillary sweating locus, essentially in the center of the axilla.[2] This procedure derived from a serendipitous observation made several years earlier of diminished axillary sweating following the removal of a large biopsy specimen from the central axilla of a young man with hyperhidrosis. Subsequent extensive study of well over 1000 sweating patterns and the effects of various local surgical procedures led them to a rational explanation of this surgical suppression of axillary sweating and to the development of an effective surgical technique based on these observations. It was determined that patterns of axillary sweating, as demonstrated colorimetrically, were constant and reproducible in a given axilla with the proper stimulus. Moreover, the ablative surgery could be selectively designed or tailored to the loci of increased sweating rather than carried out over the entire axilla. Thus evolved the present Hurley-Shelley surgical technique, the extent and topographic localization of which reflects the sweating pattern in each axilla.

A host of confirmatory reports of the efficacy of local surgical treatment of axillary hyperhidrosis have appeared over the past 20 years, using the Hurley-Shelley technique or modifications.[12-25]

Other novel local procedures employing cryosurgery,[26] subcutaneous tissue shavers,[27, 28] or curettage removal of axillary sweat glands through a small incision[29] have also been introduced. The last-mentioned method has been found by some to be inadequate,[30] and confirmation of the efficacy of the other techniques is not yet available. More radical surgery involving more or less complete excision of the entire axilla has also been advocated. Along those lines, Bretteville-Jensen recommended total excision of the axillary sweating area, without preliminary mapping of this sweating pattern, followed by Z-plasty closure.[31] Among the more recently confirmed techniques is that of Eldh and Fogdestam[23] in which a bat-shaped excision of the mapped-out hyperhidrotic area is removed and closed primarily without undermining.

In conclusion, it is apparent that in general two fundamental local surgical approaches have been employed for axillary hyperhidrosis (Table 51–1). One, as exemplified by the Skoog-Thyresson method, is intended to remove or inactivate all the sweat glands of a given axilla, without any preliminary identification of the sweating loci. The other approach, fostered by Hurley and Shelley and typified by the operation they devised, is based on preliminary mapping out of the sweating loci in each axilla and tailoring the local surgery to fit the sweating patterns. Both approaches, and most if not all of the modifications described for each, have been found to be generally successful and acceptable. The more extensive procedures are designed primarily for the plastic surgeon and carry higher morbidity, while the simpler techniques have been performed by dermatologists. The author's experience indicates that the majority of patients with axillary hyperhidrosis can be managed satisfactorily with the Hurley-Shelley operation, or variations thereof. Patients with very severe axillary hyperhidrosis, i.e., those with gravimetrically determined levels of 1200 mg or more of sweat produced during five minutes or

TABLE 51–1. Surgical Treatment of Axillary Hyperhidrosis[1–3, 12–35]

I. Local (Axillary) Surgery
  A. Total glandular removal—no preliminary sweating patterns
    1. Skoog-Thyresson technique[1]
    2. Bretteville-Jensen (Z-plasty)[31]
    3. Total excision of axilla
    4. Subcutaneous tissue shavers[27, 28]
    5. Curettage removal through skin incisions[29]
    6. Cryosurgical ablation[26]
  B. Selective glandular removal—preliminary sweating patterns
    1. Hurley-Shelley procedure[3]
    2. Eldh-Fogdestam (M or W excision)[23]
    3. Others
II. Sympathectomy
  A. "Extended" thoracic type (second to fifth ganglia)[32–35]

with heavy sweating patterns over the entire axilla would certainly be candidates for the Skoog-Thyresson or Bretteville-Jensen procedures.

A word about thoracic sympathectomy and axillary hyperhidrosis: At one time, sympathectomy was the only surgical treatment for this problem,[32, 33] but it is more formidable than local surgical ablative techniques associated with more serious complications and is not as regularly effective, even when an "extended" sympathectomy involving removal of the fourth and fifth thoracic ganglia is employed. Upper, as opposed to extended, sympathectomy in which only the second and third thoracic ganglia are removed, is not helpful in axillary hyperhidrosis but results in control of palmar hyperhidrosis. Thus, the extended type of thoracic sympathectomy was previously recommended for patients with both axillary and palmar hyperhidrosis. However, a truncal compensatory hyperhidrosis (thermal or gustatory) is more likely with the extended thoracic sympathectomy than with upper sympathectomy.[34] Accordingly, the current recommendation for the operative management of patients with coincident palmar and axillary hyperhidrosis is to combine an upper thoracic sympathectomy with a local ablative axillary surgical operation.[35]

CLINICAL FEATURES OF AXILLARY HYPERHIDROSIS

Axillary hyperhidrosis of such severity as to prompt medical consultation is an uncommon, but not rare, disorder. Its exact incidence has never been established, but it is clear that many individuals tolerate the condition without seeking professional help. In a survey of dry cleaning establishments, Hurley and Shelley found that at least 25% of the garments submitted for cleaning had large stains in the underarm areas of the apparel providing some indication of the frequency of the problem.[36] It affects both males and females, and there is no known racial variation. Our series of patients included whites and blacks, but the condition is seen in Orientals also. The onset of axillary hyperhidrosis is usually two to three years after puberty. It should be noted that eccrine sweating of the axillary area does not begin until at or near puberty,[37] unlike excessive sweating elsewhere which is seen after birth. Thus prepubertal children do not develop axillary hyperhidrosis, although volar hyperhidrosis is not uncommon in this age group. Unless treated, axillary hyperhidrosis persists indefinitely, well into late adult life. It is likely that some reduction in the axillary eccrine sweating of these individuals occurs with advancing years, but this has never been documented.

The axillary secretion produced by these patients appears watery or eccrinoid, like the eccrine sweat of other regions. In individuals with large and active axillary apocrine glands, however, it may be slightly turbid or cloudy because of contamination by milky apocrine sweat.

The excessive axillary sweating is usually intermittent, in response to emotional or mental stimulation, although an occasional individual seems to have abnormally copious axillary sweating almost constantly. However, careful examination of the sweating response after intense emotional stimulation reveals increases in activity over the "resting" level. Characteristically, the sweating diminishes or ceases altogether with sleep.

Patients with axillary hyperhidrosis do not usually have psychologic or neurotic problems that are pathogenetically related to their excessive sweating. The hypersecretion reflects increased sudomotor stimuli from the cortex, but this is not related to emotional abnormalities of significance, and psychiatric therapy with this in mind is not indicated.

It is interesting that significant seasonal variation in the axillary sweating of these patients is not observed, which emphasizes the importance of emotional, and not thermal, activation of these eccrine glands. Moreover, most patients, especially women, actually prefer summer months despite the high ambient temperatures because they can wear lightweight sleeveless apparel. Apparently, evaporative loss of the excessive axillary secretion takes place more readily under those conditions than in the colder months when heavier, more restrictive clothing is worn.

The severity of axillary hyperhidrosis varies considerably. Males tend to pour out greater quantities of axillary sweat than do females, although females seem to be affected more frequently or at least more often seek professional help for this complaint. In addition, the axillary eccrine glands of women seem to be more easily activated by emotional stimuli, producing more frequent "peaking" of their axillary eccrine responses. Both men and women with the clinical problem, however, are compromised by this condition both socially and at work, and it is not to be regarded simply as a cosmetic problem. They are unable to wear light-colored suits or dresses because of staining by the running axillary secretion (Fig. 51–1). Some appreciation of the magnitude of the axillary sweating in these patients comes with the realization that many women with the condition are insecure even while wearing two or more dress shields or pads in the axillae. A salesman whom the author later treated surgically would saturate a pack of cigarettes kept in his shirt pocket within an hour on an average working day.

About 75% of these patients have a family history of axillary hyperhidrosis, usually within the immediate family, suggesting a genetic factor in its pathogenesis.[3] If so, it appears that a dominant form of transmission, autosomal in type, is operative. A

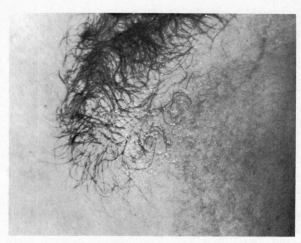

Figure 51–1. Axillary hyperhidrosis: Sweat droplets running down the lateral chest wall from the axilla of a 17-year-old student.

history of familial occurrence is noted also in volar hyperhidrosis and in some forms of gustatory hyperhidrosis.[38]

The majority of patients with axillary hyperhidrosis have concomitant volar (palmar and plantar) hyperhidrosis.[3] This association is not regularly observed, and some of the most severely affected hyperhidrotics have no excessive volar sweating. Moreover, even in those with concurrent axillary and volar hyperhidrosis, the axillary problem is often the one for which treatment is sought. Although the right axilla usually exceeds the left in sweat output, as discussed later under sweating patterns and gravimetric studies, many patients do not notice a substantial clinical difference between the two sides.

The coexistence of axillary hyperhidrosis and bromhidrosis is not to be anticipated.[3] Very few of the author's patients had concomitant axillary bromhidrosis or difficulty in easily eliminating odor with commercially available deodorants. Even in blacks, who have the largest and most productive apocrine glands, the abundant axillary eccrine sweat apparently washes away the apocrine sweat or its bacterially developed odoriferous product, thereby reducing axillary odor. Moreover, clinical examination of the axillae and study of the sweating patterns (described later) are consonant with this finding. Patients with bromhidrosis (who may at times claim hyperhidrosis or wetness also) have less visible watery sweat in their axillae or in the underarm sections of their clothing and have a different and quite distinctive sweating pattern, usually of the follicularly oriented, "large droplet" type characteristic of apocrine, not eccrine, sweating. Gravimetric study of these patients also reveals minimal axillary sweat output, customarily less than 50 mg per five minutes of sweating.

Topical aluminum, zirconium, zinc, or other antiperspirant deodorant preparations as well as oral anticholinergic drugs cannot achieve significant reduction in axillary sweating in these patients. They have usually tried most if not all of the commercially available antiperspirants without success. The only possible exception is the topical aluminum chloride hexahydrate in anhydrous ethanol preparation applied at bedtime that was discussed earlier and is described more fully later. Even when oral anticholinergic medications are administered in dosages that produce intolerable side effects, a diminution of sweating of practical value is rarely achieved.

Sweat Glands and Sweating Patterns in Axillary Hyperhidrosis

The eccrine and apocrine sweat glands of patients with axillary hyperhidrosis are indistinguishable (grossly and microscopically) from those of normal individuals.[3] Staining for Schiff-reactive materials, glycogen, lipids, and metachromasia and visualization under fluorescent microscopy and, more recently, electron microscopy have revealed no abnormalities.[39] In addition, there appears to be no variation in the innervation of these glands. The amount and localization of acetylcholinesterase is identical to that of individuals with normally responsive axillary sweat glands. Finally, in three patients so studied, serum cholinesterase levels were in the normal range.

A study of over 1000 axillary sweating patterns of patients with hyperhidrosis and of other individuals (male and female, blacks and whites) provides a rationale for the surgical procedure proposed, as discussed earlier. These sweating patterns were outlined with the Minor technique using iodine and starch, which provides a topographic semiquantitative determination of the sweating responses colorimetrically. In this method, a 3% iodine, 3% potassium iodide solution in 95% ethyl alcohol is painted on the shaved axillae and allowed to dry. Corn starch powder is then dusted over the painted areas. As the sweat droplets appear at the ductal orifices, they solubilize the iodine and react with the corn starch, producing a blue-black color at each pore. In areas of active sweating, the droplets become confluent producing solid blue-black areas (Fig. 51–2). Puddle-like accumulations appear at the sites of the highest rates of sweating.

Examination of these axillary sweating patterns in normal and hyperhidrotic patients revealed that the eccrine sweating across an axilla is not diffuse and even, as suspected originally, and it is not always most active in the center or dome of the axilla. Rather, there are usually one or two, or occasionally three, loci or zones of high sweat delivery. They vary in size and shape and in location within a given axilla. Moreover, despite some quantitative variations, reflecting differences in the intensity of stimulation, these patterns are remarkably constant and reproducible minutes, hours, or weeks later. Thus, a recorded pattern can be matched to a given axilla with subsequent stimulation of emotional sweating. These findings support the concept that a local surgical procedure that achieves removal of most or all of the sweat glands within the loci of active sweating in the axilla can significantly reduce the total axillary eccrine response. In addition, with surgical reduction of sweating in the high-delivery loci, there is no compensatory activation of eccrine glands in the rest of the axilla.

In many normal individuals, as well as some hyperhidrotics, a single major zone of sweating is seen after emotional, including mental or sensory, stimulation. Mental arithmetic, quizzing on history, geography, or current events, for example, or discussion of another medical problem about which the patient is concerned is usually an effective stimulus in these individuals. The single major locus seen is roughly circular with a diameter in the range of 3.5 to 5.0 cm and is commonly found at the apex of the axilla, i.e., the summit of the closed axillary vault. In a smaller group of patients, the major locus of sweating is at one end of the axilla, usually the inferior or thoracic pole. In others, one or two additional minor loci of sweating are seen in the center, at the thoracic or brachial (superior) pole or at both poles of the axilla. Less frequently, two nearly equal zones of sweat production may be identified, and finally, a pattern of almost equal sweating over the entire axilla is observed exceptionally. Even in these individuals, however, one or two loci showing the highest sweating rates can be detected within the diffuse sweating pattern. Pooling of the sweat on the blue-black background of the starch-iodine pattern delineates these more active loci.

The sweating patterns of the opposing axillae of a given individual are different topographically and unequal quantitatively.[3, 10] The right axilla usually exceeds the left in sweat production. This variation bears no relationship to right- or left-handedness or to any asymmetry in volar sweating. Although the difference in sweating between opposing axillae is often small, it may infrequently be extreme and dramatic. One of the blacks examined showed a single large zone of hyperhidrosis in the right axilla, but was virtually anhidrotic in the left.

It should be stressed that the primary stimulus that provokes the profuse secretion of axillary hyperhidrosis is emotional, mental, or less often, sensory in origin. Thermally induced axillary sweating produces somewhat different patterns, differing principally in that marginal, i.e., thoracic or brachial sweat glands outside the hairy axilla, are activated. Others have emphasized the difference between

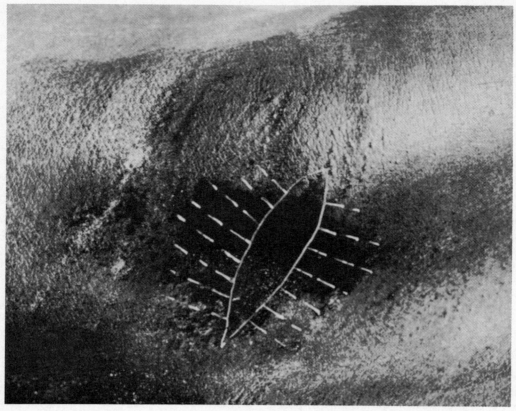

Figure 51–2. Sweating pattern in axillary hyperhidrosis. A starch-iodine colorimetric technique was used to identify confluent and isolated sweat droplets (black area). Note the single large focus of sweating in the center of this axilla. Placement of excisional ellipse is indicated by solid white line. Broken lines radiating out from this excisional site represent the zone of undercutting and subdermal glandular resection. (Reproduced with permission from H. J. Hurley and W. B. Shelley, Axillary hyperidrosis, clinical features and local surgical management. British Journal of Dermatology 78:127, 1966.)

emotional and thermogenic axillary sweating, and a classification of three major types of thermogenic axillary sweating patterns has been formulated.[40]

A point of special interest that deserves emphasis is the fact that the localization of the zone or zones of emotional eccrine sweating cannot be correlated with the density of apocrine sweat glands.[3, 40] The central or apical zone of the hairy axilla, which is palpably thicker than the rest of the axilla, can be seen grossly and histologically to contain the largest and highest concentration of apocrine glands in all patients. In many patients, however, the most active zones of sweating are at one of the poles of the axillae where fewer and smaller apocrine glands are found. Numerous actively functioning eccrine glands are found in the skin of these sweating loci, supporting the conclusion that it is the eccrine, not the apocrine, glands that are responsible for this disorder. The eccrine origin of the secretion is suggested also by its clear watery appearance, the relatively large quantities of the sweat, and the lack of any significant racial variation in the incidence of axillary hyperhidrosis. Apocrine sweat is characteristically turbid and produced in very small quantities incom-

patible with the profuse secretion of axillary hyperhidrosis. In addition, the established superiority, in numbers and functional activity, of the black person's apocrine apparatus is not reflected in any increased frequency of axillary hyperhidrosis in this racial group.

A most significant anatomic relationship exists between the axillary eccrine and apocrine glands. The smaller eccrine glands are closely attached to or wedged in between the more deeply placed and grossly visible apocrine lobules and are separated from them by faint connective tissue septae. Thus, removal of the grossly visible lobules, i.e., the apocrine glands, results in removal of part or all of the adjacent eccrine glands as well.

LOCAL SURGICAL TREATMENT OF AXILLARY HYPERHIDROSIS

The author's initial attempt at surgical management of axillary hyperhidrosis involved the excision of a large ellipse of skin (5 to 6 cm by 1.5 cm) through the center of the major sweating locus of the axilla.[2] This procedure proved effective for some patients, but certain modifications producing greater reduction in sweating were required for more severely affected patients whose sweating patterns were broader and more variable.[3] Both the original and modified procedures were based on the same fundamental principles, viz., identification of the major loci of sweating and surgical ablation of the sweat glands in these zones. In the later technique, a broader zone of anhidrosis was accomplished through excision of an elliptical wedge of skin from the primary or major sweating locus plus one or two additional fusiform excisions from the secondary loci in each axilla and subsequent resection of sweat glands on each side of each excision site.

Preoperative examination of the patient should include studies for bleeding tendencies as well as gravimetric measurement of the axillary sweating response and the axillary sweating patterns.[3] The patterns for each axilla are prepared at least twice on each patient. At the initial examination, the patterns are drawn or photographed, and then an estimate of the feasibility of the operation is possible. Obviously, the best operative result is achievable if there is only one locus of sweating or if the additional loci are small and sharply restricted. A second sweating pattern is prepared in the operating room just prior to the operation at a time when the patient's anxiety over the forthcoming surgery should provoke a maximal eccrine response. If significant sweating is not seen, mental stimulation (arithmetic or quizzing) or the production of pain by insertion of an 18-gauge needle into the palm will usually elicit a satisfactory bout of sweating. The loci of sweating are then demarcated using a sterile dye.

Preoperative preparation of the patient includes careful shaving of the axillary hair plus at least two careful washings of the axillae six to 12 hours apart with a germicidal soap or detergent. The usual preoperative administration of sedatives and anticholinergics is to be avoided since these drugs markedly alter the axillary sweating patterns necessary to define the precise sites of the surgery. Local anesthesia, with 1% to 2% lidocaine (Xylocaine) or mepivacaine (Carbocaine) without epinephrine is usually employed in this procedure. The infiltration of the anesthetic is made along the projected lines of each excision and should be superficially placed into or just below the dermis. This seems to facilitate dissection of the sweat glands. If general anesthesia or sedation-analgesia is desired, it may be administered after the sweating patterns have been established. The patient is operated on in the supine position, with the arms extended laterally or with the hand under the head in order to expose the axillary vault. Care should be taken to avoid brachial plexus injury, especially when general anesthesia is used.

The initial excisional ellipse is made through the heart of the major or primary sweating locus (Fig. 51–3A and B). It should measure 5 to 6 cm in length and approximately 1.5 cm in width at the midpoint of the ellipse. This and all subsequent excisions are made transversely across the axilla and parallel with the normal axillary lines, not in the longitudinal axis of the axilla. Excision along the long axis tends to produce contractural scarring and restriction of mobility of the limbs. In an occasional patient, because of the shape and localization of the major or primary sweating focus, it may be judicious to make an obliquely oriented excision to accomplish more complete removal of the sweat glands while sacrificing less axillary skin. The excisions should be taken down through the subcutaneous tela. At this level, removal of the elliptical section of skin leaves a base of deep fascia. Undercutting is then carried out for a distance of 2.0 to 3.0 cm on each side of the wound, roughly to the demarcated limits of the sweating locus. Reflection over the fingertip of the created skin flaps allows for dissection and removal of the lobules of sweat glands of the dermal undersurface (Fig. 51–3C and D). This is best carried out using fine curved scissors. Care should be taken to leave many of the hair follicles intact and to avoid trimming the undersurface of the dermis too closely in order not to endanger the blood supply of these skin areas. Some of the more recently introduced local techniques ignore this point and even advise close stripping of the dermal undersurface with a safety razor.[27, 28] These authors emphasize that hair follicle removal, at least in females, is desirable so that axillary shaving can be reduced or eliminated. To be confident of flap viability, however, damage to hair follicles should be minimized. Any additional minor loci of sweating are similarly treated by an initial central elliptical excision measuring 2.5 to 3.5 cm by 0.4 to 0.8 cm followed by correspondingly smaller areas of lateral undercutting and subdermal glandular resection (Fig. 51–3E and F). It should be mentioned that when more than one excision is made, undercutting at the secondary areas should not overlap that of the primary foci. Some intervening skin should be left free of undercutting between these wounds in order to avoid jeopardizing the local blood supply.

The control of bleeding in each wound is essential to smooth complete healing. Before closure, each wound should be thoroughly inspected and all significant bleeders ligated. Drains are occasionally employed, when there is concern about hemorrhage. It has not been found necessary to place deep sutures for obliteration of dead space or to facilitate wound approximation. Proper postoperative dressings tend to close the dead space and favor hemostasis, minimizing the need for insertion of drains.

Vertical mattress sutures are preferred for skin closure, with skin hooks held at each end of the

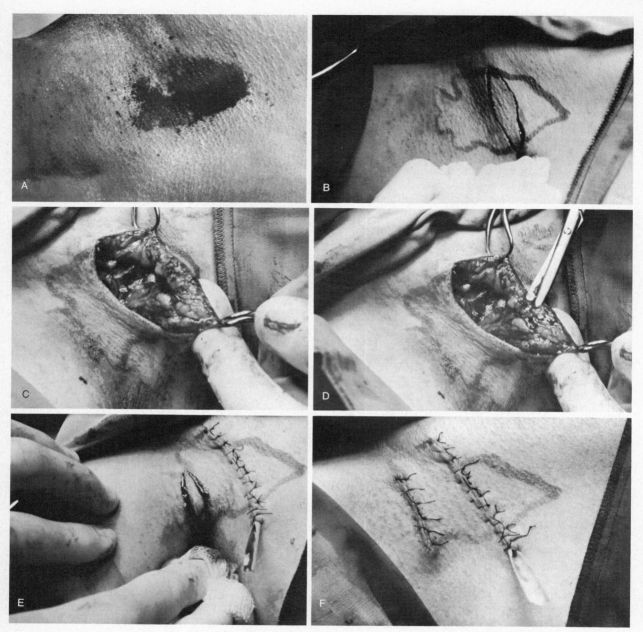

Figure 51–3. Local surgical ablation of axillary hyperhidrosis: *A,* Sweating pattern is delineated by a starch-iodine colorimetric technique. *B,* The loci of sweating are demarcated by a sterile dye, and the initial fusiform excision is made through the center of the major locus. *C,* Reflection of the undermined flap on one side of the wound. *D,* Resection of sweat glands from the dermal undersurface. *E,* After the major locus of sweating has been sutured with a drain in place, a fusiform excision is made through the secondary locus. *F,* Final operative status with both wounds closed.

wound to insure proper orientation of the wound edges. A heavy pressure dressing is applied postoperatively with a thick wad of gauze pads placed directly over the wound, and wide elastic tape, such as Elastoplast, is applied to produce pressure upward, i.e., toward the apex of the axilla. If tape is applied simply to the thorax and arm, there is insufficient pressure upward directly against the wounds, and the possibility of a hematoma is greatly

increased. Patients are instructed to keep their arms at the side postoperatively for the first 48 hours. If necessary, to assure no inadvertent raising of the arms during sleep, the arms are held at the sides with an eight-inch elastic bandage.

Half of the skin sutures are removed at one week, the remainder at 10 to 14 days, and the wound is usually left unbandaged after five to seven days. Although dressing and clerical work is allowable,

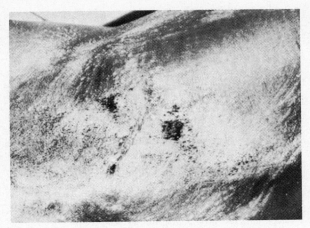

Figure 51—4. Axillary sweating pattern six weeks postoperatively. Compare with the preoperative sweating pattern of this axilla (Fig. 51—2). Single well-healed linear scar is seen in center of the axilla. (Reproduced with permission from H. J. Hurley and W. B. Shelley, Axillary hyperidrosis. Clinical features and local surgical management. British Journal of Dermatology 78:127, 1966.)

other activities involving appreciable lateral or upward extension of the arms are to be avoided until about three weeks postoperatively, when a graduated program of work and exercise may be instituted.

The scars produced by these procedures are generally soft and pliable or become so within three to six months. No undesirable sequelae, such as reduced mobility of the arms or compensatory hyperhidrosis in any skin region, have been observed following this surgery.

Axillary deodorants may be used as soon as the wounds are completely healed. Interestingly, these patients generally develop increased axillary odor postoperatively since the resultant marked reduction of axillary eccrine sweating allows accumulation of odorogenic apocrine sweat that had been regularly washed away preoperatively.

The range of reduction in axillary sweating produced by this surgical procedure varies from 60% to 90% of the original preoperative levels. In the author's series of over 130 patients, dramatically decreased sweating, very acceptable subjectively, has been achieved in 90% of the patients operated on with this technique. The reduction in axillary sweating can be readily appreciated in the postoperative sweating patterns (Fig. 51—4) and in gravimetric changes in the amount of sweat produced. An occasional patient may request a second operation for further reduction of the sweating. Sweating patterns on these individuals reveal the residual active sweating sites, and they can be easily ablated using the same basic surgery on a smaller scale.

It is to be emphasized that once a surgical reduction in axillary sweating has been achieved, topical aluminum or zirconium antiperspirant formulations can be employed to further reduce the sweating if desired. The most effective topical antiperspirant method involves the application at bedtime of 20% aluminum chloride hexahydrate in anhydrous ethanol (Drysol) under occlusion.[4] If this proves irritating, a weaker formulation containing 6.25% aluminum chloride hexahydrate in anhydrous ethanol (Xerac A.C.) may be tried. In addition, occlusion with polyvinylidine (saran) or polyethylene can be eliminated in some patients. After leaving the applied preparation on through the sleeping hours, it may be washed off on arising. This treatment can be used every night before retiring or less often, perhaps two to three times per week, as required. Control of axillary odor is also accomplished with both concentrations of the aluminum formulations.

It should be noted that the initial postoperative levels of sweating may not represent the ultimate axillary emotional response after healing is complete. Experience indicates that the result of the operation can be properly assessed gravimetrically and by sweating patterns after about six to eight weeks when postoperative edema and inflammation are fairly well resolved. Follow-up examination of patients through many months following the operation indicates that these results are permanent with no further detectable increase or decrease in sweating.

Postoperative complications of this surgery are uncommon and, to date, have been quite simple. They include only an occasional small hematoma, which may be easily evacuated, and infrequently a retrograde lymphangitis of a major brachial lymphatic vessel. This change may be identified as a cord-like thickening along the medial aspect of the arm extending downward from the axilla. It is usually mistaken for a "tendon" or "vein" by the patient and resolves without treatment within three weeks, leaving no residual change. Wound infection, which could eventuate in hidradenitis or chronically infected sinus tracts, is always a risk, but it has not been encountered so far.

It is important to realize that promising a "dry" axilla to patients undergoing this procedure is inappropriate. Complete dryness, or the absence of axillary eccrine sweat, is probably undesirable because of the possible irritation that might ensue from the friction of opposing dry axillary folds in movement of the arms. The objective is reduction of sweating to levels that are tolerable and comparable to most individuals. This would be in the range of 25 to 100 mg of sweat measured gravimetrically, although some variation due to personal psychologic needs is to be expected.

SUMMARY

Axillary hyperhidrosis is a genetically controlled hyperactivity of the eccrine sweat glands of the axillae in response to emotional stimulation. It is seen in all racial groups and in both sexes. Concomitant volar hyperhidrosis is usually, but not always, noted. Bromhidrosis does not coexist with axillary hyperhidrosis. In fact, patients with axillary hyperhidrosis usually have diminished axillary odor, possibly because the odoriferous apocrine sweat is washed away by the excessive eccrine secretion. Oral anticholinergics, sedatives, or commercially available topical antiperspirants cannot satisfactorily reduce axillary hyperhidrosis.

Surgical treatment of axillary hyperhidrosis is possible through a local operation involving elliptical excision of a wedge of axillary skin through the center of the major sweating locus and additional elliptical excisions through any secondary loci of sweating in the given axillae. Undercutting and subdermal resection of additional sweat glands on each side of each elliptical wound further reduces the axillary sweating. No significant complications have been observed after this procedure in these patients, and no compensatory emotional or thermal hyperhidrosis was observed either in the axillae or on the rest of the skin surface.

REFERENCES

1. Skoog T, Thyresson N: Hyperhidrosis of the axillae. A method of surgical treatment. Acta Chir Scand 124:531–538, 1962
2. Hurley HJ, Shelley WB: A simple surgical approach to the management of axillary hyperhidrosis. JAMA 186:109, 1963
3. Hurley HJ, Shelley WB: Axillary hyperhidrosis. Clinical features and local surgical management. Br J Dermatol 78:127, 1966
4. Savin JA: Excessive sweating of the palms and armpits. Brit Med J 286:580, 1983
5. Ellis H, Scurr JH: Axillary hyperhidrosis—topical treatment with aluminum chloride hexahydrate. Postgrad Med 55:868, 1979
6. Shelley WB, Hurley HJ: Studies on topical antiperspirant control of axillary hyperhidrosis. Acta Derm Venereol (Stockholm) 55:241, 1975
7. James WD: Personal communication
8. MacMillan FSK, Reller HH, Snyder FH: The antiperspirant action of topically applied anticholinergics. J Invest Dermatol 43:363–377, 1964
9. Juhlin L, Rollman O: Vascular effects of a local anesthetic mixture in atopic dermatitis. Acta Derm Venereol (Stockholm) 64(5):439–40, 1984
10. Levit F: Simple device for treatment of hyperhidrosis by iontophoresis. Arch Dermatol 98:505, 1968
11. Duller P, Gentry WD: Use of biofeedback in treating chronic hyperhidrosis. Brit J Derm 103:143–146, 1980
12. Holzegel K: Die Hyperhidrosis axillaris und ihre operative Behandlung. Deutsche Gesundheitswesen 21:1231, 1966
13. Preaux MJ: Le traitement chirurgical de l'hyperhidrose axillaire. Bull Soc Fr Dermatol Syphiligr 74:730, 1967
14. Tipton JB: Axillary hyperhidrosis and its surgical treatment. Plast Reconstr Surg 42:137, 1968
15. Lochovský J, Rodovský J, Rybín B: Treatment of severe hyperhidrosis by surgical removal of perspiratory glands. Cesk Dermatol 45:58, 1970
16. Petterson LO, Strombeck JO: Kirugest Behandling av Axillarhyperhidros. Lakartidningen 67:5676, 1970
17. Gillespie JA, Kane SD: Evaluation of a simple surgical treatment of axillary hyperhidrosis. Br J Dermatol 83:684, 1970
18. Gonzalez Fontana R, Alonso Ballester J, Tormo Gomez JL: Aportación al tratamiento quirúrgico de la hiperehidrosis axilar. Actas Dermosifiliogr 61:99–106, 1970
19. Weaver PC, Copeman PWM: Simple surgery for axillary hyperhidrosis. Proc R Soc Med 64:607, 1971
20. Midholn AS, Taarnhoj P: Hyperhidrosis axillae. Ugeskr Laeger 134:1528, 1972
21. Keaveny TV, Fitzgerald PA, Donnelly C, et al: Surgical management of hyperhidrosis. Br J Surg 64:570, 1977
22. Roed-Petersen AK, Andersen BL: Hyperhidrosis axillaris. The life of 107 patients before and after operative treatment of axillary hyperhidrosis. Ugesker Laeger 139:2109, 1977
23. Eldh J, Fogdestam L: The surgical treatment of hyperhidrosis axillae. Scand J Plastic Reconstr Surg 10:227, 1976
24. Rigg BOM: Axillary hyperhidrosis. Plast Reconstr Surg 59:334, 1977
25. Stenguist B: Axillary hyperhidrosis: A simple surgical procedure. J Derm Surg Oncol 11:388, 1985
26. Ashby EC, Williams JL: Cryosurgery for axillary hyperhidrosis. Brit Med J 2(6045):1173, 1976
27. Inaba M, Anthony J, Ezaki T: Radical operation to stop axillary odor and hyperhidrosis. Plast Reconstr Surg 62:355, 1978
28. Landes VE, Kappesser HJ: Zur operativen Behandlung der Hyperhidrosis axillaris. Fortschr Med 97:2169, 1979
29. Jemec, B: Abrasio axillae in hyperhidrosis. Scand J Plast Reconstr Surg 9:44, 1975
30. Ellis H: Axillary hyperhidrosis: Failure of subcutaneous curettage. Br Med J 2(6082):301, 1977
31. Bretteville-Jensen, G, Mossing N, Albrechtsen R: Surgical treatment of axillary hyperhidrosis in 123 patients. Acta Derm Venereol (Stockholm) 55:73, 1975
32. MacGregor AL: Surgery of the Sympathetic. Bristol, John Wright, 1955
33. Kux M: Thoracic endoscopic sympathectomy in palmar and axillary hyperhidrosis. Arch Surg 113:264, 1978
34. Shelley WB, Florence R: Compensatory hyperhidrosis after sympathectomy. N Engl J Med 263:1056, 1960
35. Kenawi MM, El Mofty M, Wishahy AH: The Surgical Treatment of Associated Axillary and Palmar Hyperhidrosis. J Roy Coll Surg (Edinburgh) 28:116, 1983
36. Shelley WB, Hurley HJ: Unpublished observations, 1970
37. Kuno Y: The Physiology of Human Perspiration. London, JA Churchill Ltd, 1934
38. Hurley HJ: Diseases of the eccrine sweat glands, in Moschella S, Hurley HJ (eds): Dermatology, vol 2. Philadelphia, WB Saunders, 1985
39. Richardt L, Waris T, Rintala A: Innervation of human axillary sweat glands. Scand J Plast Surg 10:107, 1976
40. Rebell G, Kirk DY: Axillary sweating patterns, in Montagna W, Ellis RA, Silver AF (eds): Eccrine Sweat Glands and Eccrine Sweating. New York, Pergamon, 1962

52

RICHARD G. BENNETT, M.D., F.A.C.C.

Treatment of Hidradenitis Suppurativa

Hidradenitis suppurativa is an inflammatory process, usually recurrent, that ordinarily develops in the apocrine gland-bearing areas of the human body, principally the axilla, the breast (especially the areola), and the anogenital region. Both the etiology and pathogenesis of this affliction are understood only vaguely. Although not rare, misdiagnosis and lack of appreciation of hidradenitis suppurativa as a distinct diagnostic entity by physicians occurs frequently. This leads not only to a delay in adequate treatment but may also eventuate in needless disability or even death for the patient. This chapter analyzes what is known about hidradenitis suppurativa so that the physician may intelligently manage patients with this condition.

SYMPTOMS

The patient initially notices a mildly erythematous, tender, firm swelling (a nodule), which occurs in one of the previously mentioned apocrine gland-bearing areas. Although this may superficially resemble a furuncle, the nodule is more deeply situated. The swelling may resolve spontaneously but commonly progresses into a larger abscess-like swelling that may drain by itself (if a physician does not incise and drain it) and form a fistulous opening to the skin surface. This process of swelling and draining usually recurs several times *in the same location* and is one of the distinguishing features of hidradenitis suppurativa. Certainly, any physician should consider a recurrent "abscess" in an apocrine gland-bearing area to be hidradenitis suppurativa until proved otherwise. Although some authors[1-3] assume that infection is *initially* present and leads to the repeated episodes of abscess formation, this may not be correct and will be discussed more fully later.

The process of swelling and draining frequently becomes chronic, burrows more deeply, and spreads laterally to involve adjacent cutaneous areas. Hidradenitis suppurativa *may not be merely a superficial* process—a fact not generally appreciated. Larger apocrine glands may extend deeply into fat, as much as 5 mm below the skin surface.[4] Furthermore, the loose alveolar tissue, especially in the axilla and perineum, predisposes to the burrowing spread of this condition.

The lateral spread of hidradenitis suppurativa evolves as additional abscess-like swellings erupt and intercommunicate by way of epithelialized tracts. This results in the formation of irregular hypertrophic scars and contractures, which may be felt as fibrous bands underneath the skin surface. As this condition progresses relentlessly and becomes more extensive, frequently involving additional apocrine gland-bearing regions of the body, the patient experiences increasing pain and disability (e.g., being unable to raise the arms or to sit comfortably). The malodor (from subsequent infection) causes social embarrassment. At this point, patients may become withdrawn, socially isolating themselves, and are even hostile, especially if several physicians have performed multiple ineffective procedures. Fever and sepsis are not uncommon as the process becomes more extensive.

The differential diagnosis of hidradenitis suppurativa includes rarer entities such as tuberculosis, syphilis, lymphogranuloma venereum, and deep fungus infections. Fortunately, these are rather remote considerations today, but the reader may refer elsewhere for a more comprehensive list.[5, 6] Hidradenitis suppurativa may be easily confused with a pilonidal cyst in the postsacral region or anal fistulae in the rectal area. Anal fistulae are reported to be rare when hidradenitis suppurativa occurs perianally[7] but may occur.[6]

INCIDENCE

Hidradenitis suppurativa usually begins in the second or third decade of life.[7-10] In the axilla, more females than males are afflicted,[11-13] but in the perianal region and perineum, the reverse is reported.[7, 9, 10] Hidradenitis suppurativa most commonly involves the axilla,[14] but it is more severe and leads to more complications when occurring in the perianal region and perineum. However, such statistics are difficult to evaluate because all apocrine gland-bearing areas may eventually be affected. Furthermore, several authors are not precise in their anatomic categorizations. For instance, the term "perineal hidradenitis" is frequently used rather loosely. What is usually meant is that the patient has involvement of the scrotum, buttocks, proximedial thighs, and the inguinal and pubic regions.

An important study in 1926 by Homma investigated autopsy skin for the presence of apocrine glands.[15] He found that *in certain locations* blacks had an increased number of apocrine glands compared with whites, especially on the abdominal, circumanal, and pubic areas. In all these areas combined, three times as many slides examined from blacks indicated that they had more apocrine glands than whites. He did not study the axilla. This may be why hidradenitis suppurativa is more common in blacks, especially in the perianal area.[9, 10]

PATHOGENESIS

Although the cause of hidradenitis suppurativa is unknown, the predilection for the apocrine gland-bearing areas of the body is certain.[8, 9, 14] The astute clinician should keep in mind that this process may occur elsewhere as well, for instance on the leg,[16] back of the neck, abdomen, face, or scalp.[7]

It is generally accepted that initially the apocrine gland orifice becomes plugged, which leads to subsequent dilatation of the apocrine duct and inflammation of the gland itself. Since this sequence of events (termed apocrinitis) was produced experimentally in only three of 12 male subjects by Shelley and Kahn,[3] there appears to be great individual susceptibility. Furthermore, subsequent infection (the next phase of the process according to these authors) was neither substantiated nor produced.

Careful pathologic studies of the various stages of hidradenitis suppurativa have not been published. One study[7] of this condition found apocrine glands in only 11% of cases, although this is at variance with other authors.[8, 17] In a recent study by Morgan and Hughes,[18] the distribution, size, and density of the apocrine glands in cases of hidradenitis suppurativa was compared with control tissues from patients operated on for other reasons. These investigators noted no significant differences compared to the controls with respect to the distribution or density of the apocrine glands. However, the size of the glands appeared to be larger in patients with hidradenitis suppurativa.

Hidradenitis suppurativa is found in individuals who have a predilection for follicular occlusive conditions. Frequently, there is a family history for such problems. Severe acne is a commonly associated problem in 30% to 70% of patients.[7, 8, 19, 20] Brunsting emphasized the occurrence of hidradenitis suppurativa with acne conglobata and dissecting cellulitis of the neck and scalp.[12] Other reported associated follicular conditions include Fox-Fordyce disease,[21] pilonidal sinus formation,[7] pityriasis rubra pilaris,[22]

and steatocystoma multiplex.[23] Other nonfollicular-associated conditions include pseudoacanthosis nigricans,[24] hay fever and allergies,[11] and interstitial keratitis.[11, 25]

Although hygiene,[1] antiperspirants,[26] and other irritants are frequently mentioned as possible contributory factors to the development of hidradenitis suppurativa, there is little data supporting this belief. Endocrine gland function has also been implicated, because this condition is rare before puberty when the apocrine glands are poorly developed. Hidradenitis suppurativa has been reported to be worse with menstruation[7] but to improve with pregnancy[12] and systemic steroids.[27] The latter effect probably underscores the importance of the inflammatory nature of hidradenitis suppurativa. Although unsubstantiated, abnormal glucose tolerance tests have also been reported.[28]

COMPLICATIONS

Infections. Whether bacteria play an essential role in the development of hidradenitis suppurativa or are merely secondary, at some point true bacterial infection is present. If cultures are performed, one usually finds *Staphylococcus aureus,* beta-hemolytic streptococcus, or *Proteus mirabilis.*[1-3, 8] In acute hidradenitis suppurativa, which lacks sinus tracts, *Staphylococcus aureus* is usually cultured; whereas in chronic hidradenitis, gram-negative bacteria are usually found in addition.[1, 20] The latter organisms are especially prevalent in perianal and perineal hidradenitis suppurativa. Frequently, mixed cultures are obtained.[8, 29] Most patients with chronic hidradenitis suppurativa have been managed with a variety of antibiotics, both orally and topically. Therefore, some organisms found on cultures may have been selected by their resistance to various drugs.

The problem of infection in hidradenitis suppurativa is important, because fever and sepsis and even death can occur.[6, 7]

One study of host defense mechanisms did not find impaired ability to respond to infections in patients with hidradenitis suppurativa.[1] However, in those impaired immunologically, recurrent axillary abscesses are common.[30]

Probably the most overlooked aspect of infection in hidradenitis suppurativa is the importance of anaerobes. Infection with these organisms promotes the subcutaneous extension of this disease. Unfortunately, most cultures are not performed anaerobically and, even if they are, are done in such a way as to be contaminated with superficially growing organisms. Also, anaerobes grow slowly and require special growth media.[32] One important study by Leach and coworkers[33] in 1979 studied cultures on patients with subareolar breast abscesses. In 15 cultures from nonpuerperal patients, eight grew anaerobes. Several of these patients had had recurrent breast abscesses (probably hidradenitis suppurativa). Metronidazole was suggested as the antibiotic of choice. In another study by the same authors of axillary abscesses,[34] 23% of the patients studied had anaerobes on culture. Of those patients with recurrent axillary abscesses, 63% grew anaerobes. Brenner and Lookingbill studied five cases of hidradenitis suppurativa and demonstrated significant growth of anaerobes (especially *Bacteroides*) in every case.[31] They were successful in bringing this infection under control with the antibiotic clindamycin, and suggested that cefoxitin or metronidazole could be used alternatively. Careful culture studies have not been done in the perineal area, but because of the large number of anaerobes in the bowel, these organisms would surely be of importance.[35]

Anemia. Not infrequently, patients with extensive chronic hidradenitis suppurativa, especially of the perineal area, have a significant anemia (hemoglobin of less than 10 gm/dl).[6, 11, 36] Although this anemia has been interpreted as being caused by chronic infection, continuous extensive serosanguineous drainage also may be contributory.

Squamous Cell Carcinoma. Squamous cell carcinoma arising in chronic hidradenitis suppurativa has been reported repeatedly.[7, 14, 37–41] All cases described arose in the perineal, perianal, or genital regions. Jackman reported an incidence of 3.2% for squamous cell carcinoma among those with hidradenitis suppurativa in the perineum or groin.[14] The fact that some of these patients died with metastatic disease underscores the importance of early adequate treatment of hidradenitis suppurativa. In those who developed squamous cell carcinoma, hidradenitis suppurativa had been present for a long time, usually 20 to 30 years. Early recognition of this complication is important, and obtaining repeated biopsies should also be emphasized, especially if one is suspicious clinically.[41]

Amyloidosis. Amyloidosis has been reported in one patient with extensive perirectal perineal disease.[6] This patient also had hypoproteinemia.

MANAGEMENT

Although each patient represents an individual problem in management, the author's personal experience and most of the literature supports the conclusion that hidradenitis suppurativa should be handled early and with surgery. Indeed, the first adequate description of hidradenitis suppurativa by Verneuil in 1854 concluded that surgical intervention should be "hardie et radicale" (daring and radical).[42]

Antibiotics. The use of antibiotics for hidradenitis suppurativa should be based on *both aerobic and anaerobic* cultures with appropriate sensitivity testing, which should always be done before surgery.

However, the physician should realize that antibiotics are a *temporizing* form of therapy and *are not curative*. Topical antibiotics have little place as the definitive treatment of hidradenitis suppurativa because they may lead to the growth of resistant organisms. However, there is some evidence to suggest that antibacterial scrubs with povodine-iodine may have a role in certain selected instances. For example, patients with granulocytopenia who are on chemotherapy are prone to develop axillary abscesses.[30]

Incision and Drainage. Although several physicians advocate the incision of acute hidradenitis suppurativa,[8, 13, 43–45] this should be viewed only as a temporizing measure to alleviate pain. The problem with hidradenitis suppurativa, as previously emphasized, is that it tends to recur. Recurrences are due to persistent, inflamed, diseased tissue that serves as a nidus of infection. The secretory portion of the apocrine gland often lies deep in the subcutaneous fat. Therefore, although this appears to be a superficial process, there may be deep foci of inflammation and infection, which must be removed to ensure a cure.

Steroids. As emphasized previously, hidradenitis suppurativa is an inflammatory process. Therefore, steroids, either local[46] or systemic,[27] have been advocated. However, recurrences with this approach are frequent in the author's experience, and physicians who use such therapy are doing so at the patient's expense.

Isotretinoin. The use of systemic retinoids has been suggested for use in patients with hidradenitis suppurativa. Isotretinoin (Accutane), also known as 13-*cis*-retinoic acid, has been found to be useful in patients with cystic acne. Because some patients with a propensity for follicular occlusion have both acne and hidradenitis suppurativa, it would seem reasonable that a drug that works for acne would also be useful for hidradenitis suppurativa as well. Although isotretinoin's specific mechanism of action is unknown, it has been shown to provide some anti-inflammatory activity.[47]

In clinical studies that have been done, the effect of isotretinoin on hidradenitis suppurativa is not uniformly successful. Jones and coworkers treated three patients who had hidradenitis suppurativa with isotretinoin at 1 mg/kg/day for 16 weeks.[48] They noted no improvement in the lesions. Dicken and colleagues, on the other hand, noted improvement in five out of eight patients given a similar dosage.[49] Perhaps the differences in these two studies can be explained by the extent of the disease in the patients treated, which was not clearly stated in either study and is difficult to quantitate. It is reasonable to expect that patients with extensive, boggy, infected sinus tracts, who are managed with medical therapy, would probably do less well than those with only a few scattered lesions.

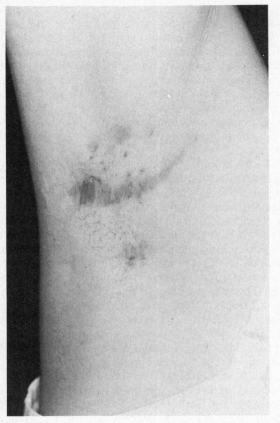

Figure 52–1. Axilla with healed surgical scar subsequent to wide transverse excision (Pollock Technique); note the residual fistulous openings.

Excision. If the area of involvement is small, excision and closure should be the primary therapy for hidradenitis suppurativa. It is helpful to have the lesion as quiescent as possible before excision in order not to contaminate the wound and extend the inflammatory, infective process. Therefore, the author uses preoperative antibiotics.

For axillary hidradenitis suppurativa, some authors[50] advocate a large en bloc excision of the axillary vault followed by a transverse primary closure (Pollock's procedure), whereas others favor a Z-plasty[2] or a modified Z-plasty.[51, 52] The problem with this approach in hidradenitis suppurativa is that as the disease process involves more and more tissue, primary excision and closure become less feasible. Surgeons will be forced to leave small foci of obvious disease to obtain direct closure (Fig. 52–1). When patients have extensive disease, high recurrence rates (up to 47%) have been reported with large areas of excision and simple closure.[7] However, in another series, a cure rate of 93% was reported on 28 patients, but the extent of the disease was not stated.[29]

Another approach mentioned by some authors is wide excision and subsequent healing by secondary intention.[9, 14, 53–55] This differs from exteriorization (mentioned later) in that the sinus tracts, characteristic of hidradenitis suppurativa, are not systemically explored and exposed. However, some surgeons[52, 53, 56] consider this to be the procedure of choice in certain locations, such as the groin.

Morgan and colleagues compared results on 10 patients operated on for bilateral hidradenitis suppurativa of the axilla.[55] In each patient, following excision, a skin graft was applied to one axilla, whereas the other was allowed to heal by granulation and epidermization. These authors noted better cosmetic results on the side allowed to heal by granulation and epidermization. In addition, the need for immobilization and secondary cutaneous defects with skin grafts was avoided. Most patients preferred the healing by secondary intention compared to the skin grafts.

One author[14] suggested excision followed by radiation therapy (200 to 300 roentgens). Although x-ray has had its champions for hidradenitis suppurativa,[57] the author feels that its use should be avoided, particularly in a condition that usually occurs under the age of 40 and in which malignant potential exists.

Skin Grafts. Skin grafts are useful in hidradenitis suppurativa[10, 18, 19, 58] and provide coverage for large areas after excisions that are too large for primary closure. Although this procedure may seem somewhat excessive, in studies of different surgical methods of therapy (including flaps), skin grafts appear to have the lowest recurrence rates,[10, 59] especially in the axilla. Problems associated with grafts include prolonged hospitalization, infection of the graft itself or donor site,[60] adequate immobilization, graft contractures, and hazardous survival. Mesh grafting[11, 61] or delayed grafting[2, 61] has been suggested to minimize problems with infection or necrosis. However, even if the graft itself is successful, the transplanted skin usually feels unnatural to the patient.

In the perineum and perianal areas, a diverting colostomy followed by skin grafting has been suggested because of the likelihood of fecal contamination.[9, 61] If the disease process is extensive, such an approach is justifiable.

Skin Flaps. An alternative to skin grafting is a skin flap. The movement of adjacent tissue with blood supply intact can provide immediate coverage of an excised defect.[17, 62] However, one is limited somewhat by the amount of tissue to be excised because the flap provides only limited coverage. The recurrence and morbidity rates in the axilla seem to be higher with flaps than grafts.[10] However, in certain selected patients, this procedure should be considered. The advantage of a skin flap is that, if sizeable blood vessels and nerves are exposed upon extirpation of diseased tissue, a flap provides thicker coverage than a graft and greater mobility may be obtained. This is particularly true if the disease

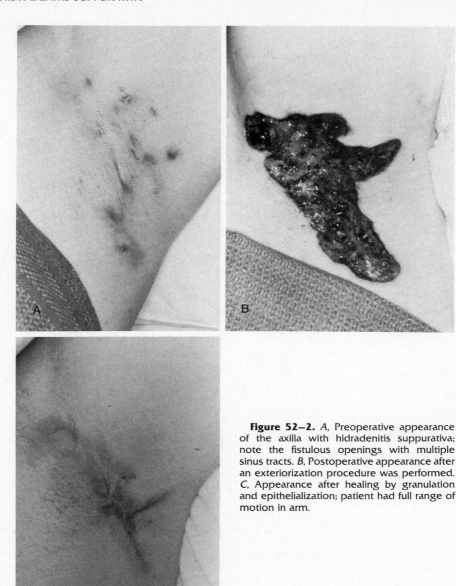

Figure 52–2. *A,* Preoperative appearance of the axilla with hidradenitis suppurativa; note the fistulous openings with multiple sinus tracts. *B,* Postoperative appearance after an exteriorization procedure was performed. *C,* Appearance after healing by granulation and epithelialization; patient had full range of motion in arm.

process has spread deeply. In the groin or perineum, where infection tends to be a problem associated with bowel contamination, flaps are likely to be associated with problems.[63]

Exteriorization. This procedure (Fig. 52–2), described in great detail by Mullins, is based upon direct visualization and exposure of the interconnecting sinus tracts.[64] The procedure, which is detailed in Figure 52–3, may be performed on an outpatient basis. The physician has the advantage of not being limited in the excision by considerations of wound coverage; the extent of the excision is determined solely by the systematic probing of sinus tracts and abscesses. Upon excision of the diseased tissue, the base is curetted and electrodessicated, to

provide hemostasis and to destroy tracts too small for a probe. The wound is then allowed to heal by granulation and epithelialization. The author usually recommends Burow's compresses three to four times a day, followed by Polysporin Ointment, until the wound has healed completely. If hypergranulation should develop during the process of wound healing, this is controlled by curettage. Depending upon the size of the wound, complete wound healing may take from four to eight weeks. The advantage of this procedure is that large amounts of diseased tissue may be treated on an outpatient basis under local anesthesia with a minimal amount of morbidity. Although high success rates associated with this exteriorization procedure are claimed,[64, 65] the pre-

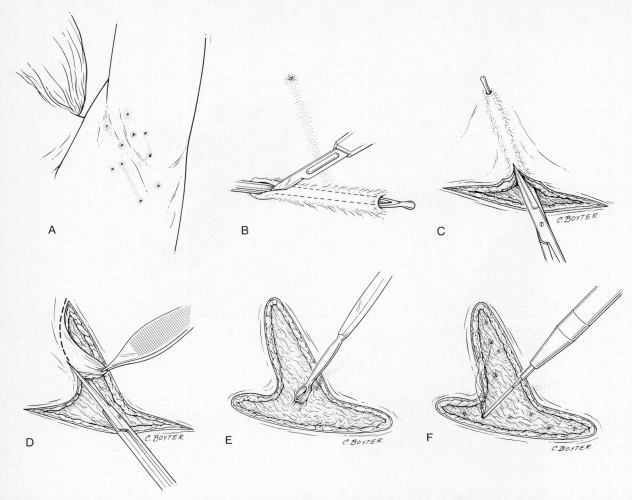

Figure 52–3. Exteriorization technique: *A*, Axilla with chronic hidradenitis suppurativa. *B*, Incision is made into a groove director in the sinus tract. *C*, Probe in an adjacent sinus tract with an incision being made by iris scissors. *D*, Redundant tissue is trimmed away at the edges so that further probing may be done if necessary and to facilitate wound healing. *E*, Curettage of the base, which is usually epithelialized. *F*, Electrocoagulation of the base for hemostasis and, more importantly, to destroy any remaining sinus tracts too small for a probe.

cise extent of the disease as well as specific cure rates are not stated.

Some physicians[65] comment that actively draining sinus tracts are easier to identify and advocate operating on patients at the time of acute infection; however, the author places the patient on appropriate antibiotics until the patient's disease is relatively quiescent. In the author's opinion, to delay the operation under such circumstances helps to reduce further infection and minimizes subsequent recurrences. Placing a probe into an infected sinus tract or abscess cavity carries the risk of perforation of the wall. This may extend the disease and thereby necessitate excision of more tissue. Where there is extensive infection, the risk of bacteremia is lessened.

Although exteriorization with subsequent granulation is said to minimize the morbidity seen with other procedures (such as graft contracture), the author has seen problems arise subsequent to the exteriorization procedure including scar contractures (especially in the axilla) and recurrences deep to the area excised. This procedure tends not to go deep into the fat, but as mentioned before, the apocrine glands may certainly go this deep.[4] Although the scar contractures may be somewhat bothersome to the patient, injections of triamcinolone and time usually ameliorate such symptoms.

SUMMARY AND CONCLUSIONS

Hidradenitis suppurativa may be an acute or chronic condition that is best managed early and with surgery. Medical forms of therapy are temporizing at best and may prevent patients from seeking an early cure. Although each patient tends to present his or her own problems, which must be dealt with individually, the physician should be firm in handling hidradenitis suppurativa. If the disease is recognized early and treated adequately as described above, the patient will have less discomfort.

One further aspect of healing with a patient with hidradenitis suppurativa is to obtain adequate follow-up. Patients should be instructed to return at regular intervals so that, if recurrences occur, they can be handled expeditiously. All too often, patients who have had multiple therapies in the past tend to neglect such recurrences in the hope that spontaneous resolution will occur.

REFERENCES

1. Dvorak VC, Rout RK, MacGregor RR: Host-defense mechanisms in hidradenitis suppurativa. Arch Derm 113:450–453, 1977
2. Greeley PW: Plastic surgical treatment of chronic suppurativa hidradenitis. Plas Reconstr Surg 7: 143–146, 1951
3. Shelley WB, Cahn MM: The pathogenesis of hidradenitis suppurativa in man. Arch Dermatol 72:562–565, 1955
4. Montagna W, Parakkal PF: The Structure and Function of Skin. New York, Academic Press, 1974
5. Gordon SW: Hidradenitis suppurativa: A closer look. J Nat Med Assoc 70:339–343, 1978
6. Moschella SL: Hidradenitis suppurativa, complications resulting in death. JAMA 198:201–203, 1966
7. Anderson JJ, Dockerty MB: Perianal hidradenitis suppurativa. Dis Colon Rectum 1:23–31, 1958
8. Brunsting HA: Hidradenitis suppurativa: Abscess of apocrine sweat glands: Study of clinical and pathological features, with report of two cases and review of literature. Arch Dermatol Syphilol 39:108–120, 1939
9. Ching CC, Stahlgren LH: Clinical review of hidradenitis suppurativa. Management of cases with severe perianal involvement. Dis Colon Rectum 8:349–352, 1965
10. Knaysi GA Jr, Cosman B, Crikelair GF: Hidradenitis suppurativa. JAMA 203:19–22, 1968
11. Bell BA, Ellis H: Hidradenitis suppurativa. J Roy Soc Med 71:511–515, 1978
12. Brunsting HA: Hidradenitis and other variants of acne. Arch Derm 65:303–315, 1952
13. Tachau P: Abscesses of the sweat glands in adults. Arch Derm Syph 40:595–600, 1939
14. Jackman RJ: Hidradenitis suppurativa: Diagnosis and surgical management of perianal manifestations. Proc R Soc Med (suppl) 52:110–112, 1959
15. Homma H: On apocrine glands in White and Negro men and women. Bull Johns Hopkins Hosp 38:365–371, 1926
16. Weiner J, Lewis JE, Samitz MH: Hidradenitis suppurativa occurring on the leg. Cutis 17:888–891, 1976
17. Paletta FX: Hidradenitis suppurativa: Pathological study and use of skin flaps. Plast Reconstr Surg 31:307–315, 1963
18. Morgan WP, Hughes LE: The distribution, size, and density of the apocrine glands in hidradenitis suppurativa. Br J Surg 66:853–856, 1979
19. Conway H, et al: Surgical treatment of chronic hidradenitis suppurativa. Surg Gynecol Obstet 94:455–464, 1952
20. Steiner K, Grayson LD: Hidradenitis suppurativa of the adult and its management. Arch Dermatol 71:205–211, 1955
21. Spiller RF, Knox JM: Fox-Fordyce disease with hidradenitis suppurativa. J Invest Dermatol 31:127–135, 1958
22. Bergeron JR: Follicular occlusion trial in a follicular blocking disease (pityriasis rubra pilaris). Dermatologica 136:362–367, 1968
23. McDonald RM, Reed WB: Natal teeth and steatocystoma multiplex complicated by hidradenitis suppurativa; a new syndrome. Arch Dermatol 112:1132–1134, 1976
24. Stone OJ: Hidradenitis suppurativa following acanthosis nigricans, report of two cases. Arch Dermatol 112:1142, 1976
25. Bergeron JR, Stone OJ: Interstitial keratitis associated with hidradenitis suppurativa. Arch Derm 95:473–475, 1967
26. Sulzberger MB: Discussion, Apocrine sweat retention in man, with Walter B. Shelley and Edwin J. Levy. Arch Derm 72:38–49, 1955
27. Danto JL: Preliminary studies of the effect of hydrocortisone of hidradenitis suppurativa. J Invest Dermatol 31:299–300, 1958
28. MacKenna RMB, Lehmann H: The glucose tolerance curve in hidradenitis suppurativa. Br J Dermat 72:142–144, 1960
29. Storino WD, Engel GH: Office surgical management of recalcitrant axillary lesions. Cutis 21:338–341, 1978
30. Murillo J, Schimoff SC, Brouillet MD: Axillary lesions in patients with acute leukemia. Cancer 43:1493–1496, 1979
31. Brenner DE, Lookingbill DP: Anaerobic microorganisms in chronic suppurative hidradenitis. Lancet 2:921, 1980
32. Smith WE, Ropes MW: Bacteroides infections. N Engl J Med 232:31–37, 1945
33. Leach RD, et al.: Anaerobic subareolar breast abscess. Lancet 1:35–37, 1979
34. Leach RD, et al.: Anaerobic axillary abscess. Br Med J 2:5–7, 1979
35. Meislin HW, et al.: Anaerobic and aerobic bacteriology and outpatient management. Ann Int Med 87:145–149, 1977
36. Tennant F, et al.: Anemia associated with hidradenitis suppurativa. Arch Dermatol 98:138–140, 1968
37. Alexander S J: Squamous cell carcinoma in chronic hidradenitis suppurativa. Cancer 43:745–748, 1979
38. Dillon JS, Spjut HJ: Epidermoid carcinoma occurring in acne conglobata. Ann Surg 159:451–455, 1964
39. Gordon SW: Squamous cell carcinoma arising in hidradenitis suppurativa. Plas Reconst Surg 60:800–802, 1977
40. Humphrey LJ, Playforth H, Leavell UW Jr: Squamous cell carcinoma arising in hidradenitis suppurativa. Arch Derm 100:59–62, 1969
41. Donsky HJ, Mendelson CG: Squamous cell carcinoma as complication of hidradenitis suppurativa. Arch Dermatol 90:488–491, 1964
42. Verneuil AS: Etudes sur les tumeurs de la peau: de quelque maladies des glands sudoripores. Arch Gen Med 94:693–705, 1854
43. Kippling HF: How I treat hidradenitis suppurativa. Postgrad Med 48:291–292, 1970
44. Lane JE: Hidrosadenitis axiliaris of Vernueil. Arch Dermato Syphilol 28:609–614, 1933
45. Paletta FX: Tumors of the skin, in Converse JM (ed): Reconstructive Plastic Surgery. Philadelphia, Saunders, 1977, pp 2879–2880
46. Arnold HL: Treatment of hidradenitis suppurativa. JAMA 223:557, 1973
47. Plewing G, Wagner A: Anti-inflammatory effects of 13-cis-retinoic acid:An in vivo study. Arch Dermatol Res 270:89–94, 1981
48. Jones DH, Cunliffe WJ, King K: Hidradenitis suppurativa—lack of success with 13-cis-retinoic acid (Letter). Brit J Dermatol 107:252, 1982
49. Dicken CH, Powel ST, Spear KL: Evaluation of isotretinoin treatment of hidradenitis suppurativa. J Am Acad Derm 11:500–502, 1984
50. Pollock WJ, Virnelli FR, Ryan RF: Axillary hidradenitis suppurativa. Plast Reconst Surg 49:22–27, 1972
51. Tasche C, Angelats J, Jayaram B: Surgical Treatment of hidradenitis suppurativa of the Axilla. Plast Reconstr Surg 55:559–562, 1975

52. Letterman G, Shurter M: Surgical treatment of hyperhidrosis and chronic hidradenitis suppurativa. J Invest Dermatol 63:174–182, 1974

53. Masson JK: Surgical treatment of hidradenitis suppurativa. Surg Clin N Am 49:1043–1052, 1969

54. Nance FC: Hidradenitis suppurativa of the perineum treated by radical excision. Am Surgeon 36:331–334, 1970

55. Morgan WP, Harding KG, Hughes LE: A comparison of skin grafting and healing by granulation following axillary excision for hidradenitis supperativa. Ann R Coll Surg Engl 65:235–236, 1983

56. Vickers MA Jr: Operative management of chronic hidradenitis suppurativa of the scrotum and perineum. J Urol 114:414–416, 1975

57. Zeligman I: Temporary x-ray epilation therapy of chronic axillary hidradenitis suppurativa. Arch Dermatol 92:690–694, 1965

58. Shaughnessy DM, et al.: Hidradenitis suppurativa, a plan for early operative treatment. JAMA 222:320–321, 1972

59. Broadwater JR, Bryant RL, Petrino et al.: Advanced hidradenitis suppurativa: Review of surgical treatment in 23 patients. Am J Surg 144:668–670, 1982

60. Gewirtz HS, Hoefflin SM, Silsby JJ: Local infection complicating in situ storage of split-skin grafts in a patient with hidradenitis suppurativa. Plast Reconst Surg 60:635–637, 1977

61. Hyland WT, et al: Surgical management of chronic hidradenitis suppurativa of the perineum. South Med J 69:1002–1004, 1976

62. Armstrong DP, Pickrell KL, Giblin TR, et al.: Axillary hidradenitis suppurativa. Plast Reconst Surg 36:200–206, 1965

63. Mladick RA, Horton CE, Adamson JE, Carraway J: Hidradenitis suppurativa of the perineum, in Horton CE (ed): Plastic and Reconstructive Surgery of the Genital Area. Boston, Little, Brown & Co, 1973, pp 515–521

64. Mullins JF, et al.: Treatment of chronic hidradenitis suppurativa: Surgical modification. Postgrad Med 26:805–808, 1959

65. Newell GB, et al.: Treatment of hidradenitis suppurativa. JAMA 223:556, 1973

53

NORMAN GOLDSTEIN, M.D., F.A.C.P.

Tattoos: Cosmetic and Therapeutic Tattooing and Removal Techniques

Tattoo (forms: tat(t)aow, tattow, tatoo, tatto, tatu) *Polynesian.* To form permanent marks or designs upon the skin by puncturing it and inserting a pigment or pigments: practiced by various tribes of low civilization, and by individuals in civilized communities.

—OXFORD ENGLISH DICTIONARY

Dermatologists are observing a wider variety of subject matter for tattoos, a broader rainbow of colors, and sizes ranging from a tiny flower on the ankle to total body tattoos. No longer the domain of the armed forces, tattoos are not restricted to covered areas and only visible to close friends or the gynecologist, proctologist, or dermatologist. Many more women are receiving "permanent body art."[1] Obviously, these tattoos are not put on only in prisons or reformatories, but in tattoo parlors across the country by professional tattoo artists—many of them very artistic women and men.

Cosmetic or therapeutic tattooing has been practiced by both tattoo artists and a limited number of physicians for several years.

Recently, because of the work of Angres[2, 3] and Fenzyl as reported in *The New York Times,*[4] cosmetic tattooing has captured the interest of dermatologists, ophthalmologists, plastic and reconstructive surgeons, and others. Eyelid tattooing has become very fashionable in some U.S. cities (Fig. 53–1). There is even an American Society of Micropigmentation Surgery being organized at this time.

The increasing interest in tattoos is actually universal and not just limited to the United States. This was clearly evidenced by the interest shown at the exhibit, "The World of Tattoos," first presented at the American Academy of Dermatology in 1979 in San Francisco, then at the California Medical Association in Los Angeles, the American Academy of Pediatrics in Toronto, and the World Congress of the International Society of Tropical Dermatology in New Orleans. Material from this exhibit is now with the Riksutstallningar, a Swedish national educational travel exhibition. Slides of interesting exotic, erotic, and artistic tattoos continue to be received by the author from dermatologists, plastic surgeons, tattoo artists, and tattoo fans from around the world.

TRENDS IN TATTOOS TODAY

Sexual preferences are clearly indicated by tattoos on buttocks, as seen in shower rooms. Less subtle preferences include small blue nevi-like tattoos on a cheek, chin, or finger of a woman. Preference for illicit drugs is indicated by H or M or the more subtle 13 (M is the thirteenth letter of the alphabet).

Decorative dental tattoos (some temporary and some permanent) are applied by a small group of cosmetic dentists.[5] The 103rd Indiana General Assembly passed the "Tattooed Teeth Bill," requiring dentists, where possible, to engrave false teeth with a patient's name or social security number.[6] (For identification of lost false teeth or perhaps lost patients?)

Small temporary tattoos on decals have been available for many years. Larger ones and more tattoo-like ones are now available. These temporary tattoos are easily removed. Not so easily removed are large total body tattoos as seen on Yakuza members and other men and women.

Even smaller tattoos almost always leave some type of cosmetic defect when removed, viz., a scar, keloid, local hyperesthesia, atrophy, or hyper- or hypopigmentation.

Eyelash Tattooing: Synonyms and Trademarks

Accents	Eyeline surgery
Blepharopigmentation	Lash augmentation
Dyelining	Lash liner
Enhancer	Lash lining
Eye enhancement	Natural eyes
Eye tattooing	Permalid Liner
Eyelash tattooing	

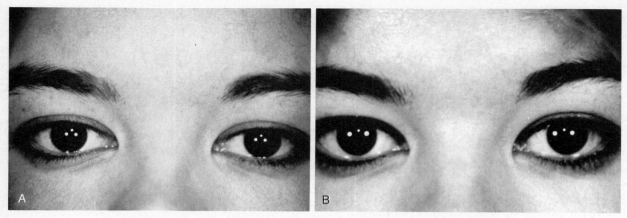

Figure 53–1. Eyelid tattooing: before (*A*) and after (*B*). (Courtesy of John Corboy, M.D.)

COSMETIC AND THERAPEUTIC TATTOOING

When Hance and coworkers[7] and Conway[8] in the 1940s reported on the use of color matching and tattooing of port-wine hemangiomas, there was minimal interest shown by physicians.

Prior to the availability of topical corticosteroids, some cases of persistent pruritus ani were treated with mercuric sulfide tattooing of the perianal area. If some of these patients accidentally or intentionally exposed the tattooed sites to sunlight or artificial ultraviolet light, they may have exacerbated their perianal pruritus from the photosensitivity reaction in the red pigment.[9] This technique is no longer used today.

There are many and varied indications and applications of cosmetic and therapeutic tattooing today,

as reported by Zwerling, Goldstein, and Christiansen in their book *Micropigmentation*.[10]

Applications for Cosmetic and Therapeutic Tattooing

A. Dermatology and Plastic/Reconstructive Surgery
1. Improvement of traumatic and surgical scars.
2. Nevus flammeus (port-wine hemangiomas).
3. Repair of lip contours.
4. Nipple and areola reconstruction after mastectomy or trauma.
5. Alopecia areata.
6. Vitiligo (Fig. 53–2).

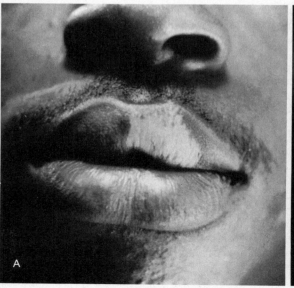
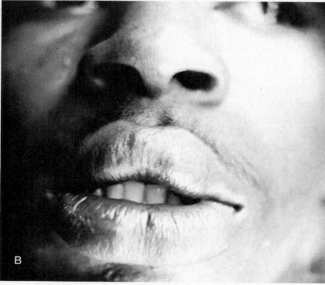

Figure 53–2. Vitiligo tattooing: before (*A*) and after (*B*). (Courtesy of Lyle Tuttle.)

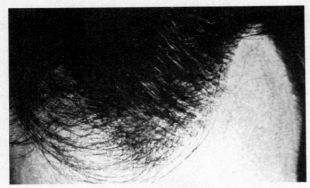

Figure 53–3. Tattooing after a hair transplant to fill in spaces between hair plugs. (Courtesy of Lyle Tuttle.)

7. Pinta.
8. Improvement of skin grafts and flaps.
9. Cryosurgery hypopigmentation.
10. Filling in spaces between hair transplant plugs (Fig. 53–3).
11. Camouflaging heroin users' needle tracks.
12. Countertattooing, i.e., a change of heart that requires covering or changing the name of a former lover or spouse and covering obscene or pornographic tattoos.

B. Ophthalmology
  1. Eyeliner
    a. Permanent eyelining.
    b. Eyelid pigmentation after cryosurgery.
  2. Eyebrows
    a. Cosmetic eyebrow enhancement.
    b. Replacement of eyebrows.
    c. Thickening of eyebrows.
    d. Outlining eyebrow edges for cosmetic pencil marking.
  3. Corneal Tattoos
    a. Congenital corneal opacities.
    b. Heterochromia.
    c. Polychromia.
    d. Congenital colobomas.
    e. Traumatic scars.
    f. Postinfection scars.
    g. Unilateral microphthalmos.
  4. Other
    a. Postoperative conjunctival flaps.
    b. Operative defects of the iris.

C. Otolaryngology
  1. Marking oral margins prior to radiation or chemotherapy.

D. Neurology
  1. Marking insertion sites for lumbar puncture needles in patients with pseudotumor cerebri.
  2. Obese patients in whom it is difficult to find repeated lumbar puncture insertion sites for therapy.

E. Oncology
  1. Preradiation marking of tumor margins. By using a superficial tattooing technique, the tattoo should usually desquamate in six to eight weeks.
  2. Marking the outer margins of tumors for Mohs' microchemosurgery.
  3. Possible tattooing of topical 5-fluorouracil for skin cancers and precancers.

F. Medical Uses
  1. Tissue typing for possible organ transplantation.
  2. Marking surgical sites.

G. Other Uses
  1. Military information was tattooed onto a shaven head (Herodotus).
  2. Tattooing of criminals and slaves for identification by the Ancient Romans.
  3. Military deserters from the British army were tattooed prior to 1879.
  4. "Enemies of the state" were tattooed in Nazi Germany.
  5. "Citizen numbers" (similar to Social Security numbers) in Denmark.
  6. Military serial numbers on American soldiers during World War II.
  7. Blood typing by the military in World War II.

H. Veterinary Uses
  1. Nasal solar dermatitis (Collie nose).
  2. Identification of laboratory animals.
  3. Identification of pets.*
  4. Wildlife identification of bears and deer.
  5. Vitiligo in show animals.
  6. Racehorse identification, usually tattooing of the lip mucous membrane.

CAVEATS TO COSMETIC TATTOOING

There are some definite cautions and contraindications to physician tattooing.

A. Legal Contraindications
  1. State laws pertaining to tattooing.[11]
  2. Potential malpractice suits from tattoo removal.[12]

B. Medical Contraindications
  1. Absolute:
    a. Psoriasis.
    b. Lichen planus.
    c. Warts.
    d. Molluscum contagiosum.
    e. Active herpes simplex.
    f. Active herpes zoster.
    g. Allergy to mercury or cadmium.
    h. Active tuberculosis.
    i. Darier's disease.

*The American Registry for Animals is active in at least 18 states.

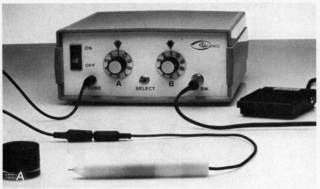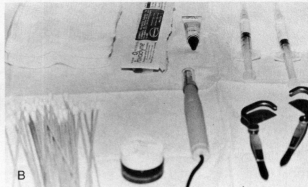

Figure 53–4. Tattoo equipment for the medical profession. *A*, Power unit with disposable handpiece. *B*, Assortment of sterile, disposable equipment. (Courtesy Dioptics Medical Products.)

j. Keloid formation.
k. Anticoagulant therapy.
l. Hemophiliacs.
2. Possible:
   a. Atopic dermatitis.
   b. Chronic pyoderma.
   c. Dermatographism.
   d. Alopecia areata.
C. Psychological Contraindications
   1. Mentally unstable patients. If in doubt, psychiatric consultation is strongly advised prior to tattooing.

TATTOO TECHNIQUES

There are several companies that supply tattoo equipment and pigment for tattoo artists, physicians, veterinarians, and other health professionals. One of the largest in the United States is Spaulding and Rogers, located in Voorheesville, New York.

Sterile, disposable, and smaller units are now available only to the medical profession (Fig. 53–4). These include Dioptics Medical Products and CooperVision Surgery (both located in Irvine, California). Penmark is manufactured in West Palm Beach, Florida. Most of the companies that sell equipment to physicians, provide an optional (or required) tattoo instruction course, given in several cities across the country.

Because of the possible transmission of serious infections—such as hepatitis (which occurred in Coney Island, New York, more than 20 years ago and was recently reported in New Jersey[13]), tuberculosis,[14] syphilis, and leprosy as well as less serious bacterial and viral infections—physicians are urged to use sterile, disposable equipment.

Though not reported as yet, the possibility of transmitting AIDS (acquired immune deficiency syndrome) via tattooing must be considered seriously.[1]

Five states (Florida, Indiana, Oklahoma, Vermont, and Virginia) permit tattooing only by physicians, dentists, veterinarians, or nurses. Thirty-five states do not have regulations or statutes pertaining to tattoos. If tattooing is legal in your state, it would be advisable to contact a tattoo artist in your community for his or her advice. Many tattoo artists are eager to cooperate with physicians and are pleased to demonstrate their techniques.

Despite some state regulations,[11] Mosaic Law (Leviticus 19:28), and Mohammed's prohibitions (nine references to tattooing in the Hadith), permanent body art by tattoo artists and physicians is increasing dramatically. It will undoubtedly increase even more because of the disposable equipment and decreasing costs of instruments.

TATTOO REMOVAL TECHNIQUES

There are as many reasons to have tattoos removed as there are reasons for getting them in the first place. A survey of dermatologists, plastic surgeons, and tattoo artists indicated the following are the most common reasons for having tattoos removed.[15]
A. Social and Cultural Reasons
   1. A change of heart (e.g., divorce, separation, or change of lovers or friends).
   2. Inability to obtain employment (a corporate image is not enhanced by a tattooed forearm).
   3. Easy identification by former prisoners or law officers who recognize certain markings (e.g., "Kill the pigs").
   4. Shame or a desire to disassociate oneself from a prison clique or other group such as a motorcycle club.
   5. Recognition by police officers who may identify a prisoner or ex-prisoner as one who can be persuaded to be an informant.

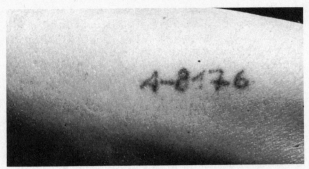

Figure 53–5. A Nazi concentration camp identification tattoo.

6. To erase the stigmata of World War II concentration camp tattoos (Fig. 53–5).
B. Medical Reasons
   1. To resolve allergic reactions in the tattoo, usually a photosensitive reaction in the red pigment.[16]
   2. To remove rare chronic infections in tattoos such as tuberculosis.
   3. To remove a neoplasm that develops in a tattoo—a very rare occurrence.[17]

There are numerous methods for removing tattoos—because there is no "best" technique. Albert Parry in his 1933 book listed the following methods as "scientifically tested and approved by chemists, physicians, and surgeons."[18] He admonished that "these methods are not to be used by the tattooed themselves or by tattoo masters, but by physicians and surgeons only."

1. The French process—tannic acid and silver nitrate.
2. Salicylic acid.
3. Monochloracetic acid or trichloracetic acid.
4. Carbolic acid (phenol).
5. Sulfuric acid (15 grains to 1 oz. of water).
6. Nitric acid (concentrated).
7. Zinc chloride.
8. Mercuric chloride.
9. Cantharides plaster (Spanish fly). Add vinegar to increase action, or open the blister formed by the Spanish fly and add a weak zinc chloride solution.
10. Glycerol of papoid (or glycerol of Caroid). A powerful organic digestant. It digests the tissue in question.
11. Zonite, a solution of sodium hypochloride, approximately twice as strong as Dakin's solution.
12. Electrolysis—similar to hair removal by electricity, feasible only on small tattooed designs.
13. Surgery—cut out mechanically, raise the flap, cut skin, scrape off the pigment from the bottom of the skin.
14. Surgery—use a grattage (a little steel scrubbing brush). Apply hydrogen peroxide.
15. Use cutaneous trephine (a surgical instrument resembling a hollow carpenter's tool).
16. When a design is superficial, use dry ice (CO_2 snow). It will freeze the skin, turn it grey, then the skin may be removed with tweezers.
17. Prolonged thin design: simple excision.
18. For larger designs: excision with grafting.

Many of the tried and true techniques summarized by Parry in his popular book are still being used, some of them by the tattooed person, some by the tattoo artist, and some by physicians. The more effective methods and some more recent ones, including cryosurgery and laser therapy, are discussed in this chapter.

METHODS USED TODAY

Do-It-Yourself Methods

The most common do-it-yourself method is salabrasion with table salt. Home tattoo kits are available; other home techniques include burning with cigarettes or hot coat hangers, scalding with steam, and picking it out.

Removal by Tattoo Artists

Many tattoo artists for legal and other reasons prefer not to remove tattoos, and many states actually prohibit them from doing so.[11] One of the most common removal methods used by tattoo artists is the Variot or French method, as described later. Other methods include counter-tattooing or retattooing. Some tattoo artists attempt to lighten a dark tattoo by using lighter pigments. Retattooing with white or pink pigments is usually not successful, because the surrounding skin color changes with sun exposure.

Removal Techniques Performed by Physicians

Imaginative and creative dermatologists and plastic surgeons have devised new techniques and modified old methods to remove tattoos. The most common are:
A. Surgery
   1. Punch removal, with or without sutures —ideal for small dark tattoos.
   2. Simple excision with primary closure for small tattoos. For larger tattoos, staging or removal in segments is recommended. Excision and grafting can also be combined.
   3. Dermatome removal with or without grafting.
   4. Abrasion:
      a. Sandpaper (CVE: Granulomas should not be abraded).
      b. Wire brush using diamond fraises.
      c. Dermabrasion with or without a skin graft.
      d. Salabrasion using coarse table salt (e.g., Hawaiian Crude or kosher salt may also be used).

B. Chemical Techniques
1. Practically every caustic chemical on the pharmacy shelf has been employed to remove tattoos. Included in this list are phenol, nitric acid, tannic acid, sulfuric acid, liquid ammonia, silver nitrate, and salicylic acid. One of the most effective chemical methods is the Variot or French method using tannic acid, silver nitrate, and dermabrasion or tattooing as modified by Dr. Penoff (described later).[19]
C. Physical Methods
1. Cold—using a Freon spray.
2. Carbon dioxide—using snow or dry ice.
3. Liquid nitrogen—employing a cotton-tipped applicator, copper applicators, or cryospray units.
4. Heat.
a. Electrocautery with or without curettage.
b. Ultraviolet light in the past has been used to produce an intense erythema with subsequent peeling of skin and some tattoo pigment.
5. Lasers—space-age technology usually employing the argon or carbon dioxide laser.

Countertattooing and Retattooing

Some physicians tattoo white opaque pigment into existing tattoos in an attempt to lighten them. The Conway tattoo attachment[8] for dermabrasion equipment may be used along with a standard electric tattooing machine or the newer type of medical tattoo units. This technique has also been used, with dubious results, in the tattooing of capillary hemangiomas.

It should be emphasized that the choice of technique depends on many factors including size, duration, and location and whether the tattoo was done by an amateur or professional. The professional tattoo artist usually puts the pigment in at the same level in the dermis (Fig. 53–6), making it easier for effective removal, where the do-it-yourself tattooer varies the levels greatly.

COMMON REMOVAL TECHNIQUES USED BY PHYSICIANS

The following methods are the ones usually employed by physicians in their attempts to remove amateur and professional tattoos. The method described is *not* necessarily the one recommended in every case.
A. Excision
1. With closure.
2. Tangential.
3. Punch.
B. Dermabrasion
1. Deep.
2. Superficial.
3. French method.
4. Toothbrush.
5. Curettage after dermabrasion.
C. Salabrasion
D. Lasers
1. Argon.
2. Carbon dioxide.
3. Ultraviolet.
4. Others.
E. Other Methods Used Today
1. Grafting.
2. Cryosurgery.
3. Mohs'.

Excision and Closure

Small tattoos may be removed simply with a punch or excised and sutured (Fig. 53–7). Unfortunately, even small tattoos, because of tension or location, may tend to spread the incision lines, leaving an unacceptable result. Staples may be employed in place of sutures (Fig. 53–8). Small tattoos, or parts of a large tattoo, may be delicately excised (Fig. 53–9). Larger tattoos may be excised in stages, removing the center, then the sides at a later date. All too often, the patient fails to return for a follow-up and excision of the original tattoo (Fig. 53–10).

Tattoos in selected locations or larger tattoos may require Z-plasty procedures (Fig. 53–11).

The following is a standard tattoo excision technique in an unusual site. A 25-year-old Japanese woman presented with a suprapubic tattoo (Fig. 53–12A). In this site, a simple horizontal excision is ideal.

A standard instrument tray is used consisting of scalpels, scissors, forceps, needle and suture mate-

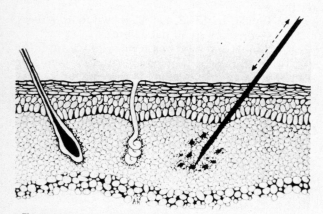

Figure 53–6. Usual depth of pigment in the skin from a tattoo machine. (Courtesy of Richard Dobson, M.D.)

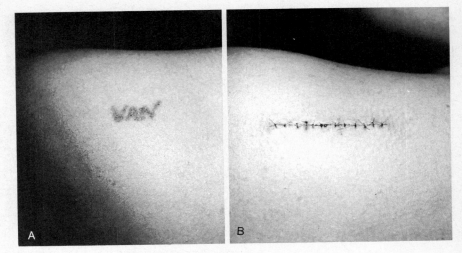

Figure 53–7. *A* and *B*, Small tattoo removed by simple excision and sutures. (Courtesy of F. Don Parsa, M.D.)

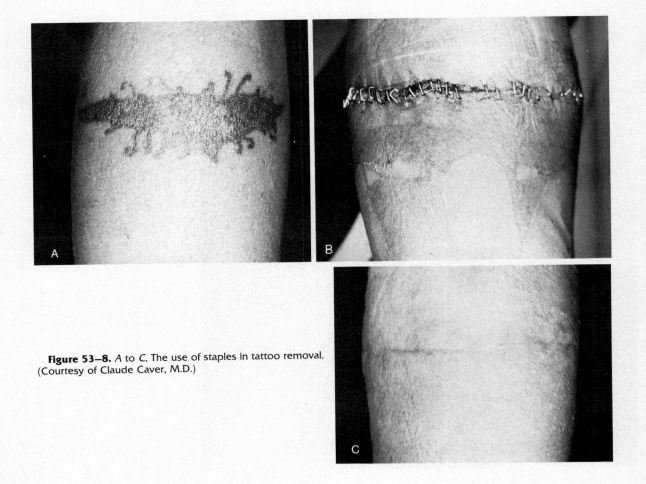

Figure 53–8. *A* to *C*, The use of staples in tattoo removal. (Courtesy of Claude Caver, M.D.)

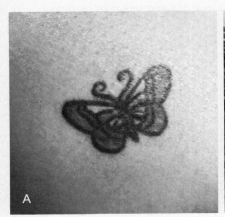

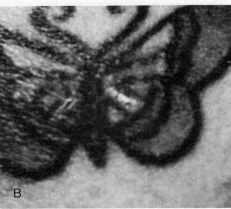

Figure 53–9. Delicate removal of the photoallergic portion of a tattoo: before (*A*) and after (*B*). (Courtesy of Bruce Chrisman, M.D.)

Figure 53–10. *A*, Incomplete removal (by a military oral surgeon) of the midportion of a tattoo. *B*, Partial removal of a tattoo by excision and flap rotation. Both patients failed to return for residual tattoo removal.

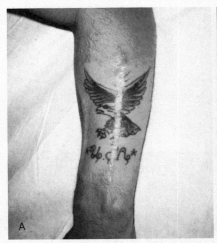

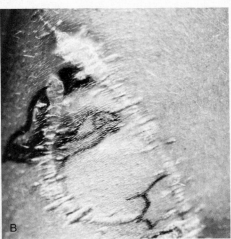

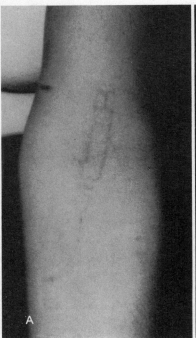

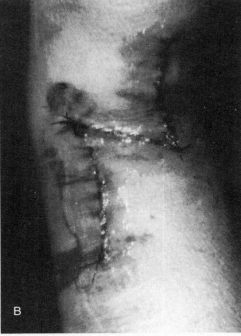

Figure 53–11. A homemade tattoo (*A*) requiring a Z-Plasty procedure for removal (*B*). (Courtesy of Steven L. Schlessinger, M.D.)

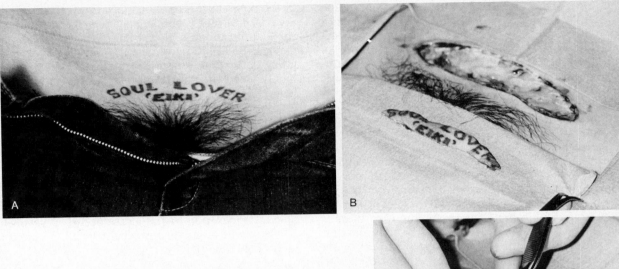

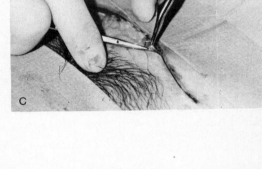

Figure 53–12. *A*, A 25-year-old Japanese woman with a suprapubic tattoo. *B*, Excision of the tattoo. *C*, Closure with over-and-over continuous sutures. (Courtesy of Victor Hay-Roe, M.D.)

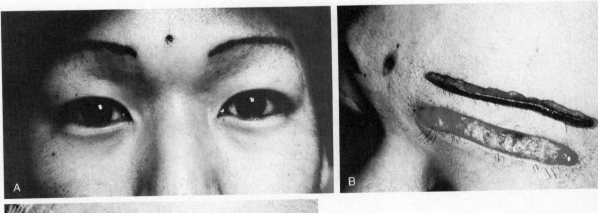

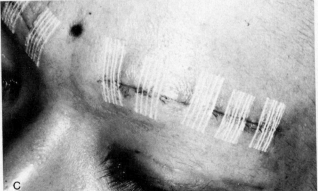

Figure 53–13. *A*, Patient with tattooed eyebrows and a nevus-like tattoo between them. *B*, Simple excision of the eyebrow tattoo. *C*, Closure with intradermal Dexon and Steri-strips. (Courtesy of Victor Hay-Roe, M.D.)

rial, local anesthetics, and syringe. A tattoo outline does not have to be marked with a dye, since sometimes the dye and the tattoo may become indistinguishable. Merely marking off the ends of the incision mark to guide the scalpel is sufficient. The entire area is infiltrated with local anesthetic and epinephrine, using a 30-gauge, 1/4 inch needle, and a Luer-Lok syringe. The area is not shaved, although some hair was removed to allow better sticking of adhesive tape. The tattoo is removed with scalpel and scissors. Minimal bleeding was controlled with an electrocautery. The wound is closed in two layers, the first a deep dermal or subcuticular stitch, just approximating the deeper layers of the dermis (Fig. 53–12B). This brings the skin edges within better approximation, so there is no tension on the skin sutures. If the tension is off the skin, the sutures can be removed very early without leaving stitch marks. The skin is closed with an over-and-over continuous suture with a knot on each end (Fig. 53–12C).

Another ideal tattoo for excision removal is demonstrated by a woman who had tattooed eyebrows which, because of a fashion change, were no longer cosmetically acceptable to her (Fig. 53–13A). Simple excisions (Fig. 53–13B) and closure with intradermal Dexon and Steri-Strips (Fig. 53–13C) gave her an acceptable result with hair regrowing after three weeks postoperatively.

Split-Thickness Tangential Excision

This method[20, 21] is particularly useful for a professional tattoo because of the uniform depth of the tattoo pigment (Fig. 53–14A). In this technique, the area is infiltrated with lidocaine without epinephrine. Infiltration is done carefully to specifically elevate the tattoo pattern. A Brown or Davol oscillating dermatome, set at approximately 15/100 of an inch is used to remove the elevated tattoo by tangential excision—similar to the process of removing a split-thickness skin graft. The wound created by the tangential excision is managed similarly to a donor site for a graft. A fine mesh cotton gauze is placed over the wound and cut to conform to the wound margins. A slightly occlusive wet dressing is applied and removed the following day. A crust forms incorporated in the overlying mesh. Healing is primarily the result of epithelialization, and spontaneous separation of the gauze occurs in seven to 10 days, with a good-to-excellent result six months later (Fig. 53–14B).

Dermabrasion

Dermabrasion has been one of the most popular methods for tattoo removal as performed by dermatologists. Because of the experience gained in acne scar removal using dermabrading units, most dermatologists feel quite at home with dermabrasion. The term "dermabrasion" was coined by Saul Blau, M.D., who perfected the dermabrading wheel used for both acne scarring and tattoo removal.[22] Dermabrasion may also be done with a toothbrush or hand brush, which is especially helpful for immediate removal of traumatic tattoos.[23]

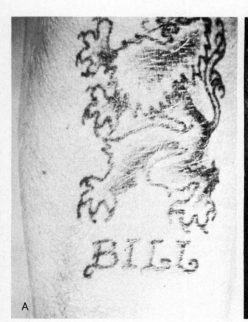
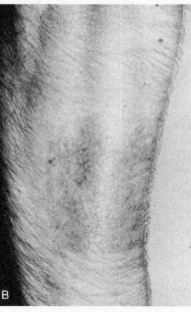

Figure 53–14. A, Patient with large professional tattoo on the forearm. B, Appearance six months later after a split-thickness tangential excision. (Courtesy of Katsusi Kubo, M.D.)

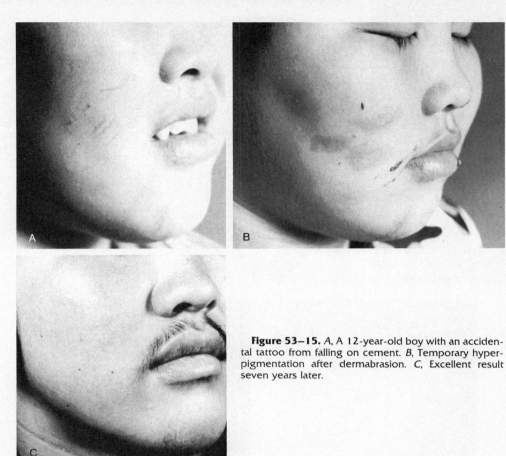

Figure 53–15. *A*, A 12-year-old boy with an accidental tattoo from falling on cement. *B*, Temporary hyperpigmentation after dermabrasion. *C*, Excellent result seven years later.

Standard Dermabrasion Technique

The standard dermabrasion technique as described by Bunke and Conway[24] and Chai[25] attempts to remove as much of the tattoo pigment as possible. Because of the deep abrasion, the precedure is often rather bloody. Skin pigment and blood splattering during the procedure requires protective operating garments and face shields. Sterile technique is not necessary, merely a clean operating room and office routines are sufficient. At least one assistant is necessary.

Technique. A small area of the tattoo is exposed using 4 × 4 gauze pads. This area is then frozen with dichlorotetrafluoroethane (Frigiderm) or similar spray or a liquid nitrogen cryospray unit. Because wire brushes tend to get caught in the gauze and adjacent drape material, most dermabraders prefer using diamond fraises and a standard Conway dermabrasion unit. Smaller, more powerful, and more adjustable units are also available. The frozen area is then physically scraped off with the dermabrader, and an Adaptic dressing is applied immediately after the dermabrasion and removed a day or two later. Serum, epidermal cells, and tattoo pigment will come out with the dressing.

If the outlines of the tattoo are followed too closely, the postdermabrasion result is not as good. Blending in of the entire tattoo or perhaps spraying the entire area at a later date with liquid nitrogen may improve the result.

Dermabrasion is also an ideal removal method for accidental tattoos. This 12-year-old boy sustained an accidental tattoo on his right cheek after falling on cement (Fig. 53–15A). A very light dermabrasion caused temporary hyperpigmentation (Fig. 53–15B). Seven years later, the postdermabrasion result was excellent (Fig. 53–15C). John Kestel, M.D., dermabraded another patient who sustained an accidental tattoo (Fig. 53–16A) from a gunshot explosion—with an excellent cosmetic result (Fig. 53–16B). Another excellent result with the standard deep dermabrasion technique was obtained by Bruce Chrisman, M.D. (Fig. 53–17).

Superficial Dermabrasion Technique

The superficial dermabrasion method, as described by West Clabaugh, M.D., does not attempt to remove all of the tattoo pigment.[26] However, in many cases, this is accomplished by natural re-

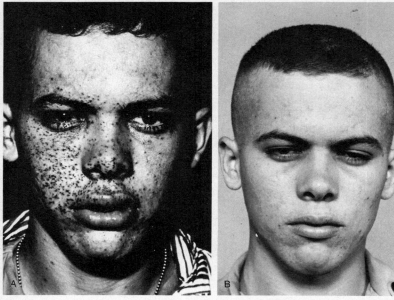

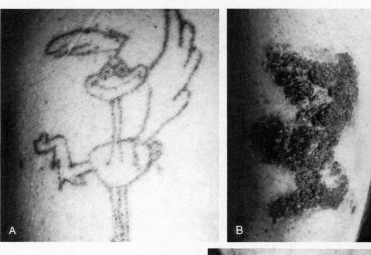

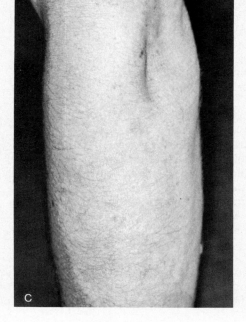

Figure 53–16. *A*, Patient with an accidental tattoo from a gunshot explosion. *B*, Excellent cosmetic result after dermabrasion. (Courtesy of John Kestel, M.D.)

Figure 53–17. *A* to *C*, Another excellent result from deep dermabrasion. (Courtesy of Bruce Chrisman, M.D.)

epithelialization. Clabaugh described 75 tattoo removals, but has now done hundreds of others. Most tattoos removed by the superficial dermabrasion technique require several procedures. Clabaugh obtained 75% to 85% good results, 10% to 15% fair results, and 5% to 10% poor results.

Technique. After the tattoo site is prepared with a surgical scrub, a small area is frozen with a refrigerant such as Frigiderm. The area is then abraded *very superficially*. Only the epidermis and parts of the papillary dermis are removed. As soon as the tattoo pigment appears in the skin scrapings, the dermabrasion should stop. It only takes a few minutes to treat an average-sized tattoo with this technique. After the bleeding subsides, the abraded site is painted with a 2% gentian violet solution, and an Adaptic dressing is applied and covered with gauze and tape. The dressings are changed daily for seven or eight days. After the dressing is removed, an outline of the tattoo can be readily seen on the Adaptic dressing.

Thus, standard or superficial dermabrasion is an easy and fast procedure with good pigment removal and usually little to no scar formation.

Dermabrasion Combined with Tannic Acid and Silver Nitrate (The French Method)

In order to increase pigment removal and reduce complications of dermabrasions, Penoff modified Variot's removal technique.[27] Variot removed tattoos by linear incisions, scratches, or punctures and then applied tannic acid and silver nitrate solution.[28] Penoff usually interrupts the integrity of the epidermis by making a grid with crisscross abrasions, using a standard dermabrading unit, or a tattoo instrument. The tannic acid solution and silver nitrate causes a flexible leathery eschar that desquamates most, if not all, of the tattoo. This is especially effective in large tattoos.

Salabrasion

It was Aëtius, the Byzantine Greek physician, who in 543 A.D. first used salt for removing tattoos. The technique consisted of applying an irritating substance to the tattoo for several days, after which salt was inoculated or rubbed into the tattoo site.[29]

In 1935, Klövekorn in Germany revived the method and rubbed salt in daily until the skin became red.[30] Crittenden first used the term "salabrasion" in 1971 for the use of salt to remove tattoos.[31, 32] Manchester then reviewed the subject and reported on more than 50 tattooed patients in 1973 and 1974.[33, 34]

Recently, Koerber and Price correlated the clinical and histologic results of salabrasions of tattoos at the VA Hospital in Palo Alto, California.[35] Their study consisted of 26 tattoos treated by salabrasion, with the salt being left on the abraded surfaces from zero to 24 hours. Catterall routinely performs up to three procedures per tattoo and feels he gets a better result than a single abrasion.[36]

Technique. The hair is shaved and the skin cleansed with povidone-iodine. The area may be anesthetized with 1% lidocaine without epinephrine, but many patients do not require a local anesthetic. The tattoo is rubbed with a slightly moistened sterile gauze dipped in salt until the skin surface is removed and a uniform glistening erosion is present (Fig. 53–18).

A variety of wooden doorknob-like devices have been used to hold the salt and gauze in order to facilitate the salabrasion (Figs. 53–19 and 53–20). Additional salt may then be applied to the abraded area and left on for varying periods of time. Gordon Sauer (personal communication) and Norman Price[37] feel the best results in most cases are obtained by removing the salt immediately after salabrasion. Treated areas may be permitted to dry uncovered, or an antibiotic ointment and occlusive

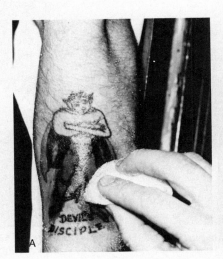
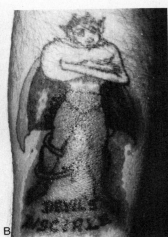

Figure 53–18. *A* and *B*, Glistening erosion obtained with salabrasion. (Courtesy of Bruce Chrisman, M.D.)

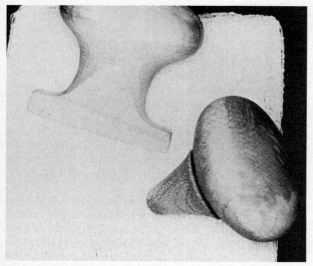

Figure 53—19. Wooden doorknob-like devices used for salabrasion. (Coutesy of Leon Goldman, M.D.)

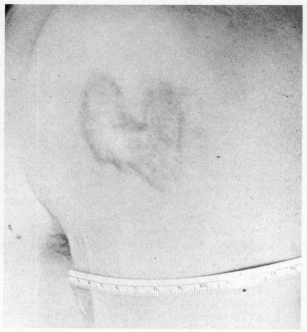

Figure 53—21. Patient who developed a keloid after a salabrasion.

dressing or Adaptic gauze may be used. The dressings are changed daily, noting the residual pigment appearing on the dressings.

Salabrasions may be performed with table salt, but most prefer a coarse type of salt such as Hawaiian Crude or kosher salt.

Complications may occur with salabrasion procedures, just as with any tattoo removal method (Fig. 53–21).

Lasers

Leon Goldman pioneered the use of lasers for tattoo removal (Fig. 53–22). In 1967, he reported his preliminary three-year clinical study.[38] Dr. Goldman continues his research and teaching activities at the University of Cincinnati Laser Center (see Chapter 25).

Lasers are optical devices that produce a unique form of light (electromagnetic) energy. This light is:
A. Monochromatic—i.e., a single wave length; however, in some laser systems, such as the argon, there are several wave lengths, but they are very close to each other (e.g., 488 nm and 514 nm) and act as though they are a single wave length.
B. Coherent—i.e., all the photons or waves of light are aligned as they are emitted and propagated, moving through space in an orderly fashion.

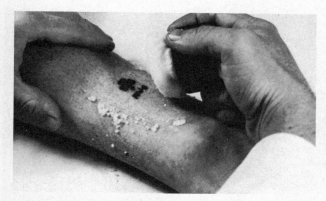

Figure 53—20. A doorknob-like device being used to facilitate salabrasion. (Courtesy of Howard Beerman, M.D.)

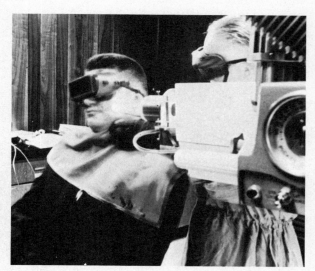

Figure 53—22. Dr. Leon Goldman treating a patient with a ruby laser in 1965.

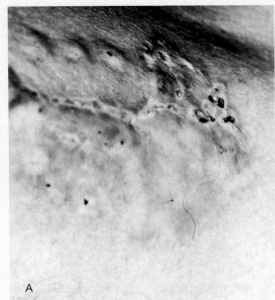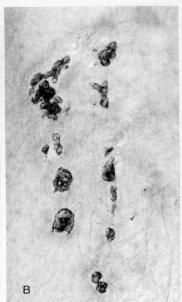

Figure 53–23. *A,* Patient who developed a keloid after argon laser therapy. Keloids frequently occur on the arm regardless of what type of treatment is used. *B,* The keloid subsided after intralesional corticosteroid injections, and the laser was used again for the residual tattoo.

C. Highly collimated, which implies the light does not diverge as it travels through space, as does normal visible light.

The laser unit requires an active medium such as a gas (carbon dioxide), a liquid (fluorescent dye), or a solid (ruby). The interactions between laser light and the skin vary greatly, depending on: wave length, optical properties of the skin, power density, energy fluence of the laser impact, length of exposure, and type of exposure.

The laser systems used most often today include argon, carbon dioxide, helium-neon, neodymium-yttrium-aluminum-garnet, ruby and tunable dye.

The use of lasers in clinical medicine and surgery is expanding at a phenominal pace, as was evidenced at the Pacific Laser International Update held in Honolulu. More than 200 representatives from 19 countries attended this multispecialty symposium. Audio tapes of the presentations are available from Sound Catchers.* In addition to a basic laser course, keynote presentations, and specialty presentations, Dr. Goldman spoke on "The Future Developments of Laser Medicine and Surgery" and presented an audiovisual discussion of laser art at the Honolulu Academy of Arts.

Early studies employing lasers to treat tattoos and other skin lesions were performed by Goldman and colleagues,[39] Laub and associates,[40] and Brady and coworkers.[41] More recently, Apfelberg and colleagues at the Palo Alto Medical Foundation in California, have performed additional studies with the argon laser.[42–47]

Strempel in Marburg, Germany,[48] Goldstein and Flores in Honolulu,[49] Saal in Los Gatos (personal communication), Dismukes in Memphis,[50] and Bailin and his associates in Cleveland[51–55] have had a great deal of experience with the use of the argon, carbon dioxide, and other lasers for tattoo removal.

There are several excellent texts dealing with the use of lasers for tattoo removal.[64–66]

While there is still some controversy concerning the best laser to use for tattoo removal, all the methods used today work. The same adverse effects of tattoo removal using dermabrasion, salabrasion, and the other physical methods also pertain to laser removal. Keloids frequently develop on the deltoid with laser treatments or any other tattoo removal methods at this site. The keloids can be injected with intralesional corticosteroids (Fig. 53–23).

Technique. Argon and carbon dioxide lasers, the two types most frequently used today, are employed in a similar manner.

Patient education and information, as in any cosmetic procedure, is vital. Proper patient selection is important for follow-up as well as for patient and physician satisfaction with the procedure. Brochures and instruction sheets are very beneficial.

Local anesthesia is usually employed. A smoke evacuator is kept near the laser site to absorb the odor of burned flesh—distracting to the physician and annoying to the patient. Antibiotic ointments and dressings are applied. Specific postoperative instruction sheets are given to the patient. The patient is advised to avoid direct sunlight and to avoid outside activities as much as possible for at least six weeks. Sun protectants with an SPF (sun

*1451 South King Street, Honolulu, HI 96814.

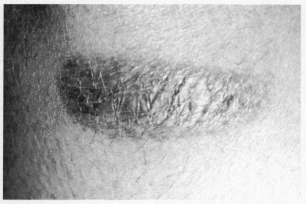

Figure 53–24. Patient with hyperpigmentation after laser treatment.

protective factor) of 15 or higher are provided, and patients are advised to apply them daily once the crust has desquamated. Postinflammatory hyperpigmentation (Fig. 53–24) is common in Hawaii—even in covered sites—perhaps because of our multiracial population and strong sunshine. Topical bleaching preparations are used to depigment the postinflammatory hyperpigmentation.

Small tattoos can be treated in one session (Fig. 53–25). Larger tattoos usually require two, three, or more sessions. (Fig. 53–26).

Patient acceptance of laser treatments for tattoo removal in the author's experience has been excellent. They prefer the space-age technology and lack of bleeding afforded by lasers. Removal of eyelid tattoos has not be done to date, but because of the possibility of allergic reactions in tattoos, this undoubtedly will become a problem in the future. Perhaps a fine laser method can be employed for this special tattoo problem.

Other Methods of Tattoo Removal

As reviewed in earlier sections of this chapter, there are many other methods employed by physicians for tattoo removal.

Cryosurgery

Cryosurgery using Freon, carbon dioxide (dry ice), liquid oxygen, and liquid nitrogen has also been used to remove tattoos. Most cryosurgeons, including Zacarian[56, 57] and Goldstein,[58] have abandoned it because of poor general results. For small and recently applied tattoos, cryosurgery with liquid nitrogen might be recommended.

Grafting

Some physicians prefer grafting of tattoos, depending on size and location. Gupta in England,[59] performed basic animal and clinical studies with grafted tattoos. However, most surgeons do not

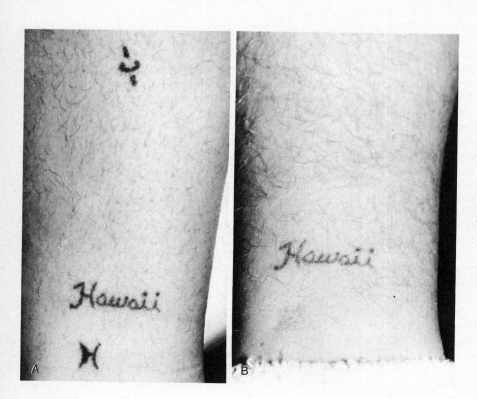

Figure 53–25. *A* and *B*, Small tattoos can be removed in one laser session. (This patient wanted to keep "Hawaii.")

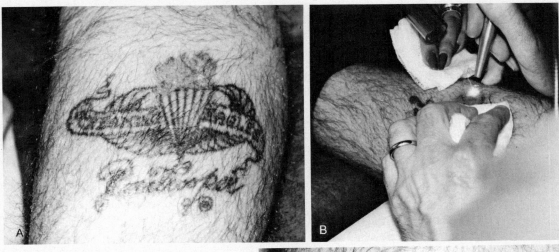

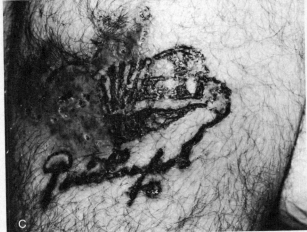

Figure 53–26. *A* to *C*, Larger tattoos usually require several sessions.

remove tattoos by grafting today because of faster, less expensive, and cosmetically better techniques.

Flaps

Transplantation, or flap procedures, are an improvement over grafting methods, since adjacent skin resembles the tattooed area more than distant donor sites. As Friederich points out, "The replacement of tattoos by pedicle flaps demands a special ability and artistic skillfulness in order to avoid scars with the contours of the tattoo."[60]

Caustics

Acids such as nitric acid are still occasionally employed for tattoo removal. Prinz obtained satisfactory results in 70% of his 120 tattoo removals in 1980.[61]

Mohs' Microsurgical Methods

Several associates have expressed interest in a modified Mohs' method for tattoo removal but, to date, have not used it.

Vitamin A Acid

Topical vitamin A acid was suggested by Albert Kligman (personal communication, 1980). An informal preliminary study of 11 patients indicated very poor results with the method employed.

Combined Techniques

A potpourri of possible combinations of removal methods have been attempted. They include (1) curettage after dermabrasion (Ceilley),[62] (2) dermabrasion followed by a split-thickness graft (Haneke),[63] and (3) salabrasion and dermabrasion by Chrisman (personal communication).

In conclusion, there is no perfect or best method for removing tattoos. The sooner the removal procedure—no matter what technique is used—the better result. Professional tattoos usually look better when removed, compared with amateur tattoos because of uniform level of pigment deposition.

With the increasing popularity of tattoos—small and large—the cosmetic surgeon will be called upon to remove more and more tattoos for a wide variety of reasons. Familiarity with several methods is highly recommended.

REFERENCES

1. Goldstein N: Tattoos today—from eyelids to ankles and some in "3-D." Arch Dermatol 121:604–605, 1985
2. Angres GG: Angres Permalid-liner method: A new surgical procedure. Ann Ophthalmol 16:145–148, 1984
3. Angres GG: Eye-liner implants: A new cosmetic procedure. Plast Recon Surg 73:833–836, 1984
4. Blumenthal D: Eyeliner by tattoo: New process debated. New York Times, Dec 29, 1984
5. Tessler S: Tattoos, "body art" goes back at least 8000 years. Detroit News, May 10, 1984
6. Anderson P: Indianapolis Sunday Herald, March 4, 1984
7. Hance G, Brown JB, Byers LT, McDowell F: Color matching of skin grafts and flaps with permanent pigment insertion. Surg Gynecol Obstet 79:624, 1944
8. Conway H: The permanent camouflage of port-wine stain of the face by the intradermal injection of insoluble pigments (tattooing). NY State J Med 48:2040, 1948
9. Goldstein N, Muller GH, Tuttle L: Modern applications of tattoos. J Dermatol Surg Oncol 5:889–891, 1979
10. Zwerling C, Goldstein N, Christensen F: Micropigmentation. Thorofare, NJ, Slack Publishing Co, 1985
11. Goldstein N: Laws and regulations relating to tattoos—an updated survey. (In preparation)
12. Zimmerman M: Suite for malpractice. Based on alleged unsightly scars resulting from removal of tattoos. J Dermatol Surg Oncol 5:911–912, 1979
13. Imtiaz R: New Jersey Department of Health. Personal communications, June 1985
14. Horney DA, Gaither JM, Lauer R, et al: Cutaneous inoculation tuberculosis secondary to jailhouse tattooing. Arch Dermatol: 121:648–650, 1985
15. Goldstein N: The World of Tattoos Exhibit. Presented at American Academy of Dermatology, 1979
16. Goldstein N: Mercury-cadmium sensitivity in tattoos. Ann Int Med 67:984–989, 1967
17. Goldstein N: Tattoo complications, in Micropigmentation. Thorofare, NJ, Slack Publishing Co, 1985
18. Parry A: Tattoo: Secrets of a Strange Art as Practiced by the Natives of the United States. New York, Simon & Schuster, 1933
19. Penoff J: Techniques of removal of tattoos. J Dermatol Surg Oncol 5:901, 1979
20. Grice KA: The removal of tattoos with a keratome. Brit J Derm 76:318, 1964
21. Wheeler MD, Miller TA: Tattoo removal by split-thickness tangential excision. West J Med 124:272–275, 1976
22. Burchfield RW (ed): Oxford English Dictionary Supplement, vol 1, p 777
23. Haneke E: Die Sofortentfernung Traumatischer Tatowierungen. Kopfklinik 2:137–138, 1978
24. Bunke HJ, Conway H: Surgery of decorative and traumatic tattoos. Plast Recon Surg 20:67–77, 1957
25. Chai KB: The decorative tattoo: Its removal by dermabrasion. Plast Recon Surg 32:559–563, 1963
26. Clabaugh W: Removal of tattoos by superficial dermabrasion. Arch Derm 98:515–521, 1968
27. Penoff J: Techniques of removal of tattoos. J Dermatol Surg Oncol 5:901, 1979
28. Variot G: Nouveau procède de destruction des tatouages. Compte rendu de la Société de Biologie (Paris) 8:836–838, 1888
29. Berechon E: Histoire Médicale de tatouage. Paris, J.B. Baillère et fils, 1869
30. Klövekorn GH: Ein Einfache Methode der Entfernung von Tatowierungen. Dermat Wochen 101:1271, 1935
31. Crittenden FR Jr: Salabrasion: Removal of tattoos by superficial abrasion with table salt. Cutis 7:295–300, 1971
32. Crittenden FR Jr: Salabrasion—removal of tattoos, in Epstein E, Epstein E Jr (eds): Skin Surgery, Ed. 5. Springfield, Ill, Charles C Thomas, 1982
33. Manchester GH: The removal of commercial tattoos by abrasion with table salt. Plast Recon Surg 53:517–521, 1974
34. Manchester GH: Tattoo removal: A new simple technique. Calif Med 118:10–12, 1973
35. Koerber WA Jr, Price NM: Salabrasion of tattoos: A correlation of the clinical and histological results. Arch Derm 114:884–888, 1978
36. Catterall MD: Removal of Tattoos (letter). Lancet 1(8175):981, 1980
37. Price N: Salabrasion technique of removal of tattoos. J Dermatol Surg Oncol 5:905, 1979
38. Goldman L, et al: Laser treatment of tattoos: A preliminary survey of three years clinical experience. JAMA 201:163–166, 1967
39. Goldman L, et al: Radiation from a Q-switched ruby laser. JID 44:69–71, 1975
40. Laub DR, et al: Preliminary histopathological observation of Q-switched ruby laser radiation on dermal tattoo pigment in man. J Surg Res 8:220–224, 1968
41. Brady SC, Blokmine A, Jewett L: Tattoo removal with a carbon dioxide laser. Ann Plas Surg 2:482–490, 1979
42. Apfelberg DB, Maser MR, Lash H: Argon laser treatment of decorative tattoos. Brit J Plas Surg 32:141–144, 1979
43. Apfelberg DB, Maser MR, Lash H: Extended clinical use of the argon laser for cutaneous lesions. Arch Derm 115:719–721, 1979
44. Apfelberg DB, et al: Pathophysiology and treatment of decorative tattoos with reference to argon laser treatment. Clinics Plas Surg 7:369–377, 1980
45. Apfelberg DB, et al: The argon laser for cutaneous lesions. JAMA 245:2073–2075, 1981
46. Apfelberg DB, et al: Progress report on extended clinical use of the argon laser for cutaneous lesions. Lasers Surg Med 1:71–83, 1980
47. Apfelberg DB, et al: Update on laser usage and treatment of decorative tattoos. Lasers in Surg & Med 2:169–177, 1982
48. Strempel H: Uber die Behandlung von Tatowierungen mit dem Argonlaser. Z Hautkr 57:335–341, 1982
49. Goldstein N, Flores JT: Clinical applications of the argon laser. Haw Med Jour 44:52–57, 1985
50. Dismukes DE: Laser therapy of cutaneous lesions with the argon and CO_2 laser. Proceedings of the 28th annual convention of the American Association of Equine Practitioners. Atlanta, GA, Dec 1982
51. Bailin PL, Ratz JL, Levine HL: Removal of tattoos by CO_2 laser. J Dermatol Surg Oncol 6:997–1001, 1980
52. Bailin PL, Ratz JL, Lutz-Nagey L: CO_2 laser modification of Mohs' surgery. J Dermatol Surg Oncol 7:621–623, 1981
53. Levine H, Bailin PL: Carbon dioxide laser treatment of cutaneous hemangiomas and tattoos. Arc Otolaryngol 108:236–238, 1982

54. Wheeland RG, Bailin PL: Dermatologic applications of the argon and carbon dioxide laser: Current concepts in skin disorders. 5–11 Summer 1984
55. Bailin PL: Lasers in dermatology. J Dermatol Surg Oncol 11:328–334, 1985
56. Zacarian SA: Cryosurgery in dermatology, in Goldsmidt H (ed): Physical Modalities in Dermatologic Therapy. New York, Springer-Verlag, 1978, pp 270–281
57. Zacarian SA: Personal communication, June 28, 1979
58. Goldstein N: Cryosurgery—techniques of removal of tattoos. J Dermatol Surg Oncol 5:905, 1979
59. Gupta SC: An investigation into a method for the removal of dermal tattoos: A report on animal and clinical studies. Plast Recon Surg 36:351–361, 1965
60. Friederich HC: Entfernung von Tatowierungen durch Hautverschiebung. Z Hautkr 57:326–333, 1981
61. Prinz Von L: Uber die Entfernung von Tatowierungen durch Salpetersaure. Dermatol Monatsschr 166:804–809, 1980
62. Ceilley RI: Curettage after dermabrasion—techniques of removal of tattoos. J Dermatol Surg Oncol 5:905, 1979
63. Haneke E: Kombinierte Spalthautlappen und Schleif Oder Exzisionsbehandlung der Tatowierungen. Dermatochirurgie Klinik und Praxis. Berlin, Springer-Verlag, 1977, pp 230–233
64. Arndt KA, Noe J, Rosen S (eds): Cutaneous Laser Therapy: Principles and Methods. New York, John Wiley & Sons, 1983
65. Dixon JA (ed): Surgical Applications of Lasers. Chicago, Year Book Medical Publishers, 1983
66. Oshiro T: Laser Treatment for Nevi. Tokyo, Japan, Medical Laser Research Co, Ltd, 1980

Progress

54

RONALD P. GRUBER, M.D.

Skin Expansion*

One of the fundamental problems of plastic surgery is obtaining skin coverage. Since the turn of the century, skin coverage has been obtained by skin grafting and flaps. In recent years, myocutaneous flaps have made it possible to bring good quality skin with essentially normal texture to various wounds that need repair and closure. More recently, free flaps of tissue have been utilized to reconstruct defects and are used in many situations in which skin and soft tissues are required. The archetypical situation occurs in breast reconstruction. All of the modalities of soft tissue come into play here including local flaps, myocutaneous flaps, and free flaps.

It is odd that it was not until the 1970s that a completely new technique of providing skin coverage should have been thought of—skin expansion. It is particularly odd because the concept of obtaining skin by expansion is as old as mankind itself. Pregnant women have had the abdominal skin stretched, the redundancy of which has been only a source of problems for them. Weight gain can result in an enormous amount of skin development and stretching, and yet this has been overlooked until recently as a potential method by which a new source of skin could be obtained for reconstruction and wound coverage. Exotic customs of various tribes, particularly those in Africa, have also demonstrated that skin expansion is possible. It is known commonly that the lips can be expanded with wooden plates, not to mention the ear lobes and other parts of the body. It was not until the 1970s that Radovan and Austad working independently came upon the idea of using a silicone inflatable implant (Fig. 54–1) that could be slowly expanded over a period of time similar to the overlying skin during pregnancy. This results in an abundance of skin that can then be used to cover an adjacent area or even the immediate area.

PHYSIOLOGY OF SKIN EXPANSION

Before proceeding with the clinical indications and technical procedures by which one can expand skin and obtain the kind of soft tissue required for reconstructive surgery, it is important to understand the microscopic and biochemical changes that happen to the skin when it is expanded by currently available skin expansion implants.

The dermis responds by initially decreasing in its overall thickness. This is not surprising simply because the physical force thins the skin, which if done to excess, is a potential complication and is discussed later. It is one of the problems of expansion done too rapidly. The papillary dermis and reticular dermis become filled with collagen fibers that form thick bundles. This is in response to constant pressure. An increased number of fibroblasts are seen also during this expansion process. Perhaps the dermis is developing a contractile function because myofibroblasts are seen in the dermis during expansion, and of course, these highly specialized cells are associated with contractility. Skin appendages such as hair follicles usually remain unchanged, and blood vessels show no significant structural alterations as a result of the pressure. However, excessive pressure may, by virtue of ischemia and interruption of the circulation, do damage to skin appendages. The latter circumstance, however, is the result of misuse of the skin expansion technique.

Muscle and fat show several interesting changes. Muscle develops a significant decrease in thickness. Its mass decreases during the process of skin expansion. This is probably related to the pressure phenomena. Fat is perhaps the most intolerant of all of the tissues to the pressure of expansion. This is manifested by decrease in the thickness of the fat layers, and by the presence of fewer fat cells during the course of skin expansion. The loss of fat cells may even be permanent. This does not necessarily imply that skin expansion is a means of causing permanent reduction in fat cells within the subcutaneous tissues, although perhaps that is a possible future research project.

Expanding the skin results in a thin layer of scar tissue that is referred to as the capsule. This capsule membrane is of varying thickness and is similar to the capsule membrane associated with silicone implants which have been used for the last 25 years for breast augmentation and reconstruction. Follow-

---

*Editor's note: This is the most important new chapter in this book. Originally, it was planned as Chapter 12, but because of a clerical error, Dr. Gruber was not asked to contribute it until after the book was already in production, He is to be congratulated for writing this excellent chapter in the very short time that he had to introduce us to this major and exciting advance in skin surgery.

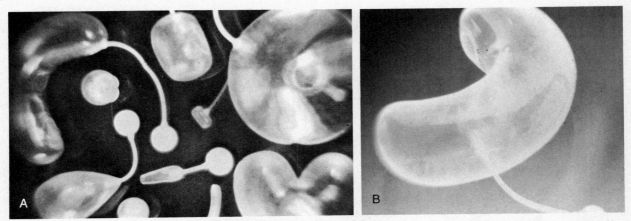

Figure 54–1. *A* and *B*, Various sizes and shapes of implants used for skin expansion. (Courtesy of Cox-Uphoff International.)

ing removal of the prosthesis when the redundant skin has been developed by the process of skin expansion, this capsular membrane rapidly thins. However, in some cases, it persists for well over a year and often a fine, barely noticeable plane remains even one year after implant removal.

Blood vessels proliferate in response to the skin expansion unless the procedure is performed too rapidly. At first, when the skin expansion technique was being developed, there was some concern that there would be less vascularization of the tissues. However, there is actually an increase in vascularity, and this phenomenon has consequently been capitalized upon by many to enhance the ultimate survival of skin flaps. For years, delaying flaps by making one or more incisions and undermining the flaps in an attempt to increase their vascularity was employed. Now, numerous surgeons are using the skin expander in an attempt to increase the vascularity without having to make these specialized incisions.

It is firmly concluded that the blood flow is increased in expanded tissue, and consequently, the surviving length of flaps made of expanded tissue is greater than their control counterparts. In one study by Cherry and colleagues, there was a 117% increase in survival length over control nondelayed flaps as a result of the skin expansion process. When comparing the skin expansion technique to that of a single surgical delay of flaps, they noticed that the conventional delay procedures only resulted in a 73% increase in survival compared to control nondelayed flaps.

There are two main reasons that skin expansion techniques are of particular interest to the field of reconstructive surgery. First and foremost, they are simpler for the patient in terms of morbidity. Unlike many of the other procedures used to obtain soft tissue coverage, there is often actually less surgical intervention. This is true particularly for myocutaneous flaps and especially for free flaps. Secondly, cost-effectiveness is a major consideration for those countries where plastic and reconstructive surgery is an absolute luxury. Skin expansion is something that can be done under local anesthesia, as discussed later with clinical examples. It is a means for obtaining soft tissue coverage for a wide variety of purposes that avoids, in most cases, the need for major operating rooms, general anesthesia, and the associated cost.

CLINICAL INDICATIONS

There are numerous situations in which skin expansion can be employed. These indications have increased since the 1970s when these procedures were first introduced. Breast reconstruction following mastectomy is the most obvious use (Fig. 54–2) and perhaps one of the more fruitful ways in which the skin expander has been employed. It is helpful for the novice surgeon who is doing skin expansion because it lends itself so well to this reconstruction. The chest after a mastectomy has a deficiency of subcutaneous tissue and skin to provide enough ptosis for the breast to assume its natural shape. It is often necessary to provide extra tissue for that purpose. Latissimus dorsi flaps, various myocutaneous flaps, and free flaps have all been used to reconstruct the breast but were fraught with considerable morbidity. Simple implants have often been all that are required, but unless the chest wall has sufficient skin, a simple silicone implant may not suffice. Consequently, the skin expander has been one of the best ways to obtain such extra skin. In particular, it is possible to insert a skin expander and stretch the skin far beyond what is ordinarily required for an implant so that there will be somewhat of a natural ptosis or sag of the breast when the skin expander is replaced with an implant that is much smaller in size. Typically, the skin expander can be used to expand tissue volume to approxi-

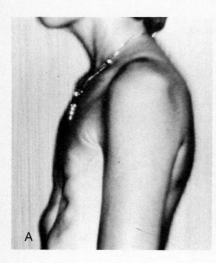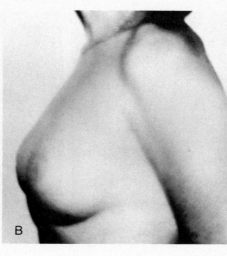

Figure 54–2. Skin expansion for a mastectomy patient. *A,* Preoperative appearance. *B,* Postoperative results. (Courtesy of Dr. John Gibney.)

mately 500 to 700 cc, at which point the implant can be replaced with an implant of 300 to 400 cc. This will produce a mound in the breast, but perhaps a more natural mound than that obtained by an implant alone because the skin is expanded enough for the breast to have a natural sag or ptosis.

An important consideration is to utilize the implant below the pectoralis muscle and possibly also the serratus muscle rather than a superficial placement. Original breast reconstruction was always performed above the muscles, but because of the extra padding afforded by the muscles of the chest wall implants and skin expanders are placed best deeply in the muscle. This often makes it more difficult to find the valve (if it is located directly on the expander) because of the increased soft tissue between the skin expander and the skin surface. However, the extra padding not only is safer during the expansion process but results in a lower incidence of a firm, hard breast (capsular contraction), which is typical of implants used in reconstructed breasts. Radovan's initial procedure used subcutaneous skin expanders. They were accompanied by a very high rate of capsular contraction. Only after the implant was placed beneath the muscle was the incidence of capsular contraction (hard breast) dramatically reduced.

After skin expansion is obtained to the desired volume, a second stage procedure is required in which the skin expander is removed and the cavity replaced with the usual silicone implant. This is usually performed at about two to three months after the expansion is complete, although some surgeons have done it immediately after the expansion. Others have even waited for as long as a year to replace the skin expander with the final implant. Finally, it should be mentioned that, in a few selected mastectomy patients, skin expanders have been placed at the time of the mastectomy followed by a gradual expansion of the soft tissues at approximately two to three weeks following the mastectomy.

One of the technical keys to breast reconstruction using the skin expander involves placing an expander just below the intended inframammary line (about 2 to 4 cm). There is a tendency for implants to rise postoperatively contrary to one's intuition and counter to the action of gravity.

It should be mentioned that capsulotomy (release of the capsule) is often performed when the expander is removed in an attempt to expand the tissues further and to achieve further advancement of the adjacent soft tissues. This additional release and advancement of soft tissues provides much more skin to give a more natural slightly sagging ptotic breast. Many surgeons feel that this additional procedure is unnecessary.

The scalp is a region of the body where the skin expander has special uses. The expander was originally used for traumatic deformities when conventional flap rotation procedures could not solve the problem. Serial excisions were one way to close large scalp defects, but it soon became apparent that this method of obtaining wound coverage was inadequate compared with the skin expander. Numerous cases have been seen in which the skin expander is placed in the subgaleal space, and skin expansion (using a distantly located valve) has resulted in stretching of the adjacent hair-bearing skin so that, when the device is removed, very large portions of the scalp can be covered. It is of interest that even galeotomies are not necessary, as one might expect, in order for the skin to expand. Starting with the first cases in Japan, the skin expander has been used to treat male pattern baldness. By placing one or more implants over the hair-bearing area that remains in the temporal regions, these portions of skin can be expanded sufficiently to cover large portions of the non–hair-bearing skin and thereby avoid the ordeal associated with hair plugs and other types of hair-bearing flap rotation procedures. One of the obvious drawbacks of using skin expanders in the scalp, whether for traumatic defects or cosmetic problems, is that the head appears unusually bulky and large for a number of weeks, if not months, prior to the final stage when the expanded skin can be set into its final location.

One of the best uses of the skin expander has been for scalp reconstruction in children who have hair loss and who would otherwise be candidates for almost any procedure in which hair-bearing skin can be brought to cover areas of alopecia. Frequently, multiple expanders placed in different locations around the scalp have been necessary to obtain a satisfactory result. The valves for these skin expanders are often located in the neck in order to provide access for filling of the expandable device.

The head and neck is another area where skin expanders are helpful. One of the earliest cases involved a large port-wine stain of the face that would be difficult to treat by any other approach. Serial incisions, which was a previous method used to treat this problem, often involves multiple anesthetics and operations. Skin grafts, which have also been employed for these problems, often lack the proper color and texture to correctly improve the deformity. The laser has recently provided improvements for patients with port-wine stains, but the color and texture can only infrequently be restored to a near-normal appearance. The skin expander, however, has made many cases of port-wine stains and other types of defects (particularly on the lateral portion of the face) amenable to complete excision. Often 300 to 400 cc of material can be gradually injected into the skin expander over a period of time so that there will ultimately be a large amount of soft tissue to cover the defect when the lesion is finally surgically extirpated.

The concept of obtaining additional skin has been helpful when trying to perform total nasal reconstruction. One of the primary problems of nasal reconstruction is inadequacy of the forehead tissue for reconstructing the entire nose. By expanding the forehead tissue prior to the usual nasal reconstruction, there is an abundance of tissue available for the nose. In addition, the donor site that remains in the forehead after transferring tissue to the nose can then be closed with less tension and without as much reduction in the overall forehead dimensions. Moreover, the skin that results from the expansion process is thinner and more suited to being contoured over the bone and cartilaginous framework giving a superior aesthetic appearance. In this instance, the thinning of the skin by the skin expander has a very beneficial effect. This well-vascularized yet thin skin that results from the expander has occasionally been enough to not only reconstruct the nose but also provide enough skin to fold it upon itself and thereby lessen the need for a skin graft or other lining on the interior of the newly reconstructed nose.

Finally, the extremities (Fig. 54–3) are yet another area of the body where skin expanders have proved themselves to be a significant and potentially useful tool in the armamentarium of the reconstructive surgeon. There have been numerous cases involving both lower and upper extremities that were not easily treatable by conventional means. In particu-

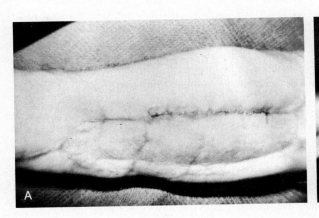
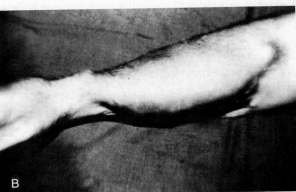
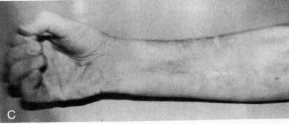

Figure 54–3. Skin expansion for a patient's forearm defects. A, Preoperative appearance. B, Inflated expander in place. C, Postoperative result after expander was removed. (Courtesy of Dr. John Gibney.)

lar, defects of the legs following automobile accidents and other trauma were not worth correcting because the new tissue was often not of the same color or texture. Even if a free flap was used, there was always a problem with a mismatch. Free flaps also leave donor defects. Skin grafts in particular are associated with this mismatch problem. Serial incision poses its own potential complications, not to mention the fact that serial incision can seldom correct all the problems, unless the defect is small. Skin expanders, on the other hand, have permitted a large piece of tissue to be harvested without creating a deformity in the donor area.

A patient with a large defect of the calf, for example, can undergo a replacement using normal tissue from the other side of the leg that has been expanded to completely cover the defect. One of the great nuisances that must be recognized with the skin expansion technique, however, is that time is required to obtain this expansion. During that time, the patient must make multiple visits to the physician for injections and expansion of the tissue. As the expander becomes full of fluid, it is conspicuous visually and causes a heavy sensation because of its location. This is especially true for skin expanders on the extremities. The more distal the expander is on the extremity and the more expansion needed, the more weight has to be carried by the patient. More recently, exciting innovations for the use of the expander have included the correction of syndactyly by expanding the adjacent skin and thereby avoiding or minimizing the need for skin grafts and other types of local flaps on the fingers.

One point of caution should be made about the lower extremities: The use of skin expanders, by virtue of the undermining and pressure, can interfere with the lymphatics causing additional edema of the lower extremity. Until improved techniques are devised, caution is urged in the use of expanders in these areas where extensive trauma has occurred, such as in degloving injuries and lower extremity injuries where good lymphatic return does not exist.

TECHNICAL DETAILS INVOLVED WITH SKIN EXPANDERS

Since the skin expander is a foreign body and since filling it with saline solution puts pressure on the overlying tissues, one of the major concerns is to avoid harm to the incision through which it is inserted. Consequently, whenever possible, the incision should be located away from the skin expander itself. Frequently, this cannot be avoided. Often, the incision is at the edge of the implant.

There are two basic types of skin expanders: one with the filling valve located directly on it and one with the valve at a distant site. The technique is slightly different in both cases. When the valve is located on the main body of the expander, there is the advantage of not having to make a separate tunnel for the tubing of a distantly located valve. However, it is often difficult to palpate the valve within the main body of the skin expander. It should be mentioned that this valve component of the implant must be secured to the subcutaneous tissues so that it will not shift and can be found easily. When using the distantly located valve, a separate tunnel often must be constructed, and in some cases, a separate incision must be made.

As a general rule, the skin expander is placed within a cavity approximately the same size as the device. At the time of surgery, the skin expander is filled with just enough soution to fill this cavity which can amount to 30 to 200 cc of saline. More solution than that is not used because tension on the suture line is undesirable whether it is directly over the skin expander or adjacent to it.

Two to three weeks later (sometimes earlier), skin expansion can be started. The amount of fluid used (by injecting a 23- or 25-gauge needle into the valve) depends strictly upon the surgeon's judgment and the nature of the tissue. The surgeon can gauge the amount of the injection by the color the overlying tissue assumes. If pallor develops, he or she has injected too much fluid. If the patient complains of pain, too much fluid has been injected. Frequently, 10 to 30 or as much as 50 cc can be injected in any one sitting for breast implants. As a general rule, it is better to underinflate than overinflate and risk causing damage by pressure to the soft tissues.

Some surgeons inject the saline on a weekly basis, some as frequently as every three days. In addition, it should be mentioned that the tissue may not initially expand very much, and this frustrates the surgeon. However, suddenly on the third or fourth office visit, there may be a change in the tissues, which respond more easily, and less pressure is required to instill the fluid through the small-gauge needle. Occasionally, the surgeon may want to use a scalp vein to avoid damage to the valve resulting from too much motion.

As a general rule, once full expansion has taken place, the actual expanded hemispheric dome of the flap can be measured by the surgeon. Advancement in centimeters is then anticipated as one half of the ultimate flap length, i.e., advancement in centimeters is equal to approximately one half of the length of the expanded flap in centimeters.

There are a number of helpful hints in the process of inserting the skin expander, performing the expansion, and obtaining the desired result. When using distant sites for valve placement, careful attention should be paid to any twisting or distortion so that the distantly located valve does not turn over. Care must also be taken to place the distantly located valve in a relatively superficial location so that it can be palpated. Placing the valve carefully and properly in a suitable pocket is important so that one does not inadvertently puncture the tubing that connects the valve to the main body of the skin expander, causing a leak.

When the skin expander is replaced with a silicone gel implant or when it is simply removed and the expanded skin used for reconstructive purposes, a separate incision is often required to remove the valve.

The pocket that is created for the skin expander should be approximately the size of the skin expander itself. This avoids kinking and distortion of the device and allows for a homogeneous expansion of all the surrounding subcutaneous tissues. The use of drains is optional depending on the surgeon's judgment about whether he or she expects the surgical field to develop a serous fluid postoperatively.

In some instances, there may be a need to make small incisions within the capsule that develops underneath the expanded skin. Although this does carry with it some risk of interfering with the circulation, some surgeons have found that the flap becomes more elastic and expansile if this release maneuver is performed. Such releasing incisions allow the surgeon to unfurl the expanded flap more completely.

COMPLICATIONS OF TISSUE EXPANSION

The complication rate has been reported at 7%, but this varies with the surgical series reviewed. Exposure of the implant is a potential but avoidable problem, as mentioned previously. Inability to complete the expansion process because the valve is no longer palpable or because a puncture of the implant has occurred is another potential problem that can also be avoided. Infection is a potential complication with the insertion of any foreign body. Preoperative intravenous antibiotics and/or oral antibiotics are prescribed frequently by surgeons using skin expansion. Mechanical failures such as deflation are fortunately uncommon. Neuropraxia is rare but has been reported when the implant was near a nerve. Apparently, pressure from the implant is responsible for this effect. Severe pain is not necessarily an actual conplication but perhaps reflects an overzealous attempt to expand the tissues too rapidly. Some

of the problems of loss of skin viability are avoided by carefully inspecting the tissues at the time of skin expansion and looking for color changes.

A disappointing result is encountered occasionally because the surgeon anticipated a harvest of more skin than what was actually obtained. This problem is often due to improperly planning the amount of possible expansion. In addition, it should be noted that at times the skin contracts after the expanded skin flap is put into place. This broadens the scar that might have been relatively narrow when the newly expanded skin flap was inserted. This occurs frequently and is similar to the scars from serial incisions that start to broaden as the tissues retract. It is for this reason that skin should be expanded to a size that is significantly larger than anticipated.

One final minor potential complication or actually undesirable effect is the time and effort required of both patient and physician. Skin expansion requires multiple office visits and at least a two-stage procedure. During that time when the skin expander is large and bulky, it may be difficult for the patient to carry it about and may be cosmetically unacceptable.

Despite these shortcomings and potential complications, skin expansion has taken its place in the armamentarium of soft tissue and skin replacement and will undoubtedly remain as one of the best means by which skin and soft tissue can be fabricated for purposes of reconstructive surgery.

SUGGESTED READINGS

Argenta LC, Marks MW, Grabb WC: Selective use of serial expansion in breast reconstruction. Ann Plast Surg 11:181, 1983.

Argenta LC: Controlled tissue expansion and reconstructive surgery. Br J Plast Surg 37:371, 1984.

Austad ED, Pasyk KA, McClatchey KD, Cherry GW: Histologic evaluation of guinea pig and soft tissues after controlled tissue expansion. Plast Reconstr Surg 70:705, 1982.

Cherry GW, Austad ED, Pasyk KA, Rohrich RJ: Increased survival and vascularity of random pattern skin flaps elevated in controlled expanded skin. Plast Reconstr Surg 72:680, 1983.

Radovan C: Reconstruction of the breast after radical mastectomy using a temporary expander. Presented at American Society of Plastic and Reconstructive Surgery Forum, Hollywood, Florida, Nov 8, 1978.

Radovan C: Breast reconstruction after mastectomy using the temporary expander. Plast Reconstr Surg 69:195, 1981.

Saski GH, Krizek TJ: Horizons in Plastic Surgery. Clinics in Plastic Surgery, April 1985.

55

C. WILLIAM HANKE, M.D.

Ideas and Innovations in Skin Surgery

Field, who wrote the chapter on "Ideas and Innovations" for the fifth edition of this book, highlighted the developments of the previous 10 years in cutaneous surgery. The present author has attempted to provide an update of Dr. Field's work. The references cited are taken largely from the *Journal of Dermatologic Surgery and Oncology*, the *Journal of the American Academy of Dermatology*, *Archives of Dermatology*, *Annals of Plastic Surgery*, *Plastic and Reconstructive Surgery*, and the *British Journal of Plastic Surgery*.

Two textbooks of basic and advanced skin surgery have recently been published by Stegman and coworkers.[1, 2] These works should be considered required reading for all who are interested in cutaneous surgery.

INSTRUMENTATION

Wearing gloves for all office surgical procedures can protect physicians and office surgical personnel from contracting hepatitis B virus (HBV).[3] Surgical tape can be applied to the tips of gloved fingers in order to prevent accidental puncture by serrated punches during hair transplantation.[4] Tiny punctures in the gloves can expose the physician to the risk of hepatitis B. The rubber-free Elastyren glove is a good substitute for rubber surgical gloves in rubber-sensitive individuals.[5]

Lewis[6] has used methoxyflurane inhalant as a preoperative analgesic for 15 years of office surgery without adverse reaction. Rounded scalpel handles are preferred by some surgeons.[7] A sterile Penrose drain can be slipped over a Birtcher Hyfrecator handle to maintain a sterile field during surgery.[8] This avoids the necessity of autoclaving the handle before every use. Alternatively, an ungloved assistant touches a bipolar electrocoagulation tip to the hinge area of the surgeon's hemostat to produce hemostasis.[9] Stegman and coworkers[10] have described an adapter tip for the Birtcher Hyfrecator which can be fitted with a disposable 30-gauge needle for treating telangiectasias relatively painlessly.

An electric scalpel has been introduced that provides instant coagulation of blood vessels as the surgeon cuts with the blade.[11] Double scalpels and double punches have been developed for more precise margin control in excising primary skin cancers.[12]

The use of surgical staples can reduce closure time in scalp reduction, split-thickness grafting, axillary vault resections, and truncal excisions.[13] The corneal shield is an easily inserted protective device for periorbital surgery.[14] The Pron Pillo is a device for obtaining proper head positioning during hair transplantation surgery.[15]

WOUND HEALING, CUTANEOUS ULCERS, AND DRESSINGS

The effects of systemic medications on wound healing have been reviewed by Pollack.[16] Modern concepts of wound healing have also been summarized.[17] Robins and coworkers[18] studied Mohs surgical wounds with multivariate analysis techniques and found the width of the wound to be the best predictor of wound-healing time. In studies of healing by second intention, wounds on concave surfaces were found to heal with better cosmesis than wounds on convex surfaces.[19]

Eighteen patients with basal cell carcinomas of the medial canthus were allowed to heal by second intention following standard excisional surgery.[20] The cosmetic and functional results were good. This was apparently new information to the authors, but Mohs has been lecturing and writing about similar observations for 50 years. Skin graft donor sites, chemically peeled skin, and excisions were irradiated with ultraviolet light in order to assess hyperpigmentation.[21] There was no evidence of ultraviolet exposure in the irradiated areas after three years. Factors other than ultraviolet light can contribute to abnormal pigmentation following surgical procedures.

Krull has reviewed the processes involved in the development of leg ulcers.[22] Stasis ulcers treated with Unna's paste boots healed faster than leg ulcers treated with elastic graded-compression stockings.[23] Gilmore and Wheeland have simplified pinch-grafting for leg ulcers by covering the pinch-grafts with a semipermeable dressing (Op-Site).[24] A 20% benzoyl peroxide lotion increased wound re-epithelialization in young domestic pigs by 33%.[25] Topical nitroglycerin ointment can be used to heal digital ulcers.[26]

Vigilon is a new wound dressing consisting of polyethylene oxide and 96% water.[27] This nonadherent occlusive dressing absorbs its weight in wound exudate and may promote more rapid healing. In studies on Yorkshire pigs, polyethylene oxide hydrogel dressings (Vigilon) promoted re-epithelialization by 44%, and copolymer starch hydrogel dressings (Bard Absorption Dressing) promoted re-epithelialization by 24%.[28] In another study, hydrocolloid dressings (DuoDerm) and polyurethane film dressings (Op-Site) accelerated epidermal wound healing by 40%.[29] Healing of ulcers under Op-Site has been found to be 2.6 times faster than controls.[30] Hydrocolloid dressings (DuoDerm) are convenient to use and can provide relief of pain in treating leg ulcers of various etiologies.[31] Alper and colleagues[32] have outlined the details of the application of vapor-permeable membranes for leg ulcers.

Angermeier and associates[33] treated two patients successfully with Op-Site for chronic ulcerations secondary to arterial insufficiency and osteomyelitis. Zitelli warns that semiocclusive dressings (e.g., Op-Site or DuoDerm) can delay wound healing if they are changed too frequently.[34]

LASER SURGERY

Bailin has reviewed the use of lasers in dermatology.[35] Moreno and coworkers studied the epidermal outgrowths from laser- and scalpel-cut explants in vitro.[36] They found that delayed onset of epidermal migration may be the factor responsible for slower epithelialization of skin wounds incised by a carbon dioxide laser.

Landthaler and colleagues reported good results in 70% of adult patients with port-wine stains treated with the argon laser.[37] Results were less satisfactory in patients under 18 years of age. Results were not good for the eradication of tattoos. Apfelberg and associates found the histologic and clinical outcomes of decorative tattoos treated with a carbon dioxide or argon laser to be similar.[38] Ratz and coworkers feel that the carbon dioxide laser may have advantages over the argon laser in treating some port-wine stains.[39]

McBurney and Rosen reported that 81% of recalcitrant-wart patients were free of lesions six months following a single carbon dioxide laser treatment.[40]

Persky treated a patient with oral florid papillomatosis on the hard palate, superior alveolar ridge, and buccal-gingival sulcus with a carbon dioxide laser with good results.[41] A patient with granuloma faciale on the nose was successfully treated with carbon dioxide laser vaporization.[42] Several authors have reported good results in treating patients with multiple trichoepitheliomas with carbon dioxide laser vaporization.[43, 44] Apfelberg and associates treated a multitude of skin lesions successfully with the argon laser including granuloma faciale, hereditary hemorrhagic telangiectasia, venous lakes, senile angiomas, pyogenic granulomas, acne rosacea, and nevus of Ota.[45]

David treated eight patients with actinic cheilitis with a carbon dioxide laser.[46] Cosmetic results were excellent and there was no recurrence of disease during a follow-up period of 27 to 34 months.

TATTOO REMOVAL

Six tattoo-removal techniques were compared in the pig model.[47] Tattoos treated by tannic acid and the carbon dioxide laser had better results than dermabrasion, split-thickness excision, and salabrasion. Serial split-thickness tangential excisions followed by polyurethane membrane dressings have been used for tattoo removal with encouraging results.[48] Robinson uses gradle scissors to excise the deep portions of tattoos immediately following dermabrasion.[49]

Pseudolymphomatous hypersensitivity reactions to tattoo pigments must be differentiated from true lymphomas.[50]

INJECTION THERAPY

Castrow and Krull surveyed 434 physicians who utilized injectable collagen (Zyderm) for the treatment of soft-tissue deficiencies.[51] The incidence of adverse reactions was very low, and their severity was not significant. Successful treatment with injectable collagen is technique-dependent.[52] Lesions most likely to be improved include soft distensible acne scars, glabellar frown lines, nasolabial lines, postrhinoplasty irregularities, and depressed skin grafts. Detailed descriptions of injection techniques have been presented by experienced investigators.[52–54]

A prospective study of 312 patients who received injectable collagen for soft-tissue deficiencies was carried out for duration of correction.[55] Patients receiving injectable collagen for scarring began to lose correction after nine to 12 months, and patients receiving injectable collagen for age-related rhytids began to lose correction after six months.

A study of positive injectable collagen skin test sites concluded that the granulomatous material was a combination of injected collagen and altered human collagen.[56] Swanson and colleagues reported that treatment site granulomas lasting several months can be seen in patients who have had a negative skin sensitivity test to injectable collagen.[57] Burke and coworkers studied injectable collagen in the pig dermis and were not able to identify the material after six weeks using multiple methods.[58] The authors felt the injected collagen had been replaced by host collagen.

Immune responses to injectable collagen are usually localized reactions that occur during the first two exposures to the material.[59] Anti-injectable collagen antibodies do not cross-react with human dermal collagen.[60]

Injectable collagen can be used for the correction of depressed scars resulting from Mohs surgery.[61] Angular cheilosis was corrected in two patients with injectable collagen treatments.[62] One patient with localized morphea on the face was treated successfully with injectable collagen with good results.[63]

Bodian has described his time-tested technique for treating sunburst varicosities with 23.4% saline (sclerotherapy).[64] This is an effective, easily learned treatment for an unsightly cosmetic problem. Other authors have used sodium tetradecyl sulfate as the sclerosing agent.[65] Green and Morgan utilized a 1:1 mixture of sodium tetradecyl sulfate and Haemaccel 3.5%.[66] The mixture is injected through a 27-gauge butterfly needle.

DERMABRASION

Six skin refrigerants used for dermabrasion were evaluated for maximum cooling temperature using thermocouple monitoring.[67] Some of the recently marketed skin refrigerants were found to be pure sources of Freon 12 or mixtures of Freon 12 and Freon 11. These newer, colder preparations are felt to be dangerous and may lead to complications following dermabrasion.

Dermabrasion may be a more easily tolerated and effective treatment than topical 5-fluorouracil for multiple actinic keratoses on the face.[68] Nine acne patients who had been treated with 13-*cis*-retinoic acid were dermabraded without complication.[69] However, the authors have encountered unusual hypertrophic scarring in several additional patients. Dermabrasion continues to be an excellent treatment for accidental tattoos from gunshot blasts.[70]

Lapins achieved a good result with dermabrasion in a patient with multiple telangiectases on the nose.[71] Facial candidosis may be an uncommon complication of dermabrasion.[72] Amniotic membranes have been used as dressings in dermabrasion patients with healing in five to seven days.[73]

If chemabrasion (i.e., chemical peel followed immediately by dermabrasion) is to be performed, 50% trichloroacetic acid is the simplest and safest peeling agent to use.[74]

HAIR TRANSPLANTATION

Alt has described the essential techniques for avoiding distortion in cutting ideal hair transplant donor grafts.[75] The essentials include firm saline infiltration and sharp carbon steel punches rotated at 5000 rpm by an electrical engine. Pinski has used similar techniques to obtain the "perfect" plug.[76]

Unger has accumulated an extensive experience in transplanting for patients with "early" androgenetic alopecia and feels it has definite advantages.[77]

Sturm performs total harvesting of donor sites followed by a two-layer closure technique. The advantages of this method are: (1) conservation of donor sites, (2) ease of donor harvesting through multiple sessions, (3) mimimal chance of postoperative hemorrhage, (4) improved cosmesis, and (5) patient preference. Disadvantages include: (1) minimally decreased quality of some of the donor grafts, (2) increased operating time, (3) increased telogen effluvium in donor sites, and (4) relative thinning of donor sites. Unger argues against total donor site harvesting (i.e., cluster harvesting) because of the inferior grafts and narrowing of the donor sites that result.[79] He proposes "collapse" closure of the donor sites with a minimum number of sutures.

Nordström and Holsti used punch grafting to treat two patients with alopecia caused by radiation exposure and had good results.[80] Occasionally, a patient may be seen with multiple pyogenic granuloma-like lesions in the recipient areas.[81] Alkyl-2-cyanoacrylates can be used as tissue adhesives in hair transplantation.[82] This avoids the necessity for bulky dressings.

After a number of reports of complications, synthetic fiber implantation has finally been banned by the FDA.[83]

Garden and Robinson treated a 26-year-old man with cutis verticis gyrata with scalp reduction; the problem was totally resolved. Similarly, McCray and Roenigk treated a patient with cutis aplasia congenita with scalp reduction surgery.[85] Scalp reduction, initially developed for cosmetic conditions, has now been extended to the treatment of certain diseases.

Unger does "mini" scalp reductions at the same time as punch hair transplants.[86] Another author advocates greater utilization of the Y-shaped scalp reduction.[87]

Nordström reports 33% to 50% "stretch-back" in the first eight to 12 months following scalp reduction.[88] He has also described a method of disguising scars in hair transplant surgery by beveling "out" the skin edges and making the hair grow through the scar.[89]

Norwood and associates have outlined the potential complications of scalp reduction and the methods of correction.[90] Scalp reduction procedures sometimes give an unnatural look to the crown area. Frechet prefers to use punch grafts in this area rather than attempt to reduce it by excision.[91] Wheeland and Bailin have utilized the carbon dioxide laser for "bloodless" scalp reduction surgery.[92]

Hair-bearing flaps are suggested for patients with fine sparse hair who desire a strong frontal hairline.[93] Bouhanna utilizes a staged postauricular transposition flap to reconstruct the frontal hairline.[94]

The subgaleal implantation of Radovan tissue expanders can effectively stretch the scalp for hair transplant surgery and other procedures.[95, 96]

MOHS SURGERY

Swanson has provided an excellent review of the Mohs surgical technique, its indications, and its applications.[97] A five-year cure rate of 93.3% was achieved with Mohs surgery in 414 cutaneous squamous cell carcinomas.[98] Abide and coworkers pointed out the nonuniformity of processing of surgical specimens by general pathologists.[99] Five of 16 plastic surgeons queried by the authors did not understand that "margins" as reported by the pathologists are merely samplings from the surgical specimens.

The use of a unique tissue-flattening device, "the Miami Special," can markedly reduce frozen section processing time in Mohs surgery.[100] Reliability data on all cryostats used in Mohs surgery has been collected.[101, 102] A nontoxic, nonflammable mixture of orange and corn oils has been developed as a substitute for xylene in the pathology laboratory.[103] The quality of the slides prepared with the mixture (Histo-Clear) is similar to that of xylene. The super widefield microscope offers the surgeon performing Mohs surgery a much larger viewing area.[104] This causes less eye strain by allowing much more of the viewer's visual fields to be utilized.

Tissue staining with monoclonal antibodies may improve the accuracy of Mohs surgery.[105]

Early reconstruction of post-Mohs surgical defects can be performed safely without complications.[106] When the periosteum requires removal during Mohs surgery, portions of the outer table of bone can be chiseled out to stimulate granulation tissue.[107] Osteomyelitis can occur occasionally in cases where exposed bone is allowed to heal over by second intention.[108]

Lateral rhinotomy can be performed to gain exposure to carcinomas that extend inside the nose.[109]

Fleishmann and associates treated a patient with an unusual microcystic adnexal carcinoma on the cheek successfully with Mohs surgery.[110] Dzubow treated two patients with sebaceous carcinomas of the eyelids with Mohs surgery and feels it is the treatment of choice.[111] Pollack and Goslen treated a patient with Merkel cell carcinoma on the scalp with Mohs surgery.[112] Cottel has described his experience in treating 13 difficult squamous cell carcinomas (with perineural invasion) with multidisciplinary Mohs surgery.[113] Dystrophic calcification secondary to radiodermatitis can be treated with fixed-tissue Mohs surgery.[114] Dermatofibrosarcoma protuberans is easily traced with Mohs surgery and has become the treatment of choice for this troublesome tumor.[115, 116]

Treatment of epithelioma cuniculatum with Mohs surgery can be performed instead of amputation.[117, 118] A large, ulcerating granular cell tumor was treated successfully with Mohs surgery.[119]

BENIGN TUMORS

Congenital smooth muscle hamartomas can masquerade as congenital pigmented nevi.[120] Liquid nitrogen cryosurgery may be more helpful than dermabrasion for some inflammatory linear verrucous epidermal nevi.[121] Hoehn uses a combination of surgical cystotomy and chemical cautery with silver nitrate for ablation of pilonidal cysts.[122] Useful surgical approaches for treating myxoid cysts of the proximal nail fold have been described.[123, 124]

Surgical excision followed by the injection of triamcinolone 40 mg/ml was successful in 20 patients with earlobe keloids.[125] The injection of keloids with syringe and needle delivers a more precise dose of triamcinolone than needleless injectors.[126] A "core" excision of earlobe keloids provides a dumbbell-shaped specimen.[127] The wound can be closed primarily and is followed by intralesional steroids. The results have been excellent. Keloids have been reported to respond poorly to cryosurgery with liquid nitrogen.[128] In contradistinction, freezing keloids with circulating N_2O may give good results.[129]

MALIGNANT TUMORS

McDaniel reported a five-year cure rate of 91.5% for basal cell carcinomas treated with curettage.[130] In another study, five-year recurrence rates for basal cell carcinomas were reported to be 26% for curettage-electrodesiccation, 9.7% for x-ray therapy, and 9.3% for surgical excision.[131] Microscopic persistence of tumor has been found in 33% of basal cell carcinomas treated with curettage and electrodesiccation three times.[132] In another study, 30% of basal cell carcinomas on the nose and in the nasolabial fold were found to contain residual tumor after being treated by curettage and electrodesiccation.[133] There does not appear to by any significant difference in cure rate between basal cell carcinomas treated three times with curettage and electrodesiccation compared with a single curettage and electrodesiccation.[134]

Solar elastosis, as one would expect, was seen as an associated finding in 93% of basal cell carcinomas.[135]

The recurrence rate was 21% when superficial basal cell carcinomas were treated with 25% 5-fluorouracil (5-FU) under occlusion for three weeks.[136] The recurrence rate dropped to 6% when light curettage preceded the topical 5-FU treatment. The temple area should be considered at high risk for basal cell carcinoma as well as the periauricular, periocular, perinasal areas, and the scalp.[137] Basal cell carcinoma rarely invades the perineural sheath. This occurs most commonly in men with recurrent basal cell carcinomas.[138] Mohs surgery provides the best chance of cure.

Metastatic basal cell carcinoma is a rare event; however, the median survival after first metastasis is only eight months.[139] Chemotherapy with cisplatin and bleomycin sulfate caused a temporary response in a keratinizing basal cell carcinoma that had metastasized to the skeleton.[140] Cristofolini and co-workers treated a patient with nevoid basal cell carcinoma syndrome with etretinate who had a regression of 83% of the tumors for one year.[141]

Lund has reviewed his experience again as a pathologist in North Carolina, and feels that metastasis from sun-induced squamous cell carcinoma is a distinctly uncommon event.[142] Epstein has warned us to be aggressive in treating sun-induced squamous cell carcinomas of the skin because of the potential for metastasis.[143]

Mora and Perniciaro found a 19.4% mortality from squamous cell carcinoma of the lip in blacks.[144] Invasive squamous cell carcinoma developed in five of 19 black patients with Bowen's disease.[145] Bowen's disease in blacks develops on non–sun-exposed sites three times more frequently than on sun-exposed sites.

To avoid problems in management, some authors feel that all keratoacanthomas should be managed by surgical excision.[146]

Hanke and associates reported three black women with plantar verrucous carcinomas.[147] Two of the patients were treated with Mohs surgery without recurrence. Four Japanese patients have been reported with metastasizing squamous cell carcinomas derived from solar keratoses.[148] An 83-year-old woman with multiple keratoacanthomas and squamous cell carcinomas was treated with oral 13-cis-retinoic acid for six months.[149] All tumors resolved and new ones were slow to develop. In this patient, the retinoid may have functioned as a chemotherapeutic agent as well as a chemopreventive agent.

Painful or blistering sunburns in childhood or adolescence have been associated with an increased risk of developing malignant melanoma.[150] Margins of greater than 3 cm for malignant melanoma excision are felt to be unwarranted.[151] Day and colleagues have provided good reasons to abandon wide excision (greater than 3 cm margins) for Stage I melanomas.[152] Many "thin" melanomas can be treated with margins of 1.5 cm or less. Fisher has recommended 1 cm margins for melanomas of less than 1.69 mm in depth, 2 cm margins for melanomas of 1.70 to 3.6 mm in depth, and 3 cm margins if the depth is greater than 3.6 mm. Certain anatomic locations for Stage I melanoma (e.g., the scalp, mandibular area, midline trunk, upper medial thighs, feet, hands, genitalia, and popliteal fossae) indicate a higher risk for recurrence.[154]

The mortality rate for blacks with Kaposi's sarcoma was 21% at Charity Hospital in New Orleans.[155] Mean survival for all patients in the study was 6.1 years. Sebaceous carcinomas have a 23% incidence of recurrence after wide excision.[156] The mortality rate at five years approaches 30%.

INFORMED CONSENT

Redden and Baker have reviewed the problem of informed consent with respect to dermatologists and other physicians who perform cosmetic surgery.[157] Wright has described the personality characteristics of the potential problem patient.[158] Her comments on patient evaluation and the dissatisfied patient provide invaluable insights for physicians and staff.

EXCISIONAL SURGERY

Stegman has devised a method for protecting buried sutures from tearing under tension by applying skin sutures over the buried sutures.[159] It is helpful to perform an intraoral submental nerve block and also to ligate the labial artery prior to doing wedge resections of the lip.[160] Harahap has reviewed the techniques for repairing split earlobes.[161]

Hill has reported good results with radical excision and reconstruction of axillae in patients with chronic hidradenitis suppurativa and severe hyperhidrosis.[162]

CHEMICAL PEEL

Resnik uses 20% to 30% trichloroacetic acid for superficial peeling.[163] The technique can be repeated weekly or monthly. Deep peels with 50% to 70% trichloroacetic acid can be done without the toxic risks of phenol peels.

Pigmentary difficulties are the most common complication of phenol face peels. Hypertrophic scarring has been encountered by 21% of plastic surgeons who perform the procedure.[164] Cardiac monitoring during phenol peels is being utilized more commonly by physicians.

Rapaport and Kamer reported four patients who developed facial herpes simplex following phenol face peels.[165] They suggest the incidence of this association may be fairly high. Phenol face peels in previously irradiated skin should be performed cautiously to avoid full-thickness skin loss.[166]

CRYOSURGERY

A cure rate of 98.8% has been reported for actinic keratoses treated with liquid nitrogen cryosurgery.[167] Zacarian reported 96.4% to 97.4% cure rates for 4228 carcinomas treated with cryosurgery.[168] Of 100 recurrences, 36 were recurrent tumors, and 86.6% appeared in the first three years following cryosurgery. Of the 20 patients with lentigo maligna treated with cryosurgery, only 10% had recurrences.[169] A case of elastosis perforans serpiginosa was treated successfully with liquid nitrogen cryosurgery.[170] Elton has reviewed the complications of cryosurgery.[171]

NAIL SURGERY

Herold and coworkers reported 339 patients who underwent radical wedge resection for ingrown toenails with excellent results.[172] Thomsen and associates have successfully treated pachyonychia congenita with curettage and electrofulguration of the matrices and nail beds.[173] The basic principles of nail surgery have been reviewed by Siegle and Swanson.[174]

AESTHETIC SURGERY

Webster recognized that reconstructive and cosmetic surgical procedures are now taught in many dermatology residency programs and that many of the procedures cross specialty lines. A monopoly cannot be granted to any single specialty "as long as the quality of care and the costs are competitive."[175]

Blepharoplasty can be done with electrosurgery instead of using a scalpel.[176] Conservative blepharoplasties can be performed on patients with palpebral deformities with low tear production.[177] Patients with Sjögren's syndrome or severe dry eye syndrome should not be treated by this surgical operation.

Transblepharoplasty brow suspension has the advantage of not producing any additional scars.[178] Small vertical wedge resections of skin at the eyelid margin can be done during blepharoplasty in order to prevent ectropion.[179]

Granulomas and cysts caused by buried eyelashes can occur occasionally following blepharoplasty.[180] Orbital abscess is a rare complication of blepharoplasty.[181] Numbness following blepharoplasty is seen in less than 1% of patients, and is caused by damage to the terminal branches of the ophthalmic division of the trigeminal nerve.[182]

Surgical transsection of the temporal branch of the facial nerve results in an inability to wrinkle the forehead and in ptosis of the eyebrow.[183] Various corrective procedures can be performed including direct brow lift, upper lid blepharoplasty, and indirect temporal or coronal brow lift.

LIPOSUCTION

Newman and Dolsky have reviewed the history and development of liposuction surgery.[184] Many dermatologists are currently using this modality of treatment. Field has provided a fine overview of the subject.[185] Liposuction was performed on fresh cadavers in order to study the effect of the procedure on the tissues microscopically.[186] Some liposuction surgeons always use general anesthesia.[187] Others prefer epidural blocks.[188] Patients become mobile as soon as they are awake. In seven years, there were no cases of infection, fat embolism, or thrombosis. Crisman and Field have used liposuction as an adjunctive technique in face-lift surgery.[189] Intravenous fluids are necessary to avoid shock when four to six pounds of fat are removed during a single liposuction procedure.[190] Courtiss utilizes suction drains for 48 hours after suction lipectomy in order to prevent ecchymoses.[191]

GRAFTS

Hill presented a helpful review of the factors responsible for the survival of full-thickness grafts.[192] Alcoholic beverages should be prohibited for two days preoperatively and five days postoperatively so as not to interfere with polymorphonuclear neutrophil function. Hill feels that the full-thickness skin graft is a more satisfactory procedure for nasal defects than flap surgery.[193]

In some cases, allowing wounds to partially heal by second intention before skin grafting improves results.[194] Delayed grafting is best done on the scalp, forehead, and nasal dorsum. Split-thickness or full-thickness grafts will "take" after removing the epidermis over traumatic scars, tattoos, and acne scars.[195]

Lipman and Roth have reviewed the factors responsible for composite earlobe graft survival.[196] The preauricular area is a good donor site for full-thickness grafts on the face.[197] Field utilized the infra-auricular area as a full-thickness skin graft donor site.[198] The donor site is closed with a V-Y closure technique.

A synthetic urethane foam pad, Reston (manufactured by the 3M Company) has intrinsic compressibility and can be used as a stent for skin grafts.[199]

FLAPS

Gormley outlined the principles of the Burow's wedge flap.[200] He utilizes double sliding flaps to close adjacent parallel elliptical wounds.[201] Forehead defects can be closed by creating a secondary defect in the frontal scalp.[202] This creates a bipedicled scalp flap. Transposition flaps from the upper eyelid can be used for reconstruction of lower eyelid defects.[203] Field described a double Z-Plasty repair of a cicatricial fold that formed at the inner canthus following cancer excision.[204]

REFERENCES

1. Stegman SJ, Tromavitch TA, Glogau RG: Basics of Dermatologic Surgery. Chicago, Year Book Medical Publishers, 1982
2. Stegman SJ, Tromavitch TA: Cosmetic Dermatologic Surgery. Chicago, Year Book Medical Publishers, 1984
3. Chalker DA, Smith JG, Rogers R: Hepatitis B: A hazard to dermatologists. J Dermatol Surg Oncol 8(6):458–459, 1982
4. Rigel DS, Albom MJ, Geronemus RG, Freedberg IM: Modification of surgical gloves to prevent exposure to hepatitis during hair transplantation. J Dermatol Surg Oncol 9(2):114–115, 1983
5. Fisher AA: Management of dermatitis due to surgical gloves. J Dermatol Surg Oncol 11(6):628–631, 1985
6. Lewis LA: Methoxyflurane analgesia for office surgery. J Dermatol Surg Oncol 10(2)85–86, 1984
7. Field LM: A new, rounded scalpel handle. J Dermatol Surg Oncol 8(11):918, 1982
8. Stoner JG, Swanson NA, Vargo N: Penrose sleeve. J Dermatol Surg Oncol 9(7):523–524, 1983
9. Sebben JE: Electrocoagulation in a sterile surgical field. J Dermatol Surg Oncol 10(8)603–604, 1984
10. Stegman SJ, Tromavitch TA, Glogau RG: The Bernsco adapter. J Dermatol Surg Oncol 10(9)680–681, 1984
11. Tromavitch TA, Glogau RG, Stegman SJ: The Shaw Scalpel. J Dermatol Surg Oncol 9(4):316–319, 1983
12. Schultz BC, Roenigk HH Jr: The double scalpel and double punch excision of skin tumors. J Am Acad Dermatol 7:495–499, 1982
13. Campbell JP, Swanson NA: The use of staples in dermatologic surgery. J Dermatol Surg Oncol 8(8):680–690, 1982
14. Robinovitz HS, Epstein G: The corneal shield. J Dermatol Surg Oncol 11(3):207–208, 1985
15. Koranda FC, Luckasen JR: Instruments and tips for dermatologic surgery. J Dermatol Surg Oncol 8(6):451–454, 1982
16. Pollack SV: Wound healing: A review. J Dermatol Surg Oncol 8(8):667–672, 1982
17. Pollack SV: Wound healing 1985: An update. J Dermatol Surg Oncol 11(3):296–300, 1985
18. Robins P, Day CL, Lew RA: A multivariate analysis of factors affecting wound-healing time. J Dermatol Surg Oncol 10(3):219–221, 1984
19. Zitelli JA: Wound healing by secondary intention. J Am Acad Dermatol 9:407–415, 1983
20. Moscona R, Pnini A, Hirshowitz B: In favor of healing by secondary intention after excision of medial canthal basal cell carcinoma. Plast Reconstr Surg 71(2):189–195, 1983
21. Wiemer DR, Spira M: Ultraviolet light and hyperpigmentation in healing wounds. Ann Plastic Surg 11(4):328–330, 1983
22. Krull EA: Chronic cutaneous ulcerations and impaired healing in human skin. J Am Acad Dermatol 12:394–401, 1985
23. Hendricks WM, Sallow RT: Management of stasis leg ulcers with Unna's boots versus elastic support stockings. J Am Acad Dermatol 12:90–98, 1985
24. Gilmore WA, Wheeland RG: Treatment of ulcers on legs by pinch grafts and a supportive dressing of polyurethane. J Dermatol Surg Oncol 8(3):177–183, 1982
25. Alvarez OM, Mertz PM, Eaglestein WH: Benzoyl peroxide and epidermal wound healing. Arch Dermatol 119:222–225, 1983
26. Wheeland RG, Gilchrist RW, Young JC: Treatment of digital ulcers with nitroglycerin ointment. J Dermatol Surg Oncol 9(7):548–551, 1983
27. Mandy SH: A new primary wound dressing made of polyethylene oxide gel. J Dermatol Surg Oncol 9(2):153–155, 1983
28. Geronemus RG, Robins P: The effect of two new dressings on epidermal wound healing. J Dermatol Surg Oncol 8(10):850–855, 1982
29. Leipziger LS, Glushko V, DiBernardo B, et al: Dermal wound repair: Role of collagen matrix implants and synthetic polymer dressings. J Am Acad Dermatol 12:409–419, 1985
30. Alper JC, Welch EA, Ginsberg M, et al: Moist wound healing under a vapor permeable membrane. Arch Dermatol 8:347–353, 1984
31. Friedman SJ, Su PW: management of leg ulcers with hydrocolloid occlusive dressing. Arch Dermatol 120:1329–1336, 1984
32. Apler JC, Welch EA, Maguire P: Use of the vapor-permeable membrane for cutaneous ulcers: Details of application and side effects. J Am Acad Dermatol 11:858–866, 1984
33. Angermeier MC, Apler JC, Urbaniak HS, Jr: Vapor-permeable membrane therapy for ulcers of osteomyelitis. J Dermatol Surg Oncol 10(5):384–388, 1984
34. Zitelli JA: Delayed wound healing with adhesive wound dressings. J Dermatol Surg Oncol 10(9):709–710, 1984
35. Bailin PL: Lasers in dermatology—1985. J Dermatol Surg Oncol 11(3):328–334, 1985
36. Moreno RA, Hebda PA, Zitelli JA, Abell E: Epidermal cell outgrowth from CO_2 laser- and scalpel-cut explants: Implications for wound healing. J Dermatol Surg Oncol 10(11):863–868, 1984
37. Landthaler M, Haina D, Waidelich W, Braun-Falco O: A three-year experience with the argon laser in dermatotherapy. J Dermatol Surg Oncol 10(6):456–461, 1984
38. Apfelberg DB, Maser MR, Lash H, et al: Comparison of argon and carbon dioxide laser treatment of decorative tattoos: A preliminary report. Ann Plastic Surg 14(1):6–15, 1985
39. Ratz JL, Bailin PL, Levin HL: CO_2 laser treatment of port-wine stains: A preliminary report. J Dermatol Surg Oncol 8(12):1039–1044, 1982
40. McBurney EI, Rosen DA: Carbon dioxide laser treatment of verrucae vulgares. J Dermatol Surg Oncol 10(1):45–48, 1984
41. Persky MS: Carbon dixoide laser treatment of oral florid papillomatosis. J Dermatol Surg Oncol 10(1):64–66, 1984
42. Wheeland RG, Ashley JR, Smith DA, Ellis DL, et al: Carbon dioxide laser treatment of granuloma faciale. J Dermatol Surg Oncol 10(9):730–733, 1984
43. Wheeland RG, Bailin PL, Kronberg E: Carbon dioxide (CO_2) laser vaporization for the treatment of multiple

trichoepithelioma. J Dermatol Surg Oncol 10(6)470–475, 1984

44. Sawchuk WS, Heald PW: CO_2 laser treatment of trichoepithelioma with focused and defocused beam. J Dermatol Surg Oncol 10(11):905–907, 1984

45. Apfelberg DB, Maser MR, Lash H, Flores J: Expanded role of the argon laser in plastic surgery. J Dermatol Surg Oncol 9(2):145–151, 1983

46. David LM: Laser vermilion ablation for actinic cheilitis. J Dermatol Surg Oncol 11(6):605–608, 1985

47. Arellano CR, Leopold DA, Shafiroff BB: Tattoo removal: Comparative study of six methods in the pig. Plast Reconstr Surg 70(6):699–703, 1982

48. Wheeland RG, Norwood OT, Roundtree JM: Tattoo removal using serial tangential excision and polyurethane membrane dressing. J Dermatol Surg Oncol 9(10):822–826, 1983

49. Robinson JK: Tattoo removal. J Dermatol Surg Oncol 11(1):14–16, 1985

50. Blumental G, Okun MR, Ponitch JA: Pseudolymphomatous reaction to tattoos. J Am Acad Dermatol 6:485–488, 1982

51. Castrow FF II, Krull EA: Injectable collagen implant—update. J Am Acad Dermatol 9:889–893, 1983

52. Klein AW: Implantation technics for injectable collagen. J Am Acad Dermatol 9:224–228, 1983

53. Tromavitch TA, Stegman SJ, Glogau RG: Zyderm collagen: Implantation techniques. J Am Acad Dermatol 10:273–278, 1984

54. Klein AW, Rish DC: Injectable collagen update. J Dermatol Surg Oncol 10(7):519–522, 1984

55. Robinson JK, Hanke CW: Injectable collagen implant: Histopathologic identification and longevity of correction. J Dermatol Surg Oncol 11(2):124–130, 1985

56. Barr RJ, Stegman SJ: Delayed skin test reaction to injectable collagen implant (Zyderm). J Am Acad Dermatol 10:652–658, 1984

57. Swanson NA, Stoner JG, Siegel FJ, Solomon AR: Treatment site reactions to Zyderm collagen implantation. J Dermatol Surg Oncol 9(5):377–380, 1983

58. Burke KE, Naughton G, Waldo E, Cassai N: Bovine collagen implant: Histologic chronology in pig dermis. J Dermatol Surg Oncol 9(11):889–895, 1983

59. Cooperman L, Michaeli D: The immunogenicity of injectable collagen II. A retrospective review of seventy-two tested and treated patients. J Am Acad Dermatol 10:647–651, 1984

60. Cooperman L, Michaeli D: The immunogenicity of injectable collagen I. A 1-year prospective study. J Am Acad Dermatol 10:638–646, 1984

61. Bailin PL, Bailin MD: Correction of depressed scars following Mohs' surgery: The role of collagen implantation. J Dermatol Surg Oncol 8(10):845–849, 1982

62. Chernosky ME: Collagen implant in management of perlèche (angular cheilosis). J Am Acad Dermatol 12:493–496, 1985

63. Stoner JG, Swanson NA, Siegle RJ: Treatment of localized morphea with Zyderm collagen implant. J Dermatol Surg Oncol 10(8):626–627, 1984

64. Bodian EL: Techniques of sclerotherapy for sunburst venous varicosities. J Dermatol Surg Oncol 11(7):696–704, 1985

65. Shields JL, Jansen GT: Therapy for superficial telangiectasias of the lower extremities. J Dermatol Surg Oncol 8(10):857–860, 1982

66. Green AR, Morgan BDG: Sclerotherapy for venous flare. Br J Plast Surg 38:241–242, 1985

67. Hanke CW, O'Brian JJ, Solow EM: Laboratory evaluation of skin refrigerants used in dermabrasion. J Dermatol Surg Oncol 11(1):45–49, 1985

68. Field LM: Dermabrasion vs 5-FU for actinic damage. J Am Acad Dermatol 6:269, 1982

69. Roenigk HH Jr, Pinski JB, Robinson JK, Hanke CW: Acne, retinoids and dermabrasion. J Dermatol Surg Oncol 11(4):396–398, 1985

70. Notaro WA: Dermabrasion for the management of traumatic tattoos. J Dermatol Surg Oncol 9(11):916–918, 1983

71. Lapins NA: Dermabrasion for telangiectasia. J Dermatol Surg Oncol 9(6):470–472, 1983

72. Siegle RJ, Chiaramonti A, Knox DW, Pollack SV: Cutaneous candidosis as a complication of facial dermabrasion. J Dermatol Surg Oncol 10(11):891–895, 1984

73. Kucan JO, Robsan MC, Parsons RW: Amniotic membranes as dressings following facial dermabrasion. Annal Plast Surg 8(6):523–527, 1982

74. Stagnone JJ, Stagnone GJ: A second look at chemabrasion. J Dermatol Surg Oncol 8(8):701–705, 1982

75. Alt TH: Evaluation of donor harvesting techniques in hair transplantation. J Dermatol Surg Oncol 10(10):799–806, 1984

76. Pinski JB: How to obtain the "perfect" plug. J Dermatol Surg Oncol 10(12):953–956, 1984

77. Unger WP: Punch transplantation in "early" androgenetic alopecia. J Dermatol Surg Oncol 10(12):945–952, 1984

78. Sturm H: The benefit of donor-site closure in hair transplantation. J Dermatol Surg Oncol 10(12):987–990, 1984

79. Unger WP: A new method of donor site harvesting. J Dermatol Surg Oncol 10(7):524–529, 1984

80. Nordström REA, Holsti LR: Hair transplantation in alopecia due to radiation. Plast Reconstr Surg 72(4):454–458, 1983

81. Sarnoff DS, Goldberg DJ, Greenspan AH, Albom MJ: Multiple pyogenic granuloma-like lesions following hair transplantation. J Dermatol Surg Oncol 11(1):32–34, 1985

82. Morrison ID: Tissue adhesives in hair transplant surgery. Plast Reconstr Surg 68(4):491–497, 1981

83. Hanke CW, Bergfeld WF: Fiber implantation for pattern baldness. J Am Acad Dermatol 4:278–283, 1981

84. Garden JM, Robinson JK: Essential primary cutis verticis gyrata. Arch Dermatol 120:1480–1483, 1984

85. McCray MK, Roenigk HH: Scalp reduction for correction of cutis aplasia congenita. J Dermatol Surg Oncol 7:655–658, 1981

86. Unger WP: Concomitant mini reductions in punch hair transplanting. J Dermatol Surg Oncol 9(5):388–392, 1983

87. Unger MG: The Y-shaped pattern of alopecia reduction and its variations. J Dermatol Surg Oncol 10(12):980–986, 1984

88. Nordström REA: "Stretch-back" in scalp reductions for male pattern baldness. Plast Reconstr Surg 73(3):422–426, 1984

89. Nordström REA: Change of direction of hair growth. J Dermatol Surg Oncol 9(2):156–158, 1983

90. Norwood OT, Shiell RC, Morrison ID: Complications of scalp reductions. J Dermatol Surg Oncol 9(10):828–835, 1983

91. Frechet P: How to avoid the principal complication of scalp reduction in the management of extensive alopecia. J Dermatol Surg Oncol 11(6):637–640, 1985

92. Wheeland RG, Bailin PL: Scalp reduction surgery with the carbon dioxide laser. J Dermatol Surg Oncol 10(7):565–569, 1984

93. Stough BD, Cates JA, Dean AJ: Updating reduction and flap procedures for baldness. Ann Plastic Surg 8(4):287–295, 1982

94. Bouhanna P: The post-auricular vertical hair-bearing transposition flap. J Dermatol Surg Oncol 10(7):551–554, 1984

95. Manders EK, Graham WP: Alopecia reduction by scalp expansion. J Dermatol Surg Oncol 10(12):967–969, 1984

96. Pierce HE: Possible use of the Radovan tissue expander in hair replacement surgery. J Dermatol Surg Oncol 11(4):413–417, 1985

97. Swanson NA: Mohs Surgery. Arch Dermatol 119:761–773, 1983

98. Dzubow LM, Rigel DS, Robins P: Risk factors for local

recurrence of primary cutaneous squamous cell carcinomas. Arch Dermatol 118:900–902, 1982

99. Abide JM, Nahai F, Bennett RG: The meaning of surgical margins. Plast Reconstr Surg 73(3):492–496, 1984

100. Hanke CW, Menn H, O'Brian JJ: Frozen section processing with the Miami special. J Dermatol Surg Oncol 9(4):260–262, 1983

101. Hanke CW: Cryostats in chemosurgery. J Dermatol Surg Oncol 8(5):346–347, 1982

102. Hanke CW, Temofeew RK: Cryostat update. J Dermatol Surg Oncol 11(6):600–602, 1985

103. Grande DJ, Phillips FW: Histo-Clear to replace xylene in the dermatopathology laboratory. J Dermatol Surg Oncol 11(2):103–105, 1985

104. Hanke CW: Super widefield microscopy in Mohs Surgery. J Dermatol Surg Oncol 10(8):588–590, 1984

105. Oseroff AR, Roth R, Lipman S, Morhenn VB: Use of a murine monoclonal antibody which binds to malignant keratinocytes to detect tumor cells in microscopically controlled surgery. J Dermatol Surg Oncol 8:616–619, 1983

106. Barton FE, Cottel WI, Walker B: The principle of chemosurgery and delayed primary reconstruction in the management of difficult basal cell carcinomas. Plast Reconstr Surg 68(5):746–757, 1981

107. Vanderveen EE, Stoner JG, Swanson NA: Chiseling of exposed bone to stimulate granulation tissue after Mohs surgery. J Dermatol Surg Oncol 9(11):925–928, 1983

108. Synder PA, Apler JC, Albom MR: Osteomyelitis complication Mohs surgery. J Am Acad Dermatol 11:513–516, 1984

109. Hanke CW, Lingeman RE, Singer MI, Maves MD, et al: Lateral rhinotomy in the treatment of nasal mucous membrane carcinomas. J Dermatol Surg Oncol 9(5):344–346, 1983

110. Fleishmann HE, Roth RJ, Wood C, Nickoloff BJ: Microcystic adnexal carcinoma treated by microscopically controlled excision. J Dermatol Surg Oncol 10(11):873–875, 1984

111. Dzubow LM: Sebaceous carcinoma of the eyelid: Treatment with Mohs surgery. J Dermatol Surg Oncol 11(1):40–44, 1985

112. Pollack MD, Goslen JB: Small-cell neuroepithelial tumor of skin: A Merkle-cell neoplasm? J Dermatol Surg Oncol 8(2):116–122, 1982

113. Cottel WI: Perineural invasion by squamous cell carcinoma. J Dermatol Surg Oncol 8(7):589–600, 1982

114. Stoner JG, Swanson NA: Chronic radiodermatitis with dystrophic calcification treated with Mohs surgery. J Dermatol Surg Oncol 11(2):160–162, 1985

115. Peters CW, Hanke CW, Pasarell HA, Bennett JE: Dermatofibrosarcoma protuberans of the face. J Dermatol Surg Oncol 8(10):823–825, 1982

116. Hess KA, Hanke CW, Estes NC, Shideler SJ: Myxoid dermatofibrosarcoma protuberans. J Dermatol Surg Oncol 11(3):268–271, 1985

117. Mora RG: Microscopically controlled surgery (Mohs chemosurgery) for treatment of verrucous squamous cell carcinoma of the foot (epithelioma cuniculatum). J Am Acad Dermatol 8:354–362, 1983

118. Padilla RS, Bailin PL, Howard WR, Dinner MI: Verrucous carcinoma of the skin and its management by Mohs surgery. Plast Reconstr Surg 73(3):442–447, 1984

119. Dzubow LM, Kramer EM: Treatment of a large, ulcerating, granular-cell tumor by microscopically controlled excision. J Dermatol Surg Oncol 11(4):392–395, 1985

120. Hanke CW, O'Brian JJ, Peters CW, Horney DA, et al: Congenital smooth muscle hamartoma masquerading as congenital pigmented nevus. J Dermatol Surg Oncol 11(7):714–717, 1985

121. Fox BJ, Lapins NA: Comparison of treatment modalities for epidermal nevus: A case report and review. J Dermatol Surg Oncol 9(11):879–885, 1983

122. Hoehn GH: A simple solution to the therapeutic dilemma of pilonidal cysts. J Dermatol Surg Oncol 8(1):56–57, 1982

123. Salasche SJ: Myxoid cysts of the proximal nail fold: A surgical approach. J Dermatol Surg Oncol 10(1):35–39, 1984

124. Bardach HG: Managing digital mucoid cysts by cryosurgery with liquid nitrogen: Preliminary report. J Dermatol Surg Oncol 9(6):455–458, 1983

125. Shons AR, Press BHJ: The treatment of earlobe keloids by surgical excision and postoperative triamcinolone injection. Ann Plast Surg 10(6):480–482, 1983

126. Berry RB: A comparison of spring and CO_2-powered needleless injections in the treatment of keloids with triamcinolone. Br J Plast Surg 34:458–461, 1981

127. Salasche SJ, Grabski WJ: Keloids of the earlobes. J Dermatol Surg Oncol 9(7):552–556, 1983

128. Shepherd JP, Dowber RPR: The response of keloid scars to cryosurgery. Plast Reconstr Surg 70(6):677–682, 1982

129. Muti E, Ponzio E: Cryotherapy in the treatment of keloids. Ann Plast Surg 11(3):227–232, 1983

130. McDaniel WE: Therapy for basal cell epitheliomas by curettage only. Arch Dermatol 119:901–903, 1983

131. Dubin N, Kopf AW: Multivariate risk score for recurrence of cutaneous basal cell carcinomas. Arch Dermatol 119:373–377, 1983

132. Suhge d'Aubermont PC, Bennett RG: Failure of curettage and electrodesiccation for removal of basal cell carcinoma. Arch Dermatol 120:1456–1460, 1984

133. Salasche SJ: Curettage and electrodesiccation in the treatment of midfacial basal cell epithelioma. J Am Acad Dermatol 8:496–503, 1983

134. Edens BL, Bartlow GA, Haghighi P: Effectiveness of curettage and electrodesiccation in the removal of basal cell carcinoma. J Am Acad Dermatol 9:383–388, 1983

135. Zayhoun S, Abi Ali L, Shaib J, Kurban A: The relationship of sun exposure and solar elastosis to basal cell carcinoma. J Am Acad Dermatol 12:522–525, 1985

136. Epstein E: Fluorouracil paste treatment of thin basal cell carcinomas. Arch Dermatol 121:207–213, 1985

137. Carruthers JA, Stegman SJ, Tromovitch TA, Glogau RG, Robertson DB: Basal cell carcinoma of the temple. J Dermatol Surg Oncol 9(9):759–762, 1983

138. Hanke CW, Wolf RL, Hochman SA, O'Brian JJ: Perineural spread of basal-cell carcinoma. J Dermatol Surg Oncol 9(9):742–747, 1983

139. Domarus HV, Stevens PJ: Metastatic basal cell carcinoma. J Am Acad Dermatol 10:1043–1060, 1984

140. Coker DD, Elias EG, Vivavathana T, et al: Chemotherapy for metastatic basal cell carcinoma. Arch Dermatol 119:44–50, 1983

141. Cristofolini M, Zumiani G, Scappini P, Piscioli F: Aromatic retinoid in the chemoprevention of the progression of nevoid basal-cell carcinoma syndrome. J Dermatol Surg Oncol 10(19):778–781, 1984

142. Lund HZ: Metastasis from sun-induced squamous-cell carcinoma of the skin: An uncommon event. J Dermatol Surg Oncol 10(3):169–170, 1984

143. Epstein E: Malignant sun-induced squamous-cell carcinoma of the skin. J Dermatol Surg Oncol 9(7):505–506, 1983

144. Mora RG, Perniciaro C: Cancer of the skin in blacks. J Am Acad Dermatol 6:1005–1009, 1982

145. Mora RG, Perniciaro C, Lee B: Cancer of the skin in blacks. A review of nineteen patients with Bowen's disease. J Am Acad Dermatol 11:557–562, 1984

146. Sanders GH, Miller TA: Are keratoacanthomas really squamous cell carcinomas? Annal Plast Surg 9(4):306–309, 1982

147. Hanke CW, Bailin PL, O'Brian JJ: Plantar verrucous carcinoma in black women. J Dermatol Surg Oncol 10(2):90–93, 1984

148. Fukamizu H, Inoue K, Matsumoto Kichiro, Okoyama H, et al: Metastatic squamous-cell carcinomas derived from solar keratosis. J Dermatol Surg Oncol 11(55):518–522, 1985

149. Levine N, Miller RC, Meyskens FL Jr: Oral isotretinoin therapy. Arch Dermatol 120:1215–1217, 1984

150. Lew RA, Sober AJ, Cook N, Marvell R, et al: Sun exposure habits in patients with cutaneous melanoma. A case control study. J Dermatol Surg Oncol 9(12):981–986, 1983

151. Day CL Jr, Lew RA: Malignant melanoma prognostic factors 3: Surgical margins. J Dermatol Surg Oncol 9(19):797–801, 1983

152. Day CL, Mihm MC, Sober AJ, et al: Narrower margins for clinical stage I malignant melanoma. New Engl J Med 306:479–481, 1982

153. Fisher JC: Safe margins for melanoma excision. Ann Plast Surg 14(2):158–167, 1985

154. Rogers GS, Kopf AW, Rigel DS, et al: Effect of anatomical location on prognosis in patients with clinical stage I melanoma. Arch Dermatol 119:644–649, 1983

155. Mora RG, Lee B: Cancer of the skin in blacks, IV: A review of nineteen black patient with Kaposi's sarcoma. J Am Acad Dermatol 11:563–567, 1984

156. Pang P, Rodriguez-Sains RS: Ophthalmic oncology: Sebaceous carcinoma of the eyelids. J Dermatol Surg Oncol 11(3):260–264, 1985

157. Redden EM, Baker DC: Coping with the complexities of informed consent in dermatologic surgery. J Dermatol Surg Oncol 10(2):111–116, 1984

158. Wright MR: How to recognize and control the problem patient. J Dermatol Surg Oncol 10(5):389–395, 1984

159. Stegman SJ: Protection of the buried suture. J Dermatol Surg Oncol 8(10):892–893, 1982

160. Sebben JE: Wedge resection of the lip: Minimizing problems. J Dermatol Surg Oncol 11(1):60–64, 1985

161. Harahap M: Repair of split earlobes. J Dermatol Surg Oncol 8(3):187–191, 1982

162. Hill TG: Radical excision and reconstruction of axillary skin. J Dermatol Surg Oncol 9(4):299–303, 1983

163. Resnik SS: Chemical peeling with trichloroacetic acid. J Dermatol Surg Oncol 10(7):549–550, 1984

164. Litton C, Trinidad G: Complications of chemical face peeling as evaluated by a questionnaire. Plast Reconstr Surg 67(6):738–744, 1981

165. Rapaport MJ, Kamer F: Exacerbation of facial herpes simplex after phenolic face peels. J Dermatol Surg Oncol 10(1):57–58, 1984

166. Wolfe SA: Chemical face peeling following therapeutic irradiation. Plast Reconstr Surg 69(5):859–862, 1982

167. Lubritz RR, Smolewski SA: Cryosurgery cure rate of actinic keratosis. J Am Acad Dermatol 7:631–632, 1982

168. Zacarian SA: Cryosurgery of cutaneous carcinomas. J Am Acad Dermatol 9:947–956, 1983

169. Zacarian SA: Cryosurgical treatment of lentigo maligna. Arch Dermatol 118:89–92, 1982

170. Rosenblum GA: Liquid nitrogen cryotherapy in a case of elastosis perforans serpiginosa. J Am Acad Dermatol 11(8):718–721, 1983

171. Elton RF: Complications of cutaneous cryosurgery. J Am Acad Dermatol 8:513–519, 1983

172. Herold HZ, Baruchin AM, Shmueli G, Daniel D, et al: Radical wedge resection for ingrown toenail: Long-term results. J Dermatol Surg Oncol 11(5):513–517, 1985

173. Thomsen RJ, Zuehlke RL, Beckman BI: Pachyonychia congenita—surgical management of the nail changes. J Dermatol Surg Oncol 8(1):24–28, 1982

174. Siegle RJ, Swanson NJ: Nail surgery: A review. J Dermatol Surg Oncol 8(8):659–666, 1982

175. Webster RC: On dermatologic plastic or cosmetic surgery. J Dermatol Surg Oncol 10(7):513–514, 1984

176. Tobin HA: Electrosurgical blepharoplasty: A technique that questions conventional concepts of fat compartmentalization. Ann Plast Surg 14(1):59–63, 1985

177. Rees TD, Jelks GW: Blepharoplasty and the dry eye syndrome: Guidelines for surgery? Plast Reconstr Surg 68(2):249–252, 1981

178. Sokol AB, Sokol TP: Transblepharoplasty brow suspension. Plast Reconstr Surg 69(6):940–944, 1982

179. Rees TD: Prevention of ectropion by horizontal shortening of the lower lid during blepharoplasty. Ann Plast Surg 11(1):17–23, 1983

180. Bennett JE, Matas JA: A minor complication of blepharoplasty. Plast Reconstr Surg 69(5):856–858, 1982

181. Rees TD, Craig SM, Fisher Y: Orbital abscess following blepharoplasty. Plast Reconstr Surg 73(1):126–127, 1984

182. Klatsky S, Manson PN: Numbness after blepharoplasty: The relation of the upper orbital fat to sensory nerves. Plast Reconstr Surg 67(1):20–22, 1981

183. Grabski WJ, Salasche SJ: Management of temporal nerve injuries. J Dermatol Surg Oncol 11(2):145–151, 1985

184. Newman J, Dolsky RL: Lipo-suction surgery: History and development. J Dermatol Surg Oncol 10(6):467–469, 1984

185. Field LM: Lipo-suction surgery: A review. J Dermatol Surg Oncol 10(7):530–538, 1984

186. Teimourian B, Adham MN, Gulin S, Shapiro C: Suction lipectomy—a review of 200 patients over a six-year period and a study of the technique in cadavers. Ann Plast Surg 11(2):93–98, 1983

187. Teimourian B, Fisher JB: Suction curettage to remove excess fat for body contouring. Plast Reconstr Surg 68(1):50–58, 1981

188. Kesselring VK: Regional fat aspiration for body contouring. Plast Reconstr Surg 72(3):610–619, 1983

189. Crisman BB, Field LM: Facelift surgery update: Suction-assisted rhytidectomy and other improvements. J Dermatol Surg Oncol 10(7):544–548, 1984

190. Illouz YG: Body contouring by lipolysis: A 5-year experience with over 3000 cases. Plast Reconstr Surg 72(5):591–597, 1983

191. Courtiss EH: Suction lipectomy: A retrospective analysis of 100 patients. Plast Reconstr Surg 73(5):780–796, 1984

192. Hill TG: Enhancing the survival of full-thickness grafts. J Dermatol Surg Oncol 10(8):639–642, 1984

193. Hill TG: Reconstruction of nasal defects using full-thickness skin grafts: A personal reappraisal. J Dermatol Surg Oncol 9(12):995–1001, 1983

194. Ceilley RI, Bumstead RM, Panje WR: Delayed skin grafting. J Dermatol Surg Oncol 9(4):288–293, 1983

195. Trimble JR: Dermal overgrafting in dermatology. J Dermatol Surg Oncol 9(12):987–993, 1983

196. Lipman SH, Roth RJ: Composite grafts from earlobes for reconstruction of defects in noses. J Dermatol Surg Oncol 8(2):135–137, 1985

197. Corwin TR, Klein AW, Habal MB: The aesthetics of the preauricular graft in facial reconstruction. Ann Plast Surg 9(4):312–315, 1982

198. Field LM: The infra-auricular full-thickness donor site with X-Y closure. J Dermatol Surg Oncol 10(5):345–346, 1984

199. Weiner LJ, Moberg AW: An ideal stent for reliable and efficient skin graft application. Ann Plast Surg 13(1):24–28, 1984

200. Gormley DE: A brief analysis of the Burow's wedge/triangle principle. J Dermatol Surg Oncol 11(2):121–124, 1985

201. Gormley DE: The "N" or reversed "N" (И) closure of adjacent, parallel, elliptical excisions. J Dermatol Surg Oncol 8(4):240–242, 1982

202. Stoner JG, Swanson NA: Use of the bipedicled scalp flap for forehead reconstruction. J Dermatol Surg Oncol 10(3):213–215, 1984

203. Field LM: The upper-to-lower eyelid transposition flap. J Dermatol Surg Oncol 9(10):809–812, 1983

204. Field LM: Repair of a cicatricial epicanthal fold by a double Z-Plasty (Spaeth). J Dermatol Surg Oncol 8(3):215–217, 1982

Index

Note: Page numbers in *italics* refer to illustrations; page numbers followed by (t) refer to tables.